a LANGE medical book

CURRENT
Diagnosis & Treatment in Family Medicine

Jeannette E. South-Paul, MD
*Professor and Chair, Department of Family Medicine
University of Pittsburgh School of Medicine, Pennsylvania*

Samuel C. Matheny, MD, MPH
*Professor and Chair, Department of Family Practice and
Community Medicine, University of Kentucky College
of Medicine, Lexington, Kentucky*

Evelyn L. Lewis, MD, MA
*Director, Regional Medical and Research Specialist, Pfizer,
Inc., Bowie, Maryland; Adjunct Associate Professor,
Department of Family Medicine, Uniformed Services
University of the Health Sciences, Bethesda, Maryland*

Lange Medical Books/McGraw-Hill
Medical Publishing Division

New York   Chicago   San Francisco   Lisbon   London   Madrid
Mexico City   Milan   New Delhi   San Juan
Seoul   Singapore   Sydney   Toronto

Current Diagnosis & Treatment in Family Medicine

2 3 4 5 6 7 8 9 0 DOC DOC 0 9 8 7 6 5 4

ISBN: 0-07-139088-X
ISSN: 1548-2189

Notice

Medicine is an ever-changing science. As new research and clinical experience broaden our knowledge, changes in treatment and drug therapy are required. The authors and the publisher of this work have checked with sources believed to be reliable in their efforts to provide information that is complete and generally in accord with the standards accepted at the time of publication. However, in view of the possibility of human error or changes in medical sciences, neither the authors nor the publisher nor any other party who has been involved in the preparation or publication of this work warrants that the information contained herein is in every respect accurate or complete, and they disclaim all responsibility for any errors or omissions or for the results obtained from use of the information contained in this work. Readers are encouraged to confirm the information contained herein with other sources. For example and in particular, readers are advised to check the product information sheet included in the package of each drug they plan to administer to be certain that the information contained in this work is accurate and that changes have not been made in the recommended dose or in the contraindications for administration. This recommendation is of particular importance in connection with new or infrequently used drugs.

This book was set in Adobe Garamond by Pine Tree Composition.
The editors were Shelley Reinhardt, Harriet Lebowitz, and Barbara Holton.
The production supervisor was Richard Ruzycka.
The illustration manager was Charissa Baker
The index was prepared by Benjamin Tedoff.
RR Donnelley was printer and binder.

This book is printed on acid-free paper.

INTERNATIONAL EDITION ISBN 0-07-121978-1
Copyright © 2004. Exclusive rights by The McGraw-Hill Companies, Inc., for manufacture and export. This book cannot be re-exported from the country to which it is consigned by McGraw-Hill. The International Edition is not available in North America.

*We would like to dedicate this book
to all family physicians who deliver care in austere environments,
especially our colleagues in uniform.*

Table of Contents

Authors

Nicole T. Ansani, PharmD
Associate Director, Drug Information Center;
    Assistant Professor, Department of Pharmacy
    and Therapeutics, University of Pittsburgh
    School of Pharmacy, Pennsylvania
ansanint@msx.upmc.edu
Pharmacotherapy

Thomas D. Armsey, MD
Associate Professor, Family and Preventive Health;
    Director, University of South Carolina Primary
    Care Sports Medicine, Columbia, South Carolina
thomas.armsey@palmettohealth.org
Common Upper & Lower Extremity Fractures

Cindy Barter, MD
Family Physician, HealthSpring, Bethlehem,
    Pennsylvania
cindy.barter@lvh.com
Abdominal Pain

Daphne P. Bicket, MD, MLS
Physician, Latterman Family Health Center,
    University of Pittsburgh Medical Center,
    McKeesport, Pennsylvania
bicketdp@upmc.edu
Common Geriatric Problems

Deborah J. Bostock, MD
Assistant Professor, Department of Family Medicine,
    Uniformed Services University of the Health
    Sciences, Bethesda, Maryland
Elder Abuse

Susan C. Brunsell, MD
Assistant Professor, Department of Family Medicine,
    Georgetown University School of Medicine, Fort
    Lincoln Family Medicine Center, Colmar Manor,
    Maryland
brunsels@georgetown.edu
Contraception

Ilene Timko Burns, MD, MPH
Renaissance Family Practice, Inc., Penn Hills
    Division, Verona, Pennsylvania
Childhood Vaccines

Peter J. Carek, MD, MS
Associate Professor, Department of Family
    Medicine, Medical University of South Carolina,
    Charleston
carekpj@musc.edu
Endocrine Disorders

Robert J. Carr, MD
Medical Director, Primary Care of Southbury,
    Southbury, Connecticut; Associate Professor
    of Family Medicine, Georgetown University
    School of Medicine, Washington, DC
carrr@georgetown.edu
Urinary Incontinence

Ronald A. Chez, MD
Deputy Director, Samueli Institute, Corona
    del Mar, California
rchez@siib.org
Complementary & Alternative Medicine

C. Randall Clinch, DO
Assistant Professor and Associate Director of Clinical
    Operations, Department of Family and
    Community Medicine, Wake Forest University
    School of Medicine, Winston-Salem, North
    Carolina
crclinch@wfubmc.edu
Evaluation & Management of Headache

Tracey D. Conti, MD
Assistant Professor, Department of Family Medicine,
    University of Pittsburgh School of Medicine,
    Pennsylvania
contitd@upmc.edu
Breast-feeding & Infant Nutrition

Kathleen A. Culhane-Pera, MD, MA
WestSide Community Family Practice Track
    Coordinator, Regions Family and Community
    Medicine Residency, St. Paul, Minnesota; Assistant
    Professor, Department of Family Practice and
    Community Health, University of Minnesota,
    Minneapolis, Minnesota
kathiecp@yahoo.com
Cultural Competence

Essam Demian, MD, MRCOG
Faculty, University of Pittsburgh Medical Center,
    McKeesport Family Practice Residency Program,
    McKeesport, Pennsylvania
demiane@upmc.edu
Preconception Care

Laura Dunne, MD
Physician, Orthopaedic Associates of Allentown,
    LTD, Allentown, Pennsylvania
lauradunne@aol.com
Abdominal Pain

William Elder, PhD
Associate Professor and Director, Behavioral Sciences,
    Department of Family Practice, University
    of Kentucky College of Medicine, Lexington
welder@email.uky.edu
*Personality Disorders; Somatoform Symptoms
    & Disorders*

Patricia Evans, MD
Assistant Professor, Department of Family Medicine,
    Georgetown University School of Medicine,
    Washington, DC
evansp@georgetown.edu
Vaginal Bleeding

Gerald A. Ferretti, DDS, MS
Professor, University of Kentucky, Colleges
    of Medicine and Dentistry, Lexington
gaferr01@email.uky.edu
Oral Health

Deborah Auer Flomenhoft, MD
Gastroenterology Fellow, Division of Gastroenterology,
    University of Kentucky College of Medicine, Lex-
    ington
drflom0@pop.uky.edu
Failure to Thrive

Ronald M. Glick, MD
Medical Director, Center for Complementary
    Medicine, UPMC University of Pittsburgh
    Medical Center, Shadyside; Assistant Professor
    of Family Medicine, Physical Medicine and Reha-
    bilitation, and Psychiatry, University of Pittsburgh
    School of Medicine, Pennsylvania
glickrm@upmc.edu
Chronic Pain Management

Wanda Gonsalves, MD
Assistant Professor, Department of Family Medicine,
    Medical University of South Carolina, Charleston
gonsalvw@musc.edu
Oral Health

Terence L. Gutgsell, MD
Medical Director, Hospice of the Bluegrass,
    Lexington, Kentucky; Medical Director,
    Palliative Care Center of the Bluegrass, Lexington,
    Kentucky
lestug@hospicebg.com
Hospice & Palliative Medicine

Jerri R. Harris, MPH
Educational Development, Department of Family
    Medicine, The Brody School of Medicine, East
    Carolina University School of Medicine,
    Greenville, North Carolina
harrisje@mail.ecu.edu
Adolescent Development & Screening

David Hilton, ThM
Chaplain, Hospice of the Bluegrass, Frankfort,
    Kentucky
dhilton@hospicebg.com
Hospice & Palliative Medicine

Robert G. Hosey, MD
Assistant Professor and Director of Primary Care
    Sports Medicine Fellowship, Department of
    Family Practice, University of Kentucky College
    of Medicine, Lexington
rhosey@email.uky.edu
Common Upper & Lower Extremity Fractures

Thomas M. Howard, MD
Chief, DeWitt Army Community Hospital,
    Ft. Belvoir, Virginia
thomas.m.howard@us.army.mil
Neck Pain

William J. Hueston, MD
Professor and Chair, Department of Family
    Medicine, Medical University of South Carolina,
    Charleston
huestowj@musc.edu
Respiratory Problems; Endocrine Disorders

Andrew Hyland, PhD
Associate Member, Department of Cancer,
    Prevention, Epidemiology, and Biostatistics,
    Roswell Park Cancer Institute, Buffalo, New York
andrew.hyland@roswellpark.org
Tobacco Cessation

Bruce E. Johnson, MD
Professor of Medicine, Division of General Internal
    Medicine, Brody School of Medicine at East
    Carolina University, Greenville, North Carolina
Arthritis: Osteoarthritis, Gout, & Rheumatoid Arthritis

Wayne B. Jonas, MD
Director, Samueli Institute, Alexandria, Virginia
    wjonas@siib.org
Complementary & Alternative Medicine

Peter J. Katsufrakis, MD, MBA
Associate Dean for Student Affairs, Keck School
    of Medicine, University of Southern California,
    Los Angeles, California
pkatsu@hsc.usc.edu
*Sexually Transmitted Diseases; Health Care Needs
    of Gay, Lesbian, Bisexual, & Transgender Patients*

Shersten Killip, MD, MPH
Assistant Professor, Department of Family Practice,
    University of Kentucky College of Medicine,
    Lexington
skill2@email.uky.edu
Urinary Tract Infections

Kenneth L. Kirsh, PhD
Assistant Director for Research, Sympton Manage-
    ment and Palliative Care; Assistant Professor
    of Medicine, University of Kentucky College
    of Medicine, Lexington
klkirsh@uky.edu
Hospice & Palliative Medicine

Mark A. Knox, MD
Associate Director, UPMC University of Pittsburgh
    Medical Center Shadyside Family Practice
    Residency Program; Clinical Associate Professor,
    University of Pittsburgh School of Medicine,
    Pennsylvania
knoxma@upmc.edu
*Common Infections in Children; Skin Diseases in
    Infants & Children*

Mary V. Krueger, DO, MPH, MAJ, MC, USA
Associate Residency Director, DeWitt Army
    Community Hospital, Family Health Center,
    Fort Belvoir, Virginia
mary.krueger@us.army.mil
Menstrual Disorders

Nancy Levine, MD
Family Practice Residency Program Director,
    Western Pennsylvania Hospital, Pittsburgh,
    Pennsylvania
nlevine@wpahs.org
Communication

Evelyn L. Lewis, MD, MA
Director, Regional Medical and Research Specialist,
    Pfizer, Inc., Bowie, Maryland; Adjunct Associate
    Professor, Department of Family Medicine,
    Uniformed Services University of the Health
    Sciences, Bethesda, Maryland
elewis@usuhs.mil
Eating Disorders

Jamee H. Lucas, MD, FAAFP
Program Director, Palmetto Health Richland Family
    Medicine Residency; Associate Professor,
    Department of Family and Preventive Medicine,
    University of South Carolina School of Medicine,
    Columbia
jamee.lucas@palmettohealth.org
Anxiety Disorders

Kiame J. Mahaniah, MD
Faculty, Lawrence Family Practice Residency
    Program, Lawrence Massachusetts
k_mahaniah@hotmail.com
Anemia

Martin C. Mahoney, MD, PhD, FAAFP
Chair, Clinical Prevention, Division of Cancer
    Prevention & Populations Sciences, Roswell Park
    Cancer Institute, Buffalo, New York; Associate
    Professor, Department of Family Medicine,
    School of Medicine and Biomedical Sciences,
    State University of New York at Buffalo
martin.mahoney@roswellpark.org
Neonatal Hyperbilirubinemia; Tobacco Cessation

Robert Mallin, MD
Associate Professor, Department of Family Medicine,
    Medical University of South Carolina, Charleston
mallinr@musc.edu
Substance Use Disorders

Dawn A. Marcus, MD
Associate Professor, Department of Anesthesiology,
    University of Pittsburgh Medical Center,
    Pennsylvania
marcusd@anes.upmc.edu
Chronic Pain Management

Samuel C. Matheny, MD, MPH
Professor and Chair, Department of Family Practice
    and Community Medicine, University of Kentucky
    College of Medicine, Lexington, Kentucky
matheny@email.uky.edu
Diseases of the Biliary Tract & Liver

Billie May, RN, MSN, APRN, BC-PCM
Clinical Nurse Specialist, Palliative Care Center
    of the Bluegrass, Saint Joseph HealthCare,
    Lexington, Kentucky
bmay@sjhlex.org
Hospice & Palliative Medicine

Scott McKay, MD
Assistant Professor, Department of Family and
    Preventive Medicine, University of South Carolina
    School of Medicine, Columbia
scott.mckay@palmettohealth.org
Anxiety Disorders

Rodrick McKinlay, MD
Clinical Fellow, Minimally Invasive Surgery,
    University of Maryland Medical Center,
    Baltimore, Maryland
rmckinlay@smail.umaryland.edu
Diseases of the Biliary Tract & Liver

Philip J. Michels, PhD
Professor and Director, Division of Behavioral
    Medicine Department of Family and Preventive
    Medicine, University of South Carolina School
    of Medicine, Columbia
phil.michels@palmettohealth.org
Anxiety Disorders

Donald B. Middleton, MD
Vice President for Family Practice Education, UPMC
    St. Margaret, University of Pittsburgh Medical
    Center, Pennsylvania
middletondb@upmc.edu
Seizures

T.A. Miller, MD
Director, Graduate Medical Education, Naval
    Medical Education and Training Command,
    Bethesda, Maryland
tmiller@nmetc.med.navy.mil
Adult Sexual Dysfunction

Karl O. Moe, PhD
Clinical Health Psychologist, Behavioral Health Care
    Service, National Naval Medical Center, Bethesda,
    Maryland
komoe@bethesda.med.navy.mil
Depression

David A. Nikovits, MD
Sports Medicine Physician, Omni HealthCare, Palm
    Bay, Florida
Common Upper & Lower Extremity Fractures

Margaret R. H. Nusbaum, DO, MPH
Associate Professor, Department of Family Medicine,
    University of North Carolina, Chapel Hill
margaret_nusbaum@med.unc.edu
Adolescent Sexuality; Adult Sexual Dysfunction

Francis G. O'Connor, MD, FACSM
Associate Professor, Department of Family Medicine;
    Director, Sports Medicine Fellowship Program,
    Uniformed Services University of the Health
    Sciences, Bethesda, Maryland
foconnor@usuhs.mil
Low Back Pain

Maureen O'Hara Padden, MD, MPH, FAAFP
Program Director, Camp Lejeune Family Medicine
    Residency, Jacksonville, North Carolina
scarlettmo@aol.com
Hypertension

Steven D. Passik, PhD
Director, Symptom Management and Palliative Care
    Program, Markey Cancer Center; Associate
    Professor of Medicine and Behavioral Science,
    University of Kentucky College of Medicine,
    Lexington
spassik@uky.edu
Hospice & Palliative Medicine

Sonia Patten, PhD
Visiting Assistant Professor, Department of
    Anthropology, Macalester College, St. Paul,
    Minnesota
patten@macalester.edu
Cultural Competence

D. Dean Patton, MD
Professor and Chairman, Department of Family
    Medicine, The Brody School of Medicine, East
    Carolina University School of Medicine,
    Greenville, North Carolina
pattondd@mail.ecu.edu
Adolescent Development & Screening

Hahn X. Pham, MD
Associate Medical Director, Hospice of the Bluegrass,
    Lexington, Kentucky
Hospice & Palliative Medicine

Brian A. Primack, MD, EdM
Assistant Professor, Department of Family Medicine
    & Clinical Epidemiology, University of Pittsburgh
    School of Medicine, Pennsylvania
primackba@upmc.edu
Anemia

Charles Privitera, MD
Associate Professor of Psychiatry and Assistant
    Professor of Family Medicine, Uniformed
    Services University of the Health Sciences,
    Bethesda, Maryland
crivitera@usuhs.mil
Depression

Goutham Rao, MD
Assistant Professor, Department of Family Medicine,
    University of Pittsburgh School of Medicine,
    Pennsylvania
raog@upmc.edu
Movement Disorders

Brian V. Reamy, MD, Col, USAF, MC
Associate Professor and Chair, Department of Family
    Medicine, Uniformed Services University of the
    Health Sciences, Bethesda, Maryland
breamy@usuhs.mil
Dyslipidemias

Charles F. Reynolds III, MD
Professor of Psychiatry, Neurology and Neuroscience,
    University of Pittsburgh School of Medicine;
    Director, Intervention Research Center for Late-
    Life Mood Disorders, Pittsburgh, Pennsylvania
reynoldscf@msx.upmc.edu
Depression in Older Patients

Richard E. Rodenberg, Jr., MD
Assistant Professor and Associate Director, Sports
    Medicine Fellowship, University of Kentucky
    College of Medicine, Lexington
rerode2@email.uky.edu
Common Upper & Lower Extremity Fractures

Jo Ann Rosenfeld, MD
Assistant Professor, Department of Medicine, The
    Johns Hopkins University School of Medicine,
    Baltimore, Maryland
jrosenfe@jhmi.edu
Evaluation of Breast Lumps

Tracy Sbrocco, PhD
Associate Professor, Department of Medical and
    Clinical Psychology, Uniformed Services
    University of the Health Sciences, Bethesda,
    Maryland
tsbrocco@usuhs.mil
Eating Disorders

Melissa A. Somma, PharmD, CDE
Assistant Professor, University of Pittsburgh School
    of Pharmacy, Pennsylvania
sommama@upmc.edu
Pharmacotherapy

Jeannette E. South-Paul, MD
Professor and Chair, Department of Family Medicine
    University of Pittsburgh School of Medicine,
    Pennsylvania
southpaulj@upmc.edu
Well Child Care; Osteoporosis; Health Disparities

Sukanya Srinivasan, MD, MPH
Assistant Professor, Department of Family Medicine,
    University of Pittsburgh School of Medicine,
    Pennsylvania
Well Child Care

Mark B. Stephens, MD, MS, FAAFP
Associate Professor, Department of Family Medicine,
    Uniformed Services University of the Health
    Sciences, Bethesda, Maryland
mstephens@usuhs.mil
Physical Activity in Adolescents

William S. Sykora, MD, Col, USAF, MC
Assistant Professor, Associate Chair for Education,
    Department of Family Medicine, Uniformed
    Services University of the Health Sciences,
    Bethesda, Maryland
wsykora@usuhs.mil
Disruptive Behavioral Disorders in Children

Andrew B. Symons, MD, MS
Clinical Instructor, Department of Family Medicine,
    SUNY Clinical Center, State University of New
    York at Buffalo
symons@buffalo.edu
Neonatal Hyperbilirubinemia

Belinda Vail, MD
Family Medicine Residency Program Director and
    Vice Chair, Department of Family Medicine,
    University of Kansas Medical Center, Kansas City
bvail@kumc.edu
Diabetes Mellitus

Charles W. Webb, DO
Director, Sports Medicine, Martin Army Community
    Hospital, Ft. Benning, Georgia; Assistant
    Professor, Family Medicine, Uniformed Services
    University of the Health Sciences, Bethesda,
    Maryland
webbo18@aol.com
Low Back Pain

Sherri Weisenfluh, LCSW
Associate Vice President Counseling, Hospice of the
    Bluegrass, Lexington, Kentucky
sweisenfluh@hospicebg.com
Hospice & Palliative Medicine

Alan L. Williams, MD
Staff Physician, Secure Medical Care, Gaithersburg,
    Maryland
Hearing & Vision Impairment in the Elderly

Cynthia M. Williams, DO
Assistant Professor, Department of Family Medicine,
    Uniformed Services University of the Health
    Sciences, Bethesda, Maryland
cwilliams@usuhs.mil
*Healthy Aging; Assessing the Vulnerable Elderly; Elder
    Abuse*

Pamela M. Williams, MD
Assistant Professor, Department of Family Medicine,
    Uniformed Services University of the Health
    Sciences, Bethesda, Maryland
pawilliams@usuhs.mil
Hearing & Vision Impairment in the Elderly

Stephen A. Wilson, MD
Assistant Director, Predoctoral Education and
    Faculty Research, University of Pittsburgh
    Medical Center St. Margaret Family Practice
    Residency; University of Pittsburgh Department
    of Family Medicine; Lincoln-Lemington Family
    Health Care Center, Pittsburgh, Pennsylvania
wilsons2@upmc.edu
Cardiovascular Disease

Cheryl E. Woodson, MD, FACP, AGSF
Director, Woodson Center for Adult HealthCare,
    Chicago Heights, Illinois
Elder Abuse

Richard Kent Zimmerman, MD, MPH
Associate Professor, Department of Family Medicine
    and Clinical Epidemiology, University of
    Pittsburgh School of Medicine, Pennsylvania
zimmer@pitt.edu
Childhood Vaccines

Preface

Current Diagnosis & Treatment in Family Medicine is the first edition of this single-source reference for house staff and practicing family physicians who provide comprehensive and continuous care of individuals of both sexes throughout the lifespan. The text is organized according to the developmental lifespan, beginning with childhood and adolescence, encompassing a focus on the reproductive years, and progressing through adulthood and the mature, senior years.

OUTSTANDING FEATURES

- Evidence-based recommendations
- Culturally related aspects of each condition
- Conservative and pharmacologic therapies
- Complementary and alternative therapies when relevant
- Suggestions for collaborations with other health care providers
- Attention to the mental and behavioral health of patients as solitary as well as comorbid conditions
- Recognition of impact of illness on the family
- Patient education information
- End-of-life issues

INTENDED AUDIENCE

Primary care trainees and practicing physicians will find this text a useful resource for common conditions seen in ambulatory practice. Detailed information in tabular and text format provides a ready reference for selecting diagnostic procedures and recommending treatments. Advanced practice nurses and physician's assistants will also find the approach provided here a practical and complete first resource for both diagnosed and undifferentiated conditions and an aid in continuing management.

Unlike smaller medical manuals that focus on urgent, one-time approaches to a particular presenting complaint or condition, this text was envisioned as a resource for clinicians who practice continuity of care and have established a longitudinal, therapeutic relationship with their patients. Consequently, recommendations are made for immediate as well as subsequent clinical encounters.

ACKNOWLEDGEMENTS

We wish to thank our many contributing authors for their diligence in creating complete, practical, and readable discussions of the many conditions seen on a daily basis in the average family medicine and primary care practice. Furthermore, the vision and support of our editors at McGraw-Hill for creating this new resource for primary care have been outstanding and critical to its completion.

Jeannette E. South-Paul, MD
Evelyn L. Lewis, MD, MA
Samuel C. Matheny, MD

SECTION I
Infancy & Childhood

Well Child Care

1

Sukanya Srinivasan, MD, MPH, & Jeannette E. South-Paul, MD

ESSENTIALS OF WELL CHILD CARE

Caring for children is an integral and enjoyable part of family practice. Although fewer family physicians provide prenatal and obstetrics services, communities still require comprehensive well child care to ensure healthy outcomes. During periodic examinations of the well child, the family physician builds a strong foundation for continuity of care with the entire family.

Although the health of children in the United States has improved significantly due to improved nutrition and immunization, children today are still at high risk for serious health problems. Barriers to health care such as lack of access and low health literacy along with societal concerns such as poverty, substance abuse, and inadequate community supports significantly affect children's health. Inadequate prenatal care, excessive lead exposure, and pediatric human immunodeficiency virus (HIV) are examples of critical issues that need to be identified and addressed. As primary care practitioners collaborate to address the needs of children, preventive care such as periodic well child examinations will play an important role.

The components of routine well child care include the following:

- interval history taking
- complete physical examination
- relevant screening tests
- developmental assessment
- tracking of growth parameters
- administration of recommended immunizations
- anticipatory guidance about child-rearing issues.

The underlying purpose of routine well child checks is to identify problems and to intervene with early treatment to prevent future complications. During the course of normal child development, family physicians need to comfortably identify the common variants as well as abnormal findings that require referral.

The proposed schedule of visits for routine well child check-ups (Table 1–1) closely mirrors the Advisory Committee on Immunization Practices (ACIP) recommended timetable of immunizations until 2 years of age. Any number of circumstances may lead to modifications of this schedule, as determined by clinicians in individual settings. In fact, any encounter, even for an acute illness, can be used as an opportunity to update health screening, provide anticipatory guidance, and administer immunizations.

Additional visits may be required in the following settings:

- The child is first born, adopted, or living with surrogate parents.
- The family is socially or economically disadvantaged.
- The child is at high risk for medical disorders, as suggested by the pregnancy, delivery, or neonatal history.
- The child may have psychological disorders as suggested by problems in areas such as toilet training, persistent temper tantrums, and school attendance.
- The parents request or require additional education or guidance.

GENERAL APPROACH

Whenever possible, prospective parents are encouraged to have a prenatal visit with the family physician. A pertinent family and genetic history can be obtained, and office policies and procedures can be reviewed. This allows the first newborn visit to be dedicated to providing guidance with child care and parenting.

Table 1–1. Proposed schedule of routine well care visits.

Newborn examination within 24 h of birth and prior to discharge from hospital
2–4 weeks 2 months 4 months 6 months 9 months 12 months 15 months 18 months 24 months
2 years 3 years 4 years 5 years 6 years 8 years 10 years
Annually, between ages of 11 and 21 years

Source: American Academy of Pediatrics, 1995.

A general principle for well child examinations is the performance of maneuvers from least to most invasive. Clinicians can first make observations, then palpate and auscultate, and finally end with the use of any specialized instruments. Although most of the communication regarding health care and decision making is between the physician and the parents, clinicians need to attempt to communicate directly with the patient. Direct communication allows the clinician to observe the child and gauge whether he or she is developmentally appropriate and also helps breed familiarity and build a rapport with the patient. This is particularly important during the adolescent years when patient trust is difficult to gain and patient compliance is difficult to assess.

Recordkeeping and good documentation in a busy practice are always challenging tasks. Children's medical records, especially immunizations, must be kept as meticulously as possible, as these records are often required for school enrollment. A checklist-based database is an efficient way to ensure completeness in physical and developmental examinations. A table or flow sheet, which can be updated on an ongoing basis, is helpful for tracking immunizations and screening tests. Finally, the use of standardized growth charts such as those developed by the Centers for Disease Control (CDC) to track the child's weight, height, and head circumference is a concise way to identify any worrisome trends.

Bright Futures, Guidelines for Health Supervision of Infants, Children and Adolescents. National Center for Education in Maternal and Child Health, HRSA, 2000.

Centers for Disease Control and Prevention: *2000 CDC Growth Charts: United States.* URL: http://www.cdc.gov/growthcharts/.

Dinkevich E, Ozuah PO: Well-child care: effectiveness of current recommendations. Clin Pediatr 2002;41(4):211. [PMID: 12041716].

Well Child Care: Reference Guide of the American Board of Family Practice, ed 8. American Board of Family Practice, 2000.

HEALTH MAINTENANCE & DISEASE PREVENTION

Well child care can begin in the preconception period. During a routine gynecological examination or a specific office visit for preconception counseling, family physicians can encourage female patients to begin optimizing their health in anticipation of bearing children. Prospective parents benefit from anticipatory guidance regarding avoidance of exposures such as tobacco and alcohol, appropriate nutrition including folic acid supplementation, and prevention of congenital infections such as rubella.

Studies show that the decision to breast-feed is often made well before the child is born and is based largely on cultural beliefs and value judgments, despite the known medical benefits of breast-feeding. As a result of passive immunity from the mother, potential benefits for the infant are numerous, including decreased incidence of otitis media, eczema, asthma, and diarrheal illness. Mothers need to be informed not only about the health benefits but also about the practical aspects of convenience and lower cost and the reported neurobehavioral advantages for the child such as improved bonding, better temperament, and even higher IQ. Family doctors can promote breast-feeding to female patients throughout the lifecycle.

The provision of preventive care, once a healthy baby is born, is an important task that all family doctors can accomplish with a systematic approach. Anticipatory guidance is needed in several areas of a child's life, in the progression from infancy to school age. The caregivers who support children through this transition depend on clinicians for appropriate and timely advice. Topics that need to be discussed with parents include nutrition, development and behavior, elimination, and oral health.

Nutrition

One of the crucial tasks of caregivers is to provide adequate nutrition to support the physical and psychological growth of children. Caregivers can expect that the needs and habits of children will evolve during the stages of normal development. During the newborn period, all mothers can be strongly encouraged to use breast milk as the primary source of nutrition. A widely accepted goal is exclusive breast-feeding for the first 6 months of life. Although breast milk is considered a complete source of nutrition for newborns, infants who are exclusively breast-fed require some supplementation. Recent guidelines from the American Academy of Pediatrics recommend supplementation of infants with vitamin D (400 U/day) starting at 2 months of age. Iron may be indicated for children with anemia starting at 6 months of age.

Breast-feeding may not be ideal for infants in certain situations. Mothers with HIV or mothers taking certain medications (eg, anticonvulsants) are cautioned about the risks in these cases. Infants who are premature, have congenital problems such as cleft lip or palate, or are at high risk for failure to thrive may require formula supplementation along with breast milk in order to meet their nutritional needs.

The mother who chooses to bottle feed her newborn has several choices in formulas but is not advised to use cow's milk, due to the risk of anemia. All commercial formulas are composed of milk protein and carbohydrates and are typically fortified with iron and vitamin D. Recently, infant formulas have been supplemented with fatty acids such as docosahexaenoic acid (DHA) and arachidonic acid (ARA), based on theories that these fatty acids, which are present in breast milk, promote nervous system development. Unless a medical indication is identified, parents should be discouraged from using soy or lactose-free formulas.

An appropriate weight gain is 1 ounce/day during the first 6 months of life and 0.5 ounce/day during the next 6 months. This weight gain requires a caloric intake of 120 kcal/kg/day during the first 6 months and 100 kcal/kg/day thereafter. Caregivers need to be questioned at every encounter about the amount and duration of the child's feedings. Initially, the child is be fed on demand, when caregivers note signs of hunger such as soft, suckling noises, hand-to-mouth movements,

and rooting movements. Breast-fed infants are expected to feed every 2–3 h about 10–15 min on each breast. Bottle-fed infants are typically fed every 3–4 h with approximately 1.5–3 ounces of formula.

Because the work of feeding is much less with a rubber nipple on a bottle, children who are given formula can easily be overfed, leading to emesis and perhaps a misdiagnosis of reflux. If height and weight parameters show appropriate interval change, parents can be cautioned against inadvertent overfeeding. Furthermore, once the child's eating patterns become more established, parents can learn to use alternative comforting and coping measures when the child starts to cry, instead of offering a bottle.

Solid foods are introduced at 6 months of age when the infant can support his or her head and when the tongue protrusion reflex has extinguished. Delaying introduction of solid foods until this time appears to limit the incidence of food sensitivities. The child can also continue breast- or bottle-feeding, limited to 30 ounces/day, since additional calories are now being provided by the solid foods. The child may receive cereals along with strained, pureed baby foods such as vegetables and fruits. Children can also tolerate some adult foods such as yogurt and mashed potatoes. With the appearance of primary teeth at 8–12 months of age, children may be introduced to more solid foods such as soft rice or pastas. Recommended dietary allowances (RDAs) of select nutrients for children of varying ages are listed in Table 1–2.

As an infant becomes a toddler, meal times may become a source of anxiety for caregivers as children who were "good eaters" exhibit a poor appetite or become finicky. During this time, the child begins to exhibit specific food preferences and is generally disinterested in food. Frustrated parents can be reassured if the child maintains an appropriate growth rate and is meeting developmental milestones. Coping strategies for parents include offering small portions of preferred items first and offering the child limited food choices. Children

Table 1–2. Recommended dietary allowances (RDAs) of select nutrients.

Category	Age	Vitamin A (µg)	Vitamin D (µg)	Vitamin E (µg)	Vitamin K (µg)	Vitamin C (mg)	Niacin (mg niacin equivalent)	Folate (µg)	Calcium (mg)	Iron (mg)
Infants	0–6 months	375	7.5	3	5	30	5	25	400	6
Infants	6 months–1 year	375	10	4	10	35	6	35	600	10
Children	1–3 years	400	10	6	15	40	9	50	800	10
Children	4–6 years	500	10	7	20	45	12	75	800	10

Source: Food and Nutrition Board, National Academy of Sciences, 2000.

can also be encouraged to self-feed finger foods since the pincer grasp is well-developed by this age. Toddlers are encouraged to eat during the family meal times so they can begin to adapt to a routine, especially in preparation for daycare and school schedules. Parents should strive to create a pleasant dinnertime atmosphere with the children involved in the conversation.

By school age, children need to have a wide variety of table foods in their diet. A well-balanced diet with appropriate table foods and low-fat milk is still optimal. However, such a diet may be difficult to enforce since children can make their own food choices at home and at school. Parents can be advised to minimize the availability and consumption of junk food. If the child's diet seems limited, vitamin or mineral supplementation can be considered. On the other hand, childhood obesity is becoming an alarming concern, with studies showing a prevalence of nearly 30%. Making the diagnosis in this population is important, since eating patterns can still be modified, with the cooperation of the caregivers. Often, the clinician may need to refer the entire family for a weight-loss program, which includes behavioral modification and nutritional counseling.

American Academy of Family Physicians (AAFP): *Position Paper on Breastfeeding.* URL: http://www.aafp.org/policy/x1641.xml.

Gartner LM, Gree FR: Prevention of rickets and vitamin D deficiency: new guidelines for vitamin D intake. Pediatrics 2000; 111:908. [PMID: 12671133].

Kramer MS, Kakuma R: Optimal duration of exclusive breastfeeding. Cochrane Database Syst Rev 2002. [PMID: 11869667].

Lawrence RA: Breastfeeding: benefits, risks and alternatives. Curr Opin Obstet Gynecol 2000;12(6):519. [PMID: 11128416].

Oddy WH: Breastfeeding protects against illness and infection in infants and children: a review of the evidence. Breastfeed Rev 2001;9(2):11. [PMID: 11550600].

Oken E, Lightdale JR: Updates in pediatric nutrition. Curr Opin Pediatr 2001;13(3):280. [PMID: 11389365].

Development & Behavior

Watching a newborn develop from a dependent being to a communicative and unique child is an amazing process that caregivers and clinicians can actively participate in and promote. Unfortunately, physicians fail to initially identify over 50% of developmental problems, even though screening tools are available. A spectrum of developmental disabilities may occur during the course of childhood, including cerebral palsy, mental retardation, learning disabilities, attention deficit disorder, behavioral disorders, and hearing or visual impairments.

The Denver Developmental Screening Test, specifically the revised version (DDST II), is one of the most commonly used screening instruments in medical prac-

tice. The test is typically administered to well children from ages of newborn to 6 years in a standardized manner by trained personnel. Because the test requires about 20 min to perform, such an assessment often requires a separate office appointment. Standard test material includes a ball of red wool, a box of raisins, a rattle with a handle, a small bottle, a bell, a tennis ball, and eight 1-inch blocks.

The DDST II screens children who are apparently normal, confirms any concerns that the clinician may have uncovered, and offers a way to monitor children at high risk for developmental delay. The test evaluates children in four domains of development: Personal-Social, Language, Fine Motor-Adaptive, and Gross Motor. Private physician practices often choose to develop a shorter, customized form of developmental milestones. Although these abridged checklists may result in increased numbers of children being screened, clinicians must be sure to follow up any abnormalities with a validated screening tool such as the DDST II.

A brief list of red flags in developmental milestones is given in Table 1–3. Because the period of most active development is in the first year, clinicians must ensure that a developmental assessment is performed and documented at each periodic visit during this time. The assessment is part of both the history taking and the physical examination of the child. Major developmental problems such as cerebral palsy and mental retardation will present in the first 6–8 months of life and will often be associated with some type of chromosomal syndrome. These children must be appropriately referred to a pediatric developmental specialist for a definitive diagnosis and long-term care.

Table 1–3. Developmental "red flags."[1]

Age (months)	Clinical Observation
2	Not turning toward sights or sounds
4–5	No social smiling or cooing
8–9	Not reaching for objects or reciprocating emotions/expressions
12	No signs of expression or sound exchange with caregivers
16	No signs of complex problem-solving interactions
24	Not using words to get needs met
36–48	No signs of using logical ideas with caregivers or pretend play with toys

Source: Brazelton TB, Greenspan SH: *The Irreducible Needs of Children: What Every Child Must Have to Grow, Learn, and Flourish.* Perseus Publishing, 2001.
[1]Serious emotional difficulties in parents or family members at any time warrant full evaluation.

More subtle problems such as speech delay and attention deficit disorder may not be elicited on a basic developmental screen. Parents of older children should be actively questioned about any concerns regarding their child's development. Parents are encouraged to read to their children on a regular basis, limit television to no more than 1 h daily, and directly engage in age-appropriate stimulating activities with their children.

Temperament, which is the way a child experiences and reacts to the environment, is influenced by several factors. Genetic influences, physical health, and psychosocial environment all contribute to the formation of a child's temperament or behavioral style. Furthermore, just like physical attributes, temperaments differ from child to child and many variants in behavior can still be considered normal. Clinicians can discuss the child's temperament with caregivers since knowledge of the child's temperament can guide future understanding and management of behavior and discipline.

As an infant becomes a toddler, temperament manifests in overall behavior as the child starts to develop independence and autonomy with daily living. The important tasks of early childhood include self-feeding, language acquisition, learning to fall asleep alone, and toilet training. Older children need to incorporate the skills gained from achieving prior tasks into new skills that prepare them for scholastic achievement. Some children are unable to succeed, however, due to an inability to concentrate, follow directions, or pay attention to the same degree as their peers. Attention-deficit/hyperactivity disorder is discussed in detail in Chapter 8.

Aylward GP: Conceptual issues in developmental screening and assessment. J Dev Behav Pediatr 1997;18(5):340. [PMID: 9349978].

Goldfarb CE, Roberts W: Developmental monitoring in primary care. Can Fam Physician 1996;42:1527. [PMID: 8792021].

Guidelines for Health Supervision, ed 3. American Academy of Pediatrics, 1997.

Elimination

The establishment of patterns for voiding and stooling provides reassurance to caregivers and clinicians that the child is developing appropriately.

Newborn infants, whose kidneys are fully functional *in utero* are expected to void within the first 24 h after birth. An infant who begins feeding (breast or bottle) is expected to urinate approximately six to eight times a day. Parents are advised to count diapers in the first few weeks to make sure the child is feeding well. As the child becomes older, voiding becomes less frequent, down to four to six wet diapers daily. Changes in voiding frequency can be used as an indicator of the child's hydration status, especially when the child is ill.

Parents of male infants who choose to have their sons circumcised require additional anticipatory guidance. Routine prophylactic circumcision of male infants is not currently advocated. Benefits and disadvantages of prophylactic circumcision need to be considered by families faced with this decision. A circumcised male has a decreased incidence of urinary tract infections (OR 3–5) and a decreased risk of phimosis and squamous cell carcinoma. However, some clinicians raise concerns about complications of the procedure such as bleeding, infection, or damage to the genitalia (incidence of 0.2–0.6%) as well as the trauma and pain the newborn may be subjected to. Therefore, the decision to have a circumcision is based primarily on parental choice and depends on cultural influences as well as personal preferences.

The procedure is usually performed after the second day of life, when the infant is physiologically stable. Contraindications for the procedure include ambiguous genitalia, hypospadius, HIV, and any overriding medical conditions. The denuded mucosa of the phallus appears red and raw for the first week after the procedure. A small amount of serosanguinous drainage on the diaper is normal, although parents are often concerned about infection, which occurs in less than 1% of cases. The penis can be cleansed along with the entire genital area during the regular baby bath. The phallus is completely healed with the scar below the corona radiata by the 2-week well child check-up. Clinicians can ask parents to observe if the infant's urinary stream is straight and forceful.

Stooling patterns also vary with the child's age. Newborns are expected to pass black, tarry meconium stools within the first 24 h of life, assuming a normally patent anus was noted during physical examination. If a baby fails to pass stool in that time period, a work-up for Hirschsprung's disease must be considered. Once the infant starts feeding, stool frequency can be highly variable. The consistency of the stool is usually semisolid and soft, with a yellow-green seedy appearance. Breast-fed infants typically stool after each time they nurse, although some children may stool only two or three times a day. Bottle-fed infants generally have a lower frequency of stooling than nursing infants. Occasionally, some babies may have only one stool every 2 or 3 days, without discomfort. Any appearance of blood in the stools is abnormal and warrants further investigation.

With the introduction of solid foods, stool consistency changes dramatically, becoming more solid and malodorous. The child should continue to be comfortable with stooling as different foods are slowly introduced. If the child is constipated, increased dietary intake of certain fruits and vegetables and water often relieves the problem. Treatment of mild to moderate constipation may include the use of karo syrup mixed in with feedings or psyllium seed tablets in older children. Children who are severely constipated may require referral to a gastroenterologist to rule out underlying organic pathology. After the second year of age, the child may start toilet training practices for both urination and defecation. At this point, it is especially important to monitor the child's intake and output, to ensure that the behavioral challenges of continence are not leading to retention or constipation.

American Academy of Family Physicians: Fact sheet for physicians regarding neonatal circumcision. Am Fam Physician 1995; 52(2):523. [PMID: 7625326].

Bright Futures, Guidelines for Health Supervision of Infants, Children and Adolescents. National Center for Education in Maternal and Child Health, HRSA, 2000.

Lerman SE, Liao JC: Neonatal circumcision. Pediatr Clin North Am 2001;48(6):1539. [PMID: 11732129].

Taddio A: Pain management for neonatal circumcision. Paediatr Drugs 2001;3(2):101. [PMID: 11269637].

Well Child Care: Reference Guide of the American Board of Family Practice, ed 8. American Board of Family Practice, 2000.

Oral Health

As other measures of health outcomes improve, the poor state of oral health in children is now emerging as an area of concern for public health officials. Furthermore, children who are medically and developmentally compromised, socially vulnerable, or come from minority groups or families with low income are disproportionately affected. All practitioners, especially those who work with these populations, need to be aware of the importance of early and periodic dental care. Primary prevention can be initiated by encouraging parents to provide children with a diet high in calcium and by prescribing fluoride supplementation, if the family lives in a community with an unfluoridated water supply (<0.3 ppm). Clinicians can strongly discourage caregivers from putting children to sleep with a bottle in order to minimize the incidence of baby-bottle tooth decay. Once primary teeth erupt, as early as 5–6 months of age, use of soft-bristled brushes with water and parental supervision may be started. A habit of daily brushing can be incorporated into the child's routine, even at this age. Parents can be encouraged to have infants drink from a cup as they approach their first birthday; infants should be weaned from the bottle at 12–14 months of age. The use of a pacifier or the child's thumb for nonnutritive sucking is discouraged after teeth have erupted.

Infants should ideally be scheduled for an initial oral evaluation within 6 months of the eruption of the first primary tooth. Primary care providers can strongly encourage families to seek annual dental appointments by 3 years of age. Older children may need to be limited on their intake of high-carbohydrate food after teeth have been brushed. If appropriate measures are applied early enough, it may be possible to totally prevent oral disease.

Sanchez OM, Childers NK: Anticipatory guidance in infant oral health: rationale and recommendations. Am Fam Physician 2000;61(1):115. [PMID: 10643953].

Sonis A, Zaragoza S: Dental health for the pediatrician. Curr Opin Pediatr 2001;13(3):289. [PMID: 11389366].

CLINICAL FEATURES

History & Physical Examination

During the immediate neonatal period, the prenatal history needs to be carefully reviewed for any concerns. In particular, the record is notable for gestational age at birth; any abnormal maternal obstetric laboratory tests; maternal illnesses such as diabetes, preeclampsia, depression, or infections that occurred during the pregnancy; and maternal use of drugs or exposure to teratogens. A social history should include the family structure and establishment of primary caregivers for the infant, number of other children, and socioeconomic status. The delivery record is also reviewed for pertinent information such as date of birth, mode of delivery, Apgar scores at 1 and 5 min, and birth weight, length, and head circumference.

A comprehensive physical examination of the newborn should include the following elements:

- General observation for evidence of birth trauma, dysmorphic facies, resting muscle tone, respiratory rate, skin discolorations, or rashes.
- Head, ears, eyes, nose, and throat (HEENT) examination for the presence of open fontanelles, bilateral retinal red reflexes, patency of nares, absence of cleft palate/lip, and palpation of clavicles to rule out fracture.
- Cardiovascular examination to include assessment of cardiac murmurs, peripheral pulses, capillary refill, and the presence of cyanosis.
- Pulmonary examination of use of accessory muscles and auscultation of breath sounds.
- Abdominal examination for masses, distention, and the presence of bowel sounds.
- Extremity examination of digits and toes and to screen for congenital dislocation of the hips using Ortolani and Barlow maneuvers.
- Genitourinary examination of genitalia and anus to document normal appearance.
- Neurological examination for the presence of newborn reflexes such as rooting, grasping, sucking, stepping, and Moro.

If clinicians are appropriately trained, a brief developmental assessment at the bedside can also be done using the Clinical Neonatal Behavioral Assessment System (CLNBAS). The CLNBAS is a neurobehavioral assessment designed to educate parents about the capacities of their new child. Developed from the Neonatal Behavioral Assessment Scale (NBAS) used in neonatal intensive care unit (NICU) settings, the CLNBAS can be used by clinicians to promote the parent–infant relationship through interactive observation and to provide anticipatory guidance to parents based on the observations. The CLNBAS is observational, consisting of 18 behavioral and reflex items designed to examine the newborn's physiological and motor states. The scale is composed of items that have an impact on parental caregiving, such as those related to sleep, feeding, crying, and consolability. For example, clinicians assess the infant's ability to habituate to stimuli or to respond to state changes (eg, from sleeping to wakefulness). Although the CLNBAS is not a formal screening tool for developmental delay, it may identify infants at risk for future problems. Furthermore, parents obtain valuable information regarding their baby's individuality and temperament and can adjust caregiving styles to better suit their infant.

Future interval well child visits in the family doctor's office provide a valuable opportunity to track the child's physical and developmental progress. A comprehensive physical examination is important at each encounter, even if the parents do not report any concerns. Furthermore, different clinicians may see the child, making a thorough examination necessary at every visit. To keep the infant as comfortable and cooperative as possible, the examination is performed from the least to the most invasive maneuvers. The child's weight (completely undressed), length, and head circumference are measured. After 3 years of age, blood pressure measurements need to be taken at each visit.

By 9 months of age, infants are at the height of stranger anxiety and they are likely to be much less cooperative with the physical examination. Clinicians can minimize the child's adverse reactions by approaching the child slowly and performing the examination while the child is in the parent's arms. Touching the child's leg or shoe first and then gradually moving up to the chest while distracting with a toy is often helpful. Reaching the first year of life is a milestone for both clinicians and parents. At this point, the pace of the infant's growth will start to plateau. At the 15–18 month visit, the infant will most likely be mobile and want to stand on the table during the examination, if the child is willing to stand still at all. The toddler may need to be distracted by a toy or the examining instrument and can be given choices about the examination. The child will become engaged if clinicians ask questions about where to do the examination or which body part to examine first.

Comprehensive examinations should continue annually from age 2–6, concentrating primarily on the child's psychological and intellectual development. Beginning at 2 years, the child's blood pressure is measured along with the growth parameters. A full eye examination needs to be done since strabismus can be treated during these years. By age 4 or 5 years, documentation of visual acuity can be attempted. Hearing can be informally assessed until age 5 when audiometry may be attempted. Speech usually rapidly improves in the child, with at least 75% of speech being intelligible in the 3 year old. Assessment of gait and spinal alignment continues to be important and physicians need to always be alert for any injuries that may signify child abuse or neglect. Table 1–4 highlights the important components of the physical examination at each age.

Hageman JR, Davis AT, Guest Editors: Care of the infant. Pediatr Clin North Am 1994;41(5).

Nasir LS, Nasir A: *Healthy Child Care: Conception to Age Two Years.* American Academy of Family Physicians Home Study Self Assessment Series Monograph 246, 1999.

Taeusch HW, Ballard RA, editors: *Avery's Diseases of the Newborn.* Saunders, 1998.

Unti SM: The critical first year of life. History, physical examination, and general developmental assessment. Pediatr Clin North Am 1994;41(5):859. [PMID: 7936777].

Screening Laboratory Tests

In every state, newborns undergo some type of serological screening for different inborn errors in order to prevent any developmental delay. Although these requirements can vary from state to state, the most commonly screened diseases along with their biochemical markers are listed in Table 1–5. Screening newborns for hearing problems is done in some institutions but the U.S. Preventative Task Force has not recommended for or against universal screening (Level I recommendation).

Several additional screening tests are part of routine health maintenance during the first year of life. One important tool for monitoring overall infant health is the tracking of the growth parameters. The weight, height, and head circumference are graphed at each age (office visit) on growth charts standardized across the U.S. population (CDC 2002) and the corresponding percentile is noted by the clinician. A child's rate of growth will usually follow one percentile (25th, 50th, etc) from birth through school age. A child may cross percentiles upward, for example, a prematurely born infant who then "catches" up, but a child who drops more than two percentiles is at risk for failure to thrive (see Chapter 2).

Table 1–4. Highlights of physical examination by age.

Age of Child	Components of Examination
2 weeks	Presence of bilateral red reflex Auscultation of the heart for murmurs Palpation of the abdomen for masses Ortolani/Barlow maneuvers for hip dislocation Assessment of overall muscle tone Reattainment of birth weight
2 months	Observation of anatomic abnormalities or congenital malformations (effects of birth trauma resolved by this point) Auscultation of the heart for murmurs
4–6 months	Complete musculoskeletal examination (neck control, evidence of torticollis) Ortolani/Barlow maneuvers for hip dislocation (limited abduction, asymmetrical buttock creases, metatarsus adductus) Vision assessment (conjugate gaze, symmetrical light reflex, visual tracking of an object to 180°)
9 months	Pattern and degree of tooth eruption Assessment of muscle tone Presence of bilateral pincer grasp
12 months	Ortolani/Barlow maneuvers for hip dislocation Range of motion of the hips, rotation and leg alignment Bilateral descent of the testes
15–18 months	Cover test for strabismus Signs of dental caries Ortolani/Barlow maneuvers for hip dislocation Gait assessment Any evidence of injuries

Table 1–5. Commonly screened components of newborn screening panels.[1]

Diseases Screened	Incidence of Disease in Live Births
Congenital hypothyroidism	1:4000
Phenylketonuria	1:14,000
Cystic fibrosis	1:44,000–1:80,000 (depending on population)
Biotinidase deficiency	1:60,000
Galactosemia	1:30,000
Congenital adrenal hyperplasia	1:10,000–1:18,000
Duchenne muscular dystrophy	1:4500

Source: Newborn Screening Fact Sheets. American Academy of Pediatrics Policy Statement. http://www.aap.org/policy/01565.html.
[1]Screening panel requirements vary in each state.

Screening for anemia with finger stick hemoglobin levels begins between the ages of 9 and 12 months. Due to the high prevalence of iron deficiency anemia in toddlers, repeat screenings have been recommended 6 months after the first screening and again at 24 months of age. Measurement of hemoglobin/hematocrit levels alone detects only those patients with enough iron deficiency to be anemic. Some sources recommend screening by ferritin levels or red cell distribution width (RDW) to identify patients earlier. A positive screening test is an indication for a therapeutic trial of iron, which remains the definitive method of establishing a diagnosis of iron deficiency. A sickle cell screen is indicated in African-American children, independent of their iron status.

Annual lead screening begins at age 9 months to 1 year if the child is considered to be at high risk. These risk factors include exposure to chipping or peeling paint in older buildings (built before 1950), frequent contact with an adult who may have significant lead exposure, having a sibling who is being treated for excessive lead levels, and location of the home near an industrial setting likely to release lead. Otherwise, most state agencies that administer early screening and detection programs require a one-time universal screening at 1 year of age, assuming the community has a low prevalence.

Tuberculosis screening using a purified protein derivative (PPD) or Mantoux test is offered to high-risk children at 1 year of age. Routine testing of children without risk factors from low prevalence communities is not indicated. Children require immediate testing if they have had contact with persons with confirmed or suspected cases of infectious tuberculosis, if they have emigrated from endemic countries such as those in Asia or the Middle East, or if they have any clinical or radiographic findings suggestive of tuberculosis.

Children who are infected with HIV need to be retested annually. Children placed at risk due to exposure to high-risk adults (HIV positive, homeless, institutionalized, etc) are retested every 2–3 years. Children without specific risk factors but who come from high prevalence communities may be tested twice: once at ages 4–6 and again at ages 11–12. Testing with the

Tine method is no longer considered accurate but may be used in settings if the PPD is unavailable.

A cholesterol level may be obtained after age 2 if the child has a notable family history of early coronary artery disease but this is not indicated for most children. The National Cholesterol Education Program (NCEP) recommends screening in a child with a parent who has a total cholesterol of 240 mg/dL or greater or a parent or grandparent with onset of cardiovascular disease before age 55 years. Clinical evaluation and management of the child are to be initiated if the low-density lipoprotein (LDL) cholesterol level is 130 mg/dL or greater.

Vision and hearing are assessed informally by the clinician at every visit until the child can cooperate with testing. Although formal audiometry and visual acuity testing begins at age 3, failure to meet developmental milestones triggers earlier referral. A screening urinalysis is obtained once between the ages of 4 and 12 to check for evidence of proteinuria or glycosuria.

Franklin FA Jr, Dashti N, Franklin CC: Evaluation and management of dyslipoproteinemia in children. Endocrinol Metab Clin North Am 1998;27(3):641. [PMID: 9785058].

Guide to Clinical Preventive Services, ed 3, 2000–2003. Report of the U.S. Preventive Services Task Force. URL: http://www.ahcpr.gov/clinic/cps3dix.htm.

Kazal LA Jr: Failure of hematocrit to detect iron deficiency in infants. J Fam Pract 1996;42(3):237. [PMID: 8636674].

Kohli-Kumar M: Screening for anemia in children: AAP recommendations—a critique. Pediatrics 2001;108(3):E56. [PMID: 11533374].

Kronn DF, Sapru A, Satou GM: Management of hypercholesterolemia in childhood and adolescence. Heart Dis 2000; 2(5):348. [PMID: 11728281].

CONCERNS IN NORMALLY DEVELOPING CHILDREN

Every child follows his or her own path for physical, mental, and psychological development. A wide variation exists in the spectrum of child behavior, with the majority of these behaviors considered normal if the child is growing normally and meeting developmental milestones. Anticipatory guidance regarding variations from ideal behavior can be very helpful and reassuring to caregivers when their child exhibits such characteristics. Selected behavioral issues that are commonly encountered include infantile colic, temper tantrums, and toilet training.

Infantile Colic

Colic is a term often used to describe an infant who is difficult to manage or fussy despite being otherwise healthy. Colic may be defined by the "rule of threes":

3 or more hours of uncontrollable crying or fussing at least 3 times a week within a 3-month period. Because the diagnosis of colic depends on parental report, the incidence of colic is unclear, varying from 5% to 20%. The underlying cause of colic has not yet been determined and organic pathology is present in less than 5% of the cases. Current research indicates that colic is likely due to multiple factors, including an immature digestive system that may be sensitive to certain proteins in food, an immature nervous system that may be sensitive to external stimuli, and other factors such as the infant's temperament and interactions with caregivers.

Colic occurs equally in male and female infants. Although anecdotal data suggest that colic occurs less frequently in breast-fed infants, the type of nutrition that the infant receives is likely not related to the incidence. The incidence peaks around 3–4 weeks of age and symptoms typically subside around 3–4 months of age. In addition to the persistent crying or fussiness, other symptoms include facial expressions of pain or discomfort, pulling up of the legs, passing flatus, fussiness with eating, and difficulty falling or staying asleep. Although the symptoms may occur at any time during the day, colic classically worsens during the evening hours.

Clinicians can provide reassurance to caregivers of children with colic. First, colicky children continue to eat and gain weight appropriately, despite the prolonged periods of crying. The syndrome is self-limited and usually dissipates once the child reaches 4 months of age. No evidence suggests long-term or serious outcomes associated with colic. Therefore, the main problem for caregivers is learning to cope with the anxiety that the crying child creates in the home environment.

Clinicians play an important role in offering anticipatory guidance since a stressed caregiver who is unable to handle the situation may be at risk for abusing a child. No definitive treatment can be offered for colic. Little evidence supports the use of Simethicone or Tylenol drops to relieve gas and pain. Switching to a hypoallergenic (soy) formula is effective in cases in which the child has other symptoms suggestive of cow's milk protein allergy. Breast-feeding mothers can attempt to make changes in their diets to see if the infant improves, such as avoidance of cruciferous vegetables (broccoli, cabbage, etc).

Many "home-remedy" strategies (Table 1–6) for attempting to calm the baby have been discussed among clinicians and caregivers. Reducing the amount of stimulation is moderately effective. Carrying or holding the infant, infant massage, or the use of a crib vibrator has been shown to be moderately effective. However, given the variations in infants and caregivers, rigorous study of any of these techniques is difficult. Therefore, clinicians can suggest any or all of these techniques since the cost and potential harm are minimal.

Table 1–6. Strategies for calming a colicky baby.

Frequent burping
Change of feeding position
Infant massage
Carrying the infant in a front sling or back pack
Snug wrapping or swaddling
Keeping the infant in motion on a bouncing seat or swing
Having background noise or vibrations from household
    appliances (dishwasher, vacuum, etc)
Going outside for a walk or car ride
Using a pacifier or helping the infant find their hands
Warm bath

Source: American Academy of Pediatrics: *Caring for Your Baby and Young Child: Birth to Age 5.* Shelov SP, Hanneman RE (editors). Bantam, Doubleday, Dell Publishing, 1998.

Temper Tantrums

Another normal part of child development is the occurrence of temper tantrums. Tantrum symptoms include crying, screaming, kicking, thrashing, head banging, breath holding, breaking or throwing objects, and being aggressive toward other people. Tantrums begin to occur between the ages of 1 and 3 years, a time period in which a child has to reconcile a growing sense of independence with the realities of physical limitations and parental controls. Unfortunately, children at this age also have limited vocabularies and therefore limited ability to talk about their feelings or experiences. This type of power struggle sets the stage for the expression of anger and frustration through a temper tantrum. Tantrums can follow minor frustrations or may occur for no obvious reason. They are mostly self-limited and are an expected part of a healthy child's life, unless they are excessively frequent, violent, or prolonged. Several predisposing factors to intense or persistent tantrums may be identified. An individual child's tendency toward impulsivity or impatience, a delay in the development of motor skills, or cognitive deficits may increase the incidence of tantrums. Parental factors include inconsistent, overly restrictive, or overly indulgent patterns of child rearing, any of which may confuse children who are testing their autonomy. Parents who react to the child's frustration in an inappropriate way, due to low tolerance or external pressures, model that behavior for their children. Tantrums that produce a desired effect for the child have an increased likelihood of recurrence.

Parents and caregivers often turn to physicians for advice on managing temper tantrums. Clinician counseling during the first year needs to include discussions on patterns of discipline and the self-limited nature of tantrums. In general, parents are encouraged to provide the child with a predictable home environment, as much as possible. Consistency in routines and rules will help the child to know what to expect. Parents can teach and praise desired behaviors but act calmly when handling negative behaviors to avoid reinforcement. Preparing children for any potentially difficult transitions from one activity to another and offering them some simple choices are effective ways to satisfy the child's growing need for control. Caregivers need to try to offer acknowledgment and empathy during the tantrum, perhaps holding the child, so the child feels supported. Physical punishment is not advised in these situations. The child learns the message that violence is an acceptable way to handle a problem, which is the opposite of what the caregiver wants the child to learn.

Most importantly, ignoring attention-seeking tantrums and not giving in to the demands of the tantrum will, in time, decrease the recurrence. Children who are disruptive enough to hurt themselves or others must be removed to a safer place and given time to calm down, in a nonpunitive manner. By school age, most children have learned to work out their frustrations by developing their own set of problem-solving and coping skills and are much less likely to have tantrums. Persistence of tantrums past age 4 or 5 years requires further investigation through referral to a behavioral pediatrician or a psychiatric professional. Families may also benefit from group-based parent education and counseling on how to handle behavioral issues.

Toilet Training

Toilet training is a developmental milestone that all parents eagerly await. Child "readiness" is considered one of the most important criteria before beginning training. Some indicators of readiness include an awareness of impending urination or defecation, prolonged involuntary dryness, ability to walk easily, and ability to pull clothes on and off easily. Therefore, training is best deferred until 18–30 months of age, when these indicators are likely to be present. Toddlers who are able to identify body parts, can follow instructions, and can imitate simple tasks are also exhibiting signs of behavioral readiness.

Once the child becomes interested in bathroom activities or in watching their parents use the toilet, a potty chair may be introduced to the child. When the child is comfortable with the chair, the idea of depositing excrement into the potty is introduced. Parents can then initiate toilet training by taking the diaper off and having the child sit on the potty at a time when she or he is likely to urinate or defecate. One opportune time is after meals when the gastrocolic reflex is naturally initiated. Routine sittings on the potty at specified times during the day may be helpful. Furthermore, if parents notice some stereotypical behaviors of elimination, such as straining or bending at the waist, the child may be escorted to the bathroom for a toileting trial. If the child eliminates in the toilet, praise or a small reward may be given, reinforcing the good behavior. The reward should never be linked to meals or promises of the parent's love, as these are important constants in the child's life. Rather, stickers or storybooks that the child enjoys can be used for motivation. Accidents need to be dealt with plainly and the child should not be punished, shamed, or made to feel guilty.

With repeated successes, diapers may be discontinued and/or transitional diapers (pull-ups) or training pants may be used until full continence is achieved. The training process may take days to months, depending on the child, and caregivers can expect accidents. Children with significant constipation can be treated medically, since that may present a barrier to training. About 80% of children achieve success at daytime continence by 30 months of age.

To avoid parental frustration over toilet training, clinicians can provide counseling about the underlying principles for success and practices to be avoided. As with many child-rearing issues, consistency and a nurturing environment are very important in giving the child a sense of security. Parents are to be cautioned about starting training too early or during times of family stress. Caregivers need to be reminded that different children may be at different stages of developmental readiness. The practices of prolonged sitting on the potty or leaving the child sitting on the potty are to be avoided due to their punitive nature. In most cases, patience and reassurance will adequately resolve toileting difficulties. For others, addressing toilet training issues involves an assessment of overall parenting concerns, which may then involve other areas of conflict in the family. Parents can be asked to describe specific scenarios so concrete anticipatory guidance may be given. Any circumstances that are identified as barriers to appropriate guidance should be discussed. Toilet training, as with most behavior modification, has a higher chance of success if positive achievements are rewarded and failures are not emphasized. When reminders about toileting stop and parental investment is minimized, the responsibility for toileting goes to the child, who looks for control at this age.

Barlow J, Stewart-Brown S: Behavior problems and group-based parent education programs. J Dev Behav Pediatr 2000;21(5): 356. [PMID: 11064964].

Gupta SK: Is colic a gastrointestinal disorder? Curr Opin Pediatr 2002;14(5):588. Review. [PMID: 12352253].

Lucassen PL et al: Effectiveness of treatments for infantile colic: systematic review. BMJ 1998;316(7144):1563. [PMID: 9596593].

Polaha J, Warzak WJ, Dittmer-Mcmahon K: Toilet training in primary care: current practice and recommendations from behavioral pediatrics. J Dev Behav Pediatr 2002;23(6):424. [PMID: 12476072].

MEDICAL PROBLEMS

Beyond the normal variations in child development, significant medical problems can be identified and treated by the family physician. Early diagnosis and referral lead to prevention of potentially serious sequelae and improved quality of life. Many abnormalities can be detected in the young child (Table 1–7), underscoring the need for regular and complete well child care visits. This section highlights four important concerns that may present in the outpatient setting: cryptorchidism, childhood anemia, lead toxicity, and amblyopia.

Cryptorchidism

Cryptorchidism or undescended testicles in male infants is one of the most significant findings on physical examination that can be made during newborn care. Potential sequelae include testicular torsion, inguinal hernia, subfertility, and testicular cancer. In addition, certain syndromes associated with cryptorchidism may be identified. At birth, a newborn male's testes are fully developed within the scrotal sac, after their hormonally mediated descent through the inguinal canal. Most diagnoses of cryptorchidism are made at birth, with 3–5% of term infant males affected. The incidence drops to 0.8% by 3 months of age and does not decrease further, even into adulthood.

Cryptorchidism can be categorized based on physical and operative findings: (1) true undescended testicles, which exist intraabdominally along the normal path of descent and have a normally inserted gubernaculum; (2) ectopic testicles, which have an abnormal gubernacular insertion; and (3) retractile testicles, which are not actually undescended. Cryptorchidism may occur unilaterally or bilaterally

Due to the cremasteric reflex, the testicles maintain the ability to be retracted into the abdomen due to

Table 1–7. Abnormalities detected during well child examinations.

Inguinal hernia
Hip dislocation/subluxation
Anal stenosis
Congenital heart disease
Strabismus/amblyopia
Undescended testes
Developmental delay
Pyloric stenosis
Failure to thrive

stimulation or outside environmental conditions. Therefore the testicles may be retracted intraabdominally when an infant is cold, such as during a physical examination. The examiner needs to palpate the inguinal canal from the hip down and also palpate the scrotum directly to detect the presence of the testicles. The location of the testicles needs to be documented by the clinician at every well child check. It is critical to distinguish the retractile testis during physical examination, because no hormone or surgical therapy is required for this condition. Approximately 20% of infants with cryptorchidism will have at least one nonpalpable testicle. Unless the presence of testes is clearly documented, examination by a pediatric urologist is indicated. Any other anatomic abnormalities such as hypospadius or ambiguous external genitalia should be carefully noted. Ultrasound is useful in the obese child to document the presence of gonads.

Once cryptorchidism is diagnosed, delaying referral beyond 6 months is not recommended. Because the incidence does not decrease beyond this time, truly undescended testicles are unlikely to spontaneously resolve. Furthermore, observation beyond 1 year is thought to impair spermatogenesis and lower surgical success rates. Most urologists recommend completion of treatment for cryptorchidism before age 2 years.

Management depends on whether the cryptorchidism is bilateral or unilateral and whether the testicles are palpable. In a phenotypically male newborn, bilateral nonpalpable testes warrant a work-up for congenital adrenal hyperplasia, including pelvic ultrasound, electrolyte measurements, and karyotyping. In an older child serum hormone levels (testosterone, luteinizing hormone, follicle-stimulating hormone, Müllerian-inhibiting substance, thyroid, cortisol) should be determined to rule out absence or lack of testicular formation. In most cases with bilateral nonpalpable testes, surgical exploration is needed. If no testicles can be found and the spermatic vessels end blindly, as in 10% of cases, the surgery is terminated. Over 50% of the time, the testicle is identified intraabdominally and is removed or brought to the scrotum.

In a newborn with palpable but undescended testis, management is initially medical, consisting of hormonal therapy to induce descent of the testicle. The only medication currently approved in the United States for this treatment is intramuscular human chorionic gonadotropin (HCG), typically given on a biweekly basis. Success rate is highest in cases in which the testicle is most distal. Side effects of HCG include enlargement of the penis, pubic hair growth, and aggressive behavior during treatment. If hormonal therapy fails, the standard surgery is inguinal orchiopexy, in which the testicle is brought to the scrotum manually. Complications of orchiopexy include testicular atrophy

(8% in the most distal cases and 25% in intraabdominal cases), failure of the procedure (ascent of the testis), infection, and bleeding. A good prognosis for the infant's long-term health can be ensured with early treatment, making the genitourinary examination extremely important in newborn males.

Docimo SG, Silver RI, Cromie W: The undescended testicle: diagnosis and management. Am Fam Physician 2000;62(9):2037. [PMID: 11087186].

Gill B, Kogan S: Cryptorchidism. Current concepts. Pediatr Clin North Am 1997;44(5):1211. [PMID: 9326959].

King LR: Undescended testis. JAMA 1996;276(11):856. [PMID: 8782621].

Childhood Anemia

Anemia (decreased hemoglobin level) can present in various stages of childhood and the clinician needs to be aware of the normal levels for different ages to make the diagnosis. In general, for children from the ages of 6 months to puberty, a hemoglobin level less than 11.0 g/dL is an indication for evaluation, since anemia is a symptom requiring a diagnosis. In addition, any inappropriate drop in hemoglobin levels must be investigated. Symptoms of severe anemia include increased heart rate, decreased appetite, and congestive heart failure. More commonly, the child may experience mild fatigue or may be asymptomatic. Physical examination may show pallor of conjunctiva or palmar creases. Before doing a work-up for a child with anemia, the clinician must first be confident of the accuracy of the laboratory value.

Pediatric anemias can be classified based on the appearance of the red blood cells (RBC) in the peripheral and the mean corpuscular volume (MCV) measurement in a complete blood count (CBC). Microcytic anemias are characterized by abnormally small RBCs and decreased MCV and are usually the result of decreased RBC production. Macrocytic anemias are characterized by an increased MCV and are associated with increased RBC destruction. Normocytic anemias usually have normal appearing RBCs on the smear and the MCV is in the normal range. Anemias may also be caused by acute hemorrhage, in the case of trauma.

The most commonly encountered childhood anemia is hypochromic microcytic anemia, due to iron deficiency. Iron deficiency anemia (IDA) is typically caused by poor nutrition, but chronic hemorrhage and malabsorption must be ruled out. IDA is most often detected in 10- to 18-month-old children, typically with a history of cow's milk consumption. The National Health and Nutrition Examination Survey, 1999–2000 (NHANES) showed the estimated prevalence of iron deficiency among toddlers 1–2 years was 7%, highest among all the subgroups in the country's population.

Unfortunately, IDA in infants and toddlers is associated with long-lasting diminished mental, motor, and behavioral functioning, although the exact relationship between IDA and the developmental effects is not well understood. However, these effects do not occur until iron deficiency becomes severe and chronic enough to produce anemia by CBC criteria. Although treatment with iron can reverse the blood and iron indices, improvement in developmental functioning is unclear. Therefore, intervention needs to focus on the primary prevention of iron deficiency.

Clinicians can aggressively counsel parents regarding prevention of anemia beginning in the child's first year of life. Parents are urged to completely avoid cow's milk, not only because of the low content of dietary iron but also because of potential gastrointestinal blood loss. Mothers of breast-fed infants are encouraged to eat diets rich in iron and may consider starting iron supplementation in their child at 4–6 months of age. An iron-fortified formula is recommended for all bottle-fed infants. In the second year of life, iron deficiency can be prevented by encouraging parents to give their toddlers a diversified diet that is rich in sources of iron and vitamin C. Consumption of cow's milk, which is typically begun after 1 year of age, is ideally limited to less than 24 ounces/day. All children may benefit from a daily iron-fortified multivitamin.

Treatment of IDA consists of oral iron replacement in the form of drops or tablets. A typical pediatric dosing is 3 mg/kg/day of elemental iron given in a single dose. Concomitant administration of vitamin C may enhance absorption. Follow-up hemoglobin and iron indices are measured 3, 6 and 12 months later. Treatment is typically discontinued after 3 months if the trend of the laboratory studies is good.

Other causes of hypochromic normocytic anemia are inherited blood disorders, such as thalassemia, and lead poisoning. Patient history along with review of the peripheral smear, CBC, and reticulocyte count is usually adequate for appropriate diagnosis. A therapeutic trial of iron can be offered prior to further investigation. However, the clinician must follow up on the patient until the blood is completely normal, since the coexistence of IDA and lead poisoning is well-documented.

Centers for Disease Control and Prevention: Recommendations to prevent and control iron deficiency in the United States. MMWR Recomm Rep 1998;47(RR-3):1. [PMID: 9563847].

Centers for Disease Control and Prevention: Iron deficiency—United States, 1999–2000. MMWR 2002;51(40):897. [PMID: 12418542].

Grantham-McGregor S, Ani C: A review of studies on the effect of iron deficiency on cognitive development in children. J Nutr 2001;131(2S-2):649S. [PMID: 11160596].

Hermiston ML, Mentzer WC: A practical approach to the evaluation of the anemic child. Pediatr Clin North Am 2002;49 (5):877. [PMID: 12430617].

Kazal LA Jr: Prevention of iron deficiency in infants and toddlers. Am Fam Physician 2002;66(7):1217. [PMID: 12387433].

Lead Toxicity

Clinicians need to be concerned about lead poisoning because of its serious and potentially life-threatening neurological sequelae. The spectrum of clinical presentation ranges from vague abdominal pain, malaise, and behavioral changes to acute encephalopathy, with rapid progression to coma and death. Lead intoxication is totally preventable, if a child is protected from exposure. Intoxication is caused by excessive environmental intake through aerosolized and oral contaminants. Flaking lead-based paint in older homes can be ingested by children but also inhaled as microparticles, leading to increased lead absorption. Contaminated water supplies resulting from old plumbing with lead soldering also contribute to poisoning. Other common sources of exposure include lead in soil, lead in dust from construction projects, lead chromate in coated electrical wire, lead-glazed ceramics, leaded crystal, and lead-soldered cans manufactured in foreign countries.

IDA is caused by the direct inhibition by lead of critical iron incorporation enzymes into hemoglobin. Despite normal levels of iron, microcytic anemia results, due to the drop in hemoglobin. Elevated lead levels can also have toxic effects on the renal system by interfering with the metabolism of vitamin D. The neurological complications of lead poisoning have been a concern for public health officials for several decades. Lead toxicity is associated with a two- to three-point decrease in IQ test scores for every increase of 10 µg/dL in the blood lead level. Elevated blood lead levels are also associated with developmental disorders, such as attention deficit disorder, behavioral disturbances, and learning disabilities. Toxic neurological effects on the central nervous system and resultant long-term neurobehavioral and cognitive deficits have been observed even with mildly elevated blood lead levels [10–25 µg/dL (0.50–1.20 µmol/L)]. At higher blood lead levels (more than 70 µg/dL), nephropathy, neuropathy, increased intracranial pressure, seizures, and death are common.

Based on CDC practice guidelines, all children in primary care practices are potential candidates for the screening questionnaire. If the questionnaire is positive, serum screening with a lead level is pursued. Universal serum screening is advocated in higher prevalence areas and clinicians can obtain recommendations for a specific geographic area from the local health department.

Once an at-risk child is identified, management is based on the degree of lead elevation. A level above

10 μg/dL is considered abnormal. All children with abnormal levels need a full clinical evaluation with a medical, environmental, and dietary history as well as a physical examination. If the level is between 10 and 25 μg/dL, the treatment consists of environmental, nonpharmacological interventions to reduce the child's exposure. Families benefit from receiving education on the health effects of lead poisoning, sources for potential lead exposure, and instructions on proper diet for children. Caregivers are encouraged to provide regular meals containing adequate amounts of calcium and iron and supplementation for iron deficiency.

For children with blood lead levels above 25 μg/dL, strategies recommended by the CDC include case management by a qualified social worker, environmental assessment, and lead hazard control. The local health department is usually notified and an exposure assessment is undertaken to try to discern the source of the lead exposure through a home inspection. Hazard control might involve the removal of residential paint and the installation of high-efficiency particulate air (HEPA) filters. Occasionally, home relocation is necessary if a nearby industrial source is the culprit. Clinicians may need to consider the use of chelation therapy in these children if elevated blood levels persist in this range despite environmental interventions.

American Academy of Pediatrics Committee on Environmental Health: Screening for elevated blood lead levels. Pediatrics 1998;101(6):1072. [PMID: 9614424].

Campbell C, Osterhoudt KC: Prevention of childhood lead poisoning. Curr Opin Pediatr 2000;12(5):428. [PMID: 11021406].

Centers for Disease Control and Prevention: *Managing Elevated Blood Lead Levels Among Young Children: Recommendations from the Advisory Committee on Childhood Lead Poisoning Prevention,* March 2002. URL: http://www.cdc.gov/nceh/lead/lead.htm.

Ellis MR, Kane KY: Lightening the lead load in children. Am Fam Physician 2000;62(3):545. [PMID: 10950212].

Wigg NR: Low-level lead exposure and children. J Paediatr Child Health 2001;37(5):423. [PMID: 11885702].

Amblyopia

Amblyopia, commonly referred to as lazy eye, is a preventable cause of vision loss if identified and referred for treatment by the primary care physician. It is defined as a decrease in visual acuity in one or both eyes not directly attributable to any structural abnormality of the eye or visual pathway. With a prevalence of 2%, it is the most common cause of uncorrectable loss of vision in children. It results from the lack of stimulation to the immature visual system by a focused retinal image due to various causes. The visual outcome can range from 20/25, or nearly normal, to worse than 20/200, or legally blind. With effective detection and early treatment, most vision loss associated with this condition can be avoided. Anisometropic amblyopia refers to unilateral involvement, which is most common, and isometropic amblyopia is the term used when the condition is bilateral. Although the first few years are the most crucial, amblyopia may occur in children as old as 4–6 years. There are several major categories of amblyopia—strabismic, refractive, and deprivation—based on the underlying cause.

Strabismic amblyopia is the most common type. Strabismus refers to a misalignment of the visual axes due to improper functioning of the extraocular muscles in one of the eyes, producing diplopia. The deviating eye may turn in (esotropia), out (exotropia), up (hypertropia), or down (hypotropia). The second image produced by the strabismic eye is suppressed by the child's immature visual system to prevent double vision. This suppression can become so effective that the affected eye loses its visual potential. The diagnosis becomes difficult when the eye deviation is subtle. Refractive amblyopia occurs if the two eyes have significantly different refractive states. The young child may rely on the sight of the more focused eye, causing the other eye to lose its visual potential. This type is the most difficult to detect since the child will appear to see normally because the normal eye is being used for visual tasks. Deprivation amblyopia, the most severe in terms of vision loss, develops because the retina does not receive a clear image. Children with unilateral or bilateral congenital cataracts are typically affected, but it also may occur in children with corneal or vitreous opacity, severe ptosis (droopy eyelid), or excessive patching.

Practitioners can play an important role in detecting these problems by performing a thorough ophthalmological examination during well child visits. In the newborn period, the ophthalmoscope is used to examine the red reflex and children with suspected media opacities, as detected by the absence or distortion of red reflex, require urgent referral. Eyelid hemangiomas or other masses, even if subtle, may cause changes in refraction, and children with these problems benefit from early referral. Children with a family history of amblyopia are noted to be at increased risk. Screening for visual acuity starts at 4–6 months of age since infants can usually track an object in horizontal and vertical planes. Clinicians can use the cover test to check for central fixation. Strabismus can be estimated using the corneal light reflex test. If there is displacement of a penlight held 1 m away, an esotropia (temporal deviation) or exotropia (nasal deviation) is present. A more accurate test to detect misalignment is the alternate cover test. Children with suspected strabismus, even if mild or intermittent, are referred for evaluation beginning at 4–6 months of age. Starting at age 3 years, quantitation of visual acuity can be attempted. Tools are available for assessment even if the child does not yet know the alphabet.

Treatment of amblyopia begins with appropriate optical correction using eyeglasses or contact lenses. In the absence of strabismus, this passive treatment may be effective after several months. The classic therapy is occlusion or patching of the normal eye. Nearly full-time occlusion is often prescribed initially. Blurring of the normal eye with atropine is used by some ophthalmologists as an alternative to patching. Follow-up evaluations are recommended at intervals that vary depending on the age of the child, being more frequent for younger children. Treatment is always most effective if started early and the importance of early vision screening cannot be overemphasized.

REFERENCES

Olitsky SE, Nelson LB: Common ophthalmologic concerns in infants and children. Pediatr Clin North Am 1998;45(4):993. [PMID: 9728197].

Simon JW, Kaw P: Commonly missed diagnoses in the childhood eye examination. Am Fam Physician 2001;64(4):623. [PMID: 11529261].

Failure to Thrive

Deborah Auer Flomenhoft, MD

 ESSENTIALS OF DIAGNOSIS

- Persistent weight loss over time.
- Growth failure associated with disordered behavior and development.
- Weight less than third percentile for age.
- Weight crosses two major percentiles downward over any period of time and continues to fall.
- Median weight for age of 76–90% (mild undernutrition), 61–75% (moderate undernutrition), or <61% (severe undernutrition).

General Considerations

Failure to thrive (FTT) is an old problem that continues to be an important entity for all practitioners who provide care to children. Growth is one of the essential tasks of childhood and is an indication of the child's general health. Growth failure may be the first symptom of serious organ dysfunction. Most frequently, however, growth failure represents inadequate caloric intake; malnutrition during the critical period of brain growth in early childhood has been linked to delayed motor, cognitive, and social development. Developmental deficits may persist even after nutritional therapy has been instituted.

FTT was first described by Holt in 1897: he describes a group of children who suddenly "ceased to thrive" and became "wasted skeletons" when weaning was necessitated after the first 4–6 weeks of life. More than 100 years later, although Holt's words continue to resonate in our own experiences, there is no consensus definition of FTT. Residents and medical students need to be familiar with several definitions of FTT. Practitioners must also recognize the limitations of each definition. Competing definitions of FTT include the following:

- ***Persistent weight loss over time.*** Children should steadily gain weight. Although weight loss beyond the setting of an acute illness is pathological, the assessment and treatment for FTT need to be addressed *before* the child has had persistent weight loss.
- ***Growth failure associated with disordered behavior and development.*** This old definition is useful because it reminds the practitioner of the serious sequelae associated with undernutrition. Currently, FTT is more commonly defined by anthropometric guidelines alone.
- ***Weight less than the third percentile for age*** is a classic definition. However, this definition includes children with genetic short stature and children whose weight transiently dips beneath the third percentile with an intercurrent illness.
- ***Weight crosses two major percentiles downward over any period of time.*** Thirty percent of normal children will drop two major percentiles within the first 2 years of life as their growth curve shifts to their genetic potential. These healthy children will continue to grow on the adjusted growth curve. Children with FTT do not attain a new curve, but continue to fall.

The above definitions comprise the classic definitions, but perhaps not the most useful. An assessment of the percentage of the child's median weight for age is the most clinically useful definition of FTT. This quick calculation enables the clinician to assess the degree of undernutrition and plan an appropriate course of evaluation and intervention. The median weight for age is determined by the United States Centers for Disease Control and Prevention (CDC) growth charts. The median should not be adjusted for race, ethnicity, or country of origin. Differences in growth that had previously been attributed to these factors are more likely due to inadequate nutrition in specific geographic or economically deprived populations. Determinations of nutritional status are as follows:

- **76–90% median weight for age represents mild undernutrition.** These children are in no immediate danger and may be safely observed over time.
- **61–75% median weight for age is moderate undernutrition.** These children warrant immediate evaluation and intervention with close follow-up in an outpatient setting.
- **<61% median weight for age is severe undernutrition.** These children may require hospitalization for evaluation and nutritional support.

FTT is one of the most common diagnoses of early childhood in the United States. It affects all socioeconomic groups, although children in poverty are more likely to be affected and more likely to suffer long-term sequelae. Failure to thrive comprises between 3% and 5% of all hospital admissions for children under 2 years. Ten percent of children in poverty meet criteria for FTT. As many as 30% of children presenting to emergency departments for unrelated complaints can be diagnosed with FTT. This last group of children is of most concern. They are least likely to have good continuity of care and most likely to suffer additional developmental insults such as social isolation, tenuous housing situations, and neglect. Because FTT is most prevalent in at-risk populations that are least likely to have good continuity of care it is crucial to address growth parameters at every visit, both sick and well. Many children with FTT may not present for well child visits: if that is the only visit at which the clinician considers growth, many opportunities for meaningful intervention may be lost.

Pathogenesis

When diagnosing FTT it is essential to consider the etiology. Historically there has been a dichotomy: organic versus nonorganic FTT. Either children had major organ dysfunction (organic) or psychosocial problems led to inadequate nutrition (nonorganic). Over the past decades FTT has been better understood as a mixed entity in which both organic disease and psychosocial factors influence each other. With this understanding, the old belief that a child who gains weight in the hospital has nonorganic FTT has been debunked.

A. ORGANIC FTT

Organic causes are identified in 10% of children with FTT. In-hospital evaluations reveal an underlying organic etiology in about 30% of children. These data are misleading, however. More than two-thirds of these children are diagnosed with gastroesophageal reflux disease (GERD). The practitioner risks one of two errors in diagnosing GERD as the source of failure to thrive: physiological reflux is found in as many as 70% of in-

fants. It may be a normal finding in an infant who is failing to thrive for other reasons. Further, undernutrition causes decreased lower esophageal segment (LES) tone, which may lead to reflux as an effect rather than a cause of FTT.

B. NONORGANIC FTT

Nonorganic FTT, weight loss in which no physiological disease is identified, constitutes 80% of cases. Historically, the responsibility for this diagnosis fell on the caretaker. Either the parent was unable to provide enough nutrition or the parent was emotionally unavailable to the infant. In either circumstance the result was unsuccessful feeding. Psychosocial stressors were thought to create a neuroendocrine milieu preventing growth even when calories were available: increased cortisol and decreased insulin levels in undernourished children were thought to hamper weight gain.

C. MIXED FTT

Most FTT is neither purely organic nor nonorganic, but rather *mixed*: there is a transaction between both physiological and psychosocial factors that creates a vicious cycle of undernutrition. For example, a child with organic disease may initially have difficulty eating for purely physiological reasons. However, over time, the feedings become fraught with anxiety for both parents and child and are even less successful. The child senses the parents' anxiety and eats less and more fretfully than before. The parents, afraid to overtax the "fragile" child, may not give the child the time needed to eat. Or they may become frustrated that they are not easily able to accomplish this most basic and essential care for their child. Parents with an ill child may also perceive that other aspects of the child's care are more important than feeding, such as strict adherence to a medication or therapy regimen.

Children with organic disease underlying FTT often gain weight in the hospital when fed by emotionally uninvolved parties such as nurses, volunteers, or physicians: these people do not feel that the child's difficulties represent personal failure and may be more patient. They are also not the sole providers for all of the child's needs. This happy circumstance (weight gain in the hospital) should not be mistaken for parental neglect in the home; rather, the primary care provider should pay close attention to the psychosocial stressors on the feeding dyad.

Conversely the child who seems to be failing to thrive for purely psychosocial reasons often has complicating organic issues. The undernourished child is lethargic and irritable, especially at feeding times. As noted above, undernutrition decreases LES tone and may worsen reflux: the undernourished child is more difficult to feed and holds down fewer calories. Poor nutrition adversely affects immunity: children with FTT often have recurrent infections that increase their caloric requirements and decrease their ability to meet them.

The mixed model reminds the clinician that FTT is an interactive process involving physiological and psychosocial elements and, more importantly, both parent and child. The child's attributes affect the relationship as surely as the parents'. A fussy child may be more difficult for a particular parent to feed. A "good" or passive baby may not elicit enough feeding. Physical characteristics also affect parent–child relationships: organic disease may not only make feeding difficult but may engender a sense of failure or disappointment in the parent. It is crucial to remember that each child is different; parents have unique relationships with each of their children. Therefore, a parent whose first child is diagnosed with FTT is not doomed to repeat the cycle with the second child. Conversely, an experienced parent who has fed previous children successfully is not immune from the specter of FTT.

D. CAUSES OF FTT

All failure to thrive is caused by undernutrition. The mechanism varies. The child may have increased caloric requirements because of organic disease. The child may have inadequate intake either because not enough food is made available or there is mechanical difficulty in eating.

Or adequate calories may be provided but the child is unable to utilize them either because the nutrients cannot be absorbed across the bowel wall or because of inborn errors of metabolism (Table 2–1).

The astute clinician will note that there may be overlap between these mechanisms. For example, a child with cystic fibrosis has increased caloric requirements associated with chronic respiratory tract infections. However, shortness of breath may make it difficult for the child to eat sufficient quantities. And finally, a child with pancreatic insufficiency will be unable to absorb the nutrients needed to grow.

Prevention

FTT may be prevented by good communication between the primary care provider and the family. The practitioner should regularly assess feeding practices and growth and educate parents about appropriate age-specific diets. As a general rule, infants who are feeding successfully gain about

- 30 g/day at 0–3 months
- 20 g/day at 3–6 months
- 15 g/day at 6–9 months
- 12 g/day at 9–12 months
- 8 g/day at 1–3 years

In addition, growth parameters need to be recorded at every visit, sick or well. Weight should be documented

Table 2–1. Causes of failure to thrive.[1]

Decreased Caloric Intake	Increased Caloric Requirement	Impaired Utilization/Loss
Neurological disorders	Sepsis	Inborn errors of metabolism
Structural anomalies	Trauma	Storage diseases
Injury or infection of mouth or esophagus	Burns	Pyloric stenosis
Chromosomal abnormalities	Congenital heart disease	GERD
Metabolic disease	Renal disease	Pancreatic insufficiency
Improper formula preparation	Cystic fibrosis	Brush border enzyme deficiency (after chronic diarrhea)
Inappropriate diet	Chronic infection: HIV; TB	Short bowel
Food allergies	Hyperthyroidism; malignancy	IBD; celiac disease
Anorexia	Cerebral palsy	Parasitic infection: *Giardia*
Parental/infant factors	Sickle cell disease	Chronic enteric infection
Asthma	Asthma	Diabetes mellitus; Addison's disease
BPD	BPD	Allergies

[1]GERD, gastroesophageal reflux disease; HIV, human immunodeficiency virus; TB, tuberculosis; IBD, inflammatory bowel disease; BPD, bronchopulmonary dysplasia.

for all children. Recumbent length is measured for children younger than 2 years old. Height is measured for children older than 3 years old. Between the ages of 2 and 3 years either height or length may be recorded. Length measurements exceed heights by an average of 1 cm. With a good growth chart in hand, the primary care provider can monitor growth and intervene early if problems arise.

Clinicians should investigate the economic stresses on families. In a family struggling with recent unemployment or underemployment, referral to a walk-in clinic or other social support programs may prevent hunger and subsequent FTT.

Clinical Findings

A. Symptoms and Signs

The importance of a complete, long-term growth curve in making the diagnosis of FTT cannot be overemphasized. Acute undernutrition manifests as "wasting"; the velocity of weight gain decreases while height velocity continues to be preserved. The result is a thin child of normal height. Chronic undernutrition manifests as "stunting"; both height and weight are affected. The child may appear proportionately small. Review of a growth curve may reveal that weight was initially affected and increase the suspicion for FTT.

B. History

The clinician's most valuable tool in the diagnosis of FTT is the history. Each aspect of the history adds invaluable information. While taking the history health care providers have the opportunity to establish themselves as the child's advocate and the parents' support. Care must be taken not to establish an adversarial relationship with the parents. It is useful to begin by asking the parents their perception of their child's health; many parents do not recognize FTT until the clinician brings it to their attention.

The history and physical examination are more valuable than any standard battery of tests in uncovering significant organ dysfunction contributing to growth failure. For example, the child who feeds poorly may have a physical impediment to caloric intake such as cleft palate or painful dental caries. Poor suck may also raise concerns for neurological disease. Recurrent upper or lower respiratory tract infections may suggest cystic fibrosis (CF), human immunodeficiency virus (HIV), or immunodeficiency. Sweating during feeding should prompt consideration of an underlying cardiac problem with or without cyanosis. Chronic diarrhea indicates malabsorption: chronic infection, allergic disease, sprue, and pancreatic insufficiency should be evaluated.

The health care provider must elicit more subtle aspects of past medical history as well: particular attention must be paid to developmental history and intercurrent illnesses. Delay in achievement of milestones should prompt a close neurological examination: inborn errors of metabolism and cerebral palsy can present with growth failure. A history of recurrent serious illness may be the only indicator of inborn errors of metabolism. Recurrent febrile illness without a clear source may also indicate urinary tract infection. A history of snoring or sleep apnea should prompt an evaluation for tonsillar and adenoidal hypertrophy, which has been identified as a cause of FTT.

Past medical history must include a complete perinatal history. Children with lower birth weights and those with specific prenatal exposures are at higher risk for growth problems. Forty percent of children with FTT have birth weights below 2500 g; only 7% of all births are below 2500 g. Low birth weights may be caused by infection, drug exposure, or other maternal and placental factors.

The child with symmetric growth retardation is of particular concern. Infants exposed *in utero* to rubella, cytomegalovirus (CMV), syphilis, toxoplasmosis, or malaria are at high risk for low birth weight, length, and head circumference. These measurements portend poor catch-up growth potential. Short stature is often accompanied by developmental delay and mental retardation.

Children with asymmetric intrauterine growth retardation (preserved head circumference) have better potential for catch-up growth and appropriate development. Fetal growth is affected by both maternal factors and exposure to toxins. Drugs of abuse such as tobacco, cocaine, and heroin have been correlated with low birth weight. Placental insufficiency caused by hypertension, preeclampsia, collagen vascular disease, or diabetes may result in an undernourished baby with decreased birth weight. And, finally, intrauterine physical factors may reduce the fetus's growth: uterine malformation, multiple gestation, and fibroids may all contribute to smaller babies.

A careful investigation of the health of the mother is warranted. Maternal HIV is a significant risk factor for FTT. Most children born to HIV-positive mothers have normal birth weights and lengths. However, children who are infected frequently develop FTT within the first year of life.

An examination of the family's relationship with the child and one another can uncover valuable information. The parents' description of the child's disposition is informative. Children described as "difficult" or "unpredictable" by their mothers have been noted to be slow or poor feeders by independent observers. Maternal depression and history of abuse are strong risk factors for FTT; addressing these issues is integral to establishing a functional feeding relationship between parent and child. Finally, a thorough assessment of economic supports may reveal that nutritious foods are unobtainable or difficult to access. Social financial supports are often inadequate to meet children's needs: WIC provides about 26 ounces of formula per day and food stamps provide three dollars per person per day. Tenuous housing or homelessness may make it impossible to keep appropriate foods readily available.

C. FEEDING HISTORY

A careful feeding history constitutes the history of present illness; it often sheds more light on the problem than a battery of laboratory tests. When assessing an infant, it is essential to know what formula the infant is taking, what volume, and how frequently. Careful attention must be paid to the mixing of formula. Pictograms on the back of powdered formulas routinely show a single scoop of formula being added to a full bottle of water: families that are non-English speaking or have low literacy skills may be inadvertently mixing dilute formula. In calculating caloric intake, the practitioner should remember that breast milk and formula have 20 cal/ounce. Baby foods range from 40 to 120 cal/jar: a good rule is 80 cal/4-ounce jar.

How the baby eats is as important as how much the baby eats. The examiner should ask how long it takes the baby to eat: slow eating may be associated with poor suck or decreased stamina secondary to organic dysfunction. Parental estimation of the infant's suck may also be helpful. Parents should be asked both if the baby is spitty and if the baby vomits frequently as they may endorse one symptom and deny the other. The clinician should inquire about feeding techniques: bottle propping may indicate a poor parent–child relationship or an overtaxed parent.

The breast-fed baby merits special mention. The sequelae of unsuccessful breast-feeding are profound. Infants may present with severe dehydration: normal infants have been neurologically devastated and even died. Parents rarely recognize that the infant is failing to thrive. Mothers are often discharged from the hospital before milk is in and may be unsure about what to expect or misinterpret their experience in the hospital as successful nursing.

The neonatal period is the most critical period in the establishment of breast-feeding. The primary care provider should educate the breast-feeding mother prior to hospital discharge. Milk should be in by Day 3 or 4. The neonate should feed at least eight times in a 24-h period and should not be sleeping through the night. A "good" baby, an infant who sleeps through the night, should rouse concerns of possible dehydration. Breast-fed babies should have at least six wet diapers a day. Whereas formula-fed infants may have many stool patterns, the successful breast-fed neonate should have at least four yellow seedy stools a day. (After 4 weeks of life stool pattern may change to once a day or less.)

Breast-fed babies should be followed up within the first week of life to evaluate infant weight and feeding success. Weight loss is expected until Day 5 of life. Infants should regain their birthweight by the end of the second week of life. Any weight loss greater than 8% should elicit concern: weight loss greater than 10–12% should prompt evaluation for dehydration, ie, serum sodium. Primary care providers should ask about the infant's suck and whether the mother feels her breasts are emptied at the feeding. The successful infant should empty the mother's breast and be contented at the end of the nursing session.

The evaluation of older children also requires a thorough diet history. An accurate diet history begins with a 24-h diet recall: parents should be asked to quantify the amount their child has eaten of each food. The 24-h recall acts as a template for a 72-h diet diary, the most accurate assessment of intake. Studies demonstrate that the first 48 h of a diet diary are the most reliable. All intakes must be recorded including juices, water, and snacks. The child who consumes an excessive amount of milk or juice may not have the appetite to eat more nutrient-rich foods: a child needs no more than 16–24 ounces of milk and should be limited to less than 12 ounces of juice per day.

It is as important to assess mealtime habits as the meals themselves. Activity in the household during mealtime may be distracting to young children. Television watching may preempt eating. Excessive attention to how much the child eats can increase the tension and ultimately decrease the child's intake. Most toddlers cannot sit for longer than 15 min: prolonging the table time in the hopes of increasing the amount eaten may only exacerbate the already fragile parent–child relationship. And although many toddlers graze throughout the day, some are unable to take in appropriate calories with this strategy.

The primary care provider should also discuss the family's beliefs about a healthy diet. Some families have dietary restrictions, either by choice or culturally, that affect growth. Many have read the dietary recommendations for a healthy adult diet, but a low-fat, low-cholesterol diet is not an appropriate diet for a toddler. Until the age of 2 years children should drink whole milk and their fats should not be limited. Only after the age of 5 years is it appropriate to move to a Step 1 diet. This may seem counterintuitive to many parents.

D. PHYSICAL EXAMINATION

In addition to reviewing the growth curve the clinician must complete a physical examination. A weight, length, or height as appropriate for the child's age, and head circumference are indicated for all children. Growth parameters may be roughly interpreted using the following guidelines:

- Acute undernutrition: low weight, normal height, normal head circumference.
- Chronic undernutrition: short height, normal weight for height, normal head circumference.
- Acute or chronic undernutrition: short height, proportionately low weight for height, normal head circumference.
- Congenital infection or genetic disorder impairing growth: short height, normal to low weight for height, small head circumference.

The general examination provides a wealth of information. Vital signs should be documented: bradycardia and hypotension are worrisome findings in the malnourished child. It is important to document observations of the parent–child interaction in the physical examination: are the parent and child responsive to one another or is the child lying unattended on the examining table? In the same vein, it is useful to note both the parent's and the child's affect: parental depression has been associated with higher risk of FTT. And, as noted above, the child's disposition is integral in shaping the parent–child relationship. Occasionally the examiner may find subtle indications of neglect such as a flat occiput indicating that the child is left alone for long periods. However, in this day of "back to sleep" a flat occiput may be a normal finding.

Children with undernutrition often have objective findings of their nutritional state. Unlike the genetically small child, children with FTT have decreased subcutaneous fat. If undernutrition has been prolonged they will also have muscle wasting: in infants it is easier to assess muscle wasting in the calves and thighs rather than in the interosseous muscles. It is also important to remember that infants suck rather than chew, therefore they will not have the characteristic facies of temporal wasting. Nail beds and hair should be carefully noted as nutritional deficiencies may cause pitting or lines in the nails. Hair may be thin or brittle. Skin should be examined for scaling and cracking, which may be seen with both zinc and fatty acid deficiencies.

The physical examination should be completed with special attention directed to the organ systems of concern uncovered in the history. However, examination of some organ systems may reveal abnormalities not elicited through history. A thorough abdominal examination is of particular importance: organomegaly in the child with FTT raises the possibility of inborn errors of metabolism and requires laboratory evaluation. The examiner should note the genitourinary (GU) examination: undescended testicles may indicate panhypopituitarism; ambiguous genitalia may indicate congenital

adrenogenital hyperplasia (CAH). A careful neurological examination may reveal subtly increased tone consistent with cerebral palsy and, therefore, increased caloric requirements. And finally, the examiner must not neglect the rectal examination: fissures and hemorrhoids can be signs of inflammatory bowel disease (IBD) in young children.

Children with undernutrition have been repeatedly shown to have behavioral and cognitive delays. Unfortunately the Denver Development Screen II is an inadequate tool to assess the subtle but real delays in these children. It has been suggested that the Bayley Test may be a more sensitive tool when assessing these children. Even with nutritional and social support, behavioral and cognitive lags may not correct. Indeed, children who have suffered FTT remain sensitive to undernutrition throughout childhood: one study found a significant decrease in fluency in children with a remote history of undernutrition when they did not eat breakfast. Children with a normal nutritional history were not found to be similarly affected.

The immune system is affected by nutritional status. Children with FTT may present with recurrent mucosal infections: otitis media, sinusitis, pneumonia, and gastroenteritis. Immunoglobulin A (IgA) production is extremely sensitive to undernutrition. With this in mind, the clinician must be sensitive to the growth parameters of children presenting frequently for intercurrent illness. Children with FTT also may be lymphopenic (lymphocyte count <1500) or anergic: both of these immune effects are found in more severe malnutrition.

Undernourished children are frequently iron deficient, even in the absence of anemia. Iron and calcium deficiencies enhance the absorption of lead. In areas in which there is any concern for lead exposure, lead levels should be assessed as part of the workup for FTT.

E. LABORATORY FINDINGS

No single battery of laboratory tests or imaging studies can be advocated in the workup of FTT. Testing should be guided by the history and physical examination. Less than 1% of "routine laboratory tests" ordered in the evaluation of FTT provide useful information for treatment or diagnosis.

Tests that had been advocated as markers of nutritional status have limitations. Albumin has an extremely long half-life (21 days) and is a poor indicator of recent undernutrition. Prealbumin, which has been touted as a marker for recent protein nutrition, is decreased in both acute inflammation and undernutrition. Retinol-binding protein reflects only the calories consumed but is unaffected by the protein content (and, by extension, the quality) of the diet.

Laboratory evaluation is indicated when the history and physical examination suggest underlying organic disease. Children with developmental delay and organomegaly or severe episodic illness should have a metabolic workup including urine organic and serum amino acids: there is a 5% yield in this subset of patients. Children with a history of recurrent respiratory tract infections or diarrhea should have a sweat chloride performed at a cystic fibrosis center. Less experienced laboratories offer unreliable results. A history of poorly defined febrile illnesses or recurrent "viral illness" may be followed up with a urinalysis, culture, and renal function to evaluate for occult urinary tract disease. In children with diarrhea it may be useful to send stool for *Giardia* antigen, qualitative fat, white blood cell (WBC) count, occult blood, ova and parasites (O&P), rotavirus, and α_1-antitrypsin. Rotavirus has been associated with a prolonged gastroenteritis and FTT. Elevated α_1-antitrypsin in the stool is a marker for protein enteropathy.

Infectious diseases need to be specifically addressed. Worldwide, tuberculosis (TB) is one of the most common causes of FTT. A Mantoux test and anergy panel must be placed on any child with risk factors for TB exposure. HIV must also be entertained. FTT is frequently a presenting symptom of HIV in the infant. Testing for HIV is not legally required in prenatal assessment: mothers may not know their children are at risk. Any suspicion of HIV merits testing. Less ominous infectious etiologies can also cause FTT: persistent giardiasis and rotavirus are two common toddler infections that cause poor growth.

Differential Diagnosis

It is essential to differentiate a small child from the child with FTT. No criterion is specific enough to exclude those who are small for other reasons. Included in the differential diagnosis of FTT are familial short stature, Turner's syndrome, normal growth variant, prematurity, endocrine dysfunction, and genetic syndromes limiting growth.

Here, too, a good growth chart is of great utility. The child with FTT has a deceleration in weight first. Height velocity continues unaffected for a time. Children with familial short stature have a simultaneous change in their height and weight curves. Height velocity slows first (it can even plateau) in endocrine disorders such as hypothyroidism. The preterm infant's growth parameters need to be adjusted for gestational age: head circumference is adjusted until 18 months, weight until 24 months, and height through 40 months.

The family history is helpful in differentiating the child with FTT from the child with constitutional growth delay or familial short stature. Midparental height, which can be calculated from the family history, is a useful calculation of probable genetic potential:

- For girls: (father's height in inches − 5 + mother's height)/2 plus or minus 2 inches
- For boys: (mother's height in inches + 5 + father's height)/2 plus or minus 2 inches.

If the child's current growth curve translates into an adult height that falls within the range of midparental height reassurance may be offered.

It is most difficult to differentiate the child with constitutional growth delay from the child with FTT. These children typically have reduced weight for height as do children with FTT. However, unlike children with FTT they ultimately gain both weight and height on a steady curve. Family history is often revealing in constitutional growth delay. Querying parents about the onset of their own pubertal signs may seem intrusive, but often gives the clinician the information needed to reassure parents about their child's growth.

Breast-feeding infants may be growing normally and not follow the CDC growth curves. After 4–6 months their weight may decrease relative to their peers. After 12 months their weight catches up to that of age-matched formula-fed infants. However, a decrease in weight in early infancy is a symptom of unsuccessful breast-feeding and should be interpreted as FTT.

Complications

Developmental delay may persist in children with FTT well past the period of undernutrition. Studies have repeatedly shown that these children, as a group, have more behavioral and cognitive problems in school than their peers, even into adolescence. One caveat about these studies is that many defined failure to thrive by that classic definition: growth failure associated with disordered behavior and development. These studies do not doom every child with FTT to scholastic and social failure: but the clinician must be vigilant and act as the child's advocate. Formal developmental screening is especially important in the child with a history of FTT. Intervention should be offered early rather than waiting "to see if the child catches up." Children with FTT can be successful but may need specific supports on the road to achieving that success.

Treatment

A. NUTRITION

The cornerstone of therapy is nutrition. The goal of treatment is catch-up growth. Children with FTT may need 1.5 to 2 times the usual daily calories to achieve catch-up growth. For an infant this is roughly 150–200 cal/kg/day. There are many formulas for calculating caloric requirements: one simple estimate is

$$kcal/kg = 120 \text{ kcal/kg} \times \text{median weight for current}$$
$$\text{height/current weight (kg)}$$

It is important that this nutrition include adequate protein calories. Children with undernutrtion require 3 g protein/kg body weight/day to initiate catch-up growth and may need as much 5 g/kg. (In the literature from the developing world some malnourished children have required as much as 12 g protein/kg/day!) High calorie diets should continue until the child achieves an age-appropriate weight for height.

It is almost impossible for any child to take in two times the usual volume of food. Some solutions are to offer higher calorie formulas (24–30 cal/ounce) to infants. For older children it is possible to replace or add higher calorie foods. Heavy cream may be substituted for milk on cereal or in cooking. Cheese may be added to vegetables. Instant breakfast drinks may be offered as snacks. It is advisable to enlist a dietician in designing a high-calorie diet for the child with FTT.

Occasionally tube feedings are indicated in the child with FTT. Some children may benefit from nighttime feedings through a nasogastric or a percutaneous endoscopic gastrostomy tube. This solution is particularly useful in children with underlying increased caloric requirements, eg, children with cystic fibrosis and cerebral palsy. Children with mechanical feeding difficulties may also require tube feeding for some period of time. The child who is primarily tube fed should have early intervention with an occupational or speech therapist. Without therapy the child may develop oral aversions or fail to develop appropriate oral–motor coordination: both issues will worsen FTT when oral feeding is reinstituted.

Parents need to be educated at the onset of nutritional therapy. Catch-up growth is expected within the first month. However, some children may not show accelerated weight gain until after the first 2 weeks of increased nutrition. Children usually gain 1.5 times their daily expected weight gains during the catch-up phase. Children's weight improves well before their height increases: parents may expect their previously skinny child to become cherubic and even plump. This change in body habitus does not indicate overfeeding but successful therapy. It does not matter how quickly the child gains; the composition of weight gain will be 45–65% lean body mass.

B. MEDICATIONS

Few medications are indicated in the treatment of FTT. Those few are nutritional supports. Children with FTT should be supplemented with iron. Zinc has also been shown to improve linear growth. It is sufficient to supplement children with a multivitamin containing zinc and iron. Vitamin D supplementation should also be considered. Vitamin D replacement is especially important in dark-skinned children and in children who are not regularly exposed to sunlight.

C. SOCIAL SUPPORT

Beyond nutritional support the importance of social support has already been alluded to. The services offered must be tailored to the family and the child. Certainly frequent visits with the primary care provider are useful: weight gain can be measured and concerns addressed. Home visits by social services have been shown to decrease hospitalizations and improve weight gain. Children with developmental delay need early assessment and intervention by the appropriate therapists.

The primary care provider plays a critical role in recognizing and assessing FTT. These seemingly simple interventions made early in childhood have lasting ramifications throughout the life span.

D. INDICATIONS FOR REFERRAL OR ADMISSION

Most FTT can and should be managed by the primary care provider. A trusting relationship between the clinician and the family is an invaluable asset in the treatment of failure to thrive. Parents struggling with the diagnosis often believe that the health care system views them as neglectful. This anxiety creates barriers to open and honest communication about the child's feeding and developmental status. However, suspicions may be allayed when primary care providers enlist themselves as allies in the treatment.

The primary indication for referral is the treatment of an underlying organ dysfunction, eg, cystic fibrosis, that requires specialized care. The clinician may also wish to reevaluate the child who fails to begin catch-up growth after 1–2 months of nutritional intervention.

Most children with FTT can be managed in the outpatient setting: a few may need hospitalization at some point during their evaluation. Indications for admission at initial evaluation are bradycardia or hypotension, indicators of severe malnutrition. As noted above, children who are less than 61% of the median weight for their age should be admitted for nutritional support. The practitioner should have a low threshold for admitting children with hypoglycemia: low serum glucose is worrisome for severe malnutrition and metabolic disease.

The majority of families of children with FTT are neither abusive nor neglectful. However, if the clinician suspects abuse or neglect the child should be admitted: about 10% of children with FTT are abused. These children ultimately experience poorer developmental outcomes than other children with FTT if left in the home. When abuse is documented social services must be involved.

The third group of children who may be considered for hospital admission are those who have failed to initiate catch-up growth with outpatient management. A brief hospital stay will allow the clinician to observe feeding practices and enable the family to internalize the plan of care. Further testing for organ dysfunction may be indicated during this hospitalization. It can also be a time to enlist other health professionals in the treatment plan: occupational therapists and social workers are often helpful allies in the treatment of FTT.

Neonatal Hyperbilirubinemia

Andrew B. Symons, MD, MS, & Martin C. Mahoney, MD, PhD, FAAFP

ESSENTIALS OF DIAGNOSIS

- Visible yellowing of the skin, ocular sclera, or both are present.
- Serum bilirubin levels are in excess of 5 mg/dL (85 μmol/L).

General Considerations

Nearly every baby is born with a serum bilirubin level that is above that of the normal adult. Approximately 60% of newborns are visibly jaundiced during the first week of life. The diagnostic and therapeutic challenge for the physician is to differentiate normal physiological jaundice from pathological jaundice, and to institute appropriate evaluation and therapy when necessary.

Table 3–1 lists several maternal and neonatal factors that are risk factors for neonatal hyperbilirubinemia. Common clinical characteristics associated with severe hyperbilirubinemia include clinical jaundice in the first 24 h, visible jaundice prior to hospital discharge, previous jaundiced sibling, gestation <37 weeks, exclusive breast-feeding, East Asian race, bruising, cephalohematoma, maternal age over 25 years, and male gender.

Pathogenesis

A. PHYSIOLOGICAL JAUNDICE

The three classifications of neonatal hyperbilirubinemia are summarized in Table 3–2 based upon mechanism of accumulation. In the newborn, unconjugated bilirubin is produced faster and removed slowly than in the normal adult due to immaturity of the glucuronyl transferase enzyme system. The main source of unconjugated bilirubin is the breakdown of hemoglobin in senescent red blood cells. Newborns have an increased erythrocyte mass at birth (average hematocrit of 50% versus 33% in the adult) and a shorter life span for erythrocytes (90 days versus 120 days in the adult). The newborn cannot readily excrete unconjugated bilirubin, and much of it is reabsorbed by the intestine and returned to the enterohepatic circulation.

Increased production and decreased elimination of bilirubin lead to a "physiological jaundice" in most normal newborns. Bilirubin is a very effective and potent antioxidant, and physiological jaundice may provide a mechanism for protecting the newborn from oxygen free-radical injury. The average full-term white newborn experiences a peak serum bilirubin concentration of 5–6 mg/dL (86–103 μmol/L), which begins to rise after the first day of life, peaks on the third day of life, and falls to normal adult levels by Day 10–12. African-American infants tend to have slightly lower peaks in serum bilirubin. In Asian infants, serum bilirubin levels rise more quickly than in white infants and tend to reach higher peaks on average (8–12 mg/dL; 135–205 μmol/L). This leads to a longer period of physiological jaundice among Asian and Native American newborns. Preterm infants (<37 weeks gestation) of all races may take 4–5 days to reach peak serum bilirubin levels, and these peaks may be twice that observed among full-term infants.

B. BREAST-FEEDING AND BREAST MILK JAUNDICE

Babies who are breast-fed may experience exaggerated bilirubin levels due to two separate phenomena: breast-feeding and breast milk. Breast-fed babies may experience relative starvation in the first few days of life due to delayed release of milk by the mother or difficulties with breast-feeding. This nutritional inadequacy can result in increased enterohepatic circulation of bilirubin leading to elevated serum bilirubin levels in the first few days of life termed "breast-feeding jaundice." This is considered abnormal and can be overcome by offering frequent feedings (10–12 times per day) and by avoiding water supplementation in breast-fed infants.

Breast milk is believed to increase the enterohepatic circulation of bilirubin; however, the specific factor(s) present in breast milk responsible for this action are unknown. "Breast milk jaundice" is a phenomenon that

Table 3–1. Risk factors for neonatal hyperbilirubinemia.

Maternal Factors	Neonatal Factors
Blood type ABO or Rh incompatibility	Birth trauma: cephalohematoma, cutaneous bruising, instrument delivery
Breast-feeding	Drugs: sulfisoxazole acetyl with erythromycin, ethylsuccinate, chloramphenicol
Drugs: diazepam, oxytocin	
Ethnicity: Asian, Native American	Excessive weight loss after birth
	Infections: TORCH
Maternal illness: gestational diabetes	Infrequent feedings
Maternal age ≥25	Male gender
	Polycythemia
	Prematurity
	Previous sibling with hyperbilirubinemia
	Jaundiced in first 24 h
	Visible jaundice upon discharge

Maternal mnemonic

A—ABO or RH incompatibility; maternal age >25 years
B—breast-feeding
C—child-induced condition → gestational diabetes
D—drugs: oxytocin, diazepam
E—ethnicity: Asian, Native American

Infant mnemonic

A—arrived early (i.e., prematurity)
B—birth trauma/bruising
B—blood → polycythemia
C—cephalohematoma
D—drugs
E—excessive weight loss
F—feeding (infrequent feedings; breast-feeding)
G—gender → male
H—history of siblings with hyperbilirubinemia
I—Infections (TORCH)
J—jaundiced within 24 h or visibly jaundiced on discharge

Adapted from American Academy of Pediatrics, Subcommittee on Neo-natal Hyperbilirubinemia: Neonatal jaundice and kernicterus. Pediatrics 2001 and Porter MI, Dennis BI: Hyperbilirubinemia in the term newborn. Am Fam Physician 2002;65:599.

occurs in breast-fed infants that begins at approximately Day 6 of life (for the first 5 days of life, serum bilirubin in breast-fed infants parallels non-breast-fed infants). Around Day 6 of life, serum bilirubin either rises a little for a few days or declines more slowly. Approximately two-thirds of breast-fed babies may be expected to have hyperbilirubinemia from 3 weeks to 3 months of age, with as many as one-third exhibiting clinical jaundice. Breast milk jaundice (unlike breast-feeding jaundice) is considered a form of normal physiological jaundice in healthy, thriving breast-fed infants.

C. PATHOLOGICAL JAUNDICE

Exaggerated physiological jaundice occurs at serum bilirubin levels between 7 and 17 mg/dL (104–291 μmol/L). Bilirubin levels above 17 mg/dL in full-term infants are no longer considered physiological, and further investigation is warranted.

The onset of jaundice within the first 24 h of life and/or a rate of increase in serum bilirubin exceeding 0.5 mg/dL/h (8 μmol/L/h) is potentially pathological and suggestive of hemolytic disease. Conjugated serum bilirubin concentrations exceeding 10% of total bilirubin or 2 mg/dL (35 μmol/L) are also not physiological and suggest hepatobiliary disease or a general metabolic disorder.

Table 3–3 summarizes factors that may indicate that jaundice is pathological as opposed to physiological, warranting further evaluation. Important historical features include family history of hemolytic disease, onset of jaundice in the first 24 h of life, a rapid rise in serum bilirubin levels, and ethnicity, as well as infant feeding patterns, stool and urine appearance, and activity levels. Clinical assessment requires careful attention to vital signs, weight loss, general appearance, pallor, and hepatosplenomegaly.

The primary concern with severe hyperbilirubinemia is the potential for neurotoxic effects as well as general cellular injury, which can occur at total serum bilirubin levels exceeding 20–25 mg/dL. "Kernicterus" refers to the yellow staining of the basal ganglia observed postmortem among infants who died with severe jaundice. (Bilirubin deposition in the basal ganglia can also be imaged used magnetic resonance techniques.) Although a common complication of hyperbilirubinemia in the 1940s and 1950s due to Rh erythroblastosis fetalis and ABO hemolytic disease, kernicterus is rare today with the use of Rh immunoglobulin and with the intervention of phototherapy and exchange transfusion. With early discharge to home, however, a small resurgence of kernicterus has been observed in countries in which this complication had essentially disappeared. For instance, although no cases of kernicterus were identified in Denmark during the 20 years preceding 1994, six cases were diagnosed between 1994 and 1998. No published data on the incidence or prevalence of kernicterus in the United States are available.

Bilirubin can interfere with DNA synthesis as well as protein synthesis and protein phosphorylation. Bilirubin can also interfere with neuroexitatory signals and impair nerve conduction, particularly in the auditory nerve. Hyperbilirubinemia may also impair cerebral glucose metabolism in the brain.

Table 3-2. Classification of neonatal hyperbilirubinemia based on mechanism of accumulation.

Increased Bilirubin Load	Decreased Bilirubin Conjugation	Impaired Bilirubin Excretion
Hemolytic causes	Characteristics	Characteristics
Characteristics	Increased unconjugated	Increased unconjugated and conjugated
Increased unconjugated	bilirubin level	bilirubin level
bilirubin level	Normal percentage of	Negative Coomb's test
>6% reticulocytes	reticulocytes	Conjugated bilirubin level of >2 mg/dL
Hemoglobin concentration <13 g/dL	Physiological jaundice	or >20% of total serum bilirubin level
Coomb's test positive	Crigler–Najar syndrome types	conjugated bilirubin in urine
Rh factor incompatibly	1 and 2	Biliary obstruction
ABO incompatibility	Gilbert syndrome	Biliary atresia
Minor antigens	Hypothyroidism	Choledochal cyst
Coomb's test negative	Breast milk jaundice	Primary sclerosing cholangitis
Red blood cell defects		Gallstones
(sphereocytosis, elliptocytosis)		Neoplasm
Red blood cell enzyme defects		Dubin–Johnson syndrome
(G6PD deficiency, pyruvate		Rotor's syndrome
kinase deficiency)		Infection
Drugs (e.g., sulfisoxazole acetyl		Sepsis
with erythromycin		Urinary tract infection
ethylsuccinate, streptomycin,		Syphilis
vitamin K)		Toxoplasmosis
Abnormal red blood cells		Tuberculosis
(hemoglobinopathies)		Hepatitis
Sepsis		Rubella
Nonhemolytic causes		Herpes
Characteristics		Metabolic disorder
Increased unconjugated		α_1-Antitrypsin deficiency
bilirubin level		Cystic fibrosis
Normal percentage of		Galactosemia
reticulocytes		Glycogen storage disease
Extravascular sources		Gaucher's disease
Cephalohematoma		Hypothyroidism
Bruising		Wilson's disease
Central nervous system		Niemann–Pick disease
hemorrhage		Chromosomal abnormality
Swallowed blood		Turner's syndrome
Polycythemia		Trisomy 18 and 21 syndromes
Fetal–maternal transfusion		Drugs
Delayed cord clamping		Aspirin
Twin–twin transfusion		Acetaminophen
Exaggerated enterohepatic		Sulfa
circulation		Alcohol
Cystic fibrosis		Rifampin
Ileal atresia		Erythromycin
Pyloric stenosis		Corticosteroids
Hirschsprung's disease		Tetracycline
Breast milk jaundice		

Adapted from Porter MI, Dennis BI: Hyperbilirubinemia in the term newborn. Am Fam Physician 2002; 65:599 and Siberry GK, Iannone R (editors): *The Harriet Lane Handbook: A Manual for Pediatric House Officers*, ed 15. Mosby, 2000: 257.

Table 3–3. Factors indicating a pathological cause of jaundice among newborns.

General considerations
  Family history of significant hemolytic disease
  Onset of jaundice before the age of 24 h
  Rise in serum bilirubin levels of more than 0.5 mg/dL/h
  Pallor, hepatosplenomegaly
  Rapid increase in the total serum bilirubin (TSB) level after
    24–48 h (consider G6PD deficiency)
  Ethnicity suggestive of inherited disease (G6PD deficiency,
    etc)
  Failure of phototherapy to lower the TSB level

Clinical signs suggesting other diseases (sepsis or galac-
tosemia) with jaundice as one manifestation
  Vomiting
  Lethargy
  Poor feeding
  Hepatosplenomegaly
  Excessive weight loss
  Apnea
  Temperature instability
  Tachypnea

Signs of cholestatic jaundice suggesting the need to rule out
biliary atresia or other causes of cholestasis
  Dark urine or urine positive for bilirubin
  Light-colored stools
  Persistent jaundice for more than 3 weeks

From American Academy of Pediatrics, Provisional Committee for Quality Improvement and Subcommittee on Hyperbilirubinemia: Management of hyperbilirubinemia in the healthy term newborn. Pediatrics 1994; 94:558.

The concentration of bilirubin in the brain as well as the duration of exposure are important determinants of the neurotoxic effects of bilirubin. Bilirubin can enter the brain when not bound to albumin, so infants with low albumin are at increased risk of developing kernicterus. Conditions that alter the blood–brain barrier such as infection, acidosis, hypoxia, sepsis, prematurity, and hyperosmolarity may affect the entry of bilirubin into the brain.

In infants without hemolysis, serum bilirubin levels and encephalopathy do not correlate well. In infants with hemolysis, serum bilirubin levels higher than 20 mg/dL are associated with poorer neurological outcomes, although some infants with concentrations of 25 mg/dL are normal. Kernicterus was detected in 8% of infants with associated hemolysis who had serum bilirubin levels of 19–25 mg/dL, 33% of infants with levels of 25–29 mg/dL, and 73% of infants with levels of 30–40 mg/dL. It should be noted that the majority of cases of kernicterus described in recent years have been among neonates who had total serum bilirubin >30 mg/dL at the time of diagnosis, which is well above the recommended treatment thresholds of 15 or 20 mg/dL.

It is estimated that up to 15% of infants with kernicterus have no obvious neurological signs or symptoms. In its acute form, kernicterus may present in the first 1–2 days with poor sucking, stupor, hypotonia, and seizures. During the middle of the first week, hypertonia of extensor muscles, opisthotonus (backward arching of the trunk), retrocollis (backward arching of the neck), and fever may be observed. After the first week, the infant may exhibit generalized hypertonia. Some of these changes disappear spontaneously, or can be reversed with exchange transfusion. In most infants with moderate (10–20 mg/dL) to severe (>20 mg/dL) hyperbilirubinemia, evoked neurological responses return to normal within 6 months. A minority of infants (ranging between 6% and 23%) exhibit persistent neurological deficits.

In its chronic form, kernicterus may present in the first year with hypotonia, active deep-tendon reflexes, obligatory tonic neck reflexes, dental dysplasia, and delayed motor skills. After the first year, movement disorders, upward gaze, and sensorineural hearing loss may develop. It has been suggested that long-term effects of severe hyperbilirubinemia on IQ are more likely in boys than in girls. Seidman et al. studied 1948 subjects from Hadaasah Hebrew University Medical Center in Jerusalem born in 1970–1971 and drafted into the army 17 years later and found a significantly higher risk of lowered IQ (<85) among males with a history of total serum bilirubin exceeding 20 mg/dL (OR 2.96, 95% CI 1.29–6.79).

Clinical Findings

The American Academy of Family Physicians offers no clinical policy on neonatal hyperbilirubinemia. However, in 1994 the American Academy of Pediatrics (AAP) issued a practice parameter for the evaluation and treatment of hyperbilirubinemia among healthy term newborns. (Note: these recommendations are currently under review.) It should be emphaszied that the AAP practice parameter applies only to the evaluation and treatment of hyperbilirubinemia in otherwise *healthy term* neonates. Elements of these recommendations are summarized below and can be accessed in full at http://www.aap.org.

A. Symptoms and Signs

Clinically, jaundice usually progresses from head to toe. The total serum bilirubin level can be estimated by the degree of caudal extension: face, 5 mg/dL; upper chest, 10 mg/dL; abdomen, 12 mg/dL; palms and soles,

>15 mg/dL. However, estimates of total bilirubin via cephalocaudal progression are considered to be reliable only to the nipple line. Transcutaneous bilirubin measurement devices are more accurate than clinical estimation and may provide an alternative to frequent blood draws for the accurate assessment of serum bilirubin. Unfortunately, transcutaneous measurement units do not currently appear to be widely available in community hospital settings.

A total serum bilirubin needs to be performed on infants noted to be jaundiced within the first 24 h of life. Clinical jaundice can be assessed by blanching the skin with digital pressure in a well-lighted room. The cephalocaudal progression may be helpful in quantifying the degree of jaundice. If available, use of a transcutaneous jaundice meter may also be helpful. Evaluation of infants who develop abnormal signs such as feeding difficulty, behavior changes, apnea, and temperature changes is recommended regardless of whether jaundice has been detected in order to rule out underlying disease.

B. Laboratory Findings

When a pathological cause for jaundice is suspected, laboratory studies should be promptly completed:

- When jaundice is noticed within the first 24 h, evaluation should include a sepsis work-up, evaluation for rubella and toxoplasmosis infection, and blood typing to rule out erythroblastosis fetalis, as well as fractionated serum bilirubin levels.
- For jaundice noted after 24 h but within the first 2 weeks of life, fractionated total serum bilirubin (TSB) should be measured. If the conjugated bilirubin is >2 mg/dL, a reason for impaired bilirubin excretion should be sought (see Table 3–2). If conjugated bilirubin is <2 mg/dL, hemoglobin levels and reticulocyte counts should be evaluated. A high hemoglobin concentration indicates polycythemia. A low hemoglobin concentration with an abnormal reticulocyte count suggests hemolysis (see Table 3–2). If the reticulocyte count is normal, the infant must be evaluated for a nonhemolytic cause of jaundice (see Table 3–2, columns 1 and 2).
- For jaundice noted after the first 2 weeks of life, laboratory evaluation should include fractionated bilirubin level, urine bilirubin level, thyroid studies, sepsis work-up, and tests for metabolic disorders.

Maternal prenatal testing should include ABO and Rh (D) typing and a serum screen for unusual isoimmune antibodies. If the mother has not had prenatal blood grouping, or is Rh negative, a direct Coomb's test, blood type, and Rh (D) type of the infant's cord blood should be performed. Institutions are encouraged to save cord blood for future testing, particularly when the mother's blood type is group O. When the family history is positive for glucose-6-phosphate dehydrogenase (G6PD) or some other cause of hemolytic disease, appropriate laboratory assessment of the infant should be performed.

C. Neonatal Jaundice after Hospital Discharge

Follow-up should be provided to all neonates discharged less than 48 h after birth. This evaluation with a health care professional should occur within 2–3 days of discharge.

Approximately one-third of healthy breast-fed infants have persistent jaundice after 2 weeks of age. A report of dark urine or light stools should prompt a measurement of direct serum bilirubin. If the history and physical examination are normal, continued observation is appropriate. If jaundice persists beyond 3 weeks, a urine sample should be tested for bilirubin, and a measurement of total and direct serum bilirubin should be obtained.

Prediction & Prevention

Shorter hospital stays after delivery limit the time for hospital-based assessment of infant feeding, instruction about breast-feeding, and the detection of jaundice. Hyperbilirubinemia and problems related to feeding are the main reasons for hospital readmission during the first week of life. Of 29,934 infants discharged between 1988 and 1994 from a large suburban hospital in Michigan, just 0.8% were readmitted by the age of 14 days. Of those readmitted, 51% were diagnosed with hyperbilirubinemia and 31% with sepsis.

Because bilirubin levels usually peak on Day 3 or 4 of life, and most newborns are discharged within 48 h, most cases of jaundice will occur at home. It is therefore important that infants be seen by a health care professional within a few days of discharge to assess for jaundice and overall well-being. This is particularly important in near-term infants (35–36 weeks gestation) who are at particular risk for hyperbilirubinemia due to both relative hepatic immaturity and inadequate nutritional intake.

It has been suggested that measuring total serum bilirubin before discharge and then applying a percentile-based nomogram (see Figure 3–1) to predict the risk of subsequent moderately severe hyperbilirubinemia (>17 mg/dL) can guide physicians in identifying neonates for whom close follow-up is warranted. In one study neonates in a high-risk group (95th percentile for TSB) at 18–72 h of life had a 40% chance of developing moderately severe hyperbilirubinemia upon discharge, whereas for those in a low-risk group (40th percentile for TSB) the probability for subsequently developing moderately severe hyperbilirubinemia was zero.

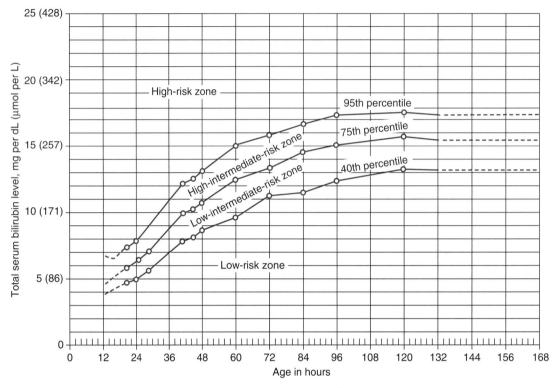

Figure 3–1. Nomogram of risk for significant hyperbilirubinemia in healthy term and near-term well newborns.
(Porter MI, Dennis BI: Hyperbilirubinemia in the term newborn. Am Fam Physician 2002;65:599.)

However, it should be noted that there are no evidence-based guidelines that endorse this approach.

Carbon monoxide is a byproduct resulting from the breakdown of heme. Measuring end-tidal carbon monoxide (ETCO) in neonates has also been proposed as a potential tool for predicting the development of severe hyperbilirubinemia, however, others have questioned the value of routine measurements of ETCO. At present, CO measurements to assess hyperbilirubinemia are not yet validated for use in clinical settings.

Treatment

A. Suspected Pathological Jaundice

The decision whether to intervene in cases of elevated bilirubin levels during the neonatal period is tempered by clinical judgment, and the physician team (including the family physician and consultants) is encouraged to discuss management options with the parents or guardians of the infant. Treatment decisions are based on TSB levels. Intensive phototherapy should produce a decline in TSB of 1–2 mg/dL within 4–6 h, and the decline should continue thereafter. If the TSB does not respond appro-

priately to intensive phototherapy, exchange transfusion is recommended. If levels are in the range that suggests the need for exchange transfusion (see Table 3–4), intensive phototherapy should be attempted while preparations for exchange transfusion are made. Exchange transfusion is also recommended in infants whose TSB levels rise to exchange transfusion levels in spite of intensive phototherapy. In any of the above situations, failure of intensive phototherapy to lower the TSB level strongly suggests the presence of hemolytic disease or other pathological processes and strongly warrants further investigation/consultation. Factors that may suggest a pathologicalal cause for jaundice appear in Table 3–3.

Table 3–4 summarizes the management strategy for hyperbilirubinemia in healthy term infants. Management decisions are based on the infant's age and TSB levels. These recommendations pertain to infants without clinical signs of illness or hemolytic disease.

B. Phototherapy and Exchange Transfusion

Phototherapy involves exposing the infant to high-intensity light in the blue-green wavelengths. Light interacts with unconjugated bilirubin in the skin, con-

Table 3–4. Management of hyperbilirubinemia in healthy term newborns.

Age (h)	TSB	Management According to Total Serum Bilirubin (TSB) Level, mg/dL (μmol/L)			
		Consider Phototherapy	**Initiate Phototherapy**	**Exchange Transfusion if Intensive Phototherapy Fails**	**Exchange Transfusion and Intensive Phototherapy**
≤24[1]	mg/dL	—	—	—	—
	(μmol/L)	—	—	—	—
25–48	mg/DL	≥12	≥15	≥20	≥25
	(μmol/L)	210	260	340	430
49–72	mg/dL	≥15	≥18	≥25	≥30
	(μmol/L)	260	310	430	510
>72	mg/dL	≥17	≥20	≥25	≥30
	(μmol/L)	290	340	430	510

From American Academy of Pediatrics, Provisional Committee for Quality Improvement and Subcommittee on Hyperbilirubinemia: Management of hyperbilirubinemia in the healthy term newborn. Pediatrics 1994; 94:558.
[1]Term infants who are clinically jaundiced at ≤24 h old are not considered healthy and require prompt evaluation and work-up.

verting it to less toxic photoisomers that are excreted in the bile and urine without conjugation. The efficacy of phototherapy is strongly influenced by the energy output in the blue spectrum, the spectrum of the light, and the surface area of the infant exposed to phototherapy. Phototherapy units contain a number of fluorescent tubes that are either free standing or are part of a radiant warming device. Fiberoptic systems have been developed that deliver light through a fiberoptic blanket. The phototherapy tubes (designated F20 T12/BB) make the babies look blue, which may be bothersome to health care workers and make clinical evaluation of jaundice difficult. However, this problem can be mitigated by using four special blue tubes and two daylight fluorescent tubes in the unit. Eye protection is placed on the infant, and the bank of lights is placed 15–20 cm from the infant. The infant is placed naked in a bassinet. Exposure is increased by placing a fiberoptic blanket under the infant, by placing lighting units all around the infant, or by putting a white sheet around the bassinet to serve as a reflecting surface. If slight warming of the infant is noted, the tubes can be moved away a bit. Phototherapy may be interrupted briefly for parental visits or breast-feeding.

In infants with TSB levels >25 mg/dL, phototherapy should be administered continuously until a response is documented, or until exchange therapy is initiated. If the TSB is not responding to conventional phototherapy (a response is defined as a sustained reduction in total serum bilirubin of 1–2 mg/dL in 4–6 h), intensity should be increased by adding more lights; increasing the intensity of the lights used is indicated

while exchange transfusion is prepared. With commonly used light sources, overdose is impossible, although the infant may experience loose stools. Phototherapy is continued until TSB is below 14–15 mg/dL. The infant may be discharged after the completion of phototherapy. Rebound of total serum bilirubin following cessation of phototherapy is usually less than 1 mg/dL.

Exchange transfusion rapidly removes bilirubin from the circulation. Circulating antibodies against erythrocytes are also removed. Exchange transfusion is particularly beneficial in neonates with hemolysis. One or two central catheters are placed. Small aliquots of blood (8–10 mL per pass) are removed from the infant's circulation and replaced with equal amounts of donor red cells mixed with plasma. The procedure is repeated until twice the infant's blood volume is replaced (approximately 160–200 mL/kg). Serum electrolytes and bilirubin are measured periodically during the procedure. In some cases the procedure must be repeated to lower serum bilirubin levels sufficiently. Infusing salt-poor albumin at a dose of 1 g/kg 1–4 h before exchange transfusion has been shown to increase the amount of bilirubin removed during the procedure.

Complications of exchange transfusion include thrombocytopenia, portal vein thrombosis, necrotizing enterocolitis, electrolyte imbalance, graft-versus-host disease, and infection. Mortality from exchange transfusion approaches 2% and an additional 12% of infants may suffer serious complications. Therefore, exchange transfusion should be reserved for neonates who have failed intensive phototherapy and should be performed by clinicians and facilities with proper experience.

C. Suspected Nonpathological Jaundice

For the management of breast-feeding jaundice, interruption of breast-feeding in healthy term newborns is generally discouraged. Recommendations for frequent breast-feeding sessions (at least 8–10 times in 24 h) are advised. However, if the mother and physician wish, they may consider using supplemental formula feedings or temporarily interrupting breast-feeding and replacing it with formula feeds. Phototherapy may be initiated depending on TSB levels.

"Breast milk jaundice," intitially seen after Day 6 of life, occurs in approximately two-thirds of breast-fed babies between ages 3 weeks and 3 months. This is a form of normal physiological jaundice in healthy, thriving breast-fed infants.

Conclusions

Because up to 60% of all newborns are noted to be clinically jaundiced, all family physicians who care for neonates will encounter this common clinical entity. In the overwhelming majority of cases, this jaundice is entirely benign. However, it is important that the family physician recognize cases in which jaundice could represent a pathological process and cases in which the infant is at risk for developing severe hyperbilirubinemia.

Like other conditions such as fever in the neonate, close monitoring and surveillance are important, and strategies for assessing risk must be utilized. Infants who are discharged prior to 48 h of age, particularly those who are born at less than 37 weeks gestation, should be seen in the office within a few days of discharge to evaluate jaundice and overall clinical status.

The possibility of jaundice should be discussed with parents prior to hospital discharge. Parents of newborns should be assured of the generally benign nature of most cases of jaundice, especially breast-feeding jaundice and breast milk jaundice. Parental education should emphasize the need to monitor the infant for jaundice and associated symptoms such as poor feeding, lethargy, dark urine, and light colored stools. Family physicians should encourage parents to contact the office with specific questions and concerns.

Agrawal VK et al: Brainstem auditory evoked response in newborns with hyperbilirubinemia. Indian Pediatr 1998;35:513.

American Academy of Pediatrics, Subcommittee on Neo-natal Hyperbilirubinemia: Neonatal jaundice and kernicterus. Pediatrics 2001;108:763.

American Academy of Pediatrics, Provisional Committee for Quality Improvement and Subcommittee on Hyperbilirubinemia: Management of hyperbilirubinemia in the healthy term newborn. Pediatrics 1994;94:558.

Bertini G et al: Prevention of bilirubin encephalopathy. Biol Neonate 2001;79:219.

Bhutani VK, Johnson L, Sivieri EM: Predictive ability of a predischarge hour-specific serum bilirubin for subsequent hyperbilirubinemia in healthy term and near-term newborns. Pediatrics 1999;103:6.

Dennery PA, Seidman DS, Stevenson DK: Drug therapy: neonatal hyperbilirubinemia. N Engl J Med 2001;344:581.

Gartner LM: Neonatal jaundice. Pediatr Rev 1994;15:422.

Halamek LP, Stevenson DK: Neonatal jaundice and liver disease. In: *Neonatal-Perinatal Medicine: Diseases of the Fetus and Infant,* ed 6, Vol 2. Fanaroff AA, Martin RJ (editors). Mosby-Year Book, 1997: 1345.

Hansen TWR: Kernicterus in term and near term infants—the specter walks again. Acta Paediatr 2000;89:1155.

Johnson LH, Sivieri E, Bhutani V: Neurological outcome of singleton greater/equal 2500g CORE Project babies not treated for hyperbilirubinemia. Pediatr Res 1999;45:203A (abstract).

Maisels MJ, Kring E: Transcutaneous bilirubinometry decreases the need for serum bilirubin measurements and saves money. Pediatrics 1997;99:599.

Maisels MJ, Kring E: Length of stay, jaundice and hospital readmission. Pediatrics 1998;101:995.

Maisels MJ, Newman TB: Predicting hyperbilirubinemia in newborns: the importance of timing. Pediatrics 1999;103:493.

Moyer VA, Ahn C, Sneed S: Accuracy of clinical judgement in neonatal jaundice. Arch Pediatric Adolesc Med 2000;154: 391.

Porter MI, Dennis BI: Hyperbilirubinemia in the term newborn. Am Fam Physician 2002;65:599.

Seidman DS et al: Neonatal hyperbilirubinemia and physical and cognitive performance at 17 years of age. Pediatrics 1991;88: 828.

Siberry GK, Iannone R (editors): *The Harriet Lane Handbook: A Manual for Pediatric House Officers,* ed 15. Mosby, 2000: 257.

Stevenson DK et al: Prediction of hyperbilirubinemia in near-term and term infants. Pediatrics 2001;108:31.

Valaes T: Problems with prediction of neonatal hyperbilirubinemia. Pediatrics 2001;108:175.

Volpe JJ: *Neonatal Neurology.* WB Saunders, 1999: 490.

Breast-feeding & Infant Nutrition

4

Tracey D. Conti, MD

General Considerations

Nutrition is a critical capstone for the proper growth and development of infants. Breast-feeding of term infants by healthy mothers is the optimal mechanism for providing the caloric and nutrient needs of infants. Preterm infants can also benefit from breast milk and breast-feeding although supplementation and fortification of preterm breast milk may be required. Barring some unique circumstances, human breast milk can provide nutritional, social, and motor developmental benefits for most infants.

Recently, there has been a resurgence of interest in breast-feeding among practitioners and their patients. Despite increased emphasis on breast-feeding education, less than 65% percent of women choose to breast-feed their children. Of these women, only 29% and 16% are still breast-feeding at 6 months and 1 year, respectively. The Department of Health and Human Services Healthy People 2010 initiative proposes to increase these numbers to 50% and 25% for infants at 6 and 12 months, respectively. Education of practitioners as well as their patients is an integral component of this initiative.

Most women presently of childbearing age were not breast-fed and report having no maternal relatives who breast-fed their children. Because evidence clearly suggests familial influences in the development of infant feeding practices, practitioners may find it difficult to encourage breast-feeding behaviors among women with no direct familial breast-feeding experience.

Efforts to alter knowledge, attitudes, and behaviors regarding breast-feeding must effectively address the numerous psychosocial barriers. Health care providers are critical conduits for maternal and familial education. All members of the health care team, including physicians, midwives, and nurses, are valuable sources of important evidence-based information as well as psychological support for mothers in search of guidance regarding infant feeding practices. Unless health care practitioners are properly educated regarding breast-feeding practices and

barriers, efforts to achieve the Healthy People 2010 objectives will remain suboptimal.

Numerous studies have shown the superiority of breast milk and the health advantages that breast-fed children have. The literature has shown that infants who are breast-fed have fewer episodes of diarrheal illness, ear infections, and allergies. There are likewise financial advantages to breast-feeding. Other somewhat controversial investigations suggest higher intelligence among breast-fed infants.

Numerous consensus recommendations advocate breast-feeding for the first 4–6 months prior to the introduction of age-appropriate solid foods and advise continued breast-feeding for the first year of life.

The American Academy of Pediatrics (AAP) Committee on Nutrition recommends breast-feeding for the first year of life with supplemental vitamin D at birth and the addition of supplemental iron at age 4 months and possible addition of fluoride at age 6 months for infants living in regions in which water is low in fluoride. Vitamin D supplementation is particularly applicable in regions with limited sunlight and for infants of mothers with decreased daily intake of cow's milk. Further recommendations include delaying introduction of cow's milk until after 1 year and delaying addition of reduced fat milk until 2 years of age. To this end, new mothers should be encouraged to continue prenatal vitamins for continued supplemental iron, calcium, and vitamin D. Supplemental solid foods should be considered at or around 6 months of age once the infant demonstrates appropriate readiness.

Anatomy of the Human Breast & Breast-feeding

Women are able to produce milk by the age they are able to bear children. There is no evidence that breast function, breast milk production, or composition is different among younger women. The principal external structures of the mature human female breast are the nipple, areola, and Montgomery's tubercles. The areola is the darker part of the breast, with the nipple being the central-most structure through which milk ducts open and milk is expressed. Within the areola are Montgomery's tubercles, through which sebaceous and sweat glands (Montgomery's glands) open, producing lubricating substances for the nipple.

Underlying structures include mammary gland cells and contractile myoepithelial cells surrounding the gland cells (allowing for milk ejection) that produce alveoli. Milk produced within the alveoli is ejected into the milk ducts, which empty into lactiferous ducts and sinuses, in which milk is stored between breast-feeding periods.

Infant breast-feeding draws the nipple and areola into the mouth, causing elongation of the nipple. The elongated nipple is compressed between the palate and the tongue and milk is expressed less than 0.05 s after the nipple has elongated. Compression of the areola between the infant's gums causes expression of milk from lactiferous sinuses. Stimulation of the areola is essential for the oxytocin-mediated hormonal cascade that controls milk ejection.

Physiology of Breast-feeding

Two principal hormones are required for breast milk production—oxytocin and prolactin—controlled by the hypothalamic–pituitary axis. Oxytocin production and secretion are under the control of the posterior pituitary and are stimulated by suckling. Oxytocin production in response to suckling is intermittent and stimulates ejection ("let down") of breast milk. Oxytocin does not appear to affect breast milk production, although numerous stressors can negatively impact breast milk let down. Evidence suggests that lactogenesis may be delayed and let down reduced following stressful vaginal delivery or cesarean section.

Milk production is controlled primarily by the release of prolactin. Prolactin secretion is through a feedback loop under dopaminergic control with the primary action on prolactin receptors on mammary epithelium. Suckling likewise stimulates prolactin release. Furthermore, prolactin acts as an inhibitor of ovulation through hormonal feedback control, although breast-feeding is considered a relatively unreliable contraceptive mechanism.

Several additional hormones are required for milk production: cortisol, human growth hormone, insulin, thyroid and parathyroid hormones, and feedback inhibitor of lactation (FIL). Not entirely understood, FIL appears to act at the level of breast tissue to inhibit continued breast milk production when the breast is not completely emptied.

Milk production begins during the postpartum period with prolactin production and concomitant decreased estrogen and progesterone production following placental delivery. Milk production will persist under this hormonal control for the first several days, however, continued milk production beyond the initial 48 h postpartum requires suckling. Although mothers will continue to produce milk between feedings once suckling has initiated the feedback loop, milk production significantly rises during breast-feeding.

Breast Milk

A. Stages of Production

Production of human breast milk among healthy mothers who deliver full-term infants occurs in three phases—colostrum, transitional milk, and mature milk. Colostrum is a thick, yellow substance produced during the first several days postpartum. Healthy mothers produce approximately 80–100 mL daily. Colostrum is rich in calcium, antibodies, minerals, proteins, potassium, and fat-soluble vitamins. This milk has immunological qualities that are vital to the infant and it possesses gastrointestinal properties to aid in secretion of meconium. Production of colostrum is followed for the next 5–6 days with transitional milk, which provides essential components more closely resembling mature breast milk. Most women will notice a significant change evidenced by the fullness of their breasts and the change in the consistency of the milk. True milk is white and sometimes has a bluish tint. The consistency is similar to cow's milk with a sweet taste. Mature breast milk, produced beginning at or near postpartum Day 10, produces key components to be discussed in the next section.

Numerous factors may affect the supply of breast milk including anxiety, medications, maternal nutritional status, sleep, exercise, breast-feeding frequency, tactile stimulation, and fluid intake. Breast-feeding mothers should be encouraged to consume generous amounts of fluids and express breast milk every 2–3 h. The hormonal feedback loop that controls the production and release of prolactin and oxytocin is initiated by suckling or other tactile stimulation of the breast. The greater the amount of suckling or other tactile breast stimulation, the greater the milk supply.

B. Components

Mature human breast milk contains protein, carbohydrate, and fat components and provides approximately 20 kcal/ounce and 1 gram % of protein. The principal protein elements of both mature and premature breast milk are casein (40%) and whey (60%). Breast milk contains approximately 2.5 g/L of casein. Also called "curds," this protein forms calcium complexes. Higher concentrations of this protein are found in cow's milk. Whey (approximately 6.4 g/L) is a protein component composed of α-lactalbumin, lactoferrin, lyzozyme, immunoglobulins, and albumin.

Free nitrogen, vital for amino acid synthesis, is also a significant component of mature breast milk and is integral for multiple biochemical pathways including production of uric acid, urea, ammonia, and creatinine. It is also a key component of insulin and epidermal growth factor.

There are approximately 70 g/L of lactose, the primary carbohydrate in mature breast milk. Composed of galactose and glucose, the lactose concentration continues to increase throughout breast-feeding. Human milk fat likewise increases with continued breast-feeding. Mature breast milk provides approximately 40 g/L and includes triacylglycerides, phospholipids, and essential fatty acids. There is no evidence that lipid levels are not affected by maternal diet, although the type of lipids may vary.

The principal electrolytes in breast milk are sodium, potassium, magnesium, and calcium. Calcium appears to be mediated through the parathyroid hormone-related protein, which allows for mobilization of calcium stores from bone in otherwise healthy women. Bone calcium levels return to normal after termination of breast-feeding. Regulation of sodium and potassium concentrations in breast milk occurs through corticosteroids.

Iron absorption is particularly high in newborns and infants, although the relative concentration of iron in mature breast milk is low. For infants under 6 months of age, the concentration of iron in breast milk is sufficient and supplementation is not necessary, however, recommendations for infants more than 6 months old include supplemental iron from green vegetables, meats, and iron-rich cereals. The recommended amount of supplemental elemental iron is 1 mg/kg/day. Iron is an essential component in the synthesis of hemoglobin.

Vitamin K, a lipid-soluble vitamin and important component in the clotting cascade, is routinely provided in the immediate postpartum period as a 1 mg intramuscular injection. There is evidence that oral vitamin K may produce similar benefit as well as maternal supplementation of 5 mg/day of oral vitamin K for 12 weeks following delivery.

Another lipid-soluble component, vitamin D, is essential for bone formation. Women who have limited exposure to sunlight or suboptimal vitamin D intake will produce little or no vitamin D in breast milk. The recommended daily intake of vitamin D is 400 IU/day. Practitioners must be cognizant of mothers with special diets (ie, vegetarian diets) whose low vitamin D intake might indicate a need for supplemental vitamin D.

Other elemental minerals in breast milk include zinc, copper, selenium, manganese, nickel, molybdenum, and chromium, as found in trace amounts, but nonetheless essential for a multitude of biochemical processes.

C. COMPOSITION OF PRETERM BREAST MILK

The composition of breast milk in mothers of preterm infants is different from that of term infants. This difference persists for approximately 4 weeks before the composition approaches that of term infant breast milk. The difference in preterm milk composition reflects the increased nutrient demands of preterm infants. Preterm breast milk contains higher concentrations of total and bound nitrogen, immunoglobulins, sodium, iron, chloride, and medium-chain fatty acids. However, it may not contain sufficient amounts of phosphorus, calcium, copper, and zinc. Preterm infants are more likely to require fortification with human milk fortifiers (HMF) to correct these deficiencies.

Breast-feeding Technique

Preparation for breast-feeding should begin in the preconception period or at the first contact with the patient. Most women choose their method of feeding prior to conception. Psychosocial support and education may encourage breast-feeding among women who might not otherwise have considered it. Evidence for this strategy, however, is anecdotal and requires further investigation.

There are numerous potential supports available to women who are considering feeding behaviors. Practitioners are encouraged to identify members of the patient's support network and provide similar education to minimize the potential barriers posed by uninformed support individuals.

One commonly perceived physical barrier is nipple inversion. Women who have inverted nipples will have difficulty with the latch-on process (which will be discussed later in this chapter). Nipple shields are relatively inexpensive devices that can draw the nipple out. Manual or electric breast pumps may also be used to draw out inverted nipples, typically beginning after delivery.

Adoptive mothers represent another group with perceived potential barriers to breast-feeding. Feeding of the infant must be discussed once the decision to adopt has been made. Adoptive mothers can be medicated to simulate pregnancy and stimulate production of milk. Despite these hormonal adjuncts, these mothers sometimes will have an inadequate response and subsequent inadequate milk supply. There are several types of supplemental feeding systems that women can wear while breast-feeding that attach to the nipple to provide additional nutrition along with the breast milk.

Breast-feeding should begin immediately after the postpartum period, ideally in the first 30–40 min after delivery. This is easier to accomplish if the infant is left in the room with the mother before being bathed and before the newborn examination is performed. It is also safe to allow breast-feeding before administration of vitamin K and erythromycin ophthalmic ointment.

Clinical situations arise that preclude initiation of breast-feeding in the immediate postpartum period (ie, cesarean section delivery, maternal perineal repair, maternal or fetal distress). In such cases breast-feeding should be initiated at the earliest time possible. Only when medically necessary should a supplemental feeding be initiated. If mothers have expressed a desire to breast-feed, the practitioner should coordinate an interim feeding plan, emphasizing that bottle feeding not be started. Acceptable alternatives include spoon, cup, or syringe feeding.

Breast-fed children commonly feed at least every 2–3 h during the first several weeks postpartum. Infants should not be allowed to sleep through feedings; however, if necessary, feeding intervals may be increased to every 3–4 h overnight. The production of breast milk is on a supply–demand cycle. Breast stimulation through suckling and the mechanism of breast-feeding signals the body to make more milk. When feedings are missed or breasts are not emptied effectively, the feedback loop decreases the milk supply. As the infant grows, feedings every 3–4 h are acceptable. Because growth spurts are common and the amount of milk needed for the rate of growth often exceeds milk production, feeding intervals often must be adjusted to growth periods until the milk supply "catches up."

Although feeding intervals may be increased during nighttime periods, a common question becomes when to stop waking the infant for night feedings. Anecdotal evidence suggests that after the first 2 weeks postpartum, in the absence of specific nutritional concerns, the infant can determine its own overnight feeding schedule. Typically, most infants will begin to sleep through the night once they have reached approximately 10 pounds.

Positioning of the infant is critical for effective feeding in the neonatal period, allowing for optimal latch-on. In general, infant and mother should face each other in one of the following three positions: the cradle, the most common, the football, or the lay/side. The cradle hold allows the mother to hold the infant horizontally across the front of the chest. The infant's head can be on the left or right side of the mother depending on which side the baby is feeding. The infant's head should be supported with the crook of the mother's arm. The football hold is performed with the mother sitting on a bed or chair, the infant's bottom against the

bed or chair and its body lying next to the mother's side, and the infant's head cradled in her hand. The side position allows the mother to lay on her left or right side with the infant lying parallel to her. Again, the infant's head is cradled in the crook of the mother's elbow. This position is ideally suited for women post-cesarean section as it reduces the pain associated with pressure from the infant on their incisions. It must be stressed that choice of position is based upon mother and infant comfort. It is not unusual to experiment with any or all positions prior to determining the most desirable. It is likewise not uncommon to find previously undesirable positions more effective and comfortable as the infant grows and the breast-feeding experience progresses. All breast-feeding positions should allow for cradling of the infant's head with the mother's hand or elbow allowing for better head control in the latch-on stage. The infant should be placed at a height (often achieved with a pillow) appropriate for preventing awkward positioning, maximizing comfort, and encouraging latch-on.

Many of the difficulties with breast-feeding result from improper latch-on. Latch-on problems are often the source of multiple breast-feeding complaints among mothers from engorgement to sore cracked nipples. Many women discontinue breast-feeding secondary to these issues. The latch-on process is governed by primitive reflexes. Stroking the infant's cheek will cause the infant to turn toward the side on which the cheek was stroked. This reflex is useful if the baby is not looking toward the breast. Tickling the baby's bottom lip will cause the baby to open its mouth wide in order to latch on to the breast. The mother should hold her breast to help position the areola to ease latch-on. It is important that the mother's fingers be behind the areola so as not to provide a physical barrier to latch-on. Once the infant's mouth is opened wide, the head should be pulled quickly to the breast. The infant's mouth should encompass the entire areola to compress the milk ducts. If this is done improperly, the infant will compress the nipple, leading to pain and eventually cracking with minimal or no milk expression. The mother should not experience pain with breast-feeding. If this occurs the mother should break the suction by inserting a finger into the side of the baby's mouth and latch the baby on again. This process should be repeated as many times as necessary until proper latch-on is achieved.

One issue that continually plagues parents is adequate amounts of breast milk. Several clinical measures can be used to determine if infants are receiving enough milk. Weight is an excellent method of assessment. Pre- and postmeasurement of an infant with a scale that is of high quality and measures to the ounce is a very accurate means of determining weight. The problem is that most families will not have this type of scale available to them. Weight can also be evaluated on a longer term basis. Infants should not lose more than about 8% of their birth weight and should gain this weight back in 2 weeks. Most infants with difficulties, however, will decompensate before this 2-week period. Breast-fed babies should be evaluated 2–3 days after discharge, especially if discharged prior to 48 h. A more convenient way to determine the adequacy of the infant's intake of milk is through clinical signs such as infant satisfaction postfeeding and bowel and bladder amounts. In most cases infants who are satisfied after feeding will fall asleep. Infants who do not receive enough milk will usually be fussy or irritable or continuously want to suck at the breast, their finger, etc. Breast-fed infants usually will stool after most feeds but at a minimum five to six times a day. After the first couple of days, the stool should turn from meconiumlike to a mustard-colored seedy type. Breast-fed infants who are still passing meconium or do not have an adequate amount of stool should alert the parents and health care team that they may not be taking in enough milk. Infants should also urinate approximately three or four times a day. This may be hard to assess with the era's superabsorbent diapers. Careful examination of the diaper should be made.

Problems Associated with Breast-feeding

An inadequate milk supply can lead to disastrous outcomes if not identified or not treated. There are two types of milk inadequacies, the inability to make milk and the inability to keep the supply adequate. The first type of milk inadequacy is quite rare but examples include surgeries in which the milk ducts are severed or Sheehan's syndrome. There is no specific treatment to initiate milk production in these individuals. The inability to maintain an adequate milk supply has numerous etiologies ranging from dietary deficiencies to engorgement. The key in preventing adverse events is early recognition and effective treatment. One of the mainstays of treatment is working with the body's own feedback loop of supply and demand to increase the supply. As more milk is needed, more milk will be produced. This is effectively done by using a breast pump. Pumping should be performed after the infant has fed.

Engorgement is caused by inadequate or ineffective emptying of the breasts. As milk builds up in the breasts they become swollen. If the condition is not relieved, the breasts can become tender and warm. A mastitis can also develop. The mainstay of treatment is emptying the breasts of milk, either by the infant or if that is not possible by mechanical means. Usually when the breast is engorged, the areola and nipple are affected and proper latch-on becomes difficult if not impossible. A warm compress may be used to help with "let down"

and the breast can be manually expressed enough to allow the infant to latch on. If this is not possible or is too painful the milk can be removed with an electrical breast pump. Between feedings a cold pack can be used to decrease the amount of swelling. There have been reports that chilled cabbage leaves used to line the bra can act as a cold pack that conforms to the shape of the breast and can reduce the pain and swelling. However, there is no evidence of any medicinal properties in the cabbage that affect engorgement. Mastitis, if occurring, is treated with antibiotics. Mothers can continue to breast-feed with the affected breast so care should be taken to choose an antibiotic that is safe for the infant.

Sore nipples is another problem that plagues breast-feeding mothers. In the first few weeks there may be some soreness associated with breast-feeding as the skin gets used to the constant moisture. There should not be pain with breast-feeding; if there is pain it is usually secondary to improper latch-on, which resolves with correction. With severe cracking there will occasionally be bleeding. Breast-feeding can be continued with mild bleeding, but if severe bleeding occurs the breast should be pumped and the milk discarded to prevent gastrointestinal upset in the infant. There are some remedies that can be used in the event of cracking. Keeping the nipples clean and dry between feedings can help prevent and heal cracking. The mother's own milk or a pure lanolin ointment can also be used as a salve. Mothers should be warned not to use herbal rubs or vitamin E because of the risk of absorption by the baby. Another cause of sore nipples is a candidal infection. This usually presents when an infant has thrush. Sometimes treating the infant will resolve the problem, but occasionally the mother will need to be treated as well. Taking the same nystatin liquid dose that the infant is using twice a day will resolve the infection. Again, keeping the nipples clean and dry can help.

Other issues with breast-feeding include medications, nutrient supplementation, and mothers returning to work. Although these issues are broad in scope we will touch on a few key elements. There have been books dedicated to the subject of breast-feeding and medications. The most important issue to understand is that limited research has been done in this area and that there is insufficient information on most medicines to advocate their use. Health care providers should try to use the safest medications possible that will allow mothers to continue breast-feeding. If this is not possible mothers should be encouraged to pump the milk and discard it to maintain the milk supply. Nutrient supplementation is another *controversial* issue. Vitamin D is recommended for supplementation in either dark-skinned women or women who do not receive much sunlight. The iron found in breast milk, although in low concentrations, is highly absorbable. Infants who are breast-fed do not need additional sources of iron until they are 4–6 months old. This is the time when most children are started on cereal. Choosing an iron-fortified cereal will satisfy the additional iron requirement. The major cause of discontinuing breast-feeding is women returning to work. Planning this return from birth and pumping milk for storage help women to continue breast-feeding. Understanding employers who provide time and a comfortable place to pump milk at work will also improve breast-feeding rates. Although the goal is to increase the number of women who begin breast-feeding and continue it throughout the first year of the infant's life, many women cannot or do not choose to breast-feed. Their decision must be supported and they must be educated on alternative methods of providing nutrition for their infant.

Vegetarian Diet

The number of Americans choosing a vegetarian diet has increased dramatically in the past decade. With these increasing numbers more research has been done in an effort to evaluate the feasibility of a vegetarian diet in infancy. A vegetarian diet is defined as a diet consisting of no meat. This definition does not encompass the variety of vegetarian diets that are consumed. A pure vegetarian or vegan consumes only plant food. In general most pure vegetarians also do not use products that result from animal cruelty such as wool, silk, etc. Lacto-ovo vegetarians consume dairy products and eggs in addition to plants and lacto vegetarians consume only dairy products with their plant diet.

There is great variety in each of these diets and therefore great variety in the type and amount of food necessary for adequate nutrition. Milk from breast-feeding mothers who are vegetarians is adequate in all nutrients necessary for proper growth and development. Although all required nutrients can be found in any vegetarian diet, in infancy the amount necessary may be difficult to provide without supplementation. The American Dietetic Association stated that a lacto-ovo vegetarian diet is recommended in infancy. If this diet is not desired by parents or is not tolerated by children then supplementation may be necessary. Vitamin B_{12}, iron, and vitamin D are nutrients that may need to be supplemented depending on environmental factors.

Contraindications to Breast-feeding

Although considered the optimal method of providing infant nutrition during the first year of life, contraindications may preclude breast-feeding among some mothers. These include mothers who actively use illicit drugs such as heroin, cocaine, alcohol, and PCP, mothers with human immunodeficiency virus (HIV) infec-tion or acquired immunodeficiency syndrome (AIDS), and mothers receiving pharmacotherapy with agents transmitted in breast milk and contraindicated in children, particularly potent cancer agents. Some immunizations for foreign travelers and military personnel may also be contraindicated in breast-feeding mothers. Infants with galactosemia should also not breast-feed.

Infant Formulas

The historical record reveals that methods of replacing, fortifying, and delivering milk and milk substitutes date back to the Stone Age. Evidence suggests that the original infant "formulas" of the early and mid-twentieth century consisted of 1:1 concentrations of evaporated milk and water with supplemental cod liver oil, orange juice, and honey. As the number of working mothers steadily increased during this time, the use of infant formulas became more popular.

In the past three decades, more sophisticated neonatal medical practices have led to the development of countless infant formula preparations to meet a wide variety of clinical situations. Formulas exist as concentrates and powders that require dilution with water and as ready-to-feed preparations. Commonly, formula preparations provide 20 calories/ounce with standard dilutions of 1 ounce concentrate/1 ounce water and 1 scoop powder formula/2 ounces water for liquid concentrates and powders, respectively. Formulas exist as cow's milk-based, soy-based, and casein-based preparations. Each will be discussed separately for indications, characteristics, and nutrient composition.

A. Cow's Milk-Based Formula Preparations

This is the preferred, standard non-breast milk preparation for otherwise healthy term infants who do not breast-feed or for whom breast-feeding has been terminated prior to 1 year of age. Cow's milk-based formula closely resembles human breast milk and is composed of 20% whey and 80% casein with 50% more protein/dL than breast milk as well as iron, linoleic acid, carnitine, taurine, and nucleotides. Approximately 32 ounces will meet 100% of the recommended daily allowance (RDA) for calories, vitamins, and minerals. These formula preparations are diluted to a standard 20 calories/ounce and are typically whey-dominant protein preparations with vegetable oils and lactose. There are also multiple lactose-free preparations. Most standard formula preparations do not meet the RDA for fluoride and exclusively formula-fed infants may require 0.25 mg/day of supplemental fluoride.

B. Soy-Based Formula Preparations

Indicated primarily for vegetarian mothers and lactose-intolerant, galactosemic, and cow's milk allergic infants, soy-based formulas provide a protein-rich formula that contains more protein/deciliter than both breast milk and cow's milk formula preparations. Because the proteins are plant based, vitamin and mineral composition is increased to compensate for plant-based mineral antagonists while supplementing protein composition with the addition of methionine. Soy-based formulas tend to have a sweeter taste owing to a carbohydrate composition that includes sucrose and corn syrup. Prosobee, Isomil, and Isoyalac are common soy-based preparations.

C. CASEIN-HYDROLYSATE-BASED FORMULA PREPARATIONS

This poor tasting, expensive formula preparation is indicated principally for infants with either milk and soy-protein allergies or intolerance. Other indications include complex gastrointestinal pathologies. This formula, which contains casein-based protein and glucose, is not recommended for prolonged use in preterm infants owing to inadequate vitamin and mineral composition and proteins that may be difficult to metabolize. Standard preparations provide 20–24 calories/ounce.

D. PREMATURE INFANT FORMULA PREPARATIONS

Indicated for use in preterm infants of less than 1800 g birth weight, and with three times the vitamin and mineral content of standard formula preparations, these formulations provide 20–24 calories/ounce. Premature infant preparations are approximately 60% casein and 40% whey with 1:1 concentrations of lactose and glucose as well as 1:1 concentrations of long- and medium-chain fatty acids. Commercially available preparations include Enfamil Premature with Iron, Similac Natural Care Breast Milk Fortifier, and Similac Special Care with Iron. Similac Neo-Care, designed for preterm infants greater than 1800 g at birth, provides 22 calories/ounce in standard dilution.

Human Milk Fortifiers for Preterm Infants

Human milk fortifiers (HMFs) are indicated for preterm infants less than 34 weeks gestation or less than 1500 g birth weight once feeding has reached 75% full volume. HMFs are designed to supplement calories, protein, phosphorus, calcium, and other vitamins and minerals.

ENFAMIL-HMF is mixed to 24 calories/ounce by adding one 3.8-g packet to 25 mL of breast milk, increasing the osmolality to greater than 350 mOsm/L. Increased osmolality may enhance gastrointestinal irritability and impact tolerance. Practitioners may recommend a lower osmolality for the first 48 h beginning with one packet of ENFAMIL-HMF in 50 mL of breast milk producing 22 calories/ounce. The maxi-

mum caloric density from this HMF is 24 calories/ounce. Practitioners may add emulsified fat blends to increase caloric needs.

Similac Natural Care is a liquid milk fortifier that is typically mixed in a 1:1 ratio with breast milk. Other alternatives may include feedings with breast milk and fortifier. The osmolality of Similac Natural Care is lower than that of ENFAMIL—280 mOsm/L. This liquid fortifier may be preferable, particularly for infants whose mothers have low milk production.

American Academy of Pediatrics. Committee on Practice and Ambulatory Medicine: Pediatrician's responsibility for infant nutrition. Pediatrics 1997;99(5):749.

American Academy of Pediatrics. Work Group on Breastfeeding: Breastfeeding and the use of human milk. Pediatrics. 1997; 100(6):1035.

American Dietetic Association: *Nutrition Management of the Infant. Manual of Clinical Dietetics,* 1997.

Bachrach VR, Schwarz E, Bachrach LR: Breastfeeding and the risk of hospitalization for respiratory disease in infancy: a meta-analysis. Arch Pediatr Adolesc Med 2003;157(3):237.

Bentley ME, Dee DL, Jensen JL: Breastfeeding among low income, African-American women: power, beliefs and decision making. J Nutr 2003;133(1):305S.

Chezem J, Friesen C, Boettcher J: Breastfeeding knowledge, breastfeeding confidence, and infant feeding plans: effects on actual feeding practices. J Obstet Gynecol Neonatal Nurs 2003;32 (1):40.

Clark FI, James EJP: Twenty-seven years of experience with oral vitamin K1 therapy in neonates. J Pediatr 1995;127(2):301.

Department of Health and Human Services. Office on Women's Health: *HHS Blueprint for Action on Breastfeeding,* 2000.

Dewey KG: Maternal and fetal stress are associated with impaired lactogenesis in humans. J Nutr 2001;131:3012S.

Dewey KG: Is breastfeeding protective against child obesity? J Hum Lact 2003;19(1):9.

Furman L et al: The effect of maternal milk on neonatal morbidity of very low-birth-weight infants. Arch Pediatr Adolesc Med 2003;157(1):66.

Greenwood K, Littlejohn P: Breastfeeding intentions and outcomes of adolescent mothers in the Starting Out program. Breastfeed Rev 2002;10(3):19.

Gross SM et al: Counseling and motivational videotapes increase duration of breast-feeding in African-American WIC participants who initiate breast-feeding. J Am Diet Assoc 1998;98 (2):143.

Howard CR et al: Randomized clinical trial of pacifier use and bottle-feeding or cupfeeding and their effect on breastfeeding. Pediatrics 2003;111(3):511.

Khoury AJ et al: Improving breastfeeding knowledge, attitudes, and practices of WIC clinic staff. Public Health Rep 2002;117(5): 453.

Lawrence RA, Lawrence RM: *Breastfeeding, a Guide for the Medical Profession,* ed 5. Mosby, 1999.

Lovelady CA, Hunter CP, Geigerman C: Effect of exercise on immunologic factors in breast milk. Pediatrics 2003;111(2): E148.

Mikiel-Kostyra K, Mazur J, Boltruszko I: Effect of early skin-to-skin contact after delivery on duration of breast-feeding: a prospective cohort study. Acta Paediatr 2002;91(12):1301.

Mizuno K, Ueda A: The maturation and coordination of sucking, swallowing, and respiration in preterm infants. J Pediatr 2003;142(1):36.

Neville MC: Anatomy and physiology of lactation. Pediatr Clin North Am 2001;48(1):13.

Oddy WH: The impact of breastmilk on infant and child health. Breastfeed Rev 2002;10(3):5.

Peaker M, Wilde CJ, Knight CH: Local control of the mammary gland. Biochem Soc Symp 1998;63:71.

WEB SITES

www.aap.org/family/brstguid.htm—"A Woman's Guide to Breast-feeding"

www.breastfeedingbasics.org

www.breastfeeding.hypermart.net

www.lalecheleague.org

www.medela.com

Common Infections in Children

5

Mark A. Knox, MD

Infectious diseases are a major cause of illness in children. The widespread use of antibiotics has greatly reduced morbidity and mortality, but infections are still one of the most common types of problems encountered by physicians who care for children.

■ FEVER WITHOUT A SOURCE

General Considerations

Fever is the primary indication of an infectious process in children of all ages. Other than fever, however, many children do not display signs or symptoms indicative of the underlying disease. Of febrile children 20%, after history and physical examination, will have fever without a source of infection (FWS). The physician's dilemma is to separate children with a serious bacterial illness (SBI) from those with a viral or nonserious bacterial illness. A serious bacterial illness is defined variably, but generally includes growth of a known bacterial pathogen from cerebrospinal fluid, blood, urine, or stool, as well as abscess or cellulitis and pneumonia with positive blood cultures. Historically, children have been divided into three groups for evaluation purposes—young children ages 3 months to 3 years, young infants ages 2–3 months, and neonates 1 month of age or less. Young children are much more likely to show outward signs of illness, and their evaluation is much easier than that of younger infants. Neonates are a separate diagnostic group, more likely to have infections with organisms seen in the newborn period and less likely to show overt clinical signs of infection.

No officially adopted, evidence-based guidelines have been published to guide physicians in the workup and management of febrile illnesses, although guidelines based on expert opinion, group consensus, and locally performed research studies have been suggested. There is also general agreement that all proposed guidelines are followed only variably, according to local practice standards. Baraff et al, in 1993, published a set of practice guidelines that is useful and that will be summarized below.

The frequency and nature of serious bacterial illness are different in the three different age groups. Neonates less than 1 month of age are the most difficult to diagnose. The rate of SBI in nontoxic febrile neonates is reported to be 8.6% and the rate of SBI overall to be 12.6%. However, existing screening protocols lacked the sensitivity and negative predictive value to identify infants at low risk for SBI. For this reason, it is generally recommended that all febrile infants less than 1 month of age be admitted to the hospital, given a complete sepsis workup, and treated with parenteral antibiotics pending the results of the workup. Of these infants, approximately 65% will have a viral infection, 13% will have an SBI, and the rest will have nonbacterial gastroenteritis, aseptic meningitis, or bronchiolitis. Viral encephalitis and pneumonia account for less than 1% of cases. Of the SBIs, roughly 7% will have a urinary tract infection, with *Escherichia coli* being the most common pathogen. Three percent will have bacteremia, with group B *Streptococcus, Enterobacter, Listeria, S pneumoniae, E coli, Enterococcus,* and *Klebsiella* all being found. Less than 2% will have meningitis, usually caused by *Klebsiella, Listeria,* and group B *Streptococcus.* Less than 1% will have bacterial gastroenteritis, and 2% will have a variety of other infections.

In evaluating infants older than 1 month of age, it is useful to first identify which infants are at low risk for SBI. The criteria for low risk are being previously healthy, having no focal source of infection found on physical examination, and having a negative laboratory evaluation. A negative laboratory evaluation is defined as having a white blood cell (WBC) count of 5000–15,000/mm^3, fewer than 1500 bands/mm^3, normal urinalysis, and if diarrhea is present, fewer than five WBCs/high-power field in the stool. Chest radiography is included in some, but not all, sets of criteria. Lumbar puncture may be done at the physician's discretion but should always be done if empiric antibiotics are to be used. Additional low-risk criteria are appearing nontoxic and having a good social situation with reliable follow-up. Low-risk, nontoxic-appearing infants may be treated as outpatients, with close follow-up. Most recommendations are to use empiric antibiotics, although antibiotics may be withheld if the infant can be followed closely. All toxic-appearing or non-low-risk infants should be hospitalized and treated with parenteral antibiotics. The risk of SBI in toxic-appearing infants in this age group is about 17%. The overall frequency of SBIs in this age group is roughly 9% overall and 1–2% in low-risk infants, with most of the infections being urinary tract infections (UTIs), bacteremia, and bacterial enteritis. Meningitis accounts for slightly more than 1% of febrile infants.

Similar criteria may be used to evaluate children age 3 months to 3 years. The most common SBIs in this group are bacteremia and UTIs. UTIs are present in nearly 5% of febrile infants less than 12 months of age. In this group, 6–8% of girls and 2–3% of boys will have UTIs. The rates are higher with higher temperatures. After 12 months of age, the prevalence of UTI is lower.

In this age group, the rate of bacteremia has been reported to be 3–11%, with a mean of 4.3% if the temperature is 39°C or higher. The most common organisms isolated are *S pneumoniae* (85%), *Haemophilus influenzae* type b (10%), and *Neisseria meningitidis* (3%). The rate of infection with *H influenzae* has fallen dramatically since the use of the influenza vaccine has become widespread, and the rate of pneumococcal bacteremia is expected to do likewise in the near future.

Occult pneumonia is rare in febrile children who have a normal WBC count and who do not have signs of lower respiratory infection, such as cough, tachypnea, rales, or rhonchi. Bacterial enteritis is unusual in children who do not have diarrhea.

As in younger infants, toxic-appearing or non-low-risk infants should be hospitalized and treated with parenteral antibiotics. The rate of SBIs in toxic-appearing children in this age group has been reported to be 10–90%, depending on the definition of toxic.

Low-risk, nontoxic-appearing children in this age group may be treated as outpatients. The use of empiric antibiotics is not necessary, although it should be considered for children who have not received pneumococcal vaccine. There is general consensus that bacteremia is a risk factor for development of infectious complications, such as meningitis. However, pneumococcal bacteremia responds well to oral antibiotics, so these drugs can be used in children who appear well despite having positive blood cultures.

Clinical Findings

A. SYMPTOMS AND SIGNS

The most important clinical decision is to decide which infants appear toxic and therefore need more aggressive evaluation and treatment. The definition of toxic is consistent with the sepsis syndrome—lethargy, signs of poor perfusion, marked hypoventilation or hyperventilation, or cyanosis. Lethargy is defined as an impaired level of consciousness as manifested by poor or absent eye contact or by failure of the child to recognize parents or to interact with people or objects in the environment.

Fever is defined as a temperature of 38°C (100.4°F) or greater. Rectal measurement is the only accurate way to determine fever. A careful, complete physical examination is necessary to exclude focal signs of infection. The skin should be examined for exanthems, cellulitis, abscesses, or petechiae. Between 2% and 8% of children with fever and a petechial rash will have an SBI, most often caused by *N meningitidis*. Meningococcemia is less likely if petechiae are not present below the nipples, and most children with meningococcal disease will not appear otherwise well. Common childhood infections, such as pharyngitis and otitis media, should be sought, and a careful lung examination should be done looking for evidence of pneumonia. The abdomen should be examined for signs of peritonitis or tenderness. A musculoskeletal examination should be done looking for evidence of osteomyelitis or septic arthritis. The neurological examination should be directed toward the level of consciousness and should look for focal neurological deficits, although most infants and children with meningitis will also appear toxic.

B. LABORATORY FINDINGS

The laboratory investigation includes WBC count and differential, urinalysis and urine culture, blood culture, lumbar puncture with routine analysis and culture, and chest x-ray. If the child has diarrhea, stool cultures should be done.

Treatment

All infants less than 1 month of age should be hospitalized. An appropriate antibiotic regimen includes ceftriaxone (50 mg/kg/day) with or without gentamicin. In the past, ampicillin has been used routinely to cover the possibility of *Listeria* infection. Although it appears that the frequency of infection with *Listeria* is decreasing, ampicillin may be added to the above regimen if the physician chooses.

Ceftriaxone is also an appropriate antibiotic for hospitalized older infants and children and for infants and children treated as outpatients. In infants 2–3 months of age, a single intramuscular dose of ceftriaxone should be given. The child should be reevaluated in 18–24 h and a second dose of ceftriaxone given. If blood cultures are found to be positive, the child should be hospitalized for further treatment. If the urine culture is positive, and the child has a persistent fever, the child should be hospitalized for treatment. If the child is afebrile and well, outpatient antibiotics may be used.

Table 5–1 presents guidelines that may be useful for investigating and treating febrile children.

Baker M, Bell L: Unpredictability of serious bacterial illness in febrile infants from birth to 1 month of age. Arch Pediatr Adolesc Med 1999;153:508. (More complete investigation of the problem in neonates. Discusses the unreliability of previously proposed evaluation protocols in children in this age group.)

Baraff L: Management of fever without source in infants and children. Ann Emerg Med 2000;36:602. (A clear and concise discussion of the issue with clear recommendations for evaluation. Not much discussion of treatment.)

Baraff L et al: Practice guidelines for the management of infants and children 0 to 36 months of age with fever without source. Pediatrics 1993;92:1. (These protocols are proposed by the authors and do not constitute official practice guidelines of the American Academy of Pediatrics. Still the most complete guidelines to be found in the literature.)

Sadow K, Derr R, Teach S: Bacterial infections in infants 60 days and younger: epidemiology, resistance, and implications for treatment. Arch Pediatr Adolesc Med 1999;153:611. (Brief discussion of the changing microbiology of infections in young infants.)

■ INFECTIONS OF THE UPPER RESPIRATORY TRACT

OTITIS MEDIA

 ESSENTIALS OF DIAGNOSIS

- *Preexisting URI (93%).*
- *Fever (25%).*
- *Ear pain (variable, depending on age).*
- *Tympanic membrane bulging, immobile.*
- *Color dull gray, yellow, or red.*
- *Perforated TM with purulent drainage (diagnostic).*

General Considerations

Acute otitis media (AOM) is the most common reason that children are brought to a physician. Among children under 1 year of age, there are almost 30 million physician visits each year. Almost all children will have

Table 5–1. Evaluation and treatment of febrile children.

Less than 1 month of age
  Admit for evaluation and treatment

Two to 3 months of age
  Toxic or non-low risk, admit
  Nontoxic, low risk
    Option 1
      Blood culture
      Urine culture
      Lumbar puncture
      Ceftriaxone 50 mg/kg intramuscularly (1 g maximum)
      Return for reevaluation within 24 h
    Option 2
      Blood culture
      Urine culture
      Careful observation
  Low-risk criteria
    Clinical
      Previously healthy, term infant with uncomplicated nursery stay
      Nontoxic appearance
      No focal bacterial infection on examination (except otitis media)
    Laboratory
      WBC count 5000–15,000/mm^3, <1500 bands/mm^3
      Negative gram stain of unspun urine (preferred), or negative urine leukocyte esterase and nitrite, or <5 WBCs/high-power field
      Cerebrospinal fluid <8 WBCs/mm^3 and negative gram stain

Three months to 3 years of age
  Toxic, admit
  Nontoxic
    Temperature <39.0°C
      No tests or antibiotics
      Symptomatic treatment for fever
      Return if fever persists more than 48 h or if condition deteriorates
    Temperature ≥39.0°C
      Urinalysis, if positive, perform culture, treat with oral third-generation cephalosporin
      If child has not received pneumococcal conjugate vaccine
      If temperature ≥39.5°C, obtain WBC count
      If WBC count ≥15,000
        Blood culture
        Ceftriaxone 50 mg/kg
    If Sao$_2$ <95%, respiratory distress, tachypnea, rales, or temperature ≥39.5°C and WBC count ≥20,000
      Chest x-ray
    Symptomatic treatment for fever
    Return if fever persists more than 48 h or if condition deteriorates

Adapted from Baraff L: Management of fever without source in infants and children. *Ann Emerg Med* 2000;36:602.

at least one episode of otitis media each year, and one-third will have three or more episodes. For reasons that are unclear, the incidence has increased, as has the frequency of recurrent infections.

Pathogenesis

The microbiology of AOM is well established. When cultures of middle ear fluid are done, *S pneumoniae* is found in about 35%, *H influenzae* in about 25%, and *Moraxella catarrhalis* in about 15%; 10% will have more than one of these bacteria. About 25% of middle ear effusions will be sterile. Viruses will be recovered in a large percentage of cases, with or without bacteria, but whether their role is causative remains unclear.

Prevention

There are several identified risk factors for otitis media, not all of which are easily modifiable for prevention of the disease. The primary risk factor is day care, which increases substantially the number of pathogens to which the child is exposed. Other risk factors include increased number of siblings in the house, exposure to tobacco smoke, pacifier use, formula feeding, and lower socioeconomic status. Children with abnormalities of the palatal architecture, such as those with cleft palate or Down's syndrome, are at greatly increased risk. Widespread use of vaccines against *H influenzae* type B and *S pneumoniae* is not expected to have much impact on the disease, as the infection is generally caused by nontypeable *Hemophilus* and by strains of pneumococcus not covered by the pediatric 7-valent vaccine.

Clinical Findings

A. SYMPTOMS AND SIGNS

Despite the frequency with which physicians see children with otitis media, the diagnostic criteria are not standardized, and the diagnosis itself is often unclear. Individual physicians and research protocols alike show considerable diversity with respect to the criteria used to diagnose this disease. Otitis media most often begins with an upper respiratory infection (URI), and as many as 93% of children with AOM have typical URI symptoms such as nasal congestion, rhinorrhea, or cough. The viral infection causes dysfunction of the eustachian tube, which leads to accumulation of secretions in the middle ear followed by colonization with bacteria. Symptoms of AOM may develop over only a few hours, or the onset may be more gradual. Ear pain is the most characteristic symptom, with a high degree of specificity and positive predictive value. Younger children do not localize pain as obviously as older children. Fever is present in only about 25% of children and is more common in younger children. The TM will bulge and

may be cloudy, yellow, or red in color. Erythema of the TM may be caused by fever or by screaming, so this sign is of questionable reliability. The drum will generally be immobile with pneumatic otoscopy or tympanometry. The infection is bilateral in 50% of affected children. Fewer than 5% of TMs rupture, but pus draining through a perforation is diagnostic.

Differential Diagnosis

As discussed above, the primary illness that may be confused with otitis media is acute URI. Many of the symptoms are identical, and findings in the TM may be subtle and nondiagnostic. Many physicians err on the side of overdiagnosis, leading to overuse of antibiotics in children with URIs.

Complications

Complications of otitis media fall into two main categories—suppurative and nonsuppurative. Suppurative complications may arise from direct extension of the infection into the surrounding bones or into the adjacent brain, such as mastoiditis, venous sinus thrombosis, and brain abscess. They may also arise from hematogenous spread of the bacteria from the middle ear, primarily sepsis and meningitis. The main suppurative complication is mastoiditis. Recent research shows that treatment of otitis media does not reduce the incidence of this complication. The bacteria responsible for hematogenous spread are principally *S pneumoniae* and *H influenzae*.

Nonsuppurative complications primarily arise from middle ear effusion and inflammation and scarring of the structures of the middle ear. Antibiotic treatment does not influence the persistence of middle ear effusions after otitis media, nor does it have any effect on long-term hearing and language development. No evidence exists to assess the effect of treatment on later development of tympanosclerosis and otosclerosis, which may cause long-term conductive hearing loss. In summary, it appears that complications of otitis media may not be preventable by antibiotic treatment.

Treatment

Antibiotic treatment has long been the standard of care for children with otitis media. However, in the past decade, research has made it clear that the benefits of antibiotics are much less clear than was believed in the past. As many as 59% of children will have resolution of symptoms within 24 h without treatment, and 80–85% will recover in 1–7 days without antibiotics. Antibiotic treatment reduces the persistence of symptoms at 2–7 days to 7%, or about a 12% reduction. In other words, about eight children will need to be treated to benefit one. The high spontaneous resolution rate makes comparison of treatments difficult. Numerous studies have been done comparing various antibiotic regimens. Narrow-spectrum antibiotics have the same success rate as broad-spectrum antibiotics, although adverse effects, primarily gastrointestinal, are more common with the latter. High-dose amoxicillin (80 mg/kg/day) is no more effective than standard-dose amoxicillin (40 mg/kg/day). Single-dose intramuscular ceftriaxone (50 mg/kg) is as effective as oral antibiotics. Regarding duration of treatment, numerous studies also document that a 5-day course of antibiotics is as effective as the standard 10-day course. The conclusion of numerous studies is that children with otitis media should be treated with a 5-day course of narrow-spectrum antibiotics. In an era of growing antibiotic resistance, the widespread use of broad-spectrum antibiotics when narrow-spectrum drugs are equally effective should be a serious concern to physicians.

It is important to note that studies have not adequately addressed the issues of treatment of children less than 2 years of age and of treatment of frequently recurrent or complicated otitis media. Physicians are left to their clinical judgment as to the best treatment for these children.

The best treatment for children with frequent recurrences of otitis media is another area of study. The best evidence is that children will benefit from daily antibiotic prophylaxis only if they have had more than three episodes in 6 months or four episodes in 1 year. The magnitude of benefit is small, with a reduction of about one episode per year. Antibiotics studied have primarily been narrow-spectrum drugs, such as erythromycin, amoxicillin, sulfisoxazole, and trimethoprim-sulfamethoxazole.

Prognosis

In general, children with otitis media recover uneventfully. About 1 in 1000 will develop mastoiditis. The effusion associated with the infection persists for a time after the clinical signs of infection have resolved. Approximately 70% of children will have a persistent middle ear effusion at 2 weeks after treatment, 50% at 1 month, 20% at 2 months, and 10% at 3 months. Repeated courses of antibiotics have no effect on these effusions and should not be used.

PHARYNGITIS

Sore throat is a common problem in pediatrics, leading to millions of physician office visits each year. However, obtaining a clear diagnosis identifying the cause of this problem is far from simple. The most important diagnosis to make is group A β-hemolytic streptococcal (GABHS) infection, which is responsible for about

15% of cases of pharyngitis. Antibiotic treatment has only a modest effect on the course of the disease, but adequate treatment with antibiotics will effectively prevent the important complication of rheumatic fever. Non-group A β-hemolytic streptococci (groups C and G) are occasional causes of pharyngitis but do not lead to rheumatic fever. Viruses of many sorts cause the vast majority of cases, including some cases of exudative pharyngitis. Adenoviruses can cause pharyngoconjunctival fever, with exudative pharyngitis and conjunctivitis. Epstein–Barr virus causes infectious mononucleosis, which commonly causes other signs, such as generalized lymphadenopathy and splenomegaly, in addition to exudative pharyngitis. Herpes viruses and coxsackie viruses can cause ulcerative stomatitis and pharyngitis. Most viruses, however, cause signs and symptoms that overlap with those of GABHS. There are numerous recommendations for diagnosis and treatment, but there is no clear consensus as to the most accurate or most cost-effective method for evaluation and treatment of the child with a sore throat.

1. Group A β-Hemolytic Streptococcal Infection

 ESSENTIALS OF DIAGNOSIS

- *Moderate to severe tonsillar swelling.*
- *Moderate to severe tender anterior cervical lymphadenopathy.*
- *Scarlatiniform rash (depending on the strain of bacteria).*
- *Absence of moderate to severe viral symptoms (cough, nasal congestion).*

General Considerations

Group A β-hemolytic streptococci cause approximately 15% of cases of sore throat in children. The disease is uncommon in children under 3–5 years of age and in adolescents over 11–15 years of age. In an effort to decrease overprescribing of antibiotics, many guidelines, with varying degrees of evidence-based support, have been proposed.

Clinical Findings

A. SYMPTOMS AND SIGNS

Clinical symptoms and signs overlap those of viral pharyngitides and URIs. The Centor criteria have been validated for adults but not for children. Attia et al have proposed a predictive model for GABHS after examining a large number of signs and symptoms (Table 5–2). This is but one possible way to interpret the data. It has not been adopted as a guideline, but it represents a logical way to interpret what may be confusing information. The findings most highly correlated with GABHS are moderate to severe tonsillar swelling, moderate to severe tender anterior cervical lymphadenopathy, scarlatiniform rash, and the absence of moderate to severe coryza. If all four of these are present, the likelihood of GABHS is 95%. Excluding scarlatiniform rash, the presence of the remaining three gives a probability of greater than 65%. In the absence of moderate to severe tonsillar enlargement, moderate to severe lymphadenopathy, and scarlatiniform rash and in the presence of moderate to severe coryza, the likelihood of GABHS is less than 15%.

B. LABORATORY FINDINGS

Rapid antigen detection tests are commonly used in practice. Although the sensitivities of these assays may be reported as very high in laboratories, in practice they may have a false negative rate of as high as 20%. The sensitivity and specificity of throat culture are dependent on technique and may also have a false negative rate of 10–20%. Another complicating factor is the inability of either rapid antigen testing or culture to distinguish between a true streptococcal infection and a viral infection in a child who is an otherwise asymptomatic carrier. Carrier rates among asymptomatic children may be as high as 17%, depending on the age of the child and the season of the year.

Complications

Complications of GABHS fall into two main categories—nonsuppurative and suppurative. The nonsuppurative complications are rheumatic fever and poststreptococcal glomerulonephritis. The main suppurative complications are peritonsillar and retropharyngeal abscess.

Acute rheumatic fever follows about 3% of cases of untreated GABHS. The cause is still not fully understood, but the prevailing theory is that there is some similarity between certain streptococcal antigens and certain myocardial proteins leading to antistreptococcal antibody recognition and interaction with the myocardial proteins. For reasons that are unclear, there is great geographic variability in the incidence of this disease. Rheumatic fever can be prevented by treatment of GABHS, even if treatment is delayed for up to 9 days, but a full 10 days of treatment is necessary for complete prevention. Poststreptococcal glomerulonephritis also seems to be caused by a poorly understood antigen–antibody reaction and is seen with certain "nephritogenic" strains of streptococci. For reasons that are unknown, the incidence of this complication has been declining over the past decade, and it is now no longer the most common cause of glomerulonephritis in children. Unlike rheumatic fever, glomerulonephritis is not prevented by treatment of GABHS.

Treatment

Treatment of GABHS may accomplish two things—quicker resolution of disease and prevention of some complications. Treatment of the acute infection may shorten the course of the disease by a small amount, although untreated disease will resolve within several days in the majority of cases. It is not clear whether immediate antibiotic treatment offers greater benefit than symptomatic treatment. It is generally believed that treatment will reduce the rate of suppurative complications, but many children present with peritonsillar abscess in whom the initial streptococcal infection would not have been recognized in its earlier stages. As mentioned earlier, adequate antibiotic treatment can prevent rheumatic fever but not glomerulonephritis.

No group A β-hemolytic streptococci are resistant to penicillin or cephalosporins. Penicillin V (25–30 mg/kg/day, divided twice a day) is the drug of choice for children who are not allergic to penicillin. A single intramuscular dose of benzathine penicillin (0.3–0.6 million units/kg if <27 kg, 900,000 units if >27 kg) is an alternative for children in whom compliance is suspected to be a problem. Erythromycin has long been the drug of choice for penicillin-allergic patients. However, in recent years, the rates of resistance to erythromycin have risen to very high levels in some areas. There is no agreement as to the best alternative to penicillin, but clindamycin is often recommended. It is well established that 10 days of treatment is necessary to achieve the maximum possibility of bacterial eradica-

Table 5–2. Decision tree for GABHS.

Presence of tender, enlarged nodes and tonsillar swelling, the absence of coryza, and the presence or absence of scarlatiniform rash
    Probability of GABHS 65–95%
        Treat
        Do not test
Absence of scarlatiniform rash plus the absence of one or more of the above three signs
    Probability of GABHS 15–65%
        Test with rapid antigen test or culture, treat if positive
Absence of scarlatiniform rash and tender, enlarged nodes and the presence of coryza
    Probability of GABHS less than 15%
        No treatment
        No testing

tion from the pharynx. However, for reasons that are unclear, streptococci will persist in the pharynx in about 10% of treated children, regardless of which antibiotic is used. There is no consensus as to the best way to deal with this phenomenon.

Prognosis

Streptococcal pharyngitis is ordinarily a benign self-limited disease. Morbidity and mortality are primarily related to the above-mentioned complications. Antibiotic treatment can eliminate many, but not all of these.

2. Peritonsilar Abscess

ESSENTIALS OF DIAGNOSIS

- *Severe sore throat.*
- *Odynophagia.*
- *High fever.*
- *Unilateral pharyngeal swelling with deviation of uvula.*

General Considerations

Peritonsillar abscess is the most common deep space head and neck infection in children, accounting for almost 50% of these infections. It is most commonly caused by infection with GABHS. The exact cause is unknown, but it is thought that the infection usually spreads from the tonsil itself into the deep spaces behind the tonsil, where it produces a collection of pus. It can occur in children of all ages, as well as in adults, but it affects older children and adolescents more than younger children. It is almost always unilateral.

Clinical Findings

A. SYMPTOMS AND SIGNS

Most children with peritonsillar abscess have had symptoms of pharyngitis, for which many will have been treated with antibiotics, for 1–7 days before presenting with symptoms related to the abscess. The most common symptoms are severe throat or neck pain, painful swallowing, high fever, and poor oral intake, sometimes with dehydration. The most common physical signs are cervical adenopathy, uvular deviation, and muffled voice with trismus. Symptoms are less clear and the ex-

amination is more difficult in younger children, and young children who cannot cooperate may have to be examined under sedation.

B. LABORATORY FINDINGS

The white blood cell count is usually elevated with a left shift. Throat cultures for streptococci are positive in only about 16% of children.

C. IMAGING STUDIES

Computed tomography and ultrasound studies of the neck will often show the abscess, but the diagnosis is generally made by history and physical examination.

Differential Diagnosis

The primary disease in the differential diagnosis is epiglottitis. This infection is uncommon in an era of widespread immunization against *H influenzae* type B, but the clinical picture may be identical in young children. Examination in the operating room under sedation may be necessary to establish the diagnosis.

Complications

Prompt treatment is necessary, as untreated abscesses may spread into other deep spaces in the head and neck. The airway may be compromised by swelling, especially in younger children. If the abscess ruptures into the throat, aspiration of pus may cause pneumonia.

Treatment

The treatment is drainage of the abscess, either by incision or by needle aspiration. This is generally done by an otolaryngologist or by a surgeon familiar with the anatomy of the neck. Tonsillectomy is often done at the discretion of the surgeon, either at the time of the acute infection or shortly thereafter. Antibiotics effective against streptococci and staphylococci, such as nafcillin and ceftriaxone, are indicated, initially intravenously. Once cultures of the pus indicate the causative organism, treatment may be focused according to its antibiotic sensitivities.

Prognosis

Children generally recover uneventfully once appropriate treatment is begun. These children may be at increased risk for a second infection, however, since in one series, 7% of children with peritonsillar abscess had been treated for this condition in the past.

SINUSITIS

ESSENTIALS OF DIAGNOSIS

- *URI symptoms (nasal congestion and drainage, cough) without improvement for longer than 10–14 days.*
- *Symptoms of more severe infection (temperature >39°C, dental pain, facial pain, facial swelling) for a shorter duration.*

General Considerations

Essentially every child who has a URI has a concomitant sinusitis, as the effects of the virus do not stop at the sinus ostia, but rather involve the entire upper respiratory tract. It is estimated that bacterial sinusitis occurs after 0.5–5% of URIs. Distinguishing bacterial sinusitis from viral rhinosinusitis is made difficult by the facts that the symptoms of the two illnesses overlap significantly, that there are no diagnostic tests that reliably distinguish the two, and that approximately 60% of cases of bacterial sinusitis will resolve spontaneously without antibiotic treatment. Chronic sinusitis is defined as the persistence of these symptoms for longer than 30 days.

Pathogenesis

The inciting event in most cases of bacterial sinusitis is thought to be a URI. Allergic rhinitis has also been implicated as a cause. Both conditions cause inflammation and edema of the sinus mucosa, which obstruct the sinus ostia, causing fluid accumulation in the sinuses, which is then infected by bacteria that normally inhabit the upper respiratory tract. Studies on fluid collected by sinus aspiration show *S pneumoniae* in 30–66%, *H influenzae,* usually nontypeable, and *M catarrhalis* each in about 20%, and viruses alone in about 10% of cases.

Clinical Findings

A. SYMPTOMS AND SIGNS

The symptoms and signs of bacterial sinusitis overlap with those of URIs. Bacterial sinusitis is considered to be more likely when the symptoms of URI persist without improvement for more than 10–14 days. The diagnosis can be entertained after a shorter period of time if more severe signs and symptoms are present, such as fever greater than 39°C, dental pain, facial pain, or facial swelling. Although widely used by physicians as a discriminating sign, the color or degree of purulence of nasal drainage does not indicate a bacterial infection and has no diagnostic value.

B. IMAGING STUDIES

Imaging studies are of little value in diagnosing bacterial sinusitis, and most physicians treat the infection without these studies. Plain films can show mucosal thickening, air–fluid levels, and opacification of the sinuses, but these findings are neither sensitive nor specific. Computed tomography (CT) is sensitive for edema of sinus mucosa, but may be negative in some children with abnormal plain radiographic studies. In addition, its specificity is extremely low. It shows soft tissue changes in the sinuses of 20–70% of children who undergo CT scanning for reasons other than sinus disease and in 100% of children who have a CT within 2 weeks of a URI. Also, the changes seen on CT can persist up to 8 weeks after a URI.

Complications

The complications of bacterial sinusitis are primarily related to direct extension of the infection into or through adjacent bone or soft tissues. Sinusitis is often found in children with periorbital cellulitis. Cerebral sinus thrombosis and brain abscess are rare complications. There are no data to show whether early treatment of sinusitis can reduce the incidence of these rare complications.

Treatment

Given the high rate of spontaneous resolution and the global concern about overuse of these medications, antibiotics should be used only for children who have a high likelihood of bacterial sinusitis. Antibiotics are superior to placebo in children who have symptoms for longer than 10 days and who have positive radiographs. Because 80% of children with symptoms that persist longer than 10 days have positive x-rays, these studies do not contribute significantly to the decision to treat. Amoxicillin is still considered to be the drug of first choice, although local antibiotic resistance patterns must be considered when choosing a medication. For patients allergic to penicillin, a similarly narrow-spectrum antibiotic should be used. There are no data to support the use of broad-spectrum antibiotics as first-line agents. The optimum duration of treatment has not been established, although many authorities recommend treatment for 7 days beyond the point at which symptoms resolve or improve substantially, usually 10–14 days. If the child has not responded significantly after 2–3 days of treatment, a broad-spectrum antibiotic, such as amoxicillin-clavulanate, or a cephalosporin effective against penicillin-resistant pneumococci should be used.

Antihistamines and decongestants are often used as adjunctive treatments. However, no strong randomized data exist to justify their routine use. One small randomized trial supports the use of intranasal steroids.

INFLUENZA

 ESSENTIALS OF DIAGNOSIS

- *Nonspecific respiratory infection in infants and young children.*
- *In older children, respiratory symptoms include coryza, conjunctivitis, pharyngitis, and dry cough.*
- *In older children, pronounced high fever, myalgia, headache, and malaise.*

General Considerations

Influenza is caused by a respiratory virus that results in a respiratory infection of variable severity in children. Although influenza itself is a benign, self-limited disease, its sequelae, primarily pneumonia, can cause serious illness and occasionally death.

Pathogenesis

Influenza is caused by a variety of influenza viruses. Types A and B cause epidemic illness, whereas type C produces sporadic cases of respiratory infections. Influenza viruses are unusual in that they undergo continuous genetic alteration, both small changes from year to year and larger, more distinctive changes every several years or longer. Infection with influenza virus confers limited immunity that lasts several years, until the virus becomes genetically distinct enough to escape this protection. Because every virus is new for infants, the attack rate is highest in infants and young children, with 30–50% showing serological evidence of infection in a normal year.

Prevention

The most effective way to prevent influenza and its complications is to immunize people of all ages at highest risk for complications. Influenza vaccine protects against both types A and B. In past years, immunization was recommended for children over the age of 6 months who lived in chronic care facilities or who had chronic illnesses of any type, based on the belief that these children had higher rates of serious complications than children without these risk factors. Studying

the complications of influenza is difficult because influenza and respiratory syncytial virus share a season of peak activity and have many of the same features. More recent studies, however, have shown that the rate of complications is similar in both groups, and that otherwise healthy children under the age of 2 years, and possibly those between the ages of 2 and 4 years as well, have a higher rate of complications than older children. For this reason, it is recommended that all children between the ages of 6–23 months be immunized. These recommendations are currently under discussion.

Children under the age of 9 years who have never been immunized against influenza should receive two doses of vaccine, 1 month apart. Children 9 years of age and older need only one dose. The unit dose for children 6–35 months of age is 0.25 mL. The unit dose for children 36 months of age and older is 0.5 mL. The vaccine must be repeated annually, as the influenza virus changes genetically from year to year. The vaccine should be given in October or November, to protect children during the peak infection months of December through February. Peak antibody levels are achieved roughly 2 weeks after immunization (2 weeks after the second dose in vaccine-naive children).

Chemoprophylaxis with a variety of drugs is an alternative to immunization, although this option is much more expensive than the vaccine. Three drugs are available—the antiviral drugs amantadine and rimantadine, which protect only against type A, and the neuraminidase inhibitor oseltamivir, which protects against both types A and B. The dose of amantadine or rimantadine for children ages 1–9 years is 5 mg/kg/day, up to 150 mg/day, in two divided doses. For children aged 10 years and older, the dose is 100 mg twice a day. These drugs are not indicated for children under 1 year of age. In some patients, amantadine and rimantadine permit subclinical infection with development of protective antibody. Oseltamivir is indicated for prophylaxis in adolescents aged 13 and older. The dose is 75 mg twice a day. The optimal duration of treatment is not known.

Clinical Findings

A. SYMPTOMS AND SIGNS

Influenza viruses types A and B cause nearly identical symptoms, except that the duration of symptoms in type A infection is usually several days, whereas symptoms usually last only 2 or 3 days in type B infection. Influenza in infants and young children causes a nonspecific respiratory infection, often indistinguishable from a URI. Occasionally the fever will be high enough and the child toxic enough in appearance to prompt hospitalization and workup for sepsis. In older children and adolescents, the disease presents with the abrupt onset of respiratory symptoms, such as URI symptoms, conjunctivitis, pharyngitis, and dry cough. The features that distinguish influenza from the usual URI are high fever and pronounced myalgia, headache, and malaise. The acute symptoms typically last for 2–4 days, but the cough and malaise may persist for several days longer. Physical findings are nonspecific, including pharyngitis, conjunctivitis, cervical lymphadenopathy, and occasionally rales, wheezes, or rhonchi in the lungs.

B. SPECIAL TESTS

Influenza is generally diagnosed based on clinical criteria. If confirmation of infection is desired, the virus can be identified by nasopharyngeal swabs sent for viral culture.

Complications

Otitis media and pneumonia are the most common complications from influenza. Up to 25% of children will have otitis media after a documented influenza infection. Influenza causes a primary viral pneumonia, but the more serious pneumonic complications are caused by bacterial superinfection.

Treatment

Treatment of established influenza infection within 2 days of the onset of symptoms can reduce the duration of symptoms by about 1 day compared to placebo. However, no drug has been shown to reduce the incidence of serious complications following the disease. Four drugs are available—the antiviral drugs amantadine and rimantadine, which protect only against type A, and the neuraminidase inhibitors oseltamivir and zanamivir, which protect against both types A and B. As for prophylaxis, the dose of amantadine or rimantadine for children ages 1–9 years is 5 mg/kg/day, up to 150 mg/day, in two divided doses. For children aged 10 years and older, the dose is 100 mg twice a day. These drugs are not indicated for children under 1 year of age. Amantadine should be given until the symptoms have been resolved for 1–2 days. Rimantidine is recommended as a 7-day course. Oseltamivir is indicated for treatment in children over 1 year of age. The dose for children ≤15 kg is 30 mg twice a day, for children 15–23 kg it is 45 mg twice a day, for children 23–40 kg it is 60 mg twice a day, and for children over 40 kg it is 75 mg twice a day. Zanamivir is indicated for treatment of children aged 7 years and older. It is an inhaled powder given in a dose of 10 mg twice a day. Oseltamivir and zanamivir are given as a 5-day course. Given the cost of these medications and their inability to prevent complications, immunization is clearly a superior alternative for controlling influenza and its sequelae.

Prognosis

Influenza is ordinarily a benign self-limited disease. Morbidity and mortality are related either to postinfluenza pneumonia or to exacerbation of underlying chronic illness caused by the virus.

Attia M et al: Multivariate predictive models for group A beta-hemolytic streptococcal pharyngitis in children. Acad Emerg Med 1999;6:8. (Good review of predictive value of signs and symptoms associated with streptococcal pharyngitis with a decision analysis model and suggestions for treatment and testing based on the model.)

Blumer J: Fundamental basis for rational therapeutics in acute otitis media. Pediatr Infect Dis J 1999;18:1130. (A good discussion of the role of antibiotics in otitis media, with a discussion of pharmacological characteristics of various antibiotics.)

Bridges C et al: Prevention and control of influenza: recommendations of the Advisory Committee on Immunization Practice (ACIP). MMWR 2002;51:1. [Extensive review of prevention and treatment of influenza, with discussion of rationale for routine immunization of children (not yet universally accepted).]

Dowell S et al: Otitis media: principles of judicious use of antimicrobial agents. Pediatrics 1998;101:165. (Relatively brief. References evidence but does not discuss in detail. Much emphasis on acute otitis media as compared to otitis media with effusion.)

Faden H, Duffy L, Boeve M: Otitis media: back to basics. Pediatr Infect Dis J 1998;17:1105. (Similar to Dowell et al, with more discussion of pathophysiology.)

Lau J, Ioannidis J, Wald E: Diagnosis and treatment of uncomplicated acute sinusitis in children. Evidence Report/Technology Assessment, 9(suppl). Agency for Healthcare Research and Quality, 2000. AHRQ Publication Number 01-E005. (Extensive evidence-based review of the subject. Illustrates the dearth of good evidence about this illness.)

Martin J et al: Erythromycin-resistant group A streptococci in schoolchildren in Pittsburgh. New Engl J Med 2002;346:1200. (Describes a new and changing resistance pattern for this illness.)

McAlister W, Kronemer K: Imaging of sinusitis in children. Pediatr Infect Dis J 1999;18:1019. (Brief review of sensitivity and specificity of imaging studies in sinusitis.)

O'Brien K et al: Acute sinusitis: principles of judicious use of antimicrobial agents. Pediatrics 1998;101:174. (Brief review of diagnostic uncertainties and management options in sinusitis.)

Schraff S, McGinn J, Derkay C: Peritonsillar abscess in children: a 10-year review of diagnosis and management. Int J Pediatr Otorhinolaryngol 2001;57:213. (Review of diagnostic features of the disease, with discussion about management options.)

Schwartz B et al: Pharyngitis: principles of judicious antibiotic use. Pediatrics 1998;101:171. (Some authors from the Centers for Disease Control and Prevention. Brief review of the disease, with opinions about diagnosis that are based on the sensitivity and specificity of tests but that are not otherwise evidence based.)

Takata G et al: Evidence assessment of management of acute otitis media: I. The role of antibiotics in treatment of uncomplicated otitis media. Pediatrics 2001;108:239. (Very good evidence-based discussion of various treatment options, including brief reviews of relevant studies and their outcomes.)

■ INFECTIONS OF THE LOWER RESPIRATORY TRACT

CROUP (ACUTE LARYNGEOTRACHEOBRONCHITIS)

ESSENTIALS OF DIAGNOSIS

- URI prodrome.
- Barking cough.
- Symptoms worst on first or second day, with gradual resolution.
- Lungs clear.
- Inspiratory stridor, respiratory distress, and cyanosis in severe cases.

General Considerations

Croup is a relatively common infection in children, causing between 27,000 and 62,000 hospitalizations each year. Most cases occur in the autumn and early winter, with most hospitalizations occurring in October and February. The peak age incidence of croup is 3 months to 5 years, with 91% of hospitalizations occurring in children under 5 years of age.

Pathogenesis

Croup is caused by an infection of the upper airways— the larynx, trachea, and the upper levels of the bronchial tree—and obstruction of these airways caused by edema produces most of the classic symptoms of the disease. Nearly all cases of croup are caused by viruses. Parainfluenza viruses, types 1, 2, and 3, cause 75% of cases, with type 1 the most common cause. Adenovirus and respiratory syncytial virus cause most of the remainder, with *Mycoplasma pneumoniae* accounting for 3–4% of cases.

Clinical Findings

A. SYMPTOMS AND SIGNS

The symptoms of croup are usually typical, and diagnosis is not difficult. Most children present with several days of prodromal URI symptoms, which are followed by the gradual onset of a barking, "seal-like" cough. Stridor is generally mild and intermittent at first, primarily with inspiration and worse when the child is agitated. Typically, respiratory distress is only mild to moderate. In most children, this is the maximum extent of the disease. The symptoms are generally worst on the first and/or second day, are usually worse at night than during the day, and gradually resolve over several days. If the symptoms progress beyond this point, the child will develop worsening respiratory distress, more pronounced and more constant stridor, and cyanosis.

The physical findings of croup are variable and depend on the severity of the illness. The lungs are usually clear. The degree of subcostal and intercostal retractions, the degree of stridor, and the presence of cyanosis are important clues to the severity of the illness. If the child is cyanotic and in respiratory distress, manipulation of the pharynx, eg, trying to examine the pharynx using a tongue depressor, may trigger respiratory arrest. This maneuver should therefore be avoided until the clinician is in a position to manage the child's airway by endotracheal intubation.

B. LABORATORY FINDINGS

Laboratory findings are generally minimal in this disease. The WBC count is usually normal or slightly elevated, with counts greater than 15,000 occurring in about 20% of cases. The blood oxygen saturation may be normal or decreased, depending on the severity of the disease.

C. IMAGING STUDIES

In a typical case of croup, the chest x-ray will be normal. In 40–50% of cases, anteroposterior soft-tissue x-rays of the neck will show subglottic narrowing, causing the classic "steeple" sign of croup.

Differential Diagnosis

Croup must be differentiated from other respiratory illnesses that have cough as the main symptom. Normally, the time course and nature of the cough are diagnostic. Spasmodic croup lacks the URI prodrome and has a more abrupt onset than typical croup. Bacterial tracheitis presents as typical croup that worsens instead of improving after a few days. Children with epiglottitis and peritonsillar abscess are acutely ill and often toxic appearing, and although they may have a cough, it is not the predominant feature of the disease. Children with bronchiolitis are usually younger than children with croup, and their lungs show diffuse fine end-expiratory wheezes. Similarly, expiratory wheezing is a prominent feature of asthma but not of croup, where inspiratory stridor may be prominent in severe disease.

Children with pneumonia usually have a looser, more productive cough, they will often have more focal pulmonary findings on examination, and chest x-ray will often show an infiltrate.

Complications

About 15% of children with croup will experience complications of varying severity. These are usually related to extension of the infection to other parts of the respiratory tract, such as otitis media or viral pneumonia. Bacterial pneumonia is unusual, but bacterial tracheitis may occur. Children with severe croup may develop complications of hypoxemia, if this is not adequately treated. Death is unusual and is generally due to laryngeal obstruction.

Treatment

Perhaps the most critical decision to make when evaluating a child with croup is which patient needs to be treated in the hospital and which will do well at home. Between 1.5% and 15% of children with croup are hospitalized for treatment, and of these, 1–5% will require intubation and ventilation. Although there are no commonly accepted scoring systems for croup severity, there are several signs and symptoms that indicate more serious illness. High fever, toxic appearance, worsening stridor, respiratory distress, cyanosis or pallor, hypoxia, and restlessness or lethargy are all symptoms of more severe disease and should prompt the physician to admit the child for inpatient treatment.

Most children with croup may be treated at home. The mainstay of treatment has long been cool, moist air, although research has not confirmed the effectiveness of this. Although corticosteroids have long been an accepted part of inpatient treatment, their role in outpatient management of this disease has only recently been addressed. A single intramuscular dose of dexamethasone, 0.6 mg/kg, may be effective in reducing the severity of moderate to severe croup in patients treated at home. Because dexamethasone requires about 6 h for onset of action, a single dose of racemic epinephrine may be given before the child is sent home. Racemic epinephrine is commonly used in hospitalized patients, but β_2-agonist bronchodilators have not been shown to be effective.

Inpatient treatment of croup has changed little in recent years. As with home treatment, the mainstay of therapy is cool, humidified air, using a croup tent instead of cruder home measures. Supplemental oxygen is generally used to correct hypoxemia. Racemic epinephrine has long been the mainstay of treatment for patients who do not respond to cool, moist air or who have respiratory distress. Numerous studies have confirmed its effectiveness. The drug is usually given in a dose of 0.25–0.5 mL of a 2.25% solution mixed with 2 mL of normal saline and administered via a nebulizer and face mask. It has a duration of action of 1–2 h. Although racemic epinephrine is the drug most commonly used, *l*-epinephrine (5 mL of 1:1000 *l*-epinephrine) is equally effective, less expensive, and more widely available. Systemic corticosteroids have for many years been an important part of inpatient treatment of croup. Dexamethasone is the most widely studied drug, and has been shown to be effective in reducing both the severity and duration of the disease and the need for intubation. Because of its long action, it can be given as a single dose, 0.6 mg/kg, intramuscularly, which remains effective for the remainder of the course of the disease. It should be given as early as possible in the course of the disease and has not been associated with any deleterious effects. Numerous studies have been done comparing the effectiveness of nebulized steroids, primarily budesonide, to dexamethasone. Nebulized budesonide is superior to placebo and equally effective as oral dexamethasone. Although both are superior to placebo, intramuscular dexamethasone is more effective than nebulized budesonide. Children hospitalized for treatment of croup should be observed carefully for any signs of respiratory distress. Intubation and mechanical ventilation are necessary in a small percentage of children with this disease.

Prognosis

The natural history of croup is that recurrences are common. However, as the child grows, his or her airways grow larger and are less affected by edema, and symptoms tend to get less severe over time.

SPASMODIC CROUP

Spasmodic croup is a disorder that is clinically similar to infectious croup, but with some important differences. It primarily affects children between 1 and 3 years of age. Unlike infectious croup, the URI prodrome is usually absent, and the disease presents with the sudden onset, at night, of a croupy cough with variable degrees of stridor and respiratory distress. These symptoms gradually decrease over several hours, only to recur each night for one to two more nights, decreasing in severity each night. Like infectious croup, the symptoms respond to cool air and racemic epinephrine. The cause of this disorder is unclear. It may be a viral infection or an allergic response to viral antigens. In fact, no good evidence exists to support the concept that this is a distinct entity from infectious croup, and it may be that they are simply different manifestations of the same disease.

EPIGLOTTITIS

 ESSENTIALS OF DIAGNOSIS

- *Acute onset, rapid progression.*
- *Child looks seriously ill.*
- *Drooling, hoarse.*
- *Croupy cough, respiratory distress.*
- *Lateral x-ray shows edema of epiglottis (50%).*

General Considerations

Epiglottitis is a life-threatening bacterial infection of the epiglottis. The infection causes edema of the epiglottis, which has the potential to cause fatal airway obstruction. Untreated, the disease has a high mortality rate, but with treatment, the mortality rate is less than 1%. Fortunately, due to widespread use of vaccines against *H influenzae* type B, the disease frequency has been reduced by approximately 80%, and retropharyngeal abscess is now a more common cause of acute respiratory distress. The disease affects children between the ages of 2 and 7 years, with a peak incidence at 3–4 years of age.

Pathogenesis

This disease is caused primarily by *H influenzae* type B, and the majority of cases occur in children who either have not been immunized or whose immunizations are incomplete. Occasional cases are caused by *Streptococcus pyogenes*.

Clinical Findings

A. SYMPTOMS AND SIGNS

The presentation of epiglottitis is dramatic and usually suggests the diagnosis, although milder cases may be confused with croup. The symptoms of high fever, hoarseness, croupy cough, stridor, and respiratory distress typically have an abrupt onset and may progress to death from airway obstruction within hours. The physical examination is likewise dramatic and distinctive. The child usually has a high fever and looks toxic. The child will usually be sitting, leaning forward, and often drooling because of dysphagia. The child often is unable to speak, but if able to talk, the voice is notably hoarse because of inflammation of the vocal cords and surrounding tissue. Respiratory distress is moderate to severe. Visualization of the epiglottis is diagnostic, with the epiglottis being erythematous and markedly enlarged. However, this maneuver has the potential to precipitate complete and fatal airway obstruction and should be attempted only by a physician who has the skill to manage acute airway obstruction, including performing an emergency tracheostomy.

B. LABORATORY FINDINGS

Laboratory tests are not generally of much value. The WBC count is usually elevated at greater than 10,000/mm^3. Blood cultures will be positive in the majority of cases but are not useful acutely.

C. IMAGING STUDIES

X-rays of the chest are normal. If epiglottitis is suspected, soft-tissue lateral x-rays of the neck may be helpful. The classic finding is an enlarged, thumb-shaped epiglottis, but these films, which should be done as portable films in the emergency department, are positive in only about 50% of cases. Children with suspected epiglottitis should not be sent to the Radiology Department, where they may sit unobserved for a period of time.

Differential Diagnosis

The primary illnesses in the differential diagnosis are peritonsillar or retropharyngeal abscess. Examination in the operating room may be necessary to distinguish these diseases. Milder cases of epiglottitis may be confused with croup, although the rapid progression of this disease will eventually allow the distinction to be made.

Complications

Untreated epiglottitis has a significant mortality rate due to laryngeal obstruction. Complications are rare if the disease is treated promptly and are usually due to hypoxemia or complications of sepsis.

Treatment

The treatment of epiglottitis depends on rapid diagnosis, airway management, and institution of appropriate antibiotic therapy. The clinical picture is suggestive of the disease, but definitive diagnosis depends on visualization of the epiglottis. All children with confirmed epiglottitis require endotracheal intubation. The mortality rate in unintubated children is as high as 6%, compared to less than 1% in intubated children. This procedure should normally be attempted, usually in the operating room, by a physician who has the skills to manage the airway and to perform an emergency tracheostomy if a failed attempt at intubation triggers airway obstruction. Aside from airway management, antibiotics directed at the primary causative organisms are essential. Due to the high proportion of β-lactamase-producing organisms, second- and third-generation cephalosporins are considered drugs of first choice and should be continued for 7–10 days. Steroids and racemic epinephrine are of no value in this disease. The child will generally remain intubated for 2–3 days, until, in the judgment of an otolaryngologist, the epiglottal edema has subsided enough that the child is no longer in danger of airway obstruction. Flexible endoscopy may be a useful tool for following the course of the disease and deciding when extubation is safe.

BRONCHIOLITIS

 ## ESSENTIALS OF DIAGNOSIS

- URI symptoms.
- Paroxysmal wheezy cough.
- Dyspnea.
- Tachypnea.
- Diffuse fine rales.

General Considerations

Bronchiolitis is a common disease of infants seen most frequently in the first 2 years of life, with a peak at age about 6 months. Up to 7% of infants are affected, leading to hospitalization in up to 1%. It is an infection that causes edema and obstruction of the small airways. Older children and adults contract the same infection, but because they have larger airways, they do not experience the same degree of obstruction. In fact, an older sibling or a parent is often the source of the infant's infection.

Pathogenesis

Bronchiolitis is most often viral in etiology. Respiratory syncytial virus (RSV) causes more than 50% of cases with other cases caused by parainfluenza and viruses, and a few cases caused by *M pneumoniae*. Adenoviruses can cause a severe necrotizing infection, called bronchiolitis obliterans. Pathologically, edema and accumulated cellular debris cause obstruction of small airways. This obstruction causes a ventilation–perfusion mismatch with wasted perfusion, a right-to-left shunt, and hypoxemia early in the course of the disease.

Prevention

Since 1999, palivizumab (Synagis) has been available in the United States for prevention of RSV disease in high-risk infants. The drug has been shown to decrease hospitalization rates among high-risk infants with and without chronic lung disease, although the death rates in the initial studies were not significantly different between the treatment and placebo groups. The decision to use this drug is based on the age of the child at the onset of RSV season and the child's medical history. The American Academy of Pediatrics recommends prophylaxis with palivizumab for children less than 2 years of age with chronic lung disease who have required medical treatment in the preceding 6 months, for infants less than 1 year of age who were born at 28 weeks gestation or earlier, for infants less than 6 months of age who were born at 29–32 weeks gestation, and for infants less than 6 months of age born between 32 and 35 weeks gestation who have other risk factors for RSV infection such as day care attendance or three or more siblings. Palivizumab is given in a dose of 15 mg/kg intramuscularly once a month beginning with the onset of the local RSV season and continuing for 4–5 months. Protective antibody levels are achieved in 66% of infants after one injection and in 86% after a second injection.

Clinical Findings

A. SYMPTOMS AND SIGNS

The typical course of bronchiolitis begins with the exposure of the infant to another person with a URI. The infant will generally have URI symptoms for several days, with or without fever. The child then experiences the gradual onset of respiratory distress, with a paroxysmal wheezy cough and dyspnea. The child may be irritable and feed poorly, but there are usually no other systemic symptoms. The temperature is often in the range of 38.5–39°C, although it may be subnormal to greatly elevated.

Physical examination shows the child to be tachypneic, with a respiratory rate as high as 60–80/min, and often in severe respiratory distress. Alar flaring, retractions, and use of accessory muscles of respiration may be evident. Examination of the lungs often shows a prolonged expiratory phase with diffuse wheezes. Diffuse fine rales at the end of expiration and the beginning of inspiration are typical findings. The lungs are often hyperinflated with shallow respirations, and breath sounds may be nearly inaudible if the obstruction is severe.

The most critical phase of bronchiolitis is the first 2–3 days of the illness. Most cases will resolve in 1–3 days without much difficulty. However, in severe cases, symptoms may develop within hours and may be protracted.

B. LABORATORY FINDINGS

The laboratory finding of most utility is the oxygen saturation. If bronchiolitis is suspected, a nasopharyngeal swab may be done for RSV culture, but this has little if any effect on the outcome of the illness.

C. IMAGING STUDIES

X-rays usually show signs of hyperinflation. In about one-third of cases, x-rays will show scattered areas of consolidation. These may represent postobstructive atelectasis or inflammation of alveoli. It may not be possible to exclude early bacterial pneumonia solely on the basis of x-ray findings.

Differential Diagnosis

An important item in the differential diagnosis of bronchiolitis is acute asthma, as there may be many similarities in history and physical examination between these two conditions. Asthma is unusual in the first year of life, whereas the incidence of bronchiolitis peaks at 6 months of age. The presence of one or more of the following favors the diagnosis of asthma: family history of asthma, sudden onset without a preceding URI, repeated attacks, a markedly prolonged expiratory phase of respiration, eosinophilia, and response to one dose of epinephrine.

Complications

Bronchiolitis is ordinarily a benign disease. Complications are related to hypoxemia and are more common and more severe in children with underlying cardiac or pulmonary disease. The mortality rate is 1–2% for all infants, 3–4% in children with underlying cardiac or pulmonary disease, and 20–67% in immunocompromised children.

Treatment

Treatment of bronchiolitis is primarily supportive. The decision to hospitalize the child is clinical and is based on the degree of respiratory distress. Placing the child in a tent with cool humidified oxygen both relieves hypoxemia and reduces water loss from tachypnea. Intravenous fluids may be necessary. Antibiotics and steroids are of no benefit in bronchiolitis but antibiotics may be given if the x-ray suggests pneumonia. The role of bronchodilators is controversial. Bronchodilators are not helpful in bronchiolitis per se, but some infants with what appears to be bronchiolitis respond to these medications, suggesting a possible link between bronchiolitis and reactive airways disease. Many physicians elect to use bronchodilators for children in whom wheezing is a prominent feature of their disease. Treatment with antiinflammatory medications such as nebulized budesonide or cromolyn sodium after an episode of bronchiolitis can reduce wheezing episodes and hospital admissions for bronchospasm. Whether such treatment is useful for all children or should be reserved only for those children with clinically apparent wheezing after bronchiolitis has not been established. Despite considerable initial interest, ribavirin has not been shown to be of benefit, and it is no longer recommended for use in this disease.

Prognosis

There appears to be a relationship between bronchiolitis and reactive airways disease, although the exact connection is unclear. Children who develop bronchiolitis do not appear to have family histories of asthma or atopy or histories of exposure to cigarette smoke that are different from children who do not develop the disease. Some, but not all studies have shown an increased incidence of airway hyperreactivity that may persist for years in children who have had bronchiolitis. However, a similar, although somewhat lesser, phenomenon can be seen in children who have been diagnosed with pneumonia in early childhood.

BRONCHITIS

Although acute bronchitis is a diagnosis commonly made in primary care, it probably does not exist as a distinct clinical entity. What is often diagnosed as bronchitis is most often a URI with a prominent component of cough. As such, these are viral infections, although numerous prescriptions for antibiotics are written each year to treat these infections. Although sputum cultures may show *S pneumoniae, H influenzae, Staphylococcus aureus,* or various other species of *Streptococcus,* it has not been shown that these are causative agents, and antibiotics have not been shown to be effective treatments.

PERTUSSIS

 ESSENTIALS OF DIAGNOSIS

- *URI symptoms.*
- *Paroxysms of coughing, often with "whoops" on inspiration.*
- *Coughing to the point of vomiting.*

- *Dyspnea.*
- *Seizures.*

General Considerations

Pertussis is a bacterial infection that affects airways lined with ciliated epithelium. It is endemic in the general population, with epidemics occurring every 3–4 years. The disease is most common in unimmunized infants and in adults, as immunity wanes 5–10 years after the last immunization. Pertussis causes serious disease in children and mild or asymptomatic disease in adults. Infants less than 6 months of age have greater morbidity than older children, and those under 2 months have the highest rates of pertussis-related hospitalization, pneumonia, seizures, encephalopathy, and death. Pertussis is highly contagious, with attack rates as high as 100% in susceptible individuals exposed at close range.

Pathogenesis

The most common cause of pertussis is *Bordetella pertussis,* but *Bordetella parapertussis* occasionally causes the disease, and adenoviruses can cause a similar disease. Pathologically, the bacteria attack ciliated epithelium in the respiratory tree, where they produce toxins and other active factors. These cause inflammation and necrosis of the walls of small airways, which lead in turn to plugging of airways, bronchopneumonia, and hypoxemia.

Prevention

The key to prevention of pertussis is immunization. However, immunization does not confer complete protection, and immunized children may be asymptomatic reservoirs for infection. Of the 7288 cases reported in 1999, 27% occurred in children less than 7 months of age, ie, in children too young to have received the full initial course of three doses of pertussis vaccine, 11% occurred in children between the ages of 1 and 4 years, and 28% were in children between the ages of 10 and 19 years.

Clinical Findings

A. Symptoms and Signs

In China, pertussis is called the "cough of one hundred days," reflecting the long duration of symptoms. High fever is unusual in all ages. Children under the age of 2 years show the most typical symptoms of the disease.

In these children, 100% will have paroxysms of coughing, with 60–70% manifesting the "whoops" that give this disease its nickname of "whooping cough," 60–80% will have vomiting induced by coughing, 70–80% will have dyspnea lasting more than 1 month, and 20–25% will have seizures. Children over the age of 2 years have lower incidences of all these symptoms and a shorter duration of disease, whereas adults often have atypical symptoms.

Pertussis has an incubation period lasting 3–12 days. After that, the disease progresses through three stages, each lasting approximately 2 weeks.

The catarrhal stage is characterized by symptoms typical of a URI. The child may have especially thick nasal discharge during this stage, but the symptoms are nonspecific, and the diagnosis of pertussis is usually not considered.

The paroxysmal stage lasts 2–4 weeks, and occasionally longer. During this stage, episodes of coughing increase in severity and number. The typical paroxysm is 5–10 hard coughs in a single expiration, followed by the classic "whoop" as the patient inspires. Facial redness or cyanosis, bulging eyes, lacrimation, and salivation are common. The paroxysms recur until the mucous plugs causing the cough are dislodged. Coughing to the point of vomiting is common, and the diagnosis of pertussis should be considered in any patient with this symptom. The paroxysms are exhausting, and the child may appear apathetic and may lose weight because the child is too weak to eat or drink. The paroxysms may be frequent enough to cause hypoxemia, which may be severe enough to cause anoxic encephalopathy. Except for the paroxysms, however, the patient may not appear to be especially sick.

During the convalescent stage, the paroxysms gradually decrease in frequency and number. The patient may experience a cough for several months after the disease has otherwise resolved.

The diagnosis of pertussis can usually be made in the paroxysmal stage, but it requires a certain level of suspicion. A cough lasting more than 2 weeks, associated with posttussive vomiting, should prompt the physician to consider the diagnosis. As a diagnostic feature, the finding of an acute cough of presumed infectious etiology that lasts for more than 14 days is highly sensitive and moderately specific for the disease. There are no specific physical findings.

B. Laboratory Findings

A high WBC count (20,000–50,000) with an absolute lymphocytosis is common but not specific to the disease. The organism can be obtained for culture or staining by a nasopharyngeal swab. The sensitivity of culture is related to the stage of the disease, being very high early in the disease, when pertussis is least suspected. Culture is about 80% sensitive during the first 2 weeks of infection, 14% after the fourth week of infection, and zero after 5 weeks. Direct fluorescent antibody staining can provide a rapid diagnosis, but it has variable sensitivity and specificity, and all suspected cases should be cultured for definitive identification. Serology is useful only for retrospective diagnosis.

Differential Diagnosis

Any illness that causes cough should be considered in the differential diagnosis. Older children and children who have been immunized against the disease may have milder, atypical symptoms, and the only clue to the disease may be the long duration of the symptoms.

Complications

Complications of pertussis are numerous and often severe. Pneumonia is the most frequent complication and is seen in almost all fatal cases. *S pneumoniae, S aureus,* and oral flora are the most common organisms involved. A high fever or absolute neutrophilia in a patient with pertussis may be the only clues to a secondary bacterial infection. The cough may be severe enough to rupture alveoli and may cause interstitial and subcutaneous emphysema or pneumothorax. The cough may also cause epistaxis, melena, subconjunctival hemorrhage, spinal epidural hematoma, intracranial hemorrhage, rupture of the diaphragm, or umbilical or inguinal hernia. Inability to eat or drink may lead to dehydration, electrolyte imbalances, or nutritional deficiencies, primarily in settings in which intravenous fluids are not available. Seizures are usually caused by anoxia but may be caused by hyponatremia secondary to inappropriate antidiuretic hormone secretion, although tetanic seizures may be caused by electrolyte imbalances. Finally, anoxia may be severe enough to lead to coma.

Treatment

Treatment of pertussis is primarily supportive, involving hydration, pulmonary toilet, and oxygen. The decision to hospitalize the patient depends on the patient's age and general condition. Essentially all children less than 3 months of age are admitted to the hospital, as are children between the ages of 3 and 6 months, unless witnessed paroxysms are not severe. Nearly all children who require ventilation are less than 3 months of age. Older children may be admitted if they experience complications of the disease or if their families are unable to provide care at home. Infants born prematurely

and those with underlying cardiac, pulmonary, or neuromuscular disorders are also at higher risk for complications. The patient should be placed in respiratory isolation until antibiotics have been given for at least 5 days. Erythromycin given for 14 days will eliminate the bacteria from the respiratory tract within 3–4 days. Clarithromycin and azithromycin may be equally effective, if more expensive. Trimethoprim-sulfamethoxazole for 14 days may be as effective as erythromycin in clearing the organism from the nasopharynx, but whether it is as effective clinically is unknown. Antibiotics given within 14 days of the onset of the disease may abort or shorten the course of the disease, but the diagnosis of pertussis is rarely made in this stage of the illness. Once the paroxysmal stage begins, erythromycin will not affect the course of the disease, although it will shorten the period of infectivity and reduce communicability. Other appropriate antibiotics should be given if pneumonia or another secondary bacterial infection is suspected. Bronchodilators and steroids are probably of no benefit, and cough suppressants are likewise not helpful.

During a pertussis epidemic, newborns should receive their first immunization at 4 weeks of age, with repeat doses given at 6, 10, and 14 weeks of age. Partially immunized children less than 7 years of age should complete the immunization series at the minimum intervals, and completely immunized children under the age of 7 years should receive one booster dose, unless they have received one in the preceding 3 years. Children over the age of 7 years do not need further immunizations. Children who have had documented pertussis at any age are exempt from further pertussis immunizations. All contacts of patients with pertussis should be given erythromycin for 14 days after the date of their last contact with the patient. Continuous contacts of the patient, eg, parents, should be given erythromycin until the patient's cough has stopped, or until the patient has received 7 days of erythromycin.

Prognosis

The prognosis of pertussis depends primarily on the age of the patient. Mortality is rare in adults and children. With proper supportive care, the mortality rate for children under 2 years of age, the group at highest risk, is approximately 1%. Most mortality is due to pneumonia and cerebral anoxia. The incidence of long-term pulmonary sequelae is not known, but it appears that infants less than 6 months of age who are hospitalized with severe disease may have minor pulmonary function abnormalities and lower respiratory tract abnormalities, including wheezing, that persist into adulthood.

PNEUMONIA

 ESSENTIALS OF DIAGNOSIS

- *Fever.*
- *Acute respiratory symptoms.*
- *Radiographic evidence of parenchymal infiltrates.*

General Considerations

Pneumonia occurs more often in young children than in any other age group, with an incidence of 34–40 cases per 1000 in children under 5 years of age. Many definitions of pneumonia have been proposed, based on several different criteria. The criteria that will be used here are the presence of fever, respiratory findings, and evidence of parenchymal infiltrates on chest radiography. Although accurate diagnosis of an infection as potentially serious as pneumonia is obviously desirable, there are significant obstacles to diagnostic certainty.

Pathogenesis

Viruses are a leading cause of pneumonia in children of all ages. Bacterial infections are more common in developing countries and in children with complicated infections.

Age is an important consideration in determining the potential etiology of pneumonia. Neonates less than 20 days of age are most likely to have infections with pathogens that cause other neonatal infection syndromes, including group B streptococci, gram-negative enteric bacteria, cytomegalovirus, and *Listeria monocytogenes.*

Children between the ages of 3 weeks and 3 months may have infections caused by *Chlamydia trachomatis,* normally acquired from exposure at the time of birth to infection in the mother's genital tract. RSV pneumonia peaks at 2–7 months of age and is difficult to distinguish from bronchiolitis. *S pneumoniae* is probably the most common cause of bacterial pneumonia in this age group. *B pertussis* usually causes bronchitis but may in severe cases cause pneumonia. Finally, *S aureus* is an uncommon cause of pneumonia but is associated with severe disease.

Respiratory viruses of many types are the most common cause of pneumonia in children between the ages of 4 months and 4 years. *S pneumoniae* and nontypeable *H influenzae* are common bacterial causes. *M pneumo-*

niae mainly affects older children in this age group. Tuberculosis should be considered in children who live in areas of high tuberculosis prevalence.

M pneumoniae is the most common cause of pneumonia in children from 5 to 15 years of age. *Chlamydia pneumoniae* has long been thought to be an important cause of pneumonia in these children, but its role is open to question, given a high rate of recovery of this organism from asymptomatic children. Pneumococcus is the most likely cause of lobar pneumonia. As in younger children, tuberculosis should be considered in areas of high prevalence.

Prevention

The only significantly effective form of prevention is immunization. With widespread immunization in the United States, pneumonia caused by *H influenzae* type B has become uncommon, and infections caused by *S pneumoniae* are likewise expected to soon become unusual.

Clinical Findings

A. SYMPTOMS AND SIGNS

Perhaps the most confounding problem in the diagnosis of pneumonia is that the symptoms and signs of pneumonia overlap significantly, and indeed are often identical to those of other cough-producing illnesses, such as those discussed previously. Young infants are particularly likely to have nonspecific signs and symptoms. Assessing the sensitivity and specificity of signs is complicated by the lack of a true gold standard for diagnosis. Tachypnea is an important finding. This is defined by a respiratory rate greater than 60/min in infants younger than 2 months, greater than 50/min in infants 2–12 months, and greater than 40/min in children older than 12 months of age. Evidence of increased work of breathing, such as subcostal or intercostal retractions, nasal flaring, and grunting, may indicate more severe disease. Auscultatory findings are variable and include decreased breath sounds, wheezes, rhonchi, and crackles. The absence of these various pulmonary findings is helpful in predicting that a child will not have pneumonia, but the presence of these is only moderately predictive of the presence of pneumonia.

B. LABORATORY FINDINGS

Laboratory findings are generally not helpful in the diagnosis of pneumonia. A WBC count of greater than 17,000/mm^3 indicates a higher likelihood of bacteremia, although blood cultures are rarely positive except in complicated infections, and oxygen desaturation indicates more severe disease. Sputum culture is the most accurate way to ascertain the cause of the infection, although the presence of bacteria in a culture does not exclude the possibility of a viral infection with bacterial colonization. Obtaining microbiological evidence is problematic, however, since children are very often unable to produce adequate sputum samples for culture.

C. IMAGING STUDIES

A positive chest radiograph is generally considered to be diagnostic evidence of pneumonia. In children, however, radiographic patterns of respiratory infections are highly variable and may not be helpful in differentiating pneumonia from bronchiolitis, or bacterial disease from infection with viruses or atypical organisms. In infants especially, bacterial pneumonia may produce infiltrates that range from lobar consolidation to interstitial infiltrates.

Differential Diagnosis

The differential diagnosis of pneumonia includes all the previously discussed illnesses in which dyspnea and cough are prominent features of the disease.

Treatment

The appropriate treatment of childhood pneumonia depends on the age of the child and on the physician's clinical judgment as to how sick the child is. Neonates should all be treated as inpatients. Infants 3 weeks to 3 months of age may be treated as outpatients if they are not febrile or hypoxemic, do not appear toxic, and do not have an alveolar infiltrate or a large pleural effusion. Older infants and children may be treated as outpatients if they do not appear seriously ill.

The choice of antibiotics depends on the age of the child and the most likely cause of infection. Neonates should be treated with ampicillin and gentamicin, with or without cefotaxime, as appropriate for a neonatal sepsis syndrome. Macrolides are appropriate first choices for children 3 weeks to 3 months and 5–15 years of age. All macrolides are equally effective. The oral dose for erythromycin is 30–40 mg/kg/day, divided four times a day for 10 days, and for azithromycin is 10 mg/kg the first day, then 5 mg/kg once a day for 4 days. In children older than 5 years, clarithromycin (15 mg/kg/day, divided twice a day for 10 days) may be used, and doxycycline (4 mg/kg/day, divided twice a day for 10 days) may be used in children older than 8 years. Children who are ill enough to require inpatient treatment should be treated with erythromycin, either orally or intravenously (40 mg/kg/day divided every 6 h) plus either cefotaxime (200 mg/kg/day divided every 8 h) or cefuroxime (150 mg/kg/day divided every 8 h).

In children between 4 months and 4 years of age, treatment may be withheld if a viral infection is considered to be the most likely cause. Otherwise, high-dose amoxicillin (80–100 mg/kg/day in three or four divided doses for 10 days) is the appropriate first-line treatment. For children sick enough to require hospitalization, intravenous ampicillin (200 mg/kg/day divided every 6 h) is appropriate. For children who appear septic or who have alveolar infiltrates or large pleural effusions, cefotaxime or cefuroxime should be used.

An important caveat in choosing an antibiotic is the consideration of the likelihood that the child has an infection with *S pneumoniae*. If this is thought to be likely, knowledge of local antibiotic resistance patterns is important. A growing rise in macrolide resistance is paralleling the rise in penicillin resistance in some parts of the United States, with important implications for antibiotic selection.

Prognosis

Worldwide, pneumonia is an important cause of death in children. In developed countries, however, the death rate for childhood pneumonia has dropped dramatically with the development of antibiotics. In 1939, the death rate from pneumonia was approximately 75 per 100,000 children. In 1996 there were 800 deaths from childhood pneumonia, or roughly 2 per 100,000 children.

American Academy of Pediatrics, Committee on Infectious Diseases and Committee on Fetus and Newborn: Prevention of respiratory syncytial virus infections: indications for the use of palivizumab and update on the use of RSV-IGIV. Pediatrics 1998;102:1211. (Position statement from the American Academy of Pediatrics.)

Baugh R, Gilmore BB: Infectious croup: a critical review. Otolaryngol Head Neck Surg 1986;95:40. (Nearly all the important literature on croup is old. This is a good review of the disease.)

Centers for Disease Control and Prevention: Summary of notifiable diseases, United States—1999. MMRW 2001;48:1.

Dowell S et al: Mortality from pneumonia in children in the United States, 1939 through 1996. New Engl J Med 2000; 342:1399. (Brief discussion of declining mortality from childhood pneumonia in the United States.)

Hueston W et al: Does acute bronchitis really exist? A reconceptualization of acute viral respiratory infections. J Fam Pract 2000;49(5):401. (Discussion of the evidence about bronchitis.)

IMpact-RSV Study Group: Palivizumab, a humanized respiratory syncytial virus monoclonal antibody, reduces hospitalization from respiratory syncytial virus infection in high-risk infants. Pediatrics 1998;102:531. (Good study of the utility of this drug.)

Johnson DW et al: A comparison of nebulized budesonide, intramuscular dexamethasone, and placebo for moderately severe croup. New Engl J Med 1998;339(8):498. (A good review.)

Klassen TP et al: Nebulized budesonide and oral dexamethasone for treatment of croup: a randomized controlled trial. JAMA 1998;279(20):1629. (A good review.)

Lee SS, Schwartz RH, Bahadori RS: Retropharyngeal abscess: epiglottitis of the new millennium. J Pediatr 2001;138(3): 435. (Good review of this illness.)

Margolis P, Gadomski A: Does this infant have pneumonia? JAMA 1998;279:308. (Brief discussion of the predictive values of symptoms and the variability of radiological findings in children with pneumonia.)

Marx A et al: Pediatric hospitalizations for croup (laryngotracheo-bronchitis): biennial increases associated with human parainfluenzavirus 1 epidemics. J Infect Dis 1997;176(6):1423. (Discussion of periodicity of infection rates in croup.)

McIntosh K: Current concepts: community-acquired pneumonia in children. New Engl J Med 2002;346:429. (Helpful summary of etiology and recommendations for treatment.)

Srugo I et al: Pertussis infection in fully-vaccinated children in day-care centers, Israel. Emerg Infect Dis 2000;6:526. (Discussion of the limitations of pertussis immunization.)

■ OTHER VIRAL INFECTIONS

INFECTIOUS MONONUCLEOSIS

ESSENTIALS OF DIAGNOSIS

- *Fever.*
- *Pharyngitis.*
- *Generalized lymphadenopathy.*

General Considerations

Infectious mononucleosis is a clinical syndrome usually caused by Epstein–Barr virus (EBV). It is ordinarily a benign illness, but there are a number of important, if unusual complications.

Pathogenesis

Although EBV is by far the most common cause of mononucleosis, 5–10% of mononucleosis-like illnesses are caused by cytomegalovirus, *Toxoplasma gondii,* or a variety of other viruses. EBV infects 95% of the world's population. It is transmitted in oral secretions by kissing and saliva to saliva transmission, as is common in children. The virus is shed for up to 6 months after the acute infection and then intermittently for the life of the person. Most infants and young children have inapparent infections or infections indistinguishable from other childhood respiratory infections. In developed countries, about one-third of infections occur in adolescence or early adulthood, and of these about 50% develop clinically apparent disease.

The infection first begins in the cells of the oral cavity, and then spreads to adjacent salivary glands and lymphoid tissue. Eventually the virus infects the entire reticuloendothelial system, including the liver and spleen.

Prevention

As the virus is ubiquitous and is shed intermittently by nearly every adult, there is no effective prevention for this illness.

Clinical Findings

A. SYMPTOMS AND SIGNS

In adolescents, the incubation period is 30–50 days, but it may be shorter in younger children. There is often a 1–2 week prodromal period of nonspecific respiratory symptoms, including fever and sore throat. Typical symptoms include fever, sore throat, myalgia, headache, nausea, and abdominal pain.

Physical findings include pharyngitis, often with exudative tonsillitis and palatal petechiae similar to streptococcal pharyngitis. Lymphadenopathy is seen in 90% of cases, most often in the anterior and posterior cervical chains and less often in the axillary and inguinal chains. Epitrochlear adenopathy is a highly suggestive finding. Splenomegaly is found in about 50% of cases and hepatomegaly in 10–25%. Symptomatic hepatitis, with or without jaundice, may occur but is unusual. Various rashes, most often maculopapular, are seen in less than 50% of patients, but nearly all patients will develop a rash if they are given ampicillin or amoxicillin.

B. LABORATORY FINDINGS

At the onset of the illness, the WBC count is usually elevated to 12,000–25,000/mm^3. Of these 50–70% will be lymphocytes and 20–40% will be atypical lymphocytes. Of patients 50–80% will have elevated hepatic transaminases, but jaundice occurs in only about 5%.

The most commonly done diagnostic test is the Monospot test. The diagnosis may be confused by the fact that this test is often negative during the first week of symptoms. This test should be used only in adolescents, as it has a sensitivity of less than 50% in children under the age of 14.

C. Imaging Studies

No imaging studies are routinely useful in this illness. Ultrasound will show splenomegaly more accurately than physical examination, but this is usually done only to assess the risk of splenic rupture in patients who are active in sports.

Differential Diagnosis

Streptococcal pharyngitis is the primary illness in the differential diagnosis. This may coexist with mononucleosis, or the child with mononucleosis may be a carrier of *Streptococcus,* so a positive throat culture does not definitively rule out mononucleosis. Likewise, a negative Monospot test in the first several days of the illness does not rule out mononucleosis. Lymphadenopathy associated with mononucleosis is usually more generalized than that associated with streptococcal infections.

Complications

Mononucleosis is normally a benign illness. The most serious complication is spontaneous splenic rupture. This occurs in less than 0.5% of patients, usually during the second week of the illness. The risk of splenic rupture with trauma is elevated, and all patients with this illness should avoid contact sports for 1 month. Those with documented splenomegaly should not return to sports until resolution has been confirmed by ultrasound.

Other complications are unusual and include rare cases of airway obstruction (<5%), symptomatic hepatitis (rare), and a variety of neurological complications (1–5%), including meningitis, encephalitis, and cranial, autonomic, or peripheral neuritides. Hemolytic anemia may occur in about 3% of cases. Aplastic anemia is rare. Mild neutropenia is common early in the disease, but severe neutropenia is rare. Likewise, mild thrombocytopenia is common, but severe thrombocytopenia is rare.

Treatment

Treatment is generally symptomatic. Steroids speed recovery, but because most patients recover uneventfully, these should be used only for severe or complicated cases. Accepted indications for the use of steroids include impending airway obstruction, severe hemolytic anemia, severe thrombocytopenia, and persistent severe disease. Evidence does not support the use of acyclovir for this illness.

Prognosis

Symptoms typically last 2–4 weeks. Relapses may occur for 6 months to 1 year.

Papesch M, Watkins R: Epstein-Barr virus infectious mononucleosis. Clin Otolaryngol 2001;26:3. (Recent review of the illness and of the evidence for treatment.)

Torre D, Tambini R: Acyclovir for treatment of infectious mononucleosis: a meta-analysis. Scand J Infect Dis 1999;31: 543. (European meta-analysis of the use of acyclovir.)

■ GASTROENTERITIS

 ESSENTIALS OF DIAGNOSIS

- *Diarrhea.*
- *Vomiting may be present or absent.*

General Considerations

Diarrheal diseases are one of the most common illnesses and perhaps the leading cause of death among children worldwide. It is estimated that there are 1 billion illnesses and 3–5 million deaths from these illnesses each year. In the United States, there are an estimated 20–35 million cases of diarrhea annually, with 2–4 million visits to physicians and over 200,000 hospitalizations but only 400–500 deaths. Gastroenteritis may be caused by any of a large number of viruses, bacteria, or parasites. Most infections are caused by ingestion of contaminated food or water.

Pathogenesis

Four families of viruses can cause gastroenteritis. All are spread easily through fecal–oral contact, and many are associated with localized outbreaks in hospitals, day care centers, and schools. Rotavirus is a common cause of gastroenteritis during winter months. It primarily affects children between 3 months and 2 years of age, and by age 4 or 5, nearly all children have serological evidence of infection. Norwalk virus is the most common cause of gastroenteritis among older children. Astroviruses and enteric adenoviruses are the other common causes of disease among children. These last three types cause year-round, often localized outbreaks of disease.

Bacteria may cause either inflammatory or noninflammatory diarrhea. Common causes of inflammatory diarrhea are *Campylobacter jejuni,* enteroinvasive or enterohemorrhagic *E coli, Salmonella* spp., *Shigella* spp., and *Yersinia enterocolitica.* Noninflammatory diarrhea may be caused by enteropathogenic or enterotoxigenic *E coli* or by *Vibrio cholerae.*

The most common parasitic cause of diarrhea in the United States is *Giardia lamblia.* Numerous other parasites, including protozoa and various types of roundworms and flatworms, may cause diarrhea. Most parasitic infections cause chronic diarrhea and are beyond the scope of this chapter.

Prevention

The most effective prevention measure is for children to have access to uncontaminated food and water. Careful hand washing and good sanitation practices also help prevent the spread of infection among children. An increased rate of breast-feeding has been shown to decrease the incidence of gastroenteritis among all children in small communities. A recent vaccine against rotavirus was withdrawn from the market shortly after its introduction after it was shown to be associated with an increased rate of intussusception.

Clinical Findings

A. Symptoms and Signs

The cardinal sign of gastroenteritis is diarrhea, with or without vomiting. Systemic symptoms and signs may include fever and malaise. Fever and severe abdominal pain are more common with inflammatory diarrhea. The degree of dehydration is important to establish before beginning treatment.

In most children with viral gastroenteritis, fever and vomiting last less than 2–3 days, although diarrhea may persist up to 5–7 days. Most cases of diarrhea caused by food-borne toxins last 1–2 days. Many, but not all bacterial infections last for longer periods of time.

B. Laboratory Findings

Most children with gastroenteritis from any cause have a short-lived illness, and the cause of the infection is rarely ascertained. Stool cultures for bacteria and examination for parasites should be done if the stool is positive for blood or leukocytes, if diarrhea persists for more than 1 week, or if the patient is immunocompromised. The presence of fecal leukocytes indicates an inflammatory infection, although not all such infections will produce a positive test. Blood indicates a hemorrhagic or inflammatory infection. In a child who appears significantly dehydrated, serum electrolytes should be tested, especially if the child is hospitalized for fluid therapy.

Complications

Diarrheal diseases are for the most part benign, self-limited infections. Mortality is primarily caused by dehydration, shock, and circulatory collapse. Bacterial pathogens may spread to remote sites and cause meningitis, pneumonia, and other infections. *E coli* 0157:H7 may cause hemolytic-uremic syndrome.

Treatment

The keys to treatment of gastroenteritis are rehydration, or avoidance of dehydration, and early refeeding. Children who are severely ($\geq 10\%$) dehydrated or who appear toxic or seriously ill should be admitted to the hospital for rehydration and treatment. Otherwise, children may be managed at home. Vomiting is the chief obstacle to rehydration or maintenance of hydration. Children who are vomiting should be given frequent (every 1–2 min) very small amounts (5 mL) of rehydration solution to avoid provoking further attacks of emesis. The idea that the gastrointestinal tract should be rested for a time by avoiding oral intake has been disproven.

Children who have diarrhea but who are not dehydrated should continue on whatever age-appropriate foods they were taking before the illness. In those who are dehydrated but not severely so, oral rehydration has been shown to be the preferred method. Juices, water flavored with drink mix, and sports drinks do not have the recommended concentrations of carbohydrates and electrolytes and should be avoided. The WHO or UNICEF rehydration solution is the preferred therapy. Recently, a reduced-osmolarity solution has been developed, that appears to be superior to older solutions. This solution is available commercially and contains the following concentrations (mmol/L): Na^+ 75, Cl^- 60, glucose 75, K^+ 20, citrate 10, with a total osmolarity of 245 mmol/L. Children who are mildly (3–5%) dehydrated should be given 50 mL/kg of solution, plus replacement of ongoing losses from stool or emesis, over each 4-h period. Children who are moderately (6–9%) dehydrated should be given 100 mL/kg, plus losses, over each 4-h period. Refeeding with age-appropriate foods should begin as soon as the child is interested in eating. The classic BRAT (bananas, rice cereal, applesauce, toast) diet is lacking in calories, protein, and fat and is no longer recommended.

Therapy with various antidiarrheal medications, including loperamide, anticholinergics, and bismuth subsalicylate has been shown to have minimal effect on the volume of diarrhea. Additionally, these drugs have an unacceptably high rate of side effects, and their use is not recommended. Antiemetic drugs, likewise, have limited effectiveness and high rates of toxicities.

Even when diagnosed, many bacterial infections do not require treatment. All *Campylobacter* (erythromycin) and *Shigella* [trimethoprim-sulfamethoxazole (TMP-SMX) or cephalosporin] infections should be treated. Infections with *Salmonella* should not be treated with antibiotics unless the child is less than 3 months of age or has evidence of bacteremia or disseminated infection. Ampicillin, chloramphenicol, TMP-SMX, and cefotaxime are appropriate choices. All *E coli* 0157:H7 infections should be treated (TMP-SMX), but other *E coli* infections should be treated only if they are severe or prolonged. *Giardia* infections should be treated with metronidazole or quinacrine.

Prognosis

With proper rehydration and refeeding, morbidity and mortality from viral gastroenteritis are minimal. Morbidity and mortality from bacterial infections are dependent on the virulence of the organism and complications from distant spread or remote effects, such as hemolytic-uremic syndrome.

Nazarian L et al: Practice guideline: the management of acute gastroenteritis in young children. Pediatrics 1996;97:424. (Well-researched, evidence-based practice guidelines from the American Academy of Pediatrics.)

Santosham M et al: A double-blind clinical trial comparing World Health Organization oral rehydration solution with a reduced osmolarity solution containing equal amounts of sodium and glucose. J Pediatr 1996;128:45. (Comparison of older and newer formulations of rehydration solutions.)

■ URINARY TRACT INFECTIONS

ESSENTIALS OF DIAGNOSIS

- *Common bacterial cause of febrile illness in young children.*
- *Symptoms often lacking or nonspecific in young children.*
- *Urinalysis not always reliable, need culture for accurate diagnosis.*

General Considerations

Urinary tract infections (UTI) are the most common serious bacterial infection in young children. The age group defined by the term "young children" varies from less than 2 years to less than 5 years, although most research that is done uses the criterion of less than 2 years. Among febrile young children, between 3% and 5% will have a UTI, and among infants less than 8 weeks of age, these account for approximately 7.5% of febrile illnesses. A UTI may be a marker for urinary tract anomalies in young children. It is generally believed that UTIs may lead to renal scarring, which may cause hypertension and renal insufficiency later in life.

Pathogenesis

In the first 8–12 weeks of life, some UTIs may be caused by hematogenous spread of bacteria from a remote source. Otherwise, the infections are caused by bacteria ascending the urethra into the bladder. From the bladder, bacteria may ascend the ureters to cause pyelonephritis.

The most common pathogens responsible for UTIs are enteric bacteria. *E coli* is found in 70–90% of infections. *P aeruginosa* is the most common nonenteric gram-negative pathogen, and *Enterococcus* spp. are the most common gram-postitive organisms seen. Group B *Streptococcus* is occasionally found in neonates. *S aureus* is rarely seen in children without indwelling catheters and suggests seeding from a distant focus, such as renal abscess, osteomyelitis, or endocarditis. Adenovirus is the only viral urinary tract pathogen.

The most important factors in the prevalence of UTIs are the patient's age and gender. In newborns, preterm infants are several times more likely to have a UTI than full-term infants. Up to 3 months of age, boys are more likely to be infected than girls, after which infections in girls predominate for the rest of childhood. The usual age at which children experience a first symptomatic infection is 1–5 years. In this age group girls are 10–20 times more likely to have a UTI than boys.

Prevention

Prevention of long-term sequelae of UTIs focuses on prevention of recurrent infection. This, in turn, involves correction, if possible, of associated urinary tract abnormalities. Widespread use of prenatal ultrasonography has led to the identification of a number of infants with intrauterine hydronephrosis. In many boys with vesicoureteral reflux (VUR), renal scarring is thought to be congenital, whereas in girls it is more highly associated with recurrent infection. The degree of VUR is important in determining appropriate treatment. Mild VUR generally improves over time as the bladder enlarges and the length of the submucosal tunnel through which the ureter passes increases. More severe degrees of reflux are unlikely to improve and more often require surgical correction. Posterior urethral valves and ureterovesical obstruction also require surgical intervention.

In children with structurally normal urinary tracts, treatment of chronic constipation has been shown to decrease the recurrence of UTI, as has behavioral correction of voiding dysfunction associated with incomplete emptying of the bladder. Improving hygiene, especially in girls, has not been shown to decrease rates of UTI. Based on retrospective studies, circumcision of boys may be associated with decreased rates of UTI, but there are no randomized controlled trials investigating this idea.

For some children with recurrent UTIs, long-term prophylactic antibiotic treatment may be effective in reducing the frequency of infections. However, there are no clear guidelines as to when this treatment should be considered.

Clinical Findings

A. SYMPTOMS AND SIGNS

Among children less than 2 years of age, symptoms are often lacking or nonspecific. Parents may become suspicious if the child appears to be in pain while urinating, but otherwise fever may be the only presenting complaint. Among children who have developed language skills, typical UTI symptoms, such as dysuria, urgency, and urinary frequency, may be seen. Fever is the only reliable clinical sign distinguishing upper tract infection (pyelonephritis) from lower tract infection (cystitis).

B. LABORATORY FINDINGS

To be reliable, urine for analysis must be collected by catheterization or by suprapubic aspiration. Urine collected in an adhesive collection bag is too often contaminated by skin flora to be useful.

Positive findings on urinalysis are positive dipstick tests for leukocyte esterase or nitrite or the microscopic finding of pyuria ($\geq$5 WBC/high-power field). However, urinalysis in young children is not sensitive enough to stand alone as a diagnostic test, and urine culture is needed for accurate diagnosis. The bacterial colony count that defines a UTI varies by collection method and by gender. In a specimen collected by suprapubic aspiration, the finding of any gram-negative organisms or of more than 10^3 gram-positive organisms indicates a 99% probability of UTI. In catheter-obtained specimens, more than 10^5 bacteria indicates a 95% probability of UTI and 10^4–10^5 is considered suspicious. The numbers are similar for clean-voided urines, although in boys, more than 10^4 bacteria indicates a probable UTI.

Blood cultures should be done as part of the workup of a young infant with fever without an apparent source.

Blood cultures are unlikely to be positive in children over the age of 2 months. Even when blood cultures are positive, they will show the same organism as the urine culture, and they contribute little if anything to the diagnosis.

C. IMAGING STUDIES

Renal cortical nuclide scanning with technetium-99m dimercaptosuccinic acid (DMSA) can show evidence of acute pyelonephritis, as well as areas of decreased uptake that suggest old cortical scars. However, this test is not universally available, and despite a substantial false-negative rate, many physicians rely on the presence of fever to distinguish pyelonephritis from cystitis.

More important than imaging renal cortical scanning is diagnosing the presence of VUR and other urinary tract anomalies that are associated with a high rate of recurrent infections. Shortly after finishing treatment for a first UTI, children should have a voiding cystourethrogram (VCUG), either with x-ray contrast dye or with a radionuclide tracer. Renal ultrasonography will show other structural abnormalities and may be considered in addition to the VCUG. VUR will be found in 30–50% of children after a first UTI, and other anomalies, such as posterior urethral valves (in boys) or duplication of the collecting system, will be found in a small number of children.

Although all boys with a first UTI should receive a full diagnostic workup, as girls grow from toddlers to school age, the likelihood of significant findings decreases. There is no clear guidance from the literature as to the age after which a girl with a first UTI should be subjected to an expensive, uncomfortable, and potentially traumatic investigation.

Differential Diagnosis

As discussed in the section on fever without source, a UTI should be considered in any child who presents with a febrile illness in whom the cause of the fever cannot be readily ascertained by physical examination.

Complications

Acute complications of UTI include sepsis, renal abscess, and disseminated infection, including meningitis. Recurrent pyelonephritis can cause renal scarring, which can lead to hypertension or renal insufficiency later in life.

Treatment

Infants under the age of 2 months with a UTI should be hospitalized and treated with intravenous antibiotics as indicated for sepsis until cultures identify the causative organism and the best antibiotic for treatment. Infants 2 months to 2 years of age may be treated as outpatients with oral antibiotics unless they appear toxic, are dehydrated, or are unable to retain oral intake, in which case hospitalization and intravenous antibiotics are necessary. Older children can usually be treated as outpatients, unless they appear seriously ill. The initial choice of antibiotic may be a sulfonamide, TMP-SMX, or a cephalosporin. Resistance of *E coli* to ampicillin is widespread enough in the United States to make ampicillin and amoxicillin poor choices for initial therapy. Nitrofurantoin, which is excreted in the urine but does not reach therapeutic blood levels, should not be used to treat febrile children with UTI. In general, the duration of treatment should be 7–10 days. Some authorities recommend 14 days of treatment, but there are no data comparing 10 days to 14 days of treatment.

If the child responds clinically to treatment within 2 days, no further immediate follow-up is needed, such as reculture of the urine or immediate imaging studies. If the child is not improving after 2 days of treatment, the urine should be recultured and renal ultrasonography should be performed immediately.

Once treatment of a first infection has been completed, the child should be continued on either full or prophylactic doses of antibiotics until imaging studies have been completed. Appropriate prophylactic antibiotics include TMP-SMX (2 mg TMP, 10 mg SMX once daily), sulfisoxazole (10–20 mg/kg, divided every 12 h), and nitrofurantoin (1–2 mg/kg, once daily).

Bachur R, Harper M: Reliability of the urinalysis for predicting urinary tract infections in young febrile children. Arch Pediatr Adolesc Med 2001;155:60. (Study of sensitivity of urinalysis compared to urine culture for diagnosis of UTI.)

Pitetti R, Choi S: Utility of blood cultures in febrile children with UTI. Am J Emerg Med 2002;20:271. (Short, well-done paper addressing this one question.)

Roberts K et al: Practice guideline: the diagnosis, treatment, and evaluation of the initial urinary tract infection in febrile infants and young children. Pediatrics 1999;103:843. (Evidence-based practice guidelines from the American Academy of Pediatrics.)

Schlager T: Urinary tract infections in children younger than 5 years of age: epidemiology, diagnosis, treatment, outcomes, and prevention. Pediatr Drugs 2001;3:219. (Complete but concise review of the disease.)

Skin Diseases in Infants & Children

6

Mark A. Knox, MD

■ INFECTIONS OF THE SKIN

IMPETIGO

ESSENTIALS OF DIAGNOSIS

- *Nonbullous: yellowish crusted plaques.*
- *Bullous: bullae, little surrounding erythema, rupture to leave shallow ulcer.*

General Considerations

Impetigo is a bacterial infection of the skin with two main types—nonbullous and bullous. More than 70% of cases are of the nonbullous variety.

Pathogenesis

Most cases of nonbullous impetigo are caused by *Staphylococcus aureus.* Group A β-hemolytic streptococci are found in some cases, most often in children of preschool age but older than 2 years. Coagulase-positive *S aureus* is the cause of bullous impetigo. Impetigo can develop in traumatized skin, or the bacteria can spread to intact skin from its reservoir in the nose.

Clinical Findings

A. SYMPTOMS AND SIGNS

Nonbullous impetigo can develop in areas where the skin integrity has been compromised, or it can develop in areas of intact skin. Typical lesions preceding impetigo include chicken pox, burns, insect bites, abrasions, and lacerations. Occasionally it will develop secondarily in infected lesions caused by fungi, viruses, or parasites such as scabies or lice. Treating the underlying infection, if

possible, is necessary for successful treatment of the impetigo. Usually, a small vesicle or pustule develops initially, followed by the classic small (less than 2 cm) honey-colored crusted plaque. The infection may be spread to other parts of the body by fingers or clothing. There is usually little surrounding erythema, itching occurs occasionally, and pain is usually absent. Regionally lymphadenopathy is seen in most cases. Without treatment, the lesions resolve without scarring in 2 weeks.

Bullous impetigo is usually seen in infants and young children. Lesions begin on intact skin on almost any part of the body. Flaccid, thin-roofed vesicles develop, which rupture to form shallow ulcers. Bullous impetigo is a localized manifestation of staphylococcal scalded skin syndrome.

B. LABORATORY FINDINGS

Laboratory investigation is rarely done in these conditions. Culture of the fluid from bullae will yield the infecting organism. In nonbullous impetigo, lifting the edge of a crusted lesion and swabbing beneath it will likewise yield the organism, but this is not normally done unless there has been no response to 7 days of antibiotic therapy.

Differential Diagnosis

Nonbullous impetigo is unique in appearance. Bullous impetigo is similar in appearance to pemphigus and bullous pemphigoid. Growth of staphylococci from fluid in a bulla confirms the diagnosis.

Complications

Cellulitis follows about 10% of cases of nonbullous impetigo but rarely follows bullous impetigo. Either type may rarely lead to septicemia, septic arthritis, or osteomyelitis. Lymphadenitis, scarlet fever, and poststreptococcal glomerulonephritis may follow streptococcal impetigo.

66

Treatment

Localized disease may be treated with mupirocin 2% ointment, applied three times a day for 5–7 days. Patients with widespread lesions or evidence of cellulitis should be treated with systemic antibiotics effective against staphylococci and streptococci. Erythromycin, dicloxacillin, and cephalexin are appropriate choices. Newer macrolides such as azithromycin and clarithromycin are equally effective, but not more effective than erythromycin. They are somewhat better tolerated but much more expensive. Seven days of treatment is adequate.

Prognosis

Except for rare complications caused by disseminated infection, impetigo is a benign, self-limited infection. Treatment with antibiotics may reduce the risk of some complications.

FUNGAL INFECTIONS

General Considerations

Fungal infections of the skin and skin structures may be caused by a variety of organisms. Fungal infections are often generically called "tinea" infections. These may be generally grouped into three categories—dermatophyte infections, other tinea infections, and candidal infections.

Pathogenesis

Dermatophytoses are caused by a group of related fungal species that requires keratin for growth and can invade hair, nails, and the stratum corneum of the skin. This group, which includes *Microsporum, Trichophyton,* and *Epidermophyton* species, causes most fungal skin infections. Some of these organisms are spread from person to person, some from animals to people, and some infect people from the soil. Other fungi can also cause skin disease, such as *Malassazia furfur* in tinea versicolor. Finally, *Candida albicans,* a common resident of the gastrointestinal tract, can cause diaper dermatitis and thrush.

Clinical Findings

A. SYMPTOMS AND SIGNS

1. Dermatophytoses—

a. Tinea corporis—Infection of the skin produces one or more characteristic gradually spreading lesions with erythematous raised borders and central areas that are generally scaly but relatively clearer and less indurated than the margins of the lesions. The central clearing helps to differentiate these lesions from those of psoriasis. Small lesions may resemble those of nummular eczema. The lesions may have a somewhat serpiginous border, but they are usually more or less round in shape, hence the common name of "ringworm." They can range in size from one to several centimeters.

b. Tinea capitis—Fungal infection of the scalp and hair is the most common dermatophytosis in children. This presents as areas of alopecia with more or less regular borders. Typically, the hair shafts break off a few millimeters from the skin surface, distinguishing this from alopecia areata. The infection may also produce a sterile inflammatory mass in the scalp, called a "kerion," which may be confused with a bacterial infection.

2. Nondermatophyte infections—

a. Tinea versicolor—Tinea versicolor is normally seen in adolescents and adults. The causative organism, *M furfur,* is part of the normal skin flora. The infection most often becomes evident during warm weather, when new lesions develop. A warm, humid environment, excessive sweating, and genetic susceptibility are important factors for developing this infection. Because treatment does not eradicate the fungus from the skin, it often recurs annually, during the summer months, in susceptible individuals. The lesions are characteristically scaly macules, usually reddish brown in whites but often hyper- or hypopigmented in people of color. They can be found almost anywhere on the body but are most commonly on the torso. Unlike adults, facial lesions are not uncommon in children. The lesions are rarely pruritic. The individual lesions may enlarge and coalesce to form larger lesions with irregular borders.

3. Candidal infections—

a. Thrush—Thrush is a common oral infection in infants. Isolated incidents of this disease are common in immunocompetent infants, but recurrent infections in infants or infections in children and adolescents may indicate an underlying immune deficiency. The infection presents as thick white plaques on the tongue and buccal mucosa. These can be scraped off only with difficulty, distinguishing them from adherent milk or formula, and the base is erythematous.

b. Candidal diaper dermatitis—This infection is most common in infants from 2 to 4 months of age. *Candida* is a common colonist of the gastrointestinal

(GI) tract, and infants with diaper dermatitis should be examined for signs of thrush. The fungus does not ordinarily invade the skin, but the warm, humid environment of the diaper area provides an ideal medium for growth. Often a small area of seborrhea or eczema is the portal of entry for the fungus. The infection is characterized by an intensely erythematous plaque with a sharply demarcated border. Advancing from the border are numerous satellite papules, which enlarge and coalesce to enlarge the affected area.

B. SPECIAL TESTS

Dermatophyte and other tinea infections are usually diagnosed clinically. Examination of potassium hydroxide preparations of scrapings from the affected area, which show hyphae, confirms the diagnosis. Woods lamp (ultraviolet light) examination of lesions is of limited value, since the most common pathogens seen in the United States do not fluoresce. However, some species of *Microsporum* that cause tinea capitis fluoresce blue-green, and lesions of tinea versicolor often fluoresce pale yellow to white. Fungal cultures are slow and expensive but may help in cases in which the diagnosis is suspected but cannot otherwise be confirmed.

Treatment

Tinea corporis is treated with topical antifungal medications. Miconazole 2%, clotrimazole 1%, ketoconazole 1%, and terbinafine 1% creams are all effective. Rarely, widespread infection requires systemic therapy.

Topical therapy is ineffective in tinea capitis. The gold standard for treatment has long been griseofulvin, but because of the 6-week duration of therapy required, other treatments of shorter duration are becoming more popular. Griseofulvin is given as a dose of 20 mg/kg/day for 6 weeks. The other medications are given for 2 weeks. If at the end of 2 more weeks without treatment, signs of infection persist, a third week of treatment can be given. Fluconazole is given as a dose of 6 mg/kg/day, itraconazole as a dose of 5 mg/kg/day, and terbinafine as follows: for weight less than 20 kg, 62.5 mg/day; 20–40 kg, 125 mg/day; and greater than 40 kg, 250 mg/day. There have been rare but serious incidents of hepatotoxicity with ketoconazole, and this drug is not recommended for this infection.

Tinea versicolor can be treated with topical selenium sulfide lotion or any of the topical creams listed above. In older children, systemic treatment can also be given either with ketoconazole or itraconazole 200 mg daily for 5 days, or with ketoconazole or fluconazole 400 mg repeated after 1 week.

Candidal infections are most often treated with nystatin. Diaper dermatitis responds well to topical nystatin cream. If intense inflammation is present, topical steroids for a few days may be helpful. Thrush is usually treated with nystatin suspension, 100,000 units/mL, 1 mL applied over each side of the inside of the mouth, four times a day. Up to 2 weeks may be needed for complete resolution of the infection. In resistant cases, the mouth may be painted with gentian violet.

Prognosis

All these infections in immunocompetent children respond well to treatment. However, left untreated, they can cause widespread and significant skin disease.

Gupta K et al: Therapeutic options for the treatment of tinea capitis caused by *Trichophyton* species: griesofulvin versus the new oral antifungal agents, terbinafine, itraconazole, and fluconazole. Pediatr Dermatol 2001;18:433. (Randomized prospective trial of antifungal agents.)

■ PARASITIC INFESTATIONS

SCABIES

 ESSENTIALS OF DIAGNOSIS

- *Intense pruritis.*
- *Small erythematous papules.*
- *Burrows are pathognomonic but may not be seen.*

Pathogenesis

Scabies is a common infestation caused by the mite *Sarcoptes scabei.* The disease is acquired by physical contact with an infected person. Transmission of the disease by contact with infested linens or clothing is less common, as the mites can live off the body only for 2–3 days. The mite that causes mange in dogs is a variant of the species and can cause disease in humans, as well. The female mite burrows through the skin, between the superficial and deeper layers of the epidermis. She lays eggs and deposits feces as she goes along. After

4–5 weeks, her egg laying is complete, and she dies in the burrow. The eggs hatch, releasing larvae that move to the skin surface, molt into nymphs, mature to adults, mate, and begin the cycle again. Pruritis is caused by an allergic reaction to mite antigens.

Clinical Findings

A. SYMPTOMS AND SIGNS

Diagnosis is based primarily on clinical suspicion, as the physical findings are highly variable. The classic early symptom is intense pruritis. The usual finding is 1- to 2-mm erythematous papules, often in a linear pattern. The finding of burrows connecting the papules is diagnostic but is not always seen. In infants, the disease may involve the entire body, including the face and scalp and the palms and soles, and pustules and vesicles are common. In older children and adolescents, the head, palms, and soles are rarely affected, and the lesions are most often seen in the interdigital spaces, wrist flexors, umbilicus, groin, and genitalia. Severe infestation may produce widespread crusted lesions, and untreated disease may lead to impetigo, cellulitis, and eczema.

B. SPECIAL TESTS

Potassium hydroxide preparations of skin scrapings may show entire mites, eggs, or fecal pellets. However, success in finding these is limited and a negative examination does not rule out the disease.

Differential Diagnosis

The differential diagnosis of scabies is extensive, as the disease can mimic a wide variety of skin conditions.

Treatment

Lindane 1% has historically been the standard treatment. However, concerns about neurotoxicity in infants and carcinogenicity have markedly diminished its use. Permethrin 5% cream, applied to the entire body (excluding the face in older children), is preferred. Recently, good results have been reported from a single oral dose of ivermectin, 150–200 μg/kg, with no adverse reactions. Treatment will kill mites and eliminate the risk of contagion within 24 h. However, the pruritis may continue for several days to 2 weeks after treatment. Treatment with topical steroids, oral hydroxyzine, or diphenhydramine is usually helpful. The entire family should be treated at the same time, and all clothing and bedding should be washed.

Prognosis

This infection responds well to treatment. However, it is difficult to diagnose accurately and, if left untreated, it can lead to widespread and significant skin disease.

LICE (PEDICULOSIS)

 ESSENTIALS OF DIAGNOSIS

- *Pruritis.*
- *Visualization of lice on body or in hair.*

Pathogenesis

Three varieties of lice cause human disease, each with its own fairly well-demarcated territory on the body. *Pediculis humanis corporis* causes infestations on the body and *Pediculis humanis capitis* causes infestation on the head. These have recently been shown to be genetically identical subspecies but with different territorial preferences. *Phthirus pubis,* or crab lice, infests the pubic area. All are spread by physical contact, either with an infested person or with clothing, towels, or hairbrushes that have been in recent contact with an infested person. Symptoms are caused by an allergic reaction to louse antigens that develops after a period of sensitization. Body lice can be a vector for other disease, such as typhus, trench fever, and relapsing fever. Infestation with pubic lice is highly correlated with infection by other sexually transmitted diseases. Nits are the eggs of the louse. They are cemented to hairs, are usually less than 1 mm in length, and are translucent. Body lice lay their nits in the seams of clothing. The nits can remain viable for up to 1 month and will hatch when exposed to body heat when the clothing is worn again.

Prevention

Body lice are associated primarily with poor hygiene and can be prevented by regular bathing and washing of clothing and bedding. There are no specific measures for prevention of infestation by other types of lice.

Clinical Findings

A. SYMPTOMS AND SIGNS

The cardinal symptom of louse infestation is pruritis. This does not occur immediately but develops as the person becomes sensitized. Excoriations in the infested area are common. The lice themselves can usually be seen easily. Body lice are present on the body only when feeding. At other times they live in the seams of clothing. Head and pubic lice are more easily seen.

Treatment

As with scabies, lindane, once the standard treatment, has fallen out of favor. Additionally, lindane resistance is rising, as is resistance to permethrin and other pediculocides. Permethrin cream, applied for 8–12 h, is the treatment of choice for body lice. Clothing and bedding should be washed, as exposure to hot water will kill the nits. Permethrin cream rinse is used to treat head and pubic lice. Thorough combing with a fine-toothed nit comb after treatment for head lice is useful in removing nits and reducing the probability of reinfestation.

Saez-de-Ocariz M, McKinster C, Orozco-Covarrubias L: Treatment of 18 children with scabies of cutaneous larva migrans using ivermectin. Clin Exp Dermatol 2002;27:264. (Report of successful treatment in a small number of children.)

■ INFECTIOUS DISEASES WITH SKIN MANIFESTATIONS

BACTERIAL INFECTIONS

1. Scarlet Fever (Scarlatina)

ESSENTIALS OF DIAGNOSIS

- *Symptoms of streptococcal pharyngitis.*
- *"Sandpaper" rash.*
- *Circumoral pallor.*
- *"Strawberry" tongue (red or white).*

General Considerations

Scarlet fever is an infection caused by strains of group A streptococci that produce one of several toxins, known as erythrotoxins. The infection most commonly begins as a typical streptococcal pharyngitis, with the expected signs and symptoms of that disease. However, it can also follow streptococcal cellulitis or infection of wounds or burns, in which case the pharyngeal signs and symptoms are absent.

Clinical Findings

A. SYMPTOMS AND SIGNS

The classic feature of scarlet fever is the rash, which develops 12–48 h after the onset of pharyngitis symptoms, usually beginning in the neck, axillae, and groin and becoming generalized within 24 h. The rash is a fine faintly erythematous exanthem that is often more easily felt than seen, giving it the name of "sandpaper" rash. Occasionally, petechiae and hyperpigmentation in the deep skin creases may be seen. The rash itself is usually not present on the face, but there is often flushing of the face except for the area around the mouth (circumoral pallor). The tongue is often erythematous and swollen. In the early stages of the disease, the tongue may have swollen papillae protruding through a white coating (white "strawberry" tongue). Later in the illness, the coating desquamates, leaving the red tongue and swollen papillae (red "strawberry" tongue).

After about 1 week, desquamation begins on the face and progresses downward over the body, finally involving the hands and feet. The duration and extent of the desquamation are proportional to the intensity of the initial rash.

Differential Diagnosis

Numerous other diseases must be considered in the differential diagnosis. Some species of *Staphylococcus* produce toxins that cause a similar rash. Kawasaki disease and any of the viral exanthems, such as measles, rubella, roseola, and enteroviruses, may be confused with scarlet fever. These are distinguished by the other features of the viral infections, and by a positive antigen test or culture in patients with scarlet fever.

Complications

Scarlet fever, although dramatic in appearance, is generally a benign disease. In severe cases, bacteremia and sepsis may occur. In these cases, the child will appear seriously ill and will generally be admitted to the hospital for appropriate diagnostic tests and antibiotic treatment. In addition, rheumatic fever and glomerulonephritis may follow an untreated infection.

Treatment

Treatment of scarlet fever is no different from treatment of the primary streptococcal infection, whether it is a pharyngeal or a skin infection.

VIRAL INFECTIONS

1. Roseola (Exanthem Subitum)

ESSENTIALS OF DIAGNOSIS

- *Sudden onset of high fever.*
- *No diagnostic signs.*
- *Development of rash as fever breaks after 3–4 days.*

Pathogenesis

Roseola is an infection caused primarily by human herpesvirus 6 (HHV 6). Although about 90% of children are seropositive for HHV 6 by age 2 years, only about one-third of children will experience clinical disease. HHV 6 causes the vast majority of cases of clinical roseola, although enteroviruses and other viruses cause some cases, as well. It is rare in infants under 3 months and over 2 years of age, with most cases occurring between ages 6 and 12 months. Infections occur year round.

Clinical Findings

A. SYMPTOMS AND SIGNS

The hallmark of roseola is the abrupt onset of high fever, often 103–106°F. Febrile seizures occur in up to one-third of cases. Despite the high fever, children usually look relatively well. Mild signs of upper respiratory infection may be seen, but there are no diagnostic signs. After 3–4 days, the fever breaks suddenly, followed by the appearance of a rash. This is usually a macular or maculopapular rash that starts on the trunk and spreads to the arms and neck and then often to the face and legs. The rash resolves within 3 days, but it may be more transient. Rare cases of fever without rash or rash without fever have been reported.

B. LABORATORY FINDINGS

The white blood cell (WBC) count is usually normal, although there may be a significant lymphocytosis. Laboratory findings are otherwise normal.

Differential Diagnosis

Roseola usually presents in retrospect as a typical clinical picture. However, in the early days of high fever, often with seizures, many children are admitted to the hospital for workup of suspected meningitis or sepsis.

Complications

Rare cases of encephalitis or fulminant hepatitis have been reported.

Treatment

Treatment is entirely symptomatic.

Prognosis

Unless the patient develops one of the rare complications listed above, roseola is a benign, self-limited infection.

2. Varicella (Chickenpox)

ESSENTIALS OF DIAGNOSIS

- *Upper respiratory infection (URI) prodrome.*
- *Rash consists of small vesicles on an erythematous base.*
- *Vesicles rupture with crusting.*

General Considerations

Varicella infection (chickenpox) is a common childhood disease. Approximately 90% of adults in the United States have serological evidence of infection, whether they have had clinically apparent disease or not. Although some important complications have been described, it is ordinarily a benign infection. With the recent implementation of widespread immunization in the United States, it should soon become a rare disease.

Pathogenesis

The varicella-zoster virus (VZV) is a herpes virus. After resolution of the initial infection, the virus produces a latent infection in the dorsal root ganglia. Reactivation produces herpes zoster (shingles), which is unusual in children but common in adults.

Prevention

Childhood immunization should prevent most disease, although general use of the vaccine is too recent a phenomenon to know how complete or how durable the protection conferred by the vaccine will be. The vaccine is given as a single dose between 12 and 18 months of age. Varicella-zoster immune globulin can help prevent infection in immunocompromised children, in nonimmune pregnant women who are exposed to the virus, and in newborns exposed to maternal varicella.

Clinical Findings

A. SYMPTOMS AND SIGNS

The usual incubation period of varicella is about 14 days. Most children will experience a prodromal phase of URI-like symptoms lasting 1–2 days before the onset of the rash. Fever is usually moderate but may be high in some cases. Almost all infected children will develop a rash. The extent of the rash is variable, with as few as 10 lesions or more than 1000. Lesions usually begin on the trunk or head, but eventually can involve the entire body. The classic lesion is a pruritic erythematous macule that develops a clear central vesicle ("a dew drop on a rose petal"). After 1–2 days, the vesicle ruptures, forming a crust. New lesions develop daily for 3–7 days, and typically there are lesions scattered over the body in various states of evolution at the same time. Ulcerative lesions on the buccal mucosa are common. The infection is contagious from the onset of the prodrome until the last of the lesions has crusted over.

Differential Diagnosis

Varicella usually presents as an unmistakable clinical picture, but the rash may be missed in children with mild disease, and the infection may be confused with any nonspecific viral illness.

Complications

In immunocompetent children, the most common complication is bacterial superinfection of the lesions, causing cellulitis or impetigo. Other, more serious complications are most common in children less than 5 years or adults over 20 years of age. Meningoencephalitis and cerebellar ataxia can occur. These normally resolve within 1–3 days without sequelae. Viral hepatitis is common but is normally subclinical. Varicella pneumonia is uncommon in healthy children. This usually resolves after 1–3 days but may progress to respiratory failure in rare cases.

Treatment

Treatment is ordinarily symptomatic, including antipruritic medications if needed. Aspirin should be avoided to prevent development of Reye's syndrome.

Patients with signs of disseminated varicella, such as encephalitis and pneumonia, should be treated with intravenous acyclovir. Oral acyclovir may be effective in reducing the severity and duration of the disease if started within 24 h of the appearance of the rash, but treatment of uncomplicated varicella is not necessary in this otherwise benign disease.

Prognosis

Varicella is normally a benign self-limited disease. Complications in immunocompetent children are rare.

3. Rubeola (Measles)

ESSENTIALS OF DIAGNOSIS

- *Prodromal phase of coryza, conjunctivitis, cough, and lesions on the buccal and pharyngeal mucosa.*
- *Maculopapular rash involving the entire body, associated with high fever, lasting 7–10 days*

General Considerations

Measles is a highly contagious infection that is endemic throughout most of the world. With nearly universal immunization in the United States, the infection has become rare. If measles is suspected, acute and convalescent antibody titers should be drawn to confirm the disease.

Pathogenesis

Measles is caused by a paramyxovirus. It is highly contagious, and over 90% of nonimmune household contacts will develop the disease. The disease is spread by droplets and becomes contagious near the beginning of the prodromal phase.

Prevention

Measles immunization provides nearly complete protection against infection. The vaccine is given in two doses, the first between 12 and 18 months of age and the second at about age 5 years. Nonimmune infants and children with chronic illnesses who are exposed to measles can be given immune serum globulin (γ-globulin). This should be given as soon as possible after exposure, as its effectiveness declines significantly 7 days after exposure, and it is nearly ineffective once the infection has become clinically apparent.

Clinical Findings

A. SYMPTOMS AND SIGNS

The incubation period is usually 10–12 days, although it can be as short as 6 days. The prodromal phase lasts 3–5 days and is characterized by coryza, a progressively worsening cough, conjunctivitis, and mild to moderate fever. Cough is nearly universal, and the disease should not be diagnosed in the absence of cough. Koplik's spots are pathognomonic of measles. There is usually an enanthem or mottling of the buccal and pharyngeal mucosa. Koplik's spots are small grayish-white dots, usually with an erythematous halo, that appear on the buccal and occasionally on the pharyngeal mucosa. They appear and disappear quickly, usually within 12–18 hours.

As the rash appears, a high fever appears, often as high as 104°F. The rash begins as red macules on the head and face, which then become maculopapular. The maculopapular lesions often coalesce to form the typical morbiliform rash. The lesions spread downward over the entire body and reach the feet after 2–3 days. When the rash reaches the feet, the fever usually breaks, and the patient rapidly feels better. At the same time, the lesions on the face begin to fade, and the lesions clear from the body in the same order in which they developed. The entire process normally takes 7–10 days.

Differential Diagnosis

Because measles is rare in the United States, other viral exanthems, including roseola, coxsackievirus, echovirus, and adenovirus, must be considered as more likely causes of this illness. Scarlet fever, drug rash, and Kawasaki disease must also be considered.

Complications

Pneumonia and encephalitis are the main complications of measles. Pneumonia may be caused by the virus itself or by bacterial superinfection, and it may be mild to severe.

Encephalitis occurs in 1–2 of every 1000 cases. The severity of encephalitis is not related to the severity of the measles infection. Encephalitis may be mild, it may be severe with permanent sequelae, or it may even be fatal.

Treatment

Treatment of measles is supportive, with antipyretics and antipruritics. In developing countries, oral vitamin A, 400,000 IU, has been shown to decrease morbidity and mortality in children with severe measles, and it is recommended for all children with the disease in these countries.

Prognosis

In the absence of severe complications, measles is benign. Morbidity and mortality are primarily related to pneumonia and encephalitis.

4. Rubella

 ESSENTIALS OF DIAGNOSIS

- *Mild prodromal phase of coryza symptoms.*
- *Prominent postauricular, posterior cervical, and occipital lymphadenopathy.*
- *Maculopapular rash involving the entire body, associated with minimal to mild fever, lasting 3 days.*

General Considerations

Like measles, rubella is a highly contagious infection that is endemic throughout most of the world. With nearly universal immunization in the United States, the infection has become rare. If rubella is suspected, acute and convalescent antibody titers should be drawn to confirm the disease. Unlike measles, complications are infrequent. The primary danger of rubella is transplacental passage from mother to fetus, which results in congenital rubella syndrome.

Pathogenesis

Rubella is caused by a togavirus. It is highly contagious, and nearly 100% of nonimmune close contacts will become infected. The disease is spread by droplets and is contagious from about 7 days before the onset of the rash to about 7 days after the rash clears. It is most common during the spring months.

Prevention

Rubella immunization provides nearly complete protection against infection. The vaccine is given in two doses, the first between 12 and 18 months of age and the second at about age 5 years. Women who are discovered during prenatal care to be nonimmune should be immunized shortly after delivery. Nonimmune infants and children with chronic illnesses who are exposed to rubella can be given immune serum globulin (γ-globulin). This is effective if given within 7–8 days after exposure, but the effectiveness of this treatment is highly variable.

Clinical Findings

A. Symptoms and Signs

Rubella is often subclinical, with perhaps twice as many inapparent infections as clinically evident cases. The incubation period of rubella is 14–21 days. The prodromal phase of coryza symptoms lasts 3–4 days or less and may be mild or inapparent. Lymphadenopathy begins about 1 day before the rash and lasts for 7 days or more. Postauricular, posterior cervical, and occipital lymphadenopathy are striking features of this illness and are present to a degree rare in any other illness. The rash is a maculopapular rash. The lesions are usually discrete but may be confluent. The rash begins on the face and spreads downward to involve the entire body. It clears in the order in which it develops and is usually resolved within 3 days. There may be mild associated pharyngitis and conjunctivitis. Fever is absent to mild, rarely higher than 101°F.

Differential Diagnosis

Because rubella is rare in the United States, other viral exanthems, including roseola, coxsackievirus, echovirus, and adenovirus, must be considered as more likely causes of this illness. Scarlet fever, drug rash, and Kawasaki disease must also be considered.

Complications

Complications are unusual in children. Encephalitis occurs in about 1 in every 6000 cases, and about 70% of affected children have some neurological sequelae. Arthritis is an occasional complication.

The most feared complication of rubella is congenital rubella infection. This is now rare in the United States. The consequences of this infection depend on the severity of the infection and on the stage of development of the fetus at the time of infection. During the first trimester, about 80% of fetuses of infected mothers will become infected, and nearly all of them will have sequelae. Transmission and sequelae are less frequent later in gestation. The virus affects nearly all organs in the fetus. The most common complication is growth retardation. Congenital cataracts, with or without microphthalmia, are common. Structural cardiac defects, meningitis, mental retardation, and congenital hearing loss may occur.

Treatment

Treatment is entirely asymptomatic, as no effective treatments have been developed.

Prognosis

In children who do not develop encephalitis, rubella is a benign illness. Infants born with congenital rubella may have mild to severe impairments.

5. Erythema Infectiosum (Fifth Disease)

ESSENTIALS OF DIAGNOSIS

- *Mild URI prodrome.*
- *Rash begins as erythema of cheeks.*
- *Rash becomes more generalized, macular at first, then reticular.*
- *Rash lasts 1–3 weeks*

General Considerations

Erythema infectiosum (fifth disease) is a common childhood infection that rarely causes clinically significant disease.

Pathogenesis

Erythema infectiosum is caused by parvovirus B 19. It appears sporadically but often in epidemics in communities. Children are infectious during the prodromal stage, which is inapparent or mild and usually indistinguishable from a URI. The rash is an immune-mediated phenomenon that occurs after the infection. Children with the rash are not infectious and should not be restricted from school or other activities.

Prevention

There are no effective prevention measures for this disease.

Clinical Findings

A. Symptoms and Signs

Erythema infectiosum begins with a prodromal stage of URI symptoms, headache, and low-grade fever. This stage may be clinically inapparent.

The rash occurs in three phases, but any one phase may be transient enough to go unnoticed. The first stage is facial flushing, described as a "slapped cheek" appearance. Shortly afterward, the rash becomes generalized over the body, initially as a faint erythematous, often confluent, macular rash. In the third stage, the central regions of the macules clear, leaving a distinctive faint reticular rash. The rash comes and goes evanescently over the body. Often, the area of the body affected by the rash when the parent calls for an appointment for the child has cleared and a new area has become affected by the time the child comes to the physician's office. The rash can last from 1 to 3 weeks. There are rarely any other associated findings, although lymphadenopathy and atypical rashes have been reported.

Differential Diagnosis

Erythema infectiosum is usually recognizable as a distinct clinical illness, but it may be confused with other viral exanthems.

Complications

Arthritis is rare in children but may occur in adolescents. Thrombocytopenic purpura and aseptic meningitis are rare complications.

Fetal hydrops and fetal demise may be seen in fetuses whose mothers contract the infection. Because the primary infection is often inapparent, it is difficult to know who has been infected, and the frequency of transmission to the fetus is unknown. It is estimated that 5% or fewer of infected fetuses will be affected by the virus.

Treatment

There is no known treatment for this disease.

Prognosis

Except for rare complications in children, this is a benign infection. Fetal complications are unusual.

■ INFLAMMATORY DISORDERS OF THE SKIN

ATOPIC DERMATITIS

 ESSENTIALS OF DIAGNOSIS

- *Pruritis is the cardinal symptom.*
- *Lesions are excoriated, scaly, and may become lichenified.*

General Considerations

Atopic dermatitis is a common skin disorder in children, affecting 10–15% of the population. It appears during the first year of life in 60% and during the first 5 years in 85% of cases. By the age of 5 years, the dis-

ease usually becomes less prominent, although it often persists at some level into adulthood.

Pathogenesis

The cause of atopic dermatitis is unclear. It has a strong association, both in the individual and in families, with allergic rhinitis and asthma, and it is classified as an atopic disorder. Immunoglobulin E (IgE)-mediated cutaneous allergy may be a factor in some cases, but it is felt to be primarily a disorder of T cell hypersensitivity. Food allergies, primarily to cow's milk, wheat, eggs, soy, fish, and peanuts, have been implicated in 20–30% of cases.

Clinical Findings

A. SYMPTOMS AND SIGNS

The diagnosis is based on the presence of three of the following major criteria: pruritis, lesions with typical morphology and distribution, facial and extensor involvement in infants and children, chronic or chronically relapsing dermatitis, and personal or family history of atopic disease. Numerous minor criteria have also been proposed, but they are all so nonspecific as to be of little help in diagnosis.

Pruritis is the hallmark of the disease, usually preceding the skin lesions, which most often develop as a reaction to scratching. The skin becomes excoriated, develops weeping and crusting, and later may become scaly or lichenified. Secondary bacterial infection is common. In infants, the lesions usually involve the face, but may appear in a generalized pattern over much of the body. In young children, the extensor surfaces of the extremities are often involved. In older children and adults, the disease often moves to involve the flexion areas of the extremities instead. The disease typically is chronic, although remissions and relapses are common.

Differential Diagnosis

Atopic dermatitis may be confused with seborrheic dermatitis, especially in infants, where facial lesions are common. Atopic dermatitis does not usually follow the distribution of oil glands, as is typical with seborrheic dermatitis. However, the two disorders may coexist. Atopic dermatitis may also be confused with psoriasis, contact dermatitis, scabies, and cutaneous fungal infections.

Complications

The most common complication is secondary bacterial infection, which can result in impetigo or cellulitis. Low-grade bacterial infection should be considered as a factor in lesions that do not respond well to the usual therapies.

Treatment

Nonpharmacological measures are important in the treatment of this disease. Long baths and bathing in hot water exacerbate dryness of the skin and should be avoided. Use of soaps that do not contain fragrances may help, or it may be necessary to use nonsoap cleansers instead. Moisturizers that contain fragrances and other irritants will aggravate the problem. Petrolatum is ideal as a moisturizer. If secondary infection is suspected, systemic antibiotics effective against streptococci and staphylococci should be given.

Topical corticosteroids are the mainstay of treatment. The lowest potency preparation that is effective should be used, especially on the face and on the diaper area, which are more sensitive to the skin atrophy associated with the prolonged use of higher-potency steroids. Systemic steroids are useful for severe acute flares, but their use should be restricted to once or twice a year, if possible. Antipruritic medications, such as hydroxyzine, may be useful, but these all have significant sedative side effects. Tacrolimus and pimecrolimus, new topical immune modulators, are effective, although less so than high-potency topical steroids. Whether they are as effective as or less effective than medium-potency steroids is unclear. Because these new drugs do not cause skin atrophy, they may be useful for prolonged treatment of facial lesions. Doxepin, a tricyclic antidepressant with strong antihistaminic effects, is often useful in severe cases. Finally, there are reports that cyclosporine and azathioprine have been effective in some of the most refractory cases.

Prognosis

Although it is usually fairly easily controlled, atopic dermatitis is a chronic skin disorder. It often becomes less severe as children grow into school age, but relapses and persistence of some disease into adulthood are common.

SEBORRHEIC DERMATITIS

ESSENTIALS OF DIAGNOSIS

- Lesions may be localized or generalized.
- Inflamed lesions with yellowish or brownish crusting.

General Considerations

Seborrheic dermatitis is a common inflammatory disorder of the skin. It is most common in infancy and adolescence, times when the sebaceous glands are more active. It generally resolves or lessens in severity after infancy, but localized lesions or mild, generalized scalp disease may be seen throughout adulthood.

Pathogenesis

The cause of seborrheic dermatitis is unknown. The fungus *Pityrosporum ovale* has been implicated, but whether it is causative in all cases is not known.

Clinical Findings

A. SYMPTOMS AND SIGNS

The typical lesions of seborrheic dermatitis are inflammatory macular lesions, usually with brownish or yellowish scaling. It may begin during the first month of life, and it usually becomes evident within the first year. In infants, the lesions may be generalized, but in older children, lesions are most common in areas in which sebaceous glands are concentrated, such as the scalp, face, and axillae. Marginal blepharitis may be seen. Cradle cap is a common variant seen in infants, either by itself or associated with other lesions. This is seen as scaling and crusting of the scalp, often with extremely heavy buildup of scale in untreated infants.

Differential Diagnosis

Atopic dermatitis is the main element in the differential diagnosis. The disease may also be confused with psoriasis and other cutaneous fungal infections.

Complications

Secondary infection, either bacterial or fungal, is a common complication.

Treatment

Seborrheic dermatitis usually responds more readily to treatment than does atopic dermatitis. Topical corticosteroids are the main treatment for inflammatory lesions. Medium- and high-potency preparations are usually not necessary. Scalp lesions usually respond to antiseborrheic shampoos, such as selenium sulfide. Topical treatment with antifungal creams or shampoo may also be helpful. Cradle cap is treated by soaking the scales with mineral oil and then gently debriding them with a toothbrush or washcloth. Following debridement, cleaning with baby shampoo is normally adequate for control, and antiseborrheic or antifungal shampoos are usually not necessary.

Prognosis

Seborrheic dermatitis generally resolves or lessens in severity after infancy, but localized lesions or mild, generalized scalp disease may be seen throughout adulthood.

The Medical Letter 2001;43:33.
The Medical Letter 2002;44:48.

Childhood Vaccines

Richard Kent Zimmerman, MD, MPH, Donald B. Middleton, MD, & Ilene Timko Burns, MD, MPH

The development of effective immunizations is one of the greatest achievements of the twentieth century. Routine vaccination has greatly reduced suffering from childhood diseases. This chapter discusses the routine childhood vaccines indicated by age and vaccination procedures. Important considerations in routine use of vaccines includes disease burden, vaccine efficacy, and adverse reactions.

HEPATITIS B VACCINE

Disease Burden

Before routine vaccination, between 128,000 and 320,000 persons in the United States were infected annually with hepatitis B virus (HBV). The number of persons chronically infected with HBV, each of whom is potentially infectious, is estimated at 1.25 million, and the lifetime risk for acquiring HBV infection has been estimated at 5%. Approximately 6000 persons in the United States die annually of HBV-related liver disease, mostly due to cirrhosis or primary hepatocellular carcinoma. HBV infection is the second leading cause of cancer worldwide.

HBV infection is much more likely to become chronic when acquired earlier in life than when acquired later in life. Chronic HBV infection develops in 90% of those infected as infants, 30–60% of those infected before the age of 4 years, and only 5–10% of those infected as adults. Therefore although most acute HBV infections in the United States occur in adulthood because of high-risk behaviors, 36% of all persons in the United States with chronic HBV infection contracted the infection during childhood. Up to 25% of individuals infected with HBV as infants will die of HBV-related chronic liver disease as adults.

HBV can be contracted from persons acutely or chronically infected with HBV. Transmission of HBV occurs primarily through blood exchange (eg, via shared needles during injection drug use) and by sexual contact, but the source of infection is not identified in 30–40% of hepatitis B cases. These cases may result from (1) underreporting of injection drug use or sexual activity and (2) inapparent contamination of skin lesions or mucosal surfaces [hepatitis B surface antigen (HbsAg) has been found in impetigo lesions and saliva of persons chronically infected with HBV, and on toothbrush racks and coffee cups in their homes].

Vaccines

The childhood hepatitis B vaccines currently produced in the United States, Recombivax HB and Engerix-B, are manufactured by recombinant DNA technology using Bakers' yeast and do not contain human plasma or thimerosal. Preexposure vaccination results in protective antibody levels in almost all infants and children (>95%).

A. IMMUNITY

The duration of immunity in healthy persons is based on immunological memory. Although antibody levels may slowly diminish with time following vaccination, the immunological memory and long incubation period of hepatitis B infection allow most immunized persons who have low titers to mount an anamnestic immune response if challenged by HBV. Although a few persons in the United States who adequately responded to hepatitis B vaccine have developed HBV subclinical infection following exposure years after vaccination, none of these people has become chronically infected or developed serious complications such as chronic liver disease.

B. EFFICACY

When given to susceptible infants, children, and adults, efficacy, ie, protection against HBV infection, is 80–95% for hepatitis B vaccines licensed in the United States.

Adverse Reactions

The most common adverse event after administration of hepatitis B vaccine is pain at the injection site, which occurs in 3–9% of children. Mild, transient systemic adverse events such as fatigue and headache have been reported in 8–18% of children. Recombinant hepatitis B vaccine is not linked to multiple sclerosis.

Recommendations

Hepatitis B vaccine is given in a three-dose schedule, 0.5 mL intramuscularly in the anterolateral thigh or deltoid. The infant hepatitis B vaccination schedule depends on the mother's HBsAg status and the birth weight. For infants born to mothers with positive surface antigen status, postexposure prophylaxis, consisting of both hepatitis B immune globulin (HBIG) and vaccine, should be initiated within 12 h of birth, regardless of gestational age. These infants should receive their second and third doses of vaccine at ages 1–2 months and 6 months, respectively. If the mother is chronically infected with HBV, the infant should be tested for HBsAg and anti-HBs at 9–15 months of age to determine the success of vaccination.

For infants born to mothers whose HBsAg status is unknown, vaccine should be given within 12 h of birth and maternal blood should be drawn at the time of delivery to determine HBsAg status. If the test result is positive, HBIG should be given as soon as possible (no later than 1 week of age).

For infants born to HbsAg-negative mothers, the schedule is 0–2 months for the first dose, 1–4 months for the second dose, and 6–18 months for the third dose (Figure 7–1).

Seroconversion rates are lower in infants born prematurely. Therefore, infants weighing less than 2 kg at birth whose mother is known to be HBsAg negative should have the first dose of hepatitis B vaccine delayed until the infant weighs 2 kg. For newborns weighing more than 2 kg at birth whose mother is known to be HBsAg negative, the first dose of hepatitis B vaccine can be given at or before the time of hospital discharge or delayed up until 2 months of age. Premature infants whose mother is HBsAg positive should be vaccinated and given HBIG within 12 h of birth, as described previously.

Ascherio A et al: Hepatitis B vaccination and the risk of multiple sclerosis. New Engl J Med 2001;344(5):327.

PERTUSSIS VACCINE

Disease Burden

Most hospitalizations for and serious complications of pertussis occur in infants. About one-third (29%) of reported cases of pertussis occur in infants, and half (41%) occur in children younger than 5 years of age. Most (63%) reported cases of pertussis in infants younger than 6 months of age require hospitalization. Females are somewhat more likely to exhibit clinical pertussis than males, probably due to smaller airway size.

Complications of pertussis include pneumonia, seizures, encephalopathy, permanent brain damage, and death. Pneumonia occurs in about 12% of pertussis cases in infants less than 6 months of age and is the leading cause of death from pertussis. Encephalopathy, perhaps due to hypoxia or minute cerebral hemorrhages, is fatal in approximately one-third of cases and causes permanent brain damage in another one-third.

Pertussis is highly contagious: 70–100% of susceptible household contacts and 50–80% of susceptible school contacts will become infected following exposure to a person who is contagious. A person is contagious from 7 days after exposure to 3 weeks after the onset of the symptoms. Pertussis is transmitted by respiratory droplets or occasionally by contact with freshly contaminated objects. Adults and adolescents are the primary source of pertussis infection for young infants. The incubation period ranges from 5 to 21 days and is most typically from 7 to 10 days. Immunity following pertussis disease lasts for many years and is possibly lifelong. Transplacental immunity wanes rapidly following birth.

Vaccines

International cooperative efforts resulted in the production of acellular pertussis vaccines to replace whole cell vaccines, which were effective but had a number of adverse effects. Analysis of the pathogenesis resulted in identification of the components of *Bordetella pertussis* that are important in the organism's ability to cause disease and therefore might be important in an acellular vaccine. These include (1) tracheal cytotoxin that destroys cilia, making it difficult to clear thickened mucus; (2) pertussis toxin (also called lymphocytosis-promoting factor), which interferes with immune cell function, contributes to ciliary damage, and aids attachment to respiratory epithelium; (3) filamentous hemagglutinin, which helps the bacteria attach to cilia of the respiratory tract; (4) pertactin (also called 69-kDa protein), which also aids bacterial attachment to cilia; and (5) agglutinogens, which may aid persistent attachment to cilia. Acellular vaccines use one or more of these components (Table 7 –1).

A. EFFICACY

In studies conducted in the United States, diphtheria toxoid, tetanus toxoid, and whole-cell pertussis (DTP) vaccination was found to be 70–90% effective in preventing pertussis disease. In studies conducted in Europe, diphtheria toxoid, tetanus toxoid, and acellular pertussis (DTaP) vaccines demonstrated efficacies between 59% and 89% while DTP vaccines had efficacies

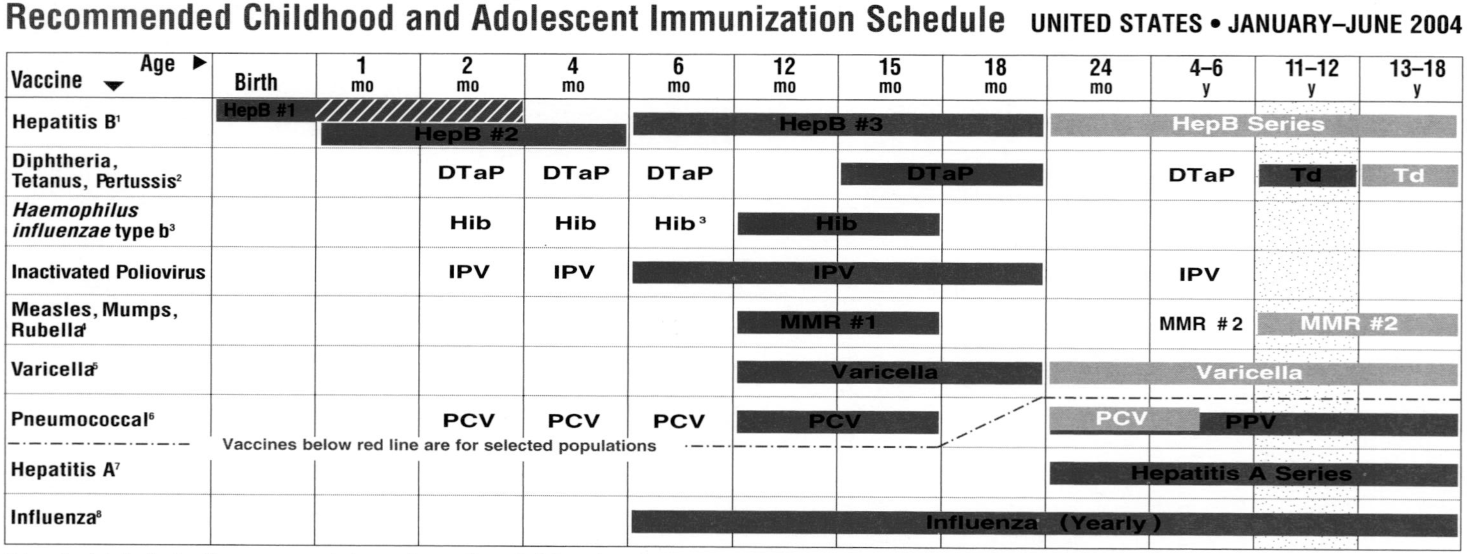

Recommended Childhood and Adolescent Immunization Schedule · UNITED STATES · JANUARY–JUNE 2004

Vaccine ▶ Age ▶	Birth	1 mo	2 mo	4 mo	6 mo	12 mo	15 mo	18 mo	24 mo	4–6 y	11–12 y	13–18 y
Hepatitis B[1]	HepB #1	HepB #2			HepB #3						HepB Series	
Diphtheria, Tetanus, Pertussis[2]			DTaP	DTaP	DTaP		DTaP	DTaP		DTaP	Td	Td
Haemophilus influenzae type b[3]			Hib	Hib	Hib[3]	Hib						
Inactivated Poliovirus			IPV	IPV	IPV	IPV				IPV		
Measles, Mumps, Rubella[4]						MMR #1				MMR #2	MMR #2	
Varicella[5]						Varicella			Varicella			
Pneumococcal[6]			PCV	PCV	PCV	PCV			PCV	PPV		
Hepatitis A[7]									Hepatitis A Series			
Influenza[8]						Influenza (Yearly)						

Vaccines below red line are for selected populations

Range of recommended ages
Preadolescent assessment
Only if mother HBsAg(–)
Catch-up vaccination

This schedule indicates the recommended ages for routine administration of currently licensed childhood vaccines, as of December 1, 2003, for children through age 18 years. Any dose not given at the recommended age should be given at any subsequent visit when indicated and feasible. ▓ Indicates age groups that warrant special effort to administer those vaccines not previously given. Additional vaccines may be licensed and recommended during the year. Licensed combination vaccines may be used whenever any components of the combination are indicated and the vaccine's other components are not contraindicated. Providers should consult the manufacturers' package inserts for detailed recommendations. Clinically significant adverse events that follow immunization should be reported to the Vaccine Adverse Event Reporting System (VAERS). Guidance about how to obtain and complete a VAERS form can be found on the Internet: *www .vaers.org* or by calling 800-822-7967.

Figure 7-1. Recommended childhood immunization schedule, United States, 2003.

1. Hepatitis B (HepB) vaccine. All infants should receive the first dose of hepatitis B vaccine soon after birth and before hospital discharge; the first dose may also be given by age 2 months if the infant's mother is hepatitis B surface antigen (HBsAg) negative. Only monovalent HepB can be used for the birth dose. Monovalent or combination vaccine containing HepB may be used to complete the series. Four doses of vaccine may be administered when a birth dose is given. The second dose should be given at least 4 weeks after the first dose, except for combination vaccines which cannot be administered before age 6 weeks. The third dose should be given at least 16 weeks after the first dose and at least 8 weeks after the second dose. The last dose in the vaccination series (third or fourth dose) should not be administered before age 24 weeks.

Infants born to HBsAg-positive mothers should receive HepB and 0.5 mL of Hepatitis B Immune Globulin (HBIG) within 12 hours of birth at separate sites. The second dose is recommended at age 1 to 2 months. The last dose in the immunization series should not be administered before age 24 weeks. These infants should be tested for HBsAg and antibody to HBsAg (anti-HBs) at age 9 to 15 months.

Infants born to mothers whose HBsAg status is unknown should receive the first dose of the HepB series within 12 hours of birth. Maternal blood should be drawn as soon as possible to determine the mother's HBsAg status; if the HBsAg test is positive, the infant should receive HBIG as soon as possible (no later than age 1 week). The second dose is recommended at age 1 to 2 months. The last dose in the immunization series should not be administered before age 24 weeks.

2. Diphtheria and tetanus toxoids and acellular pertussis (DTaP) vaccine. The fourth dose of DTaP may be administered as early as age 12 months, provided 6 months have elapsed since the third dose and the child is unlikely to return at age 15 to 18 months. The final dose in the series should be given at age ≥4 years.

Tetanus and diphtheria toxoids (Td) is recommended at age 11 to 12 years if at least 5 years have elapsed since the last dose of tetanus and diphtheria toxoid-containing vaccine. Subsequent routine Td boosters are recommended every 10 years.

3. *Haemophilus influenzae* type b (Hib) conjugate vaccine. Three Hib conjugate vaccines are licensed for infant use. If PRPOMP (PedvaxHIB or ComVax [Merck]) is administered at ages 2 and 4 months, a dose at age 6 months is not required. DTaP/Hib combination products should not be used for primary immunization in infants at ages 2, 4 or 6 months but can be used as boosters following any Hib vaccine. The final dose in the series should be given at age ≥12 months.

4. Measles, mumps, and rubella vaccine (MMR). The second dose of MMR is recommended routinely at age 4 to 6 years but may be administered during any visit, provided at least 4 weeks have elapsed since the first dose and both doses are administered beginning at or after age 12 months. Those who have not previously received the second dose should complete the schedule by the 11- to 12-year-old visit.

5. Varicella vaccine. Varicella vaccine is recommended at any visit at or after age 12 months for susceptible children (i.e., those who lack a reliable history of chickenpox). Susceptible persons age ≥13 years should receive 2 doses, given at least 4 weeks apart.

6. Pneumococcal vaccine. The heptavalent **pneumococcal conjugate vaccine (PCV)** is recommended for all children age 2 to 23 months. It is also recommended for certain children age 24 to 59 months. The final dose in the series should be given at age ≥12 months. **Pneumococcal polysaccharide vaccine (PPV)** is recommended in addition to PCV for certain high-risk groups. See *MMWR* 2000;49(RR-9):1-38.

7. Hepatitis A vaccine. Hepatitis A vaccine is recommended for children and adolescents in selected states and regions and for certain high-risk groups; consult your local public health authority Children and adolescents in these states, regions, and high-risk groups who have not been immunized against hepatitis A can begin the hepatitis A immunization series during any visit. The 2 doses in the series should be administered at least 6 months apart. See *MMWR* 1999;48(RR-12):1-37.

8. Influenza vaccine. Influenza vaccine is recommended annually for children age ≥6 months with certain risk factors (including but not limited to children with asthma, cardiac disease, sickle cell disease, human immunodeficiency virus infection, and diabetes; and household members of persons in high-risk groups [see *MMWR* 2003;52(RR-8):1-36]) and can be administered to all others wishing to obtain immunity. In addition, healthy children age 6 to 23 months are encouraged to receive influenza vaccine if feasible, because children in this age group are at substantially increased risk of influenza-related hospitalizations. For healthy persons age 5 to 49 years, the intranasally administered live-attenuated influenza vaccine (LAIV) is an acceptable alternative to the intramuscular trivalent inactivated influenza vaccine (TIV). See *MMWR* 2003;52(RR-13):1-8. Children receiving TIV should be administered a dosage appropriate for their age (0.25 mL if age 6 to 35 months or 0.5 mL if age ≥3 years). Children age ≤8 years who are receiving influenza vaccine for the first time should receive 2 doses (separated by at least 4 weeks for TIV and at least 6 weeks for LAIV).

Table 7–1. Study sites, vaccines, vaccination schedules, and efficacy estimates used in the evaluation of the efficacy of acellular pertussis vaccine licensed in the United States when administered in infancy.[1]

Site of Study	Acellular Pertussis Vaccine	Vaccine Composition				Studied Trial Type	Schedule DTaP (%) (Months)	Vaccine Efficacy against ≥21 Days of Cough	
		PT	FHA	Pn	Fim			DTP[2] (%) (95% CI)	(95% CI)
Italy	SKB-3P (Infanrix)	X	X	X		Randomized double blind	2, 4, 6	84 (76–90)[3]	36 (14–52)
Germany	SKB-3P (Infanrix)	X	X	X		Household contact with passive surveillance	3, 4, 5	89 (77–95)[3]	98 (83–100)
Stockholm, Sweden	DAPTACEL (CLL-4F2)	X	X	X	X (types 2 & 3)	Randomized double-blind	2, 4, 6	85 (81–89)	48 (37–58)
Munich, Germany	CB-2 (Tripedia)	X	X			Case–control study with passive surveillance	3, 5, 7	80 (59–90)[4]	95 (81–99)

Modified from CDC: Pertussis vaccination: use of acellular pertussis vaccines among infants and young children. Recommendations of the ACIP. MMWR 1997;46 (No. RR-7):6. Public domain.

[1]PT, pertussis toxin; FHA, filamentous hemagglutinin; Pn, pertactin; DTaP, pediatric dose of diphtheria toxoid and tetanus toxoid and acellular pertussis vaccine; DTP, pediatric dose of diphtheria toxoid and tetanus toxoid and whole-cell pertussis vaccine.
[2]The whole-cell vaccines differed; some are not available in the United States.
[3]Efficacy against ≥21 days of paroxysmal cough with culture or serological confirmation.
[4]Efficacy against ≥21 days of any cough and confirmation by culture or link to culture; positive household contact.

from 36% to 98%. However, comparing the results of various studies is difficult because of differences in (1) study type, (2) degree of blinding, (3) case definition of pertussis, (4) criteria for confirmation of pertussis infection, (5) ethnicity of study population, (6) number of children studied, (7) timing of the vaccine schedule, and (8) manufacturer of whole-cell vaccine used for comparison. The protection afforded by pertussis vaccination wanes with time.

Adverse Reactions

DTaP vaccines cause approximately 25–50% the common adverse reactions associated with DTP vaccines; furthermore, the rates of adverse reactions are similar for DTaP and DT. Minor adverse reactions associated with DTaP vaccination include localized edema at the injection site, fever, and fussiness; edema is more common after the fourth or fifth dose.

Uncommon adverse reactions after whole-cell DTP are persistent crying for 3 h or more, an unusual high-pitched cry, seizures, and hypotonic–hyporesponsive episodes. Most seizures that occur after DTP vaccination are simple febrile seizures that do not have any permanent sequelae. On rare occasions, a child may have an anaphylactic reaction to DTP, which is a contraindication to further doses of DTP or DTaP. Allegations of other serious adverse reactions, such as permanent neurological damage, after a dose of DTP vaccine are controversial and have been discussed elsewhere in depth.

Administration of DTaP vaccine has also been associated with seizures, persistent crying, and hypotonic–

hyporesponsive episodes but at lower rates than for DTP vaccine. Acellular pertussis vaccines currently produced in the United States have either no thimerosal or the amount has been reduced to only a trace.

Recommendations

DTaP is recommended for all children because of the reduced risk of adverse reactions when compared with DTP. Although five doses of pertussis vaccine, 0.5 mL intramuscularly, are recommended, persons who receive their fourth dose on or after their fourth birthday do not need the fifth dose. Premature infants should be vaccinated with full doses at the appropriate chronological age.

Other combination vaccines that include acellular pertussis vaccine are being developed. The first combination licensed was TriHIBit, in which the *Haemophilus influenzae* type b (Hib) vaccine ActHIB is reconstituted with the Tripedia acellular pertussis vaccine. TriHIBit is currently licensed only for use as the fourth dose of the series and should not be used earlier unless so licensed. Pediarix is a combination of DtaP, IPV, and hepatitis B vaccine that is licensed for the three doses of the primary series.

Tetanus Wound Prophylaxis

Administration of tetanus toxoid with or without immunoglobulin is indicated (after the wound has been cleaned, debrided if necessary, and dressed) if the patient did not complete an initial tetanus vaccination series or has not had a tetanus booster in the last

Table 7–2. Tetanus wound prophylaxis.

	Previous Immunization History[1]		
	Uncertain or Less Than Three Doses		Three or More Doses[2]
Type of Wound	**Give Td?**	**Give TIG?**	**Give Td? (No TIG Needed)**
Clean, minor wounds	Yes	No	No, unless ≥10 years since previous dose
Wounds contaminated with dirt, feces, or saliva	Yes	Yes	No, unless >5 years since previous dose
Puncture or missile wounds	Yes	Yes	No, unless >5 years since previous dose
Burns, frostbite, or crush injury	Yes	Yes	No, unless >5 years since previous dose

Modified from MMWR 1991;40 (No. RR-10):16. Public domain.

[1]Td, adult tetanus and diphtheria toxoids; TIG, tetanus immune globulin.

[2]If the individual has only had three doses of the nonabsorbed (fluid) tetanus toxoid, administer a fourth dose of Td or tetanus toxoid. Nonabsorbed (fluid) vaccine was available only as single antigen tetanus toxoid; diphtheria and tetanus toxoids and pertussis vaccine (DTP), Td, and pediatric diphtheria and tetanus toxoids (DT) all use absorbed preparations.

5–10 years (see Table 7–2, which lists indications for tetanus toxoid and tetanus immunoglobulin administration). When tetanus toxoid is indicated, administration of adult tetanus and diphtheria toxoids (Td) is preferred over monovalent tetanus toxoid. The typical dose of tetanus immune globulin is 250 mg, administered intramuscularly at a separate site from tetanus toxoid.

Centers for Disease Control and Prevention: Update: vaccine side effects, adverse reactions, contraindications, and precautions—recommendations of the Advisory Committee on Immunization Practices (ACIP). MMWR 1996;45(RR-12):1.

Centers for Disease Control and Prevention: Pertussis vaccination: use of acellular pertussis vaccines among infants and young children. MMWR 1997;46:1.

Centers for Disease Control and Prevention: Pertussis—United States, 1997–2000. MMWR 2002;51(4):73.

HAEMOPHILUS INFLUENZAE TYPE B VACCINES

Disease Burden

Before the development of effective vaccines, *Haemophilus influenzae* type b (Hib) caused invasive disease in about 1 of every 200 children younger than 5 years of age in the United States. Hib was the most common cause of bacterial meningitis in this age group, with a peak incidence between 6 and 12 months of age. Hib meningitis, the illness in about two-thirds of cases of invasive Hib disease, carries a 2–5% mortality rate, even with appropriate treatment. Neurological sequelae (including hearing loss, vision loss, mental retardation, seizures, and motor and speech delays) are seen in 15–30% of survivors. Other manifestations of invasive Hib disease include epiglottitis (with its 5–10% mortality rate due to airway obstruction), cellulitis (especially facial, periorbital, and orbital locations), pneumonia, osteomyelitis, septic arthritis, bacteremia, and pericarditis.

Vaccines

To develop a vaccine immunogenic in infants, the polysaccharide antigen of the Hib capsule had to be linked to a protein that would improve recognition by the immature immune system. Since 1990, four Hib vaccines immunogenic in infants as young as 6 weeks of age have been licensed: HibTITER (HbOC) links Hib polysaccharide to a mutant diphtheria protein, ActHIB and OmniHIB (PRP-T) use tetanus toxoid, and PedvaxHIB (PRP-OMP) uses meningococcal group B outer membrane protein. Conjugate Hib vaccines by themselves do not result in protection against the protein used in conjugation (ie, PRP-T by itself does not protect against tetanus).

A. EFFICACY

Conjugate Hib vaccines are estimated to be 95–100% efficacious. The incidence of invasive Hib disease dropped by 97% in the first 10 years of conjugate vaccine use (1987–1997).

Adverse Reactions

No serious adverse reactions have been linked to Hib vaccine. Local reactions (tenderness, swelling, erythema) occur in 5–30% of recipients. Fever occurs in 1–less than 5% of recipients.

Recommendations

The schedule for Hib vaccination, 0.5 mL intramuscularly, varies by product: 2, 4, 6, and 12–15 months for

HbOC (HibTITER) and PRP-T (ActHib) and 2, 4, and 12–15 months for PRP-OMP (PedvaxHIB). Hib-containing vaccines should **not** be administered to children younger than 6 weeks of age as immune tolerance to the antigen can be induced. If the combination Hib–hepatitis B vaccine is used, the schedule for PRP-OMP Hib should be followed, ie, no dose is required at 6 months of age for a child who has received doses at 2 and 4 months, and the series is completed on or after the first birthday.

Centers for Disease Control and Prevention: Progress toward eliminating *Haemophilus influenzae* type b disease among infants and children 1987–1997. MMWR 1998;47:993.

Centers for Disease Control and Prevention: *Epidemiology and Prevention of Vaccine-Preventable Diseases,* ed 6. Public Health Foundation, 2000.

PNEUMOCOCCAL CONJUGATE VACCINE

Disease Burden

Streptococcus pneumoniae is a gram-positive diplococcus with a polysaccharide capsule that helps protect it from host defense mechanisms; 90 capsular serotypes have been identified. Infection is spread by droplets from respiratory tract secretions. *S pneumoniae* causes approximately 2600 cases of meningitis, 63,000 cases of bacteremia, 100,000–135,000 cases of pneumonia requiring hospitalization, and 7 million cases of otitis media annually in the United States. Prior to the introduction of pneumococcal vaccination, among children younger than 5 years of age, *S pneumoniae* annually caused about 17,000 cases of invasive disease, including 200 deaths. Invasive disease consists of bacteremia, meningitis, or infection in a normally sterile site, excluding the middle ear. *S pneumoniae* is the most common bacterial cause of community-acquired pneumonia, sinusitis, and acute otitis media in young children. Since the tremendous success of Hib vaccines in reducing meningitis, *S pneumoniae* now has become the leading cause of bacterial meningitis in the United States.

Heightening the importance of immunizations is the increasing proportion of *S pneumoniae* that is resistant to antibiotics. In 1998, based on cases of invasive pneumococcal disease detected in the surveillance areas for the Active Bacterial Core, 24% of isolates had intermediate susceptibility or were resistant to penicillin. Some isolates are resistant to multiple antibiotics.

Vaccines

Two vaccines are currently available against pneumococcus: the older 23-valent polysaccharide vaccine, given 0.5 mL intramuscularly or subcutaneously, and the 7-valent conjugate (Prevnar) vaccine licensed in 2000, given 0.5 mL intramuscularly.

The older pneumococcal polysaccharide vaccine (PPV) contains T-independent antigens that stimulate mature B-lymphocytes to produce effective antibody but do not stimulate T-lymphocytes. T-independent immune responses do not produce an anamnestic response upon challenge and may not be long lasting. The vaccine is effective among older children and adults but not in children less than 2 years of age as they do not respond well to such antigens.

A 7-valent pneumococcal conjugate vaccine (PCV) was licensed in 2000 in the United States. The vaccine was designed to cover the seven serotypes (4, 6B, 9V, 14, 18C, 19F, and 23F) most common in children. These serotypes account for about 80% of invasive infections in children less than 6 years of age, but only 50% of infections in those aged 6 and older. Obviously, PCV covers fewer serotypes than the 23-valent PPV. However, for the serotypes in PCV, it is more immunogenic than PPV. PCV elicits a T-dependent immune response that leads to an anamnestic response on challenge and is effective in infants. PCV reduces nasopharyngeal carriage of *S pneumoniae* and theoretically could create herd immunity.

A. EFFICACY

A randomized, double-blind controlled trial was conducted in Northern Kaiser Permanente, California. In the primary efficacy analysis, the efficacy against invasive disease was 100%. In the follow-up analysis done 8 months later, vaccine efficacy against invasive disease was 94% for serotypes included in the vaccine in the intent-to-treat analysis and 97% for serotypes in the vaccine among the fully vaccinated. The efficacy against all serotypes including nonvaccine types was 89%, suggesting some cross-protection among related serotypes. In the intent-to-treat analyses, which are clinically more meaningful, the efficacy was 11% against clinical pneumonia, 33% against clinical pneumonia supported with any radiographic evidence of infiltrate, and 73% against pneumonia with radiographic evidence of consolidation ≥2.5 cm. Of course, radiographic evidence of consolidation is more typical of pneumococcal pneumonia whereas clinically diagnosed pneumonia is often viral. The number needed to vaccinate ("treat") is 411 to prevent an episode of invasive disease, 239 to prevent pneumonia, and 151 to prevent invasive disease or pneumonia.

Published analyses show that the vaccination of healthy infants would prevent more than 12,000 cases of meningitis and bacteremia and 53,000 cases of pneumonia. The break-even price is $46 per dose from the societal perspective and $18 per dose from the health care payer's perspective. The manufacturer's list price is about $58 per dose, making it the most expensive routine infant immunization series to date. At this price, infant vaccination costs $80,000 per year of life saved and $3200 per pneumonia case prevented.

Adverse Reactions

No serious adverse reactions are associated with PCV. When given with DTaP but at another site, fever $\geq 38°C$ occurred in 15–24% of those vaccinated with PCV compared to 9–17% of those receiving the control vaccine (experimental meningococcal conjugate vaccine). Among PCV vaccinees, 15–23% develop tenderness at the injection site.

Recommendations

The Advisory Committee on Immunization Practices (ACIP), American Academy of Family Physicians (AAFP), and American Academy of Pediatrics (AAP) recommend PCV for routine infant immunization and catch-up vaccination of children 23 months of age or younger. The ACIP, AAP, and AAFP all recommend catch-up vaccination of children 24–59 months of age at high risk for invasive disease. Children at highest risk are those with sickle cell disease, asplenia, human immunodeficiency virus (HIV) infection, or immunocompromise. In addition to the aforementioned PCV recommendations, these children should have both a dose of PPV at least 2 months after the PCV series and a single revaccination with PPV (see ACIP recommendations for details). Catch-up vaccination with PCV is also recommended for children at high risk due to chronic illness (eg, diabetes mellitus, chronic bronchopulmonary dysplasia, or congenital heart disease); a single dose of PPV is also recommended for these children at least 2 months after the last dose of PCV. Penicillin prophylaxis should continue for children with sickle cell disease after vaccination with PCV.

Black S et al: Efficacy, safety and immunogenicity of heptavalent pneumococcal conjugate vaccine in children. Pediatr Infect Dis J 2000;19:187.

Centers for Disease Control and Prevention: Active Bacterial Core Surveillance (ABCs) Report, Emerging Infections Program Network, *Streptococcus pneumoniae,* 1998. www.cdc.gov/ncidod/dbmd/abcs/survreports/spneu98.pdf and www.cdc.gov/ncidod/dbmd/diseaseinfo/drugresisstreppneum_t.htm.

Centers for Disease Control and Prevention: Preventing pneumococcal disease among infants and young children: Recommendations of the Advisory Committee on Immunization Practices (ACIP). MMWR 2000;49(RR-9):1.

Kellner JD, Ford-Jones EL: *Streptococcus pneumoniae* carriage in children attending 59 Canadian child care centers. Arch Pediatr Adolesc Med 1999;153:495.

Lieu TA et al: Projected cost-effectiveness of pneumococcal conjugate vaccination of healthy infants and young children. JAMA 2000;283(11):1460.

Schuchat A et al: Bacterial meningitis in the United States in 1995. New Engl J Med 1997;337(14):970.

POLIOVIRUS VACCINE

Disease Burden

Poliomyelitis was a dreaded disease in the twentieth century. Over 18,000 paralytic cases occurred in 1954 in the United States. An outbreak of poliomyelitis occurred recently in the Dominican Republic and Haiti that was caused by a revertant virus (ie, mutated so no longer attenuated) from oral poliovirus vaccine strain 1. This outbreak demonstrates the need for continued vigilance to maintain high rates of vaccination. Wild poliovirus is quite infectious, and transmission to susceptible household contacts occurs in 73–96% of infections, depending on the contact's age. Transmission occurs primarily by the fecal–oral route, although oral–oral transmission can occur. After the virus enters the mouth it multiplies in the pharynx and gastrointestinal tract before invading the bloodstream and, potentially, the central nervous system. The incubation period ranges from 3 to 35 days.

The results of poliovirus infection, in decreasing order of likelihood, are subclinical infection (up to 95% of cases), nonspecific viral illnesses with complete recovery (about 5% of cases), nonparalytic aseptic meningitis (1–2% of cases), and paralytic poliomyelitis (less than 2% of cases). The ratio of inapparent to paralytic illness is about 200:1 (range 50:1 to 1000:1). The case-fatality rate for paralytic poliomyelitis is 2–5% in children and 15–30% in adults.

Poliovirus vaccination programs have resulted in dramatic decreases in disease incidence. Circulation of indigenous wild polioviruses ceased in the United States in the 1960s and the last case of wild poliomyelitis contracted in the United States was reported in 1979. The last case of poliomyelitis due to indigenous virus in the Americas occurred in 1991 in Peru, and in 1994 the Americas were declared free of indigenous poliomyelitis.

Vaccines

Two vaccines have been used in the United States: inactivated poliovirus vaccine (IPV) and oral polio virus vaccine (OPV). IPV, also known as the Salk vaccine, was licensed in 1955. An enhanced-potency IPV formulation became available in 1988 and is the formulation in use in the United States today. IPV is inactivated, cannot cause vaccine-associated paralytic poliomyelitis (VAPP), and thus is safe for immunocompromised persons and contacts of immunocompromised persons. Almost all immunocompetent persons develop protective antibody levels after three doses. The disadvantages of IPV include administration by injection and less gastrointestinal immunity. OPV has the advantage of easier administration, and induces early intestinal immunity. The main disadvantage of OPV is that the oral polioviruses can revert to a more virulent form and cause VAPP.

Adverse Reactions

Minor local reactions occur following IPV. On rare occasions, VAPP occurs after OPV.

Recommendations

The all IPV, 0.5 mL subcutaneously or intramuscularly, schedule is recommended for the United States. OPV is recommended by the World Health Organization for global eradication efforts. Prior to school entry, four doses of poliovirus vaccine are generally recommended; any combination of IPV and/or OPV is acceptable.

Centers for Disease Control and Prevention: Poliomyelitis prevention in the United States: introduction of a sequential vaccination schedule of inactivated poliovirus vaccine followed by oral poliovirus vaccine: recommendations of the Advisory Committee on Immunization Practices (ACIP). MMWR 1997;46(RR-3):1.

Centers for Disease Control and Prevention: Progress toward global eradication of poliomyelitis. MMWR 1997;46:579.

MEASLES, MUMPS, & RUBELLA VACCINE (MMR)

Disease Burden

From the middle years of the twentieth century until now, the burden of disease due to measles, mumps, and rubella ("German measles") has been largely eliminated through widespread vaccination against these three viruses. In the United States the annual number of reported cases dropped from 503,000 to below 100 for measles, 152,000 to below 700 for mumps, and 50,000 to below 400 for rubella. Measles outbreaks occurred because the virus is highly contagious, with an attack rate among unvaccinated household contacts of 90% or higher. Infected persons may transmit the disease from 4 days prior to until 4 days after the appearance of the rash.

Vaccine

The live, highly attenuated measles vaccine currently used in the United States is from the Enders–Edmonston strain. Following measles vaccination, seroconversion rates are 95% for children vaccinated at 12 months of age and 98% for children vaccinated at 15 months of age. Antibody persists for at least 17 years and probably life-long in almost all vaccinated persons who initially seroconvert. Of the few whose antibody level wanes, most are probably still immune because they have secondary immune responses upon revaccination.

Two factors may contribute to inadequate protection from the first dose of measles vaccine: lack of initial seroconversion and waning immunity. Lack of initial seroconversion is usually due to the presence of higher initial titers of passively acquired antibody. Mothers whose immunity was acquired actively rather than passively (by vaccination) confer higher initial levels of immunity to their children, resulting in longer periods of protection for the infant. When most mothers had actively acquired immunity to measles infection, the immunity in their infants lasted until an average age of 11 months or more, and seroconversion rates were optimal when administration of MMR vaccine was delayed until children were 15 months of age.

Because the usual source of maternal immunity to measles is now vaccination, the duration of immunity in infants decreased, to about 9 months, resulting in a higher proportion of children experiencing a period of inadequate protection from measles. This window in coverage probably accounts for the fact that in 1990, 26% of measles cases occurred in children under 16 months of age. In response to these findings, in 1994 the ACIP changed the recommendation for the first dose of MMR from 15 months of age to 12–15 months of age. Failure of seroconversion after the initial dose of measles vaccine occurs at a rate of 2–5%. In comparison, the rate of secondary vaccine failure, also known as waning immunity, has been reported to be less than 0.2%.

A. EFFICACY

MMR vaccine is 95% efficacious against measles disease at age 12 months for all three diseases and 98% at age 15 months. After two doses more than 99% of persons are immune. Vaccination of already immune individuals is not harmful.

Adverse Reactions

Pain, irritation, and redness at the site of injection are common but mild. Delayed reactions to measles vaccine include fever that is usually below 38.8°C (102°F) or rash of 2–5 days duration, occurring 5–20 days later. Adverse reactions to rubella vaccine include generalized lymphadenopathy and arthralgia in young women, with no reported long-term arthritis. Adverse reactions to mumps vaccine include transient orchitis in young men. Concern that the measles vaccine is linked to autism appears to be erroneous. Rarely, thrombocytopenia is reported.

Recommendations

The MMR vaccine, 0.5 mL subcutaneously, is routinely given to all healthy children at age 12–15 months, with a second dose at age 4–6 years.

American Academy of Pediatrics: Measles. In: *2000 Red Book: Report of the Committee on Infectious Diseases.* Pickering LK (editor). AAP, 2000: 385.

Dales L, Hammer SJ, Smith NJ: Time trends in autism and in MMR immunization coverage in California. JAMA 2001; 285(9):1183.

VARICELLA VACCINE

Disease Burden

During childhood, the highly contagious varicella-zoster virus (VZV) most often causes chickenpox, which is generally a self-limited and benign illness. Prior to varicella vaccine, roughly 4 million cases of VZV infection occurred annually in the United States with a hospitalization rate of five cases per 1000 population and a death rate of 0.7 per 100,000. Because secondary attack rates are as high as 90% and because communicability by aerosol droplet begins 1–2 days prior to the rash, prevention of spread requires a universal vaccination program. Complications include secondary bacterial skin infection (both impetigo and invasive group A streptococcal disease), pneumonia, Reye syndrome, and encephalomeningitis. The lifetime risk of the late complication of herpes zoster is 10%.

VZV is most severe in neonates and in adults. However, the largest numbers of hospitalizations occur in the 1–4 year age group because VZV is so common at those ages. Most hospitalized individuals are immunologically normal but many develop the secondary complications mentioned above, sometimes with fatal outcomes. Routine vaccination is a cost-effective measure to reduce VZV morbidity and mortality. Each $1 spent on universal immunization of children avoids approximately $5 in costs.

Vaccine

The current varicella vaccine contains live attenuated virus (Oka strain) and is 97% effective against moderately severe and severe disease and 85% protective for any infection for at least 7 years. When vaccinees do get disease, it is mild, with fewer than 30 pox lesions.

Because varicella vaccine is less immunogenic in older children and adults, a second dose is required in those aged 13 years and older. The seroconversion rate in these individuals is 67–85% after one dose and 94–100% after the second dose, given 4–8 weeks later.

The long-term duration of vaccine-induced immunity is unknown. The concern that widespread vaccination of children would shift the disease burden to adults with waning antibody levels remains unsettled. However, recent surveillance data show that cases have declined in all age groups. One expert panel estimated that a child given one dose of varicella vaccine might have a 15% chance of eventual inadequate immunity over a lifetime. Furthermore, repeated exposure to wild varicella in the community should at least in the immediate future boost antibody levels. Continued surveillance of vaccine-induced antibody levels is in progress. Protective antibody levels have persisted for longer than 20 years in Japan. Mathematical models show that the overall numbers of hospitalizations would decrease with varicella vaccination on a national basis, even if immunity fails more rapidly than expected.

Adverse Reactions

Local pain and erythema occur in 2–20% of children and 10–25% of adults after the first dose. Up to 47% develop local reactions with the second dose. From 4% to 10% develop a few (median of five) varicella-like lesions 5–41 days after administration; these last 2–8 days. Low-grade fever develops in 12–30% of vaccinees up to 42 days later and is of brief duration. Vaccine virus has been rarely transmitted to healthy immunocompetent siblings and parents, especially if the vaccinee developed a varicelliform rash or had leukemia, but no major ill effects have resulted. To date, the risk for zoster is less among vaccinees than those who had natural infection.

Recommendations

The ACIP, AAFP, and AAP recommend that children age 12 months up to 13 years be given one dose, 0.5 mL subcutaneously, unless they have a history of prior varicella infection. Vaccine is also approved for persons 13 years of age and older without a history of chickenpox on a two-dose schedule spaced 4–8 weeks apart. Because about 70–90% of adults without a history of chickenpox are actually immune, serological tests may be cost efficient, but are not required because the vaccine is well tolerated in these individuals. Testing may also make sense in 9- to 12-year-old children with uncertain VZV histories who are often already immune. Varicella vaccine is effective in preventing or modifying varicella if given within 3 days (and possibly up to 5 days) of exposure to wild varicella.

Salicylate therapy should theoretically be avoided for 6 weeks after vaccination due to the association between aspirin use and Reye syndrome following varicella. Households with immunocompromised persons require no special precautions unless the vaccinee develops a rash, after which direct contact should be avoided. Immunocompromised contacts who develop a rash may require antiviral therapy.

Arvin AM: Varicella vaccine—the first six years. New Engl J Med 2001;(344):1007.

Centers for Disease Control and Prevention: Prevention of varicella: recommendations of the Advisory Committee on Immunization Practices (ACIP). MMWR 1996;45:1.

Salzman MB, Garcia C: Postexposure varicella vaccination in siblings of children with active varicella. Pediatr Infect Dis J 1998;17(3):256.

Seward JF et al: Varicella disease after introduction of varicella vaccine in the United States, 1995–2000. JAMA 2002;287(5):606.

Vazquez M et al: The effectiveness of varicella vaccine in clinical practice. New Engl J Med 2001;344:955.

HEPATITIS A VACCINE

Vaccinations for children at high risk due to medical conditions, environmental risks, or life-style are a complex topic that is covered elsewhere. In 1999, the ACIP recommended routine hepatitis A vaccination of children in states, counties, or communities with hepatitis A rates that are twice the 1987–1997 national range or greater (ie, 20 or more cases per 100,000 population). Consideration should be given to routine vaccination of children in states, counties, or communities with rates exceeding the 1987–1997 national average (ie, at least 10 but not more than 20 cases per 100,000 population). The Centers for Disease Control and Prevention (CDC) has a map with hepatitis A rates at www.cdc.gov/ncidod/diseases/hepatitis/a/vax/index.htm.

INFLUENZA VACCINE

Annual influenza vaccination is recommended for routine use in children 6–23 months of age. Annual influenza vaccination with trivalent inactivated influenza vaccine is also recommended for children 2 or more years of age with specific risk factors, including asthma and other chronic diseases and close contacts of high risk persons.

Previously unvaccinated children under 9 years of age should receive two doses, at least 1 month apart. Children who have received vaccine in prior years require only one dose in subsequent years. Dosage of inactivated vaccine varies by age: 0.5 mL intramuscularly for persons 3 years of age and older and 0.25 mL intramuscularly for children 6–35 months of age. In 2003, live attenuated influenza vaccines were licensed for healthy persons 5–49 years of age.

Centers for Disease Control and Prevention: Prevention of hepatitis a through active or passive immunization: recommendations of the Advisory Committee on Immunization Practices (ACIP). MMWR 1999;48(RR12):1.

Zimmerman RK, Middleton DB, Smith NJ: Vaccines for persons at high risk due to medical conditions, occupation, environment or lifestyle. J Fam Pract 2001;50:S21.

VACCINATION PROCEDURES

Late Vaccinations & Interrupted Schedules

If the childhood vaccination schedule is started late, or if the child is more than 1 month late receiving a dose of vaccine, then the catch-up vaccination schedule should be used (Tables 7–3 and 7–4). Because the number of doses varies by age and by the presence of high-risk medical conditions, special schedules exist for catch-up vaccination when the series is started late for Hib vaccine (Table 7–5) and for pneumococcal conjugate vaccine (PCV) (Table 7–6), or when a lapse in PCV immunization has occurred (Table 7–7). If the vaccination schedule is interrupted, it need not be restarted. Instead, the schedule should be resumed using minimal intervals (see Tables 7–3 and 7–4).

Minimal Intervals & Interference

Doses of a particular vaccine that are given too close together or at less than the minimum age may be less immunogenic than appropriately spaced doses. However, because doses given a few days early are likely to be immunogenic, national authorities allow a 4 day grace period. Doses given ≥5 days earlier than the minimum interval should not be counted as valid and, thus, should be repeated. The repeat dose should be spaced by at least the minimum interval from the invalid dose.

The potential for interference between licensed vaccines is not a problem either for different inactivated vaccines or for inactivated vaccines given simultaneously with live viral vaccines. However, interference has occurred if the parentally administered live viral vaccines MMR and varicella are not administered on the same day or at least 4 weeks apart. If this occurs, the vaccine administered second should be considered invalid and should be repeated at an interval of at least 4 weeks from the invalid dose. Live attenuated influenza vaccine should not be administered within 4 weeks of other live-viral vaccines until more data are available.

Simultaneous Vaccination & Combination Vaccines

Simultaneous administration of routine vaccines (eg, administering MMR vaccine and varicella vaccine at

Table 7–3. Catch-up schedule for children age 4 months through 6 years.

Dose One (Minimum Age)	Minimum Interval between Doses			
	Dose One to Dose Two	Dose Two to Dose Three	Dose Three to Dose Four	Dose Four to Dose Five
DTaP (6 weeks)	4 weeks	4 weeks	6 months	6 months[1]
IPV (6 weeks)	4 weeks	4 weeks	4 weeks[2]	
HepB[3] (birth)	4 weeks	8 weeks (and 16 weeks after first dose)		
MMR (12 months)	4 weeks[4]			
Varicella (12 months)				
HIB[5] (6 weeks)	4 weeks: if first dose given at age <12 months 8 weeks (as final dose): if first dose given at age 12–14 months No further doses needed: if first dose given at age ≥15 months	4 weeks[6] if current age <12 months 8 weeks (as final dose)[6]: if current age ≥12 months and second dose given at age <15 months No further doses needed: if previous dose given at age ≥15 months	8 weeks (as final dose): this dose necessary only for children age 12 months–5 years who received three doses before age 12 months	
PCV[7] (6 weeks)	4 weeks: if first dose given at age <12 months and current age <24 months 8 weeks (as final dose): if first dose given at age ≥12 months or current age 24–59 months No further doses needed: for healthy children if first dose given at age ≥24 months	4 weeks: if current age <12 months 8 weeks (as final dose): if current age ≥12 months No further doses needed: for healthy children if previous dose given at age ≥24 months	8 weeks (as final dose): this dose necessary only for children age 12 months–5 years who received doses before age 12 months	

From General Recommendations on Immunization, Centers for Disease Control and Prevention, Atlanta, GA.

[1]DTaP: The fifth dose is not necessary if the dose was given after the fourth birthday.

[2]IPV: For children who received an all-IPV or all-OPV series, a fourth dose is not necessary if the third dose was given at age ≥4 years. If both OPV and IPV were given as part of a series, a total of four doses should be given, regardless of the child's current age.

[3]HepB: All children and adolescents who have not been immunized against hepatitis B should begin the hepatitis B vaccination series during any visit. Providers should make special efforts to immunize children who were born in, or whose parents were born in, areas of the world in which hepatitis B virus infection is moderately or highly endemic.

[4]MMR: The second dose of MMR is recommended routinely at age 4–6 years, but may be given earlier if desired.

[5]Hib: Vaccine is not generally recommended for children age ≥5 years.

[6]Hib: If current age <12 months and the first two doses were PRP–OMP (PedvaxHIB or ComVAX), the third (and final) dose should be given at age 12–15 months and at least 8 weeks after the second dose.

[7]PCV: Vaccine is not generally recommended for children age ≥5 years.

Table 7–4. Catch-up schedule for children age 7 through 18 years.

Minimum Interval between Doses		
Dose One to Dose Two	**Dose Two to Dose Three**	**Dose Three to Booster Dose**

Td: 4 weeks	Td: 6 months	Td[1]:
		  6 months: if first dose given at age <12 months and current age <11 years
		  5 years: if first dose given at age ≥12 months and third dose given at age <7 years and current age ≥11 years
		  10 years: if third dose given at age ≥7 years

IPV[2]: 4 weeks	IPV[2]: 4 weeks	IPV[2]
HepB: 4 weeks	HepB: 8 weeks (and 16 weeks after the first dose)	
MMR: 4 weeks		
Varicella[3]: 4 weeks		

From General Recommendations on Immunization, Centers for Disease Control and Prevention, Atlanta, GA.
[1]Td: For children age 7–10 years, the interval between the third and booster dose is determined by the age when the first dose was given. For adolescents age 11–18 years, the interval is determined by the age when the third dose was given.
[2]IPV: Vaccine is not generally recommended for persons age ≥18 years.
[3]Varicella: Give two-dose series to all susceptible adolescents age ≥13 years.

Table 7–5. Detailed vaccination schedule for *Haemophilus influenzae* type b conjugate vaccines including when starting the series late.

Vaccine[1]	**Age at First Dose (Months)**	**Primary Series**	**Booster**
HbOC or PRP-T	2–6	Three doses, 2 months apart	12–15 months
	7–11	Two doses, 2 months apart	12–18 months
	12–14	One dose	2 months later
	15–59	One dose	—
PRP-OMP	2–6	Two doses, 2 months apart	12–15 months
	7–11	Two doses, 2 months apart	12–18 months
	12–14	One dose	2 months later
	15–59	One dose	—
PRP-D	15–59	One dose	—

Modified from Centers for Disease Control and Prevention. National Immunization Program: *Epidemiology and Prevention of Vaccine-Preventable Diseases*, ed 4. Centers for Disease Control and Prevention, 1997: 110. Public domain.
[1]Hib, *Haemophilus influenzae* type b; HbOC, Hib vaccine conjugated with diphtheria toxoid; PRP-T, Hib vaccine conjugated with tetanus toxoid; PRP-OMP, Hib vaccine conjugated with *Neisseria meningitidis* group B; PRP-D, Hib vaccine conjugated with diphtheria toxoid.

Table 7–6. Schedule for administration of pneumococcal conjugate vaccine in unvaccinated infants and children including catch-up for those starting late.

Age at First Dose (Months)	Primary Series	Booster Dose
2–6	Three doses, 2 months apart[1]	One dose at 12–15 months[2]
7–11	Two doses, 2 months apart[1]	One dose at 12–15 months[2]
12–23	Two doses, 2 months apart	—

24–59
   Healthy children[3]
   Children with sickle cell disease, asplenia, HIV infection, chronic illness, or immunocompromising condition[4,5]
	
	 One dose
	 Two doses, 2 months apart
		
		 —
		 —

Adapted from Preventing Pneumococcal Disease Among Infants and Young Children, Recommendations of the Advisory Committee on Immunization Practices: MMWR 2000;49 (No. RR-9):24. Public domain.
[1] For the primary series in children vaccinated prior to 12 months of age, the minimum interval between doses is 4 weeks.
[2] The booster dose should be administered at least 8 weeks after the primary series is completed.
[3] With priority given to the following populations at higher risk for invasive pneumococcal disease: children aged 24–35 months, children of Alaska Native or American Indian descent, children of African-American descent, and children who attend group day care centers.
[4] Recommendations do not include children who have undergone bone marrow transplant.
[5] Pneumococcal polysaccharide vaccine is also recommended for high-risk children.

the same visit) is both immunogenic and safe and is, therefore, recommended to increase vaccination rates and avoid missed opportunities to vaccinate.

To reduce the number of injections and costs of stocking and administering separate vaccines, combination vaccine products are preferred over separate products. Extra doses of an antigen are permitted when the benefits are felt to outweigh the risk. Thus, an office that stocks the Hib– hepatitis B combination vaccine instead of monovalent Hib vaccine could give the Hib–hepatitis B combination for all doses of Hib. This is permissible even though some children receive a dose of hepatitis B vaccine at birth and thus would have received four doses, one dose more than required. Hib vaccine and Hib–hepatitis B combination vaccines should not be given earlier than 6 weeks of age because of decreased response to the Hib component.

Table 7–7. Vaccination schedule for pneumococcal conjugate vaccine (PCV) when a lapse in immunization has occurred.

Age at Presentation (Months)	Previous PCV Immunization History	Recommended Regimen
7–11	One dose	One dose PCV at 7–11 months followed by a booster dose at 12–15 months of age with a minimal interval of 2 months
	Two doses	One dose PCV at 7–11 months followed by a booster dose at 12–15 months of age with a minimal interval of 2 months
12–23	One dose before age 12 months	Two doses of PCV, at least 2 months apart
	Two doses before age 12 months	One dose of PCV, at least 2 months following the most recent dose
24–59	Any incomplete schedule	One dose of PCV[1]

Adapted from Preventing Pneumococcal Disease Among Infants and Young Children, Recommendations of the Advisory Committee on Immunization Practices: MMWR 2000;49 (No. RR-9):24. Public domain.
[1] Children with certain chronic diseases or immunosuppressing conditions should receive two doses at least 2 months apart (see Tables 7–3 and 7–4).

Interchangeability of Vaccines from Different Manufacturers

Vaccines from different manufacturers to prevent the same disease may be interchanged when a particular antibody is known to protect against disease (called the serologic correlate of immunity) and when these vaccines result in protective antibody titers. Protective titers occur when hepatitis B, hepatitis A, and conjugate Hib vaccines from different manufacturers are used in series. PRP-OMPC Hib vaccine requires only two doses in the first year of life at 2 and 4 months of age if it is the only Hib vaccine given (a third dose is recommended at 12–15 months of age). However, if PRP-OMPC and Hib vaccine from another manufacturer are interchanged in the first year of life, then three doses are recommended for the infant series (a fourth dose is recommended at 12–15 months of age).

For diseases in which the serologic correlate of immunity is unknown, such as pertussis, use of a vaccine from a single manufacturer is preferred until studies confirm that good protection occurs when vaccines from different manufacturers are given in series. If for a child's previous dose the manufacturer is unknown or that manufacturer's product is not available, any product may be used, rather than miss the opportunity to vaccinate.

Contraindications

There are two permanent contraindications to administering a dose of vaccine: (1) severe allergy to a vaccine component or anaphylactic reaction to a previous dose of the vaccine and (2) encephalopathy without a known cause within 7 days of a dose of pertussis vaccine. Contact dermatitis from neomycin is a delayed-type, cell-mediated immune response and is not a contraindication to vaccination. Egg allergy is not a contraindication to MMR, because the vaccine does not contain egg albumin; previous anaphylactic reactions following MMR may be due to gelatin. If the pertussis component is withheld because of a contraindication or precaution, pediatric DT should be administered instead, except in the case of true anaphylaxis, in which the diphtheria and pertussis components are permanently contraindicated. In such cases, referral may be made to an allergist to assess whether tetanus toxoid can be given or for possible desensitization to tetanus toxoid.

There are four conditions generally considered temporary contraindications to vaccination: (1) severe acute illness, (2) immunosuppression, (3) pregnancy, and (4) recent receipt of blood products.

Severe acute illness (eg, pneumonia requiring antibiotics and bronchodilators) usually warrants postponement of vaccination until the patient has recovered from the acute phase of illness. Fever itself is not a contraindication to vaccination.

Immunosuppression (due to an immune deficiency disease, malignancy, or therapy with high-dose corticosteroid drugs, alkylating agents, antimetabolites, or radiation) is generally a contraindication to administration of a live vaccine. Inactivated vaccines lacking live organisms that can replicate may be given to immunosuppressed persons. However, immunosuppression may decrease the response to vaccination. There are two exceptions to this general principle: (1) HIV-infected persons who are not severely immunosuppressed should receive MMR vaccine when otherwise indicated based on age; and (2) although varicella vaccine remains contraindicated in cellular immunodeficiencies, it now may be given to those with humoral immunodeficiencies. Children infected with HIV are at increased risk for morbidity from varicella and herpes zoster (ie, shingles) compared with healthy children. The ACIP recommends that after weighing potential risks and benefits two doses of varicella vaccine spaced 3 months apart should be considered for asymptomatic or mildly symptomatic HIV-infected children in CDC class N1 or A1 with age-specific CD4$^+$ T-lymphocyte percentages of ≥25% (see ACIP recommendations for details). Because persons with impaired cellular immunity may be at greater risk for complications after vaccination with a live-virus vaccine, these vaccinees should return for evaluation if they experience a postvaccination reaction such as a varicella-like rash.

Pregnancy is a contraindication to administration of live-virus vaccines such as live attenuated influenza vaccine because of the theoretical risk that the live virus could damage the fetus. Furthermore, women should avoid becoming pregnant within 28 days of receiving MMR, measles, mumps, rubella, or varicella vaccine. Inadvertent administration of a live-virus vaccine during pregnancy is not an indication for termination of pregnancy because no data link live-virus vaccination to an increased risk of fetal malformations. Inactivated influenza vaccine and Td may be used in pregnancy. Unless otherwise contraindicated, all vaccines may be given to breast-feeding mothers.

Recent administration of blood products can interfere with development of an immune response to a live-virus but not to an inactivated vaccine. For instance, MMR may not be effective if given within 6 months after receipt of whole blood and within 8–10 months of receipt of large doses of intravenous immunoglobulin. Tables have been published that describe when various vaccines may be administered in such cases.

Precautions

Precautions for vaccination are conditions that *may* increase the risk for a serious adverse event or may compromise the ability of the vaccine to produce immunity.

Whether to vaccinate in such cases involves weighing the individual patient's risk of acquiring the disease against the risk of the adverse event or the inability to produce immunity. Generally, the vaccine is withheld or postponed in high adverse risk situations. Certain infrequent adverse events occurring after pertussis vaccination are precautions to further doses: (1) temperature of $\geq 40.5°C$ (105°F), not due to another identifiable cause, within 48 h of a previous dose, (2) collapse or a shock-like state (hypotonic–hyporesponsive episode) with 48 h of a previous dose, (3) persistent, inconsolable crying lasting 3 h or more, occurring within 48 h of a previous dose, or (4) convulsions within 3 days of a previous dose.

DTaP vaccination should be postponed for infants with an evolving neurological disorder, unevaluated seizures, or a neurological event between doses of DTaP. Vaccination should be resumed after evaluation and treatment of the condition.

Vaccine Information Statements for Patients

Patients or their legal guardians should receive information that is easy to understand about the benefits and risks of vaccination. Under the Public Health Service Act, health care providers who administer any routine childhood vaccine are required to provide a copy of the relevant Vaccine Information Statements (VISs) to the patient or guardian prior to vaccination, even if the patient is an adult. These VISs may be viewed and downloaded from the following web sites in multiple languages: http://www.cdc.gov/nip/vistable.htm or http://www.immunize.org/vis/index.htm. If a VIS is not available, the physician should provide information about the disease risk, the protection afforded by vaccination, the risk of adverse events to a vaccine, and what to do if a serious adverse event occurs.

Adverse Reaction Reporting

Health care providers are required to report certain adverse reactions and may report any adverse reactions following vaccination to the Vaccine Adverse Event Reporting System (VAERS). VAERS forms and instructions can be obtained by calling 1-800-822-7967.

Vaccine Injury Compensation Program

The Vaccine Injury Compensation Program (VICP) is a system under which no-fault compensation can be awarded for specified injuries that are temporally related to administration of specified vaccinations, typically the vaccines for children. For vaccines covered by the VICP, the program has reduced the risk of litigation for both providers and vaccine manufacturers following adverse advents. Information about specific adverse events that are covered is available from the Health Resources and Services Administration by telephoning 1-800-338-2382.

Providers who administer vaccines covered by the VICP are required to record, either in an office log or the recipient's permanent medical record, the date of vaccine administration; the vaccine's manufacturer and lot number; and the name, address, and title of the person administering the vaccine.

American Academy of Pediatrics Committee on Infectious Diseases: *Red Book 2000: Report of the Committee on Infectious Diseases,* ed 25. AAP, 2000.

Centers for Disease Control and Prevention: Prevention of varicella: updated recommendations of the Advisory Committee on Immunization Practices (ACIP). MMWR 1999;48(RR-6):1.

Centers for Disease Control and Prevention: General recommendations on immunization: recommendations of the Advisory Committee on Immunization Practices and the American Academy of Family Physicians. MMWR 2002;51(RR-2):1.

Disruptive Behavioral Disorders in Children

8

William S. Sykora, MD, Col, USAF, MC

We expect our children to be active and energetic. They bounce from one activity to another as they explore and learn about their environment. Children get bored easily with tasks they do not enjoy and they react naturally, emotionally, and without forethought to the events around them. We anticipate and celebrate this *joie de vivre*. But when children exceed the norms for their age in their displays of activity, or their lack of impulse control, or their inability to focus their attention, they are likely to experience a number of problems in their social, familial, academic, and emotional interactions. Overly active, inattentive, and impulsive children find themselves less able than their peers to be organized, self-sufficient, reflective, responsible, and productive. They are often seen as lazy, unmotivated, selfish, immature, irresponsible, and "out-of-control." Society can be unkind to these children, handing out judgments, punishments, and outright rejection. Self-esteem is adversely affected and these individuals are at greater risk of developing antisocial disorders, substance abuse disorders, academic failure, employment failure, and secondary mood and anxiety disorders. These behavioral variants, therefore, cause a significant social burden and are often brought to the attention of primary care physicians. This chapter will address three Axis I childhood behavioral problems likely to be encountered in the primary care setting—attention deficit/hyperactivity disorder (ADHD), oppositional defiant disorder (ODD), and conduct disorder (CD).

These diagnoses represent a spectrum of increasing societal dysfunction. The essential feature of ADHD is "a persistent pattern of inattention and/or hyperactivity-impulsivity that is more frequently displayed and more severe than is typically observed in individuals at a comparable stage of development." The essential features of ODD are a persistent pattern of "negativistic, defiant, disobedient and hostile behavior towards authority figures" that leads to a significant impairment. The essential features of CD are a repetitive and persistent pattern of "behavior in which the basic rights of others and major age-appropriate societal norms are violated." The comorbidity of these conditions is significant with up to a third of ADHD children also having ODD and a quarter of ADHD children having CD.

This overlap has a great effect on overall prognosis and outcome. It is therefore appropriate to look at these conditions together.

History and literature have been filled with stories of "hyperactive" and "bad" children. They were almost all boys and they almost always came to a sad end. In 1937, neurostimulants were, surprisingly, shown to have a calming effect on many of these children. This led to interest in the hyperactive and impulse control aspects of the disorders, resulting in the concept of the "hyperactive child syndrome" of the 1960s. In the 1970s, the emphasis shifted to the inattentive problems and impulse control and in 1980 the *Diagnostic and Statistical Manual of Mental Disorders—III (DSM-III)* labeled the conditions as attention deficit disorder (ADD) and conduct disorder and introduced oppositional disorder. This was also the first time a distinction was made between the hyperactive and inattentive types of ADD. In *DSM-III-R* (revised) the current label of ADHD was given. Further clarification of the diagnostic criteria of these three behavioral conditions was made in the *International Classification of Diseases (ICD-10)* in 1993 by the World Health Organization and in *DSM-IV* in 1994 by the American Psychiatric Association. There are minor differences in the International and American criteria and, in the United States, the *DSM-IV* criteria form the basis for diagnostic and treatment guidelines.

There has been controversy as to whether these problems are really valid disorders and not just the inattentive and disruptive end of the normal continuum of human behaviors. This situation is not unique as many conditions, such as hypertension and depression, are continuous in our population yet their diagnosis and treatment are well established in modern medicine. Because there is no single independent valid and reliable test for these behavioral conditions, their existence has been questioned. Controversy has also surrounded the use of controlled substances in the routine treatment of these conditions and the dramatic increase in the manufacture (500% increase in Ritalin production during the 1990s) and use of neurostimulants. These debates are irrelevant to the individuals who exhibit the patterns of behavior that define these conditions. Parents,

94

teachers, and patients continue to come to their physicians to seek help. The object of this chapter is to provide current information on the diagnosis and treatment of these behavioral disorders in children.

ATTENTION DEFICIT/HYPERACTIVITY DISORDER

 ESSENTIALS OF DIAGNOSIS

- *A persistent pattern of inattention and/or hyperactivity. More frequent and severe displays of impulsivity.*
- *Academic underachievement and behavioral problems.*

General Considerations

Up to 20% of school-age children in the United States have behavioral problems and at least half of these involve difficulties with attention or hyperactivity. Attention deficit/hyperactivity disorder is the most common and well-studied of the childhood behavioral disorders. We have all noticed classically hyperactive children and their beleaguered parents and teachers in our practices and in our social interactions, but have also totally missed the quiet but inattentive "daydreamer." The seeming dichotomy between the hyperactive and the inattentive types of ADHD can be confusing to both clinicians and the public. Family physicians and pediatricians should be familiar with the features of this disorder and are ideally positioned to evaluate and treat the majority of children and families dealing with this condition.

Pressures from frustrated parents and teachers for a "quick fix" to these problems should not prevent a thoughtful analysis of the situation and consideration of the differential diagnosis for ADHD. Proper evaluation and treatment for ADHD can result in very rewarding success in helping these children cope with symptoms that for two of three represent a lifelong condition. The physician must understand the spectrum of this condition, the common comorbidities, and both behavioral and medical treatment modalities to maximize the potential of those affected. To empower patients and their families, the treating physician must also be familiar with the school system as well as community and national resources. Dealing with this condition in many ways defines the true spirit of family medicine and the full spectrum of patient advocacy.

Many of the controversial issues surrounding ADHD were addressed by the 1998 NIH Consensus Conference and its resulting Consensus Statement. The conclusions were that ADHD is a valid diagnosis with established criteria that has a significant impact on individuals and society, that effective therapies exist, that stimulant medication was the most effective therapy, and that proper use of stimulants was safe but longer term studies were needed. This Consensus Statement provided a framework for further work in this complicated field.

Pathogenesis

To date neurophysiological data suggest that there is no single cognitive or behavioral deficit common to all individuals with ADHD. The problem may be more with response inhibition and other executive functions than with attention and hyperactivity. Emerging data suggest that individuals with ADHD have abnormalities in the frontal-striatal circuits, but the exact problem has not been isolated. Morphological and functional imaging studies implicate the prefrontal cortex, which usually exhibits inhibitory control over motor functions, and the basal ganglia as possible sites for the etiology of ADHD but are yet inconclusive. Dopamine and catecholamine systems also appear to be affected in this area of the brain, but the exact role or defect is unknown. Therefore, imaging studies and blood testing are of little utility to the clinical evaluation of ADHD without comorbidity.

Based on current behavioral models for ADHD the primary defect is a lack of behavioral inhibition, which then affects four executive functions: (1) prolongation and working memory, (2) self-regulation of affect/motivation/arousal, (3) internalization of speech, and (4) reconstitution. These executive functions then affect motor control and fluency. This model helps to provide some conceptual framework to the behaviors seen in ADHD and areas in which medications or cognitive and behavior modification therapy may play a role.

There is good evidence that ADHD is *not* caused by too much television (although patients may be attracted and distracted by it), by food allergies (although the rare child may display inattention secondary to such allergies), by excess sugar, artificial flavorings, colorings, or preservatives in food, by poor home life or parenting skills (although the behaviors characteristic of ADHD do set up the classic parent–child confrontation seen in ODD and account for some of that common comorbidity), or by poor schools or teachers. Data suggest that maternal smoking and use of cocaine and alcohol during pregnancy could contribute to the development of ADHD in some children. Fetal alcohol syndrome results in similar problems with hyperactivity, inattention, and impulsivity.

Epidemiology/Cultural Demographics

Prevalence estimates for ADHD vary depending on methodology. The estimate of prevalence in school-aged children in *DSM-IV* is 3–5%. Other studies show prevalence in approximately 20% of the school-aged population. The male to female ratio is estimated at 4 to 1 for the hyperactive type of ADHD and 2 to 1 for the inattentive type. However, teachers identify fewer girls than boys and even females identified as having symptoms of ADHD are less likely to be labeled with the diagnosis or given treatment. This gender bias of teachers has yet to be studied or explained. For ADHD alone, without comorbid factors such as conduct disorder, there is no difference along socioeconomic classes. Cultural variations in prevalence are difficult to interpret as the ranges of prevalences in different cultures are also very wide. Prevalences as high as 22% were found in school-aged boys in New Zealand and 29% in India. Among ethnic groups in the United States, teacher ratings, which always run the highest, had prevalence rates of 24% for African-American children and 16% for white and Latino-American children. These minor differences seem to disappear when controlled for behavioral prejudices. It would seem that ADHD arises across ethnic groups and, although cultural and ethnic factors may cause variations in the diagnosis, there is no cultural or ethnic component to the etiology and true prevalence of ADHD.

Studies of adopted children support a substantial genetic contribution to ADHD. Studies show that siblings have a two to three times higher risk of having ADHD than normal controls. Concordance is higher in full siblings than half siblings and higher in identical twins than dizygotic twins. The parents of children with ADHD have a higher than average incidence of the condition and a higher incidence of other psychiatric problems. Relatives of children with ADHD but without CD have a higher incidence of mood problems, anxiety disorders, and learning disabilities. Relatives of children with both ADHD and CD are more likely to have CD, antisocial personality disorder, substance abuse problems, depression, and marital dysfunction.

ADHD was long considered a problem of school-aged children. Evidence now favors a lifelong process and struggle. It has even been suggested that hyperactivity starts in the womb. Preschoolers who are likely to develop symptoms of ADHD once in school are being identified with great predictability. Of children with ADHD up to 80% have features of the disorder into adolescence and 65% into adulthood. The family physician is ideally placed to help across the spectrum.

Clinical Findings

A. SYMPTOMS AND SIGNS

There is no single diagnostic test or tool for ADHD. The diagnosis in children is dependent on adults' reports of symptoms and behaviors. The diagnostic criteria established in *DSM-IV* by the American Psychiatric Association in 1994 are the current basis for the identification of individuals with ADHD. Meeting these criteria (Table 8–1) does not exclude the possibility of other conditions and the full differential diagnosis must be considered by the evaluating physician.

The American Academy of Child and Adolescent Psychiatry and the American Academy of Pediatrics (AAP), with input from members of the American Academy of Family Physicians, have formulated evidence-based practice guidelines to aid in the improvement of current diagnostic and treatment practices as identified in the NIH Consensus Statement. The AAP partnered with the Agency for Healthcare Research and Quality along with the Evidence-based Practice Center at McMaster University, Ontario, Canada, to produce these guidelines. The diagnosis is made by parent interview, by direct observation, by the use of standardized and scored behavioral checklists that are specific for ADHD, and by input from both the parents and the teachers. The standard for diagnosis on the checklists is two standard deviations above the mean in the number of ADHD symptoms displayed. Broader based scales are not recommended for diagnosis, secondary to the high prevalence of comorbid conditions that may be responsible for the scores, but can be useful for follow-up and management.

ADHD was once considered a disorder of hyperkinesis, but with the *DSM-IV* criteria inattention and hyperactivity are equally emphasized as core features. Three subtypes of ADHD are recognized (see Table 8–1): predominantly inattentive (which accounts for 20–30% of ADHD individuals), predominantly hyperactive–impulsive (which accounts for less than 15%), and the combined subtype (the most common, which accounts for 50–75% of cases). This differentiation has significant prognostic implications. Individuals with the inattentive subtype have fewer behavioral problems but are subject to mood fluctuations. They also have more academic problems than those with the hyperactive subtype. Individuals with the combined subtype have the most comorbid psychiatric problems, the most problems with substance abuse, and are the most impaired.

Table 8–1. *DSM-IV-TR* diagnostic criteria for attention-deficit/hyperactivity disorder.

A. Either (1) or (2):

(1) Six (or more) of the following symptoms of **inattention** have persisted for at least 6 months to a degree that is maladaptive and inconsistent with developmental level:

Inattention

(a) often fails to give close attention to details or makes careless mistakes in schoolwork, work, or other activities

(b) often has difficulty sustaining attention in tasks or play activities

(c) often does not seem to listen when spoken to directly

(d) often does not follow through on instructions and fails to finish schoolwork, chores, or duties in the workplace (not due to oppositional behavior or failure to understand instructions)

(e) often has difficulty organizing tasks and activities

(f) often avoids, dislikes, or is reluctant to engage in tasks that require sustained mental effort (such as schoolwork or homework)

(g) often loses things necessary for tasks or activities (eg, toys, school assignments, pencils, books, or tools)

(h) is often easily distracted by extraneous stimuli

(i) is often forgetful in daily activities

(2) six (or more) of the following symptoms of **hyperactivity-impulsivity** have persisted for at least 6 months to a degree that is maladaptive and inconsistent with developmental level:

Hyperactivity

(a) often fidgets with hands or feet or squirms in seat

(b) leaves seat in classroom or in other situations in which remaining seated is expected

(c) often runs about or climbs excessively in situations in which it is inappropriate (in adolescents or adults, may be limited to subjective feelings of restlessness)

(d) often has difficulty playing or engaging in leisure activities quietly

(e) is often "on the go" or often acts as if "driven by a motor"

(f) often talks excessively

There are some limitations to the *DSM-IV* definition of ADHD. Although six is the current consensus, there are no clear empirical data indicating the number of items needed to support the diagnosis. Current criteria do not take gender or developmental differences into account. The behavioral characteristics are subjective and open to interpretation. Therefore the diagnosis remains a clinical one with input from parents and schools on the true impact of the symptoms on the achievement and relationships of the child. Other criteria exist, such as those for hyperkinetic disorders in the ICD-10 from the World Health Organization. They are similar to *DSM-IV* but allow for behaviors observed in the office and exclude children with anxiety, developmental, and depressive disorders. These differences in criteria may account for the differences in prevalence rates around the world.

Some children may not fully meet *DSM-IV* criteria. A useful reference for these children has been supplied by the AAP in their *Diagnostic and Statistical Manual for Primary Care (DSM-PC), Child and Adolescent Version*. The *DSM-PC* considers environmental and developmental influences on the more common variations in behavior to help in the diagnosis and management of children with ADHD.

B. LABORATORY FINDINGS

There is rarely a need for extensive laboratory analysis but screening for iron deficiency and thyroid dysfunction is reasonable.

C. COMORBIDITIES

ADHD is often associated with other Axis I diagnoses, especially in referred populations, which are represented in the majority of the studies. Of referred ADHD children 35–60% have ODD and 25–50% will develop CD. Of these 15–25% will progress to antisocial personality disorder in adulthood. Indeed, ADHD can be used as a reliable early predictor of disruptive behavior disorders. A family history of conduct problems helps with this prediction. It does appear that among children with ADHD, those who are most hyperactive–impulsive are at greatest risk for development of ODD. Nevertheless, it is possible to distinguish between the two disorders. ODD symptoms, such as "loses temper," "actively defies," and "swears," are less characteristic of children with ADHD.

Anxiety disorders seem to be more common in the predominantly inattentive type of ADHD, occurring in 25–40% of referred children. As many as 50% of referred ADHD children eventually develop a mood disorder, most commonly depression, and, most commonly, diagnosed in adolescence. There seems to be an association between the early diagnosis of ADHD and the risk of developing bipolar disease later in life. The diagnosis of bipolar disease in childhood increases the risk of the concurrent label of ADHD because of the overlap of behaviors. About 50% of children with Tourette's Syndrome have ADHD and the symptoms of ADHD usually precede the other symptoms of Tourette's. The medical treatment of Tourette's and ADHD is complicated by the effects of stimulant medications on tics. The determination of the coexistence of ADHD and Tourette's is vital in obtaining appropriate social and educational services for these children.

There appears to be a strong correlation between sleep disorders and ADHD. Children who snore are almost twice as likely to meet diagnostic criteria for ADHD than their nonsnoring counterparts and for younger (under age 8) males the risk is three times higher. Whether this is a cause and effect phenomenon needs further study, but this link should be kept in mind when taking a history.

There is a definite association between ADHD, academic problems, and learning disabilities. Between 20% and 50% of children with ADHD have at least one type of learning disorder. The large discrepancy in incidence is due to differences in the definition of a learning disability. If the criterion of two grades below grade level is used then up to 80% of ADHD children 12 and older could be defined as having learning disorders. In any child with ADHD, where academic achievement seems to lag behind intelligence, testing should be done for learning disabilities. The documentation of a learning disability makes it easier to obtain academic accommodations and modifications through individual educational plans as protected by the Individuals with Disabilities Education Act (IDEA). ADHD individuals have a higher risk of difficulties with reading, arithmetic, and writing. They are often very poor spellers and have poor handwriting. These are associated with difficulties with the executive functions of integration of working memory and motor coordination and fluency, all mediated by the lack of intact inhibitory processes.

There does not seem to be an association between intelligence and ADHD, although the verbal scores, mental arithmetic scores, and digital span scores in many IQ tests can be lower due to problems with working memory. These differences are gone when hyperactive behavior is factored out of the testing and are thought to be due to the methodology rather than true differences in intelligence. The true impact of ADHD is on the application of intelligence in everyday functioning and academic work.

Differential Diagnosis

See Table 8–2 for the differential diagnosis of ADHD.

Treatment

A. AAP Practice Guidelines

The American Academy of Pediatrics Committee on Quality Improvement again teamed with the Agency for Healthcare Research and Quality and the Evidence-based Practice Center at McMaster University, Ontario, Canada, to systemically review the literature on the treatment of ADHD and to formulate evidence-based clinical practice guidelines. Those guidelines are intended for the treatment of children aged 6 through 12, but the underlying principles are applicable to all age groups.

B. Pharmacological

1. Stimulants—In 1937 it was first reported that *dl*-amphetamine seemed to calm hyperactive children. Over the past 60 years these medications have become the most studied of any psychotropic agents used in children. Their efficacy in controlling some of the manifestations of ADHD has been proven, but they are not

Table 8–2. Differential diagnosis of ADHD.

General Medical Conditions	Neurological Conditions	Psychiatric Conditions	Environmental Conditions
Hearing impairment	Learning disability[1]	Conduct disorder[1]	Improper learning environment
Visual impairment	Tic disorders (eg, Tourette's)	Oppositional defiant disorder[1]	(eg, unsafe, disruptive)[1]
Medication effects (eg,	Seizures disorder	Substance abuse	Mismatch of school curriculum
antihistamine decongestants,	Mental retardation (eg,	Anxiety[1]	with child's ability (eg, gifted,
β-agonists, anticonvulsants)	fetal alcohol syndrome,	Obsessive–compulsive	learning-disabled)
Asthma	fragile X syndrome,	disorder[1]	Family dysfunction or stressful
Allergic rhinitis	phenylketonuria)	Posttraumatic stress	home environment[1]
Eczema	Developmental delays	disorder	Poor parenting (eg, inappro-
Enuresis[1]	Brain injury	Depression[1]	priate, inconsistent, punitive)[1]
Encopresis	Sleep disorders		Child neglect or abuse[1]
Malnutrition			Parental psychopathology[1]
Hypothyroidism			
Lead toxicity			

From Smocker, WD, Hedayat M: Evaluation and treatment of ADHD. Am Fam Physician 2001;64(5):817.
[1]Common comorbid and associated conditions.

a "cure." The fact that the stimulants are controlled substances (Schedule II) with an abuse potential justifies close scrutiny of their use. About 65% of children with ADHD will show improvement in the core symptoms of hyperactivity, inattention, and impulsivity with their first trial of a stimulant and up to 95% will respond when given appropriate trials of the various stimulants. The use of this class of medication for treatment of ADHD is therefore one of the most efficacious of all psychiatric interventions. The management of these medications can be complex and treatment failures may result more from improper treatment strategies than from ineffective medication.

The central mechanism of action of the psychostimulants remains unclear. Current theories of ADHD focus on the prefrontal cortex and the control of executive functions. Stimulants seem to have putative effects on central dopamine and norepinephrine pathways involved in frontal lobe function. By binding to the dopamine transporter, which results in increased synaptic dopamine, they may enhance the executive functions in the prefrontal cortex and improve inhibitory control and working memory. The pharmacokinetics of the stimulants are characterized by rapid absorption, low plasma protein binding, and rapid extracellular metabolism. Up to 80% may be excreted in the urine unchanged or deesterized. Therefore half-lives are short and frequent dosing or sustained release preparations are necessary. Response does not seem to be weight dependent so weight-dependent dosing strategies are not as helpful as with other medications. Plasma levels of these agents are not useful in determining optimal dosing.

Successful management of the stimulants in children with ADHD requires a systematic approach. This is an area that the NIH Consensus Conference found to be inconsistent among American physicians. The following model is one reasonable approach to initiate and follow stimulant therapy. It involves a (1) counseling phase, (2) titration phase, (3) maintenance phase, and (4) potential termination phase. Integrated into this model is a discussion of the various agents and the side effects of stimulants with their management.

a. Counseling phase—This phase begins with the decision to use stimulant medications and involves incorporating the parents and child in the process. The goals are to explain the rationale for the trial of the medication as well as both the expected positive and potential negative effects. Children must understand that the medication is coming from the physician in an effort to help them control the inattention and impulsivity that makes it hard for them to perform to everyone's expectations. They should know that the doctor

and not their parents or teachers is responsible for the treatment. The details of the treatment should also be discussed including the choice of medication, the dosage, and the expected frequency of follow-up. Parents should be told which behaviors to monitor, what side effects to expect, and how they will be dealt with. This session should also explain the expected changes in dosing, the timing of medications, and the anticipated eventual shift from short-acting to sustained-release preparations. An important aspect of this session is to determine the targeted symptoms, which will be unique for each child and family. The physician and parents need to review the child's symptoms and prioritize them based on their effect on the child's performance. Responders have shown specific effects outlined below.

Motor Effects
- Reduced hyperactivity
- Decreased excessive talking and disruption
- Improved handwriting
- Improved fine motor control

Social Effects
- Reduced off-task behaviors
- Improved ability to play and work independently
- Decreased intensity of behavior
- Reduced anger
- Improved (but not normalized) peer social interaction
- Improved mother–child interactions
- Reduced verbal and physical aggression

Cognitive Effects
- Increased sustained attention
- Reduced distractibility
- Improved short-term memory
- Increased work completed
- Increased accuracy of academic work

Perhaps the most important step at this phase is the choice of medications. The current choices include methylphenidate and dexmethylphenidate, dextroamphetamine, and methamphetamine, plus a combination of mixed amphetamine salts. Pemoline (Cylert) had been used in the past, but concerns about liver toxicity have made it a treatment of final resort. Its use requires biweekly monitoring of liver enzymes and the signing of an informed consent. Most of these agents are available in short- (2–4 h) and long-acting (6–8 h) formulations. Among available agents there appears to be little difference in the number of children who respond initially or in the side effect profiles. Each child will react differently to the various stimulants and finding the optimal agent and dose is a matter of trial and error. A combination of short- and long-acting medications is often necessary for best coverage of periods of peak target symptoms. The patient and parents must be aware of this and should be active participants in the decisions that will follow.

Absolute contraindications to the use of stimulants include concomitant use of monoamine oxidase (MAO) inhibitors, psychosis, glaucoma, underlying cardiac conditions, existing liver disorders, and a history of stimulant drug dependence. Most manufacturers do not recommend the use of stimulants in children under age 6, although several are approved for use in children as young as 3. Check the manufacturer's recommendations prior to the initiation of drug therapy. Most practitioners initiate treatment with a stimulant with which they are comfortable, and have an alternative in case the first does not succeed. The goals of the counseling phase are to explain the procedures of the trial to both the child and the parents.

b. Titration phase—Management of medication requires close monitoring of behaviors and frequent modifications in timing and strength of dosing to achieve optimal results. Titration usually lasts several months and should be monitored by the physician weekly. There are no levels or laboratory tests to determine appropriate dosing and there is wide variation in response and side effects. Patients and families should be counseled that the initial dose may be ineffective and that establishing an effective regimen will take time. Table 8–3 outlines the basic principles of the titration

Table 8–3. Basic principles of titration phase.

1. Weight-based dosing is ineffective. Begin with the lowest reasonable dose (Table 8–4) and increase weekly until positive response to target symptoms or significant side effects (Table 8–5).
2. Begin with short-acting agents then switch to longer acting agents once dosage is established (see Table 8–6). Consider combinations to best cover peak periods (not unlike insulin therapy for diabetes).
3. Distinguish between inadequate dosage, medication effects, or rebound effects by monitoring the timing of symptoms and medication.
4. Administer as frequently as needed to modify all target symptoms. This means afternoon, weekend, and summer dosages.
5. Minimize side effects by adjusting the timing and/or the form of the medication (see Table 8–5).
6. If one stimulant is not effective or has intolerable side effects, begin the titration process with another stimulant.

period and Table 8–4 offers some guidelines for starting dosages, increments of increase, and highest dosages for the currently available short-acting and intermediate-acting medications.

The most common side effects from stimulants are appetite suppression, which may be accompanied by nausea or stomach pain (but usually not), difficulty falling asleep, irritability, and sadness. There may also be a rebound in hyperactive behaviors as the medication wears off. Side effects are the most common reason for discontinuation of these medications. Table 8–5 lists common side effects of stimulants and strategies to manage them.

Most of the short-acting agents affect symptoms for about 3–4 hours. The mixed amphetamine salts (Adderall) have an intermediate length of action of 4–6 h. Long-acting medications, which have a delayed onset of action (usually about an hour compared to 20 min for the shorter acting agents), are preferable to shorter acting agents because they have less rebound phenomenon and do not require a noontime dose in school. The effects of the longer acting agents on the target symptoms must be compared to the effects established by the shorter agents.

The final part of the titration phase is an attempt to convert from the shorter acting agents to longer acting agents or to combine them to obtain the maximum benefit. It is possible to use a lower dose of the long-acting agent as a baseline and to use shorter acting agents for periods in which control of symptoms is needed the most. This is an individual process and requires a great deal of communication between the patient, parents, teacher, and prescribing physician. Table 8–6 lists conversion factors for some common medications.

c. Maintenance phase—Once the dosage of a long-acting agent is established and target symptoms are controlled, the frequency of visits between the physician and the patient can decrease. Because the stimulants are Schedule II controlled substances, prescriptions with no refills are usually written monthly, although several states allow 3-month prescriptions. In the large MTA cooperative study in 1999, the children who did the best had monthly 30-min medication visits. Growth and vital signs should be checked and documented. Because children grow and their situations are constantly changing, it is vital to monitor the effects of the medication and the child's progress. Issues to address include (1) the adequacy and the timing of the dosage, (2) compliance with the regimen, (3) changes in school or out-of-school activities that may affect medical therapy, and (4) maintenance of appropriate growth. There is usually some initial drop-off in weight

Table 8–4. Starting dosage guidelines for short-acting agents.

Medication	Starting Dose (mg twice a day)		Increments (mg)		Highest Dose (mg/day)	
	5–8 years	9–12 years	5–8 years	9–12 years	5–8 years	9–12 years
Methylphenidate 5, 10, 20 mg tablets (Ritalin, Methylin)	5	10	5	5	40	60
Dexmethylphenidate 2.5, 5, 10 mg tablets (Focalin)	2.5	5	2.5	2.5	20	30
Dextroamphetamine 5, 10, 15 mg tablets (Dexedrine, Dextrostat)	2.5	5	2.5	5	15	30
Methamphetamine 5 mg tablet (Desoxyn)	2.5	5	2.5	5	15	30
Mixed amphetamine salts 5, 10, 20, 30 mg (Adderall)	5	10	5	5	30	50

gain in the titration phase, but this reverses over 2 years and there is no long-term sustained growth suppression from stimulant use. Drug holidays are no longer standard procedure, but parents may opt for periods off the medications to minimize potential unknown drug effects or to assess the continuing need for the medication.

d. Termination of stimulant medication—Stopping stimulant medication is based on a clinical trial off the medication and close monitoring of target symptoms. If there is an immediate return of targeted behaviors when medication is accidentally forgotten the child is not ready for such a trial. A trial off medication is best done in less stressful periods such as school vacations. Two weeks without return of symptoms warrants an extended trial. The child's behavior should be monitored for about a year before deciding to permanently discontinue stimulant therapy.

2. Nonstimulants—Many nonstimulant medications are being used for ADHD, alone and in combination with the neurostimulants. They have been studied less extensively and are summarized here to provide the physician with knowledge about their use. Generally these medications are used when comorbidities are involved and they may best be managed in partnership with a pediatric psychiatrist with close follow-up. They vary from established effective treatments such as the tricyclic antidepressants to potentially effective treat-

ments such as the newer highly selective catecholamine reuptake inhibitors, eg, the Food and Drug Administration (FDA)-approved atomoxetine (Strattera), which is discussed below. They are often used to treat both the ADHD and the comorbid states and their effectiveness alone is generally less than that of the neurostimulants. Fear and misunderstanding of the neurostimulants make these medications attractive to parents. The rationale for the use of these agents, their theoretical effectiveness, and their potential adverse effects are summarized in Table 8–7. These agents are categorized by their efficacy, safety, and effectiveness.

The FDA approval of atomoxetine-HCl for the treatment of ADHD in children over age 6 and in adults provides a noncontrolled medication. Testing has shown it to be effective in children and adults with both predominantly inattentive and predominantly hyperactive forms of ADHD for up to 10 weeks. Although less effective than the neurostimulants, its lack of potential for addiction and abuse makes it attractive to many parents and physicians. Because of this, a body of evidence about its true effectiveness will develop quickly. Like the stimulants, atomoxetine should not be used as a diagnostic trial. Warnings have been given about allergic reactions and delayed growth. Adverse effects include abdominal pain, decreased appetite, nausea, vomiting, somnolence, cardiovascular effects (increases in blood pressure and heart rate), and problems with urinary retention and sexual side effects in adults.

Table 8–5. Side effects of stimulants and their management.

Appetite suppression
Will decrease with time (why stimulants eventually fail as "diet pills")
Try to time meals when medication effect is minimal or worn off
Make breakfast a major meal, prior to dosing
Make favorite foods for lunch
Offer substantial meal at bedtime

Delayed sleep onset
Determine if problem was preexisting, in which case an afternoon dose may actually help
If real, consider decreasing afternoon dosing
Usual sleep hygiene maintenance (same bedtime routine, bed just for sleep, etc)
Rarely consider second agent such as clonidine or trazadone (usually with consultation)

Rebound or "wearing-off" phenomenon
Check dosing, consider a 4 PM dosing of a short-acting agent
Switch to longer acting agents (pharmacokinetics decrease withdrawal)

Tics
Check child for emergence of Tourette's syndrome
Simple tics are common and not necessarily associated with stimulants; they can be observed
If troublesome or irretractible, stop stimulant and consider adding or substituting another agent (such as a centrally acting α-agonist) with consultation

Depression
Check timing of symptoms; if they concur with medication timing consider a different agent
Make sure that attention problems were not really a mood problem
Consider consultation

Social withdrawal
Uncommon effect of "zombie-like" behavior due to excessive dosing
Check timing of symptoms and dosing; decrease dose or increase intervals

---

Dosing of atomoxetine is by weight at an initial dose of 0.5 mg/kg/day, increasing every 3 days to a target dosage of 1.2 mg/kg/day. It is dosed once daily and is believed to have effects for 16 h. The total daily dose should not exceed 1.4 mg/kg/day or 100 mg total, whichever is less. It is supplied in 5, 10, 18, 25, 40, and 60 mg strengths. Like other selective neurotransmitter

Table 8–6. Guidelines for the conversion of short-acting agents to long-acting agents.[1]

Previous Short Dose	Recommended Long Dose
Dextroamphetamine (Dextrostat)	Dexedrine Spanule 0 mg
5 mg twice a day	15 mg and 5 mg tablet
10 mg twice a day	or 20 mg
Methylphenidate (Ritalin)	Methylphenidate (Ritalin SR)
5 mg twice a day	20 mg/day
10 mg twice a day	20 mg and 10 mg tablet
15 mg twice a day	40 mg/day
Methylphenidate (Ritalin)	Methylphenidate (Concerta)
5 mg orally twice a day	18 mg orally/day
5 mg twice a day	36 mg/day
10 mg twice a day	54 mg/day
Dexmethylphenidate (Focalin)	Methylphenidate (Concerta) 18 mg/day
2.5 mg twice a day	36 mg/day
5 mg twice a day	54 mg/day
10 mg twice a day	Mixed amphetamine salt
Methylphenidate (Ritalin)	(Adderall)
5 mg twice a day	10 mg AM, 5 mg PM
10 mg twice a day	15 mg twice a day
15 mg twice a day	20 mg twice a day
Methylphenidate (Metadate ER)	Methylphenidate (Metadate CD)
5 mg twice a day	0 mg
10 mg twice a day	20 mg/day
20 mg twice a day	40 mg/day

[1]Adderall to Adderall XR at the same total daily dose only once a day; Ritalin to Ritalin LA at the same daily dose once a day; a 27 mg dose of Concerta is also available.

reuptake inhibitors, it may take several weeks to see the full effects. For now, this agent could be considered when patients fail to respond to proper titrated stimulants, cannot tolerate stimulants, or refuse to try stimulants.

C. BEHAVIOR MODIFICATION

Whereas stimulant medications reduce inattention, hyperactivity, and impulsivity, behavioral modifications are designed to improve specific behaviors, social skills, and performance in specific settings. Behavioral approaches require the detailed assessment of the child's responses and the conditions that elicited them. Strategies are then developed to change the environment and the behaviors while maintaining and generalizing the behavioral changes. The most prudent approach to the treatment of ADHD is multimodal, and combination therapy with psychosocial interventions and medications shows the best results.

Table 8–7. Additional medications considered for ADHD.

Medication	Rationale	Evidence of Effectiveness	Adverse Effects
Established effective therapies			
Tricyclic antidepressants	Increase in neurotransmitors, useful as second line or in ADHD associated with enuresis or bulimia	Equal to stimulants for behavior, inferior for cognitive improvement, not very effective in inattentive type ADHD	Cardiac conductive slowing, anticholinergic effects, overdose potential, *unexplained deaths reported*
Bupropion	Dopaminergic and noradrenergic effects, may be effective in hostility and conduct comorbid states	Less effective than stimulants for core ADHD symptoms, better than placebo	Skin rashes in children, seizures in bulimics, possibly aggravates tics
Efficacious but usually *inadvisable* due to potential toxicity			
Pemoline	Neurostimulant with proven efficacy similar to other stimulants	Improves hyperactivity, aggressive behaviors and attention	"Black box" warning for liver toxicity, must have informed consent and monitor liver function tests
Carbamazepine	Anticonvulsive and mood stabilization properties	Improves impulsive and aggressive behaviors but not attention	Agranulocytosis, behavioral destabilization
Monoamine oxidase inhibitors	Accumulation of neurotransmittors and bioamines in the central nervous system	General improvement in core symptoms of impulsivity and attention	Risk of hypertension and headaches with tyramine-containing foods, overdose potentially fatal
Conventional neuroleptics	Sedative effects, antipsychotic effects	Improvement in aggression and impulsivity	Neuroleptic malignant syndrome, tardive dyskinesia
Newer neuroleptics	Sedative effects, antipsychotic effects	Improves severe agitation and psychotic symptoms	Extrapyramidal side effects, agranulocytosis, weight gain
Nicotine	Nicotine receptor agonists affect catecholamine levels	Improves attention, learning, and memory in nonsmokers	Nicotine addiction, risks of smoking
Probably effective			
Venlafaxine	Selective inhibition of neuronal uptake of seratonin and norepinephrine	Therapeutic benefits on behavior but not attention and cognition, useful for obsessive–compulsive disorder and depression	Gastrointestinal (GI) side effects, possible hypertension
Clonidine	Reduces noradrenergic transmission through α-adrenergic receptor agonism	Best results with sleep problems, impulsivity, and hyperexcited states, little effect on attention	Somnolence, cognitive decrease, hypotension, cardiac effects including conduction disorders; *fatalities reported in combination with stimulants*
Guanfacine	Weaker α-adrenergic receptor agonist than clonidine	Shows promise for attention, impulsivity, and tics	Less severe effects than clonidine, some sedation and hypotension, reported hypomania
Possible efficacy			
β-blockers	β-adrenergic receptor antagonists	Useful in combination with stimulants to decrease agitation and rage	Can worsen depression and asthma, has cardiac effects
Speculative effectiveness			
Donepezil (Aricept)	Anticholinesterase can increase acetylcholine levels	Limited study shows "sharper thinking," awareness of detail, and organizational skills	GI side effects and cost

(continued)

Table 8–7. Additional medications considered for ADHD. (Continued)

Medication	Rationale	Evidence of Effectiveness	Adverse Effects
Modafinil (Provigil)	Stimulation of α receptors and reduction in γ-aminobutyric acid (GABA) release	Limited use with mixed results, not studied in children	Cardiovascular side effects, psychosis
Selective catecholamine agents: reboxetine, tomoxetine, ropinirole, pramipexole	Norepinephrine reuptake inhibition or selective dopamine receptor agonists	Initial studies show 50% response rates	Side effects similar to selective serotonin reuptake inhibitors (SSRIs)
Antiseizure agents	Inhibit reuptake of dopamine, norepinephrine, and GABA	Valproate has a methylphenidate effect on arousal: further study pending, especially with gabapentin	Can induce neurocognitive impairment, may induce autoimmune reactions
Piracetam	GABA derivative	No changes in arousal but improves learning in reading disorders	Unstudied in the United States
Probably ineffective Selective serotonin reuptake inhibitors	Increase serotonin in the central nervous system	Only benefits have been in combination with stimulants without additive effects	Motor hyperactivity and restlessness, SSRI-induced mania, SSRI amotivational syndrome

Adapted from Popper CW: Pharmacologic alternatives to psychostimulants for ADHD. Child Adolesc Psychiatr Clin North Am 2000;9(3):605.

One approach to the design of behavioral therapy is to identify the positive and negative environmental inputs that increase or decrease targeted behaviors and then modify those inputs to increase adaptive behaviors and minimize problematic ones. The "token economy" uses points, stars, or tokens for positive behaviors (or lack of negative ones). These are then exchanged for "reinforcers," which may be money, food, toys, or time with an adult in fun activity. The most effective programs involve consistency between home and school and focus on targeted behaviors. They provide punishments and rewards that follow behavior quickly and consistently and incorporate novelty to keep interest. This may require intensive and prolonged programs that are fairly time consuming.

Behavioral therapy alone is less effective than protocol-based medication alone and combining it with medication use has resulted in little additional improvement in inattention, impulsivity, and hyperactivity. The efficacy of behavioral modification comes from enhanced academic and social successes, which are hard to measure and generalize. Intensive behavioral therapy alone was shown to have equal efficacy to the usual care in the community, even if medications were given to the community care group. This confirms the viability of specialized behavioral treatment for parents who prefer nonpharmacological therapy for ADHD.

D. EDUCATIONAL INTERVENTIONS

Teachers and schools play a huge role in the identification and subsequent management of ADHD. The goal of educational interventions should be to build the child's competence. Success depends on the parents, schools, and physicians working together. Educational strategies for ADHD that can be shared with teachers include the following:

1. Classes need to highly ordered and predictable. Rules and expectations must be clear and consistent.
2. Enclosed classrooms reduce distractions. ADHD children should be seated away from distractions and near peers who can role model behaviors. A quiet work area should be available on request.
3. Plan more rigorous subjects for the morning, provide regularly scheduled breaks, and use attention-getting devices.
4. Reduce the amount of work assigned, modify assignments, or allow more time to complete assignments or tests. Use a mixture of high and low interest tasks.
5. Create learning partnerships in which an active child is paired with a calm or advanced student to help with new concepts and practice established

skills. Try to give each student at least one task a day that he or she can do successfully.

The education of children with ADHD is covered by three federal statutes: the Individuals with Disabilities Education Act (IDEA), Section 504 of the Rehabilitation Act of 1973, and the Americans with Disabilities Act (ADA) of 1990. The diagnosis of ADHD alone is not enough to qualify a child for special educational services. The ADHD must impair the child's ability to learn. Based on a 1991 Department of Education Policy Clarification Memorandum, ADHD children may be eligible for special education if they (1) are health impaired (or have another documented condition such as Tourette's), (2) have a specific learning disability (this could be ADHD alone if there is a significant discrepancy between a child's cognitive ability or intelligence and academic performance), and (3) are seriously emotionally disturbed. It is therefore vital to document all comorbid conditions in these children. For children who qualify, the accommodation strategies and specific goals should be outlined in the student's Individualized Education Plan (IEP), which is mandated under IDEA and is usually put together by teachers and parents along with school psychologists and administrators. Occasionally parents will ask for physician input into this process as they advocate for their children. Physician documentation of the diagnosis and management of ADHD is necessary to obtain accommodations for college entry examinations and other testing.

E. PARENT EDUCATION AND TRAINING

Parental understanding of ADHD is vital to successful treatment. Parents must know the difference between noncompliance and inability to perform. They need to understand that ADHD is not a choice but a result of nature. Physicians are in the position to defuse parental feelings of guilt that arise from thinking that their child's behavior is due to bad parenting. Unfortunately, there is a fair amount of disinformation in the general population that reinforces these beliefs. Parent education can be frustrating at times because parents of children with ADHD often have features of it themselves. Many parents respond well to referral to local and national support groups such as Children and Adults with Attention Deficit/Hyperactivity Disorder (CHADD—www.chadd.org) or the Attention Deficit Disorder Association (ADDA—www.add.org). They need to know their child is not the only one affected and that other caring parents have similar problems and they need to learn how to become educated advocates for their children. Parental strategies for coping and home adaptation are provided by these organizations.

Formal parental behavior modification may be necessary for noncompliant, oppositional, and aggressive chil-

dren. The most effective of these training programs use written materials, verbal instruction in social learning principles, modeling by the clinician (usually a psychologist), and role playing. These strategies are discussed in more detail in the ODD section of this chapter.

Some families will require formal family therapy to treat the dysfunction that is caused or aggravated by raising a child with ADHD. The basic strategies are to help the family solve problems together.

F. OTHER BEHAVIORAL APPROACHES

Other behavioral approaches utilized for ADHD include social skills training, academic skills training, cognitive–behavioral modification, therapeutic recreation, and individual psychotherapy. These approaches must be individualized for each situation and require a trained therapist to work with the physician. They require time and, in many cases, financial commitment.

Social skills training is difficult with ADHD children because their social problems are so variable. Individual training is not very successful due to lack of self-observation. Group training using modeling, practice, feedback, and reinforcement in natural environments such as schools is best. Peer-mediated conflict resolution skills can decrease aggressive behaviors and improve problem-solving skills.

Academic skills training is essentially tutoring in organizational and study skills. These services are available professionally or through the schools.

Cognitive–behavioral modification is problem-solving therapy and can be group or individual. It can directly address deficits in impulsivity and problem solving and has resulted in improvements in cognitive impulsivity, social behavior, and coping strategies.

Therapeutic recreation uses play and sports programs to teach cooperation and social skills. Success at recreational and sports activities can greatly enhance ADHD children's self-esteem.

Individual psychotherapy is hampered by the lack of insight into ADHD but can be used to address comorbid states such as anxiety and depression. This therapy works well in forming therapeutic alliances, especially in adolescents assuming control of their own medications.

G. ALTERNATIVE TREATMENTS

Because ADHD has no easily understood etiology and no pharmacological "magic" cure, and because of the stigma associated with the use of stimulant medications, there exists an eager market for alternative therapies. However, caution must be exercised when evaluating all alternative modalities. Caution should be used when a remedy is said to work for everybody with ADHD, when evidence is based on testimonials only and only one study is cited for support, and when the active ingredients of the product are not listed or the remedy is said to be based on a "secret formula" or is described as harmless because it is "natural." However, physicians should be careful not to alienate patients who find a certain remedy is working for them and seems responsible for social and academic success. Their role is to advocate, educate, and protect patients in making decisions about alternative therapies.

In spite of strong claims from prestigious backers and some good reviews, there is little or no evidence of the efficacy of these therapies. Some therapies, such as elimination diets, have shown promise with a very small subset of patients (enough to allow for some outstanding testimonials) but have never been proven better than placebo in controlled studies. Sugar has often been labeled as the cause of all behavioral problems in children, but studies have either been inconclusive or have shown no correlation between sugar intake and attention and learning. Vitamin therapy has shown efficacy only in proven deficiency states and megadoses can be potentially dangerous.

Prognosis

Follow-up studies of children with ADHD show that the adult outcomes can vary greatly. About 30% of affected children will function well in adulthood and have no more difficulty than controlled normal functioning adults. The largest group, about 50–60%, will continue to have problems with concentration, impulsivity, and social relationships leading to workplace problems, troubled relationships, poor self-esteem, and emotional lability. The final group, about 10–15%, continue to have significant psychiatric or antisocial problems in adulthood. Predictors for bad outcomes include comorbid conduct disorder, low IQ, and concurrent parental pathology. Treatment for all groups has been shown to be effective for the core symptoms over the short term and the continuation of treatment may be necessary to maintain gains and improve the quality of life for the patients and their families. Long-term treatment and outcome studies have yet to be performed.

The consequences of ADHD are impressive. Up to 40% of children with ADHD will get some form of special education by adolescence, 25–35% will have been retained in grade at least once, 10–25% will be expelled from school, and 10–35% never finish high school. Proneness to accidents is greatly increased, with 15% of ADHD children having four or more serious accidents, including accidental poisoning and auto accidents. Adolescents with ADHD are also at increased risk for cigarette use and substance abuse, especially true when ADHD is combined with CD.

The association with accidents, automobile incidents, conduct problems, crime, substance abuse, and risk-taking behavior should result in a lowered life expectancy. Studies are limited, but one follow-up study of highly intelligent children with impulsive, uncontrolled personality characteristics showed an 8-year decrease in life expectancy.

Studies have shown that the annual per capita health care costs for ADHD children are twice as high as for children without ADHD. The total financial impact of ADHD is unknown. However, with its increased morbidity and mortality, it is clear that ADHD imposes a huge burden on society. Successful recognition and proper treatment can make a difference in many lives. The well-informed family physician is in a unique position to have a profound positive impact on the quality of the lives of these individuals and their families.

American Academy of Pediatrics: Clinical practice guideline: diagnosis and evaluation of the child with attention deficit/hyperactivity disorder. Pediatrics 2000;105:1158.

American Academy of Pediatrics: Clinical practice guideline: treatment of the school-aged child with attention deficit/hyperactivity disorder. Pediatrics 2001;108:1033. www.aap.org/policy/s0120.html.

Dulcan M: Practice parameters for the assessment and treatment of children, adolescents, and adults with attention-deficit/hyperactivity disorder. American Academy of Child and Adolescent Psychiatry. J Am Acad Child Adolesc Psychiatry 1997;36: 85S. www.aap.org/policy/ac0002.html.

Ingerstoll B: *ADD and LD—Realities, Myths and Controversial Treatments.* Doubleday, 1993.

Jadad AR et al: Treatment of attention-deficit/hyperactivity disorder. Agency of Health Care Policy and Research (AHCPR) Pub. #99-E017, Rockville, MD, 2003.

Mash E, Barkley R (editors): *Child Psychopathology.* The Guilford Press, 1996

Medical Letter 2003;45(1149).

MTA Cooperative Group: A 14 month randomized clinical trial of treatment strategies for attention-deficit/hyperactivity disorder. The Multimodal Treatment Study of Children with ADHD. Arch Gen Psychiatry 1999;56:1073.

National Institutes of Health: Diagnosis and treatment of attention deficit hyperactivity disorder. Consensus Development Conference Statement 1998;16(2):1. http://odp.od.nih.gov/consensus/cons/110/110_statement.htm.

Ravenel SD: Practice parameter for the use of stimulant medications in the treatment of children, adolescents, and adults. J Am Acad Child Adolesc Psychiatry 2002;41(2):1146.

Spencer T, Biederman J, Wilens T: Attention-deficit/hyperactivity disorder and comorbidity, Pediatr Clin North Am 1999; 46(5):915.

Wender EH: Managing stimulant medication for attention-deficit/hyperactivity disorder 2001;6(6):183.

WEB SITES

American Academy of Child and Adolescent Psychiatry
www.aacap.org
American Psychiatric Association

www.psych.org

Children and Adults with Attention Deficit/Hyperactivity Disorder

www.chadd.org

National Alliance for the Mentally Ill

www.nami.org

National Institute of Mental Health Information Resources and Inquiries Branch

www.nimh.org

National Mental Health Association

www.nmha.org

OPPOSITIONAL DEFIANT DISORDER

 ESSENTIALS OF DIAGNOSIS

- A persistent pattern of negative, defiant, disobedient, and hostile behavior toward authority figures that is not part of a psychotic, mood, or conduct disorder.
- Age-inappropriate display of angry, defiant, irritable, and oppositional behaviors that have occurred for at least 6 months.

General Considerations

Originally called oppositional disorder, oppositional defiant disorder (ODD) emerged as a defined disruptive behavior disorder in the 1988 revision of *DSM-III*. ODD is defined by an age-inappropriate display of angry, defiant, irritable, and oppositional behaviors that has occurred for at least 6 months. Although many teenagers seem to fit this diagnosis, the object is to define and help those individuals whose behavior is clearly impairing their functioning. The diagnosis is not made if the behaviors are part of a psychotic or mood disorder, nor can it be made if the criteria of CD are met. The diagnosis is based on aggressive and antisocial behaviors that are exhibited in early and middle childhood and do not reach the severity of the behavior seen in CD. Children with ODD do not usually have significant problems with the law and are not physically aggressive. The validity of ODD as a separate diagnostic entity is debated by some as its symptoms can be considered within the range of normal developmental actions. The majority of children with ODD do not progress to CD if action is taken to treat the disorder. Although there is much overlap and comorbidity with ADHD, there is clear evidence of divergence from attention deficit syndromes. The problem is more one of inability to inhibit moody outbursts and less with exec-

utive functioning. Due to its recent emergence as a separate diagnostic entity, ODD has not been extensively studied and is usually linked to CD.

The manifestations of this disorder include persistent stubbornness, resistance to directions, and unwillingness to negotiate and compromise with others. Defiant behaviors include persistent testing of limits, arguing, ignoring orders, and denying blame for misdeeds. Hostility usually takes the form of verbal abuse and aggression. Because the most common setting is the home ODD may not be evident to teachers or others in the community. And because the symptoms of the disorder are most likely to be manifested toward individuals that the patient knows well, ODD will rarely be apparent during clinical examination. These children do not see themselves as the problem but rather view their own behavior as a reasonable response to unreasonable demands. They have problems with low self-esteem, lability of mood, and a low tolerance of frustration and are more likely to be involved with substance abuse. These are difficult children to live with and difficult homes to live in and families will frequently turn to their physicians for help.

Psychopathology

ODD is seen as a behavioral disorder and is not associated with any known physical or biochemical abnormality. There is some evidence that oppositional children have higher levels of androgen than normal control subjects but this finding is not conclusive. The cause is generally related to social, parental, and child factors.

A. SOCIAL FACTORS

There is a correlation between ODD and living in crowded conditions, such as high-rise buildings with inadequate play space, and between ODD and social class (although more commonly found in lower income neighborhoods this does not hold when other factors are controlled), but no correlation to paternal or maternal employment. There does seem to be some correlation with the quality of the daycare if the mother is employed.

B. PARENTAL FACTORS

It is difficult to determine whether parental behavior causes ODD or ODD causes the parental behavior, but there are strong correlations between the way parents act and oppositional behavior. Parents of ODD children (not all, but certainly in pattern) tend to be critical, rejecting, lacking in warmth, passive, and unstimulating. Mothers, especially, show high levels of anxiety and depression. Family relationships, especially the marital relationship, tend to be strained. This sets up a vicious cycle as the child becomes more insecure and more difficult to handle and the parents react with greater rejection.

C. CHILD FACTORS

It has been impossible to determine if the adverse temperamental factors that contribute to ODD are present from birth. ODD children are more likely to have language delay and a higher incidence of enuresis than age-controlled peers.

D. PRESENTATION

The presentation of oppositional behaviors is highly variable. During the preschool years, transient oppositional behavior is normal. However, when these behaviors are of a persistent nature and last beyond the preschool years, the development of more disruptive behaviors is likely. On the basis of research data, two possible developmental trajectories have been suggested. In most oppositional children, especially those who are not physically aggressive, oppositional behaviors peak around age 8 and decrease beyond that. In a second group of children, delinquent behaviors follow the onset of oppositional behaviors. Early physical aggression is a key element of this group, with physically aggressive children being more likely to progress to the violation of others' property and rights that categorizes CD.

Prevalence/Demographics

The prevalence of ODD has varied from 2% to 16% of the school-aged population. These differences are due to the methodology of the studies and the difference in diagnostic criteria between *DSM-III* (which required five of nine symptoms) and *DSM-IV* criteria (which require four of eight symptoms). Studies show an increasing rate of diagnosis from grade school to middle school to high school and then a decrease in the college-aged groups. Unlike CD and ADHD, gender differences are minimal, with boys only slightly more likely to be diagnosed than girls. Good data on racial or cultural differences do not exist, but worldwide ODD (and CD) is more prevalent among low socioeconomic status families who tend to live in closer quarters. Differences in the prevalence of ODD in rural and urban environments are mixed. The early onset of disruptive behaviors in which others' rights are violated (as in CD), which has a worse prognosis and the highest social burden, seems to be concentrated in cities in the United States.

There are usually familial situations that play into the diagnosis. ODD is more common when at least one parent has a history of a mood disorder, conduct disorder, antisocial personality disorder, or substance-related disorder (18% of children with ODD have alcoholic fathers). Mothers with depression are more likely to have oppositional children. Family adversity scores in children with ODD are usually intermediate between those of children with CD and normal children. Whether this is a cause or effect in unknown, but the family physician is ideally suited to help address and untangle these complex issues.

Clinical Findings

A. SYMPTOMS AND SIGNS

DSM-IV has specific diagnostic criteria for ODD (Table 8–8). The clinical features that bring children to physicians' offices are based on control issues, aggression, and activity. Control issues start early with battles over bedtime and mealtime at age 3 and 4. These children begin to be verbally aggressive toward their parents almost as soon as they can talk. This may progress to physical aggression, which is usually directed at the parents or caretakers and rarely at strangers. Activity levels are variable and may depend on the common comorbid condition of ADHD. Other features include anxiety and an increased incidence of temper tantrums and breath-holding attacks.

Table 8–8. *DSM-IV* diagnostic criteria for 313.81 oppositional defiant disorder.

A. A pattern of negativistic, hostile, and defiant behavior lasting at least 6 months, during which four (or more) of the following are present:
(1) often loses temper, (2) often argues with adults, (3) often actively defies or refuses to comply with adults' requests or rules, (4) often deliberately annoys people, (5) often blames others for his or her mistakes or misbehavior, (6) is often touchy or easily annoyed by others, (7) is often angry and resentful, (8) is often spiteful or vindictive.

Note: Consider a criterion met only if the behavior occurs more frequently than is typically observed in individuals of comparable age and developmental level.

B. The disturbance in behavior causes clinically significant impairment in social, academic, or occupational functioning.
C. The behaviors do not occur exclusively during the course of a psychotic or mood disorder.
D. Criteria are not met for conduct disorder, and, if the individual is age 18 years or older, criteria are not met for antisocial personality disorder.

From Loeber R et al: Oppositional defiant and conduct disorder: a review of the past 10 years, part 1. J Am Acad Child Adolesc Psychiatry 2000; 39:1468.

DSM-IV does not establish an age of onset for the diagnosis other than younger than 18. The average age of onset of ODD behaviors is 6, with the behaviors tending to peak at age 8. Diagnosis is made by parental, patient, or teacher history and by direct observation. Behavioral checklists that can pick up the pattern of ODD include the *Child Behavioral Checklist* and the *Rochester Adaptive Behavior Inventory*. A structured interview such as the *Diagnostic Interview for Children and Adolescents* or the *Child and Adolescent Psychiatric Assessment* may be helpful. Medical testing or neuropsychiatric testing is rarely necessary unless there are comorbid states.

B. Comorbidities

ODD is common among those with ADHD. The disruptive behaviors of ADHD tend to bring out the parental behaviors associated with ODD. The combination of ADHD, ODD, family adversity, and low verbal IQ are predictors of progression to more serious conduct disorders and antisocial behaviors as adults. However, although up to 50% of ADHD children have ODD behaviors, only about 15% of those diagnosed with ODD have ADHD.

About 15% of ODD children have anxiety disorders and approximately 10% have depression or mood disorders. Addressing these problems can often help with the oppositional behaviors.

Differential Diagnosis

Because all the behaviors of ODD are present in CD, ODD is not diagnosed in the presence of CD. Although there is comorbidity with mood disorders, the diagnosis of ODD should not be made if there is a major mood disorder or if there is a psychotic disorder. ODD should be distinguished from ADHD although both can be present in many children, in which case both diagnoses should be given. Physical causes for oppositional behavior must be considered, especially if hearing or auditory comprehension is impaired. The diagnosis of ODD in those with mental retardation is difficult and can be made only if the behaviors exceed those usually seen at that severity of cognitive function and age. Bipolar disease can be confused with ODD. Any of the social or medical conditions listed in Table 8–2 could also be confused with ODD.

Treatment

Management of ODD depends on the extent of the behavioral problem. The majority of these patients and their families can be managed with behavioral therapies, especially parental training and family therapy.

Parental-controlled behavioral modification is based on the social learning theory and uses naturally occurring consequences to teach social skills and self-evaluation. Parents are taught to minimize emotional reactions to oppositional behaviors, to give clear instructions and limits, to positively reinforce good behaviors, and to use punishment selectively. Parent training is usually conducted by psychologists or trained social workers and can be conducted in groups. Parents need to communicate with each other to avoid the child playing one parent against the other. Communication with teachers and principals is also important. Parents need to be advised to make sure that they are healthy themselves. Children who watch 4–6 h of television a day are more violent, more likely to use drugs, and more preoccupied with sex. The American Academy of Pediatrics recommends that television viewing should be limited to 1–2 h/day. Likewise, video games can be addictive and children who play violent video games are more physically aggressive and not as intelligent as control children.

Unfortunately, many families of ODD children are characterized by low socioeconomic status, parental psychopathology, and marital conflict. These issues also need to be addressed by counseling or medication if any behavioral modification techniques are to be successful with the child. Family therapy may be indicated to address family dysfunction from the oppositional behavior or from primary parental or marital problems. Behavioral intervention can be performed in which the family learns how to negotiate together. One technique for adolescents is parent–child contracting, which involves written agreements for behavioral changes in both based on specified contingencies.

There is no accepted pharmacological treatment for oppositional behaviors, but it is important that comorbid conditions such as ADHD or depression be addressed and treated appropriately. For severe cases that do not respond to nonmedical interventions or that involve extreme impairment, it is best to consult a pediatric psychiatrist. Medications used for ODD include clonidine, lithium, carbamazepine, valproic acid, and risperidone. These medications all have significant risks and their use should be monitored carefully.

Prognosis

The most serious consequence of ODD is the development of more dangerous conduct problems. A diagnosis of CD supersedes ODD because approximately 90% of children with CD also meet criteria for ODD. Although the majority of children with ODD will not develop CD, in some cases ODD appears to represent a developmental precursor of CD. This seems to be truer in boys than girls. ADHD also plays a role. In cases in which ODD precedes CD, the onset of CD is typically before age 10 years (childhood-onset CD). Age 8 is an important milestone. This is when ODD symptoms normally peak and if they decrease with maturity the prognosis is good. If the behaviors progress and start to involve the violation of others' rights, the child will probably progress to CD. Children with ODD demonstrate lower degrees of impairment and are more socially competent compared with children with CD. Furthermore, children with CD come from less advantaged families and, by definition, have greater conflict with school and judicial systems compared with children with ODD. These can be used to predict which children may need more aggressive intervention. The family physician is, again, ideally positioned to identify these individuals and coordinate their care.

Lavigne JV et al: Oppositional defiant disorder with onset in preschool years: longitudinal stability and pathways to other disorders. J Am Acad Child Adolesc Psychiatry 2001;40:1393.

CONDUCT DISORDER

 ESSENTIALS OF DIAGNOSIS

- A repetitive and persistent pattern of behavior in which the basic rights of others and major age-appropriate societal norms are violated.
- Behavior characterized by aggression toward people and animals, destruction of property, deceitfulness or theft, and serious violation of rules.

General Considerations

The most serious disruptive behavioral problem of childhood seen in primary care is conduct disorder (CD). These cases come to the attention of physicians when parents bring their children in for a variety of reasons. Younger children may present with outright refusal to cooperate with examinations or immunizations and with frequent instances of running away from their parents. Older children may be referred by teachers or school administrators, who request a medical evaluation prior to allowing a suspended student back into school. Adolescents may present after they have been arrested for violent or destructive behaviors. These behaviors are not only disruptive but involve blatant breaking of societal rules and violation of the rights of others. Many normal children will have lapses in judgment and break rules or hurt others. Conduct disorder represents a persistent or repetitive pattern of such behaviors. These children represent a significant problem for the patients,

their family, and society in general and often physicians are consulted to help.

Social norms tend to be culture specific and there may be significant differences in categorizing specific behavior as antisocial. Oriental cultures put a high value on conformity not found in western society. As a result, in some schools, fighting in the playground is taken for granted and, in others, it is a matter of grave concern. University students turning over cars after a big sports victory are viewed differently than a group of youths engaged in the same behavior after being refused entry into a nightclub. Physicians and professionals must be aware that their judgments of abnormality will be affected by the values of their particular society.

Because of some significant differences in the two groups, CD is subtyped by age of onset before or after age 10 years. There are four main groupings of behaviors in conduct disorder: (1) aggression to people or animals, (2) destruction of property, (3) deceitfulness or theft, and (4) serious violation of rules. Due to the diversity of disruptive behaviors, *DSM-IV* has included "specifiers" that classify behaviors into mild, moderate, and severe. These are useful in trying to predict the nature of the presenting problems, the developmental course, and the outcomes.

American society seems to be experiencing an increase in youth crime and sensational incidents in which children act as the perpetrators of aggression, assault, and even mass murder. CD is a condition in which the expertise and potential for intervention of the family physician have implications for society in general as well as individual patients and their families. It is also a condition that is a referral diagnosis for most primary care physicians and may be best addressed by working in conjunction with specialized pediatric and adolescent psychiatrists and therapists. Family physicians may be called upon for brief behavioral counseling and sometimes for pharmacotherapy. Their biggest role may be the determination and treatment of the many comorbid conditions found in these individuals. There is also a public health concern with CD contributing to school and gang violence, weapon use, substance abuse, and high drop-out rates. It is therefore important to identify these behaviors and intervene as early as possible.

Psychopathology

The etiology of conduct disorder is unknown but certainly seems to involve an interaction of genetic and constitutional factors with familial and environmental factors.

A. CONSTITUTIONAL FACTORS

The risk of CD is higher in children with biological or adoptive parents with antisocial personality disorder or with biological parents with ADHD, CD, alcohol dependence, mood disorders, and schizophrenia. Siblings of children with CD have a higher risk for developing it also. Studies of the physiological factors involved in CD have centered around a decreased autonomic response to various stimuli. Essentially, it seems to take a lot to get an autonomic and visceral response in those with CD, especially in early-onset individuals. Hormonal factors have been studied, especially the influence of testosterone on aggression and cortisol on anxiety. There are trends but no distinct cause and effect relationship. Neurotransmitters also play a role in aggression with current research pointing to serotonin.

B. ENVIRONMENTAL FACTORS

There is no doubt that the caretaker–child interaction contributes to disruptive behavior. Exposure to antisocial behavior in a caretaker as well as child abuse (especially sexual abuse in females) increase the risk of CD. Divorce was thought to play a role but does not seem to if one controls for parental pyschopathology. There is a bidirectional influence of the parents' behavior on the child and the child's behavior on the parents. Factors in these relationships include (1) low levels of parental involvement in their child's activities, (2) poor supervision, and (3) harsh and inconsistent discipline practices. Behavior problems are seen as strategies by the child to get attention and get closer to the caretaker or parent. There are neighborhood and peer factors also. Being poor, living in crowded conditions in a high crime neighborhood, and having "deviant" peer groups all increase the risk of CD.

Prevalence/Demographics

The prevalence of CD varies from 1% to 10% overall depending on the population studied with ranges of 6–16% in boys and 2–9% in girls under age 18. CD tends to increase from middle childhood to adolescence. Certain behaviors decrease with age such as physical fighting. The most serious aggressive behaviors such as robbery, rape, and murder increase during adolescence. The difference between the sexes (boys with a 3–4 risk ratio) does not seem to occur until after age 6. Males exhibit more fighting, stealing, vandalism, and problems with school discipline. Females are more likely to lie, be truant, run away, and engage in substance abuse.

The incidence of CD does not seem to have racial or ethnic differences if one controls for socioeconomic group and for high crime neighborhoods. CD had been on the rise, as evidenced by substantial increases in juvenile arrests for violent crimes in the decade from 1984 to 1994; however, the numbers have declined since. It is generally felt that differences between generations are due to recall bias in the older population.

Clinical Findings

A. SYMPTOMS AND SIGNS

Cases of CD are referred to physicians either by parents or by authorities. Physicians must distinguish normal adolescent risk-taking and antisocial behaviors from CD. Normal experimentation usually does not harm others and does not recur persistently. Screening questions might include asking about troubles with police, involvement in physical fights, suspensions from school, running away from home, sexual activity, and the use of tobacco, alcohol, and drugs.

DSM-IV states that the diagnosis of CD should not be made when behaviors are in response to the social context and stresses that there should be three specific CD behaviors within at least 6 months to make the diagnosis. The full *DSM-IV* criteria are given in Table 8–9.

It has become more common to make use of standardized interviews to make the diagnosis. These include the NIMH Diagnostic Interview Schedule for Children Version IV, the Child and Adolescent Psychiatric Assessment, the Schedule for Affective Disorders and Schizophrenia for School-Age Children, and the Diagnostic Interview for Children and Adolescents. These interviews are time consuming but yield more information than behavioral checklists. Pictorial instruments are available for very young children. Because parents and authorities usually do not know the full extent of the child's behavior, it is useful to interview the child as well.

The key to the diagnosis of CD is the disregard for the rights of others and the rules of society. *DSM-IV* also allows for a broad range of behaviors and makes a clear distinction between early-onset and later-onset CD. This is useful as the prognosis is much better if the onset of these behaviors is after age 10. Most primary care physicians refer cases of CD to pediatric psychiatrists, but may be involved in the initial workup. Special tests are rarely necessary.

Comorbidities

A majority of children (75%) with CD have at least one other psychiatric diagnosis. The relationship between ADHD and CD has been studied the most. ADHD can be conceptualized as a cognitive–developmental disorder, with an earlier age of onset than CD. Children with ADHD more frequently show deficits on measures of attention and cognitive function, have hyperactivity, and have greater neurodevelopmental abnormalities. Children with CD tend to be characterized by higher levels of aggression and greater familial dysfunction.

A significant proportion of children (30–50%) present with symptoms of both ADHD and CD, and both conditions should be diagnosed when this occurs. Co-

Table 8-9. *DSM-IV diagnostic criteria for conduct disorder.*

A. A repetitive and persistent pattern of behavior in which the basic rights of others or major age-appropriate societal norms or rules are violated, as manifested by the presence of three (or more) of the following criteria in the past 12 months, with at least one criterion present in the past 6 months:

Aggression to people and animals
(1) often bullies, threatens, or intimidates others
(2) often initiates physical fights
(3) has used a weapon that can cause serious physical harm to others (eg, a bat, brick, broken bottle, knife, gun)
(4) has been physically cruel to people
(5) has been physically cruel to animals
(6) has stolen while confronting a victim (eg, mugging, purse snatching, extortion, armed robbery)
(7) has forced someone into sexual activity

Destruction of property
(8) has deliberately engaged in fire setting with the intention of causing serious damage
(9) has deliberately destroyed others' property (other than by fire setting)

Deceitfulness or theft
(10) has broken into someone else's house, building, or car
(11) often lies to obtain goods or favors or to avoid obligations (ie, "cons" others)
(12) has stolen items of nontrivial value without confronting a victim (eg, shoplifting, but without breaking and entering; forgery)

Serious violations of rules
(13) often stays out at night despite parental prohibitions, beginning before age 13 years
(14) has run away from home overnight at least twice while living in parental or parental surrogate home (or once without returning for a lengthy period)
(15) is often truant from school, beginning before age 13 years
B. The disturbance in behavior causes clinically significant impairment in social, academic, or occupational functioning.
C. If the individual is age 18 years or older, criteria are not met for antisocial personality disorder.
Code based on age at onset:
312.81 Conduct Disorder, Childhood-Onset Type: onset of at least one criterion characteristic of conduct disorder prior to age 10 years
312.82 Conduct Disorder, Adolescent-Onset Type: absence of any criteria characteristic of conduct disorder prior to age 10 years
312.89 Conduct Disorder, Unspecified Onset: age at onset is not known
Specify severity:
Mild: few if any conduct problems in excess of those required to make the diagnosis and conduct problems cause only minor harm to others
Moderate: number of conduct problems and effect on others intermediate between "mild" and "severe"
Severe: many conduct problems in excess of those required to make the diagnosis or conduct problems cause considerable harm to others

morbid ADHD and CD is consistently reported to be more disabling than either disorder alone. These children have the problems found in both disorders and tend to show increased levels of aggressive behaviors at an early age, which remain remarkably persistent. This is in contrast to the more typical episodic course seen in children who have CD alone. They tend to do bad things impulsively and tend to get caught. Finally, children with comorbid ADHD and CD appear to have a much poorer long-term outcome than children with either disorder alone. In children who have late-onset CD, symptoms of ODD and ADHD are usually not present during early childhood.

Other psychiatric diagnoses commonly associated with CD include substance abuse, mania, schizophrenia, somatoform disorder, and obsessive–compulsive disorder. This is not surprising as these diagnoses are more common in the parents of children with CD. Anxiety disorders and mood disorders are also commonly diagnosed with CD (25%), especially in females.

Differential Diagnosis

All of the social or medical conditions listed in Table 8–2 could cause behaviors that resemble CD.

Oppositional defiant disorder is often thought of as a precursor of CD with the line being crossed when others' rights or societal rules are broken. If a child meets the criteria for both, the diagnosis of CD takes precedence.

ADHD children have disruptive and impulsive behavior, but their behavior does not violate age-appropriate societal norms and rarely hurts others. If the criteria for both diagnoses are met, the child is given both.

Major depression may present with acting out behaviors. Mood disorders are usually associated with affective symptoms, sleep disturbances, and appetite disruption. Having CD and depression puts one at great risk for impulsive suicidal behavior. Bipolar disease can manifest in irrational behavior and conduct problems but the episodic nature of the behaviors and other symptoms of mania are usually apparent. It is possible to have both disorders.

Intermittent explosive disorder features sudden aggressive outbursts that are usually unprovoked. These individuals do not intend to hurt anyone but say they "snapped" and, without realizing it, attacked another person. These are distinguished from CD in that these episodes are the only signs of behavioral problems and these individuals do not engage in other rule violations.

Late onset of CD may be associated with substance abuse or dependence, especially in the previously normal child. There may be a large overlap with CD. Repeated use of alcohol at an early age (10–13 years) is a marker for development of CD.

Treatment

The family physician is usually the first health professional consulted by parents of children with CD. A key element in the initial treatment of these individuals is parental involvement. Although many of these parents have problems themselves, they do not want their children to follow their path. All parties need to be aware of the possibility of a poor prognosis without the interventions of the caregiver.

Behavioral interventions are similar to those with ODD. Parents need to monitor their child's activities and friends and to structure those activities and set consistent behavioral guidelines with consistent and clear consequences. Referral to family counseling can help with communication problems. In children whose symptoms are mild this may be all that is needed, but in those whose symptoms are moderate to severe it is best to refer to a subspecialist who can devote the time necessary to these patients. Individual psychotherapy seems to be more effective in CD than in ODD.

Pharmacotherapy should be considered an adjunct to behavioral therapies or can be directed at specific comorbid states. Medications target specific symptoms as there is no approved medication for CD. These should be prescribed in collaboration with a specialist unless the primary physician is very familiar and comfortable with the medication and the condition.

Prognosis

About 40% of children with early-onset CD will become adults with antisocial personality disorder or psychopathy. Overall about 30% of CD children will continue with a repetitive display of illegal behaviors. Antisocial behavior rarely begins in adulthood. It is therefore critical that early-onset CD be caught and appropriate interventions made to avoid a lifetime of criminal activity and/or prison. Furthermore, there is a family cycle of antisocial behaviors that is difficult to break. The social burden and public health concerns make this condition very important. As with all the disruptive behaviors of childhood, family physicians can make a significant impact with screening, recognition, treatment, and referral.

Loeber R et al: Oppositional defiant and conduct disorder: a review of the past 10 years, part 1. J Am Acad Child Adolesc Psychiatry 2000;39:1468.

Mash E, Barkley R (editors): *Child Psychopathology*. Guilford Press, 1996.

Searight HR et al: Conduct disorder: diagnosis and treatment in primary care. Am Fam Physician 2001;63:1579.

Seizures

Donald B. Middleton, MD

ESSENTIALS OF DIAGNOSIS

- *Abnormality on neuroimaging.*
- *Diagnostic electroencephalogram.*
- *Mood or behavioral changes.*
- *Occurrence of an aura.*
- *Alteration in or impaired consciousness.*
- *Confusion, lethargy, sleepiness.*
- *Fever in children.*

General Considerations

Few events in life are more dramatic or frightening than a seizure, yet despite an alarming appearance, a single seizure rarely causes permanent sequelae. The lifetime risk of having a seizure is 10%. About 3% of the population develops epilepsy, which is defined as spontaneous or unprovoked, recurrent seizures. These numbers translate into an annual incidence of 50,000–150,000 new seizures in children and adolescents, 15,000–30,000 of whom have epilepsy. Therefore, during childhood the majority of seizure victims will not have a recurrence or develop epilepsy.

Epilepsy has an annual incidence of 50/100,000 population with a prevalence of 5–10/1000. Its incidence is high in childhood, decreases in midlife, then peaks in the elderly. Generally seizures must be repetitive to be classified as epilepsy, but even a single seizure coupled with a significant abnormality on neuroimaging or a diagnostic electroencephalogram (EEG) signifies epilepsy.

Each year about 3% of 6-month-old to 6-year-old children suffer from a febrile seizure, the most common seizure entity. Of the 10% of children who have one seizure, only about 30% go for medical evaluation. In contradistinction, more than 80% of children with a second seizure seek medical assistance. Persons at the lowest risk for seizure recurrence are those with recognizable treatable seizure etiologies, normal EEG, negative family histories, normal physical examinations, lack of head trauma, and normal neuroimaging studies.

Leppik IE: *Contemporary Diagnosis and Management of the Patient with Epilepsy,* ed 5. Handbooks in Health Care, 2000.

Pathogenesis

A seizure is the reflection of an abnormal, transient outburst of involuntary neuronal activity. Anoxic degeneration, focal neuron loss, hippocampal sclerosis (the major pathological finding in temporal lobe epilepsy), and neoplasia are examples of pathological central nervous system (CNS) changes that can produce seizures. Why a seizure spontaneously explodes is unclear, but most antiepileptic drugs (AED) alter ion flow, suggesting abnormal ion flow as the event producing a seizure. For example, phenytoin and carbamazepine inhibit the rapid discharge phase in neuronal sodium channels. Other drugs, notably gabapentin, enhance γ-aminobutyric acid (GABA) activity, reducing neuronal excitability. Hence seizures appear to be the result of abnormally discharging neurons.

Seizures are either generalized, meaning a simultaneous discharge from the entire cortex, or partial (focal), meaning a discharge from a focal point within the brain. Generalized seizures impair consciousness and, with the exception of some petite mal (absence) spells, cause abnormal motor movements. Convulsions are the intense motor contractions that reflect underlying seizures. Because generalized convulsions occur most commonly in the absence of a focal defect, the initiating mechanism of a generalized seizure is less well understood than that of a partial seizure, which arises from a focal CNS lesion. Partial seizures may either impair (complex) or not impair (simple) consciousness and can present with almost any neurological complaint or aura including abnormal smells, visions, movements, feelings, or behaviors. Partial seizures can progress to and thus mimic generalized seizures, a fact that sometimes obscures the true nature of the problem because of the trauma of the convulsion.

During childhood the majority of seizures are reactive, ie, due to an inciting event. Although specific events such as head trauma, CNS infection, drug ingestion, or metabolic abnormalities like hypoglycemia or hyponatremia provoke some seizures, the cause of many reactive seizures remains unknown. Nonspecific etiologies like stress or sleep deprivation are often blamed without specific pathophysiology. Most probably a genetic predisposition to seize is distributed throughout the population. When some stressor changes the threshold for neuronal discharge, a seizure occurs. Unlike reactive seizures, the etiology for the majority of epilepsies remains obscure. These are termed the cryptogenic epilepsies. When an identifiable cause for epilepsy is evident, that epilepsy is called symptomatic. If genetic inheritance is at fault, the epilepsy is idiopathic. For instance, possible etiologic factors for a complex partial seizure include inheritance (idiopathic), head injury or CNS infection (symptomatic), or unknown cause (cryptogenic).

Genetic predisposition to seizures has been clearly defined for some types of epilepsy. Juvenile myoclonic epilepsy is linked to a specific gene location. Some inherited diseases with an increased incidence of seizures such as tuberous sclerosis are also secondary to specific chromosomal defects.

Table 9–1 presents a useful scheme of seizure description which is used to guide treatment and predict outcome. Some forms of epilepsy do not fall into this seizure classification and so receive special categorization as epilepsy syndromes. Examples include infantile spasms

Table 9–1. Classification of seizures.

I. Generalized
  A. Convulsive: tonic, clonic, tonic–clonic
  B. Nonconvulsive: absence (petit mal), atypical absence, myoclonic, atonic
II. Partial (focal or localization related)
  A. Simple (consciousness preserved): motor, somatosensory, special sensory, autonomic, psychic
  B. Complex (consciousness impaired): at onset, progressing to loss of consciousness
  C. Evolving to secondary generalized
III. Unclassified
  A. Syndrome: West's syndrome (infantile spasms), Lennox–Gastaut syndrome, neonatal seizures, others
  B. Other

From Commission on Classification and Terminology of the International League Against Epilepsy: Proposal for the classification of epilepsy and epilepsy syndromes. Epilepsia 1989;30:389.

(West's syndrome) or benign childhood epilepsy with centrotemporal spikes (rolandic epilepsy). Unprovoked seizures are more likely to be epilepsy. Table 9–2 lists a general classification of epilepsy. Other sources present detailed lists of various epilepsy syndromes.

Hirtz D et al: Practice parameters: evaluating a first nonfebrile seizure in children. Neurology 2000;55:616.

Prevention

Primary prevention equates to attentive provision of preventive health services. During pregnancy, mothers must avoid addictive drug use (alcohol, cocaine, benzodiazepines), trauma (automobile safety), and infection (young kittens with risk for toxoplasmosis infection). Appropriate obstetrical techniques should minimize birth trauma to reduce the hazard of cerebral anoxia, which leads to cerebral palsy. Family history may reveal significant inborn errors of metabolism (Gaucher's disease) or chromosomal abnormalities (Down syndrome), some of which are amenable to treatment. Strict attention to childhood immunizations (prevention of sepsis and meningitis, especially for pneumococcus and *Haemophilus influenzae* type b), safety during childhood activities (wearing bicycle helmets, supervision when swimming or in the bathtub) and for adolescents (wearing seatbelts), and avoidance of addictive drugs (cocaine, phencyclidine) are examples of appropriate, primary seizure preventives. Regular adequate sleep and exercise and a well-rounded diet are extremely important to good growth and development in general and to the primary prevention of seizures.

Secondary prevention requires attention to the triggers of seizures, such as drugs that lower seizure threshold or cause seizures *de novo* (Table 9–3). The role of caffeine is unclear. Some children develop seizures after prolonged lack of eating, possibly induced by hypoglycemia. An example of this phenomenon is the unfed infant who seizes on Sunday morning when the parents have overslept after a late Saturday night out, the so-called "Saturday night seizure." In some forms of epilepsy stimulation from light or noise, startle responses, faints, fever, or metabolic derangements can worsen underlying tendencies for seizure or cause repetitive seizures. Therefore, strict adherence to regular, healthy activities and avoidance of any known prior precipitant of seizure are required to reduce likelihood of seizure. Known epileptics should not drive until seizure free for 6 months, swim or take baths alone, or engage in any potentially dangerous activity. Steps should be taken to decrease the potential for febrile illnesses (eg, annual influenza vaccination reduces the likelihood of high fever with resultant loss of seizure control).

Table 9–2. Classification of epilepsies and epileptic syndromes.

I. Localization-related (focal, local, partial) epilepsies and syndromes
  A. Idiopathic (genetic) with age-related onset
    1. Benign childhood epilepsy with centrotemporal spikes (rolandic)
    2. Childhood epilepsy with occipital paroxysms
    3. Primary reading epilepsy
  B. Symptomatic (remote or preexisting cause)
  C. Cryptogenic (unknown etiology)
II. Generalized epilepsies and syndromes
  A. Idiopathic with age-related onset in order of age at onset
    1. Benign neonatal familial convulsions
    2. Benign neonatal convulsions
    3. Benign myoclonic epilepsy in infancy
    4. Childhood absence epilepsy (pyknolepsy)
    5. Juvenile myoclonic epilepsy (impulsive petit mal)
    6. Epilepsy with grand mal seizures on awakening
    7. Other
  B. Cryptogenic and/or symptomatic epilepsies in order of age at onset
    1. Infantile spasms (West's syndrome)
    2. Lennox–Gastaut syndrome
    3. Epilepsy with myoclonic–astatic seizures
    4. Epilepsy with myoclonic absences
  C. Symptomatic
    1. Nonspecific etiology
      a. Early myoclonic encephalopathy
    2. Specific syndromes
      a. Diseases presenting with or predominantly evidenced by seizures
III. Epilepsies and syndromes undetermined as to whether they are focal or generalized
  A. With both types
    1. Neonatal seizures
    2. Severe myoclonic epilepsy in infancy
    3. Epilepsy with continuous spike waves during slow wave sleep
    4. Acquired epileptic aphasia (Landau-Kleffner syndrome)
  B. Without unequivocal generalized or focal features
    1. Sleep-induced grand mal
IV. Special syndromes
  A. Situation-related seizures
    1. Febrile convulsions
    2. Related to other identifiable situations: stress, hormonal changes, drugs, alcohol, sleep deprivation
  B. Isolated, apparently unprovoked epileptic events
  C. Epilepsies characterized by specific modes of seizure precipitation
  D. Chronic progressive epilepsia partialis continua of childhood

---

From Leppik IE: *Contemporary Diagnosis and Management of the Patient with Epilepsy,* ed 5, Handbooks in Health Care, 2000; Commission on Classification and Terminology of the International League Against Epilepsy: Proposal for the classification of epilepsy and epilepsy syndromes. Epilepsia 1989;30:389; and Guberman AH, Bruni J: *Essentials of Clinical Epilepsy,* ed 2. Butterworth Heinemann, 1999.

Clinical Findings

A. Symptoms and Signs

The primary tool for seizure assessment is the history, which should include (1) age at onset, (2) family history, (3) developmental status, (4) behavior profile, (5) health at seizure onset including fever, vomiting, diarrhea, or illness exposure, (6) precipitating events including exposure to toxin or trauma, (7) sleep pattern, and (8) dietary pattern. Whether an aura occurred prior to the seizure is a critical piece of information. Because 20% of childhood seizures occur only at night, description of early morning behavior including transient neurological dysfunction or disorientation is especially important. Any symptom can be an aura, which may indicate a focal CNS lesion, which in turn requires further evaluation. Therefore, preictal behavior must be elucidated. Specific areas for investigation are summa-

Table 9–3. Drugs linked to seizures.

A. Over-the-counter
  1. Antihistamines: cold remedies
  2. Ephedrine: common in diet supplements
  3. Insect repellents and insecticides: benzene hexachloride
  4. "Health" and "diet" drugs
B. Prescription
  1. Antibiotics: penicillins, imipenem, fluoroquinolones; acyclovir; metronidazole; mefloquine; isoniazid
  2. Asthma treatments: aminophylline, theophylline, high-dose steroids
  3. Chemotherapeutic agents: methotrexate, tacrolimus
  4. Mental illness agents: tricyclics, selective serotonin reuptake inhibitors, methylphenidate, lithium, antipsychotics, bupropion
  5. Anesthetics and pain relievers: meperidine, propoxyphene, tramadol; local (lidocaine) or general anesthesia
  6. Antidiabetic medications: insulin and oral agents
  7. Miscellaneous: some β-blockers, immunizations, radiocontrast
C. Drugs of abuse
  1. Alcohol
  2. Cocaine
  3. Phencyclidine
  4. Amphetamine
  5. LSD
  6. Marijuana overdose
D. Drug withdrawal
  1. Benzodiazepines: diazepam, alprazolam, chlordiazepoxide
  2. Barbiturates
  3. Meprobamate
  4. Pentazocine may precipitate withdrawal from other agents
  5. Alcohol
  6. Narcotics
  7. Antiepileptic drugs: rapid drop in levels

From Leppik IE: *Contemporary Diagnosis and Management of the Patient with Epilepsy*, ed 5. Handbooks in Health Care, 2000; Menkes JH, Sankar R: Paroxysmal disorders. In *Child Neurology*, ed 6. Menkes JH, Sarnat HB (editors). Lippincott Williams & Wilkins, 2000; and Guberman AH, Bruni J: *Essentials of Clinical Epilepsy*, ed 2. Butterworth Heinemann, 1999.

Table 9–4. Historical evaluation of possible seizure.

I. Behavior: mood or behavior changes before and after the seizure
II. Preictal symptoms or aura
  A. Vocal: cry or gasp, slurred or garbled speech
  B. Motor: head or eye turning, chewing, posturing, jerking, stiffening, automatisms (eg, purposeless picking at clothes or lip smacking), jacksonian march, hemiballism
  C. Respiration: change in or cessation of breathing, cyanosis
  D. Autonomic: drooling, dilated pupils, pallor, nausea, vomiting, urinary or fecal incontinence, laughter, sweating, swallowing, apnea, piloerection
  E. Sensory changes
  F. Consciousness alteration: stare, unresponsiveness, dystonic positioning
  G. Psychic phenomena: delusion, déjà vu, daydreams, fear, anger
III. Postictal symptoms
  A. Amnesia
  B. Paralysis: up to 24 hours, may be focal
  C. Confusion, lethargy, or sleepiness
  D. Nausea or vomiting
  E. Headache
  F. Muscle ache
  G. Trauma: tongue, head, bruising, fracture, laceration
  H. Transient aphasia

From Hirtz D et al: Practice parameters: evaluating a first non-febrile seizure in children. Neurology 2000;55:616.

rized in Table 9–4. Reports of preictal, ictal, and postictal symptoms and actions from both the seizure victim and witnesses help to clarify the seizure type and lead to appropriate choice of therapy.

Unlike adults, children and adolescents with seizures tend to have fewer correctable associated conditions. The majority of seizures are reactive and are not epileptic. For example, following head trauma the 5-year risk for epilepsy is only 2%, despite the fact that after impact seizures are common. On the other hand 15–30% of children with depressed skull fractures develop epilepsy. Syncopal episodes often result in minor twitching or even major tonic–clonic seizures. These seizures do not reflect epilepsy but are an example of the result of transiently diminished CNS perfusion.

The most common associated conditions are mental retardation and cerebral palsy. Multiple other conditions that influence CNS structure or function need to be considered in children with repetitive seizures. Associated psychological difficulties are common and often make recognition and/or control of seizure disorders difficult. Cognitive deficiencies linked to epilepsy include attention deficit, memory difficulties, and learning disorders. In adolescents, psychosis and eating disorders (anorexia nervosa) should be considered. Psychoses and anxiety disorders including panic attacks are rare in younger children, but affective problems such as depression or personality disorders are occasionally present.

Abnormalities that lead to seizures in the normal population include transient stress or injury such as sleep deprivation or hypoglycemia. Reflex seizures follow numerous stimulants: visual (photic stimulation, television, video games, colors, eye fluttering), auditory (music, loud noises, specific voice or sound), somatosensory (tap, touch, immersion in hot water, tooth brushing), cognitive (math problems, card games, drawing), motor (movement, swallowing, eye convergence), and combinations of stimulants (reading, eating, exercise, startle). Seizures are also associated with genetic disorders (neurofibromatosis, Klinefelter syndrome), structural problems (hippocampal sclerosis, neoplasia), congenital lesions (hamartoma, porencephalic cyst), cerebrovascular disorders (arteriovenous malformation, stroke), collagen vascular disease (systemic lupus erythematosus), demyelinating disorders (multiple sclerosis), blood dyscrasias (sickle cell disease, idiopathic thrombocytopenia), eclampsia, metabolic disorders [porphyria, phenylketonuria, electrolyte abnormality (hypoglycemia, hypocalcemia, hypomagnesemia), hyperosmolality], mental diseases (autism), trauma, or infection (syphilis, tuberculosis, human immunodeficiency virus). This myriad of possibilities creates an extremely large differential diagnosis that requires diligence to elucidate. Inciting events such as infection can also precipitate seizures in epileptic patients. The etiologies of childhood epilepsy differ markedly from those of adult epilepsy, especially with regard to tumor and cardiovascular risks. Epilepsy in childhood is 68% idiopathic, 20% congenital, 5% traumatic, and 4% postinfectious, but only 1% each vascular, neoplastic, and degenerative, which are much more common in adulthood. These etiologies present 21% of the time as complex partial seizures, the most difficult to control; 19% as generalized tonic–clonic, the easiest to control; 12% as absence, which almost universally ceases prior to adulthood; 11% as simple partial seizures; 11% as other generalized; 7% as simultaneous multiple types, often syndrome associated; 14% as myoclonic, often difficult to recognize because of limited motor activity; and 5% as other.

1. Generalized seizures—Major motor seizures with tonic–clonic (grand mal) movements, apnea, and cyanosis are both the most common and the most readily recognized. A short cry just before the seizure is usual. The majority of these seizures are reactive and nonrecurrent. Convulsions usually last less than 3 min but may last up to 15 min. Survival with normal mental functioning indicates that cardiopulmonary function is maintained during the bulk of seizures.

Other generalized seizures may be more difficult to identify. About 10% of epileptic children have typical absence (petit mal) spells: brief (10–30 s) losses of consciousness without collapse. Absence spells are characterized by a blank, unresponsive stare with occasional chewing or lip smacking, all without aura or postictal change. Normal activity is interrupted only briefly. These spells are common from ages 3 to 20 years and can be precipitated by photic stimulation or hyperventilation. Unfortunately up to 50% of individuals with absence spells develop tonic–clonic seizures later in life, especially if the onset of absence was during adolescence. Another 10% of epileptic children have atypical absence spells with some motor activity of the extremities, duration greater than 30 s, and postictal confusion. Many children with atypical absence spells are mentally handicapped. Both types of absence spells can occur up to hundreds of times per day and so can create havoc with school performance or be dangerous in recreational activities. Hence school failure or repetitive trauma may indicate the presence of absence spells.

Another generalized epilepsy syndrome, juvenile myoclonic epilepsy, affects 1–3/1000 persons. It is genetically linked to chromosome 6 but is not fully penetrant, so that a family history of similar seizures is present in only 40% of patients. The onset of myoclonic, tonic–clonic, and absence seizures begins between ages 8 and 18 years in otherwise normal children. Triggering events include sleep deprivation, photostimulation, alcohol intake, and stress. Unlike typical absence spells, prospects for permanent remission are poor: about 90% relapse when AED treatment is stopped.

2. Partial seizures—Partial seizures in childhood include benign epilepsy with centrotemporal spikes (BECTS or rolandic epilepsy), which accounts for 15% of all epilepsies. With an onset between ages 2 and 14 years, BECTS presents with guttural noises, paresthesias, and tonic or clonic face or arm contractions. Daytime BECTS presents with an aura of numbness or tingling in the mouth that precedes motor arrest of speech and excessive salivation in an otherwise conscious child. Nocturnal BECTS may generalize into grand mal convulsions. The annual incidence is 10–11/100,000 children. These seizures often occur in the early morning, with the child screaming, drooling, falling, or confused. Although causing great concern, they are not usually dangerous. About 20% of these children have only one episode whereas 25% develop repetitive seizures unless treated. By age 16 years almost all of these children are seizure free.

The classic, albeit rare, simple partial seizure is the jacksonian march, which is an orderly progression of clonic motor activity, distal to proximal, indicating a focal motor cortex defect. Much more common is the versive seizure, in which the eyes and/or head turn away from the side of the seizure focus. The arm on the side to which the head turns may be extended and the opposite arm may flex, creating the classic fencer's posture. Many of these seizures generalize into clonic–tonic convulsions. Unlike in adults, Todd's postictal paralysis in childhood following these convulsions usually does not suggest an underlying structural lesion.

Other simple partial seizures include myoclonic jerks consisting of single or repetitive contractions of a muscle or muscle group. Myoclonic convulsions account for 7% of seizures in the first 3 years of life. Benign occipital epilepsy has an onset between ages 1 and 14 years with a peak incidence between ages 4 and 8 years. These otherwise normal children develop migraine-like headaches with vomiting, loss of vision, visual hallucinations, or illusions. Seizures may be oculoclonic, hemiclonic, photosensitive, and/or suppressed by eye closure. These episodes usually stop during adolescence.

Complex partial seizures usually last 1–2 min, and 50–75% are accompanied by automatisms. Postictal confusion is usual. These seizures usually begin after age 10 years. Consciousness may be lost at seizure onset or gradually over time. The myriad of manifestations of complex partial seizures makes it difficult to determine which child is likely to benefit from epilepsy evaluation. Behavior alteration, including numbing, hissing, random walking or wondering, sleepwalking, irrelevant or incoherent speech, affective change such as fearfulness or anger, daydreaming, aggression, searching behavior, or ideational blocking, demonstrates this variety. Nausea, vomiting, abdominal pain, pallor, flushing, enuresis, falling, illusions, and drooling can all be signs of complex partial seizures, which should be considered for children with repetitive episodes. Especially common are changes in body or limb position, confusion during activities, and a dazed expression. The child will always exhibit amnesia for these events upon recovery. Syndromes such as Lennox–Gastaut usually present with several different types of seizures closely linked in time. Myoclonic jerks, grand mal seizures, and absence spells in the same, usually mentally deficient individual should suggest this syndrome.

Guberman AH, Bruni J: *Essentials of Clinical Epilepsy,* ed 2. Butterworth Heinemann, 1999.

Menkes JH, Sankar R: Paroxysmal disorders. In: *Child Neurology,* ed 6. Menkes JH, Sarnat HB (editors). Lippincott Williams & Wilkins, 2000: 919.

B. PHYSICAL FINDINGS

Vital signs should be assessed and steps taken to correct abnormalities. Because 3% of children have simple febrile convulsions, fever is by far the most important physical finding. A stiff neck coupled with a fever mandates further study, usually including a lumbar puncture to detect meningitis. Focal infection such as pneumonia can also cause febrile seizures. For all types of seizure, preexisting focal deficits, mental deficiency, abnormal neurological findings, and postictal focal deficits are clues to CNS pathology, which may point to the need for imaging studies. Failure to return to baseline alertness should trigger more intensive evaluation. The head should be closely examined for asymmetry and signs of trauma, generally absent if a problem such as syncope rather than a seizure is at fault.

Definitive evidence of seizure activity should be sought. For example, a tongue can be bitten intentionally by those faking seizures, but a fractured tooth is strong evidence of a true clonic–tonic seizure. Scars can reflect past seizure-induced injury. Because excessive salivation occurs in true seizures, malingering patients often use soap to simulate frothing at the mouth. Although frequent with a true seizure, incontinence of urine or stool is not definite evidence of such, as malingerers may urinate or defecate voluntarily.

Fluid leak from the nose suggests cribriform plate fracture. The skin should be examined for café au lait spots, adenoma sebaceum and hypopigmented spots (tuberous sclerosis), portwine stain (Sturge–Weber), or cutaneous telangiectasia (Louis–Bar). The eyes may show similar syndrome-related findings (cherry red spots).

The lungs can reveal signs of aspiration pneumonia, or the heart cardiac rhythm disturbances or murmurs. Lacerations or fractures of the extremities or elsewhere are much more definitive proof of seizure-related trauma, but can also suggest child abuse. Shaken baby syndrome with CNS hemorrhage can present with a seizure. Significant complications of seizures include oral lacerations, fractures, dislocations, bruises, cuts, burns, concussion, arrhythmias, pulmonary edema, myocardial infarction, drowning, and death. Many of these problems arise from well-intentional but misdirected bystander assistance that leads to trauma from attempts to stop the seizure or stop the tongue from "being swallowed." Sudden unexpected death in epilepsy occurs in 1–2 persons/1000 per year. Tonic–clonic seizures, treatment with three or more AEDs, and an intelligence quotient (IQ) of less than 70 are risk factors for sudden death, whereas choice of AED and serum level are not. Sudden death, which is uncommon in childhood, peaks at age 50–59 years.

Walczak TS et al: Incidence and risk factors in sudden unexpected death in epilepsy. Neurology 2001;56:519.

C. LABORATORY FINDINGS

The decision to perform laboratory or radiographic evaluations is based on (1) the patient's age (age below 6–12 months requires action); (2) history of preceding illness, especially gastroenteritis and dehydration; (3) history of substance abuse or drug exposure; (4) the type of seizure, eg, complex partial seizures generally require evaluation; (5) failure to return to a normal state following a seizure; and (6) an abnormal neurological examination upon recovery from the seizure. Table 9–5 lists the usual battery of examinations, which should be augmented with cardiac, pulmonary, or liver testing or arterial blood gases when the history or physical examination suggests problems with these organ systems. The vast majority of evidence fails to support routine testing, which is especially unwarranted for first time, tonic–clonic seizures. Although the first EEG is abnormal in 50% of those later proven to have epilepsy, obtaining an EEG may not be worthwile. The EEG fails to accurately predict who will have a seizure recurrence and about 2% of normal children have abnormal EEGs. Similar criticism can be leveled at neuroimaging. The clinical presentation should serve as a guide to who needs an EEG or neuroimaging.

In children and adolescents a linkage between a seizure and an underlying brain tumor is extremely rare in the absence of other abnormalities. Brain tumors in childhood are rare, seizures are not. In an international review of 3291 children with brain tumors, only 35 (1%) otherwise normal children had a seizure as the initial difficulty. However, for adults, 1–2% of computed tomography (CT) scans reveal tumors, numbers that are even higher for those with risk factors such as smoking. The key is to perform a complete neurological examination to detect other abnormalities, obtain reassurance of the benign nature of the seizure, and provide adequate follow-up.

Magnetic resonance imaging (MRI) is preferred to a CT scan. Although abnormalities are detected in up to one-third of MRIs, only 1–2% of these findings influence either treatment or prognosis, especially in otherwise normal children. Only about 1% of these tests point to a correctable lesion. Table 9–6 lists recommended evaluations for neuroimaging for each seizure type. Neuroimaging is primarily useful for those who have focally abnormal neurological examinations or a

Table 9–5. Recommendations for evaluation of a first seizure.

Study	Recommendation	Strength of Recommendation[1]
Electroencephalogram	All patients[2]	A[3–5]
Blood tests [electrolytes, glucose, blood urea nitrogen (BUN), creatinine, calcium, magnesium]	Individual basis: especially indicated for age 6 months or less; continued illness; history of vomiting, diarrhea, or dehydration	A[6]
Toxicology screening	If any possibility of drug or substance of abuse exposure	C[6]
Lumbar puncture	If possibility of meningitis or central nervous system (CNS) infection; continued CNS dysfunction	B[7]
CNS imaging		
Computed tomography (CT)	Value limited largely to head trauma	A[6,8]
Magnetic resonance imaging (MRI)	Best performed for	A[6]
	Prolonged postictal paralysis or failure to return to baseline	
	Persistent significant cognitive, motor, or other unexplained neurological abnormality	
	Age under 12 months	
	Perhaps with partial seizures	
	An EEG indicative of nonbenign seizure disorder	
Prolactin level	Variable benefit; 15 to 30 min after a seizure	B[6]
Creatine kinase level	Variable benefit	C[6]

[1]A, supported by clinical studies and expert opinion; B, expert opinion; limited evidence for support; C, limited to specific situations; insufficient evidence for or against this evaluation.
[2]Somewhat in debate.
[3]Martinovic Z, Jovic N: Seizure recurrence after a first generalized tonic clonic seizure, in children, adolescents and young adults. Seizures 1997;6:461.
[4]Shinnar S et al: The risk of seizure recurrence following a first unprovoked afebrile seizure in childhood: an extended follow-up. Pediatrics 1996;98:216.
[5]Stroink H et al: The first unprovoked, untreated seizure in childhood: a hospital based study of the accuracy of diagnosis, rate of recurrence, and long term outcome after recurrence. Dutch study of epilepsy in childhood. J Neurol Neurosurg Psychiatry 1998;64:595.
[6]Hirtz D et al: Practice parameters: evaluating a first nonfebrile seizure in children. Neurology 2000;55:616.
[7]Rider LG et al: Cerebrospinal fluid analysis in children with seizures. Pediatr Emerg Care 1995;11:226.
[8]Garvey MA et al: Emergency brain computed tomography in children with seizures: who is most likely to benefit. J Pediatr 1998;133:664.

Table 9–6. Imaging recommendations for childhood seizures.

Seizure Type	Imaging Study[1]
Neonatal	Cranial ultrasound preferred
	CT acceptable
Partial	MRI preferred
	CT acceptable
Generalized	
Neurologically normal	MRI or CT but low yield
Neurologically abnormal	MRI preferred
	CT acceptable
Intractable or refractory	MRI preferred
	SPECT acceptable
	PET acceptable
Febrile	"No study" recommended
Posttraumatic (seizures	CT preferred
within 1 week of trauma)	MRI acceptable

From Strain JD et al: Imaging of the paediatric patient with seizures. American College of Radiology Appropriateness Criteria 1999;787.
[1]CT, computed tomography without contrast; MRI, magnetic resonance imaging without gadolinium; SPECT, single-photon emission tomography; PET, positron emission tomography. Other studies also acceptable in some instances.

history suggesting deteriorating behavior or school function, infection, or trauma; the extremely young infant; those with persistent, focal seizures except for BECTS; focal EEG abnormalities; or in persons over 18 years of age. Patients presenting with status epilepticus (SE), 27% of whom have abnormal MRIs, deserve study.

Other sometimes helpful evaluations include pregnancy tests in young women and psychometric studies to detect focal mental defects or psychiatric disease. Prior to CNS surgery, MRI or cerebral angiography and positron emission tomography (PET) scans are needed to assess the extent of the surgical procedure.

Routine blood tests are more often abnormal in patients with isolated seizures than in those with epilepsy, with the caveat that those on carbamazepine can develop hyponatremia. Glucose, magnesium, calcium, blood urea nitrogen (BUN), creatinine, electrolytes, and complete blood counts (CBC) usually are normal. A high creatine phosphokinase or prolactin level may indicate prior seizure activity. A toxicology screen is useful if drug exposure or ingestion is elicited during the history. Lumbar puncture is required only if meningitis is suspected, an unusual problem in a fully immunized child, especially in one given pneumonococcal and *H influenzae* type b vaccines. Meningococcal meningitis still remains a hazard and is most likely to affect the young infant or college freshman residing in a dormitory room. The latter may benefit from meningococcal vaccine.

An EEG is diagnostic in 30–50% of first-time seizure victims, but its accuracy improves to 90% with repetitive testing. The EEG can also localize an abnormality in the CNS, eg, a frontal lobe tumor, suggesting the need for neuroimaging. Most importantly, among patients suspected clinically to have epilepsy, the EEG has a 95% positive predictive value. Unfortunately, up to a third of those individuals with normal EEGs eventually are proven to have epilepsy. Many experts advise that an EEG is indicated for evaluation of all patients with first nonfebrile seizures and repetitive febrile seizures, about 5% of whom develop epilepsy. Awake, asleep, hyperventilation, and photic-stimulated EEG tracings give the best chance of uncovering an abnormality. Prediction of risk of seizure reoccurrence is about 50% with an abnormal EEG and only 25% with a normal nonepileptic EEG. Unfortunately 2% of normal children have epileptiform spikes on EEGs, thus limiting its accuracy. Because tracings within 48 h of a seizure may be falsely abnormal, the optimal timing for an EEG is unclear. EEG patterns are particularly diagnostic in absence spells, BECTS, and juvenile myoclonic epilepsy. When doubt exists as to the veracity of a seizure diagnosis, video-EEG recording can be diagnostic, especially in detecting psychogenic seizures. Twenty-four-hour EEG monitoring often reveals a seizure frequency much greater than otherwise suspected.

Berg AT et al: Neuroimaging in children with newly diagnosed epilepsy: a community-based study. Pediatrics 2000;106:527.

Gilbert DL, Buncher CR: An EEG should not be obtained routinely after first unprovoked seizure in childhood. Neurology 2000;54:635.

Strain JD et al: Imaging of the pediatric patient with seizures. American College of Radiology Appropriateness Criteria 1999;787.

Differential Diagnosis

Many entities resemble seizures. Gastroesophageal reflux, brief shuddering, benign nonepileptic myoclonus, or the Moro reflex in infants can mimic seizures. Breath-holding spells, night terrors, and benign paroxysmal vertigo in toddlers can raise concern about epilepsy. Tics and behavior problems can precede true seizures or act as seizure mimics. Children and adolescents who suffer from psychogenic seizures (pseudoseizures) must be carefully evaluated for underlying psychiatric disturbances or suicidal ideation. Video-EEG should clarify the diagnosis, but psychogenic seizures, which account for 20% of referrals to epilepsy centers, often coexist with true seizures. Hysteria, panic attacks, transient global amnesia, and hyperventilation can mimic a seizure disorder. Malingering to avoid stressful situations such as school or true conversion reactions are uncommon during childhood but can occur in adolescents.

Drugs of abuse, narcolepsy, and migraine can cause seizure-like episodes. Syncopal seizures are best treated with efforts to control syncope, not seizures. Cough-induced or vasovagal syncopal convulsions often occur in childhood. Cardiac entities such as prolonged QT interval (electrocardiogram), aortic stenosis (ECHO cardiogram), or hypertrophic cardiomyopathy (ECHO cardiogram) should be considered in those with a family history of fainting or appropriate physical findings. Shuddering attacks, hereditary tremors, and Tourette's syndrome can masquerade as epilepsy. However, in all of these conditions patients usually have normal EEGs and few improve with AED treatment. In difficult situations, neurological consultation, video-EEG recording, 24-h EEG recording, and watchful waiting almost always provide the correct diagnosis.

Austin JK et al: Behavior problems in children before recognized seizures. Pediatrics 2001;107:115.

Gudmundsson O, Prendergast M: Outcome of pseudo-seizures in children and adolescents: a 6-year symptom survival analysis. Dev Med Child Neurol 2001;43:547.

Treatment

A. First Aid and Initial Care

Acute assistance for a seizure requires placing the patient prone, removing eyeglasses, loosening clothing and jewelry, clearing the area of harmful objects, and **not** putting any object into the patient's mouth or attempting to apply any restraint. After the seizure, the patient should be placed on one side and observed until awake. Families should call for medical assistance if a seizure lasts longer than 3 min, the patient requests assistance or is injured, or a second seizure occurs. After a tonic–clonic seizure, vigorous stimulation may reduce postictal apnea and perhaps sudden death. To avoid aspiration, patients with epilepsy should be encouraged to sleep in the supine position. Hospitalization is necessary only if the patient is at high risk, lives alone without appropriate supervision, or remains ill. Following a seizure, a patient appreciates an explanation of what transpired and information as to how to avoid further difficulties. Follow-up arrangements need to be definite. Avoidance of seizure-provoking activities, provocative drugs, or other seizure-inducing behaviors is adequate treatment for reactive seizures.

B. Drugs

Persons with correctable etiologies that provoke seizures or with unprovoked seizures that are not likely to be dangerous or frequent do not require antiepileptic medications. Most experts do not treat for a single seizure.

Side effects of medication include worsening seizure severity or frequency, organ damage, or even death. AEDs do not always provide seizure control. In fact, 20–30% of those on AEDs still have significant seizure activity. Nor do AEDs appear to affect long-term prognosis positively.

Nonetheless, all primary care physicians should have a command of basic AED use and side effect profiles. Table 9–7 provides information on the most useful AEDs. Other drugs used during childhood usually require specialist help. These include ACTH, nitrazepam, pyridoxine (vitamin B_6), and vigabatrin (which may damage the eyes) for infantile spasms, acetazolamide for absence spells, felbamate (highly toxic and rarely used) for Lennox–Gastaut syndrome, levetiracetum for refractory partial seizures, oxcarbazepine for partial (both simple and complex) seizures, tiagabine for complex partial epilepsy, topiramate for generalized tonic–clonic and partial (both types) epilepsy, and zonisamide for myoclonus. Lamotrigine is approved for children above the age of 2 years for treatment of generalized tonic–clonic epilepsy and partial epilepsy. When valproic acid is part of the patient's AED regimen lamotrigine is given at 0.15 mg/kg/day, divided up in two doses, and is increased in dose 0.15 mg/kg every 2 weeks to a maintenance dose of 1–5 mg/kg/day (maximum 200 mg/day). The dose is three to four times greater when valproic acid is not in the regimen (maximum 400 mg/day).

The selection of AED is based on the seizure type, which unfortunately is inaccurately identified at least 25% of the time. The least toxic AED, usually carbamazepine, valproic acid, or phenytoin, is initiated. Primary generalized seizures respond best to valproate, which controls seizures in 80% of patients when given as monotherapy. Divalproex produces fewer side effects, especially of the gastrointestinal tract. Lamotrigine, carbamazepine, and phenytoin are also good choices to control tonic–clonic convulsions. If no other seizure types are present, ethosuximide is an ideal choice for absence spells. Lamotrigine is also effective. Although juvenile myoclonic epilepsy responds well to valproate, it is unlikely to respond to other agents and is therefore sometimes difficult to control. Partial seizures are best treated with carbamazepine or phenytoin. Lamotrigine or gabapentin can be added when control is inadequate. However, these drugs have a limited role in control of childhood epilepsy. Side effects are sometimes serious and usually unfamiliar to primary care physicians. For example, lamotrigine can cause a life-threatening rash in up to 1 in 50 children. Many of the newer agents are also expensive. If not for the cost, oxcarbazepine at 8–10 mg/kg/day, divided twice a day (maximal starting dose 300 mg, twice a day), offers a significant reduction in side effects and may become an excellent substitute for carbamazepine.

Table 9-7. Drugs for the treatment of seizures.[1]

Drug	Seizure Type	Pediatric Dosage (mg/kg)				Therapeutic Level (μg/ml)	Dosage Forms		Notes
		Starting Dose	Usual Daily Dose	Maximal Dose	Number of Daily Doses		Pill (mg)	Liquid	
Phenytoin	GM, CPS, SPS	5 orally, 10–20 intravenously	5–15	700 mg daily 1000 mg loading	1–3	10–20	C:100 EC: 30,100 CT: 50	S: 125 mg/5 ml (use not recommended)	Gen/Tr (some forms)
Carbamazepine	GM, CPS, SPS	5–10	15–30	2000	2–4	4–12	T: 200; CT: 100; ET: 100, 200, 300 400	S: 100 mg/5 ml	Gen/Tr (some forms)
Valproic acid	GM, PM, CPS, SPS, M	10–15	15–60	3000	2–4	50–120	C:250 CS:125 ET: 500 DT: 125, 250, 500	SY: 250 mg/5 ml	Gen/Tr (some forms)
Ethosuximide	PM	10–20	10–40	2000	1–2	40–100	C: 250	SY: 250 mg/5 ml	Gen/Tr (some forms)
Clonazepam	M	0.01–0.03	0.025–0.2	20	2–3	18–80	T: 0.5, 1, 2	—	Gen/Tr
Gabapentin	Additive only; GM, CPS, SPS	10–15	25–50	4800	3	>2	C: 100, 300, 400 T: 600, 800	SOL: 50 mg/5 ml	Tr
Primidone	GM, CPS, SPS	10	10–30	1500	2–4	5–15	T: 50, 250	S: 250 mg/5 ml	Gen/Tr (some forms)

[1]GM, grand mal; PM, petit mal; CPS, complex partial seizures; SPS, simple partial seizure; M, myoclonic; C, capsule; EC, extended release capsule; T, tablet; CT, chewable tablet; S, suspension; ET, extended release tablet; SY, syrup; CS, capsule sprinkles; DT, delayed release tablet; SOL, solution; Gen, generic; Tr, trade.

One drug pushed to control seizures, to its maximum or to just below toxicity, is best. If one drug proves ineffective, it should gradually be withdrawn at the same time another AED is started. Medication, especially phenobarbital, must be withdrawn slowly to avoid precipitation of seizures or even SE. Polytherapy is fraught with drug side effects and often loss of seizure control. However, in 25% of patients, seizures require two drugs to achieve satisfactory control. Withdrawal of an old AED with institution of a new AED should be accomplished slowly over at least 7 days. Newer drugs generally cause unfamiliar side effects, so often a superior choice to random new drug selection is neurological consultation.

Levels of AEDs, especially ethosuximide, phenytoin, and carbamazepine, help to guide dosage, but valproic acid levels often fail to predict toxicity or seizure control. Serum AED levels should be obtained (1) at initiation to set a baseline dose; (2) as a check on compliance; (3) to detect toxicity, especially for those on multiple agents or who are too young or mentally handicapped to communicate their symptoms; (4) when the overall drug regimen is changed; (5) when seizure control is poor; and (6) when a new problem develops that can affect drug levels. Whether seizure-free children require periodic drug levels is unclear. Unlike adults, children are rapidly growing, so levels of AEDs lessen over time. As children grow they will require larger doses of AED to maintain a therapeutic level. Some advise allowing a child to "grow out" of the AED as a slow taper-off medication to see if a seizure recurs. If this path is chosen, patients and parents must be informed about the plan. Whether routine checks of hematological or liver functions can prevent organ damage is even more unclear. Certainly all patients and parents should be warned to be alert for fever, jaundice, itching, bruising, bleeding, and other signs of bone marrow or liver toxicity. Many physicians choose to follow CBCs, liver and renal tests, and serum AED levels periodically, once or twice a year. In special circumstances (pregnancy, uremia, hypoalbuminemia, or concurrent drug use with agents that displace AED off protein, ie, salicylate), serum-free AED levels may be a better guide to dosing. This situation is especially true for phenytoin and valproate, both highly bound to protein.

Because all AEDs can cause fetal malformations during pregnancy, the drug that has best controlled seizures should be continued. Folic acid up to 4 mg daily before and throughout pregnancy and vitamins D and K given during the last 4 weeks should minimize problems for the fetus. Sonographic evaluation of the fetus helps to identify trouble early. Pregnancy can alter serum AED levels, especially with phenytoin, which must often be increased in dose during pregnancy and slowly decreased after the delivery.

Some AEDs, especially carbamazepine, felbamate, oxcarbazepine, phenobarbital, phenytoin, primidone, and topiramate may interfere with oral contraceptives (OCP). Midcycle bleeding indicates possible OCP failure. This problem can be avoided with alternative contraceptive methods, a higher estrogen content OCP, or prescription of a noninteracting AED such as gabapentin or lamotrigine. Breast-feeding for women on AEDs is considered to be safe.

Despite the low cost and ease of administration, side effects of phenytoin prohibit its use for everyone. Dose-related problems include nystagmus (an excellent marker for overdose), hypotension, ataxia, blurred vision, dysarthria, and drowsiness. With prolonged use, folate-deficiency-related anemia, osteomalacia, neuropathy, coarseness of facial features, gingival hyperplasia (preventable with dental flossing and regular dental cleaning), acne, hirsutism, lymphadenopathy, and mental dullness can occur. Some of these problems are idiosyncratic. Rarely, bone marrow suppression, toxic rash, or hepatic failure develops. Drugs that increase phenytoin levels include warfarin, isoniazid, disulfiram, alcohol acutely ingested, benzodiazepines, and other anticonvulsants. Decreased levels occur with chronic alcohol use, amiodarone, rifampin, folic acid, or certain chemotherapies. Phenytoin can change serum levels of warfarin, lithium, acetaminophen, oral contraceptives, thyroid hormone, quinidine, and insulin. Therefore, whenever any agent is added to or withdrawn from the drug regimen of a patient on phenytoin, a serum level should be obtained at steady state, which is usually 5–7 days later. Phenytoin dosing does not follow first-order kinetics. When its dose is changed, a wise rule is to increase the amount less than appears necessary and decrease the amount more than appears necessary. Thus, a dose increase of 50 mg may raise the serum level by 5–7 µg/mL. A patient with a highly toxic serum level should not continue to take phenytoin at a reduced level but should stop the drug for several days until the serum level is satisfactory and then restart the phenytoin at a reduced dose.

Carbamazepine causes gastrointestinal upset, sleepiness, blurred vision, impaired performance, and, rarely, hepatic or bone marrow failure or allergic rash. It also causes hyponatremia in up to 10% of patients. Drugs that raise or lower carbamazepine levels include selective serotonin reuptake inhibitors, verapamil, diltiazem, erythromycin, clarithromycin, isoniazid, cimetidine, and tricyclic antidepressants (and a multitude of others). Hence a change in drug regimen should trigger a serum level check.

With the exceptions of gabapentin and levetiracetam, most AEDs have multiple drug interactions. Any time a new drug is prescribed to a patient taking an AED, references such as product circulars or drug interaction computer programs must be cross-checked. All AEDs have serious side effects, usually decreased CNS function, as all these agents suppress neurological activity, or gastrointestinal upset. Phenobarbital causes personality changes, precluding its routine use. Patients on phenobarbital may "outgrow" the dose, resulting in a slow taper off the drug. If seizures do not recur, it should not be restarted. When given, dosage ranges from 4 to 8 mg/kg once or divided twice a day. Serum levels should be between 10 and 40 µg/mL. Valproate can cause hair loss, weight gain, pancreatitis, edema, or thrombocytopenia. Topiramate and zonisamide can produce renal stones, ethosuximide can cause abdominal pain or abnormal behavior, and lamotrigine can cause rash or Steven–Johnson syndrome. Any new symptom or sign in a patient on AEDs must trigger a search in a standard reference for AED side effects.

For home treatment of acute repetitive seizures, rectal diazepam given at 0.2–0.5 mg/kg appears to be safe and effective. Rectal diazepam is available as a gel in doses of 2.5, 5, 10, 15, and 20 mg.

No specific seizure-free time interval fits all situations. A single seizure type, normal neurological examination, normal IQ, and normal EEG all predict good outcomes if AED is stopped. In 1013 patients who had been seizure free for 2 years, 40% had a recurrence following drug withdrawal compared to 12% of those who maintained AED treatments. Freedom from drug side effects and daily medication must be weighed against this 28% increased probability of recurrence with potential loss of job or driving ability or possible injury. Certainly a recently abnormal EEG would make a decision to stop therapy more difficult. If stopped, phenytoin, carbamazepine, and valproate should be slowly withdrawn over at least 6–10 weeks. Once children grow into young adulthood, assuming a 2- to 5-year period without seizures, an attempt to stop AED treatment ought to be strongly considered.

Leppik IE: Monotherapy and polypharmacy. Neurology 2000;55 (suppl 3):S25.

Pellock JM: Managing pediatric epilepsy syndromes with new antiepileptic drugs. Pediatrics 1999;104:1106.

Willmore LJ: Clinical pharmacology of new antiepileptic drugs. Neurology 2000;55(suppl 3):S17.

C. Referral or Hospitalization

Although care of seizure disorders lies within the purview of family physicians, poorly controlled or complicated seizures should receive prompt neurological consultation. Developmental delay may also be a sign that referral is required. In addition to issues mentioned under First Aid, hospitalization is necessary for prolonged or complicated seizures, status epilepticus, inadequate family resources, or parental or physician anxiety. In general, seizures are not dangerous, but children with repetitive seizures must be guarded against injury and other complications. Available guidelines for seizure evaluation and management follow the general outline in this chapter.

D. Surgery

Because 20% of epilepsy is inadequately controlled with AEDs alone, other therapies have arisen. Surgery for epilepsy, including severing of the corpus callosum or temporal lobe resection, results in 80% seizure-free outcomes. Candidates for surgery should have recurrent uncontrolled seizures, focal EEGs, and consistent focal abnormalities on neuroimaging. MRIs may be normal in a patient with abnormal metabolism as revealed on PET. Vagal nerve stimulation is less invasive and controls seizures in about 40% of cases of previously refractory epilepsy. The ketogenic diet reduces episodes by about 50%. These treatments all require referral and extensive evaluation prior to institution.

Tatum WO IV, Benbadis SR, Vale FL: The neurosurgical treatment of epilepsy. Arch Fam Med 2000;9:1142.

E. Family Counseling

Family members, teachers, and other caregivers need instruction in proper seizure first aid. Helpful information and group support are available from the American Epilepsy Society (web site: www.aesnet.org) and the Epilepsy Foundation of America (web site: www.efa.org) or local epilepsy foundations. Vocational help and assistance to defray medical costs are often needed. To serve the interests of the patient and family, a close physician–patient relationship must be fostered. All patients must have adequate sleep and exercise, reduce stress, and avoid alcohol or sedative drug use.

The physician should reassure patients and family that seizures do not lower IQ or cause brain damage. Psychologically, dealing with epilepsy is difficult. The negative consequences of a seizure disorder to daily life should not be underestimated, but most otherwise normal patients with epilepsy lead full, productive lives. In fact only 25% of untreated epilepsy is debilitating. Hence reassurance that in general an individual can lead a normal existence despite the epilepsy is warranted. Scheduled activities for each day may help. Some children do better with home schooling until seizures are controlled. For those who develop psychological dysfunction, especially depression, psychiatric consultation or medication is usually extremely helpful.

Centers for Disease Control and Prevention: Health-related quality of life among persons with epilepsy—Texas, 1998. MMWR 2001;50:24.

Wiegarty P et al: Co-morbid psychiatric disorder in chronic epilepsy: recognition and etiology of depression. Neurology 1999;54(suppl 2):S3.

F. Alternative Therapies

Few of the commonly utilized alternative therapies have evidence-based support. Some such as pyridoxine (vitamin B_6) and magnesium have scientific grounding for use in specific seizure disorders. Multiple web sites present information that must be recommended with caution if at all. Commonly advised are a diet high in fat, low in protein, and low in carbohydrates. Food allergies are occasionally blamed for seizures, again without scientific proof. Most alternative therapy sources advise avoidance of alcohol, caffeine, and aspartame, the first two of which are at least logical. Proof that taurine, folic acid, vitamin B_{12}, manganese, zinc, dimethylglycine, or megavitamins reduce seizure frequency or medication requirements is absent or marginal. Herbs such as passionflower, skullcap, or valerian are recommended without study. Homeopaths may prescribe belladonna, causticum, cicuta, or cuprum metallicum, none of which has been adequately studied. Whether acupuncture, chiropractic, or naturopathic manipulation helps children with seizures is open to question.

On the other hand, any nontoxic technique to reduce stress and bring order to a child's life may help. Some patients have learned to control seizures with self-relaxation or special techniques such as looking at a particular piece of jewelry as an aura comes on. Hence, those families who wish to augment medical treatment with noninvasive treatments may be encouraged to do so after physician review for safety and if the treatments appear to help over time.

Additional information is available at multiple web sites such as http://home.mdconsult.com or http://healthcare.micromedex.com. The veracity of advice on these sites is left to the user to investigate.

Febrile Convulsions

Febrile convulsions are the most common seizure disorder, affecting 3% of children between ages 6 months and 6 years. Children up to age 14 years may have febrile seizures. Despite a recurrence rate of 30%, only 3% of these individuals develop epilepsy, but those with a family history of epilepsy, abnormal neurological or developmental status prior to the seizure, or a prolonged (greater than 15 min) focal seizure have at least a 15% chance of later epilepsy. Commonly the young toddler with an upper respiratory infection suddenly seizes during an afternoon nap. Viral infection such as nonpolio enterovirus or roseola has been implicated as a common etiology. Although these are usually short tonic–clonic convulsions, seizures are multiple in one-third of cases. Postictal sleepiness can last several hours.

Generally laboratory tests are unnecessary unless meningitis is suggested by failure to arouse, continued focal seizures, suggestive physical findings (stiff neck, bulging fontanel, rash), or age under 9 months. Seizures that occur in the office or emergency department can also be more indicative of serious infection.

Treatment consists of reassurance to worried parents that the worst has passed and that these seizures leave no permanent brain damage. Parents want to prevent these episodes. Controlling fever with warm baths; acetaminophen, 10–15 mg/kg, every 4 h; or ibuprofen, 5–10 mg/kg, every 6 h may reduce immediate risk of recurrence. If begun at the onset of fever, oral or rectal valproate, 20 mg/kg, every 8 h, or diazepam, 0.5 mg/kg, every 8 h, for 1–3 days can reduce recurrence. Intravenous diazepam or lorazepam is the drug of choice for prolonged febrile seizures. Hospitalization is best if seizures are prolonged beyond 30 min or are recurrent or complicated, if follow-up is inadequate, or if parents or the physician are overly frightened. Chronic treatment is advised only for the child with multiple recurrences, persistent neurological abnormality, or a worrisome EEG.

Baumann RJ: Prevention and management of febrile seizures. Paediatr Drugs 2001;3:585.

Baumann RJ, Duffner PK: Treatment of children with simple febrile seizures: the AAP practice parameter. Pediatr Neurol 2000;23:11.

Gordon KE et al: Treatment of febrile seizures: the influence of treatment efficacy and side-effect profile on value to parents. Pediatrics 2001;108:1080.

Status Epilepticus

Any recurrent or prolonged seizure uninterrupted by consciousness for more than 30 min is termed SE. About 5% of children with febrile convulsions and 20% of those with epilepsy have SE at least once. Newly diagnosed epileptics often develop SE. These children run a low risk of residual brain damage, which can be minimized through rapid treatment. Although all seizure types including simple partial seizures can present in SE, most commonly consciousness is severely impaired. A generalized persistent grand mal seizure is usually readily identified as SE, but myoclonic SE with preserved consciousness is more difficult to recognize. Perhaps the most difficult is the patient in SE who has no abnormal motor movement but is comatose. Confused but moving children may be in absence or complex partial epilepsy SE. Diagnosis is based on clinical presentation with typical EEG findings. Permanent intellectual impairment is possible following prolonged SE. Death is usually related to a serious underlying etiology for the SE rather than the SE itself.

Management requires vital stabilization of vital signs. Adolescents should be given 100 mg of thiamine followed by 50 mL of 50% glucose (children 2–4 mL/kg of 25% glucose) intravenously coupled with naloxone (0.1 mg/kg up to 2 mg) repeated as necessary. Lorazepam 0.1 mg/kg (maximum 4 mg) intravenous push at 2 mg/min is successful in stopping 80% of SE episodes in 2–3 min. A second dose in 10 min is frequently successful in the remaining 20%. An alternative is diazepam 0.5 mg/kg (maximum 20 mg) intravenous push at 5 mg/min. Poorly controlled SE responds to phenytoin 20 mg/kg, intravenous push at 50 mg/min, while monitoring the electrocardiogram and blood pressure, or its more safe prodrug, fosphenytoin, given at 30 mg/kg intravenous push at 150 mg/min. Other alternatives are phenobarbital and propofol. Immediate serum AED levels define adequacy of therapy. Some SE in children under 18 months of age responds to pyridoxine, 50 mg intravenously. Other drugs for SE are reviewed elsehwere. Once the SE is controlled, a search for the underlying cause should be conducted to minimize the risk of recurrence.

Sabo-Graham T, Seay AR: Management of status epilepticus in children. Pediatr Rev 1998;19:306.

Neonatal Seizures

In the first month of life, clonic–tonic seizure activity is uncommon. Hence, most neonatal seizures are difficult to recognize. Focal rhythmic twitches, recurrent vomiting, unusual high-pitched crying, posturing, chewing, apnea, cyanosis, and excessive salivation should raise alarm. Diligent inquiry into family history, prenatal history, and maternal habits is warranted. Definitive diagnosis rests on neurological consultation and EEG tracings. These seizures are also often difficult to control and may have a dismal outcome. Appropriate treatment for maternal drug addiction with resultant neonatal drug withdrawal seizures, which often leave no residual defects, includes paregoric, methadone, chlorpromazine, and phenobarbital. Table 9–8 lists suggested evaluations. An ultrasound is of critical importance to rule out intracranial hemorrhage.

Moshe SL: Seizure early in life. Neurology 2000;54:635.

Prognosis

Overall, after one seizure about one-third of patients have a second seizure. Of these about 75% experience a third seizure. However, no adverse outcomes are likely even with up to 10 untreated seizures. A study of

Table 9–8. Evaluation of neonatal seizures.

I. History
 A. Pregnancy related
  1. Infection: toxoplasmosis, rubella, cytomegalovirus, herpes, syphilis (TORCHS); immunoglobulin M level
  2. Maternal addiction: smoking, alcohol, cocaine, heroin, barbiturates
  3. Maternal behavior: inadequate prenatal care, lack of folic acid
 B. Delivery related
  1. Anoxia
  2. Trauma
 C. Family history: chromosomal disorders, errors of metabolism
II. Physical findings
 A. Recognizable patterns of malformation: eyes, ears, hands, facies, head shape
 B. Neurological evaluation: motor, sensory, cranial nerves
 C. Odor: phenylketonuria
 D. Dermatological signs: crusted vesicles, abnormal creases, hypopigmentation, nevi
 E. Ocular: chorioretinitis, cataracts, coloboma, cherry red spot
III. Laboratory evaluation
 A. Neuroimaging: cranial ultrasound, magnetic resonance imaging (MRI), computed tomography (CT) scan
 B. Chest radiograph
 C. Cerebral spinal fluid: culture, cell count, gram stain, India ink, VDRL, glycine, glucose, protein, xanthochromia
 D. Blood test: cultures, complete blood count, electrolytes, renal function, glucose, magnesium, calcium, karyotype, glycine, lactate, ammonia, long-chain fatty acid levels
 E. Urine: culture, glucose, protein, cells

From Hill A: Neonatal seizures. Pediatr Rev 2000;21:117 and Moshe SL: Seizure early in life. Neurology 2000;54:635.

220 children indicated that 92% of those treated for idiopathic seizures remain seizure free for as long as 5 years. The same was true for 62% of cryptogenic epileptics. However, over 25% of patients off all medicine had no seizures for 5 years, but unfortunately many of those with severe CNS damage died. This information reaffirms the need to carefully consider AED treatment before institution and before discontinuation. Eventually 60% of epileptic children become seizure free.

Shinnar S et al: Predictors of multiple seizures in a cohort of children prospectively followed from the time of their first unprovoked seizure. Ann Neurol 2000;48:140.

SECTION II

Adolescence

Adolescent Development & Screening

10

D. Dean Patton, MD, & Jerri R. Harris, MPH

Family physicians are in a unique position among medical professionals to provide health care for adolescents. Family practice encompasses care of patients throughout all life stages, attending to biopsychosocial issues through every stage. Adolescence, along with the period from ages 0 to 3, is one of the most concentrated periods of developmental change in a person's life. Care and management of patients in the transition from child to adult require knowledge, skills, and attitudes specific to the physical, psychological, and social development of this population. Behaviors and attitudes developed during this period shape the health of adulthood, and thus can have profound long-range implications for individuals and society.

Among primary care specialists, family physicians provide health care for more than half of all adolescents, and, according to the American Academy of Family Physicians (AAFP), for about two-thirds of all adolescents obtaining health care. Family physicians who also provide health care for parents of adolescents can begin to establish a relationship of trust early in the child's life, and begin anticipatory guidance in a family context to ease the transition for both children and their parents. Family history also is essential in recognizing individual development and growth norms determined by genetic factors and allaying concerns of parents and adolescents if development does not occur as they might expect.

Growth & Development

Physical (puberty), psychosocial, and cognitive development characterize adolescence, although all do not occur at the same time or at the same rate. Develop-

mental age (preadolescent, mid-adolescent, or postadolescent) is more descriptive of when growth and development occur than is chronological age (Table 10–1).

Puberty

All the prepubertal mechanisms contributing to the onset of puberty are not well known. Most likely, the trigger for the release of gonadotrophin-releasing hormone (GnRH), which stimulates secretion of pituitary gonadotrophins, is associated with bone age and body composition. Gonadotrophins stimulate synthesis and secretion of follicle-stimulating hormone (FSH) and luteinizing hormone (LH). About 6 months after pubertal levels of FSH and LH are reached, the child begins to show signs of sexual maturation. FSH stimulates growth of the ovarian follicle and production of estrogenic hormones; LH is associated with ovulation, corpus luteum formation, progesterone production, theca cell androgen production, and regulation of estradiol production after ovulation. In males, LH by way of the Leydig cells stimulates testicular maturation and production of testosterone. The combination of LH and FSH stimulates the last stage of spermatogenesis.

Androgens in males and estrogens in females increase serum growth hormone (GH) and insulin-like growth factor 1 (IGF-1) during puberty. For girls the adolescent growth spurt takes place usually between ages 12 and 13, and for boys, usually between ages 14 and 15. Most skeletal and muscular systems are involved, but not to an equal degree, and not at the same time. Height growth occurs primarily through the trunk; muscle growth takes place about 3 months and

Table 10–1. Characteristics of Early, Middle, and Late Adolescence.

Characteristics	Early Adolescence	Mid-Adolescence	Late Adolescence
Growth	Secondary sexual characteristics have begun to appear Growth rapidly accelerating; reaches peak velocity	Secondary sexual characteristics well advanced Growth decelerating; stature reaches 95% of adult height	Physically mature; statural and reproductive growth virtually complete
Cognition	Concrete thought dominant Existential orientation Cannot perceive long-range implications of current decisions and acts	Rapidly gaining competence in abstract thought Capable of perceiving future implications of current acts and decisions but variably applied Reverts to concrete operations under stress	Established abstract thought processes Future oriented Capable of perceiving and acting on long-range options
Psychosocial self	Preoccupation with rapid body change Former body image disrupted	Reestablishes body images as growth decelerates and stabilizes Preoccupation with fantasy and idealism in exploring expanded cognition and future options Development of a sense of omnipotence and invincibility	Emancipation completed Intellectual and functional identity established May experience "crisis of 21" when facing societal demands for autonomy
Family	Defining independence–dependence boundaries No major conflicts over parental control	Major conflicts over control Struggle for emancipation	Transposition of child–parent dependency relationship to the adult–adult model
Peer group	Seeks peer affiliation to counter instability generated by rapid change Compares own normality and acceptance with same sex/age mates	Strong need for identification to affirm self-image Looks to peer group to define behavioral code during emancipation process	Recedes in importance in favor of individual friendships
Sexuality	Self-exploration and evaluation Limited dating Limited intimacy	Multiple plural relationships Heightened sexual activity Testing ability to attract opposite sex and parameters of masculinity or femininity Preoccupation with romantic fantasy	Forms stable relationships Capable of mutuality and reciprocity in caring for another rather than former narcissistic orientation Plans for future in thinking of marriage, family Intimacy involves commitment rather than exploration and romanticism
Age range	Initiates between ages 11 and 13 and merges with mid-adolescence at 14–15 years	Begins around 14–15 years and blends into late adolescence about age 17	Approximately 17–21 years; upper end particularly variable; dependent on cultural, economic, and educational factors

From Hofmann AD: Adolescent growth and development. In *Adolescent Medicine,* ed 3. Hofmann AD, Greydanus DE (editors). Appleton & Lange, 1997. Reproduced with permission of the McGraw-Hill Companies.

weight peak velocity about 6 months after the height peak.

The heart and other organs also have growth spurts during this period. Whether brain growth also is accelerated at this time is not clear. The facial profile straightens, incisors are more upright, and the nose becomes more prominent. Changes in facial structure are greater in boys than in girls. Boys also develop larger hearts, skeletal muscles, and lungs, as well as higher systolic blood pressure, lower resting heart rate, greater capacity for carrying oxygen in the blood, and greater capacity for neutralizing the chemical products of exercise.

Sexual Maturation

Much of the work on sexual maturation was done by James Tanner in 1962. Tanner classified sexual maturation into five developmental stages, from the prepubertal state (Stage 1) to the adult state (Stage 5). The sexual maturation rating (SMR) is more useful in defining the health care needs and developmental issues of adolescence than is chronological age.

Understanding the stages of sexual maturation enables the physician to provide anticipatory guidance to both parents and adolescents. Important in that understanding is recognizing that developmentally, adolescents may be more or less mature than they appear. Although most adolescents progress through the stages with no more than one stage difference, a two-stage difference can still be within the normal distribution range of maturation. Knowing this can help adolescents understand that accelerated or delayed maturation can still be normal and that, perhaps sooner or later than their peers, they will reach and pass through Stage 5.

Development of Pubic Hair, Genitalia, & Breasts

Tanner stages are defined by development of pubic hair and breasts for girls and pubic hair and genitalia for boys (Tables 10–2, 10–3, and 10–4). Progression through the five stages is predictable. Lack of this predictable progression could be an indication of pubertal disorder and might require further examination and possible referral to an endocrinologist. Figures 10–1, 10–2, and 10–3 illustrate development by stage.

Features & Common Concerns of Male & Female Development

Tanner stages span an average of 4.5 years (Table 10–5). Features of male development include onset of Stage 1 between 9 and 13 years of age; peak height velocity between Stages 3 and 4, with an average height

Table 10–2. Development of pubic hair through Tanner Stages 1–5.

Stage	Girls	Boys
1	No coarse pubic hair, vellus only	Vellus hair over the medial pubic bones
2	Sparse growth of long, straight, or slightly curly hair along the labia only; the hair is usually pigmented	Sparse growth of curled or straight, slightly pigmented hair at the base of the penis, mainly on the sides
3	Hair is more coarse, darker, and spreads upward to sparsely cover the mons pubis	Extension of darker, coarser, and more curled hair to the mons pubis
4	Hair is adult in appearance, but the area covered is slightly less; no extension of hair to the medial thigh	Adult type hair, but not as extensive, and not spread to the medial thigh
5	Adult type hair and area covered, with spread to the medial thigh	Adult type hair and area covered, with spread to the medial thigh

gain of 5–7 inches; first ejaculations typically during Stage 3; and strength peaks between Stages 4 and 5. A common concern of male adolescents is perceived delayed puberty. This is often ruled out by a normal history and physical, as well as growth records indicating normal patterns. Often there is a family history of "delayed" puberty.

Features of female development include onset of Stage 1 between 8 and 13 years of age and growth spurt during Stage 2, with an average height gain of 4 inches. Menarche occurs at about age 12, and acne is common during Stages 3 and 4. Common concerns of female adolescents include isolated breast development associated with premature thelarche and isolated pubic hair development associated with premature adrenarche.

Table 10–3. Female breast development.

Stage	Description
1	Elevation of papilla only
2	Breast bud stage: elevation of the breast and papilla as a single mound; enlargement of the areola
3	Further enlargement with no separation of contour
4	A secondary mound is formed by the elevation of the areola and papilla as a separate contour
5	Mature adult with protrusion of only the nipple

Table 10–4. Male genital development.

Stage	Penis	Testes
1	Preadolescent	Preadolescent (<1.5 mL)
2	Slight enlargement	Slight enlargement, slight darkening of scrotum (1.56 mL)
3	Longer	Larger (6–12 mL)
4	Longer and broader	Larger, scrotum darker (12–20 mL)
5	Adult size	Adult size (> 20 mL)

From Brook CGD: *Growth Assessment in Childhood and Adolescence.* Blackwell Scientific Publications, 1982.

Neither is usually associated with significant pathology. Concerns can be alleviated for the patient by placing the finding in context with normal ranges and familial patterns.

Gynecomastia is a common condition occurring in approximately 60% of adolescent males. It is most often bilateral, begins about 6 months after the onset of sexual development, is more prevalent at about age 14, and usually resolves without treatment by about age 17. Gynecomastia can cause anxiety and extreme embarrassment for parents and adolescents. Discussion of gynecomastia should be a routine part of anticipatory guidance with male adolescents. They may feel reassured also by the information handout available through the AAFP and *American Family Physician* on the World Wide Web. Causes of gynecomastia range from benign and temporal conditions related to puberty to more serious pathology related to drugs, adrenal disorders, or chronic disease. Evaluation of the history of the disorder during routine examinations will determine whether treatment or even surgery may be required. Patients should be cautioned against squeezing the tissue, which in rare instances stimulates lactation.

Cognitive Development

Intellectual and emotional development is associated to some degree with advancement in skeletal maturity. Growth rate and timing are determined mostly by biological factors, not by social interaction. The child who is developing more slowly may need to be evaluated for potential problems. Normally, the gradual shift from concrete to abstract thinking begins around age 12 and continues to full development at about age 16, enabling most adolescents to apply concepts and experiences to different situations. Competence in applying abstract thinking seems to be related to the degree to which students have opportunities to practice and apply reasoning, analytic, and decision-making skills in school. Of note is that about 30% of the normal population do not fully develop the ability to think abstractly. Nevertheless, abstract thinking plays a major role in psychosocial development, including the adolescent's search for identity and the formulation of personal values.

In stressful situations such as conflicts at home or school (or visits to the doctor), adolescents may revert to concrete thinking, although they are developing abstract thinking skills, just as many adults may do. For example, under the potentially stressful situation of a clinical encounter, the adolescent may appear to be uncommunicative or uncooperative. Physicians may need to adjust their communication styles to accommodate either concrete (immediate consequences or benefits of behaviors) or abstract (long-range consequences or benefits of behaviors) processes. For example, reasons not to smoke might relate to athletic performance or social issues for concrete thinkers or to long-term effects on morbidity and mortality for abstract thinkers.

Male and female adolescents may have problems related to development that could affect adjustment in school. For example, girls who develop breasts early or boys who develop late may still be within the norm, but feel embarrassed or humiliated among their peers if they appear to be different.

Psychosocial Development

Adolescent development includes the psychological progression from dependent child to independent, self-reliant adult. Emancipation, forming a sexual, intellectual, and moral identity, as well as the focus on life goals can all be stressful for adolescents and their families. Because of expectations about education or training and earlier maturation over the past several generations, physiological development may be 95% complete up to 10 years before adolescents become self-reliant. When reproductive maturity precedes cognitive and psychological maturity, high-risk behaviors become even more challenging for teens and parents, and consequently also for physicians.

Cultural conflicts can also arise in the process of promoting adolescent health and development. Adolescents from minority cultures within the United States may face conflicts resulting from differences in culture between their family and society. Psychological development may be complicated by discrepancies between societal expectations and family cultures that emphasize the importance of family, respect for elders, gender differences, and interdependence of extended families. Western cultures are more likely to emphasize independence, autonomy, a youth culture, individualism, and competition. Differences exist within Western cultures as well, potentially creating tension between a family's

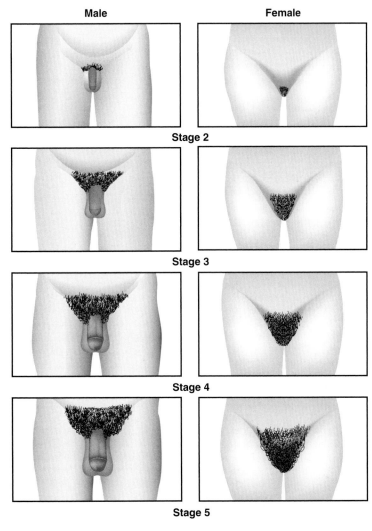

Male   **Female**

Stage 2

Stage 3

Stage 4

Stage 5

MALE	FEMALE
Stage 1 Preadolescent: no pubic hair present; a fine vellus hair covers the genital area.	Preadolescent: no pubic hair present; a fine vellus hair covers the genital area.
Stage 2 A sparse distribution of long, slightly pigmented hair appears at the base of the penis.	A sparse distribution of long, slightly pigmented straight hair appears bilaterally along medial border of the labia majora.
Stage 3 The pubic hair pigmentation increases; the hairs begin to curl and to spread laterally in a scanty distribution.	The pubic hair pigmentation increases; the hairs begin to curl and to spread sparsely over the mons pubis.
Stage 4 The pubic hairs continue to curl and become coarse in texture. An adult type of distribution is attained, but the number of hairs remains fewer.	The pubic hairs continue to curl and become coarse in texture. The number of hairs continues to increase.
Stage 5 Mature: the pubic hair attains an adult distribution with spread to the surface of the medial thigh. Pubic hair will grow along linea alba in 80% of males.	Mature: pubic hair attains an adult feminine triangular pattern, with spread to the surface of the medial thigh.

Figure 10–1. Maturational stages of pubic hair development. [From Hofmann AD: Adolescent growth and development. In: *Adolescent Medicine.* Hofmann AD, Greydanus DE (editors). Appleton & Lange, 1997. Reproduced with permission of McGraw-Hill Companies.]

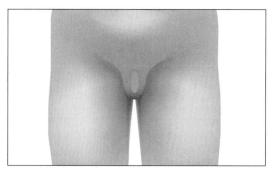

Stage 1

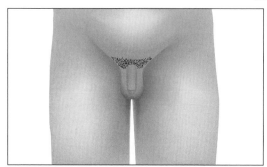

Stage 2

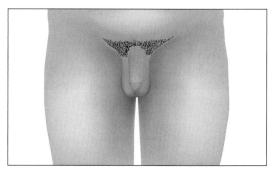

Stage 3

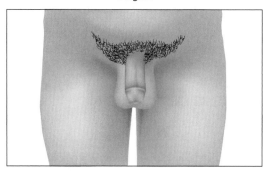

Stage 4

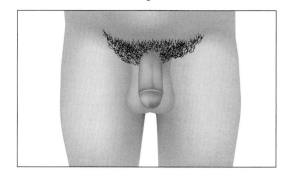

Stage 5

Stage 1   Preadolescent: testes, scrotum, and penis identical to early childhood.
Stage 2   Enlargement of testes as result of canalization of seminiferous tubules. The scrotum enlarges, developing a reddish hue and altering its skin texture. The penis enlarges slightly.
Stage 3   The testes and scrotum continue to grow. The length of the penis increases.
Stage 4   The testes and scrotum continue to grow; the scrotal skin darkens. The penis grows in width, and the glans penis develops.
Stage 5   Mature: adult size and shape of testes, scrotum, and penis.

Figure 10–2. Male genital development. [From Hofmann AD: Adolescent growth and development. In: *Adolescent Medicine*. Hofmann AD, Greydanus DE (editors). Appleton & Lange, 1997. Reproduced with permission of McGraw-Hill Companies.]

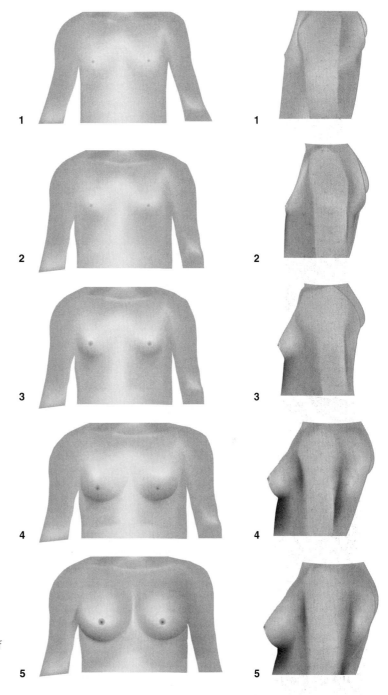

Figure 10–3. Female breast development. (Courtesy of JM Tanner, MD, Institute of Child Health, Department of Growth and Development, University of London, London, England.)

Table 10–5. Mean age of secondary characteristics.

Male	Age (Years)	Female	Age (Years)
Testicular and penile changes begin	11.6	Thelarche	11.2
Adrenarche	13.4	Adrenarche	11.7
Pubarche	14.1	Pubarche	12.3
Tanner Stage 5 pubic hair	15.2	Menarche	13.5
		Tanner Stage 5 pubic hair	14.4
		Tanner Stage 5 breast	15.3

From Brook CGD: *Growth Assessment in Childhood and Adolescence.* Blackwell Scientific Publications, 1982.

values regarding issues such as sex education, counseling, and confidentiality and a physician's goal of promoting health, which could be seen by the family as usurping their roles and responsibilities. As with other aspects of caring for adolescents, a long-term relationship with the family, as well as clarification of the goals of providing health care and screening, will aid in caring for teens who find themselves between two cultures.

Issues of Consent & Confidentiality

Adolescents do not seek or may delay seeking health care for a number of reasons. In addition to lack of access, finances, and awareness of clinical services are concerns about confidentiality. They are more likely to seek care about sensitive issues if they feel the provider will not disclose that information to their parents. Trust in the relationship usually is best developed over time. Therefore, the physician is more likely to have opportunities to assess developmental issues within a relationship that has been fostered through contact in the prepubertal period.

Laws governing confidentiality issues in treating minors have been based on the recognition that (1) adolescents are more likely to seek care about sensitive and potentially harmful behaviors if they feel their care will be confidential and (2) mature minors have a right to give informed consent to health care. Laws deal with circumstances in which minors are not required to have parental consent (reproductive health care, treatment of sexually transmitted diseases, rape or incest, health-risk behaviors, and emergency health care). Other laws are based on emancipation status, whether a minor is a parent, is or has been married, lives away from home, is in the armed forces, is a high school graduate, or is mature as determined by age. In most states age of maturity is

considered to be 18, although in a few states it is younger (14 in Alabama, 15 in Oregon, and 16 in South Carolina except for surgery). In Nebraska the age of consent is 19.

Confidentiality statutes have been subject to change in recent years by state and federal legislation guided by beliefs about parental involvement in children's health care. Because statutes differ across states, physicians need to clarify what is and is not required. Sources for this information are local and state medical societies, departments of health and social services, and legal authorities on health care laws. Whether the institution or organization is primarily concerned with patient rights or provider risk will influence how the laws will be interpreted.

The position of the American Academy of Family Physicians (AAFP) on confidentiality (Compendium of AAFP Positions on Selected Health Issues) recognizes the need to balance the "rights of the parents and what is necessary to maintain and promote the health and well-being of the adolescent." The AAFP maintains that it is both "proper and ethical for the family physician to protect an adolescent's confidentiality." Further, the position states that it may be appropriate to withhold information from third parties, including parents, "when it pertains to but is not limited to contraception, pregnancy, sexually transmitted diseases and physical and/or sexual abuse by a parent."

Issues of confidentiality and consent usually are most easily managed in the context of a long-term physician–family relationship. Beginning in late childhood to talk about the anticipated day when the child will see the physician without the presence of a parent lays the groundwork. A private conversation with a parent or parents informing them of the physician's intent to develop a relationship with their adolescent that will respect the privacy of the adolescent sometimes can relieve parental anxiety. It may be preferable to have the first "private" visit while the child is still prepubertal.

It is almost always preferable to treat adolescents in the context of family. Open communication between parents and adolescents is the ideal situation and should be encouraged and sometimes facilitated by the family physician. Because the framework for the ideal family relationship does not always exist for the adolescent seeking health care, it is imperative that health care providers understand the issues related to consent for care, as well as the issues related to the right to privacy versus the parents' right to know. Consent and confidentiality issues do not bind the physician to provide care that may violate the physician's own moral code.

Privacy of the medical and billing records is yet another issue to be addressed with staff, patients, and their parents. Separate notes can be kept as part of, but apart from, medical records. Nevertheless, adolescents should be aware that records or billing statements may reveal information that may concern them. In addition, they should be aware of the physician's legal responsibility to report situations in which patients are at risk for suicide or homicide, or are victims of sexual or physical abuse.

Guidelines for Adolescent Preventive Services

The Guidelines for Adolescent Preventive Services (GAPS) are recommendations developed by the American Medical Association's Department of Adolescent Health that were first published in 1993. They emphasize the value of annual visits for health promotion both for adolescents and their parents, and outline screening and prevention protocols for all patients ages 11–21 years. The guidelines serve to organize health care delivery for adolescents and are useful in helping to identify patients at risk during early, mid, and late stages of adolescent growth and development. In addition to addressing common medical problems that occur in this age group, the guidelines incorporate screening for the social and behavioral health risks most responsible for morbidity and mortality among adolescents.

Concerns have been raised about the quality of evidence supporting the guidelines, the appropriateness of adopting some recommendations previously developed for adult patients, and the cost effectiveness of annual health maintenance visits for adolescents. Stickler challenges the need for annual screening visits for adolescents. His review of 12 studies (a total of 20,047 examinations) found that yearly physical examinations revealed few problems not previously known, and that the examinations were not cost effective. He concludes that a comprehensive examination could be done in early adolescence, mid-adolescence (the start of high school), and late adolescence, using screening questionnaires and testing for height, weight, vision, and blood pressure, in addition to performing the physical examination and inspecting for scoliosis. He acknowledges, however, that "special risk groups," such as those who are sexually active or who are known to engage in substance abuse, should have examinations more often. Stickler also states that emotional problems of adolescents likely are "better recognized by teachers, parents, and counselors," given that office visits do not provide enough time to detect them. Nevertheless, the GAPS screening recommendations do incorporate questions regarding family, peer, and school relationships that can screen for potential biomedical, psychosocial, and behavioral problems that affect health and development, and indicate situations that need referral.

Longitudinal epidemiological and descriptive studies conducted during the past decade, such as the National Longitudinal Study on Adolescent Health, and cumulative data from risk behavior surveys by the Centers for Disease Control and Prevention and other national surveys indicate substantial increases in serious health risks for many adolescents in the United States. Among African-American, Native American, and Hispanic adolescents, the rates can be even higher for problems such as early sex, sexually transmitted diseases, unintended pregnancies, violence, and substance abuse. Also higher among minority adolescent populations are rates of diabetes, including increases in type 2 diabetes, and obesity. (See other chapters in the section on Adolescence for more detailed discussions of nutrition, obesity, eating disorders, sexuality, and sexually transmitted diseases.) Because adolescent development involves more than biomedical issues, cost-effectiveness studies that rely on medical diagnoses per dollar spent will not reflect the potential long-term costs of care for high-risk behavior or chronic diseases. Until those data are available, physicians may prefer to consider the more aggressive GAPS recommendations.

GAPS Recommendations

GAPS recommendations are organized into four categories: (1) delivery of health care services, (2) the use of health guidance to promote health and well-being, (3) screening for conditions common during adolescence that have the potential to cause current and future suffering, and (4) the use of immunizations to prevent infectious diseases. Topics and health conditions addressed by GAPS are shown in Table 10–6.

Table 10–6. GAPS health promotion and prevention topics and conditions.

Promoting	Preventing
Parents' ability to respond to the health needs of their adolescents	Hypertension
Adjustment to puberty and adolescence	Hyperlipidemia
Safety and injury prevention	Use of tobacco products
Physical fitness	Use and abuse of alcohol and other drugs
Healthy dietary habits	Eating disorders and obesity
Healthy psychosocial adjustment	Negative health consequences of sexual behaviors
	Severe or recurrent depression and suicide
	Physical, sexual, and emotional abuse
	Learning problems
	Infectious diseases

Recommendations indicate that health care services should be provided regularly and tailored to individual patients, and that information should be shared with the adolescent and be kept confidential. Recommendations for health guidance are designed to help adolescents approach development with greater knowledge and understanding, particularly as they develop cognitively and psychologically. Health guidance for parents or guardians is suggested to help them respond more effectively to the health needs of their adolescents. Guidelines for screening include recommendations for biomedical, behavioral, and emotional conditions. From initial screenings, physicians can determine whether to continue assessment and management or refer the patient to another provider. Immunization recommendations are based on guidelines from the Advisory Committee on Immunization Practices convened by the federal government and include hepatitis B recommendations and indications for hepatitis A.

Along with the GAPS recommendations, the American Medical Association (AMA) also developed screening questionnaires in both English and Spanish. One questionnaire is designed for parents or guardians to complete; two other questionnaires are designed for younger adolescents and middle to older adolescents to complete. Also available through the AMA web site is a Parent Package of information sheets covering 15 topics. Each handout contains facts, tips, and other resources to help parents provide guidance for their adolescents. The handouts can supplement anticipatory guidance provided by the physician.

American Academy of Family Physicians: Recommended Curriculum Guidelines for Family Practice Residents. Adolescent Health. AAFP Reprint 278, 1999. www.aafp.org/edu/guide/rep278.html. Downloaded 3/2002.

American Medical Association: Guidelines for Adolescent Preventive Services. Parent/Guardian Questionnaire, 1997. Available on the AMA web site, www.ama·assn.org. Downloaded 3/2002.

American Medical Association: Guidelines for Adolescent Preventive Services. Younger Adolescent Questionnaire, 1997. Available on the AMA web site, www.ama·assn.org. Downloaded 3/2002.

American Medical Association: Guidelines for Adolescent Preventive Services. Younger Adolescent Questionnaire, 1998. Available on the AMA web site, www.ama·assn.org. Downloaded 3/2002.

American Medical Association: Medicine and Public Health. The Parent Package, 2001. Available on the AMA web site, www.ama·assn.org. Downloaded 3/2002.

Blum RW et al: The effects of race/ethnicity, income, and family structure on adolescent risk behaviors. Am J Public Health 2000;90(12):1879.

Fagot-Campagna A et al: Type 2 diabetes among North American children and adolescents: an epidemiologic review and a public health perspective. J Am Pediatrics 2000;136(5):665.

Friedman HL: Culture and adolescent development. J Adolescent Health 1999;25:1.

Guidelines for Adolescent Preventive Services (GAPS): Recommendations Monograph, 1997. Available on the AMA web site, www.ama·assn.org. Downloaded 3/2002.

Gynecomastia: when breasts form in males. Patient information. Am Fam Physician 1997;55(5):1849.

Hofmann AD: Adolescent growth and development. In: *Adolescent Medicine,* ed 3. Hofmann AD, Greydanus DE (editors). Appleton & Lange, 1997: 10–21.

Hofmann AD: Consent and confidentiality. In: *Adolescent Medicine,* ed 3. Hofmann AD, Greydanus DE (editors). Appleton & Lange, 1997: 61–73.

Neuman JF: Evaluation and treatment of gynecomastia. Am Fam Physician 1997;55(5):1835.

Proimos J: Confidentiality issues in the adolescent population. Curr Opin Pediatr 1997;9:325.

Resnick MD et al: Protecting adolescents from harm: findings from the National Longitudinal Study on Adolescent Health. JAMA 1997;278(10):823.

Stevens N: Adolescent guidelines: should we use them? Am Fam Physician 1998;57(9):2060.

Stickler GB: Are yearly physical examinations in adolescents necessary? JABFP 2000;13(1):172.

Tanner JM: *Growth at Adolescence.* Blackwell, 1962.

Physical Activity in Adolescents

Mark B. Stephens, MD, MS, FAAFP[1]

"Regular physical activity enhances both personal health and the vitality of our society. Establishing such activity as a habit for all our citizens must be a national priority."

—*Former President Jimmy Carter*

General Considerations

The United States is in the midst of a growing epidemic of physical inactivity and obesity. During the past two decades, physical inactivity has played a major role in the staggering rise of obesity among children and adolescents. Longitudinal data from the National Health and Examination Surveys show that the percentage of overweight adolescent females has increased from 5% to 10% and the percentage of overweight adolescent males has increased from 5% to 12% of the population (Figure 11–1). Currently, one in four adolescents in the United States is either overweight or at risk for becoming overweight. Overweight youth are much less likely to engage in physical activity and are much more likely to report chronic health problems compared with normal weight peers.

During adolescence, levels of spontaneous physical activity drop precipitously from childhood levels. One-third of U.S. high-school students are not regularly active (Figure 11–2). One-half of high school seniors are not enrolled in physical education classes, and 70% of all high school students watch at least one hour of television every day of the week. For those students enrolled in physical education, the actual amount of class time spent engaged in physical activity has dropped significantly over the past decade. Students spend a majority of time in physical education class standing around, waiting for instructions, or socializing.

Individuals who are overweight during adolescence are far more likely to be overweight as adults. Teens spend a majority of their days engaged in sedentary activities, averaging a mere 12 min/day of vigorous physical activity. Behaviors also tend to consolidate during adolescence. Health-related behaviors, such as dietary habits and physical activity patterns, solidify during adolescence and persist into adulthood. Therefore, recognition of individuals who are insufficiently active, overweight, or obese during adolescence is important.

Lowry R et al: Recent trends in participation in physical education among US high school students. J Sch Health 2001;71(4): 145.

U.S. Department of Health and Human Services: *Promoting Better Health for Young People through Physical Activity and Sports.* U.S. Department of Health and Human Services and the Centers for Disease Control, 2000.

U.S. Department of Health and Human Services Centers for Disease Control and Prevention: Youth risk behavior surveillance—United States, 1999. MMWR. 2000;49(SS-5):1.

Definitions

The following definitions apply to the discussion of physical activity and obesity (Table 11–1). *Physical fitness* refers to a general state of well-being that allows an individual to perform most activities of daily living in a vigorous manner. Physical fitness is further described in terms of health-related characteristics and skill-related characteristics. Health-related components of physical fitness include cardiorespiratory endurance, muscular strength, muscular endurance, flexibility, and body composition. Skill-related components of physical fitness include power, speed, agility, and balance. Historically, more attention has been given to skill-related activities and athletic ability. From a public health perspective, however, the health-related characteristics of physical fitness are more relevant in terms of overall morbidity and mortality from chronic diseases related to physical inactivity.

Physical activity refers to any bodily movement that results in the expenditure of energy. Physical activity occurs in a broad range of settings. Leisure-time activities, occupational activities, routine activities of daily

---

[1]The opinions herein are those of the author. They do not represent official policy of the Uniformed Services University, the Department of the Navy, or the Department of Defense.

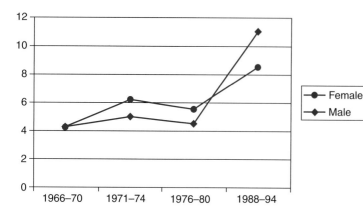

Figure 11–1. Rates of overweight among U.S. adolescents 1966–1994. (National Health and Nutrition Examination Surveys.)

living, and dedicated exercise sessions are all valid forms of physical activity. Activity varies along a continuum of intensity from light (eg, housework) to moderate (eg, jogging) to more vigorous (eg, strenuous bicycling). *Exercise* is a structured routine of physical activity specifically designed to improve or maintain one of the components of health-related physical fitness. To date, society has emphasized exercise programs as the primary means of achieving physical fitness rather than promoting physical activity in a more general sense.

Body mass index (BMI) is currently the anthropometric measurement of choice for assessing body composition in children, adolescents, and adults. BMI is calculated by dividing an individuals weight (in kilograms) by the square of the individual's height (in meters). Charts and digital tools for the office (http://www.cdc.gov/nccdphp/dnpa/bmi/calc-bmi.htm) and for handheld computers (http://hin.nhlbi.nih.gov/bmi_palm.htm) are available for rapid calculation of BMI. Normative values for underweight, normal weight, overweight, and obesity for adolescents have been established, and are presented in Table 11–2. BMI-for-age charts have replaced standard weight-for-height charts

as the preferred mechanism for tracking weight in children and adolescents (Figures 11–3 and 11–4).

U.S. Department of Health and Human Services Public Health Service, Centers for Disease Control and Prevention, National Center for Chronic Disease Prevention and Health Promotion, Division of Nutrition and Physical Activity: *Promoting Physical Activity: A Guide for Community Action.* Human Kinetics, 1999.

Risk Factors Associated with Physical Inactivity/Benefits of Physical Activity

Physical inactivity is a primary risk factor for cardiovascular disease and all-cause mortality. A sedentary lifestyle also contributes to increased rates of diabetes, hypertension, hyperlipidemia, osteoporosis, cerebrovascular disease, and colon cancer. Adolescents who are less physically active are more likely to smoke cigarettes, less likely to consume appropriate amounts of fruits and vegetables, less likely to routinely wear a seat belt, and more likely to spend time watching television.

Physical activity serves numerous preventive functions. In addition to preventing chronic diseases such as

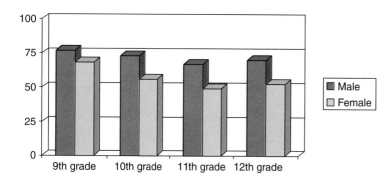

Figure 11–2. Percentage of adolescents attaining recommended levels of vigorous physical activity on a regular basis by age. (Centers for Disease Control, Youth Risk Behavior Survey.)

Table 11–1. Definitions of physical activity, physical fitness, and exercise.

Physical activity	Any bodily movement that results in the expenditure of energy
Physical fitness	A general state of overall well-being that allows individuals to conduct the majority of their activities of daily living in a vigorous manner
Health-related physical fitness	Aerobic capacity (cardiorespiratory endurance) Body composition Muscular strength Muscular endurance Flexibility
Skill-related physical fitness	Power Agility Speed Balance Coordination Reaction time
Exercise	A structured routine of physical activity specifically designed to improve or maintain one of the components of health-related physical fitness

hypertension, diabetes, and cardiovascular disease, individuals who engage in physical activity on a regular basis have lower rates of mental illness. Physically active adolescents have lower levels of stress and anxiety and have higher self-esteem than sedentary peers. Active adolescents also have fewer somatic complaints, are more confident about their own future health, and have a better body image.

Table 11–2. Definitions of overweight and obesity for adolescents and adults.

Definition	Clinical Parameter
Obesity (adults)	BMI > 30
Overweight (adults)	BMI 25.1–29.9
Overweight (adolescents)	BMI > 95th percentile for age
At risk for overweight (adolescents)	BMI > 85th percentile for age
Underweight (adolescents)	BMI < 5th percentile for age

Source: Centers for Disease Control (http://www.cdc.gov/nccdphp/dnpa/bmi/bmi-for-age.htm).

U.S. Department of Health and Human Services: *Physical Activity and Health: A Report of the Surgeon General.* U.S. Department of Health and Human Services, Centers for Disease Control and Prevention, National Center for Chronic Disease Prevention and Health Promotion, 1996.

Why Aren't More Youth Physically Active?

Despite the overwhelming evidence supporting the health-related benefits of physical activity, young Americans are increasingly sedentary. A complex interaction of social, cultural, gender-based, environmental, and familial factors associated with "modern living" has contributed to decreased rates of physical activity.

A. SOCIAL FACTORS

Socioeconomic status is one of the strongest predictors of physical activity in both adolescents and adults. Lower levels of socioeconomic status are associated with lower levels of spontaneous physical activity. Youth of higher socioeconomic status engage in more spontaneous physical activity, are more frequently enrolled in physical education classes, and are more active during physical education classes compared with peers of lower socioeconomic status. This relationship persists when controlling for age, gender, and ethnicity.

Social mobility also plays an important role in shaping levels of physical activity. Specifically, achieved levels of social positioning are more strongly associated with positive health behaviors and increased levels of physical activity than the social class of origin. Youth with active friends are more likely to be active and youth with sedentary friends are more likely to be sedentary. Differences also exist in patterns of physical activity between youth attending public and private secondary schools. In the public school system, individuals are more likely to enroll in physical education classes. In private schools, adolescents are more likely to participate in organized team sports.

Finally, all Americans have become increasingly reliant upon automated transportation. This has negatively impacted the simplest form of physical activity: walking. Historically, walking was the way most youth got to school. This is no longer the case. It is estimated that of all trips Americans take under one mile in distance, 75% are made via automobile or some other form of automated transportation. This reliance upon the automobile has become a significant barrier to physical activity.

B. CULTURAL AND ETHNIC FACTORS

Cohort studies consistently suggest that there are inherent cultural differences in levels of spontaneous physical activity. Data from the Youth Risk Behavior Survey and the National Longitudinal Study of Adolescent

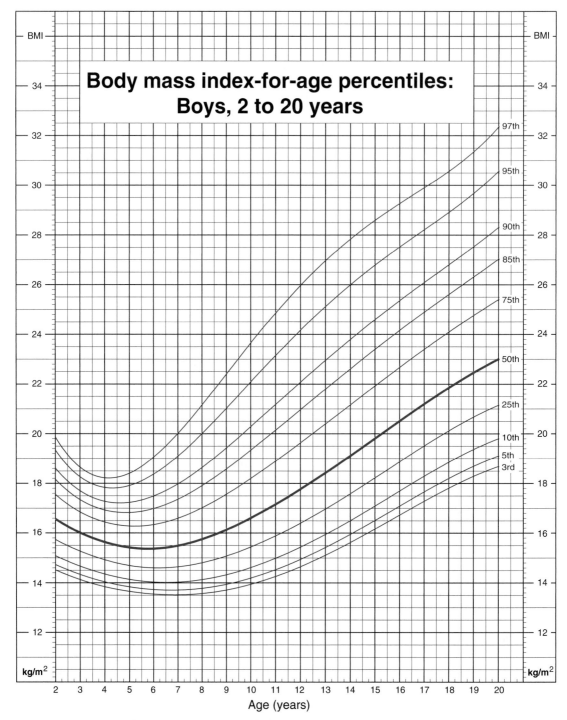

Body mass index-for-age percentiles:
Boys, 2 to 20 years

Published May 30, 2000.
SOURCE: Developed by the National Center for Health Statistics in collaboration with
the National Center for Chronic Disease Prevention and Health Promotion (2000).

Figure 11–3. Body mass index for age—males.
(http://www.cdc.gov/nchs/about/major/nhanes/growthcharts/set1/chart15.pdf. Centers for Disease Control and Prevention.)

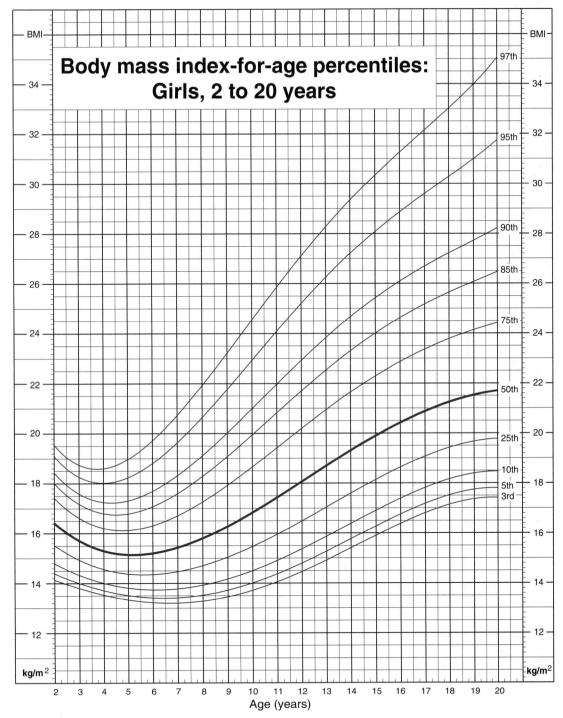

Published May 30, 2000.
SOURCE: Developed by the National Center for Health Statistics in collaboration with the National Center for Chronic Disease Prevention and Health Promotion (2000).

Figure 11–4. Body mass index for age—females. (http://www.cdc.gov/nchs/about/major/nhanes/growthcharts/set1/chart16.pdf. Centers for Disease Control and Prevention.)

Health show that minority adolescents engage in the lowest levels of physical activity (Figure 11–5). These findings are consistent for both leisure-time physical activity and activity during physical education class.

Currently, 25% of adolescents view themselves as being "too fat." Hispanic youth are more likely to view themselves as overweight when compared to African-Americans and non-Hispanic whites (Figure 11–6). Those adolescents who view themselves as overweight are significantly less physically active than their normal-weight peers and are less likely to engage in health-promoting behaviors. When compared with non-Hispanic whites, African-American and Hispanic youth are at significantly higher risk for being overweight and obese.

There are important cultural differences in perceptions about the inherent value of exercise. Not all cultures encourage using time for fitness activities. In fact, dedicating time for exercise as an isolated activity can be viewed as either selfish or a poor use of time. Cultural and ethnic differences also exist in television viewing habits. Hispanic and African-American adolescents spend significantly more time watching television than do non-Hispanic whites.

C. GENDER-SPECIFIC FACTORS

There are significant differences in levels of spontaneous physical activity between male and female adolescents. Males are more active than females from childhood through adolescence. Levels of physical activity decline for both males and females during adolescence, but there is a disproportionate decline in females. The reasons for this are unclear. Factors that are positively associated with an increased likelihood of physical activity among female adolescents include perceived competence at a particular activity, perceived value of the activity, favorable physical appearance during and after the activity, and positive social support for the activity.

D. ENVIRONMENTAL FACTORS

Many of the barriers to physical activity are environmental. Of these, television is the most important. It is estimated that between the ages of 8 and 18, youth spend an average of 4.5 h/day watching television or video tapes. This translates to over 25% of waking hours being spent in front of the television. By contrast, adolescents spend less than 1% of their time (an estimated 12–14 min/day) engaged in vigorous physical activity. The impact of television on the activity levels of youth is so significant that the American Academy of Pediatrics has released a position statement recommending that youth watch a maximum 1–2 h of television per day.

Television is not the only environmental issue contributing to adolescent inactivity and obesity. Adolescents are more reliant than ever on labor-saving devices. Elevators and escalators take precedence over staircases and high-technology tools such as the Internet have further reduced the incentive to get up and get moving. Automated transportation often represents the pinnacle of adolescence with the acquisition of a driver's license providing an excuse to drive everywhere. Poor community planning has resulted in a paucity of safe gymnasiums or playing fields for adolescents to use during their leisure time. In addition, there is an abundance of readily available, inexpensive, calorically dense foodstuffs. Many schools now routinely have vending machines in their hallways.

E. FAMILIAL FACTORS

Finally, there are factors inherent within individual families that shape how active young individuals will be. Children and adolescents with overweight parents are more likely to be overweight themselves. Interestingly, parental levels of physical activity do not correlate with their children's levels of physical activity. Children and youth from larger families are more active

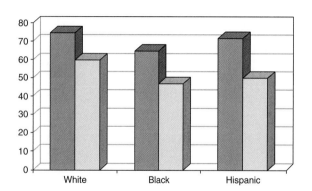

Figure 11–5. Percentage of youth engaging in recommended levels of vigorous physical activity by gender and ethnicity. (Centers for Disease Control and Prevention: Youth risk behavior surveillance—United States, 1999.)

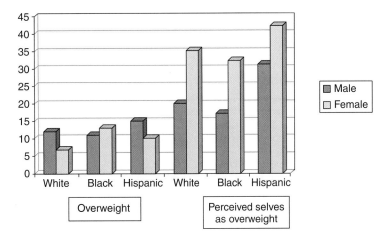

Figure 11–6. Differences in percentage of overweight youth and self-perceptions of weight by gender and ethnicity.

than children from small families. Children whose parents are available to provide transportation to activities are more likely to be physically active. Individuals who are forced to exercise as children are less likely to be physically active as adults. Thus, although it is important for parents to model physical activity, clearly there are external forces at work in an adolescent's life shaping individual patterns of health-related behaviors.

Allison KR, Adlaf EM: Age and sex differences in physical inactivity among Ontario teenagers. Can J Public Health 1997;88 (3):177.

Gordon-Larsen P, McMurray RG, Popkin BM: Determinants of adolescent physical activity and inactivity patterns. Pediatrics 2000;105(6):E83.

Koivusilta LK, Rimpela AH, Rimpela MK: Health-related lifestyle in adolescence—origin of social class differences in health? Health Educ Res 1999;14(3):339.

Taylor WC et al: Childhood and adolescent physical activity patterns and adult physical activity. Med Sci Sports Exerc 1999; 31(1):118.

Assessment

There are three ways to assess physical activity levels in adolescents: (1) direct observation, (2) activity monitors or heart rate monitors, and (3) self-report questionnaires. Of these, direct observation is the gold standard. It is also the most labor intensive. Therefore, several attempts have been made to provide valid, accurate, and rapid clinical tools for assessing physical activity levels in adolescents.

The Patient-Centered Assessment and Counseling for Exercise Plus (PACE+) Nutrition program has been developed to assist clinicians in assessing physical activity levels and to counsel patients regarding appropriate levels of physical activity and proper nutrition. As part of this program, a rapid screening tool has been developed specifically to screen levels of adolescent physical activity (Table 11–3). This simple two-question survey provides clinicians with a valid assessment of whether adolescents are achieving recommended levels of physical activity on a regular basis. The combination of BMI and the PACE+ activity measure allows for a rapid clinical assessment of adolescents' physical activity status, weight status, and potential health risk.

Sirard JR, Pate RR: Physical activity assessment in children and adolescents. Sports Med 2001;31(6):439.

Guidelines & Clinical Interventions

Because it is known that risk factors for chronic disease track from childhood into adolescence and into adulthood, overweight adolescents are more likely to become overweight adults, and levels of obesity are rising sharply among adolescents and levels of physical activity are declining, there is an acute need for interventions to promote physical activity in childhood and adolescence. The following guidelines can assist clinicians in providing activity counseling for their adolescent patients (Table 11–4).

A. AMERICAN COLLEGE OF SPORTS MEDICINE

The American College of Sports Medicine (ACSM) published the initial set of guidelines for physical activity in adults in 1978. Recommendations call for 15–60 min of exercise, 3–5 days/week at an intensity of 60–90% of an individual's maximum heart rate. These guidelines emphasize physical training as opposed to physical activity. In 1990, this position was modified to include conditioning for muscular strength and endurance.

Table 11–3. Sixty-minute screening measure for moderate-to-vigorous physical activity in adolescents: PACE + (Patient-Centered Assessment and Counseling for Exercise plus Nutrition).

Physical activity is any activity that increases your heart rate and makes you get out of breath some of the time

Physical activity can be done in sports, playing with friends, or walking to school

Some examples of **physical activity** include running, brisk walking, rollerblading, biking, dancing, skateboarding, swimming, soccer, basketball, football, and surfing.

Add up all the time you spend in physical activity each day (don't include your physical education or gym class).

1. Over the past 7 days, on how many days were you physically active for a total of at least 60 minutes per day?
   _1_2_3_4_5_6_7
2. Over a typical or usual week, on how many days are you physically active for a total of at least 60 minutes per day?
   _1_2_3_4_5_6_7

Scoring: Add the value from question 1 and question 2 and divide by 2 (Q1 + Q2/2). If this score is less than 5, the individual is not meeting current physical activity guidelines

From Prochaska JJ, Sallis JF, Long B: A physical activity screening measure for use with adolescents in primary care. Arch Pediatr Adolesc Med 2001;155(5):554. Reproduced with permission of the authors.

B. HEALTHY PEOPLE 2000

In 1991, the U.S. Department of Health and Human Services released a series of national public health goals. The number one priority in this report was promoting physical activity. Of the 13 health objectives outlined in *Healthy People 2000,* five were specifically targeted to promote physical activity in adolescents. Unfortunately, in the decade between 1991 and 2001, these objectives fell significantly short of the desired targets.

C. INTERNATIONAL CONSENSUS CONFERENCE ON PHYSICAL ACTIVITY GUIDELINES FOR ADOLESCENTS

Convened in 1993, this expert panel recommends that adolescents be physically active on most if not all days of the week. Adolescents should strive for activity 3–5 days/week for 20 min or more at levels requiring moderate to vigorous exertion. Activity should routinely occur as part of play, games, sporting activities, work, recreation, physical education, or planned exercise sessions. These guidelines also emphasize the importance of considering family, school, and community factors when counseling adolescents about physical activity.

D. ACSM/CDC CONSENSUS STATEMENT

This 1995 statement serves as a consensus for several national societies, and calls for all Americans to engage in regular physical activity according to their individual abilities. Simply stated, adolescents should strive to obtain 30 min of moderate to vigorous physical activity on most, if not all days of the week.

E. SURGEON GENERAL'S REPORT: PHYSICAL ACTIVITY AND HEALTH

In 1996, the surgeon general released a report summarizing available medical evidence relating to the health benefits of regular physical activity. This report emphasizes that even modest amounts of physical activity have important health benefits for sedentary individuals. It also states physical activity need not be overly strenuous to be beneficial.

F. HEALTHY PEOPLE 2010

Given the modest achievements of *Healthy People 2000,* the U.S. Department of Health and Human Services restated the importance of physical activity by making it the primary leading health indicator for *Healthy People 2010.* Objectives relating specifically to physical activity in adolescents are presented in Table 11–3.

G. DIETARY GUIDELINES FOR AMERICANS

Now in its fifth edition, these guidelines are the cornerstone for providing clinical nutritional advice. Emphasizing the inherent relationship between physical activity, dietary choices, and resultant weight issues, the current edition of the *Guidelines* is the first to specifically recommend physical activity as a part of routine dietary practice. Individuals should aim to accumulate 60 min or more of moderate physical activity on a daily basis.

H. SURGEON GENERAL'S CALL TO ACTION

Recognizing the need for further action, the surgeon general has recently released an additional report recommending that individuals, families, schools, worksites, health care providers, and communities work together to combat the increasing problem of physical inactivity, overweight, and obesity in the United States.

American College of Sports Medicine: The recommended quantity and quality of exercise for developing and maintaining fitness in healthy adults. Med Sci Sport Exerc 1978;10:vii.

Pate RR et al: Physical activity and public health: A recommendation from the Centers for Disease Control and Prevention and the American College of Sports Medicine. JAMA 1995; 273(5):402.

Sallis JF, Patrick K: Physical activity guidelines for adolescents: consensus statement. Pediatr Exer Sci 1994;6:302.

U.S. Department of Health and Human Services: *Healthy People 2010: Understanding and Improving Health.* U.S. Department of Health and Human Services, Government Printing Office, 2000.

Table 11–4. Guidelines for physical activity in adolescence.

Guideline Source	Recommendation
American College of Sports Medicine	Fifteen to 60 min of exercise per day Exercise 3–5 days/week Intensity of 60–90% of maximal heart rate
Healthy People 2000	Reduce overweight among adolescents to no more than 15% Increase to at least 30% the number of adolescents who engage in regular, preferably daily light to moderate physical activity for at least 30 min Increase to at least 75% the proportion of adolescents who engage in vigorous physical activity 3 or more days/week for 20 min or more Reduce to no more than 15% the number of adolescents who engage in no leisure-time physical activity Increase to at least 50% the number of adolescents who participate in daily physical education
International Consensus Conference on Physical Activity Guidelines for Adolescents	Physical activity 3–5 days/week Activity sessions of 20 min or more requiring moderate to vigorous physical exertion Emphasis on consideration of familial, social, and community factors when promoting activity
ACSM/CDC Consensus Statement	All Americans should strive to be physically active on most, preferably all days of the week according to individual abilities Goal of accumulating 30 min of moderate to vigorous physical activity each day
Surgeon General's Report	Sedentary individuals benefit from even modest levels of physical activity Sufficient levels of activity can be accumulated through independent bouts of activity throughout the day
Healthy People 2010	Increase the proportion of adolescents who engage in moderate physical activity for at least 30 min on 5 or more days/week Increase the proportion of adolescents who engage in vigorous activity 3 or more days/week for 20 min or more per occasion Increase the proportion of adolescents participating in daily physical education Increase the proportion of adolescents who spend at least 50% of class time during physical education engaged in physical activity Increase the proportion of adolescents who walk to school (less than 1 mile) Increase the proportion of adolescents who bicycle to school (less than 2 miles)
Dietary Guidelines for Americans	Accumulate 60 min of moderate activity per day
Surgeon General's Call to Action	Clinicians, schools, communities, and families should work together to promote physical activity and healthy life-style choices for all individuals

U.S. Department of Health and Human Services: *The Surgeon General's Call to Action to Prevent and Decrease Overweight and Obesity.* U.S. Department of Health and Human Services, Public Health Service, Office of the Surgeon General, 2001.

U.S. Department of Health and Human Services Public Health Service, Centers for Disease Control and Prevention, National Center for Chronic Disease Prevention and Health Promotion, Division of Nutrition and Physical Activity: *Healthy People 2000: Final Review.* Centers for Disease Control, 2001.

U.S. Department of Health and Human Services; U.S. Department of Agriculture: *Nutrition and Your Health: Dietary Guidelines for Americans,* ed 5. U.S. Department of Agriculture and U.S. Department of Health and Human Services, Government Printing Office, 2000.

U.S. Public Health Service: *Healthy People 2000: National Health Promotion and Disease Prevention Objectives.* U.S. Department of Health and Human Services, Public Health Service, 1991. Publication No. (PHS) 91-212.

Promoting Success: What Can We Do to Improve?

Health care professionals play a central role in promoting physical activity among adolescents. Adolescents have the lowest utilization of health care services of any segment of the population. They do, however, rely on their physician as a reliable source of health care information. Clinicians must, therefore, take the opportunity to provide preventive advice at each adolescent visit in accordance with the guidelines established by the U.S. Preventive Services Task Force. During each adolescent visit "appropriate counseling to promote physical activity and a healthy diet should be provided."

Unfortunately, however, this has not been the case. Very few visits with adolescents actually document preventive counseling. In a study of overweight individuals, only one in four received specific advice from their provider regarding physical activity. When reviewing guidelines or recommending life-style changes with adolescent patients, it is important to promote the concept of physical activity as opposed to physical fitness. Adolescents should be aware that cumulative bouts of physical activity are just as effective as sustained periods of exercise in attaining health-related benefits. For changes to be effective in adolescence, physical activity must be enjoyable and there should be social support for the activity either from family or from peers. Using established guidelines within the context of social, cultural, familial, and environmental factors, clinicians must improve preventive counseling services to adolescents.

Feldman E: Risks, resilience, prevention: the epidemiology of adolescent Health. Clin Fam Pract 2000;2(4):767.

U.S. Preventive Services Task Force: *Guide to Clinical Preventive Services,* ed 2. Williams & Wilkins, 1996.

Special Considerations Relating to Physical Activity in Adolescents

A. PERFORMANCE-ENHANCING SUPPLEMENTS

Over the past decade, the use of performance-enhancing supplements has exploded. One-half of the U.S. population consumes some form of nutritional supplement on a regular basis, resulting in over $15 billion in annual sales. Reasons cited for the use of dietary nutritional supplements include ensuring good nutrition, preventing illness, improving performance, warding off fatigue, and enhancing personal appearance.

Estimates suggest that 1 million adolescents have used performance-enhancing nutritional supplements with creatine being the most common. Creatine is reported to increase energy during short-term intense exercise, increase muscle mass, increase strength, increase lean body mass, and decrease lactate accumulation during intense exercise. Although it is clear that supplementation with exogenous creatine can raise intramuscular creatine stores, it is not clear how effective creatine is as a performance aid. In general, creatine supplementation may be useful for activities requiring short, repetitive bouts of high-intensity exercise. There is conflicting evidence, however, as to whether it is effective in increasing muscle strength or muscle mass. There are no scientific data regarding the safety or effectiveness of long-term use of creatine in adolescents.

Anabolic-androgenic steroids (AAS) are another important category of performance-enhancing substances used by adolescents. Testosterone is the prototypical androgenic steroid hormone. Many synthetic modifications have been made to the basic molecular structure of testosterone in an attempt to promote the anabolic, muscle-building effects of testosterone while minimizing androgenic side effects. Androstenedione is one of several oral performance-enhancing supplements that are precursors to testosterone. It is metabolized *in vivo* to testosterone, and therefore has been marketed as a "prohormone" under the Dietary Supplement Health and Education Act of 1994. Its use increased significantly after the success of Mark McGwire during the 1998 major league baseball season. Despite this popularity, the effectiveness of androstenedione as a performance-enhancing supplement is debatable. To date, the largest controlled trial examining its effectiveness showed no significant gains in muscular strength compared with a standard program of resistance training. Additionally, the *in vivo* metabolism of androstenedione to estrogen-related compounds leads to predictable side effects (eg, gynecomastia). Its use is banned by most sporting communities.

Although androstenedione has been marketed as a prohormone, many other more potent testosterone derivatives are available. These products have been classified as Schedule III (nonnarcotic) compounds under the Anabolic Steroid Control Act of 1990. Their use is prohibited. Despite this ban, it is estimated that 3–10% of adolescents have used anabolic steroids. Importantly, adolescents who use anabolic steroids have been shown to be more likely to engage in high-risk personal health behaviors such as tobacco use and excessive alcohol consumption. Users of other nutritional performance-enhancing supplement have also been shown to engage in similar predictable high-risk behaviors.

Clinicians should be aware of the prevalence of performance-enhancing supplement use in the adolescent population. They should also be aware of health-related behaviors that often accompany the use of these products and provide preventive counseling accordingly. The preparticipation physical examination represents an excellent opportunity for clinicians to provide information about performance-enhancing products to young athletes. When counseling adolescents about the use of performance-enhancing products it is helpful to ask the following questions: (1) Is the product safe to use? (2) Why does the adolescent want to use a particular product? (3) Is the product effective in helping to meet the desired goal? (4) Is the product legal? Many adolescents will either try or continue to use performance-enhancing products regardless of the information or advice they receive. Nevertheless, they should be aware of potential health risks or bans from competition that accompany use of performance-enhancing products. The use of performance-enhancing supplements in adolescents should be discouraged.

American Academy of Pediatrics: Position Statement of the American Academy of Pediatrics. Paper presented at a Conference on the Science and Policy of Performance-Enhancing Products, 2002.

Blue Cross Blue Shield Healthy Competition Foundation: Survey projects 1 million youths aged 12-17 use potentially dangerous sports supplements and drugs. Blue Cross Blue Shield. Available at www.healthycompetition.org. Accessed January 11, 2002.

National Institutes of Health—Office of Dietary Supplements; Center for Responsible Nutrition: Patterns of use. Paper presented at a Conference on the Science and Policy of Performance-Enhancing Products, 2002.

B. FEMALE ATHLETE TRIAD

Although many adolescents engage in too little physical activity, there is a segment of the population for whom too much exercise leads to specific physiological side effects. The female athlete triad refers to the combination of disordered eating, amenorrhea, and osteoporosis that can accompany excessive physical training in young female athletes. Athletes particularly at risk include those who participate in gymnastics, ballet, figure skating, distance running, or any other sport that emphasizes a particularly lean physique.

The preparticipation physical examination represents an excellent opportunity for clinicians to screen for and to prevent the female athlete triad. During this examination, screening questions for female athletes should include careful menstrual, dietary (including a history of disordered eating practices), and exercise histories. When elicited, a history of amenorrhea (particularly in a previously menstruating female) should be taken seriously. The American College of Sports Medicine recommends that that these women be considered at risk for the female athlete triad and that a formal medical evaluation should be undertaken within 3 months.

Hobart JA, Smucker DR: The female athlete triad. Am Fam Physician 2000;61(11):3357.

C. EXERCISE AND SUDDEN DEATH

Another small segment of the adolescent population is at risk during exercise. These individuals are predisposed to sudden cardiac death during physical activity. Highly publicized events among well-known athletes have further focused attention on this issue. Although the incidence of sudden cardiac death in young athletes is fortunately quite low, proper screening is still important. Here again, the preparticipation physical examination represents an excellent clinical opportunity for prevention.

When screening for sudden death in young athletes, the medical history should include questions about exercise-related syncope or near-syncope, shortness of breath, chest pain, or palpitations. The clinician should ask about a family history of premature death or premature cardiovascular disease. Any prior history of a cardiac murmur or specific knowledge of an underlying cardiac abnormality (either structural, valvular, or arrhythmic) in the athlete should be elicited as well. If the examining clinician has any suspicion that the athlete might have a symptomatic arrhythmia, that individual should be withheld from physical activity pending consultation with a cardiologist.

On physical examination, blood pressure should be recorded. The precordial fields should be auscultated in the supine, squatting, and standing positions. Murmurs that increase with moving from the squatting to standing position or that increase with the Valsalva maneuver are of potential concern and merit further evaluation. The equality of the femoral pulses should be noted. If any abnormalities are noted on the initial preparticipation history or physical examination, a more detailed evaluation is warranted.

O'Connor FG, Kugler JP, Oriscello RG: Sudden death in young athletes: Screening for the needle in a haystack. Am Fam Physician 1998;57(11):2763.

Eating Disorders

Evelyn L. Lewis, MD, MA, & Tracy Sbrocco, PhD

General Considerations

Since the 1950s and 1960s there has been a concomitant recognition of eating disorders as clinical syndromes and a drive for thinness as individuals, particularly by women, as they strive to attain a thin beauty ideal. Anorexia nervosa and bulimia nervosa first appeared in the *Diagnostic and Statistical Manual of Mental Disorders (DSM-III)* of the American Psychiatric Association under "Disorders First Evident in Childhood and Adolescence." Anorexia is characterized by the refusal to eat anything but minimal amounts of food resulting in low body weight, whereas bulimia is characterized by the attempt to restrict food intake that eventually leads to out-of-control eating episodes followed by inappropriate compensatory behaviors (eg, vomiting). Over the ensuing decades, the increased clinical recognition and the research focus on the problem have led to a substantial increase in our understanding of eating disorders, their treatment, and, more recently, preventive strategies. In addition, these syndromes have been further defined and now appear in a separate section in the *DSM-IV* entitled "Eating Disorders." Currently, there is an increased focus on the binge eating disorders as well as the overlap among obesity, eating disorders, and other mental disorders. The commonalities among the eating disorders include disturbance in body image, including both body shape and body weight, as well as a drive for thinness. In part, these themes are present in the population as a whole.

There is a great deal of dieting that occurs in our culture as part of "normal eating." In fact, estimates suggest that anywhere from 15% to 80% of the population may be dieting at any given time. Despite this prevalence, over 60% of the adult population and 13% of children and adolescents are considered overweight or obese (22% of African-American and Hispanic children compared to 12% of non-Hispanic white children). Women are most likely to restrict their food intake to control their weight or lose weight, but men are also increasingly engaging in dieting behavior. Most disconcerting is the prevalence of dieting among adolescents and even children. Dieting is a factor to consider in the prevention of eating disorders, particularly among adolescents, who may feel pressure to lose weight. Lastly, the acceptance of dieting as "normal" may hamper the ability of the clinician to recognize problem eating.

The prevalence and incidence rates for the eating disorders vary significantly. Much depends on the type of disorder and the population. However, generally speaking, of patients with classic signs and symptoms of anorexia or bulimia, 90% are female, 95% are white, and 75% are adolescent when they develop the disorder. These data are substantiated by several cross-cultural studies that report few, if any cases of eating disorders in non-Western countries, with the exception of Japan.

Anorexia nervosa (AN) has been implicated as a "culture-bound syndrome" as certain cultural mores are reflected in the signs and symptoms of the disorder. In the United States, the frequency of AN among young Hispanic women appears to be about as common as that seen in whites, more common among Native Americans, and less common among African-Americans and Asians. However, several studies have shown that there may be many eating disorder behaviors that are more common to African-American women such as purging by laxatives versus vomiting. Black women are also more likely to develop bulimia nervosa or binge eating disorder than anorexia nervosa. Contributing elements appear to be increased influence by the media, such as television and commercials that depict thin beauty ideals, the rise in standard of living, the lack of physical activity, and increased food availability, which makes weight gain common.

Most patients are from middle to upper socioeconomic status (SES). Age-specific and sex-specific estimates suggest that about 0.5–1% of adolescent girls develop AN, whereas about 5% of older adolescent and young adult females develop bulimia nervosa (BN). There is also a high frequency of coexistence between AN and BN: as many as 50% of AN patients may exhibit bulimic behaviors whereas 30–80% of patients with BN have a history of AN. Male adolescents constitute a small segment of patients with eating disorders, with most diagnosed with BN or binge eating disorder (BED). Estimates suggest that approximately 4% of community samples have BED. The most prevalent eating disorder (ED) falls into the category of eating disorder not otherwise specified (EDNOS) and affects 6–10% of young women.

Bemporad JR: Self-starvation through the ages: reflections on the pre-history of anorexia nervosa. Int J Eating Disord 1996;19 (3):217.

Dolan B: Cross cultural aspects of anorexia and bulimia: a review. Int J Eating Disord 1991;10:67.

Langer L, Warheit G, Zimmerman R: Epidemiological study of problem eating behaviors and related attitudes in the general population. Addict Behav 1992;16:167.

Nasser M: *Culture and Weight Consciousness.* Routledge, 1997.

Pathogenesis

The origins of eating disorders (anorexia nervosa, bulimia nervosa, and binge eating disorders) are extremely complex and poorly understood. However, biological, psychological, cultural, and societal factors are likely contributors to the predisposition, precipitation, and perpetuation of these disorders. In particular, mounting data support substantial biological predispositions to AN and BN. Mothers and sisters of probands who had AN were eight times more likely to develop an eating disorder as compared to the general population. Genetic studies are also lending strong support to the underlying biological supposition regarding eating disorders. Twin studies have shown heritability estimates in the 50–90% range for AN and 35–50% range for BN, with monozygotic twins having higher concordance than dizygotic twins. A strong association between AN and BN in families has also been found in the Virginia Twin Registry.

Eating disorders may also be precipitated by psychosocial factors in vulnerable individuals. These precipitating factors often relate to developmental tasks of adolescence and include fear of maturation, particularly related to sexual development, peer group involvement, independence and autonomy struggles, family conflicts, sexual abuse, and identity conflicts. Because sexual trauma and depression figure prominently in the pathogenesis of BN or BED, it is important to note the presence of depression or history of sexual trauma during the initial patient assessment. Overall, eating disorders present an unusual challenge for the physician. Much of the denial, resistance, and anger of the patient and occasionally the family may now be directed at you. However, being aware that patients with disorders are frequently ambivalent, desire but are often afraid of recovery, and make you the target of their emotions and their inner conflict serves to facilitate the building of a trusting relationship, the foundation of effective therapy.

Kreipe RE, Dukarm CP: Eating disorders in adolescents and older children. Pediatr Rev 1999;20(10).

Strober M, Freeman R, Morrell W: The long-term course of severe anorexia nervosa in adolescents: survival analysis of recovery, relapse and outcome predictors over 10-15 years in a prospective study. Int J Eating Disord 1997;22:339.

Prevention

The evidence clearly shows that the eating disorders are serious and complex problems and the earlier an eating disorder is identified, the better the chance for recovery. This makes a compelling argument for targeted screening of at-risk groups (males and females), which include gymnasts, runners, body builders, wrestlers, dancers, rowers, and swimmers. These groups warrant close monitoring because their sports and/or livelihood dictate weight restriction. The populations at highest risk for AN and BN are adolescents and young adult females and screening should occur at about ages 14 and 18. This correlates with the transition to high school and college with their associated stressors. Almost all individuals seeking treatment for weight control should be screened for BED because of its high incidence in this group. Although they may fall short of meeting the full criteria, the problematic attitudes associated with BED will likely be uncovered. The tools used for screening can be very sophisticated and vary with the population being assessed. However, there are some that are easily incorporated into the routine primary care office visit (Table 12–1). These questions are very helpful for the early detection of BN and BED, as these individuals can be uncovered using self-report alone. Those with AN, on the other hand, are resistant to self-reporting and usually require reporting by others (ie,

Table 12–1. Screening questionnaire.

1. Has there been any change in your weight?
2. What did you eat yesterday?
3. Do you ever binge?
4. Have you ever used self-induced vomiting, laxatives, diuretics, or enemas to lose weight or compensate for overeating?
5. How much do you exercise in a typical week?
6. How do you feel about how you look?
7. Are your menstrual periods regular?

From Powers PS: Initial assessment and early treatment options for anorexia nervosa and bulimia nervosa. Psychiatr Clin North Am 1996;19(4):639.

parents, friends). Therefore, it is imperative that parents, friends, teachers, family, dentists, and physicians become educated about the signs and symptoms associated with these difficult-to-manage disorders to facilitate prevention or early management.

Clinical Findings

A. SYMPTOMS AND SIGNS

The multiple symptoms experienced by the patient and signs noted by the physician are related to the numerous methods used to manipulate weight. When initially screening a patient, a symptom checklist can facilitate taking a history (Table 12–2). The questions are generally answered honestly except in the case of anorectics, who are usually reticent to be seen or report any problem with their weight.

An initial screening that reveals primarily positive results may be indicative of a significant problem for the patient. Most commonly, AN patients complain of amenorrhea, depression, fatigue, weakness, hair loss, and bone pain (which may be indicative of a pathological fracture secondary to osteopenia). Constipation and/or abdominal pain occur frequently but may be commonly mistaken as symptoms of endometriosis or pelvic inflammatory disease (PID), which are disorders common to both anorexia and bulimia. Unlike AN, BN may be missed initially by the inexperienced clinician because the patients may present with normal or near normal body weight or be only slightly underweight. In addition to constipation and gastrointestinal pain, bulimics may likely present with menstrual irregularity, food and fluid restrictions, abuse of diuretics and laxatives (causing dizziness and bloody diarrhea), misuse of diet pills (leading to palpitations and anxiety), frequent vomiting (resulting in throat irritation and pharyngeal trauma), sexually transmitted diseases (which appears to be related to impulsive, risk-taking behaviors associated with this disorder), and bone pain. Mouth sores, weakness, dental caries, heartburn, muscle cramps and fainting, hair loss, easy bruising, and intolerance to cold are some of the more obvious presenting complaints.

1. Anorexia nervosa—The diagnostic criteria are defined and listed in the *DSM-IV* (Table 12–3). AN is

Table 12–2. Evaluation of eating disorders: the history.

History should include questions on the following:
  Weight (minimum/maximum, as well as ideal)
  Menstrual history and pattern (if applicable: age of menarche, date of last period)
  Body image (thin, normal, heavy; satisfaction/dissatisfaction with current weight)
  Exercise regimen (amount, intensity, response to inability to exercise)
  Eating habits
  Sexual history [if applicable, a history of current sexual activity, number of partners, review of health habits and sexual practices that might place the patient at risk for sexually transmitted diseases (STD)]
  Current and past medication
  Laxative/diuretic/diet pill use, ipecac, cigarettes, alcohol, drugs
  Substance abuse (eg, cigarettes, alcohol, drugs)
  Binge-eating and purging behavior (identify a binge: how much, what kinds of food; presence of triggers: foods, time of day, feelings; frequency of binge eating; identify vomiting methods: finger, toothbrush)
  Psychiatric history (substance abuse, mood/anxiety/personality disorders)
  Suicidal ideation

Table 12–3. DSM-IV criteria for anorexia nervosa.

A. Refusal to maintain body weight at or above a minimally normal weight for age and height (eg, weight loss leading to maintenance of body weight less than 85% of that expected, or failure to make expected weight gain during period of growth, leading to body weight less than 85% of that expected).

B. Intense fear of gaining weight or becoming fat, even though underweight.

C. Disturbance in the way in which one's body weight or shape is experienced, undue influence of body weight or shape on self-evaluation, or denial of the seriousness of the current low body weight.

D. In postmenarcheal females, amenorrhea, ie, the absence of at least three consecutive menstrual cycles. (A woman is considered to have amenorrhea if her periods occur only following hormone, eg, estrogen, administration.)

Restricting Type: During the current episode of anorexia nervosa, the person has not regularly engaged in binge eating or purging behavior (ie, self-induced vomiting or the misuse of laxatives, diuretics, or enemas).

Binge Eating/Purging Type: During the current episode of anorexia nervosa, the person has regularly engaged in binge eating or purging behavior (ie, self-induced vomiting or the misuse of laxatives, diuretics, or enemas).

From *Diagnostic and Statistical Manual of Mental Disorders* [ed 4 (*DSM-IV*), text revision]: American Psychiatric Association, 2000: 326. Copyright 2000 by the American Psychiatric Association.

characterized by the refusal to maintain minimum body weight defined as maintenance of 85% of expected weight or body mass index (BMI) >17.5 k/m^2 or failure to make appropriate weight gains with growth. These patients exhibit an intense fear of weight gain and body image disturbance that may include any or all of three components: emotional (eg, self-disgust), perceptual (eg, my thighs are too fat), and cognitive (eg, people will hate me if I'm fat). Amenorrhea (albeit occasionally controversial) is also a defining element. In prepubertal females, menarche is delayed, and in postmenarcheal females, it is the absence of at least three consecutive cycles. The amenorrhea is attributed to low follicle-stimulating hormone (FSH) and luteinizing hormone (LH) and may eventually precede weight loss in up to 20% of patients. Two subtypes of AN have been identified. The binge eating/purging subtype includes patients who engage in diuretic–laxative abuse, vomiting, and overuse of enemas to eliminate calories. The restrictive subtype includes patients who do not engage in either binge eating or purging behaviors. The AN binge eating/purging subtype can be distinguished from BN by weight criteria, the size of the binge, which is usually smaller, and the consistency of purging, which is less frequent.

2. Bulimia nervosa—BN or "hunger of an ox" is more common than AN and is largely confined to collegiate women, although it usually starts in the late teen years. The characteristic of this illness is the patient's attempt to restrict food intake. This results in out-of-control eating followed by inappropriate compensatory behaviors. These patients may be slightly more difficult to identify initially, as 10% are within normal weight for age and height.

The *DSM-IV* defined criteria for BN (Table 12–4) include recurrent episodes of binge eating in which more food than normal is consumed in a discrete period of time followed by recurrent inappropriate compensatory behaviors. Both criteria occur an average of two times per week for at least 3 months. BN is also divided into two subtypes. The purging subtype requires regular engagement in self-induced vomiting and abuse of laxatives, diuretics, or enemas. The nonpurging subtype emphasizes other inappropriate behaviors such as fasting and excessive exercise, but does not include vomiting or the abuse of laxatives, enemas, or diuretics. About two-thirds of patients are purgers and they have been found to exhibit more severe pathology, including more frequent binging and higher comorbidity of other psychological disorders.

3. Binge eating disorder—The most recent ED diagnostic category is BED. The evidence suggests that BED affects women and men more evenly, affects a broader

Table 12–4. *DSM-IV* criteria for bulimia nervosa.

A. Recurrent episodes of binge eating. An episode of binge eating is characterized by both of the following:
  (1) Eating, in a discrete period of time (eg, within any 2-h period), an amount of food that is definitely larger than most people would eat during a similar period of time and under similar circumstances.
  (2) A sense of lack of control over eating during the episode (eg, a feeling that one cannot stop eating or control how much one is eating).
B. Recurrent inappropriate compensatory behavior in order to prevent weight gain, such as self-induced vomiting, misuse of laxatives, diuretics, enemas, or other medications; fasting, or excessive exercise.
C. The binge eating and inappropriate compensatory behaviors both occur, on average, at least twice a week for 3 months.
D. Self-evaluation is unduly influenced by body shape and weight.
E. The disturbance does not occur exclusively during episodes of anorexia nervosa.

From *Diagnostic and Statistical Manual of Mental Disorders* [ed 4 (*DSM-IV*), text revision]. American Psychiatric Association, 2000: 328. Copyright 2000 by the American Psychiatric Association.

age range of individuals (20–50), and likely affects African-Americans as frequently as whites. Most of the people with BED are obese and have a history of "yo-yo" dieting. This disorder is characterized by binge eating in the absence of compensatory behaviors. These individuals report feeling a "loss of control" as they consume larger amounts of food than typical for most people in a discrete period of time. The episodes are associated with rapid eating, eating until uncomfortable, eating large amounts when they are not hungry, and eating alone. Other diagnostic markers and criteria include feeling depressed, disgusted, or guilty (regarding their binging behavior), and the presence of these behaviors 2 days per week for at least 6 months.

4. Eating disorders not otherwise specified—In general, common examples of EDNOS include individuals who meet all the criteria for AN but have regular menses, normal range weight, and less frequent binges (Table 12–5). With this in mind, it is easy to understand the importance of identifying and treating these individuals. Nonetheless, many are frequently not treated by their clinician because they fail to meet full AN criteria. Other unique features of this disorder not seen in AN or BN include regular use of compensatory behaviors after consuming small amounts of food and chewing and spitting out of their food before swallowing.

Table 12–5. *DSM-IV* criteria for eating disorder not otherwise specified.

The eating disorder not otherwise specified category is for disorders of eating that do not meet the criteria for any specific eating disorder. Examples include:

1. For females, all of the criteria for anorexia nervosa are met except that the individual has regular menses.
2. All of the criteria for anorexia nervosa are met except that, despite significant weight loss, the individual's current weight is in the normal range.
3. All of the criteria for bulimia nervosa are met except that the binge eating and inappropriate compensatory mechanisms occur at a frequency of less than twice a week or for a duration of less than 3 months.
4. The regular use of inappropriate compensatory behaviors by an individual of normal body weight after eating small amounts of food (eg, self-induced vomiting after the consumption of two cookies).
5. Repeatedly chewing and spitting out, but not swallowing, large amounts of food.
6. Binge eating disorder: recurrent episodes of binge eating in the absence of the regular use of inappropriate behaviors characteristic of bulimia nervosa.

From *Diagnostic and Statistical Manual of Mental Disorders* [ed. 4 (*DSM-IV*), text revision]. American Psychiatric Association, 2000: 330. Copyright 2000 by the American Psychiatric Association.

Table 12–6. Physical examination.

Physical examination, including:
  Assessment of vital signs
    Body temperature (hypothermia: <96°F)
    Heart rate (bradycardia: <50)
    Blood pressure (hypotension: 90/50 mm Hg)
Weight (taken with the patient dressed in a hospital gown) and height assessment should take into account previous height and weight percentiles, anticipated growth, and average weights of healthy adolescents of the same sex, height, and sexual maturation [prepared from National Center for Health Statistics (NCHS) data]
Evaluation of body mass index (BMI):
  Quetelet's BMI (weight-to-height relationship: defined as weight in kilograms divided by height in meters squared; this BMI is then compared to reference data; percentile tables for BMI for age and sex based on NCHS data have been developed for children and adolescents)
Gynecological examination (if applicable):
  Pelvic evaluation (atrophic vaginitis)
  Breast evaluation (atrophy)
  Pregnancy testing (where appropriate)
  Sexually transmitted disease testing (where appropriate)

From Fisher M et al: Eating disorders in adolescents: a background paper. J Adolesc Health 1995;16:420.

B. PHYSICAL EXAMINATION

Whenever there is reason for concern about eating disorders, a detailed physical and dental examination should be conducted (Table 12–6). The "good looking" or "normal-weight" patient may delay diagnoses by even the most astute physician. In today's world, the multilayered baggy clothing worn by adolescents may be representative of the latest fads in fashion or of a significant eating disturbance. Just as baggy clothing may be used to conceal cachexia, patients also use increased fluid consumption and hidden weights to normalize their weights prior to weigh-ins.

A thorough physical examination may indicate the presence of another condition such as Crohn's disease or a central nervous system lesion (papilledema), or emphasize to the patient that the body is adapting to an unhealthy state, particularly since the use of scare tactics to motivate healthy behaviors is unusually futile.

One of the most significant disturbances associated with patients undergoing evaluation for eating disorders will be detected by assessing pulse, resting, and other static measurements at the initial evaluation and at each follow-up. Anorectic patients often have significant bradycardia (<60 beats/min in up to 91% of patients in various series). Eighty-five percent of anorectics may have hypotension with pressures below

90/60–90/50 secondary to a chronic volume-depleted state. Symptomatic orthostatic hypotension has been suggested as a reason for hospitalization. Cardiac arrhythmias are also common and it is critical to listen for them. Laxative and diuretic abuse cause the most serious damage for bulimic patients. The misuse of syrup of ipecac to induce vomiting is extremely dangerous in this population and often results in irreversible cardiomyopathy. Assessment of vital signs is critical and often leads to the detection of cardiac arrhythmia due to hypokalemia, metabolic acidosis, hypotension, and faint pulse. Height, weight, and BMI should also be recorded regularly and at each visit. This is helpful in establishing the patient's weight trends, as few anorectic patients are overweight prior to the onset of their disease. These weight trends also help to identify the patient's failure to gain weight during normal adolescent growth spurts. It is vitally important to obtain accurate readings. Therefore, patients should be weighed in a hospital gown, not in personal clothing, because of the various strategies they employ to disguise their weight loss. Careful examination of the patient's body should also be performed. Signs of anorexia such as brittle hair and nails, dry scaly skin, loss of subcutaneous fat, fine facial and body hair (lanugo hair), carotene pigmentation, breast atrophy, and atrophic vaginitis may be readily observable. Findings on physical examination more representative of the bulimic patient would include the callused finger (Russell's sign) used to induce vomiting, erosion, dry skin, and dull hair. Peridontal diseases are well recognized sequelae of bulimia and may present as erosion of tooth enamel, mouth sores, dental caries, green inflammation, chipped teeth, and sialadenosis (swelling of the parotid glands).

C. LABORATORY FINDINGS

There are no confirmatory laboratory tests specific to the diagnosis of eating disorders. Nonetheless, screening or baseline evaluations are recommended and should include a complete blood count with differential, urinalysis, blood chemistries (electrolytes, calcium, magnesium, and phosphorus), thyroid function test, an amenorrhea evaluation, and baseline electrocardiogram (EKG) as indicated. Generally speaking, laboratory abnormalities are due to the weight control habits or methods used by the patient, or the resulting complications. In the early stages of anorexia, laboratory findings are usually normal except for an elevated blood urea nitrogen (BUN), which may be secondary to dehydration. In addition, low circulatory levels of LH and FSH, osteopenia and osteoporosis, deficiency of gonadotropin-releasing hormone (GNRH), low estradiol, elevated cortisol, low triiodothyronine (T_3) and free thyroxine (T_4), an increase in reverse T_3, and hypoglycemia with diminished circulating insulin levels may be observed. Laboratory testing in bulimic patients is also usually normal. However, when an abnormality is present (ie, metabolic alkalosis), it is usually due to the effects of binge eating and purging. Significant hypokalemia due to purging places the patient at high risk for cardiac arrythmias, the most common cause of death in bulimics. Hypophosphatemia, metabolic acidosis (secondary to laxative abuse), and osteopenia and osteoporosis (in BN patients with a past history of AN) are also possible findings. Laboratory findings in male patients with AN are characterized by low testosterone, diminished LH + FSH9, and decreased testicular volume. Likewise, libido and sexual functioning are diminished in males during the starved state. Also of note is the presence of osteopenia in males with eating disorders. Although it is relatively common, it is generally an unrecognized clinical problem.

Carvey CP, Andersen AE: Eating disorders guide to mental evaluation and complications. Psychiatr Clin North Am 1996;19(4).

Davis AJ, Grace E: *Dying to Be Thin: Patients with Anorexia and Bulimia.* Continuing Education Monograph of the North American Society for Pediatric and Adolescent Gynecology, 1999.

Kreipe RE, Dukarm, CP: Outcome of eating disorders among children and adolescents. Pediatr Rev 1999;16.

Kreipe RE, Uphoff M: Treatment and outcome of adolescents with anorexia nervosa. Adolesc Med State Art Rec 1992;3:519.

Powers PS: Initial assessment and early treatment options for anorexia nervosa and bulimia nervosa. Psychiatr Clin North Am 1996;19(4):639.

Differential Diagnosis

In patients presenting with weight loss, other differential diagnoses, medical and psychiatric, must be considered (Table 12–7). Symptoms of ED may be caused by medical disorders such as brain tumors, cancer, connective tissue disease, malabsorption syndrome, hyperthyroidism and infection, gastrointestinal disease [inflammatory bowel disease (IBD), Crohn's disease, ulcerative colitis], mental irregularities, and cystic fibrosis. Psychiatric differential diagnoses include affective and major depressive disorders, schizophrenia, obsessive-compulsive disorder, and somatization disorder. However, the diagnosis of eating disorder is made by confirming, through history and mental state examination, the core psychopathology of a morbid fear of fatness and not by ruling out all conceivable medical causes of weight loss or binge–purge behavior. Because eating disorders and affective disorders have an increased incidence among individuals who are first-degree relatives of anorectics, a thorough family history should be performed.

Complications

Complications of eating disorders are listed in Table 12–8.

Treatment

A. EARLY STAGE MANAGEMENT

Although it is well documented that the number of girls and boys in elementary, middle, and high schools engaging in dieting and disordered eating behaviors is alarmingly high, most do not progress to classic eating disorders. In fact, many of these individuals fall into the *DSM-IV* category of eating disorders not otherwise specified. This includes patients who have one or two

Table 12–7. Differential diagnosis of eating disorders.

Psychiatric disorders (eg, affective and major depressive disorders, schizophrenia)
Substance abuse (eg, cocaine, amphetamines)
Brain tumor
Gastrointestinal disease [eg, inflammatory bowel disease (IBD), Crohn's disease, ulcerative colitis]
Cystic fibrosis
Menstrual irregularity

From Davis AJ, Grace E: *Dying to Be Thin: Patients with Anorexia and Bulimia.* Continuing Education Monograph of the North American Society for Pediatric and Adolescent Gynecology, 1999.

Table 12–8. Complications of eating disorders.

Cardiovascular	Constipation
Bradycardia	Delayed gastric emptying
Congestive heart failure	Esophageal or gastric rupture
Dysrhythmias	Esophagitis
Electrocardiographic	Fatty infiltration and focal
abnormalities	necrosis of liver
Ipecac-induced	Gallstones
cardiomyopathy	Intestinal atony
Mitral valve prolapse	Mallory-Weiss tears
Pericardial effusion	Parotid hypertrophy
Orthostatic hypotension	Perforation/rupture of the
	stomach
Dermatological	Perimolysis and increased
Acrocyanosis	incidence of dental caries
Brittle hair and nails	Superior mesenteric artery
Carotene pigmentation	syndrome
Edema	
Hair loss	**Hematological**
Lanugo hair	Bone marrow suppression
Russell's sign	Impaired cell-mediated
	immunity
Endocrine	Low sedimentation rate
Amenorrhea	
Diabetes insipidus	**Neurological**
Growth retardation	Cortical atrophy
Hypercortisolism	Myopathy
Hypothermia	Peripheral neuropathy
Low T_3 syndrome	Seizures
Pubertal delay	
	Skeletal
Gastrointestinal	Osteopenia
Acute pancreatitis	Osteoporosis
Barrett's esophagus	Osteoporotic fracture
Bloody diarrhea	

disordered eating habits and display subthreshold attitudes, behaviors, or signs.

Management of the early or mild stages of an eating disorder begins with assessing weight loss or weight control and the methods used to accomplish this and establishing a working relationship/rapport with patients and their families. This opens the door to educating the patient on the importance of maintaining good health, including a discussion about normal eating, nutrition, and exercise, and assisting the patient in establishing a goal weight that serves to set a boundary for excessive weight loss.

In addition to the institution of an appropriate diet and weight goal, patients should be instructed on beginning and maintaining a food diary. This assists the physician in identifying patterns and triggers for their dysfunctional habits and gives patients a way of exerting some control over their eating behavior.

Another important component of treatment is to acknowledge the possibility of relapse and have a plan in place to deal with it. Discussing some of the potential triggers of relapse [relationship problems, family issues (divorce, separation), examination and peer pressure] and the strategies to cope with them can help to avoid feelings of hopelessness when they are experienced. The patient should then be reevaluated within 3–6 weeks. Information obtained on the follow-up visit is helpful in determining if weight is changing precipitously, if there are changes in the physical examination, or, most important, if the dysfunctional eating habits are more entrenched. These markers help to determine if the patient will require referral.

B. Moderate Stage Management

Patients who clearly meet the criteria for an established eating disorder typically require management by a multidisciplinary team that includes a physician (family physician, pediatrician, or internist), nutritionist or dietician, nurse, mental health professional, and other support staff.

A family physician who is not an integral part of an established eating disorder treatment team may act to coordinate and facilitate transfer. This role is critical, because the trust in the primary care physician may not be readily transferred to the team of specialists. The physician can also remain involved in the patient's treatment by providing regular medical assessments, supporting the patient and family, clarifying the tasks performed by each of the team members, reinforcing the importance of the referral, and preventing premature discontinuation of treatment.

There are various treatment approaches to the management of eating disorders including family therapy, cognitive–behavioral therapy, behavior modification, and psychoactive medications. Based on the condition of the patient (Table 12–6) they may be applied in the inpatient or outpatient setting.

C. Anorexia Nervosa

The primary treatment goal for anorexia nervosa is to develop a trusting relationship with patients and to restore them to a healthy weight. In females, this means a weight at which ovulation and menses can occur, in males this means a return to normal hormone levels and sexual drive, and in adolescents and children this means a return to normal physical and sexual maturation. Other goals include treating medical and physical complications, motivating the patient to cooperate and participate in treatment, educating the patient regarding healthy nutrition and eating patterns, treating comorbid psychiatric conditions, encouraging and supporting family participation, and, ultimately, preventing relapse. Because of the variation and severity of symptoms presented, a comprehensive approach to available services and their clinical dimensions must be considered by the multidisciplinary team.

The cornerstone of the multidisciplinary approach to treatment is inpatient versus outpatient psychiatric management. These mental health professionals target treatment of the underlying psychological causes and symptoms of eating disorders, including distorted cognitions, body image issues, self-image and ego strength problems, and comorbid conditions (ie, mood and anxiety disorders). They employ a variety of behavioral/psychological therapies including individual dynamic therapy, family therapy, behavior modification, and cognitive–behavioral therapy. It is important to recognize that although these interventions are viewed as distinctly separate treatments, they frequently overlap. For example, the primary responsibility of the nutritional program rests on reestablishing normal eating and meeting nutritional requirements for normal maturation. To rehabilitate these patients they combine emotional nurturance and any one of a variety of behavioral interventions. These behavioral interventions typically combine reinforcers that link exercise, bed rest, and privileges to target weight and desired behaviors. As the patient improves (plus weight gain) other types of individual psychotherapeutic modalities may be employed.

The chronic and complex characteristics of AN are inherent problems in the use of psychosocial modalities for treatment. Although behavior modification and family therapy are often effective during the acute refeeding program, psychodynamic and cognitive–behavioral therapies (CBT) are not. However, psychotherapy is thought to be very helpful once malnutrition is corrected. Clinicians use the CBT approach to restructure or modify distorted beliefs and attitudes regarding strict food rituals and dichotomous thinking (viewing their world in "black or white" or "all or none"). Individual psychodynamic and group therapy is also used by many therapists to address underlying personality disturbances after the acute phase of weight restoration has occurred.

The treatment services available range from intensive inpatient settings, to partial hospital and residential programs, to varying levels of outpatient care. The pretreatment patient evaluation (weight, cardiac, and metabolic status) is essential in determining where treatment will occur. For example, patients who are significantly malnourished, weighing less than 75% of their individually estimated ideal body weight, are likely to require a 24-h hospital program. For these patients, hospitalization should occur before the onset of medical instability (ie, marked orthostatic hypotension, bradycardia of <40 bpm, tachycardia over 110 bpm, hypothermia, seizures, cardiac dysrhythmia, or failure) because this may result in greater risks when refeeding and a more

problematic prognosis overall. In these cases, hospitalization is based on psychiatric and behavioral grounds such as acute food refusal, uncontrollable binge eating and purging, failure of outpatient management, and comorbid psychiatric diagnosis (Table 12–9).

Successful alternatives to intensive inpatient programs have been partial hospitalization and day treatment programs for milder cases of AN. These programs typically involve a high level of parental participation and are indicative of the patient's motivation to participate in treatment. Initially, these programs may require the patient's presence and participation for 14 h a day. However, as they approach their target weight, they can be seen in outpatient sessions three times per week. Once the target weight is reached, follow-up is less frequent.

The least intrusive treatment arena is the outpatient setting. Patients selected for treatment in this setting are highly motivated and have brief symptom duration, cooperative supportive families, no serious medical complications, and BMI >17.5. Their management should also be orchestrated by a multidisciplinary team that includes a primary care physician (family practitioner, pediatrician), nutritionist, psychotherapist, family therapist, and support staff, because success is highly dependent on careful monitoring of weight obtained in a hospital gown and after voiding, orthostatic vital signs, temperature urine specific gravity, and the patient's eating disorder symptoms and behaviors. As an initial step, a clearly and concisely written behavioral contract with the patient and family (if appropriate)

Table 12–9. Criteria for hospitalization.

Any one or more of the following would justify hospitalization:
Severe malnutrition (weight, 75% ideal body weight)
Dehydration
Electrolyte disturbance
Cardiac dysrhythmia
Physiological instability (eg, severe bradycardia, hypotension, hypothermia, orthostatic changes)
Arrested growth and development
Failure of outpatient treatment
Acute food refusal
Uncontrollable binge eating and purging
Acute medical complications of malnutrition, such as syncope, seizures, cardiac failure
Acute psychiatric emergencies, such as suicidal ideation or acute psychosis, and any comorbid diagnosis that interferes with treatment, such as severe depression, obsessive-compulsive disorder, or severe family dysfunction

From Fisher M et al: Eating disorders in adolescents: A background paper. J Adolesc Health 1995; 16:420.

can be established. The contract is an agreement to maintain an acceptable minimum weight and vital signs or be hospitalized. Criteria for treatment failure and hospitalization are also included. However, it should be noted that although behavioral contracts are encouraged, they might not be as effective in the outpatient setting because they are more difficult to monitor. Nonetheless, it is helpful in achieving the goal of outpatient management, which is to get the patient to self-monitor and assume responsibility for appropriate eating.

In the anorectic patient, structure is key and should include three meals and several snacks each day. Parents should ensure that healthy foods are readily available and that mealtimes are planned. Although this results in a gradual increase in caloric intake, it may still be necessary to limit physical activity to facilitate weight gain of up to a pound per week. This incremental weight increase prevents the gastric dilation, edema, and congestive heart failure experienced by patients who have restricted their eating for a prolonged period of time.

In anorexia nervosa, psychotropic medications are not useful when patients are in a malnourished state. However, they are frequently used after sufficient weight restoration has occurred for maintenance and the treatment of other associated psychiatric symptoms. Psychotropic medications other than selective serotonin reuptake inhibitors are most often used. They include neuroleptics for obsessive-compulsive symptoms and anxiety disorders, and acute anxiety agents to reduce anticipatory anxiety associated with eating.

D. BULIMIA

Most patients with uncomplicated bulimia nervosa do not require hospitalization (less than 5% require inpatient care). Indications for the few bulimia patients requiring hospitalization (Table 12–9) include severe disabling symptoms that have not responded to outpatient management, binge–purge behavior causing severe physiological or cardiac disturbances (ie, dysrhythmias, dehydration, metabolic abnormalities), psychiatric disturbances (ie, suicidal ideation or attempts, substance abuse, major depression). If hospitalization is warranted, the treatment focus is on metabolic restoration, nutritional rehabilitation, and mood stabilization. These patients may also require assistance with laxative, diuretic, and illicit drug withdrawal. Hospitalization is usually brief and management then transfers to partial hospitalization programs or outpatient treatment facilities. Partial hospitalization programs usually require the patient to be present 10 h/day for 5 days a week. Support is usually provided in a group format and family participation is often required. Many of the treatment modalities for bulimia resemble those for anorexia.

However, the primary focus differs significantly. Although some bulimia patients may be slightly underweight, most are of normal weight, hence nutritional rehabilitation targets the patient's pattern of binging and purging in weight restoration. Therefore, nutritional counseling serves as an adjustment to other treatment modalities and has been noted to enhance the effectiveness of the overall treatment program.

Interventions targeting the psychosocial aspects surrounding bulimia attend to the issues of binging and purging behavior, food restriction, attitudes related to eating patterns, body image, and developmental concerns, self-esteem and sexual difficulties, family dysfunction, and comorbid conditions (ie, depression). The psychosocial approach that has been shown to be most efficacious is CBT. CBT is a relatively short-term approach specifically focused on the eating disorder symptoms and underlying cognitions (ie, low self-esteem, body image concerns) of bulimic patients. Patients managed with CBT demonstrate profound decrements in three very characteristic behaviors: binge eating, vomiting, and laxative abuse. However, the percentage of patients who can achieve total abstinence from binge–purge behavior is invariably small.

Other individual psychotherapy approaches used in clinical practice are interpersonal, psychodynamic, and psychoanalytic. These may be helpful in treating some of the underlying causes of BN, including comorbid mood, anxiety, trauma, and abuse. BN can also be treated using group psychotherapy. Success is moderate, but symptom improvement and alleviation have been maintained at the 1-year follow-up. The efficacy of this approach is increased when it is combined with nutritional counseling and frequent clinic visits. Family and/or marital therapy should be considered in conjunction with other treatment modalities for adolescents living at home, older patients from dysfunctional homes, and patients experiencing marital discord.

Another important aspect of eating disorder management is pharmacotherapy with antidepressants, ie, the selective serotonin reuptake inhibitors (SSRIs). They were first used in the acute phase of treatment for BN because of their well-established comorbid association with clinical depression. It was later reported that nondepressed patients also responded to these medications. Multiple clinical studies have shown that the SSRIs have an antibulimic (reduction in binge eating and vomiting rates) effect independent of their antidepressant effect. Therapists have also noted an improvement in mood and a decrease in symptoms of anxiety. Other antidepressant medications used in the treatment of BN include the tricyclic antidepressants (imipramine-desepranine) and the monoamine oxidase inhibitors (MAOIs) (phenelzine and isocarboxazid). The MAOIs, however, should be used with great caution and only in patients with severe BN. At this time, fluoxetine is the only SSRI approved by the Food and Drug Administration for the treatment of BN. A 20 mg/day dose is used to initiate treatment with doses of 40–60 mg required for maintenance.

E. BINGE EATING PROBLEMS

Although most individuals with binge eating problems are obese, normal-weight people are also affected. Therefore, treatment usually focuses on the distress experienced by individuals rather than on their weight problem. There are several treatment modalities available, including CBT, antidepressants, behavior and group therapy, and self-help groups. All have been shown to be effective to varying degrees. However, CBT (a form of short-term psychotherapy) teaches techniques to monitor eating habits and alternative responses to difficult situations. It was originally used with bulimic patients but has been adapted for binge eaters and appears to be the most effective approach to date. The great majority of those affected can be treated as outpatients and hospitalization is rarely needed.

American Psychiatric Association Clinical Guidelines for Eating Disorders: www.psychorg/clin_res/quide.bk_2.cfm.

Crisp AH et al: Long-term mortality in anorexia nervosa: a 20-year follow-up of the St George's and Aberdeen cohorts. Br J Psychiat 1992;161:104.

Fairburn CG, Marcus MD, Wilson GT: Cognitive behavioral therapy for binge eating and bulimia nervosa: a comprehensive treatment manual. In: *Binge Eating: Nature: Assessment and Treatment.* Fairburn CG, Wilson GT (editors). Guilford Press, 1993: 361.

Hsu I: *Eating Disorders.* Guilford Press, 1990.

Kreipe RE et al: Eating disorders in adolescents: a position paper for the Society for Adolescent Medicine. J Adolesc Health 1995;16:476.

Robin Al, Gilroy M, Dennis AB: Treatment of eating disorders in children and adolescents. Clin Psychol Rev 1998;18(4):421.

Wilhellm, KA, Clarke SD: Eating disorders from a primary care perspective. MJA 1998;168:458.

Prognosis

The prognosis for full recovery of patients with anorexia nervosa is modest. Many individuals demonstrate symptomatic improvement over time, but a substantial portion have persistent problems with body image, disordered eating, and psychological challenges. A review of multiple carefully conducted follow-up studies of hospitalized populations (at least 4 years after onset of illness) showed that the outcomes for 44% could be rated as good (weight restored to within 15% of recommended weight for height; regular menses established), 24% were poor (weight never reached 15% of recommended weight for height; menses absent or sporadic), about 28% fell between the good and poor groups, and about 5% had died (early mortality). About two-thirds of patients continued to have morbid food and weight preoccupation and psychiatric symptoms, and about 40% continued to have bulimic symptoms. Lower initial weight, previous treatment failure, vomiting, family dysfunction, and being married have all been associated with a poorer prognosis. Adolescents have better outcomes than adults and younger adolescents have better outcomes than older adolescents.

The outcomes for bulimia are less certain. Generally speaking, studies of the short-term success rate for patients treated with psychosocial modalities and medication have reported success rates in the 50–70% range, with relapse rates between 30% and 50% after 6 months to 6 years of follow-up. There are also data suggesting that slow, steady progress continues when the follow-up period is extended 10–15 years.

Characteristically, bulimic patients who have onset at an early age, milder symptoms at start of treatment, and a good support system, and those more likely to be treated as outpatients, often have a better prognosis. In summary, bulimics typically have one or more relapses during recovery and anorectics generally have a more protracted and arduous course requiring long-term, intensive therapy.

Garfinkel PE, Garner DM: *The Role of Drug Treatments for Eating Disorders.* Brunner/Mazel, 1987.

Halmi KA et al: Comorbidity of psychiatric diagnosis in anorexia nervosa. Arch Gen Psychiatr 1991;48:712.

Herzog DB, Nussbaum KM, Mamor AK: Comorbidity and outcome in eating disorders. Psychiatr Clin North Am 1996;19: 843.

Adolescent Sexuality

Margaret R. H. Nusbaum, DO, MPH

General Considerations

Although nearly 90% of parents want their children to have it, 23 states require it, 13 other states encourage its teaching, and over 90 national organizations believe that all children should have it, only 5% of children in America receive sex education.

Adolescence is a time of tremendous physical and emotional turmoil. Family and cultural values, as well as personal experiences, including fears, lead to different sex education needs, such as understanding their bodies and body functions, exploring personal values, and setting sexual limits with partners. Unfortunately not only parents but many clinicians are ill prepared to discuss health issues related to sex with adolescents. Additionally, teens may be uncomfortable discussing sexual issues with their peers and adults. This leaves adults with the responsibility for facilitating the discussion.

Lack of comprehensive sex education programs as well as differences in cognitive and physical maturity put adolescents at increased risk for unwanted or unhealthy consequences of sexual activity. This includes increased susceptibility for contracting sexually transmitted illnesses and increased risk for morbidity associated with sexual activity.

Sexuality Information and Education Council of the United States: *SIECUS Guidelines for Comprehensive Sexuality Education,* ed 2. National Guidelines Task Forces, 1996.

Scope of the Problem

A. Unwanted and Unhealthy Consequences of Sexual Activity

About 50% of U.S. adolescents have begun having sexual intercourse between the ages of 15 and 18, with over 50% of adolescent girls and nearly 75% of adolescent boys having had sexual intercourse by the time they graduate from high school, and nearly 90% having had sexual intercourse by age 22. About 40% of all 15–19 year olds have had sexual intercourse in the past 3 months. For adolescents who wanted to have intercourse, the primary reasons given were sexual curiosity (50% of boys and 24% of girls) and affection for their partner (25% of boys and 48% of girls). For adolescents who agreed to have intercourse but did not really want to, the primary reasons given were peer pressure (about 30%), curiosity (50% of boys and 25% of girls), and affection for their partner (>33%). With little sex education, adolescents are poorly prepared to openly discuss their need for contraception, negotiate safe sex, and negotiate the types of behavior in which they are willing to participate. Sexual behavior that contradicts personal values is associated with emotional distress and lower self-esteem. As adolescents are learning to develop appropriate interpersonal skills, damage to self-esteem can be significant when sexual activity is exchanged for attention, affection, peer approval, or reassurance about their physical appearance. Furthermore, early unsatisfactory sexual experiences can set up patterns for repeated unsatisfactory sexual experiences into adulthood.

B. Unintended Pregnancy

Nearly 50% of all pregnancies in the United States are not planned, with the highest rates of unintended pregnancies occurring among adolescents, lower-income women, and black women. About 10% of 15–19 year olds become pregnant every year and more then 40% become pregnant before age 20. Despite similar rates of adolescent sexual activity, the United States has the highest rate of adolescent pregnancy among developed nations.

Unintended pregnancy is socially and economically costly. Medical costs include lost opportunity for preconception care and counseling, increased likelihood of late or no prenatal care, increased risk for a low birth weight infant, and increased risk for infant mortality. The social costs include reduced educational attainment and employment opportunity, increased welfare dependency, and increased risk of child abuse and neglect. In addition to being confronted with adult problems prematurely, adolescent parents' ability to lead productive and healthy lives and to achieve academic and economic success is compromised.

Although abortion rates are higher for women in their 20s, accounting for 80% of total induced abortions, a greater proportion of adolescent pregnancies end in abortion (29%) than do pregnancies for women over 20 years of age (21%). Adolescents who terminate pregnancies are less likely to get pregnant over the next 2 years, more likely to graduate from high school, and more likely to show lower anxiety, higher self-esteem, and more internal control. For an adolescent, postponement of childbearing appears to improve social, psychological, academic, and economic outcomes of life (see Chapter 17).

C. SEXUALLY TRANSMITTED DISEASES

Adolescents (10–19 years old) and young adults (20–24 years old) have the highest rate of sexually transmitted diseases, with chlamydia and gonorrhea rates being highest among women aged 15–19 years. Additionally, one in five cases of acquired immunodeficiency syndrome (AIDS) in the United States is diagnosed in the 20–29 year age group, with the likelihood that human immunodeficiency virus (HIV) was acquired up to 10 years earlier (see Chapter 15).

D. SEXUAL ABUSE

There are an estimated 104,000 child victims of sexual abuse per year. Sexual abuse contributes to sexual and mental health dysfunction as well as public health problems such as substance abuse. Victims of sexual abuse may have greater difficulty with identity formation as well as problems establishing and maintaining healthy relationships with others. Additionally, they may engage in premature sexual behavior, frequently seeking immediate release of sexual tension, and have poor sexual decision-making skills, attempting to create intimacy through sex.

Although only a relatively small proportion of rapes are reported, a major national study found that 22% of women and approximately 2% of men had been victims of a forced sexual act. Unfortunately, adolescent boys are more likely to believe that sexual coercion is justifiable.

Delinquency and homelessness are associated with a history of physical, emotional, and sexual abuse, as well as negative parental reactions to sexual orientation. Homelessness is associated with exchanging sex for money, food, or drugs. Additionally, homeless adolescents are at high risk for repeated episodes of sexual assault.

Fleming PS, editor: *Youth and HIV/AIDS: An American Agenda.* A Report to the President. Washington, DC, 1996.

Institute of Medicine: *The Best Intentions: Unintended Pregnancy and the Well-Being of Children and Families.* Brown SS, Eisenberg L (editors). National Academy Press, 1995.

Institute of Medicine: *The Hidden Epidemic: Confronting Sexually Transmitted Diseases.* Eng TR, Butler WT (editors). National Academy Press, 1997.

Michael R et al: *Sex in America—a Definitive Survey.* Little, Brown, 1994.

U.S. Department of Health and Human Services: *Child Maltreatment 1998: Reports from the States to the National Child Abuse and Neglect Data System.* US Government Printing Office, 2000.

Development

Adolescence is a time of complex physical, psychosocial, sexual, and cognitive changes. With earlier onset of puberty, physical changes occur in advance of cognitive changes. Not until maturity is reached in all of these realms does the adolescent acquire mature decision-making skills and the ability to make healthy decisions regarding sexual activity. Sexuality is more then just anatomic gender or physical sexual behavior; it is how individuals view themselves as male or female, how they relate to others, and their ability to enter and maintain an intimate relationship on a giving and trusting basis. Adolescents who are sexually active before having achieved the capacity for intimacy are at risk for unwanted or unhealthy consequences of sexual activity. Adolescent sexual development forms the basis for further adult sexuality and future intimate relationships. The child's successful achievements during each stage have major implications for both physical and psychosocial development, positive self-concept, and, ultimately, healthy sexuality.

A. PHYSICAL

Adolescents often feel uncomfortable, clumsy, and self-conscious because of the rapid changes in their bodies. Disproportionate physical development among girls and boys contributes additionally to the awkwardness of adolescence. Adolescents must adapt to a new physical identity, which includes hormonal changes, menstruation (often irregular or unpredictable for the first 18–24 months), unpredictable spontaneous erections, nocturnal ejaculations ("wet dreams"), growth of pubic and axillary hair, and even the odors from maturing apocrine glands necessitating deodorant use.

As adolescents are learning to adjust and grow comfortable with their changing bodies, questions concerning body image are common: penis size, breast size and development, distribution of pubic hair, and changing physique in general. In addition to adapting to a new body, adolescents must develop social skills and learn to interact with peers and adults.

B. PSYCHOSOCIAL

Adolescent psychosocial development necessitates that the adolescent develop a realistic and positive self-image and identity. Adolescent identity includes the development of physical, cognitive, and social skills, emotional and spiritual maturity, and sexual identity, including sexual orientation. Adolescents must develop the ability to not only view themselves realistically but also to relate to others. This necessitates successfully achieving independence from the family. Successfully acquiring a stable sense of self allows the adolescent to move on to face the task of the young adult: achieving intimacy by developing openness, mutual trust, sharing, self-abandon, and commitment to another. Core developmental tasks of adolescence include the following:

1. developing independence: becoming emotionally and behaviorally independent rather than dependent, in particular, developing independence from the family;

2. acquiring educational and other experiences needed for adult work roles and developing a realistic vocational goal;

3. learning to deal with emerging sexuality and to achieve a mature level of sexuality;

4. resolving issues of identity (essentially being reborn) and achieving a realistic and positive self-image; and

5. developing interpersonal skills, including the capacity for intimacy, and preparing for intimate partnering with others.

This development includes both internal/introspective as well as external forces. Peers, parents/guardians, teachers, and coaches have an important influence on adolescent expectations, evaluations, values, feedback, and social comparison. Failure to accomplish the developmental tasks necessary for adulthood results in identity or role diffusion: an uncertain self-concept, indecisiveness, and clinging to the more secure dependencies of childhood. With physical, cognitive, and social changes, it is natural for adolescents to explore sexual relationships and sexual roles in their social interactions, which contributes to self-identity. The adolescent's task is to successfully manage the conflict between sexual drives and the recogniton of the emotional, interpersonal, and biological results of sexual behavior.

C. SEXUAL

Gender identity forms a foundation for sexual identity. Gender identity, the sense of maleness or femaleness, is established by age 2, solidifying as adolescents experience and integrate sexuality into their identity.

Sexual identity is the erotic expression of self as male or female and the awareness of self as a sexual being who can be in a sexual relationship with others. The task of adolescence is to integrate sexual orientation into sexual identity. Heterosexual orientation is taken

for granted by society. For lesbian and gay individuals, this creates a clash between outside cultural expectations and their inner sense of self. Currently in our society, the primary developmental task of the gay adolescent is to adapt to a socially stigmatized sexual role. Same-sex orientation emerges during adolescence, but is far more subtle and complex; it includes behavior, sexual attraction, erotic fantasy, emotional preference, social preference, and self-identification—felt to be a continuum from completely heterosexual to completely homosexual (see Chapter 56).

Sexual orientation is typically determined by adolescence, or earlier, and there is no valid scientific evidence that sexual orientation can be changed. Nonetheless, our culture often stigmatizes homosexual behavior, identity, and relationships. These antihomosexual attitudes are associated with significant psychological distress for gay, lesbian, and bisexual (GLB) persons and have a negative impact on mental health, including a greater incidence of depression and suicide (as many as a third have attempted suicide at least once), lower self-acceptance, and a greater likelihood of hiding sexual orientation. When GLB adolescents disclose their orientation to their families, they often experience overt rejection at home as well as social isolation. GLB adolescents lack role models and access to support systems. They frequently run away and become homeless, which places them at higher risk for unsafe sex, drug and alcohol use, and exchanging sex for money or drugs. Although the research is limited, transgendered persons are reported to experience similar problems. Negative attitudes within society toward gay, lesbian, bisexual, and transgendered (GLBT) individuals lead to antigay violence. Media coverage of the Mathew Shepard case brought such violence to greater public awareness. Data from over two dozen studies indicate that 80% of gay men and lesbians have experienced verbal or physical harassment on the basis of their orientation, 45% have been threatened with violence, and 17% have experienced a physical attack.

Adolescents with questions or concerns about sexual orientation need the opportunity to talk about their feelings, their experiences, and their fears of exposure to family and friends. GLBT adolescents need reassurance about their value as a person, support regarding parental and societal reactions, and access to role models. Parents, Families and Friends of Lesbians and Gays (PFLAG) is a nationwide organization whose purpose is to assist parents with information and support (see Chapter 56).

Problems with sexual identity may manifest in extremes—sexually acting out or repression of sexuality. Frequent sexual activity and a variety of sexual partners, negative risk factors for physical or psychological health, suggest poor integration of sexual identity in adolescents. Sexual behavior might be used to gain a sense of security in terms of gender and sexual identity or to gain acceptance or status in a peer group.

D. COGNITIVE

Cognitively, the shift from concrete thinking to abstract thinking (the cognitive development of formal operations) starts developing in early adolescence (11–12 years old) and usually reaches full development by 15–16 years—so 10–14 year olds should not be expected to function with full capacity for abstract thinking. In contrast to younger children, adolescents

- show an increased ability to generate and hold in mind more than one complex mental representation;
- show an appreciation of the relativity and uncertainty of knowledge;
- tend to think in terms of abstract rather than only concrete representations: they think of consequences and the future (abstract) versus a sense of being omnipotent, invincible, infallible, and immune to mishaps (concrete);
- show a far greater use of strategies for obtaining knowledge, such as active planning and evaluation of alternatives;
- are self-aware in their thinking, being able to reflect on their own thought processes and evaluate the credibility of the knowledge source;
- understand that fantasies are not acted out; and
- have the capacity to develop intimate, meaningful relationships.

Adolescents have the task of figuring out what should and should not be done sexually. In concrete thinking risks of sexual behavior are not completely understood or thought out. Abstract thinking allows the capacity for responsible sexual decision making. The concept of relationship is abstract. Sexual intimacy includes not only eroticism but also a sense of commitment: emotional closeness, mutual caring, vulnerability, and trust. The level of intimacy and cognitive development influences sexual decision making. It is estimated that a third of the adult population may never have fully achieved operational thinking.

American Psychiatric Association: *Position Statement on Therapies Focused on Attempts to Change Sexual Orientation (Reparative or Conversion Therapies)*. American Psychiatric Association, 2000.

Berrill KT: Anti-gay violence and victimization in the United States: an overview. In: *Hate Crimes: Confronting Violence against Lesbians and Gay Men.* Herek GM, Berrill KT (editors). Sage, 1992: 19.

Brown RT, Kromer BA: Adolescent Sexuality. In: *Pediatric and Adolescent Gynecology.* Sanfilipo JS (editor). WB Saunders, 1994: 278.

Grant LM, Demetriou E: Adolescent sexuality. Pediatr Clin North Am 1988;35:1271.

Sexual Behavior & Initiation of Sexual Activity

Adolescents often learn about sexuality from a wide range of sources outside of school (family, friends, television, movies, advertising, magazines, the internet, partners, church, and youth organizations). In addition to physical changes, early to middle-stage adolescents begin to experience sexual urges that may be satisfied by masturbation. Masturbation is the exploration of the sexual self and provides a sense of control over one's body and sexual needs. Masturbation starts in infancy, providing children with enjoyment of their bodies. Parents are typically uncomfortable observing this behavior. Compared to younger children, in adolescents masturbation is accompanied by fantasies. In early adolescence, masturbation is an important developmental task, allowing the adolescent to learn what self-stimulation is pleasurable and integrating this with fantasies of interacting with another. Sexual curiosity intensifies. Typical reasons for sexual activity in early to mid-adolescence are curiosity, peer pressure, seeking approval, physical urges, and rebellion. Sexual activity can be misinterpreted by the adolescent as evidence of independence from the family or individuation. With older adolescents, the autoeroticism of masturbation develops into experimentation with others, including intercourse.

Adolescent girls may misinterpret sexual activity as a measure of a meaningful relationship. When sexual activity is used to meet needs such as self-esteem, popularity, and dependency, it delays or prevents developing a capacity for intimacy and is associated with casual and less responsible sexual activity. The adolescent must emerge from the transitional stage of sexual development into relational sexual intimacy by participating in sexual activities in a mature and responsible manner. Sexual activity then becomes an expression of the depth and meaningfulness of the relationship. Sexual activity is not used to satisfy social or personal needs, is neither coercive nor exploitive, and occurs in an atmosphere of trust and respect in which each individual feels free to engage or refuse to engage. Sexual intimacy typically includes identity as a "couple."

Appropriate education, parental support, and a positive sexual self-concept are associated with a later age of first intercourse, a higher consistent use of contraceptives, and a lower pregnancy rate. Sexual self-concept seems to improve with age.

Parental supervision and limit setting, living with both parents in a stable environment, high self-esteem, higher family income, and orientation toward achievement are associated with delayed initiation of sexual activity.

Commitment to a religion or affiliation with certain religious denominations appears to have an effect on sexual behavior. For example, an adolescent's frequent attendance at religious services is associated with a greater likelihood of abstinence. On the other hand, for adolescents who are sexually active, frequency of attendance is associated with decreased contraceptive use by girls and increased use by boys.

Evidence suggests that school attendance reduces adolescent sexual risk-taking behavior. Worldwide, as the percentage of girls completing elementary school has increased, adolescent birth rates have decreased. In the United States, adolescents who have dropped out of school are more likely to initiate sexual activity earlier, fail to use contraception, become pregnant, and give birth. Among those who remain in school, greater involvement with school, including athletics for girls, is related to less sexual risk taking, including later age of initiation of sex and lower frequency of sex, pregnancy, and childbearing.

Schools structure students' time, creating an environment that discourages unhealthy risk taking—particularly by increasing interactions between children and adults. They also affect selection of friends and larger peer groups. Schools can increase belief in the future and help adolescents plan for higher education and careers, and they can increase students' sense of competence, as well as their communication and refusal skills. Parents vary widely in their own knowledge about sexuality, as well as their emotional capacity to explain essential health issues related to sex to their children. Schools often have access to training and communications technology and also provide an opportunity for the kind of positive peer learning that can influence social norms.

Evaluation of school-based sex education programs that typically emphasize abstinence, but also discuss condoms and other methods of contraception, indicates that the programs either have no effect on, or, in some cases, result in a delay in the initiation of sexual activity. There is strong evidence that providing information about contraception does not increase adolescent sexual activity, either by hastening the onset of sexual intercourse, increasing the frequency of sexual intercourse, or increasing the number of sexual partners. More importantly, providing this information results in increased use of condoms or contraceptives among adolescents who were already sexually active.

Early age of first intercourse and lack of contraceptive use are associated with early pubertal development, a history of sexual abuse, lower socioeconomic status, poverty, lack of attentive and nurturing parents, single-parent homes, cultural and familial patterns of early sexual experience, lack of school or career goals, and dropping out of school. Additional factors include low self-esteem, concern for physical appearance, peer group pressure, and pressure to please partners.

Compared to those not sexually active, sexually active males used more alcohol, engaged in more fights, and were more likely to know about HIV/AIDS. Similarly sexually active females used more alcohol and cigarettes. Both sexually active males and females had higher levels of stress. Alcohol and drug use is associated with greater risk taking, including unprotected sexual activity.

Coyle KK et al: Short-term impact of Safer Choices: a multi-component school-based HIV, other STD and pregnancy prevention program. J School Health 1999;69(5):181.

Darroch JE et al: Age differences between sexual partners in the United States. Fam Plan Perspect 1999;31(4):160.

Kirby D: Reducing adolescent pregnancy: approaches that work. Contemp Pediatr 1999;16:83.

Main DS et al: Preventing HIV infection among adolescents: evaluation of a school-based education program. Prevent Med 1994;23:409.

Manlove J: The influence of high school dropout and school disengagement on the risk of school-age pregnancy. J Res Adolesc 1998;8:187.

Resnick MD et al: Protecting adolescents from harm: findings from the National Longitudinal Study on Adolescent Health. JAMA 1997;278:823.

St Lawrence JS et al: Cognitive-behavioral intervention to reduce African American adolescents' risk for HIV infection. J Consult Clin Psychol 1995;63(2):221.

Werner-Wilson RJ: Gender difference in adolescent sexual attitudes: the influence of individual and family factors. Adolescence 1998;33:519.

White SD, DeBlassie RR: Adolescent sexual behavior. Adolescence 1992;27:183.

Sources of Information

A. The Family

Although not the most important source of information about sexuality, parents exert more influence on sexual attitudes. Furthermore, parent–adolescent communication mediates the strength of peer influence on sexual activity. Adolescents need stable environments, parenting that promotes healthy social and emotional development, and protection from abuse. They also need education, the development of skills, experiences that promote self-esteem, and access to sex health information and services, along with positive expectations and sound preparation for their future roles as partners in committed relationships and as parents.

A number of family factors are known to be associated with increased adolescent sexual behavior and the risk of pregnancy. These include living with a single parent, having older siblings who have had sexual intercourse, have become pregnant, or have given birth, and, for girls, the experience of sexual abuse in the family. Family factors associated with decreased sexual activity and use of contraception include parents with higher education and income, close, warm parent–child relationships, and parental supervision and monitoring of children. However, parental control can be associated with negative effects if it is excessive or coercive.

The developmental task of adolescence includes the transition from dependence on family to establishing an independent identity. The stresses of families tend to peak during adolescence, which is attributed to the desire among adolescents for an independent identity, the parents' own unresolved parent–child conflicts, and possible changing gender role identities. Additionally, adolescent sexuality can be very threatening to adults, who may not have resolved their own issues concerning

Table 13–1. How to talk to your child about sex.

1. **Be available.** Watch for clues that show they want to talk. Remember that your comfort with the subject is important. They need to get a feeling of trust from you. If your child doesn't ask, look for ways to bring up the subject. For example, you may know a pregnant woman, watch the birth of a pet, or see a baby getting a bath. Use a TV program or film to start a discussion. Libraries and schools have good books about sex for all ages.
2. **Answer their questions** honestly and without showing embarrassment, even if the time and place do not seem appropriate. A short answer may be best for the moment. Then return to the subject later. It's OK to say, "I don't know." Not being able to answer a question can be an opportunity to learn with your child. Tell your child that you'll get the information and continue the discussion later, or do the research together. Be sure to do this soon. Answer the question that is asked. Respect your child's desire for information. But don't overload the child with too much information at once. Try to give enough information to answer the question clearly, yet encourage further discussion.
3. **Use correct names** for body parts and their functions to show that they are normal and OK to talk about.
4. **Practice talking about sex** with your partner, another family member, or a friend. This will help you feel more comfortable when you do talk with your child.
5. **Talk about sex more than once.** Children need to hear things again and again over the years to really understand, because their level of understanding changes as they grow older. Make certain that you talk about feelings and not just actions. It is important not to think of sex only in terms of intercourse, pregnancy, and birth. Talk about feeling oneself as man or woman, relating to others' feelings, thoughts, and attitudes, and feelings of self-esteem.
6. **Respect their privacy.** Privacy is important, for both you and your child. If your child doesn't want to talk, say, "OK, let's talk about it later," and do. Don't forget about it. Never search a child's room, drawers, or purse for "evidence." Never listen in on a telephone or private conversation.
10. **Listen to your children.** They want to know that their questions and concerns are important. The world they're growing up in is different from what yours was. Laughing at or ignoring a child's question may stop them from asking again. They will get information, accurate or inaccurate, from other sources. When the problem belongs to your child, listen, watch their body language to know when they are ready for you to talk, repeat back to them what you think you heard, listen, respond, and guide them through solving their problem. Talk to your children, trust them, have confidence in them, and respect their feelings.
11. **Share your values.** If your jokes, behaviors, or attitudes don't show respect for sexuality, then you cannot expect your child to be sexually healthy. They learn attitudes about love, caring, and responsibility from you, whether you talk about it or not. Tell your child what your values are about sex and about life. Find out what they value in their lives. Talk about your concern for their health and their future.
12. **Make it easier for your children to talk with you.** Choose words wisely to keep communication open. Use "I" statements because "you" statements can sound accusatory or like a put-down. Instead of telling them what to do, share your values but don't try to control your children. If you act in a controlling manner by telling them what to do, your reaction is likely to lead to their being resentful, insecure, or even rebellious. But you don't want to give them freedom without responsibility for their actions as they are likely to become self-centered, demanding, or even anxious. Teach your child how to make decisions: (a) have your child identify the problem, (b) analyze the situation, (c) search for options or solutions, (d) think about possible consequences to these options, (e) choose the best option, (f) take action, and then (g) watch for the results.

From Facts of Life Netline: Planned Parenthood of Toronto. Web site: http://home-netinc.ca/~sexorg/Facts/Facts1.html); and *Adolescent Sexuality: A Guide for Parents.* Tape #5. Adolescent Wellness Series by Health Learning Systems, Inc., Lyndhurst, NJ, 1990.

sexuality. With escalating stresses, the self-esteem of parents may decline, making them either highly impulsive or overly controlling or rigid. Heightening levels of anxiety contribute to blocked communication.

Both parental lack of rules and discipline as well as very strict discipline have been strongly associated with adolescent sexual activity, whereas parents who supervised their children's dating and insisted on reasonable curfews were least likely to have adolescents who exhibited irresponsible sexual behaviors.

Because many parents are uncomfortable discussing sexuality with their children, family physicians must be proactive in initiating and facilitating conversations about the topic.

B. The Family Physician

Adolescents, in a developmental phase between childhood and adulthood, are often uncomfortable with body changes. Encouraging open communication at home is crucial. Making a handout (Table 13–1) available to parents might help facilitate discussions about sexuality. The quality of discussions at home about sexual matters is the most important factor of family life affecting the risk of teenage pregnancy. If information is not available at home, the family physician, uniquely positioned to serve as a resource, should take a proactive approach by creating the proper environment for discussion, initiating the topic of sexuality, and providing anticipatory guidance for both adolescents and their family (Table 13–2).

1. Creating the environment—The physician should provide a confidential place that fosters open and nonjudgmental communication, which augments or fulfills the parental role. The individuation of the adolescent should be supported by having a separate discussion with parents/guardians and adolescent. Ensuring confidentiality for the preadolescent or adolescent helps create a trusting environment. An office letter to the parent can outline policies regarding confidentiality and clearly communicate the desire to work with parents in making the office as accessible to adolescents as possible. Many states have particular laws regarding the ability of adolescents to seek health care for specific issues—such as contraception, mental health, substance abuse, and pregnancy—without parental presence or approval. Family physicians need to be familiar with the nuances of these laws in their practicing state.

2. Proactive approach—Physicians should recognize opportunities to provide anticipatory guidance, such as to adults who are seeing them for their health needs and mention having a preteen or teen at home. They should cue the preteen positively about upcoming physical changes and cue the parent/family by recommending

Table 13–2. Office approach to adolescent health care.

1. Establish comfortable, friendly relationships that permit discussion in an atmosphere of mutual trust well before sensitive issues arise. Ensure confidentiality before the need arises. Establish separate discussions with parents and adolescents as a matter of routine.
2. Take a firm, proactive role to initiate developmentally appropriate discussions of sexuality. Recognize and use teachable moments regarding sexuality.
3. Provide anticipatory guidance and resources to facilitate family discussions about sexuality and cue families and preteens about upcoming physical and psychosocial developmental changes.
4. Enhance communication skills. Use reflective listening. With a nonjudgmental manner, accept what adolescents have to say without agreeing or disagreeing.
5. Use a positive approach when discussing developmental changes and needed interventions, complimenting pubertal changes.
6. Increase knowledge of family systems and the impact physicians can have on the family.
7. Discuss topics about sexuality incrementally over time to improve assimilation and decrease embarrassment. Avoid scientific terms. Keep answers to questions thorough yet simple. Be cautious about questions that might erode trust.
8. Know your limitations. Use other professional staff and referrals when necessary.

From Croft CA, Asmussen L: A developmental approach to sexuality education: implications for medical practice. Adolesc Health 1993;14(2):109.

that issues concerning sex be discussed with the adolescent at home. In the office and at home sexuality should be discussed incrementally over time. Parents are more influential in early adolescence whereas peer groups are more influential in later adolescence; the extent to which adolescents can balance these two factors influences their risk-taking behavior.

3. Asking the question—Family physicians should initiate the topic of sexuality with adolescents during health maintenance or perhaps even acute care visits. Questions might include: Are you dating? Who are you attracted to? Conversations about sexuality should be tailored to the adolescent's stage of physical, social, and emotional development (Table 13–3). Because abstract thinking is still undergoing development, adolescents need explicit examples to understand ideas. History taking must be specific and directive. Instructions should be concrete. Answers to questions should be simple and thorough.

Table 13–3. Adolescent sex development.

	8–12 years	13 years and older
Sexual knowledge	Knows correct terms for sexual parts, commonly uses slang. Understands sexual aspects of pregnancy. Increasing knowledge of sexual behavior: masturbation, intercourse. Knowledge of physical aspects of puberty by age 10.	Understands sexual intercourse, contraception, and sexually transmitted illnesses (STIs).
Body parts and function	Should have complete understanding of sexual, reproductive, and elimination functions of body parts. All need anticipatory guidance on upcoming pubertal changes for both sexes, including menstruation and nocturnal emissions.	Important to discuss health and hygiene, as well as provide more information about contraceptives, STIs/HIV, and responsible sexual behaviors. Access to health care, especially gynecological care, is important.
Gender identity	Gender identity is fixed. Encouragement to pursue individual interests and talents regardless of gender stereotypes is important.	Discuss men and women in social perception. Males tend to perceive social situations more sexually than females and may interpret neutral cues (eg, clothing, friendliness, etc) as sexual invitations.
Sexual abuse prevention	Assess their understanding of an abuser and correct misconceptions. Explain how abusers, including friends, relatives, and strangers, may manipulate children. Help them to identify abusive situations, including sexual harassment. Practice assertiveness and problem-solving skills. Teach them to trust their body's internal cues and to act assertively in problematic situations.	Teach them to avoid risky situations (eg, walking alone at night, unsafe parts of town). Discuss dating relationships and, in particular, date/acquaintance rape and its association with alcohol and drug use, including date rape drugs. Encourage parents to make themselves available for a ride home anytime their teenager finds himself or herself in a difficult or potentially dangerous situation. Consider a self-defense class for children.
Sexual behavior	Sex games with peers and siblings: role-play and sex fantasy, kissing, mutual masturbation, and simulated intercourse. Masturbation in private. Shows modesty, embarrassment: hides sex games and masturbation from adults. May fantasize or dream about sex. Interested in media sex. Uses sexual language with peers. Talk about making decisions in the context of relationships. Provide information about contraceptives, STIs/HIV, and responsible sexual behaviors.	Pubertal changes continue: most girls menstruate by 16, boys capable of ejaculation by 15. Dating begins. Sexual contacts are common: mutual masturbation, kissing, petting. Sexual fantasy and dreams. Sexual intercourse may occur in up to 75% by age 18. Encourage parents to share attitudes and values. Provide access to contraceptives. Respect need and desire for privacy. Set clear rules about dating and curfews.
Developmental issues:[1] most sexual concerns are related to the development tasks.	Early adolescence (Tanner I and II): Physical changes including menstruation and nocturnal emissions. Often ambivalent over issues of independence and protection and family relationships. Egocentric. Beginning struggles of separation and emerging individual identity. Seemingly trivial concerns to adults can reach crisis proportions in young adolescents. Common concerns include fears of too slow or too rapid physical development, especially breasts and genitalia; concern and curiosity about their bodies; sexual feelings; and sexual behavior of their peer group as well as adults around them. Although masturbation is very healthy and	Middle adolescence (Tanner III and IV): Peer approval. Experimentation and risk-taking behavior arise out of the developmental task of defining oneself socially. Sexual intercourse may be viewed as requisite for peer acceptance. Curiosity, need for peer approval, self-esteem, and struggle for independence from parents can lead to intercourse at this stage. Feelings of invincibility lead to sexual activity that is impulsive and lacking discussion about sexual decision making, such as contraception, preferences for behavior, relationship commitment, or safe sex. Increasing insistence on control over decisions. Increasing conflict with parents.

(continued)

Table 13–3. Adolescent sex development. (Continued)

	8–12 years	13 years and older
	normal, reassurance may be needed given persistence of myths and mixed messages. Developmental tasks: 1. Independence and separation from the family. 2. Development of individual identity. 3. Beginning to shift from concrete to abstract thinking.	Developmental tasks: 1. Development of adult social relationships with both sexes. 2. Continued struggle for independence. 3. Continued development of individual identity. 4. Continued shifting from cognitive to abstract thinking. Late adolescence (Tanner V): With cognitive maturation, issues regarding peer acceptance and conflicts with parents regarding independence lessen. Intimacy, commitment, and life planning, including thoughts of future parenthood. Self-identity continues to solidify, moral and ethical values, exploration of sexual indentity. Crises over sexual orientation may surface at this stage. Increasing ability to recognize consequences of own behavior. Developmental tasks: 1. Abstract (futuristic) thinking. 2. Vocational plans. 3. Development of moral and ethical values. 4. Maturation toward autonomous decision making.

From Gordon BN, Schroeder: *Sexuality: A Developmental Approach to Problems.* Plenum Press, 1995; and Alexander B, McGrew MC, Shore W: Adolescent sexuality issues in office practice. Am Fam Physician 1991;1273.
[1]These are general categories; adolescents vary in their physical, psychosocial, and cognitive development.

Concerns in early adolescence typically relate to body image and what is "normal," both physically and socially. Information and reassurance about pubertal changes are critical parts of physical examinations. Conversations may include addressing concerns about obesity, acne, and body image that affect self-perception of acceptability and attractiveness. Discussions about how to handle peer pressure may always be helpful. The adolescent's understanding of safe sexual practices as well as the ability to negotiate the behavior in which they are willing or not willing to participate should be explored. Giving the adolescent the opportunity to role-play the discussion regarding these issues may contribute to confidence in successfully negotiating with a current or future partner.

Although it is important not to make assumptions about sexual orientation, an adolescent who presents with depression and suicidal ideation should be questioned about this. Hiding one's orientation increases stress. It is important to be aware of community resources for GLB adolescents such as psychologists and counselors, GLB community support groups, and organizations such as PFLAG.

Caring for adolescents can be exciting and challenging. Physicians should recognize that their own projections of unfinished sexual issues from their adolescence may surface in caring for adolescent patients. This can make discussions, particularly around sensitive subjects such as drugs, alcohol, nicotine, and sex, difficult. Recognizing and addressing these issues or referring adolescents to colleagues with greater experience and comfort with these matters would be appropriate.

The role of family physicians is to provide a supportive, sensitive, and instructive environment in which they neither ignore nor judge adolescent sexual activity but reassure, listen, clarify, and provide correct information about this important aspect of adolescent development. Consultation or referral is appropriate when it is in the best interest of the patient. Open and frank communication, ensuring confidentiality, nonjudgmental listening, and the provision of clear, accurate information help develop a successful doctor–patient relationship. Ideally the goal should be to delay sexual activity until adolescents have the knowledge and tools needed to make healthy decisions about sex. However, identifying adolescents at risk, educating about safer sex, establishing sexual limits, and providing information about support and educational resources for adolescents who are currently sexual activity are critical activities for the family physician.

Miller BC: *Families Matter: A Research Synthesis of Family Influences on Adolescent Pregnancy.* National Campaign to Prevent Teen Pregnancy, 1998.

Ryan C, Futterman D: Caring for gay and lesbian youth. Contemp Pediatr 1998;15(11):107.

WEB SITES

AAFP: Information from Your Family Doctor: Sex: Take Time to Make the Right Decision, 2000

http://www.familydoctor. org/handouts/276.html.

Gay and Lesbian Medical Association (GLMA)

http://www.glma.org

Parents, Families and Friends of Lesbians and Gays (PFLAG) http://www.pflag.org

Menstrual Disorders

Mary V. Krueger, DO, MPH, MAJ, MC, USA

Menstrual disorders are a heterogeneous group of conditions that are both physically and psychologically debilitating. Though once considered nuisance problems, it is now recognized that menstrual disorders take a significant toll on society, both in days lost from work as well as in the pain and suffering experienced by individual women. Many women consider the occurrence of their monthly cycle as evidence that their body is functioning properly, and are disturbed when irregularities in this cycle occur. These disorders may arise from physiological (ie, pregnancy), pathological (ie, endocrine abnormalities), or iatrogenic (ie, secondary to contraceptive use) conditions.

Irregularities in menstruation may manifest as complete absence of menses, dysfunctional uterine bleeding, dysmenorrhea, or premenstrual syndrome. Establishing an accurate diagnosis is essential for appropriate treatment and avoidance of potential complications. Because it is essential to know what is normal in order to define what is abnormal, normal menstrual parameters are listed in Table 14–1. This chapter will discuss the evaluation, diagnosis, and treatment of patients whose menses fall outside these parameters.

THE MENSTRUAL CYCLE

The normal menstrual cycle relies on the action and interaction of hormones released from the hypothalamus, pituitary, and ovaries and their effect on the endometrium. A disease state that affects any of these organs, or that interferes with the timing of hormone release, may result in a menstrual disorder. It is important to understand the interplay between these organs and the hormones they release to intelligently evaluate, diagnose, and treat patients with menstrual disorders.

The hypothalamus is the metronome of the menstrual cycle, keeping cadence with its release of gonadotropin-releasing hormone (GnRH). GnRH neurons originating in the arcuate nucleus accomplish this function by transforming signals received from the brain into pulsatile GnRH signals that control the rhythm of the menstrual cycle. It is through these neural messages and their control of GnRH secretion that environmental inputs such as stress, extreme weight loss, and excessive exercise are thought to exert their influences on the menstrual cycle. GnRH has a short half-life of only 5 min, so the amplitude and frequency of its release precisely control blood levels and send specific information to the pituitary, its target organ.

The pituitary responds to the GnRH pulses by secreting the gonadotropins, follicle-stimulating hormone (FSH), and luteinizing-hormone (LH), which act in concert to promote ovulation. The FSH stimulates the growth and development of several ovarian follicles in the first days of the menstrual cycle. By Day 12, the process of selection has occurred, resulting in the atresia of all but one dominant follicle. Layers of both thecal and granulosa cells surround the dominant follicle. The thecal cells produce androgens under the influence of LH, and the granulosa cells, under the influence of FSH, aromatize these androgens to estrogens. The negative feedback on the pituitary by the estrogens from the dominant follicle leads to a decrease in circulating levels of FSH, which results in involution of the remaining antral follicles. The dominant follicle continues to grow in the face of declining FSH as a result of up-regulation of its FSH receptors. The estradiol acts on the pituitary in a positive feedback loop at this stage of the cycle to increase concentrations of LH, which causes the ovary to produce progesterone. The progesterone alters the pituitary response to the circulating estradiol, LH, and FSH, resulting in an LH surge that occurs 34–36 h before ovulation. Ovulation marks the end of the follicular phase and the beginning of the luteal phase, with the formation of the corpus luteum cyst. The corpus luteum cyst, the structures remaining of the dominant follicle after ovulation, secretes progesterone and estrogen, preparing the endometrium for implantation. In the absence of fertilization and implantation of an egg, this will continue for 14 days before the corpus luteum involutes and hormone levels fall sharply.

Table 14–1. Normal menstrual parameters.

Age of menarche	<16 years old
Age of menopause	>40 years old; mean age 52
Length of menstrual cycle	22–45 days
Length of menstrual flow	3–7 days
Amount of menstrual flow	≤80 mL

The endometrium responds to these hormonal fluxes in two main phases. During the proliferative phase, the endometrium responds to the estrogen from the ovary by forming glands, vascular elements, increasing numbers of both estrogen and progesterone receptors, and proliferating. As progesterone levels increase right before ovulation, the secretory phase begins where the endometrium differentiates and secretes glycogen in preparation for implantation. If implantation occurs, chorionic gonadotropin feeds back to the corpus luteum, which will produce progesterone to maintain the pregnancy until the placenta can take over. In the absence of pregnancy, estrogen and progesterone levels drop sharply, resulting in sloughing of the endometrium with ensuing menstrual bleeding. This complex cycle is depicted pictorially in Figure 14–1. Understanding of this cycle and its complex interactions will serve the clinician well in evaluation and diagnosis of menstrual disorders.

AMENORRHEA

 ESSENTIALS OF DIAGNOSIS

- *Primary amenorrhea is the absence of menses by 16 years of age in a patient with secondary sex characteristics or the absence of menses by 14 years of age in a patient without secondary sex characteristics.*
- *In secondary amenorrhea a woman with previously normal menses goes at least 6 months without a period or a woman with previously irregular menses goes at least 12 months or at least six cycles without a period.*

Amenorrhea is the natural result of menopause, pregnancy, and lactation, but can be very distressing when it occurs outside of these conditions. Amenorrhea is a symptom, not a diagnosis, and may occur secondary to a number of endocrine and anatomic abnormalities. Classifying amenorrhea into primary and secondary amenorrhea can aid in evaluation and simplify diagnosis.

Primary Amenorrhea

General Considerations

Primary amenorrhea is defined as the absence of menses by 16 years of age in a patient with secondary sex characteristics or the absence of menses by 14 years of age in a patient without secondary sex characteristics. The most common causes are gonadal dysgenesis and physiological delay of puberty.

Clinical Findings

A. SYMPTOMS AND SIGNS

The patient with primary amenorrhea is often brought to the physician by her mother who is concerned about the patient's delay in reaching developmental milestones. The clinician should be aware that the adolescent may be uncomfortable discussing her sexuality, especially in the presence of a parent. The adolescent's rights as a patient must be respected. Important elements of the history include (1) the time of menarche in the patient's mother and sisters, (2) a history of psychosocial deprivation or abuse, (3) the presence of chronic diseases such as diabetes, juvenile rheumatoid arthritis, inflammatory bowel disease, cancer, or chronic infection, (4) anosmia (Kallman's syndrome), (5) a history of head trauma (damage to the hypothalamic–pituitary axis), (6) sexual activity (possibility of pregnancy), (7) the timeline of development of secondary sexual characteristics (if any), (8) a family history of gonadal dysgenesis, (9) medication or supplement use, and (10) a history of weight loss and the amount of regular physical activity. This targeted history will help to narrow the differential and eliminate unnecessary testing.

B. PHYSICAL FINDINGS

Assessment should focus on appearance of secondary sexual characteristics (axillary and pubic hair), breast development, external genitalia, height percentile, female body shape, and pelvic examination findings—specifically the presence or absence of a uterus. The clinician should be careful to allay patient fears, as this will often be her first pelvic examination. Body mass index (BMI) should also be calculated and compared with prior visits to assess both for anorexia or rapid weight loss. Presence or absence of breast development and presence or absence of the uterus and cervix are decision points for further testing and diagnostic categories. Table 14–2 lists causes of primary amenorrhea.

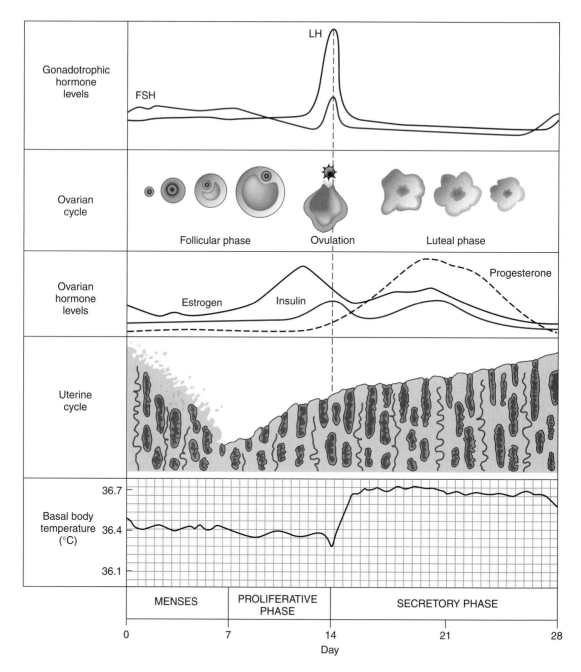

Figure 14–1. The menstrual cycle.

Table 14–2. Etiologies of primary amenorrhea.

Physiological
  Constitutional delay
  Pregnancy
Pathological
  Absent breast development, normal pelvic examination
    findings
    Hypothalamic failure
      Anorexia nervosa, excessive weight loss, excessive
        exercise, stress
      Chronic illness (juvenile rheumatoid
        arthritis, diabetes, irritable bowel syndrome)
    Gonadotropin deficiency
      Kallman's syndrome (associated with anosmia)
      Pituitary dysfunction after head trauma or shock
      Infiltrative or inflammatory processes
      Pituitary adenoma
      Craniopharyngioma
    Gonadal failure
      Gonadal dysgenesis (ie, Turner's syndrome)
  Normal breast development, normal pelvic examination
    findings
    Hypothyroidism
    Hyperprolactinemia
  Normal breast development, abnormal pelvic examination
    findings
    Testicular feminization
    Anatomic abnormalities (uterovaginal septum, imperfo-
      rate hymen)

---

1. Absent breast development with normal pelvic examination findings—

a. Hypothalamic failure—This is the common pathway for amenorrhea resulting from constitutional delay, anorexia nervosa, excessive exercise, severe stress (ie, due to abuse or psychosocial deprivation), chronic infection, cancer, or systemic illness. All these conditions are believed to suppress hypothalamic GnRH secretion through neuronal pathways in the arcuate nucleus. Patients with constitutional delay will display delayed but otherwise normal secondary sexual characteristics and there may be a history of the mother or sisters also being "late bloomers."

b. Pituitary failure—Pituitary failure results in hypogonadotropic hypogonadism. This may result from inadequate GnRH stimulation secondary to Kallman's syndrome (where the GnRH neurons fail to migrate from the olfactory bulb) and can be identified by its association with anosmia. Head trauma, severe hypotension (shock), infiltrative or inflammatory processes, pituitary adenoma, or craniopharyngioma may damage the pituitary, resulting in decreased or absent gonadotropin (LH and FSH) release. These patients will often display symptoms relating to deficiency of other pituitary hormones as well.

c. Gonadal dysgenesis—Resulting from chromosomal anomalies, this is the most common cause of primary amenorrhea, responsible for 45% of cases. Turner's syndrome (45,XO) is the most familiar type and is associated with short stature, widely spaced nipples, a webbed neck, and sexual infantilism. Ovaries are vestigial "streak gonads" and produce little to no estradiol. Mosaic variants may also occur, which can result in both subtle abnormalities as well as more striking ambiguous genitalia.

2. Normal breast development and normal pelvic examination findings—

a. Hypothyroidism and hyperprolactinemia—These can both suppress the secretion of GnRH, FSH, and LH resulting in suppression of the menstrual cycle. Pubarche and thelarche should progress normally in this setting. Conversely, profound hypothyroidism can result in precocious puberty due to the FSH-like effect of high levels of circulating thyroid-stimulating hormone (TSH).

b. Polycystic ovarian syndrome—This may cause primary amenorrhea, though it is more commonly thought of as a cause of secondary amenorrhea. Acne, hirsuitism, and obesity are commonly seen in patients with this disorder.

3. Normal breast development with abnormal pelvic examination findings—

a. Testicular feminization—Androgen resistance prevents the influence of testicular androgens on a chromosomally male (XY) fetus, resulting in female external genitalia. The testes secrete a Müllerian duct inhibitory hormone to which the fetus does respond, thus preventing development of the upper vagina and uterus.

b. Anatomic abnormalities—Failures of uterovaginal communication due to either uterovaginal septum or imperforate hymen are anatomic causes of primary amenorrhea. They are often accompanied by cyclic pelvic pain and hematocolpos. Rokitansky–Kuster–Hauser syndrome, failure of uterine development, is associated with renal anomalies.

C. LABORATORY FINDINGS

Choices of laboratory examination should be guided based on history and physical findings and are listed here based on etiology. A pregnancy test should be performed on all individuals presenting for primary amen-orrhea who have secondary sexual characteristics and functional anatomy. Though the initial cycles after menarche are often anovulatory, pregnancy can occur before the first recognized menstrual cycle. A sensitive discussion of this subject is necessary to facilitate under-standing and avoid conflict with the patient and/or her mother.

Patients with a normal pelvic examination but ab-sent breast development should have serum FSH mea-sured to distinguish peripheral (gonadal) from central (pituitary or hypothalamic) causes of amenorrhea. A high FSH suggests gonadal dysgenesis. A karyotype should be performed to identify patients who are 46,XY, as these individuals have a high peripubertal risk for gonadoblastoma and dygerminoma.

If the uterus is absent, serum testerone and kary-otype should be performed. Elevated testosterone in the presence of a Y chromosome indicates the presence of functional testicular tissue that should be excised to prevent later neoplastic transformation.

In patients with both normal breast development and a normal pelvic examination, serum prolactin and TSH should be measured to rule out hyperprolactine-mia and hypothyroidism. If these values are in the nor-mal range, investigation should proceed according to the secondary amenorrhea algorithm.

D. IMAGING STUDIES

Radiographic studies are targeted toward the diagnosis suggested by the history and by physical and laboratory studies. Magnetic resonance imaging (MRI) is indi-cated in patients in whom pituitary pathology is sus-pected. Computerized visual field testing may be added if examination or MRI indicates optic chiasm compres-sion. Pelvic ultrasound should be performed in patients with suspected pelvic anomalies.

Treatment

Successful treatment of primary amenorrhea is based on correct diagnosis of the underlying etiology. The goals of treatment are to establish a firm diagnosis, to restore ovulatory cycles and treat infertility, to treat hypoestro-genemia and hyperandrogenism, and to assess and ad-dress risks associated with a persistent hypoestrogene-mic state.

A. COUNSELING

Patients with hypothalamic failure due to anorexia, rapid weight loss, excessive exercise, abuse, or stress should re-ceive counseling to address the underlying cause of these problems. Because anorexia and associated eating disor-

ders have high rates of recidivism, providers experi-enced in the treatment of these conditions should be involved in the care of these patients. A team approach may enlist the assistance of a registered dietician to as-sist in weight gain, an exercise physiologist to assist with modified exercise, and a psychologist or a psychia-trist to manage the complex psychosocial issues in-volved. In cases of abuse, the provider should inform the patient about local support groups, safe houses, and professional counseling.

B. MEDICAL THERAPY

Pituitary adenomas, resulting in hyperprolactinemia, can be treated with either bromocriptine or cabergo-line. Bromocriptine may be used in pregnancy and has the best established safety record of all the dopamine agonists. Cabergoline is longer acting and may be more efficacious in some patients. Tumors that are large enough to affect vision or produce a mass effect should be surgically removed through transsphenoidal exci-sion. Initial success rates are high, but late recurrence rates may approach 20%.

Patients with gonadal dysgenesis should be given hormone replacement therapy to prevent the negative effects of a hypoestrogen state. Patients with an intact uterus may undergo induction of menstruation with cyclic progesterone and estrogen therapy.

C. SURGICAL THERAPY

If testing reveals a 46,XY karyotype, surgical removal of the gonads is necessary, as gonadal dysgenesis with this karyotype is associated with a high peripubertal risk of dygerminoma or gonadoblastoma.

Structural anomalies should be addressed surgically. In patients with congenital absence of a uterus, investi-gation should be undertaken for associated renal anom-alies.

Only providers experienced in this field should per-form induction of puberty in patients with constitu-tional delay. Estrogen is responsible for epiphyseal clo-sure as well as the adolescent growth spurt; mistimed administration could have significant effects on the final achieved height in these patients.

Secondary Amenorrhea

General Considerations

The most common type of amenorrhea, secondary amenorrhea, is diagnosed when a woman with previ-ously normal menses goes at least 6 months without a period or when a woman with previously irregular menses goes at least 12 months or at least six cycles without a period. It can have either physiological or pathological etiologies and can be a topic of great concern for the patient. The causes of secondary amenorrhea can be broken down into those with and those without evidence of hyperandrogenism.

Clinical Findings

A. SYMPTOMS AND SIGNS

Pertinent history in the evaluation of secondary amenorrhea includes (1) previous menstrual history (timing and quality of menses), (2) pregnancies (including terminations and complicated deliveries), (3) symptoms of endocrine disease, (4) medication history, (5) weight loss or gain, (4) exercise level, and (5) masculinizing characteristics noticed by the patient or family.

B. PHYSICAL FINDINGS

General examination should assess pubertal development and secondary sexual characteristics while looking for evidence of hyperandrogenism. These latter findings may include oily skin, acne, and hirsutism. The pelvic examination should note clitoral size, with clitorimegaly defined as a length × width product of greater than 40 mm^2. Evidence of hyperandrogenism assists in classifying etiologies of secondary amenorrhea.

1. Evidence of hyperandrogenism on examination—
a. Polycystic ovarian syndrome (PCOS)—Responsible for 30% of secondary amenorrhea, PCOS is the most common reproductive endocrine disorder in women. It is characterized by androgen excess, of ovarian origin, which results in chronic ovulatory failure. Symptoms include irregular or absent menses, hirsutism, acne, and virilization. Dysfunctional uterine bleeding and increased rates of endometrial carcinoma may occur secondary to endometrial hyperstimulation by the continuous secretion of estrogen and progesterone. There is no cyclical decrease of these hormones due to anovulation and the failure of a dominant ovarian follicle to develop. Comorbidities associated with PCOS include abdominal obesity, insulin resistance, impaired glucose tolerance, hypertension, hypertriglyceridemia, and premature vascular disease.

b. Autonomous hyperandrogenism—Tumors of adrenal or ovarian origin may secrete androgens. Virilization is more pronounced than in PCOS and may manifest as frontal balding, increased muscle bulk, deep voice, clitorimegaly and severe hirsutism.

c. Late-onset or mild congenital adrenal hyperplasia—This rare condition may be confirmed by an increased level of 17-hydroxyprogesterone in the setting of secondary amenorrhea and hyperandrogenism.

2. No evidence of hyperandrogenism on examination—
a. Medication use—History should be reviewed for use of contraceptives, particularly progesterone-only preparations. These may take the form of oral contraceptives (OCPs), implants, injectables, or intrauterine devices. Amenorrhea secondary to OCP use may lead to patient concern and discontinuation. It is important to make women aware that 20% of patients on progestin-only pills will become amenorrheic within the first year of use. Rates are even higher for those using injectable progesterone: 55% of women at 1 year and 68% of women at 2 years report amenorrhea.

b. Functional hypothalamic amenorrhea—Patients who are significantly underweight, who have experienced recent, rapid weight loss, who exercise rigorously, or who are under emotional stress may experience amenorrhea due to a functional suppression of GnRH. Careful history taking will aid in detection of these factors.

c. Hypergonadotropic hypogonadism—Premature ovarian failure (cessation of ovarian function before 40 years of age) may be autoimmune, idiopathic, or occur secondarily due to radiotherapy or chemotherapy (cyclophosphamide is associated with destruction of oocytes). A history of Addison's disease, autoimmune thyroid disease, or type I diabetes should raise suspicion of an autoimmune cause, whereas a history of treatment for Hodgkin's lymphoma, breast cancer, or Wilm's tumor points to cytotoxic drugs as a primary etiology.

d. Hyperprolactinemia—Pituatary adenomas may be associated with amenorrhea and galactorrhea, and are responsible for 20% of cases of secondary amenorrhea. Prolactin secreted by these tumors acts directly on the hypothalamus to suppress secretion of GnRH. Dopamine receptor blocking agents, hypothalamic masses, and hypothyroidism are less common causes of hyperprolactinemia.

e. Thyroid disease—Profound hypothyroidism or hyperthyroidism affects the feedback control of LH, FSH, and estradiol on the hypothalamus, causing menstrual irregularities.

f. Hypogonadotropic hypogonadism—Head trauma, severe hypotension (shock), infiltrative or inflammatory processes, pituitary adenoma, or craniopharyngioma may damage the pituitary, resulting in decreased or absent gonadotropin (LH and FSH) release. These patients will often display symptoms relating to deficiency of other pituitary hormones as well.

C. LABORATORY FINDINGS

Initial tests should include a pregnancy test, fasting glucose, TSH, and prolactin levels. In the absence of significant abnormalities in these values, a progestin challenge test should be performed to assess the patient's estrogen status. The patient is given medroxyprogesterone, 5–10 mg orally, daily for 5–7 days. Women with adequate levels of circulating estrogen should experience withdrawal bleeding within 2 weeks of administration. Some patients who do not respond to oral administration will respond to intramuscular injection. FSH should be measured for women who do not experience withdrawal bleeding within the designated time period. A high FSH value (greater than 30 IU/L) is indicative of ovarian failure, whereas normal or low values indicate either an acquired uterine anomaly (Asherman's syndrome) or hypothalamic–pituitary failure. Ovarian failure is confirmed by a low serum estradiol level, less than 30 pg/mL. A serum LH and FSH should be drawn on women who do not experience withdrawal bleeding after the progesterone challenge and have a normal estrogen level. An elevated LH value is highly suggestive of PCOS, especially in a woman with clinical features of virilization. If the LH level is normal, an LH to FSH ratio should be determined. This ratio is elevated, >2.5, in women with PCOS even when FSH and LH values are within normal limits. This diagnosis can be confirmed by measurement of serum testosterone and dehydroepiandrosterone sulfate (DHEA-S), which should be normal or just mildly elevated in women with PCOS. An increased testosterone to DHEA-S ratio is suggestive of an adrenal source. This finding warrants further study with determination of 17-hydroxyprogesterone. This level is elevated in late-onset congenital adrenal hyperplasia and Cushing's syndrome. Cushing's syndrome may be excluded with a 24-h urinary free cortisol and dexaminationethasone suppression testing.

D. IMAGING STUDIES

Computed tomographic (CT) scanning of the adrenal glands and ultrasound of the ovaries should be performed in women with clinical features of virilization and increased testosterone (greater than 200 ng/dL) or DHEAS-S (greater than 7 μg/mL). Although these are the most sensitive imaging modalities, normal ovarian ultrasound does not exclude neoplasm. Surgical exploration may be necessary in situations in which this is still a concern. A CT or MRI of the pituitary should be performed if pituitary pathology is suspected.

Treatment

Treatment depends on correct diagnosis of the underlying etiology. As in primary amenorrhea, the goals of treatment are to establish a firm diagnosis, to restore ovulatory cycles and treat infertility (when possible), to treat hypoestrogenemia and hyperandrogenism, and to assess and address risks associated with a persistent hypoestrogenemic state.

A. MEDICAL THERAPY

Treat the underlying causes of amenorrhea. Patients with identified hypothyroidism should be treated with thyroxine replacement. Patients with hyperprolactinemia secondary to prolactinoma may be treated with either surgical resection or dopamine agonist therapy. Although there are strong proponents for each therapy, many authorities currently favor a medical approach. Treatment with a dopamine agonist can suppress prolactin secretion, induce ovulation, and decrease tumor size while maintaining the pituitary reserve. Bromocriptine is often used in women who want to conceive, as there is no increased incidence of congenital malformations secondary to its use. Its main side effects are nausea, vomiting, and postural hypotension. These can be minimized by starting treatment at a low dose, 0.625 mg/day, and increasing to the target dosage over several weeks time. The lowest usual target dose is 2.5 mg or one tablet. Therapy can be monitored by checking the level of prolactin every month for the first 3 months, then once every 3 months until it is within the normal range. Cabergoline, also a dopamine agonist, is administered weekly and may be more effective in treating prolactinomas, although there are fewer data on its safety in pregnancy.

Patients found to have empty sella or Sheehan's syndrome should be treated with replacement of pituitary hormones.

Women under 40 years of age whose amenorrhea is secondary to absent ovarian function have premature ovarian failure. Those who experience ovarian failure before the age of 30 years should undergo karyotype testing to screen for Y chromosome elements, which are associated with cancer. These patients are at a high risk of osteoporosis and cardiovascular disease due to their hypoestrogenemic state. Estrogen replacement should be undertaken, with progesterone for those patients with an intact uterus, to prevent these sequelae. Assisted reproduction technology with a donor oocyte can make it possible for women desiring pregnancy to give birth.

Patients with PCOS may achieve resumption of menses with weight loss. The assistance of a registered dietician should be sought to improve success rates. Newer agents that are being used with some success in PCOS are metformin and troglitazone, although they have not yet received FDA approval. They are thought to address the underlying metabolic defects in patients with PCOS.

B. SURGICAL THERAPY

Women with adrenal or ovarian androgen-secreting tumors should undergo appropriate surgical intervention. Likewise, women for whom Asherman's syndrome is a cause for their amenorrhea should undergo lysis of adhesions followed by endometrial stimulation with estrogen. These patients are at increased risk of placenta accreta in subsequent pregnancies.

McIver B, Romanski S, Nippoldt T: Evaluation and management of amenorrhea. Mayo Clin Proc 1997;72(12):1161.

Nestler JE: Role of hyperinsulinemia in the pathogenesis of the polycystic ovary syndrome, and its clinical implications. Semin Reprod Endocrinol 1997;15(2):111.

Raymond JP et al: Follow-up of children born of bromocriptine-treated mothers. Horm Res 1985;22(3):239.

Schwallie P: Contraceptive use efficacy study utilizing medroxy-progesterone acetate administered as an intramuscular injection once every 90 days. Fertil Steril 1973;24:331.

Speroff L, Darney P: *A Clinical Guide for Contraception.* Williams & Wilkins, 1992.

Thorner M: Medical treatment of prolactinomas. J Clin Endocrinol Metab 1997;82:997.

Webster J, Piscitelli G, Polli A: A comparison of cabergonline and bromocriptine in the treatment of hyperprolactinemic amenorrhea. New Engl J Med 1994;331:904.

DYSFUNCTIONAL UTERINE BLEEDING

ESSENTIALS OF DIAGNOSIS

- *Vaginal bleeding caused by hormonal abnormalities.*
- *The absence of pregnancy, tumor, infection, or coagulopathy.*
- *Menses that are too heavy (>80 mL per cycle), too frequent (occurring every 22 days or less), or too long (>7 days of flow).*

General Considerations

Vaginal bleeding caused by hormonal abnormalities, in the absence of pregnancy, tumor, infection, or coagulopathy, is termed dysfunctional uterine bleeding. Vaginal bleeding attributed to causes other than menstrual dysfunction are addressed in Chapter 32. Dysfunctional uterine bleeding may include menses that are too heavy (>80 mL per cycle), too frequent (occurring every 22 days or less), or too long (>7 days of

flow). The most frequent cause is continuous estrogen production associated with anovulation, a common condition in adolescents, which carries significant physical, psychological, cultural, and societal morbidity. Women losing more than 60 mL of blood per month are at risk of developing iron deficiency anemia with the attendant lethargy, decreased immune function, and restriction in activities of daily living. Some cultures view menstruating women as "unclean," and therefore unable to prepare food, participate in daily activities, or have sexual intercourse. For all these reasons, it is important for the family physician to be familiar with assessment diagnosis and treatment of dysfunctional uterine bleeding.

Clinical Findings

A. SYMPTOMS AND SIGNS

Initial history should include a detailed description of menstrual bleeding as well as age of onset of menses, length of cycles, length of menses, presence of clots, number of pads or tampons used per day, and change in character or timing of menses. A symptom diary is helpful in obtaining this information. A sexual history including number of partners, form of contraception, number and timing of pregnancies, number and timing of elective terminations, and history of sexually transmitted diseases should also be documented. Patients using an intrauterine device (IUD) for contraception should be questioned about the onset of dysfunctional uterine bleeding in relation to the insertion of their IUD. Symptoms of anemia including fatigue, lethargy, and lightheadedness may be present. The patient should also be asked about both personal and family history of bleeding disorders.

B. PHYSICAL EXAMINATION

The physical examination should include an initial evaluation of hemodynamic stability followed by a pelvic examination with cervical smear and cultures. IUD placement should be confirmed in patients using this method of contraception. Special note should be made of pallor, tachycardia, hypotension, or excessive bruising. Uterine size should be noted, as enlargement may indicate fibroids, a common cause of heavy menstrual bleeding.

C. LABORATORY FINDINGS

A pregnancy test should be performed on all patients with dysfunctional uterine bleeding, especially if onset is recent, as this may represent an ectopic pregnancy. A complete blood count (CBC) should also be undertaken in all women, as hemoglobin is a surrogate assessment for excessive menstrual loss, white blood cell count may indicate chronic infection, and indices can provide an assessment of whole body iron stores. Coagulation screens, thyroid function tests, endometrial sampling, and other endocrine investigations should be performed only as indicated by the history and physical examination.

D. IMAGING STUDIES

Pelvic ultrasound should be performed only in the evaluation of pelvic disorders discovered during clinical examination, in women who weigh ≥90 kg or in women 45 years of age or older.

Treatment

A. MEDICAL THERAPY

The treatment strategy described in this section assumes that the clinician has ruled out infection, neoplasm, pregnancy, trauma, and coagulopathy as the cause for abnormal vaginal bleeding. Adolescents with irregular menstrual bleeding that does not involve excessive blood loss should be counseled on the possible etiologies and all available treatment options. If the patient is within 2 years of menarche, anovulatory cycles are the most likely cause for dysfunctional uterine bleeding, and OCPs may be used to regulate cycles. This may not be an acceptable option to all patients because of the stigma associated with OCP. Expectant management may be a preferable choice in these situations.

Patients with dysfunctional uterine bleeding due to underlying endocrine disorders should have the underlying disorder addressed.

If menorrhagia is the primary complaint, and no underlying pathology is suspected, OCPs, nonsteroidal antiinflammatory drugs (NSAIDs), levonorgestrel IUDs, luteal phase progesterone, and danazol are all medical therapies that have shown efficacy in reducing regular heavy menstrual bleeding. Clinicians must be aware of contraindications for these treatments and tailor therapy to the individual patient. NSAIDs, OCPs, progesterone IUDs, and luteal phase progesterone are equally effective at reducing heavy menstrual bleeding, although none is as effective as danazol. Use of danazol is limited by adverse androgenic side effects that include weight gain, acne, deepened voice, and hirsutism. NSAIDs have the added benefit of decreasing accompanying dysmenorrhea.

B. SURGICAL THERAPY

Surgical therapy should be limited to those patients in whom a structural cause for dysfunctional uterine bleeding exists such as fibroids, polyps, or neoplasm. Although endometrial ablation and hysterectomy are common surgical treatments for menorrhagia unresponsive to medical therapy, their use should be balanced against the associated morbidity and mortality, as well as the patient's wishes for fertility. Dilatation and curettage (D&C) is generally not therapeutic in cases of heavy menstrual bleeding.

Lethaby A, Augood C, Duckitt K: Nonsteroidal anti-inflammatory drugs for heavy menstrual bleeding. Cochrane Database Systemat Rev 2001(4):20.

Royal College of Obstetrics and Gynaecology Menorrhagia Guideline Development Group: *The Management of Menorrhagia in Secondary Care. Evidence-Based Clinical Guidelines.* RCOG Press, 1999.

Stabinsky SA, Einstein M, Breen JL: Modern treatments of menorrhagia attributable to dysfunctional uterine bleeding. Obstet Gynecol Surv 1999;54(11):251.

Stubblefield P: The role of hormonal contraceptives; menstrual impact of contraception. Am J Obstet Gynecol 1994;170(5S):1513.

Working Party for Guidelines for the Management of Heavy Menstrual Bleeding: Guideline for the management of heavy menstrual bleeding. NZ Med J 1999;112(1088):174.

DYSMENORRHEA

 ESSENTIALS OF DIAGNOSIS

- *Primary dysmenorrhea is the presence of painful menses in the absence of pelvic disease.*
- *Secondary dysmenorrhea is the occurrence of painful menses caused by pelvic disease.*

General Considerations

Dysmenorrhea, painful menstruation, is one of the most common gynecological problems seen by the family physician. It affects 50% of all adult and between 20% and 90% of all adolescent women. Approximately 1% of all adult and 15% of all adolescent women describe their dysmenorrhea as severe. It is a leading cause of morbidity in female high school students, resulting in absence from school and nonparticipation in sports. For diagnostic purposes, dysmenorrhea is classified as either primary or secondary, with primary dysmenorrhea being defined as the presence of painful menses in the absence of pelvic disease and secondary dysmenorrhea being the occurrence of painful menstruation caused by pelvic disease.

Pathogenesis

Primary dysmenorrhea is thought to be caused by the release of prostaglandin $F_{2\alpha}$ from the endometrium at the time of menstruation. The endometrium, stimulated by estrogen and progesterone released from the dominant follicle, releases large amounts of prostaglandins as the cells lyse with menstruation. This explains why younger adolescents who are often anovulatory, and do not develop a dominant follicle, experience less dysmenorrhea. Prostaglandins induce smooth muscle contraction in the uterus, as well as in the intestine, bronchi, and vasculature, which may account for the systemic symptoms of diarrhea, asthma exacerbation, hypertension, and headache experienced by women with primary dysmenorrhea. As contractions cause the pressure within the uterus to exceed that of the systemic circulation, ischemia ensues, causing an anginal equivalent in the uterus.

The cause of **secondary dysmenorrhea** varies with the underlying disease. Causes of secondary dysmenorrhea include adenomyosis, myomas, polyps, infection, endometriosis, tumors, adhesions, leiomyomas, intrauterine devices, blind uterine horn (rare), obstructed outflow of menstrual blood secondary to anatomic causes, bladder pathology, and gastrointestinal pathology.

Clinical Findings

A. SYMPTOMS AND SIGNS

Patients with a history of primary dysmenorrhea often report pain beginning with the onset of menstruation and lasting for 12–72 h. Their pain is characterized as crampy and intermittent in nature. Pain is often most intense in the lower abdomen, and may radiate to the low back or upper thighs. Headache, nausea, vomiting, diarrhea, and fatigue may accompany the pain. Symptoms are most often worst on the first day of menses and then gradually resolve. The patient may report that her dysmenorrhea began gradually, with the first year of menses, and then became worse as her periods became regular. Conversely, patients with secondary amenorrhea report symptoms beginning after age 20, lasting for 5–7 days, and progressive worsening of pain with time. These patients may also report pelvic pain that is not associated with menstruation.

B. PHYSICAL FINDINGS

A pelvic examination with cervical smear and cultures should be performed in all patients presenting with a chief complaint of dysmenorrhea. Findings of cul-de-sac induration and uterosacral ligament nodularity on pelvic examination are indicative of endometriosis. Adnexal masses could indicate endometriosis, neoplasm, hydrosalpinx, or scarring from chronic pelvic inflammatory disease (PID). Likewise uterine abnormalities or tenderness should raise the examinationiner's index of suspicion for underlying pathology as the cause for dysmenorrhea.

C. LABORATORY FINDINGS

Any woman with acute onset of pelvic pain should have a pregnancy test. Women with a history consistent with primary dysmenorrhea do not require initial laboratory work. In those who fail to respond to therapy for primary dysmenorrhea or in those in whom a diagnosis of secondary dysmenorrhea is suspected, a CBC and an erythrocyte sedimentation rate (ESR) may help to detect underlying infection or inflammation.

D. IMAGING STUDIES

Patients with abnormal findings on pelvic examination who do not respond to therapy for primary dysmenorrhea or who have a history suggestive of pelvic pathology should undergo pelvic ultrasound. In those in whom endometriosis is suggested, diagnostic laparoscopy may be indicated. Because of high rates of treatment and diagnostic failure with laparoscopy, empirically treating patients with a presumptive diagnosis of endometriosis with GnRH analogues for 3 months has been recommended. Proponents argue this provides both diagnostic and therapeutic functions, while forgoing surgical complications.

Treatment

A. MEDICAL THERAPY

Treatment for primary dysmenorrhea focuses on reducing endometrial prostaglandin production. This can be accomplished with medications that either inhibit prostaglandin synthesis (Table 14–3) or with oral contraceptives suppress ovulation.

Ibuprofen 400 mg orally four times a day is the first-line therapy based on its favorable risk–benefit ratio. In women who can predict the onset of their menses, treatment should begin the day before menstruation and be continued for 3–4 days. Patients who do not respond to this therapy can be tried on second-line agents (listed in Table 14–3). Patients are most satisfied with medications with rapid onset of action. Patients unable to tolerate the gastrointestinal side effects of traditional NSAIDs may alternatively try the cyclooxygenase-2 inhibitor rofecoxib.

For patients who do not desire fertility, combination oral contraceptives (those containing both estrogen and progesterone) are an effective treatment for primary dysmenorrhea, although most studies were done on

Table 14–3. Prostaglandin inhibitors for the treatment of primary dysmenorrhea.

Drug Class	Drug	Standard Dosage	Time to Peak Levels (h)	Half-life (h)
Fenamates	Mefenamic acid	500 mg loading; 250 mg orally four times a day	2–4	2–4
	Meclofenamate	100–200 mg orally three times a day	0.5–1	2
Phenylpropionic acid	Ibuprofen	400 mg orally four times a day	1–2	1.8–2.5
	Naproxen sodium	550 mg loading; 275 mg orally four times a day	1–2	12–13
	Ketoprofen	50 mg orally three times a day	0.5–2	2–4
Cyclooxygenase-2 inhibitor	Rofecoxib	50 mg initially, then 25 mg every 24 h	2–3	17

older formulations containing more than 35 μg of estrogen. They suppress ovulation, inhibiting endogenous progesterone production, and prevent normal endometrial growth, actions that dramatically reduce prostaglandin release. An adequate trial of OCPs for 3–6 months should be undertaken to evaluate their efficacy.

B. Behavioral Modification

Strenuous exercise and caffeine intake are both life-style factors that can modulate prostaglandin-induced uterine contractions. Strenuous exercise can increase uterine tone, resulting in increased periods of uterine "angina" with accompanying increases in prostaglandins. Decreasing strenuous exercise in the first few days of a woman's menses may reduce her dysmenorrhea. Conversely, caffeine decreases uterine tone by increasing uterine levels of cyclic adenosine monophosphate.

C. Surgical Therapy

If a patient continues to have significant dysmenorrhea with this treatment, further testing for causes of secondary dysmenorrhea should be considered. Women with chronic pelvic pain that does not respond to supportive therapy often have adhesions, endometriosis, or chronic PID discovered on diagnostic laparoscopy. Patients with secondary dysmenorrhea should undergo treatment for their underlying condition. This care often involves gynecological consultation.

Barbieri RL: Primary gonadotropin-releasing hormone agonist therapy for suspected endometriosis: a nonsurgical approach to the diagnosis and treatment of chronic pelvic pain. Am J Managed Care 1997;3(2):285.

Davis AR, Westhoff CL: Primary dysmenorrhea in adolescent girls and treatment with oral contraceptives. J Pediatr Adolesc Gynecol 2001;14(1):3.

Klein J, Litt I: Epidemiology of adolescent dysmenorrhea. Pediatrics 1981;68(5):661.

Kresch AJ et al: Laparoscopy in 100 women with chronic pelvic pain. Obstet Gynecol 1984;64(5):672.

Proctor ML et al: Combined oral contraceptive pill as treatment for primary dysmenorrhea. Cochrane Database Systemat Rev 2001(4).

Zhang WY, Po AL: Efficacy of minor analgesics in primary dysmenorrhea: a systematic review. Br J Obstet Gynaecol 1998; 105(7):780.

PREMENSTRUAL SYNDROME

ESSENTIALS OF DIAGNOSIS

- *Occurs during the luteal phase of the menstrual cycle.*
- *Symptoms include irritability, bloating, depression, food cravings, aggressiveness, and mood swings.*

General Considerations

Premenstrual syndrome (PMS) is a group of disorders and symptoms occurring during the luteal phase of the menstrual cycle that includes premenstrual dysphoric disorder (PMDD), affective disturbances, alterations in appetite, cognitive disturbances, fluid retention, and pain. Forty percent of women experience symptoms significant enough to interfere with daily life and relationships, whereas 5% of women experience severe impairment. Onset may occur at any time during the reproductive years, but once established, PMS tends to persist until menopause. Evaluation, diagnosis, and treatment of PMS should be undertaken prudently, as it is often mistaken for other disorders, and sometimes treated with counterproductive and even harmful approaches. The clinician must be sensitive in addressing issues of reduced self-worth, frustration, and depression that may be present in women suffering from this condition.

Clinical Findings

A. SYMPTOMS AND SIGNS

PMS is a cluster of affective, cognitive, and physical symptoms that occurs before the onset of menses, and not at other times during the month. Symptoms may include irritability, bloating, depression, food cravings, aggressiveness, and mood swings. Abraham's classification of PMS (Table 14–4) helps the clinician to organize history taking for affected patients.

Factors associated with an increased risk of PMS include stress, alcohol use, exercise, smoking, and the use of certain medications. It is not clear whether some of these factors are causative or are forms of self-medication used by sufferers. A prospective symptom diary kept for at least 2 months is helpful in assessing the relation of symptoms to the luteal phase of menses. The absence of a symptom-free week early in the follicular

Table 14–4. Abraham's classification of symptoms of premenstrual syndrome.

A: Anxiety
  Nervous tension
  Mood swings
  Irritability
  Anxiety

C: Cravings
  Headache
  Craving for sweets
  Increased appetite
  Heart pounding
  Fatigue
  Dizziness or faintness

D: Depression
  Depression
  Forgetfulness
  Crying
  Confusion
  Insomnia

H: Water-related symptoms
  Weight gain
  Swelling of extremities
  Breast tenderness
  Abnormal bloating

phase, the time period just after menses, suggests that a chronic psychiatric disorder may be present. Symptoms that are temporally clustered before menses and that decline or diminish 2–3 days after the start of menses are highly suggestive of PMS.

B. PHYSICAL FINDINGS

Patients with PMS experience fluid retention and fluctuating weight gain in relation to their menses. Mild edema may or may not be evident on physical examination.

C. LABORATORY FINDINGS

There are no laboratory tests that are useful in the diagnosis of PMS. Nutrient deficiency tests are not recommended, as they do not adequately assess the patients' physiological state.

D. IMAGING STUDIES

There are no radiological studies recommended in the assessment of PMS.

Treatment

The treatment goals for PMS are to minimize symptoms and functional impairment and to optimize the patient's overall health and sense of well-being. Therapy should take an integrative approach, including education, psychological support, exercise, diet, and pharmacological intervention, if necessary. The provider should begin by reassuring the patient and displaying genuine empathy. By providing education about the prevalence and treatability of PMS, the clinician can destigmatize the disease and encourage the patient to take responsibility for the treatment plan. Providers should be familiar with alternative therapies so they can adequately advise patients who are interested in pursuing these treatments.

Many first-line treatments for PMS, although not based on well-designed prospective trials, also have general health benefits, are inexpensive, and have few side effects. These include dietary modifications, similar to those recommended by the American Heart Association, and moderate exercise at least three times a week. Patients should begin to see the results of these life-style changes 2–3 months after initiation. Patients should be counseled to expect improvement in their symptoms, rather than cure. They should know that multiple approaches may be required before finding the optimal treatment.

For patients with continued symptoms, secondary treatment strategies may be employed. Dietary supplements, specifically vitamin B_6, calcium, and magnesium, may correct possible deficiencies. Current therapies are listed in Table 14–5, along with their levels of

Table 14–5. Selected pharmacological and supplemental therapies for PMS.

Medication	Mechanism of Action	Indication(s) for Use in PMS	Dosing	Primary Side Effects/Complications	Evidence Supporting Use
Mefenamic acid	Inhibits prostaglandin synthesis Competes for prostaglandin-binding sites	Pain relief	500 mg loading dose then 250 g orally four times a day for up to 7 days	Diarrhea, nausea, vomiting, drowsiness; with prolonged use decreased renal blood flow and renal papillary necrosis	RCCT[1]
GnRH agonists (nafrelin, leuprolide)	LH and FSH transient stimulation then prolonged suppression	Severe PMS; relief of all symptoms in 50% of patients	Nafrelin: 200 mg intra-nasal twice a day Leuprolide: 3.75 mg depot intramuscularly every 4 weeks or 0.5 mg sub-cutaneously every day	Vaginal dryness, accelerated bone loss, hot flashes	Controlled clinical trial[2]
Danazol	Supresses LH and FSH	Severe PMS	200 mg orally every day in the luteal phase	Acne, weight gain, hirsutism, virilization	RCCTs[3,4]
Alprazolam	Depressant effect on central nervous system	Anxiety caused by PMS	0.25 mg orally three times a day during the late luteal phase of the cycle	Drowsiness, increased appetite; discontinue if patient exhibits withdrawal symptoms	RCCT[5]
Fluoxetine	Serotonin reuptake inhibitor	Depression, anger, and anxiety caused by PMS	20 mg/day orally all month or just during the luteal phase	Nervousness, insomnia, drowsiness, nausea, anorexia	EBM review[6]
Diuretics (metolazone, spironolactone)	Reduction in retained fluid	Bloating, edema, breast tenderness (especially in women with >1.5 kg premenstrual weight gain)	Metolazone: 2.4 mg/day orally Spironolactone: 25 mg orally four times a day	Electrolyte imbalance	EBM review[7]

Bromocriptine	Dopamine agonist	Breast tenderness and fullness	2.5 mg orally twice a day or three times a day	Postural hypotension, nausea	Use not supported by RCCTs
Oral contraceptives	Suppression of estrogen and progesterone	General symptoms	Varies by formulation	Varies by formulation	Use not supported by RCCTs for treatment of PMS
Vitamin B_6	Precursor in coenzyme for the biosynthesis of dopamine and serotonin	Depression and general symptoms	50 mg orally every day or twice a day	Ataxia, sensory neuropathy	EBM review[8]
γ-Linoleic acid	Prostaglandin E_1 precursor that inhibits prostaglandin production and metabolism	Breast tenderness, bloating, weight gain, edema	3 g/day in the late luteal phase of menstrual cycle	Headache, nausea	Efficacy not supported[9]
Calcium	Restoration of calcium homeostatsis	Depression, anxiety and dysphoric states	800–1600 mg/day in divided doses	Bloating, nausea	RCCT[10]

[1]Gunston KD: Premenstrual syndrome in Cape Town. Part II. A double-blind placebo-controlled study of the efficacy of mefenamic acid. South African Med J 1986;70(3):159.

[2]Brown CS, et al: Efficacy of depot leuprolide in premenstrual syndrome: effect of symptom severity and type in a controlled trial. Obstet Gynecol 1994;84(5):779.

[3]Sarno AP Jr., Miller EJ Jr, Lundblad EG: Premenstrual syndrome: beneficial effects of periodic, low-dose danazol. Obstet Gynecol 1987;70(1):33.

[4]O'Brien PM, Abukhalil IE: Randomized controlled trial of the management of premenstrual syndrome and premenstrual mastalgia using luteal phase-only danazol. Am J Obstet Gynecol 1999;180(1, Pt. 1):18.

[5]Freeman EW et al: A double-blind trial of oral progesterone, alprazolam, and placebo in treatment of severe premenstrual syndrome. JAMA 1995;274(1):51.

[6]EBM Reviews—ACP Journal Club: Review: selective serotonin reuptake inhibitors reduce symptoms in the premenstrual syndrome. ACP J Club 2001;134(3):83.

[7]Vellacott ID, O'Brien PM: Effect of spironolactone on premenstrual syndrome symptoms. J Reprod Med 1987;32(6):429.

[8]EBM Reviews ACP Journal Club: Review: vitamin B6 is beneficial in the premenstrual syndrome. ACP J Club 1999;131(60].

[9]Budeiri D, Li Wan Po A, Dornan JC: Is evening primrose oil of value in the treatment of premenstrual syndrome? Control Clin Trials 1996;17(1):60.

[10]Thys-Jacobs S et al: Calcium carbonate and the premenstrual syndrome: effects on premenstrual and menstrual symptoms. Premenstrual Syndrome Study Group. Am J Obstet Gynecol 1998;179(2):444.

183

supporting evidence, primary benefits, and potential side effects. Pharmacological therapy, if utilized, should be tailored to the patient's symptom complex.

Numerous alternative therapies exist for premenstrual symptoms. These include herbal medicine, dietary supplements, relaxation, massage, reflexology, manipulative therapy, and biofeedback. Although some small trials have shown promising results, there is no compelling evidence from well-designed studies that supports the use of any of these therapies in the treatment of PMS.

Abraham GE: Nutritional factors in the etiology of the premenstrual tension syndromes. J Reprod Med 1983;28(7):446.

Barbieri R, Ryan K: The menstrual cycle. In: *Kistner's Gynecology & Women's Health.* Mosby, 1999: 23.

Deuster PA, Adera T, South-Paul J: Biological, social, and behavioral factors associated with premenstrual syndrome. Arch Fam Med 1999;8(2):122.

Stevinson CM, Ernst EF: Complementary/alternative therapies for premenstrual syndrome: a systematic review of randomized controlled trials. Am J Obstet Gynecol 2001;185(1):227.

Sexually Transmitted Diseases

Peter J. Katsufrakis, MD, MBA

15

General Considerations

Sexually transmitted diseases (STDs) include sexually transmitted infectious agents and the clinical syndromes they cause. Based on estimates there are up to 15 million new sexually transmitted infections in the United States annually, with rates in the United States being the highest in the developed world. In the United States the cost of treating STDs [excluding human immunodeficiency virus (HIV)] exceeds $10 billion.

Although all sexually active individuals are susceptible to infection, adolescents and young adults are most commonly affected. This is because of (1) their biological susceptibility to increased morbidity, eg, cervical cancer in adolescent girls exposed to human papillomavirus (HPV); (2) an attitude of invincibility; and (3) lack of knowledge about the risks and consequences of STDs. International travelers may be another population at increased risk for STDs and may benefit from pretravel counseling.

This chapter will emphasize the clinical presentation, diagnostic evaluation, and treatment of STDs commonly found in the United States. Readers of this chapter should be able to

- differentiate common STDs on the basis of clinical information and laboratory testing;
- treat STDs according to current guidelines; and
- intervene in patients' lives to reduce risk of future STD acquisition.

This chapter draws greatly from the most recent Centers for Disease Control and Prevention (CDC) Guidelines for Treatment of Sexually Transmitted Diseases and we are indebted to the individuals who worked to develop these.

Federal and state laws create disease-reporting requirements for many STDs. Gonorrhea, syphilis, and acquired immunodeficiency syndrome (AIDS) are reportable in every state. *Chlamydia* is reportable in most states, and HIV and other viral STDs are reportable in some but not all states. Because reporting requirements for other diseases vary by state, clinicians should contact their local health department for pertinent information.

Privacy and confidentiality concerns are different for STDs than for general medical information. Patients generally experience greater anxiety about information pertaining to a possible diagnosis of an STD, and this may limit their willingness to disclose clinically pertinent information. Conversely, legal requirements for disease reporting and health department programs of partner notification can inadvertently compromise patient confidentiality if not handled with the utmost professionalism. Furthermore, although minors generally require parental consent for nonemergent medical care, minors with STDs may be able to provide legal consent for diagnosis and treatment, subject to state laws. Finally, in some parts of the country recently enacted legislation permits physicians to prescribe treatment for partners of patients with *Chlamydia* without examining the partner. Thus, laws in different jurisdictions create additional options and complexity in treating STDs, and practitioners therefore need to be familiar with local requirements.

CDC: 1998 Guidelines for treatment of sexually transmitted diseases. MMWR 1998;47:1.

Vermillion ST, Holmes MM, Soper DE: Adolescents and sexually transmissible diseases. Obstet Gynecol Clin North Am 2000; 27:163.

Prevention

Intervening in patients' lives to reduce their risk of disease due to sexually transmitted infections is no less important than reducing disease due to smoking, inadequate exercise, poor nutrition, and other health maintenance issues. Risk assessment should prompt providers to undertake risk reduction, and thus disease prevention. Physicians' effectiveness depends on their ability to obtain an accurate sexual history employing effective counseling skills. Specific techniques include creating a trusting, confidential environment; obtaining permission to ask questions about STDs; demonstrating a nonjudgmental, optimistic attitude; and combining information collection with patient education, using clear mutually understandable language (see Chapter 18).

A. COUNSELING

Recommendations for changes in behavior should be tailored to the patient's specific risks and needs. Brief counseling using personalized risk reduction plans and culturally appropriate videos can significantly increase condom use and prevent new STDs, and can be conducted even in busy public clinics with minimal disruption to clinic operations. Effective interventions to reduce STDs in adolescents may need to extend beyond the examination room to include school-based and community-based education and programs for behavioral change. Although abstinence has been advocated by some, research suggests that this may not be the most effective intervention to prevent STD transmission.

B. CONDOMS

For sexually active patients, both male and female condoms are available and both appear effective in reducing transmission of many STDs. Effectiveness depends on correct, consistent use. Patients should be instructed to use only water-based lubricants, and providers should consider demonstrating how to place a condom on the penis via a suitable model, especially for adolescent patients or others who may be inexperienced with condom use. Condoms substantially reduce STD risk, but are not foolproof. In particular, condoms probably provide little protection against transmission of HPV.

Use of condoms with spermicide has not been shown to be more effective at reducing HIV transmission than use of condoms without spermicide. Without condoms, a vaginal spermicide alone will reduce the risk of gonorrhea and *Chlamydia,* but does not appear effective against HIV and should not be considered sufficient protection against STDs. Some patients confuse contraception with disease prevention. Nonbarrier methods of contraception such as hormonal contraceptives or surgical sterilization do not protect against STDs. Women employing these methods should be counseled about the role of condoms in prevention of STDs.

C. VACCINATION

Vaccination for hepatitis B virus (HBV) is indicated for all nonimmune patients undergoing evaluation for an STD, as well as for persons with multiple sex partners, sex partners of individuals with chronic HBV infection, and illegal drug users. Prevaccination testing of adolescents is not cost effective and may reduce compliance. The prevalence of past exposure to HBV in homosexual

men and injection drug users (IDU) may render prevaccination testing cost effective, although it may lower compliance. For this reason, if prevaccination testing is employed, patients should receive their first vaccination dose when tested. If employed, HBV core antibody testing is an effective screen for immunity

Vaccination for hepatitis A virus (HAV) is indicated for homosexual or bisexual men and persons who use illegal drugs. In cases of accidental sexual or household contact with someone with HAV, immune globulin given within 2 weeks of exposure is effective in preventing HAV infection in >85% of people.

Much attention is focused on developing vaccines to control or prevent HIV infection. Experimental vaccines are also being explored for other STDs, including *Chlamydia,* herpes, and HPV.

D. PARTNER TREATMENT

Following treatment of an individual patient, "epidemiological treatment" of asymptomatic partners of a diagnosed patient is commonly employed in STD treatment. For patients with multiple partners, it may be difficult to identify the source of infection. Partner treatment should be recommended for sexual contacts occurring prior to diagnosis within the time intervals indicated for each disease:

- Chancroid, 10 days
- Granuloma inguinale, 60 days
- Lymphogranuloma venereum, 30 days
- Syphilis, up to 90 days, even if the partner is seronegative
- *Chlamydia,* 60 days
- Gonorrhea, 60 days
- Epididymitis, 60 days
- Pelvic inflammatory disease, 60 days
- Pediculosis pubis, 30 days
- *Sarcoptes scabiei,* 30 days

These are generally "best guess" estimates, and for at least some organisms evidence suggests that infection may persist for even longer periods.

Although in general physicians must examine a patient directly before prescribing treatment, patient-delivered partner treatment has been implemented in at least one state. This permits physicians to prescribe for the partners of a woman diagnosed with *Chlamydia trachomatis* without examining the partner. Repeat diagnostic testing as a "test of cure" (TOC) following treatment is generally not indicated. TOC may be indicated if spectinomycin, due to its high failure rate, is used to treat gonorrhea. If TOC is employed using nucleic acid-based tests, up to 1 month may need to elapse to eliminate false positives due to the presence of dead organisms.

Patients should also be instructed to avoid sexual contact for the duration of therapy to ensure no further transmission occurs. Patients taking single-dose azithromycin should be instructed to avoid sexual contact for 7 days, as the medication's long half-life makes actual duration of effect much longer than the duration of medication ingestion. Patients must also be instructed to avoid contact with their previous partner(s) until they are treated.

E. Screening

Some form of screening such as questions asked during the history interview or included in routine history forms should be a universal practice for *all* patients, with periodic and regular updating. Content, frequency, and additional screening should be determined by individual patient circumstances, local disease prevalence, and research documenting effectiveness and cost–benefit. Barriers exist to talking about sexuality and STDs with most patients, especially adolescents. Effective counseling skills and techniques are needed to help adolescents manage the health consequences of their sexual behavior.

1. *Chlamydia*—Annual laboratory screening for *Chlamydia* may be indicated for all sexually active adolescents, and has been recommended in areas in which the prevalence of infection is 2% or higher. Both the CDC and the United States Preventive Services Task Force (USPSTF) recommend screening all sexually active women ages 25 years and younger and other asymptomatic women at increased risk for infection (defined as women with more than one sexual partner who have had a sexually transmitted disease in the past or who do not use condoms consistently and correctly). The argument and data supporting screening in girls and young women are convincing. Screening women has been shown to reduce pelvic inflammatory disease, and screening sexually active women up to age 25 has been shown to be cost effective. To date there is less compelling cost–benefit data supporting screening in boys and young men, although clearly men infect most women with *Chlamydia*. The CDC supports screening asymptomatic sexually active men ages 25 years and younger, but the USPSTF believes there is insufficient evidence to make such a recommendation.

2. Pregnancy—Recommendations for screening pregnant women vary somewhat depending on the source. According to the CDC, pregnant women should receive a rapid plasma reagin (RPR) test at the onset of prenatal care, again at the third trimester, and at delivery for high-risk women. Hepatitis B surface antigen (HBsAg) should be performed at the onset of prenatal care and repeated late in pregnancy for women at high risk. Providers of obstetric care should test for *Neisseria gonorrhoeae* at the onset of care if local prevalence of gonorrhea is high or if the woman is at increased risk, and testing should be repeated in the third trimester if the woman is at continued risk. Providers should test for *Chlamydia* in the third trimester for patients 25 years of age or younger who have multiple partners or who have a partner with multiple partners. Women with a past history of preterm delivery should also be tested for bacterial vaginosis.

3. HIV—Testing for HIV is indicated for any patient with a diagnosed STD, with a history of behaviors that could expose her or him to HIV, or who presents with a history and findings consistent with the acute retroviral syndrome (ARS). Appropriate testing regimens include an HIV-1 screening antibody test such as enzyme immunoassay, with a confirmatory test such as the Western blot. HIV-2 prevalence in the United States is very low, so routine testing is not indicated; it should be considered for persons coming from areas of high HIV-2 prevalence (eg, parts of West Africa, Angola, Mozambique, France, and Portugal).

Early diagnosis of ARS may present a very narrow window of opportunity to dramatically and enduringly alter the course of HIV infection in the recently infected patient. Symptoms are common and nonspecific, making diagnosis difficult without a high index of suspicion; they include fever, malaise, lymphadenopathy, pharyngitis, and skin rash. Appropriate testing should include a nucleic acid test for HIV such as HIV-RNA polymerase chain reaction (PCR) or b-DNA; routine HIV antibody tests are not sufficient, because they generally will not have become positive during ARS. Individuals with positive HIV tests should be referred immediately to an expert in HIV care.

HIV-positive individuals pose particular challenges for STD risk reduction. Reducing high-risk behaviors of known HIV-infected patients is a top priority, both to decrease the further spread of HIV and to limit the exposure of HIV patients to additional STDs. Persons with HIV also have substantial medical, psychological, and legal needs that are beyond the scope of this text.

4. Other STDs—Accepted national guidelines directing screening for gonorrhea, syphilis, and other STDs do not exist. If undertaken, additional screening should be guided by local disease prevalence and an individual patient's risk behaviors.

CDC: HIV prevention through early detection and treatment of other sexually transmitted diseases—United States recommendations of the Advisory Committee for HIV and STD Prevention. MMWR 1997;47:1.

CDC: *Epidemiology and Prevention of Vaccine-Preventable Diseases,* 2000.

Kamb ML et al: Efficacy of risk-reduction counseling to prevent human immunodeficiency virus and sexually transmitted diseases: a randomized controlled trial. Project RESPECT Study Group. JAMA 1998;280:1161.

Leung DT, Sacks SL: Current recommendations for the treatment of genital herpes. Drugs 2000;60:1329.

Maurice WL: *Sexual Medicine in Primary Care.* Mosby, 1999.

Stanberry LR: Control of STDs—the role of prophylactic vaccines against herpes simplex virus. Sexually Transmit Infect 1998;74:391.

WEB SITES

HIV InSite Knowledge Base

http://hivinsite.ucsf.edu/InSite.jsp? page=KB

U.S. Public Health Service: Guidelines for the Use of Antiretroviral Agents in HIV-Infected Adults and Adolescents.

http://www. hivatis.org/trtgdlns.html

■ SEXUALLY TRANSMITTED INFECTIONS & SYNDROMES

STD patients rarely present with accurate knowledge of their microbiological diagnosis. More commonly, patients present with clinical syndromes consistent with one or more diagnoses, so that providers frequently employ syndromic evaluation and treatment. This approach, useful for several reasons, including the fact that more than one disease may be present, has been employed most commonly in resource-poor settings with limited access to advanced diagnostic technology.

The following recommendations for testing strategies and use of empiric treatment pending laboratory results should be adapted to take into consideration local availability of specific tests, the probability of the diagnosis based upon the history and examination, and the likelihood that an untreated patient will return for laboratory test results and treatment. Treatment information is summarized in Table 15–1 and additional treatment information appears within the text description of specific diseases where applicable.

GENITAL ULCER DISEASES

In the United States, herpes simplex is the most common cause of genital ulcer diseases (GUD). Other causes such as syphilis, chancroid, lymphogranuloma venereum, and granuloma inguinale are much less common. Because this is not true throughout the world, physicians treating international travelers or recent arrivals to the United States may need to consider a broad spectrum of potential etiologies. The approach to diagnosis needs to include consideration of the likelihood of the different etiologies based on the patient's history, physical examination, and local epidemiology. Furthermore, all types of GUD are associated with increased risk of HIV transmission, making HIV testing a necessary part of GUD evaluation.

1. Herpes Simplex

Serological studies suggest that 45 million people in the United States are infected with herpes simplex virus type 2 (HSV-2). Data on genital HSV-2 seroprevalence from the National Health and Nutrition Examination Survey (NHANES) III survey conducted in 1988–1994 reveal HSV-2 seroprevalence among persons at least 12 years of age was 21.9%, 30% higher than the age-adjusted HSV-2 seroprevalence from NHANES II conducted a decade earlier. Increases in seroprevalence occurred primarily in persons aged 12–39 years.

Clinical Findings

A. SYMPTOMS AND SIGNS

A first episode of genital herpes classically presents with blisters and sores, with local tingling and discomfort. Visible lesions may be preceded by a prodrome of tingling or burning. Some patients also report dysesthesia or neuralgic-type pain in the buttocks or legs and malaise with fever. The clinical spectrum of disease can include atypical rashes, fissuring, excoriation and discomfort of the anogenital area, cervical lesions, urinary symptoms, and extragenital lesions. Recent data, however, suggest that only 37% of patients who acquire HSV-2 have symptoms, although overt disease may follow. Atypical genital herpes can present as large, chronic, hyperkeratotic ulcers. It is seen in immunocompromised patients and is sometimes due to Acyclovir-resistant HSV.

Both HSV-1 and HSV-2 cause genital disease, although HSV-1 produces fewer clinical recurrences. Previous HSV-1 infection is partially protective against subsequent HSV-2 infection. Symptoms during recurrences are generally less intense and shorter in duration. Infectious virus is shed intermittently and unpredictably in some asymptomatic patients. Patients with HSV should be counseled to use condoms during all sexual contact with new or uninfected individuals.

B. LABORATORY FINDINGS

Diagnosis of HSV is based on either Tzank smear of vesicle base or ulcer, culture of the vesicle base or ulcer, or type-specific serological testing that reveals past history of infection. Serological testing alone generally cannot conclusively confirm HSV as the etiology of a specific illness episode. The role of HSV serological testing as a screening tool remains to be determined.

Table 15–1. STD treatment guidelines for adults and adolescents.

Disease	Recommended Regimens	Dose /Route	Alternative Regimens
Chlamydia			
Uncomplicated infections in adults/adolescents[1]	Azithromycin **or** Doxycycline[2]	1 g po 100 mg po bid × 7 d	Erythromycin base 500 mg po qid × 7 d **or** Erythromycin ethylsuccinate 800 mg po qid × 7 d **or** Ofloxacin[3] 300 mg po bid × 7 d
Pregnant women[4]	Amoxicillin **or** Azithromycin **or** Erythromycin base	500 mg po tid × 7 d 1 g po 500 mg po qid × 7 d	Erythromycin base 250 mg po qid × 14 d **or** Erythromycin ethylsuccinate 800 mg p qid × 7 d **or** Erythromycin ethylsuccinate 400 mg po qid × 14 d
Gonorrhea[5]			
Uncomplicated infections in adults/adolescents	Cefixime[6] **or** Ceftriaxone **or** Levofloxacin[3] **or** Ciprofloxacin[3] **or** Ofloxacin[3] **plus** a *Chlamydia* recommended regimen listed above	400 mg po 125 mg IM 250 mg po 500 mg po 400 mg po	Spectinomycin[7] 2 g IM plus[5] a *Chlamydia* recommended regimen
Pregnant women	Ceftriaxone **or** Cefixime[6] plus[5] a *Chlamydia* recommended regimen listed above	125 mg IM 400 mg po	Spectinomycin[7] 2 g IM **plus**[5] a *Chlamydia* recommended regimen

Pelvic inflammatory disease	**Parenteral**[8]
	  Cefotetan **or**
	  Cefoxitin **plus**
	    Doxycycline[2] **or**
	  Clindamycin **plus**
	    Gentamicin
	
	Oral treatment
	  Ofloxacin[3] **plus**
	    Metronidazole **or**
	  Ceftriaxone **plus**
	    Doxycycline **or**
	  Cefoxitin and
	    Probenecid **plus**
	    Doxycycline[2]
		2 g IV q 12 h
		2 g IV q 6 h
		100 mg po or IM q 12 h
		900 mg IV q 8 h
		2 mg/kg IV or IM followed by
		1.5 mg/kg IV or IM q 8 h
		
		400 mg po bid × 14 d
		500 mg po bid × 14 d
		250 mg IM
		100 mg po bid × 14 d
		2 g IM
		1 g po
		100 mg po bid × 14 d
			Parental ofloxacin[3] 400 mg IV q 12 h **plus**
			  Metronidazole 500 mg IV q 8 h **or**
			  Ampicillin/sulbactam 3 g IV q 6 h **plus**
			    Doxycycline[2] 100 mg po or IV q 12 h **or**
			  Ciprofloxacin[3] 200 mg IV q 12 h **plus**
			    Doxycycline[2] 100 mg po or IV q 12 h **plus**
			    Metronidazole 500 mg IV q 8 h

Mucopurulent cervicitis[9]	Azithromycin **or** Doxycycline[2]	1 g po 100 mg po bid × 7 d	Erythromycin base 500 mg po qid × 7 d **or** Erythromycin ethylsuccinate 800 mg po qid × 7 d **or** Ofloxacin[3] 300 mg po bid × 7 d

(continued)

Table 15–1. STD treatment guidelines for adults and adolescents. (*Continued*)

Disease	Recommended Regimens	Dose / Route	Alternative Regimens
Nongonococcal urethritis[9]	Azithromycin **or**	1 g po	Erythromycin base 500 mg po qid × 7 d **or**
	Doxycycline[2] **or**	100 mg po bid × 7 d	Erythromycin ethylsuccinate 800 mg po qid × 7 d **or**
	Levofloxacin[3]	250 mg po	Ofloxacin[3] 300 mg po bid × 7 d
Epididymitis	Likely due to gonorrhea or *Chlamydia*		
	Ceftriaxone **plus**	250 mg IM	
	Doxycycline	100 mg po bid × 10 d	
	Likely due to enteric organisms		
	Ofloxacin[3]	300 mg po bid × 10 d	
Trichomoniasis	Metronidazole	2 g po	Metronidazole 500 mg po bid × 7 d
			If low-level resistance, 2 g daily × 5–14 d
			If high-level resistance, 3 g po daily × 10–14 d **plus** intravaginal metronidazole therapy
Vulvovaginal candidiasis	Butoconazole cream[10]	2%, 5 g intravaginally × 3 d	Fluconazole 150 po once
	Clotrimazole cream[10]	1% 5 g intravaginally × 7 d	
	Clotrimazole vaginal tablet[10]	100 mg intravaginally × 7 d	
		200 mg intravaginally × 3 d	
		500 mg intravaginally once	
	Miconazole cream[10]	2% 5 g intravaginally × 7 d	
	Miconazole vaginal suppository[10]	100 mg intravaginally × 7 d	
		200 mg intravaginally × 3 d	
	Tioconazole ointment[10]	6.5% 5 g intravaginally once	
	Terconazole cream[10]	0.4% 5 g intravaginally × 7 d	
		0.8% 5 g intravaginally × 3 d	
	Terconazole vaginal suppository[10]	80 mg intravaginally × 3 d	
Bacterial vaginosis			
Adults/adolescents	Metronidazole **or**	500 mg po bid × 7 d	Metronidazole 2 g po **or**
	Clindamycin cream[10] **or**	2%, one full applicator (5 g) intravaginally at bedtime × 7 d	Clindamycin 300 mg po bid × 7 d
	Metronidazole gel	0.75%, one full applicator (5 g) intravaginally, bid × 5 d	
Pregnant women	Metronidazole	250 mg po tid × 7 d	Metronidazole 2 g po **or**
			Clindamycin 300 mg po bid × 7 d

Chancroid	Azithromycin **or**	1 g po
	Ceftriaxone **or**	250 mg IM
	Ciprofloxacin[3] **or**	500 mg po bid × 3 d
	Erythromycin base	500 mg po qid × 7 d
Lymphogranuloma venereum	Doxycycline[2]	100 mg po bid × 21 d	Erythromycin base 500 mg po qid × 21 d
Human papillomavirus External genital/perianal warts	**Patient applied** Podofilox[11] 0.5% solution or gel **or** Imiquimod[12] 5% cream **Provider administered** Cryotherapy **or** Podophyllin[11] resin 10–25% in tincture of benzoin **or** Trichloroacetic acid (TCA) **or** Bichloroacetic acid (BCA) 80–90% **or** Surgical removal		Intralesional interferon or laser surgery
Vaginal warts	Cryotherapy **or** TCA or BCA 80–90% **or** Podophyllin[11] 10–25% in tincture of benzoin		
Urethral meatus warts	Cryotherapy **or** Podophyllin[11] 10–25% in tincture of benzoin		
Anal warts	Cryotherapy **or** TCA or BCA 80–90% **or** Surgical removal		
Herpes simplex virus[12] First clinical episode of herpes	Acyclovir[13] **or** Acyclovir[12] **or** Famciclovir[13] **or** Valacyclovir[13]	400 mg po tid × 7–10 d 200 mg po 5 × q d × 7–10 d 250 mg po tid × 7–10 d 1 g po bid × 7–10 d	

(continued)

Table 15–1. STD treatment guidelines for adults and adolescents. (*Continued*)

Disease	Recommended Regimens	Dose /Route	Alternative Regimens
Herpes simplex virus[12] Episodic therapy for recurrent episodes	Acyclovir[12] **or** Acyclovir[13] **or** Acyclovir[12] **or** Famciclovir[13] **or** Valacyclovir[12]	400 mg po tid × 5 d 200 mg po 5 × qd × 5 d 800 mg po bid × 5 d 125 mg bid × 5 d 500 mg po bid × 5 d	
Supressive therapy	Acyclovir[12] **or** Famciclovir[12] **or** Valacyclovir[12] **or** Valacyclovir[13]	400 mg po bid 250 mg po bid 500 mg po qd 1 g po qd	
Syphilis Primary, secondary, and early latent	Benzathine penicillin G	2.4 million units IM	Doxycycline[2] 100 mg po bid × 2 weeks **or** Tetracycline[2] 500 mg po qid × 2 weeks
Late latent and unknown duration	Benzathine penicillin G	7.2 million units, administered as 3 doses of 2.4 million units IM, at 1 week intervals	Doxycycline[2] 100 mg po bid × 4 weeks **or** Tetracycline[2] 500 mg po qid × 4 weeks
Neurosyphilis[14]	Aqueous crystalline penicillin G	18–24 million units daily, administered as 3–4 million units IV q 4 h × 10–14 d	Procaine penicillin G, 2.4 million units IM qd × 10–14 d **plus** Probenecid 500 mg po qid × 10–14 d
Pregnant women[14] Primary, secondary, and early latent[15]	Benzathine penicillin G	2.4 million units IM	None
Late latent and unknown duration	Benzathine penicillin G	7.2 million units, administered as 3 doses of 2.4 million units IM, at 1 week intervals	None
Neurosyphilis[14]	Aqueous crystalline penicillin G	18–24 million units daily, administered as 3–4 million units IV q 4 h × 10–14 d	Procaine penicillin G, 2.4 million units IM qd × 10–14 d **plus** Probenecid 500 mg po qid × 10–14 d

Congenital syphilis	Procaine penicillin G	50,000 U/kg IM daily for 10–14 d	Aqueous crystalline penicillin G 100,000–150,000 U/kg/day in doses of 50,000 U/kg IV q 12 h for 7 days then q 8 h for 3–7 days
Children: early (primary)	Benzathine penicillin G	50,000 U/kg IM once (max. 2.4 million units)	
Children: latent >1 year late	Benzathine penicillin G	50,000 U/kg IM for 3 doses at 1 week intervals, to max. total dose of 7.2 million units	
HIV infection			
Primary, secondary, and early latent	Benzathine penicillin G	2.4 million units IM	Doxycycline[2] 100 mg po bid × 2 weeks **or** Tetracycline[2] 500 mg po qid × 2 weeks
Late latent and unknown duration[14] with normal CSF examination	Benzathine penicillin G	7.2 million units, administered as 3 doses of 2.4 million units IM, at 1 week intervals	None
Neurosyphilis[14]	Aqueous crystalline penicillin G	18–24 million units daily, administered as 3–4 million units IV q 4 h × 10–14 d	Procaine penicillin G, 2.4 million units IM qd × 10–14 d **plus** Probenecid 500 mg po qid × 10–14 d
Pediculosis pubis[16] "crab lice"	Permethrin creme rinse	1% applied to affected areas, rinsed after 10 min	
	Pyrethrins with piperonyl butoxide	Apply to affected area, wash after 10 min	
	Lindane shampoo	1% applied to affected areas, wash after 4 min[2,17]	

(continued)

Table 15–1. STD treatment guidelines for adults and adolescents. (*Continued*)

Disease	Recommended Regimens	Dose /Route	Alternative Regimens
Scabies[16]	Permethrin cream	5% applied to entire body below neck, washed off after 8–14 h	Lindane 1% 1 oz lotion or 30 g cream applied thinly to entire body below neck, washed off after 8 h[2,17] Sulfur 6% precipitated in ointment applied thinly to entire body below neck for 3 nights, washed off before each new application and 24 h after last treatment

Adapted from the 1998 CDC STD Treatment Guidelines, the Region IX Infertility Clinical Guidelines, and the Los Angeles County Department of Health Services Sexually Transmitted Disease Program.

Abbreviations: po, orally; bid, twice a day; tid, three times a day; qid, four times a day; IM, intramuscularly; IV, intravenously; q, every; qd, every day; d, day; h, hours.

[1]Screen adolescents annually and women 20–24 years, especially if new or multiple partners.
[2]Contraindicated for pregnant and nursing women.
[3]Contraindicated for pregnant and nursing women and children < 18 years of age.
[4]Test-of-cure follow-up recommended because the regimens are not highly efficacious (amoxicillin and erythromycin) or the data on safety and efficacy are limited (azithromycin).
[5]Cotreatment for *Chlamydia* infection is indicated if coinfection rates are high (>20%), less sensitive or no *Chlamydia* test is done, or follow-up is uncertain.
[6]Not recommended for pharyngeal gonococcal infection.
[7]For patients who cannot tolerate cephalosporins or quinolones; not recommended for pharyngeal gonococcal infection.
[8]Discontinue 24 h after patient improves clinically and continue with oral therapy for a total course of 14 days.
[9]Testing for gonorrhea and *Chlamydia* is recommended because a specific diagnosis may improve compliance and partner management and these infections are reportable by CA State Law.
[10]Might weaken latex condoms and diaphragms because oil based.
[11]Contraindicated during pregnancy.
[12]Counseling especially about natural history, asymptomatic shedding, and sexual transmission is an essential component of herpes management.
[13]Safety in pregnancy has not been established.
[14]Patients allergic to penicillin should be treated with penicillin after desensitization.
[15]Some experts recommend a second dose of 2.4 million units of benzathine penicillin G administered 1 week after the initial dose.
[16]Bedding and clothing should be decontaminated (machine washed, machine dried, or dry cleaned) or removed from body contact for >72 h.
[17]Contraindicated for children <2 years of age.

Treatment

Treatment of HSV is either episodic, ie, in response to an episode of disease, or suppressive, with daily medication continuing for months or years. Treatment for an initial outbreak consists of 7–10 days of oral medication (see Table 15–1). Episodic treatment is effective when medication is started during the prodrome or on the first symptomatic day. No benefit will be seen if treatment of recurrences is delayed until lesions are vesicular. Patients should be given a prescription to have available for use when needed.

Suppressive therapy is traditionally indicated for patients with six or more recurrences in 12 months, although this may be adjusted based on the stress and disability caused by recurrences. Available experience suggests that long-term suppression is safe and is not associated with development of antiviral resistance. Suppressive therapy seems to reduce but not eliminate asymptomatic shedding. Whether this results in reduced transmission among discordant couples remains to be determined. Suppression does not change the natural history of a patient's infection, although, because the frequency of recurrences diminishes with time, suppression may be particularly useful during the time period immediately following initial infection. Available therapies appear to be safe in pregnant women.

2. Syphilis

General Considerations

Syphilis cases reported to the CDC declined in number since the early 1950s until a peak in 1990 at 135,043. The CDC then launched "The National Plan to Eliminate Syphilis from the United States." In 2000, 31,575 total cases and 5979 cases of primary and secondary syphilis were reported. Although national numbers continue to decline, recent resurgences of syphilis in some populations and geographic areas indicate the need for continued vigilance.

Clinical Findings

SYMPTOMS AND SIGNS

Syphilis infection is characterized by stages, and accurate staging of syphilis infection is vital to determine appropriate therapy. Primary syphilis is characterized by the appearance of a painless, indurated ulcer—the chancre—occurring 10 days to 3 months after infection with *Treponema pallidum.* The chancre usually heals in 4–6 weeks, although associated painless bilateral lymphadenopathy may persist for months.

Secondary syphilis has variable manifestations, but usually includes symmetrical mucocutaneous macular, papular, papulosquamous, or pustular lesions with generalized nontender lymphadenopathy. In moist skin areas such as the perianal or vulvar regions, papules may become superficially eroded to form pink or whitish condyloma lata. Constitutional symptoms such as fever, malaise, and weight loss occur commonly. Less common complications include meningitis, hepatitis, arthritis, nephropathy, and iridocyclitis.

Latent syphilis occurs in patients with serological evidence of syphilis infection *without* other current evidence of disease. "Early" latent syphilis is alternately defined as less than 1 year or less than 2 years duration, depending on the source. Because current Public Health Service (PHS) treatment guidelines use the 1-year definition, it will be employed in this text. A diagnosis of early latent syphilis is demonstrated by either seroconversion or a definitive history of primary or secondary syphilis findings within the past year. Asymptomatic patients with known infection of more than 1 year or in whom infection of less than 1 year cannot be conclusively demonstrated are classified as having late latent syphilis or latent syphilis of unknown duration, respectively. These two categories of syphilis are treated equivalently. The magnitude of serological test titers cannot reliably differentiate early from late latent syphilis.

Neurosyphilis is diagnosed by positive cerebrospinal fluid (CSF) Veneral Disease Research Laboratories (VDRL) test. It is suggested by positive CSF fluorescent treponemal antibody absorption (FTA-ABS), although false positives occur in the absence of neurosyphilis, and is suggested by CSF pleocytosis [>5 white blood cells (WBCs)/mm^3], although HIV infection and other conditions may also cause increased WBCs in the CSF.

Tertiary syphilis is diagnosed in patients with syphilitic aortitis, and in patients with one or more gummas, a syphilitic granuloma. Patients are infectious during primary, secondary, and early latent stages of syphilis.

B. LABORATORY FINDINGS AND TESTS

Positive darkfield examination or direct fluorescent antibody tests of lesion exudates definitively substantiate a diagnosis of primary syphilis. More typically, syphilis is diagnosed by positive results of both a nontreponemal test (VDRL or RPR) and a treponemal test [microhemagglutination assay—*T pallidum* (MHA-TP) or FTA-ABS].

Nontreponemal tests are sometimes falsely positive due to other medical conditions, eg, some collagen vascular diseases. When positive due to syphilis, their titers generally rise and fall in response to *T pallidum* infection and treatment, respectively, and usually return to normal (negative) following treatment, although some individuals remain "serofast" and have a low positive titer for the remainder of their lives. Treponemal tests usually yield persistent positive results throughout the patient's life following infection with *T pallidum.* Treponemal test titers do not correlate with disease activity.

Lumbar puncture is indicated for (1) any patients with signs or symptoms suggestive of neurosyphilis, ie, neurological or ophthalmological signs or symptoms, (2) other tertiary syphilis, (3) treatment failure (a four-fold increase in titer or a failure to decline four-fold or more within 12–24 months), or (4) patients with late or unknown duration latent syphilis and coexisting HIV infection.

Treatment

Treatment for syphilis as described in Table 15–1 is based on current USPHS guidelines, derived from available research and expert opinion. Follow-up testing of patients diagnosed with syphilis is a vital part of care, as it determines the effectiveness of therapy and provides useful information to differentiate potential future treated versus recurrent infection.

The 6-month posttreatment, nontreponemal test titer should have fallen four-fold or more, eg, from 1:32 to 1:8 or less. If it does not, consider this a treatment failure or an indication of reinfection. In evaluating such a potential treatment failure, the patient should, at minimum, receive continued serological follow-up, and repeat HIV serology if previously negative. Lumbar puncture should also be considered, and if the results are normal, try 2.4 million units benzathine penicillin weekly for 3 weeks.

3. Chancroid

Although very common in other parts of the world, in 2000 a total of 78 cases of chancroid were reported in the United States. These data should be interpreted with caution, however, in view of the fact that *Haemophilus ducreyi* is difficult to culture, and thus this condition may be substantially underdiagnosed.

Definitive diagnosis is difficult. It requires identification of *H ducreyi* on special culture medium that is generally not easily available. Presumptive diagnosis rests on the presence of painful genital ulcer(s) with a negative HSV test and negative syphilis serology, with or without regional lymphadenopathy.

Treatment consists of oral antibiotics as listed in Table 15–1. Healing of large ulcers may require more than 2 weeks. However, if patients do not show clinical improvement after 7 days consider the accuracy of the diagnosis, medication nonadherence, and/or antibacterial resistance. Fluctuant lymphadenopathy may require drainage via aspiration or incision.

Although definitive diagnosis generally rests on laboratory testing, history and examination often lead to a presumptive diagnosis. Table 15–2 summarizes findings for herpes simplex, syphilis, and chancroid.

4. Other Causes of GUD

Granuloma inguinale or Donovanosis is caused by *Calymmatobacterium granulomatis,* endemic in some tropical nonindustrialized parts of the world. Only four cases were reported in the United States in 2000. The bacterium does not grow on standard culture media; diagnosis rests on demonstration of "Donovan bodies" in a tissue specimen. Infection causes painless, progressive beefy red, highly vascular lesions without lymphadenopathy. Treatment is often prolonged, and relapse can occur months after initial treatment and apparent cure.

Lymphogranuloma venerum is caused by serovars L1, L2, and L3 of *C trachomatis.* Forty-two cases were reported in the United States in 2000, although this remains a more significant problem in other parts of the world. The small ulcer arising at the site of infection is often unnoticed or unreported. Patients typically present with painful unilateral lymphadenopathy. Diagnosis rests on finding positive serology. In addition to antibiotics, treatment may require aspiration or incision and drainage of buboes, and despite this patients may still experience scarring.

Drake S et al: Improving the care of patients with genital herpes. Br Med J 2000;321:619.

Rosen T, Brown TJ: Genital ulcers. Evaluation and treatment. Dermatol Clin 1998;16:673.

Table 15–2. Differentiation of common causes of genital ulcers.

	Herpes	Syphilis	Chancroid
Ulcer(s) Appearance	Often purulent	"Clean"	Purulent
Number	Usually multiple	Single[1]	Often multiple
Pain	Yes	No	Yes
Preceded by	Papule, then vesicle	Papule	Papule
Adenopathy	Painful with primary outbreak	Painless	Painful; may suppurate
Systemic symptoms	Often with primary outbreak	Usually not	Occasionally

[1]Up to 40% of patients with primary syphilis have more than one chancre.

Singh AE, Romanowski B: Syphilis: review with emphasis on clinical, epidemiologic, and some biologic features. Clin Microbiol Rev 1999;12:187.

Stanberry L et al: New developments in the epidemiology, natural history and management of genital herpes. Antivir Res 1999; 42:1.

URETHRITIS

Sexually transmitted infections causing urethritis are typically diagnosed in men, although women may also experience urethritis as a consequence of STD. For clinical management, urethritis can be divided into "nongonococcal urethritis" (NGU) and urethritis due to *N gonorrhoeae* infection.

1. Nongonococcal Urethritis

Although not all states track cases of NGU, one frequent cause is *C trachomatis* (CT), and 137,049 *Chlamydia* cases were reported in males in 2000. Female cases were more than four-fold greater at 563,206, and, although significant, these numbers likely dramatically underestimate actual cases of CT. The spectrum of CT-caused disease includes extragenital manifestations, including ophthalmic infection and a reactive arthritis.

The majority of NGU cases are due to causes other than CT and include *Mycoplasma genitalium, Ureaplasma urealyticum, Trichomonas vaginalis,* herpes simplex, and enteric bacteria. Diagnosis of NGU can be based on (1) mucopurulent or purulent urethral discharge, (2) urethral secretions with >5 WBCs/HPF and no Gram-negative intracellular diplococci (which if present would indicate gonorrhea), (3) first-void urine with positive leukocyte esterase or >10 WBCs/HPF, or (4) a positive DNA amplification-based test performed on a urine specimen. DNA-based tests offer greater convenience and better sensitivity than culture and represent the best tests currently available to diagnose CT or gonorrhea.

2. Gonorrhea

General Considerations

In 2000, reports of 358,995 cases of gonorrhea were evenly divided among males and females.

Clinical Findings

SYMPTOMS AND SIGNS

If symptomatic, gonorrhea typically causes dysuria and a purulent urethral discharge, however, it may cause disseminated systemic disease, including skin lesions, septic arthritis, tenosynovitis, arthralgias, perihepatitis, endocarditis, and meningitis. In these cases, there is usually minimal genital inflammation.

Clinical differentiation between CT and gonorrhea (GC) may be difficult. Characteristically, urethral exudate in gonorrhea is thicker and more purulent in appearance than the exudate caused by CT, which is often watery with mucus strands. However, differentiation of etiology based on clinical appearance is notoriously unreliable.

B. LABORATORY FINDINGS

DNA amplification technology has largely supplanted urethral swab for culture due to enhanced sensitivity, excellent specificity, and greater patient acceptance. Tests can be performed on a urine specimen, eliminating more invasive specimen collection.

Diagnostic evaluation identifies disease etiology and may facilitate the public health missions of contact tracing and disease eradication. For an individual patient, however, the physician might ignore testing for *Chlamydia* and gonorrhea and treat for both empirically. Decisions about diagnostic testing should consider both public health goals and how information obtained will influence patient (and partner) treatment.

In patients presenting with recurrent urethritis, diagnostic evaluation may be necessary to identify the etiology. In evaluating recurrent urethritis, assess medication compliance and potential reexposure, perform wet mount and/or culture for *T vaginalis,* and treat as indicated by findings, or empirically as per Table 15–1.

Treatment

Treatment of nongonococcal urethritis generally employs azithromycin or doxycycline, with alternatives as listed in Table 15–1. If findings of urethritis are present, treatment is generally indicated pending results of diagnostic tests. Because diagnostic testing typically does not look for all potential causes of urethritis, patients with negative tests for GC and CT may also benefit from treatment. Empiric treatment for both *Chlamydia* and gonorrhea is particularly indicated in patients in whom follow-up may be unlikely, eg, adolescents, the homeless, and the mentally ill. If treatment is not offered at the initial visit, diagnostic testing should be done with additional treatment as indicated by test results and symptom persistence.

When treating for GC, treat also for CT, as coinfection is common and treatments for GC are generally inadequate for CT. Quinolone-resistant GC exists. Providers should be aware of local trend data (available from public health departments) and use a non-quinolone-containing regimen in patients suspected of contracting GC in Asia or other areas with high prevalence of quinolone resistance.

Treatment failures should be followed by repeat culture and sensitivity testing, and any resistance should be reported to the public health department.

Erbelding EJ, Quinn TC: Urethritis treatment. Dermatol Clin 1998;16:735.

EPIDIDYMITIS

The etiology of epididymitis varies with age. It is most commonly due to GC or CT in men 35 years of age or younger or to Gram-negative enteric organisms in men 35 years of age or older who engage in unprotected insertive anal intercourse, who have undergone recent urologic surgery, or who have anatomic abnormalities. Patients usually present with unilateral testicular pain and inflammation with onset over several days. The clinician must differentiate epididymitis from testicular torsion, a surgical emergency requiring immediate correction. The laboratory evaluation of suspected epididymitis is essentially the same as for urethritis, and includes gram stain, culture or antigen test, and serological testing for HIV and syphilis.

PROCTITIS, PROCTOCOLITIS, & ENTERITIS

Proctitis, proctocolitis, and enteritis may arise from anal intercourse or oral–anal contact. Depending on organism and anatomic location of infection and inflammation, symptoms can include pain, tenesmus, rectal discharge, and diarrhea. Etiological agents include CT, GC, *T pallidum*, HSV, *Giardia lamblia, Campylobacter, Shigella,* and *Entamoeba histolytica.* In HIV-infected patients, additional etiological agents include cytomegalovirus, *Mycobacterium avium* intracellular, *Salmonella, Cryptosporidium, Microsporidium, Isospora,* and symptoms arising as a primary effect of HIV infection.

Diagnosis involves examination of stool for ova, parasites, occult blood, and white blood cells; stool culture; and anoscopy or sigmoidoscopy. If the patient's clinical situation permits, diagnostic evaluation may proceed in a stepwise fashion, delaying endoscopy until other tests prove nondiagnostic.

Treatment should generally be based on results of diagnostic studies. However, if the onset of symptoms occurs within 1–2 weeks of receptive anal intercourse, and there is evidence of purulent exudates or polymorphonuclear neutrophils on gram stain of anorectal smear, the patient can be treated presumptively for GC and CT, reserving additional evaluation and treatment for patients who fail to respond to this therapy.

VAGINITIS

Patients with vaginitis may present with vaginal discharge, vulvar itching, and/or irritation, and sometimes with complaints of abnormal vaginal odor. This is generally not an STD, although patients may believe it to be sexually transmitted and vaginitis is often diagnosed during evaluation for a potential STD. Common etiologies include *C albicans, T vaginalis,* and bacterial vaginosis. Diagnostic evaluation typically includes physical examination and evaluation of a saline wet mount and KOH prep. Differences between common causes of vaginitis are summarized in Table 15–3, and are described below.

1. Vulvovaginal Candidiasis (VVC)

VVC is typically caused by *C albicans,* although occasionally other species are identified. More than 75% of all women will have at least one episode of VVC during their lifetime. The diagnosis is presumed if the patient has vulvovaginal pruritus and erythema with or without a white discharge, and is confirmed by wet mount or potassium hydroxide (KOH) preparation showing yeast or pseudohyphae or culture showing a yeast species.

VVC can be classified as uncomplicated, complicated, or recurrent. Uncomplicated VVC encompasses sporadic, nonrecurrent, mild to moderate symptoms, due to *C albicans,* that, in an otherwise healthy patient, are sensitive to routine therapy. Complicated VVC implies recurrent or severe local disease in a patient with

Table 15–3. Common causes of vaginitis.

	Findings Characteristic of		
Diagnostic Test	***Candida albicans***	***Trichomonas vaginalis***	**Bacterial Vaginosis**
pH	<4.5		>4.5
KOH to slide	Yeast or pseudohyphae		Amine or "fishy" odor
Saline to slide	Yeast or pseudohyphae	Motile *T vaginalis* organisms	"Clue" cells
Culture	Yeast species	*T vaginalis*	Nonspecific (not recommended)

impaired immune function, eg, diabetes or HIV, or infection with resistant yeast species. Recurrent VVC is defined as four or more symptomatic episodes annually.

Treatment is summarized in Table 15–1. Uncomplicated candidiasis should respond to short-term or single-dose therapies as listed. Complicated VVC may require 10–14 days of treatment. Treatment of women with recurrent vulvovaginal candidiasis should begin with an intensive regimen for 10–14 days followed by 6 months of maintenance therapy to reduce the likelihood of subsequent recurrence. Treatment of sex partners is generally not indicated. Treatment of symptomatic male sex partners, eg, those with ballanitis, with a topical antifungal agent may be indicated, as may treatment of partners of women with recurrent infections.

2. Trichomoniasis

Vaginitis due to *T vaginalis* presents with a thin, yellow or yellow-green frothy malodorous discharge with vulvar irritation that may worsen following menstruation. Diagnosis can often be made via prompt examination of a freshly obtained wet mount, which reveals the motile trichomonads. Although culture is more sensitive, it is also more costly and may not be as readily available, and results are delayed. Partners of women with trichomonas infection require treatment; although men are usually asymptomatic, they will reinfect female partners if untreated.

3. Bacterial Vaginosis (BV)

BV arises when normal vaginal bacteria are replaced with an overgrowth of anaerobic bacteria and *Gardnerella vaginalis.* Although not thought to be an STD, it is associated with having multiple sex partners. The cause of microbiological change is uncertain.

Diagnosis can be based on the presence of three of four clinical criteria: (1) a thin, homogeneous vaginal discharge, (2) a vaginal pH value of more than 4.5, (3) a positive KOH test, and (4) the presence of clue cells in a wet mount preparation.

Culture is generally not indicated. "The detection of G. vaginalis or other bacteria associated with BV by culture or other means only produces misleading results and is wasteful of time and resources" (Taylor-Robinson and Renton, 1999). Treatment of the male partner does not affect symptoms in the female patient.

Treatment of BV relieves symptoms and may also reduce the incidence of preterm delivery in pregnant women with asymptomatic BV. If treated, consider TOC 1 month later, as recurrence in both pregnant and nonpregnant women is common.

4. Mucopurulent Cervicitis (MPC)

MPC is characterized by purulent or mucopurulent discharge from the endocervix, which may or may not be associated with vaginal discharge and/or cervical bleeding. The diagnostic evaluation should include testing for *Chlamydia* and gonorrhea, although often no etiological agent is found. Absence of symptoms should not preclude additional evaluation and treatment, as approximately 70% of *Chlamydial* infections and 50% of gonococcal infections in women are asymptomatic.

Any positive test results require treatment. Empiric treatment should be considered in areas with high prevalence of GC or CT or if follow-up is unlikely.

Taylor-Robinson D, Renton A: Diagnostic tests that are worthwhile for patients with sexually transmitted bacterial infections in industrialized countries. Int J STD AIDS 1999;10:1.

PELVIC INFLAMMATORY DISEASE (PID)

PID is defined as inflammation of the upper genital tract, including pelvic peritonitis, endometritis, salpingitis, and tuboovarian abscess due to infection with GC, CT, or vaginal and/or bowel flora. Diagnosis is challenging due to often vague symptoms, lack of a single diagnostic test, the invasive nature of technologies needed to make a definitive diagnosis, and the need to balance underdiagnosis with overtreatment. Lower abdominal tenderness with both adnexal and cervical motion tenderness without other explanation of illness is sufficient to diagnose PID. Other criteria enhance the specificity of the diagnosis (but reduce diagnostic sensitivity):

- Fever >101°F
- Abnormal cervical or vaginal discharge
- Elevated sedimentation rate
- Elevated C-reactive protein
- Cervical infection with GC or CT

Definitive diagnosis rests on techniques that are not always readily available and that are not generally used to make the diagnosis. These include laparoscopic findings consistent with PID, evidence of endometritis on endometrial biopsy, and ultrasonographic findings showing thickened fluid-filled tubes with or without free pelvic fluid or tuboovarian complex.

Determination of appropriate therapy should consider pregnancy status, severity of illness, and patient compliance. Less severe disease can generally be treated with oral antibiotics in an ambulatory setting, whereas pregnant patients and those with severe disease may need to initiate therapy as inpatients. Options are listed in Table 15–1.

Paavonen J: Pelvic inflammatory disease. From diagnosis to prevention. Dermatol Clin 1998;16:747.

EXTERNAL GENITAL WARTS (EGW)

General Considerations

It is estimated that over 24 million Americans are infected with HPV, with one million new infections and 250,000 initial visits to physicians for genital warts occurring annually. Over 80 types of HPV have been identified, and over 20 types cause genital lesions. Types 6, 11, and others typically produce benign exophytic warts, whereas types 16, 18, 31, 33, 35, and others are associated with dysplasia and neoplasia. Thus cervical and anogenital squamous cancer can be considered STDs, and other cancers may also be sexually transmitted.

Clinical Findings

Diagnosis is almost always based on physical examination with bright light and magnification, and rarely requires biopsy. If the diagnosis is uncertain, consider referral to a physician with extensive EGW experience. Biopsy should be considered for warts that are >1 cm in size; indurated, ulcerated, or fixed to underlying structures; atypical in appearance; pigmented; or resistant to therapy. Application of 3–5% acetic acid as an aid to visualization is generally not useful, and the resulting nonspecific acetowhite reaction may lead to overdiagnosis of EGWs.

Cancer screening via cervical Papanicolaou (Pap) smear, if not done in the past 12 months, is indicated for women undergoing STD evaluation, and may be collected after other specimens, eg, cervical culture swabs. Regular cervical Pap smears are also indicated for women who have sex with women, a population sometimes erroneously felt to have limited risk for cervical cancer. EGWs are not an indication for screening more frequently than every 12 months. Type-specific HPV DNA probes may have utility in cancer screening programs although at present there are insufficient data to justify their routine use. Abnormal Pap results should be managed according to current recommendations.

The prevalence of HPV infection and squamous intraepithelial lesions in homosexual and bisexual men and high-risk women indicates that these patients should receive periodic anal Pap smears. Pending additional research, practitioners collecting anal Pap smears generally use collection devices employed for obtaining cervical specimens, although optimal collection techniques and management of abnormalities remain areas of further research.

Treatment

The therapeutic goal in EGW treatment is elimination of warts, *not* elimination of HPV infection. Treatment strives to eliminate symptoms, and a potential theoretical benefit is reduced likelihood of transmission. Clinicians should be certain of the diagnosis prior to instituting therapy, and should not apply EGW treatments to skin tags, pearly penile papules, sebaceous glands, or other benign findings that do not require (and will not respond to) EGW treatment.

Ideal EGW therapy has not yet been identified; current recommendations represent options based upon available research and expert opinion. The possibility of spontaneous resolution can justify no treatment, if that is the patient's wish. Treatments can be categorized as external or internal and as provider applied or patient applied. Physicians should familiarize themselves with at least one or two treatments in each category, as described in Table 15–1.

Most treatments work via tissue destruction. Imiquimod uses a different mechanism; by inducing production of interferon, it may be more effective than other therapies in treating some genital warts or other skin conditions, including molluscum contagiosum. Patients unresponsive to an initial course of treatment may require another round of treatment, more aggressive treatment, or referral to a specialist.

Patients with HPV need to understand the chronic nature of this infection, its natural history, and treatment options, and should receive adequate education and counseling to achieve optimal treatment outcomes. The chronic nature of HPV infection combined with the serious, albeit relatively infrequent, complication of cancer creates significant challenges to patient coping and provider counseling.

Beutner KR et al: External genital warts: report of the American Medical Association Consensus Conference. AMA Expert Panel on External Genital Warts. Clin Infect Dis 1998; 27:796.

Maw RD: Treatment of anogenital warts. Dermatol Clin 1998; 16:829.

MOLLUSCUM CONTAGIOSUM (MC)

MC appears in individuals of all ages and from all races, but has been reported more commonly in the white population and in males. Lesions are due to infection with poxvirus, which is transmitted through direct skin contact, as occurs among children in a nursery school and among adults during sexual activity. Diagnosis is typically based upon inspection, which reveals dimpled or umbilicated flesh-colored or pearly papules several millimeters in diameter; if needed, a smear of the core stained with Giemsa reveals cytoplasmic inclusion bodies. Lesions usually number less than 10–30, but may exceed 100, especially in HIV-infected patients who may have verrucous, warty papules, as well as mollusca greater than 1 cm in diameter. Lesions usually resolve spontaneously within months of appearance, but can be treated with cryotherapy, cautery, curettage, or removal of the lesion's core, with or without local anesthesia.

Smith KJ, Yeager J, Skelton H: Molluscum contagiosum: its clinical, histopathologic, and immunohistochemical spectrum. Int J Dermatol 1999;38:664.

HEPATITIS

Vaccines for prevention of viral hepatitis and indications have been previously described. Diagnostic and treatment considerations of viral hepatitis are beyond the scope of this chapter.

Braunwald E, Harrison TR: *Harrison's Principles of Internal Medicine.* McGraw-Hill, 2001.

ECTOPARASITES

Pediculosis pubis results from infestation with "crab lice" or *Phthirus pubis.* Affected patients usually present with pubic and/or anogenital pruritus, and may have identified lice and/or nits. The physician should be able to identify lice or nits with careful examination, and their absence calls into question the diagnosis despite compatible history.

Sarcoptes scabiei or scabies usually presents with pruritus not necessarily limited to the genital region. The intensity of pruritus may be increased at bedtime, and may be out of proportion to modest physical findings of erythematous papules, burrows, or excoriation from scratching. A classic finding on physical examination is the serpiginous burrow present in the web space between fingers; this finding is frequently absent in individuals with scabies.

Scabies can be sexually transmitted in adults, although sexual contact is not the usual route of transmission in children. Pruritus may persist for weeks after treatment. Retreatment should be deferred if intensity of symptoms is diminishing and no new findings appear. In HIV patients with uncomplicated scabies, treatment is the same as for HIV-negative patients. However, HIV patients are at risk for a more severe infestation with Norwegian scabies, which should be managed with expert consultation.

Ambroise-Thomas P: Parasitic diseases and immunodeficiencies. Parasitology 2001;122:S65.

■ GENERAL PRINCIPLES OF THERAPY FOR STDS

Treatments may be empirically targeted to agents most likely causing the presenting clinical syndrome or targeted to a specific infection diagnosed definitively. Regardless, there are overarching concerns affecting STD treatment that pertain to adherence and treatment success, HIV status, partner treatment, test-of-cure, and pregnancy.

Adherence considerations may favor shorter or single-dose regimens. For example, although single-dose azithromycin is more expensive than 7 days of doxycycline, lower cure rates attributed to reduced medication compliance and attendant costs of follow-up evaluation for patients treated with doxycycline can favor the use of azithromycin.

With HIV coinfection, treatments are generally the same as for uninfected patients unless stated otherwise. One potential difference is that HSV often causes more significant and prolonged symptoms in HIV-infected than in uninfected patients, so that HIV-infected patients may require longer treatment and/or higher medication dosages. Syphilis treatment may be the same as for HIV-uninfected patients, although some experts recommend three weekly injections of benzathine penicillin for primary, secondary, and early latent syphilis. Careful follow-up is even more important, as treatment failure and/or progression to neurosyphilis may be more common in the presence of HIV.

STD treatment will reduce HIV transmission, although the benefit of STD treatment with respect to HIV transmission may diminish as HIV prevalence increases. Ulcerative and nonulcerative STDs increase the risk of HIV transmission approximately three- to five-fold.

Pregnancy imposes constraints and special considerations for therapy. Where applicable, these are noted in the treatment recommendations in Table 15–1.

As previously described, patients often present with a clinical syndrome potentially attributable to more than one infectious agent, and optimally focused therapy depends on microbiological identification. However, delaying therapy may prolong symptoms, result in untreated infection or continued spread (if the patient fails to return for follow-up or heed advice to avoid sexual contact until cured), and contribute to increased long-term morbidity. Consequently, it may be desirable to "overtreat" upon initial presentation to avoid these undesirable sequelae, or at least discuss with patients the risks and benefits of immediate presumptive treatment versus delayed targeted treatment. This syndromic management has been employed in other countries as a strategy to reduce HIV transmission with variable success. However, even where successful, generalization from studies performed elsewhere may not be appropriate. It appears that for several STDs, prevalence and patient presentation in African cohorts may be different than in studies of patients in industrialized countries.

Brocklehurst P: Update on the treatment of sexually transmitted infections in pregnancy—1 and 2. Int J STD AIDS 1999; 10:571 and 636.

Hayes R et al: Randomised trials of STD treatment for HIV prevention: report of an international workshop. HIV/STD Trials Workshop Group. Genitourinary Med 1997;73:432.

Hudson CP: Syndromic management for sexually transmitted diseases: back to the drawing board. Int J STD AIDS 1999; 10:423.

WEB SITES

American Social Health Association (ASHA)

http://www.ashastd.org/

CDC STD Treatment Guidelines

http://www.cdc.gov/nchstp/dstd/1998_STD_Guidlines/98m1633.pdf

Infectious Diseases Society of America (IDSA)

http://www.idsociety.org/

◼ SEXUAL ASSAULT

Management of victims of sexual assault encompasses much more than treatment or prevention of STDs. Providers must heed legal requirements, effectively manage the psychological trauma, but not compromise the best course of medical care.

Proper medical management of sexual assault victims includes collection of evidence, diagnostic evaluation, counseling, and medical therapies to treat infection and unintended pregnancy. The diagnostic evaluation should include the following:

- Culture or nonculture tests, ie, nucleic acid-based tests, for GC and CT of affected sites, including throat, vagina, and anus.

- Vaginal wet mount and culture for *T vaginalis.*
- Serum tests for syphilis, hepatitis B, and HIV

Repeat wet mount and cultures should be obtained 2 weeks after initial evaluation to detect organisms that may have been present initially in small numbers and thus were undetected, unless the patient was treated prophylactically. Providers should also consider a late screen for hepatitis C virus, transmission of which has been documented following sexual assault.

Prophylactic treatment for STDs may be offered or recommended. Hepatitis B vaccine should be administered according to the routine schedule; hepatitis B immune globulin is not necessary. Azithromycin 1 g orally plus ceftriaxone 125 mg intramuscularly plus metronidazole 2 g orally may be offered for CT, GC, BV, and *Trichomonas,* respectively. Gastrointestinal side effects, especially when combined with postcoital oral contraceptive pills, may make this regimen intolerable, and alternative therapies or watchful waiting may be preferable.

Need for and benefit from HIV postexposure prophylaxis is difficult to predict. If instituted, the greatest benefit results from initiation of therapy as soon after exposure as possible. For guidance in deciding whether to begin postexposure HIV prophylaxis and in selecting appropriate treatment and monitoring, providers may contact the The National Clinician's Post-Exposure Prophylaxis Hotline (PEPline) at 888-HIV-4911 (888-448-4911).

After the neonatal period, STDs in children most commonly result from sexual abuse. In addition to vaginal gonococcal infection, pharyngeal and anorectal infection are common and often asymptomatic. Diagnostic techniques should rely only on Food and Drug Administration-approved tests due to the legal ramifications of the results, and ideally will include confirmatory tests using different methodologies, with specimen preservation for future testing when needed.

Beck-Sague CM, Solomon F: Sexually transmitted diseases in abused children and adolescent and adult victims of rape: review of selected literature. Clin Infect Dis 1999;28:S74.

Lamba H, Murphy SM: Sexual assault and sexually transmitted infections: an updated review. Int J STD AIDS 2000;11:487.

SECTION III

Adults

Preconception Care

Essam Demian, MD, MRCOG

There were 4,025,933 births in the United States in 2001, 1% less than the previous year. Although most babies are born healthy, of critical importance is that the infant mortality rate in the United States ranks 28th among developed nations. Preconception care has been advocated as a measure to improve pregnancy outcomes. Its components parallel those of prenatal care: risk assessment, health promotion, and medical and psychosocial interventions. Preconception care can be provided most effectively as part of ongoing primary care. It can be initiated during visits for routine health maintenance, during examinations for school or work, at premarital or family planning visits, after a negative pregnancy test, or during well-child care for another family member.

Jack BW, Culpepper L: Preconception care. Risk reduction and health promotion in preparation for pregnancy. JAMA 1990; 264(9):1147.

Martin JA et al: Births: final data for 2001. National Vital Statistics Reports. 2002;51(2):1.

NUTRITION

A woman's nutritional status before pregnancy may have a profound effect on reproductive outcome. Obesity is the most common nutritional disorder in developed countries. Obese women are at increased risk for prenatal complications such as hypertensive disorders of pregnancy, gestational diabetes, and urinary tract infections. They are also more likely to deliver large-for-gestational age infants and, as a result, have a higher incidence of intrapartum complications. Because dieting is not recommended during pregnancy, obese women should be encouraged to lose weight prior to conception.

On the other hand, underweight women are more likely than women of normal weight to give birth to low birth weight infants. Low birth weight may be associated with an increased risk of developing cardiovascular disease and diabetes in adult life (the "fetal origin hypothesis").

At the preconception visit, the patient's weight and height should be assessed and inquiries should be made regarding anorexia, bulimia, pica, vegetarian eating habits, and use of megavitamin supplements.

Vitamin A is a known teratogen at high doses. Supplemental doses exceeding 5000 IU/day should be avoided by women who are, or who may become, pregnant. The form of vitamin A that is teratogenic is retinol, not β-carotene, so large consumption of fruits and vegetables rich in β-carotene is not a concern.

Folic acid supplementation: Neural tube defects (NTDs) including spina bifida, anencephaly, and encephalocele affect approximately 4000 pregnancies each year in the United States. Although anencephaly is almost always lethal, spina bifida is associated with serious disabilities including paraplegia, bowel and bladder incontinence, hydrocephalus, and intellectual impairment.

Over the past 30 years, multiple studies conducted in various countries have shown a reduced risk of NTDs in babies whose mothers used folic acid supplements. The strongest evidence was provided by the Medical Research Council Vitamin Study in the United Kingdom, which showed a 72% reduction of recurrence of NTDs with a daily dose of 4 mg of folic acid started 4 weeks prior to conception and continued through the first trimester of pregnancy. Additionally, other studies showed a reduction in the incidence of first occurrence NTD with lower doses of folic acid (0.36–0.8 mg). Since 1992, the Centers for Disease

Control and Prevention (CDC) has recommended that all women of childbearing age who are capable of becoming pregnant take 0.4 mg of folic acid daily to reduce the risk of NTDs in pregnancy. It is also recommended that patients who had a previous pregnancy affected by an NTD take 4 mg of folic acid daily starting 1–3 months prior to planned conception and continuing through the first 3 months of pregnancy.

Despite the recommendations, compliance has been poor. As of 1998 and in an effort to ensure an increased intake of folic acid, the U.S. Food and Drug Administration (FDA) mandated the fortification of cereals and grains with folic acid at doses of 0.14 mg per 100 g of grain, an amount estimated to increase folic acid consumption by an average of 0.1 mg/day. By reducing plasma homocysteine levels, folic acid fortification could also have a beneficial effect on the rates of cerebrovascular and coronary heart disease in the general population.

The American College of Preventive Medicine advocates fortification at the higher level of 0.35 mg folic acid per 100 g product. It could be argued that this level of food fortification may mask the megaloblastic anemia associated with vitamin B_{12} deficiency and allow the progression of neurological symptoms. This is unlikely to occur in women of childbearing age, but can develop in the elderly who are at high risk for vitamin B_{12} deficiency.

Centers for Disease Control and Prevention: Recommendations for the use of folic acid to reduce the number of cases of spina bifida and other neural tube defects. MMWR 1992;41(RR-14):1.

Centers for Disease Control and Prevention: Knowledge and use of folic acid by women of childbearing age—United States, 1997. MMWR 1997;46(31):721.

MRC Vitamin Study Research Group: Prevention of neural tube defects: results of the Medical Research Council Vitamin Study. Lancet 1991;338(8760):131.

EXERCISE

More and more women wish to continue with their exercise programs during pregnancy. Among a representative sample of U.S. women, 42% reported exercising during pregnancy. Walking was the leading activity (43% of all activities reported), followed by swimming and aerobics (12% each).

Available data suggest that moderate exercise is safe for pregnant women who have no medical or obstetric complications. A meta-analysis review of the literature on the effects of exercise on pregnancy outcomes found no significant difference between active and sedentary women in terms of maternal weight gain, infant birth weight, length of gestation, length of labor, or Apgar scores.

Exercise may actually reduce pregnancy-related discomforts and improve maternal fitness and sense of self-esteem. The American College of Obstetricians and Gynecologists recommends that exercise in the supine position and any activity that increases the risk of falling (gymnastics, horseback riding, downhill skiing, and vigorous racquet sports) be avoided during pregnancy. Contact sports (such as hockey, soccer, and basketball) should also be avoided as they can result in trauma to both the mother and the fetus. Scuba diving is contraindicated during pregnancy because the fetus is at risk for decompression sickness. Absolute contraindications to exercise during pregnancy are significant heart or lung disease, incompetent cervix, premature labor or ruptured membranes, placenta previa or persistent second- or third-trimester bleeding, and preeclampsia or pregnancy-induced hypertension.

ACOG Committee on Obstetric Practice: ACOG Committee opinion, Number 267. Exercise during pregnancy and the postpartum period. Obstet Gynecol 2002;99(1):171.

MEDICAL CONDITIONS

Diabetes

Congenital anomalies occur two to six times more often in the offspring of women with diabetes mellitus and have been associated with poor glycemic control during early pregnancy. Preconceptional care with good diabetic control during early embryogenesis has been shown to reduce the rate of congenital anomalies to essentially that of a control population.

In a recent meta-analysis of 18 published studies, the rate of major anomalies was lower among preconception care recipients (2.1%) than nonrecipients (6.5%). According to the American Diabetes Association recommendations, the goal for blood glucose management in the preconception period and in the first trimester is to reach the lowest A1c level possible without undue risk of hypoglycemia to the mother. A1c levels that are <1% above the normal range are desirable. Suggested pre- and postprandial goals are as follows: before meals, capillary whole-blood glucose 70–100 mg/dL; 2 h after meals, capillary whole-blood glucose <140 mg/dL.

Prior to conception, a baseline dilated eye examination is recommended as diabetic retinopathy can worsen during pregnancy. Hypertension, frequently present in diabetic patients, needs to be controlled. Angiotensin-converting enzyme inhibitors and diuretics should be avoided as they have been associated with adverse effects on the fetus. Oral hypoglycemic agents should be discontinued because they may cause fetal anomalies and neonatal hypoglycemia, and insulin should be prescribed for patients with either type 1 or type 2 diabetes.

Epilepsy

Epilepsy occurs in 1% of the population and is the most common serious neurological problem seen in pregnancy. There are approximately one million women of childbearing age with epilepsy in the United States, of whom around 20,000 deliver babies every year. Much can be done to achieve a favorable outcome of pregnancy in women with epilepsy. Ideally, this should start before conception. Menstrual disorders, ovulatory dysfunction, and infertility are relatively common problems in women with epilepsy and should be addressed.

Women with epilepsy must make choices about contraceptive methods. Certain antiepileptic drugs (AEDs) such as phenytoin, carbamazepine, phenobarbital, primidone, and topiramate induce hepatic cytochrome P-450 enzymes, leading to an increase in the metabolism of the estrogen and progestin present in the oral contraceptive pills. This increases the risk of breakthrough pregnancy. The American Academy of Neurology recommends the use of oral contraceptive formulations with at least 50 µg of ethinyl estradiol or mestranol for women with epilepsy taking enzyme-inducing AEDs.

Both levonorgestrel implants (Norplant) and the progestin-only pill have reduced efficacy in women taking enzyme-inducing AEDs. Other AEDs that do not induce liver enzymes such as valproic acid, lamotrigine, vigabatrin, gabapentin, and felbamate do not cause contraceptive failure.

Because many AEDs interfere with the metabolism of folic acid, all women with epilepsy who are planning a pregnancy should receive folic acid supplementation at a dose of 4–5 mg/day. Withdrawal of AEDs can be considered in any woman who has been seizure free for at least 2 years and has a single type of seizure, normal neurological examination/intelligence quotient, and an electroencephalogram that has normalized with treatment. Because the risk of seizure relapse is greatest in the first 6 months after discontinuing AEDs, withdrawal should be accomplished before conception. If withdrawal is not possible, monotherapy should be attempted to reduce the risk of fetal malformations. The risk of major birth defects for the offspring of women with epilepsy is 4–6%, up from the background level of 2%. Phenytoin, phenobarbital, and primidone have been linked to congenital cardiac defects and cleft lip or palate. Valproic acid and carbamazepine have been associated with neural tube defects. All standard AEDs can cause a similar group of minor abnormalities (the fetal anticonvulsant syndrome) that includes craniofacial and digital anomalies. The new AEDs (gabapentin, lamotrigine, and vigabatrin) appear to be safer but human data are still limited.

Phenylketonuria

Phenylketonuria (PKU) is one of the most common inborn errors of metabolism. It is associated with deficient activity of the liver enzyme phenylalanine hydroxylase, leading to an accumulation of phenylalanine in the blood and other tissues. If untreated, PKU can result in mental retardation, seizures, microcephaly, delayed speech, eczema, and autistic-like behaviors.

All states have screening programs for PKU at birth. When diagnosed early in the newborn period and when treated with a phenylalanine-restricted diet, affected infants have a normal development and can expect a normal life span.

Dietary control is recommended for life in individuals with PKU and especially in women planning conception. Studies have shown a strong relationship between high maternal phenylalanine levels and mental retardation, microcephaly, and congenital heart disease in the offspring.

Recently, the Maternal Phenylketonuria 12-Year Collaborative Study has demonstrated that the institution of a phenylalanine-restricted diet before conception or by 8–10 weeks gestation can significantly reduce the incidence of congenital heart disease. Their preliminary data, however, suggest that optimum intellectual status in the offspring is achieved only when dietary treatment is started prior to conception.

American Diabetes Association: Preconception care of women with diabetes. Diabetes Care 2002;25(suppl 1):S82.

Platt LD et al: The International Study of Pregnancy Outcome in Women with Maternal Phenylketonuria: Report of a 12-year study. Am J Obstet Gynecol 2000;182(2):326.

Practice parameter: Management issues for women with epilepsy (summary statement). Report of the Quality Standard Subcommittee of the American Academy of Neurology. Neurology 1998;51(4):944.

GENETIC COUNSELING

The ideal time for genetic counseling is before a couple attempts to conceive, especially if the history reveals advanced maternal age, previously affected pregnancy, consanguinity, or family history of genetic disease.

Certain ethnic groups have a relatively high carrier incidence for certain genetic disorders. For example, Ashkenazi Jews have a 1:25 chance of being a carrier for Tay–Sachs disease, a severe degenerative neurological disease that leads to death in early childhood. Carrier status can easily be determined by a serum assay for the level of the enzyme hexosaminidase A. Screening for Tay–Sachs disease is recommended prior to conception, as testing on serum is not reliable in pregnancy, and the enzyme assay on white blood cells that is used in pregnancy is more extensive and labor intensive. Ashkenazi Jews are at risk not only for Tay–Sachs disease, but also for Canavan disease, Gaucher disease, and cystic fibrosis, all of which can be screened for by DNA analysis.

Cystic fibrosis is the most common autosomal recessive genetic disorder among whites in the United States, with a carrier rate of 1:22–25. It is characterized by the production of thickened secretions throughout the body, but particularly in the lungs and the gastrointestinal tract. In 1997, the National Institutes of Health recommended that cystic fibrosis carrier screening be offered to all couples planning a pregnancy or seeking prenatal testing. However, this recommendation has not yet been implemented. The complete text of the consensus statement can be found online at http://consensus.nih.gov/cons/106/106_statement.pdf.

Other common genetic disorders for which there is a reliable screening test for carriers are sickle cell disease in African-Americans, β-thalassemia in individuals of Mediterranean descent, and α-thalassemia in Southeast Asians. Sickle cell carriers can be detected with solubility testing for the presence of hemoglobin S (Sickledex). However, the American College of Obstetricians and Gynecologists recommends hemoglobin electrophoresis screening in all patients considered at risk for having a child affected with a sickling disorder. Solubility testing is described as inadequate because it does not identify carriers of abnormal hemoglobins such as the β-thalassemia trait or the HbB, HbC, HbD, or HbE traits. A complete blood count with indices is a simple screen test for the thalassemias and will show a mild anemia with a low mean corpuscular volume.

Fragile X syndrome is the most common cause of mental retardation (MR) after Down syndrome and is the commonest inherited cause of MR. It affects approximately 1 in 4000 men and 1 in 8000 women and results from a mutation in a gene on the long arm of the X chromosome. The X-linked inheritance is atypical in that unaffected males can transmit the disorder and up to 30% of female carriers are affected.

In addition to MR, fragile X syndrome is characterized by physical features such as macroorchidism, large ears, a prominent jaw, and behavioral problems such as hyperactivity and avoidance of eye contact. Preconception screening should be offered to women with a known family history of fragile X syndrome or a family history of unexplained MR, and to women who have learning disabilities or MR.

ACOG Committee on Genetics: ACOG Committee opinion, Number 238. Genetic screening for hemoglobinopathies. Int J Gynaecol Obstet 2001;74(3):309.

National Institutes of Health: Genetic testing for cystic fibrosis. NIH Consensus Statement 1997;15(4):1.

Turner G et al: Prevalence of fragile X syndrome. Am J Med Genet 1996;64(1):196.

IMMUNIZATIONS

The preconception visit is an ideal time to screen for rubella immunity as rubella infection in pregnancy can result in miscarriage, stillbirth, or a baby with congenital rubella syndrome (CRS). The risk of developing CRS abnormalities (hearing impairment, eye defects, congenital heart defects, and developmental delay) is greatest if the mother is infected in the first trimester of pregnancy. From 1990 through 1999, 117 cases of CRS were reported in the United States. Mothers of infants with CRS tended to be young, Hispanic, and foreign born.

Immunization should be offered to any woman with a negative rubella titer and advice given to avoid conception for 3 months due to the theoretic risk to the fetus. Inadvertent immunization of a pregnant woman with rubella vaccine should not be a reason to consider termination of pregnancy as there is no evidence that the vaccine causes any malformations or CRS.

If a pregnant woman acquires varicella before 20 weeks of gestation, the fetus has a 1–2% risk of developing fetal varicella syndrome, which is characterized by skin scarring, hypoplasia of the limbs, eye defects, and neurological abnormalities. Infants born to mothers who manifest varicella 5 days before to 2 days after delivery may experience a severe infection and have a mortality rate as high as 30%.

At the preconception visit, patients who do not have a prior history of chickenpox and who are seronegative should be offered vaccination. In 1995, the live attenuated varicella vaccine was introduced and the recommended regime for patients older than 13 years is two doses 4 weeks apart. Patients should avoid becoming pregnant for at least 4 weeks after the second dose.

Since 1988, the CDC has recommended universal screening of pregnant women for hepatitis B. Although hepatitis B vaccine can be given during pregnancy, women with social or occupational risks for exposure to hepatitis B virus should ideally be identified and offered immunization prior to conception.

Reef SE et al: The changing epidemiology of rubella in the 1990s: on the verge of elimination and new challenges for control and prevention. JAMA 2002;287(4):464.

LIFE-STYLE CHANGES

Caffeine

Caffeine is present in many beverages, in chocolate, and in over-the-counter medications such as cold and headache medicines. One cup of coffee contains approximately 120 mg of caffeine, a cup of tea has 40 mg of caffeine, and soft drinks such as cola contain 45 mg of caffeine per 12 oz serving. Consumption of caffeine during pregnancy is quite common, but its metabolism is slowed. Cigarette smoking increases caffeine metabolism, leading to increased caffeine intake.

Several epidemiological studies have suggested that caffeine intake may be associated with decreased fertility, increased spontaneous abortions, and decreased birth weight. As a result in 1980 the FDA advised pregnant women to avoid caffeine during pregnancy. However, a recent extensive literature review of the effects of caffeine concluded that pregnant women who consume moderate amounts of caffeine ($\leq$5–6 mg/kg/day) spread throughout the day and do not smoke or drink alcohol have no increase in reproductive risks.

Tobacco

Between 12% and 22% of pregnant women smoke during pregnancy, subjecting themselves and their infants to a number of adverse health effects. Smoking during pregnancy has been associated with spontaneous abortion, prematurity, low birth weight, intrauterine growth restriction, placental abruption, placenta previa, as well as an increased risk for sudden infant death syndrome. Accumulating evidence also indicates that maternal tobacco use is associated with birth defects such as oral clefts and foot deformities. Paradoxically, smoking during pregnancy has reportedly been associated with a reduced risk of preeclampsia. However, the smoking-related adverse outcomes of pregnancy outweigh this benefit.

The use of nicotine replacement products to help with smoking cessation has not been sufficiently evaluated during pregnancy to determine its safety. Nicotine gum was contraindicated during pregnancy when it was initially approved, ie, category X. In 1992, the FDA downgraded the contraindication to pregnancy category C (risk cannot be ruled out). Transdermal nicotine systems are graded as pregnancy category D (positive evidence of risk).

Women who are contemplating pregnancy should be advised to quit smoking prior to conception and nicotine replacement could then be prescribed. Smoking cessation either before pregnancy or in early pregnancy is associated with improvement in maternal airway function and an infant birth weight comparable to that observed among nonsmoking pregnant women.

Alcohol

In 1981, the surgeon general of the United States recommended that women abstain from drinking alcohol during pregnancy and when planning a pregnancy, because such drinking may harm the fetus. Despite that, approximately 15% of pregnant women report drinking alcohol.

The most severe consequence of exposure to alcohol during pregnancy is fetal alcohol syndrome (FAS), characterized by a triad of prenatal or postnatal growth retardation, central nervous system neurodevelopmental abnormalities, and facial anomalies (short palpebral fissures, smooth philtrum, thin upper lip, and midfacial hypoplasia). FAS is the largest preventable cause of birth defects and mental retardation in the western world. The most recent prevalence rate of FAS in the United States is 0.97/1000 births.

Some ethnic groups are disproportionately affected by FAS. American Indians and Alaska Native populations have a prevalence of FAS 30 times higher than white populations. It also appears that binge drinking produces more severe outcomes in offspring than more chronic exposure, possibly because of *in utero* withdrawal and its concomitant effects.

At the preconception visit, physicians should counsel their patients that there is no safe level of alcohol consumption during pregnancy and that the harmful effects on the developing fetal brain can occur at any time during pregnancy. High alcohol consumption in women has also been associated with infertility, spontaneous abortion, increased menstrual symptoms, hypertension, and stroke. Mortality and breast cancer are also increased in women who report drinking more than two drinks daily.

Illicit Drugs

Illicit drug use during pregnancy remains a major health problem in the United States. The National Institute on Drug Abuse estimates that about 5.5% of women used an illicit drug while pregnant. Marijuana was used by 2.9%, cocaine by 1.1%, and heroin by 0.1%. At the preconception visit, all patients should be questioned about drug use and offered counseling, referral, and access to recovery programs.

Marijuana is the most frequently used illicit drug in pregnancy. It does not appear to be teratogenic in humans and there is no significant association between marijuana usage and preterm birth or congenital malformations. A recent study, however, reported that prenatal exposure to marijuana was associated with increased hyperactivity, impulsivity, and inattention symptoms in children at age 10.

Cocaine use during pregnancy has been associated with spontaneous abortion, premature labor, intrauterine growth restriction, placental abruption, microcephaly, limb reduction defects, and urogenital malformations. Initial reports that suggested "devastating" outcomes for prenatal exposure to cocaine, have not been substantiated. A recent meta-analysis concluded that cocaine exposure *in utero* has not been demonstrated to affect physical growth and that it does not appear to independently affect developmental scores from infancy to age 6 years.

Maternal use of heroin and other opiates is associated with low birth weight due to both premature delivery and intrauterine growth restriction, preeclampsia, placental abruption, fetal distress, and sudden infant death syndrome.

Babies born to heroin-dependent mothers often develop a syndrome of withdrawal known as neonatal abstinence syndrome within 48 h of delivery. Neonatal withdrawal is characterized by central nervous system hyperirritability, respiratory distress, gastrointestinal dysfunction, poor feeding, high-pitched cry, yawning, and sneezing. Methadone has long been used to treat opioid dependence in pregnancy because of its long half-life. It has been associated with increases in birth weight. However, the use of methadone is controversial because more than 60% of neonates born to methadone-maintained mothers require treatment for withdrawal. Also, a substantial number of patients on methadone maintenance continue to use street narcotics and other illicit drugs. Buprenorphine, a recently developed partial opiate agonist, may have important advantages over methadone, including fewer withdrawal symptoms and a lower risk of overdose.

Bradley KA et al: Medical risks for women who drink alcohol. J Gen Intern Med 1998;13(9):627.

Christian MS, Brent RL: Teratogen update: evaluation of the reproductive and developmental risks of caffeine. Teratology 2001;64(1):51.

Frank DA et al: Growth, development, and behavior in early childhood following prenatal cocaine exposure: a systematic review. JAMA 2001;285(12):1613.

Goldschmidt L, Day NL, Richardson GA: Effects of prenatal marijuana exposure on child behavior problems at age 10. Neurotoxicol Teratol 2000;22(3):325.

National Institute on Drug Abuse: Pregnancy and drug use trends. Available online at http://nida.nih.gov/Infofax/pregnancytrends.html.

U.S. Department of Health and Human Services, Public Health Services Office of the Surgeon General: *Women and Smoking: A Report of the Surgeon General.* U.S. Department of Health and Human Services, 2001.

SEXUALLY TRANSMITTED DISEASES

The latest estimates suggest that there are 15 million new cases of sexually transmitted diseases (STDs) in the United States each year. The preconception visit is a good opportunity to screen for genital infections such as *Chlamydia,* gonorrhea, syphilis, and human immunodeficiency virus (HIV).

Chlamydia and gonorrhea are two of the most prevalent STDs and both are often asymptomatic in women. In pregnancy, both *Chlamydia* and gonorrhea have been associated with premature rupture of membranes, preterm labor, postabortion and postpartum endometritis, and congenital infection.

Infants whose mothers have untreated *Chlamydia* infection have a 30–50% chance of developing inclusion conjunctivitis and a 10–20% chance of developing pneumonia. Inclusion conjunctivitis typically develops 5–14 days after delivery and is usually mild and self-limiting. Pneumonia due to *Chlamydia* usually has a slow onset without fever and can have a protracted course if untreated. Long-term complications may be significant. Ophthalmia neonatorum is the most common manifestation of neonatal gonococcal infection. It occurs 2–5 days after birth in up to 50% of exposed infants who did not receive ocular prophylaxis. Corneal ulceration may occur, and unless treatment is initiated promptly, the cornea may perforate, leading to blindness.

Untreated syphilis during pregnancy may lead to spontaneous abortion, nonimmune hydrops, stillbirth, neonatal death, as well as serious sequelae in liveborn infected children. In 1999, the CDC launched the National Plan to Eliminate Syphilis in the United States and CDC officials believe syphilis can be almost completely eradicated before the end of this decade.

Women are becoming increasingly affected by HIV. In untreated HIV-infected pregnant women, the risk of mother-to-child transmission varies from 16% to 40%. However, it is possible to dramatically reduce the transmission rates by using highly active antiretroviral therapy (HAART) during pregnancy, by offering elective cesarean section at 38 weeks if the viral load at term is >1000 copies/mL, and by discouraging breast-feeding. In developed countries, transmission rates as low as 1–2% have been achieved.

Centers for Disease Control and Prevention: Congenital syphilis— United States, 2000. MMWR 2001;50(27):573.

MEDICATIONS

Therapeutic regimens for chronic illnesses are best modified, when possible, in the preconception period to include those drugs that have been used the longest and have been determined to pose the lowest risk.

Antihypertensives

Women with chronic hypertension who are receiving angiotensin-converting enzyme inhibitors should be advised to discontinue them before becoming pregnant or as soon as they know they are pregnant because of the possible hazards to the fetus. This class of drugs can result in fetal renal impairment, anuria leading to oligohydramnios, intrauterine growth restriction, hypocalvaria, persistent patent ductus arteriosus, and stillbirth. In the absence of congestive heart failure or pulmonary edema, diuretics are best avoided during pregnancy because they reduce maternal plasma volume, which may diminish uteroplacental perfusion. Methyldopa is the drug of choice for treatment of hypertension during pregnancy, with proven maternal and fetal safety.

Anticoagulants

Warfarin (coumadin) readily crosses the placenta and is a known human teratogen. The critical period for fetal warfarin syndrome is exposure during weeks 6–9 of gestation. This syndrome primarily involves nasal hypoplasia and stippling of the epiphyses. Later drug exposure may also be associated with intracerebral hemorrhage, microcephaly, and mental retardation. In patients who require prolonged anticoagulation therapy, discontinuing warfarin in early pregnancy and substituting heparin will reduce the incidence of congenital anomalies as heparin does not cross the placenta.

Antithyroid Drugs

Both propylthiouracil and methimazole are effective in the management of hyperthyroidism in pregnancy. Propylthiouracil is generally the preferred agent because in addition to inhibition of tetraiodothyronine (T_4) synthesis, it also inhibits the peripheral conversion of T_4 to triiodothyronine (T_3). Methimazole crosses the placenta in larger amounts and has been associated with aplasia cutis, a congenital defect of the scalp. If the patient is taking methimazole, it is reasonable to switch to propylthiouracil prior to conception.

Oral Hypoglycemics

As discussed earlier, patients with diabetes who are on oral hypoglycemic agents should be on insulin before pregnancy.

Risk Categories

The FDA has defined five risk categories (A, B, C, D, and X) that are used by manufacturers to rate their products for use during pregnancy.

A. CATEGORY A

Controlled studies in women fail to demonstrate a risk to the fetus in the first trimester (and there is no evidence of risk in later trimesters), and the possibility of fetal harm appears remote, eg, folic acid and thyroxine.

B. CATEGORY B

Either animal reproduction studies have not demonstrated fetal risk but no controlled studies in pregnant women have been conducted, or animal reproduction studies have shown an adverse effect (other than a decrease in fertility) that was not confirmed in controlled studies in women in the first trimester (and there is no evidence of risk in later trimesters), eg, acetaminophen, penicillins, and cephalosporins.

C. CATEGORY C

Either studies in animals have revealed adverse effects on the fetus (teratogenic, embryocidal, or other) but no controlled studies in women have been reported, or studies in women and animals are not available. Drugs should be given only if the potential benefit justifies the potential risk to the fetus, eg, acyclovir and zidovudine.

D. CATEGORY D

Positive evidence of human fetal risk exists, but the benefits from use in pregnant women may be acceptable despite the risk, especially if the drug is used in a life-threatening situation or for a severe disease for which safer drugs cannot be used or are ineffective, eg, tetracycline and phenytoin.

E. CATEGORY X

Studies in animals or humans have demonstrated fetal abnormalities, or evidence of fetal risk exists based on human experience, or both, and the risk of using the drug in pregnant women clearly outweighs any possible benefit. The drug is contraindicated in women who are or may be pregnant, eg, isotretinoin, misoprostol, warfarin, and statins.

OCCUPATIONAL EXPOSURES

There is an increasing number of women entering the workforce worldwide, and most are in their reproductive years. This has raised concerns for the safety of pregnant women and their fetuses in the workplace. The preconception visit is the best time to identify and control exposures that may affect parental health or pregnancy outcome. The three most common occupational exposures reported to affect pregnancy are video display terminals, organic solvents, and lead.

Video Display Terminals (VDTs)

In 1980, a cluster of four infants with severe congenital malformations was reported in Canada. The cluster was linked to the fact that the mothers had all worked with VDTs during their pregnancy, at a newspaper department in Toronto. Many epidemiological studies have since investigated the effects of electromagnetic fields emitted from VDTs on pregnancy outcome. Most studies found only equivocal or no associations of VDTs with birth defects, preterm labor, and low birth weight. Thus, it is reasonable to advise women that there is no evidence that using VDTs will jeopardize pregnancy.

Organic Solvents

Organic solvents comprise a large group of chemically heterogeneous compounds that are widely used in industry and common household products. Occupational exposure to organic solvents can result from many industrial applications, including dry cleaning, painting, varnishing, degreasing, printing, and production of plastics and pharmaceuticals. Smelling the odor of organic solvents is not indicative of a significant exposure, because the olfactory nerve can detect levels as low as several parts per million, which are not necessarily associated with toxicity. A recent meta-analysis of epidemiological studies demonstrated a statistically significant relationship between exposure to organic solvents in the first trimester of pregnancy and fetal malformations. There was also a tendency toward an increased risk for spontaneous abortion. Women planning on becoming pregnant should minimize their exposure to organic solvents by routinely using ventilation systems and protective equipment.

Lead

Despite a steady decline in average blood levels of lead in the U.S. population in recent years, approximately 0.5% of women of childbearing age may have blood levels of lead >10 μg/dL. The vast majority of exposures to lead occur in artists using glass staining and in workers involved in paint manufacturing for the automotive and aircraft industries. Other occupational sources of exposure to lead include smeltering, printing, and battery manufacturing. The most worrisome consequence of low to moderate lead toxicity is neurotoxicity. A review of the literature suggested that low-dose exposure to lead *in utero* may cause developmental deficits in the infant. However, these effects seem to be reversible if further exposure to lead is avoided. It is crucial to detect

and treat lead toxicity prior to conception because the chelating agents used (Dimercaprol, ethylenediaminetetraacetate, and penicillamine) can adversely affect the fetus if used during pregnancy.

Bentur Y, Koren G: The three most common occupational exposures reported by pregnant women: an update. Am J Obstet Gynecol 1991(2);165:429.

DOMESTIC VIOLENCE

Domestic violence (DV) is increasingly recognized as a major public health issue. Findings from the 1998 National Violence Against Women Survey showed that in the United States 1.5 million women are raped or physically assaulted by an intimate partner every year. DV crosses all socioeconomic, racial, religious, and educational boundaries. Even physicians are not immune to DV: in a survey, 17% of female medical students and faculty had experienced abuse by a partner in their adult life, an estimate comparable to that of the general population. Victims of DV should be identified preconceptionally as the pattern of violence may escalate during pregnancy. The prevalence of DV during pregnancy ranges from 0.9% to 20.1%, with most studies identifying rates between 3.9% and 8.3%. Whereas violence in nonpregnant women is directed at the head, neck, and chest, the breasts and the abdomen are frequent targets during pregnancy. Physical abuse during pregnancy is a significant risk factor for low birth weight and maternal complications of low weight gain, infections, anemia, smoking, and alcohol or drug usage. If it is identifed that a patient is the victim of DV, the physician should assess her immediate safety and make timely referrals to local community resources and shelters.

Tjaden P, Thoennes N: *Prevalence, Incidence and Consequences of Violence Against Women: Findings from the National Violence Against Women Survey.* U.S. Department of Justice: National Institute of Justice and Centers for Disease Control and Prevention, 1998.

Contraception

Susan C. Brunsell, MD

In the United States, 49% of pregnancies are unintended and 54% of these end in abortion. These rates remain higher than rates of many other industrialized countries. Addressing family planning and contraception is an important issue for providers of care to reproductive-age women. An increasing number of contraceptive options are becoming available on the U.S. market. It is incumbent on physicians and other health care providers to maintain currency with the recent advances in information concerning counseling, efficacy, safety, and side effects.

COMBINED ORAL CONTRACEPTIVES

Hormonal contraception is used by over 100 million women worldwide and by over 12 million women in the United States. The year 2000 marked the fourth decade of oral contraceptive use. The introduction of lower dose combination oral contraceptives (COCs) (<50 μg ethinyl estradiol) has provided many women with a highly effective, safe, and tolerable method of contraception.

COCs suppress ovulation by diminishing the frequency of gonodotropin-releasing hormone pulses and halting the luteinizing hormone surge. They also alter the consistency of cervical mucus, affect the endometrial lining, and alter tubal transport. Most of the antiovulatory effects of COCs derive from the action of the progestin component. The estrogen doses are not sufficient to produce a consistent antiovulatory effect. The estrogenic component of COCs potentiates the action of the progestin and stabilizes the endometrium so that breakthrough bleeding is minimized. When administered correctly and consistently, they are greater than 99% effective at preventing pregnancy. However, the 1995 National Survey of Family Growth (NSFG) estimated that the failure rates of COCs were as high as 8.3% during the first year of typical use. Noncompliance is the primary reason cited for the difference between these rates, frequently secondary to side effects such as abnormal bleeding and nausea.

Hormonal Content

The estrogenic agent most commonly used in COCs is ethinyl estradiol (EE), in doses ranging from 20 to 35 μg. Mestranol, which is infrequently used, is less potent than EE (a 50 μg dose of mestranol is equivalent to 30–35 μg of EE). It appears that decreasing the dose of estrogen to 20 μg reduces the frequency of estrogen-related side effects but increases the rate of breakthrough bleeding. In addition, there may be less margin for error with low-dose preparations such that missing pills may be more likely to result in breakthrough ovulation.

Multiple progestins are used in COC formulations. Biphasic and triphasic oral contraceptives, which vary the dose of progestin over a 28-day cycle, were developed to decrease the incidence of progestin-related side effects and breakthrough bleeding, although there is no convincing evidence that multiphasics indeed cause fewer adverse effects. The most commonly used progestins include norgestrel, levonorgestrel, and norethindrone. As with estrogens, some progestins (norethindrone and levonorgestrel) are biologically active, whereas others are prodrugs that are activated by metabolism. Norethindrone acetate is converted to norethindrone and norgestimate is metabolized into several active steroids including levonorgestrel. Progestins that do not require hepatic transformation tend to have better bioavailability and a longer serum half-life. For example, levonorgestrel has a longer half-life than norethindrone. In the 1990s COCs with different progestins, norgestimate and desogestrel, were introduced to decrease the incidence of androgenic side effects.

Drospirenone, a derivative of spironolactone, is the newest progesterone to be marketed, approved by the Food and Drug Administration (FDA) in May 2001. It is available, combined with EE, under the trade name Yasmin. Drospirenone differs from other progestins in having mild antimineralocorticoid activity. Contraceptive efficacy, metabolic profile, and cycle control are comparable to other COCs. Drospirenone has pharmacological properties similar to those of spironolactone; therefore, this progestin may reduce fluid-related weight gain, bloating, breast tenderness, and swelling. Because of its antimineralocorticoid effects and the potential for hyperkalemia, drospirenone should not be used in women with severe renal disease or hepatic dysfunction.

Most COCs are designed with 21 days of hormone and 7 days of placebo during which a withdrawal bleed occurs. An exception is Mircette (Organon), which is formulated with 21 days of 150 μg of desogestrel and 20 μg of EE, 2 days of placebo, then 5 days of 10 μg of EE in a 28-day pack. This formulation is meant to decrease breakthrough ovulation and decrease early cycle bleeding. The belief that a monthly period is normal and healthy for women is being challenged. The "tricycle" regimen in which women take 42–84 active pills in a row was first described over 20 years ago. Monophasic COCs are usually used. Skipping the pill-free week has been prescribed to treat menstrual headache and estrogen withdrawal symptoms, and to suppress endometriosis. This regimen has been shown to be safe, effective, and acceptable to women.

Side Effects

Side effects may be due either to the estrogen component, the progestin component, or both. Side effects attributable to progestin include androgenic effects, such as hair growth, male-pattern baldness, and nausea. Switching to an agent with lower androgenic potential may decrease or resolve these problems. Estrogenic effects include nausea, breast tenderness, and fluid retention. Weight gain is commonly thought to be a side effect of COCs; however, multiple studies have failed to confirm a significant effect. Weight gain can be managed by switching to a different formulation; however, appropriate diet and exercise should be emphasized.

Bleeding irregularities is the side effect most frequently cited as the reason for discontinuing COCs. Patients should be counseled that irregular bleeding/spotting is common in the first 3 months of COC use and will diminish with time. Spotting is also related to missed pills. Patients should be counseled regarding the importance of taking the pill daily. If the bleeding does not appear to be related to missed pills, the patient should be evaluated for other pathology such as infection, cervical disease, or pregnancy. If this evaluation is negative the patient may be reassured. Another approach would be to change the pill formulation to increase the estrogen or progestin component. The doses can be tailored to the time in the cycle when the bleeding occurs. If the bleeding precedes the menses, consider a triphasic pill that increases the dose of estrogen (Estrostep) or progestin (eg, Ortho-Novum 7/7/7) sequentially through the cycle. If the bleeding follows the menses consider Mircette, which has only two hor-

mone-free days. Increase the estrogen and/or the progestin midcycle for midcycle bleeding (eg, Triphasil).

Combined oral contraceptives may cause a small increase in blood pressure in some patients. The risk increases with age. The hypertension usually resolves within 3 months if the COC is discontinued. Both estrogens and progestins are known to affect blood pressure. Therefore, switching to a lower estrogen formulation or a progestin-only pill may not resolve the problem.

Major Sequelae

Use of most oral contraceptives with less than 50 μg of estrogen approximately triples the risk of venous thromboembolism. Before 1995, the progestin component of COCs was not generally thought to contribute to the risk of thrombosis. However, more recent studies with formulations containing gestodene (not available in the United States) or desogestrel have shown an approximately seven-fold increased risk of thrombosis compared with nonusers of COCs. Bias and confounding in these studies do not explain the consistent epidemiological findings of an increased risk. Obesity and increasing age are contributing risk factors. The identification of the factor V Leiden mutation in 1993 introduced another risk factor. As compared with the baseline risk for women who do not use COCs and who do not carry the mutation, the risk of venous thromboembolism is increased by a factor of 35 in women who carry the mutation and also use COCs. The best approach to identify women at higher risk of venous thromboembolism before taking COCs is controversial. Universal screening for factor V Leiden is not cost effective. Furthermore, a family history of venous thromboembolism has unsatisfactory sensitivity and positive predictive value for identifying carriers of other common defects.

The risk of thrombotic or ischemic stroke among users of COCs appears to be relatively low. There is no evidence that the type of progestin influences risk or mortality associated with ischemic stroke. The risk of ischemic stoke does appear to be directly proportional to estrogen dose, but even with the newer low-estrogen preparations there is still a slightly increased risk compared with nonusers. Hypertension, cigarette smoking, and migraine headaches interact with COC use to substantially increase the risk of ischemic stroke. The risk of hemorrhagic stroke in young women is low and is not increased by the use of COCs in the absence of risk factors. The major risk factors are hypertension and cigarette smoking.

Current use of COCs is associated with an increased risk of acute myocardial infarction (AMI) among women with known cardiovascular risk factors (diabetes, cigarette smoking, and hypertension) and among those who have not been effectively screened for risk factors, particularly for blood pressure. There is no increased risk for AMI with increasing duration of use or with past use of COCs.

In 1990, more than 20 studies that evaluated changes in carbohydrate metabolism associated with 6 or more months of low-dose COC use were reviewed. It was concluded that most studies demonstrated a low degree of alterations in carbohydrate metabolism, that most changes observed were not statistically significant, and that clinical relevance of those minimal statistically significant differences was unlikely.

Many epidemiological studies reported an increased risk of breast cancer among COC users. A meta-analysis was published in 1996 to address the concerns expressed in earlier publications. For current users of COCs, the relative risk of breast cancer compared with never-users was 1.24. This small risk persisted for 10 years, but essentially disappeared after this time period. Although COC users have a modest increase in risk of breast cancer, the disease tends to be localized. The pattern of disappearance of risk after 10 years coupled with the tendency toward localized disease suggests that the overall effect may represent detection bias or perhaps a promotional effect. A population-based, case–control study with over 8000 women enrolled was conducted to evaluate risk of breast cancer in COC users later in life when the risk of cancer is higher. This study, reported in 2002, showed that among women from 35–64 years of age, current or previous contraceptive use was not associated with a significantly increased risk of breast cancer).

Noncontraceptive Health Benefits

Most studies evaluating the relationship between COCs and ovarian cancer have shown a protective effect for oral contraceptives. There appears to be a 40–80% overall decrease in risk among users, with protection beginning 1 year after starting use, with a 10–12% decrease annually in risk for each year of use. Protection persists 15–20 years after discontinuation. The mechanisms by which COCs may produce these protective effects include suppression of ovulation and suppression of gonadotropins.

The use of COCs conveys protection against endometrial cancer as well. The reduction in risk of up to 50% begins 1 year after initiation, and persists for up to 20 years after COCs are discontinued. The mechanism of action is likely reduction in the mitotic activity of endometrial cells because of progestational effects.

A number of epidemiological studies demonstrate that the use of COCs will reduce the risk of salpingitis

by 50–80% compared with the risk to women not using contraception or who use a barrier method. There is no protective effect against the acquisition of lower genital tract sexually transmitted diseases (STDs). The purported mechanisms for protection include progestin-induced thickening of the cervical mucus, so that ascent of bacteria is inhibited, and a decrease in menstrual flow, resulting in less retrograde flow to the fallopian tubes. Other noncontraceptive benefits of COCs include decreased incidence of benign breast disease, relief from menstrual disorders (dysmenorrhea and menorrhagia), reduced risk of uterine leiomyomata, protection against ovarian cysts, reduction of acne, improvement in bone mineral density, and a reduced risk of colorectal cancer.

Burkman RT: Oral contraceptives: current status. Clin Obstet Gynecol 2001;44:62.

Collaborative Group on Hormonal Factors in Breast Cancer: Breast cancer and hormonal contraceptives; collaborative reanalysis on individual data on 53,297 women with breast cancer and 100,239 women without breast cancer from 54 epidemiologic studies. Lancet 1996;347:1713.

Fu H et al: Contraceptive failure rates; new estimates from the 1995 National Survey of Family Growth. Family Planning Perspect 1999;31:56.

Gaspard UJ, Lefebvre PJ: Clinical aspects of the relationship between oral contraceptives, abnormalities in carbohydrate metabolism, and the development of cardiovascular disease. Am J Obstet Gynecol 1990;163:334.

Huezo CM: Current reversible contraceptive methods: a global perspective. Int J Gynaecol Obstet 1998;62(suppl 1):3.

Jensen JT, Speroff L: Health benefits of oral contraceptives. Obstet Gynecol Clin North Am 2000;27:705.

Marchbanks PA et al: Oral contraceptives and the risk of breast cancer. New Engl J Med 2002;346:2025.

WHO Collaborative Study of Cardiovascular Disease and Steroid Hormone Contraception: Acute myocardial infarction and combined oral contraceptives: results of an international, multicentre, case-control study. Lancet 1997;349:1202.

TRANSDERMAL CONTRACEPTIVE SYSTEM

A transdermal contraceptive patch containing norelgestromin, the active metabolite of norgestimate, and EE is marketed by Ortho-McNeil under the trade name Ortho-Evra. The system is designed to deliver 150 μg of norelgestromin and 20 μg of EE daily directly to the peripheral circulation. The treatment regimen for each cycle is three consecutive 7-day patches (21 days) followed by one patch-free week so that withdrawal bleeding can occur. The patch can be applied to one of four sites on a woman's body: the abdomen, buttocks, upper outer arm, or torso (excluding the breast).

Ortho-Evra's efficacy is comparable to that of COCs. Compliance with the patch is much higher than with COC, which may result in fewer pregnancies overall. However, pregnancy is more likely to occur in women weighing more than 198 pounds. Breakthrough bleeding, spotting, and breast tenderness are slightly higher for Ortho-Evra than COCs in the first two cycles, but there is no difference in later cycles. Amenorrhea occurs in only 0.1% of patch users. Patch-site reactions occur in 2–3% of women.

Initiation of patch use is similar to initiation of COC use. Women apply the first patch on Day 1 of their menstrual cycle. Another option is to apply the first patch on the Sunday after their menses begins. This becomes their patch change day. Subsequently, they change patches on the same day of the week. After three cycles they have a patch free week during which they can expect their menses. A back-up contraceptive should be used for the first 7 days of use.

Audet MC et al: Evaluation of contraceptive efficacy and cycle control of a transdermal contraceptive patch vs. an oral contraceptive. JAMA 2001;285:2347.

INTRAVAGINAL RING SYSTEM

NuvaRing vaginal contraceptive ring, marketed by Organon, Inc., was approved by the FDA in October 2001. It is a flexible, transparent ring made of ethylene vinylacetate copolymers, delivering an average of 120 μg of etonorgestrel and 15 μg of EE per day. A woman inserts the NuvaRing herself, wears it for 3 weeks, then removes and discards the device. After one ring-free week, during which withdrawal bleeding occurs, a new ring is inserted. Rarely, NuvaRing can slip out of the vagina if it has not been inserted properly or while removing a tampon, moving the bowels, straining, or with severe constipation. If the NuvaRing has been out of the vagina for more than 3 h, breakthrough ovulation may occur. Patients may be counseled to check the position of the NuvaRing before and after intercourse.

Peak serum concentrations of etonorgestrel and EE occur about 1 week after insertion and are 60–70% lower than peak concentrations produced by standard COCs. The manufacturer recommends using back-up birth control for the first 7 days of use if not switching from another hormonal contraceptive. NuvaRing prevents pregnancy by the same mechanism as COCs. Pregnancy rates for users of NuvaRing are between one and two per 100 women-years of use.

The side effects of NuvaRing are similar to those of COC pills with the main adverse effect being disrupted bleeding. Breakthrough bleeding/spotting occurs in 2.6–11.7% of cycles and absence of withdrawal bleed-

ing occurs in 0.6–3.8% of cycles. Fewer than 1–2% of women experience discomfort or reported discomfort from their partners with NuvaRing. NuvaRing is associated with increased vaginal secretions, which is a result of both hormonal and mechanical effects. Twenty-three percent of ring users reported vaginal discharge; however, the normal vaginal flora appears to be maintained. The contraindications to NuvaRing are similar to those of COCs. In addition, the ring may not be an appropriate choice for women with conditions that make the vagina more susceptible to irritation or that make expulsion of the ring more likely to occur, such as vaginal stenosis, cervical prolapse, cystocele, or rectocele.

Ballagh SA: Vaginal ring hormonal delivery systems in contraception and menopause. Clin Obstet Gynecol 2001;44:106.

PROGESTIN-ONLY PILL

Progestin-only oral contraceptives (POPs), sometimes called the "minipill," are not widely used in the United States. Their use tends to be concentrated in select populations, notably breast-feeding women and those with contraindications to estrogen. Two formulations of POPs are available: one containing norgestrel and the other containing norethindrone. POPs appear to prevent conception through several mechanisms including suppression of ovulation, thickening of cervical mucus, alteration of the endometrium, and inhibition of tubal transport. The efficacy of POPs depends on consistent administration. The pills should be taken at the same time every day without interruption (no hormone-free week). If a pill is taken more than 3 h late, a back-up method of contraception should be used for the next 48 h. No increase in the risk for thromboembolic events has been reported for POPs. The World Health Organization has deemed this contraceptive method to be acceptable for use in women with a history of venous thrombosis, pulmonary embolism, diabetes, obesity, or hypertension. Vascular disease is no longer considered a contraindication to use. The most common side effects of POPs are menstrual cycle disruption and breakthrough bleeding. Other common side effects include headache, breast tenderness, nausea, and dizziness. In general, POP use protects against ectopic pregnancy by lowering the chance of conception. If POP users do get pregnant, an average of 6–10% of pregnancies are extrauterine—higher than in women not using contraception. Therefore POP users should be aware of the symptoms of ectopic pregnancy.

Progestin-only oral contraceptives: an update. The Contraception Report 1999;10.

INJECTABLE CONTRACEPTIVES

Injectable long-acting contraception offers users convenient, safe, and reversible birth control as effective as surgical sterilization. In the United States, there are two available options: Depo-Provera (DMPA), a 3-month progestin-only formulation containing 150 mg medroxyprogesterone acetate per injection, and Lunelle (MPA/ E2C), a monthly contraceptive injection containing medroxyprogesterone acetate 25 mg and estradiol cypionate 5 mg/0.5 mL suspension. Both are marketed by Pharmacia. They are both administered by deep intramuscular injection into the gluteus or deltoid muscle. MPA/E2C can also be injected into the anterior thigh.

Depo-Provera acts primarily by inhibiting ovulation. With typical use, the failure rate of DMPA is 0.3 per 100 woman-years, which is comparable to that of levonorgestrel implants, copper intrauterine devices, or surgical sterilization. Neither varying weight nor use of concurrent medications has been noted to alter efficacy, apparently because of high circulating levels of progestin. The progesterone component of MPA/E2C suppresses ovulation and provides high contraceptive efficacy, whereas the E2C component contributes to a regular bleeding pattern. The failure rate of MPA/E2C is estimated at 0.1 failures per 100 woman-years, comparable to other highly effective contraceptives. In addition, body weight does not appear to impact contraceptive efficacy.

The first injection of both DMPA and MPA/E2C should be administered within 5 days of the onset of menses or within 5 days of a first-trimester abortion. If a woman is postpartum and breast-feeding then neither drug should be administered until at least 6 weeks post-delivery. When switching from COCs, the first injection may be given any time the active pills are being taken or within 7 days of taking the last active pill. Repeat injections of DMPA should be administered every 12 weeks. If a patient presents at 13 weeks or later, the manufacturer recommends excluding pregnancy before administering a repeat injection. Subsequent injections of MPA/E2C are given within 28–33 days. They may be given as early as 23 days, but this timing may change menstrual patterns.

Use of DMPA has no permanent impact on fertility; however, return of fertility may be delayed after cessation of use. Fifty percent of women who discontinue DMPA to get pregnant will have conceived within 10 months of the last injection. In a small proportion of women fertility is not reestablished until 18 months after the last injection. In contrast, return to fertility occurs rapidly after discontinuation of MPA/E2C. Pregnancy rates within 60 days after the last injection are similar to women not using contraception.

Menstrual changes are the most common side effects reported by users of both DMPA and MPA/E2C. After 1 year of use, approximately 75% of women receiving DMPA report amenorrhea with the remainder reporting irregular bleeding or spotting. Some women, especially adolescents, view amenorrhea as a potential benefit of use. Women who voice concern over this side effect can be reassured that the amenorrhea is not harmful. Patients with persistent bleeding or spotting should be evaluated for genital tract neoplasia and infection as appropriate. If these are excluded and the symptoms are bothersome to the patient, a 1–3 month trial of low-dose estrogen can be considered. Options include conjugated equine estrogen (0.625, 1.25, or 2.5 mg), EE 20 μg, or a combined oral contraceptive. Early reinjection (eg, every 8–10 weeks) does not seem to decrease bleeding. In contrast to DMPA, the majority of MPA/E2C users report regular menses. Similar to COC, women on MPA/E2C may experience irregular bleeding during the first 3 months of use. Subsequently, 80% of users report having a single withdrawal bleed without any breakthrough bleeding or spotting. Cycle length is more variable in MPA/E2C users than in COC users, but this is attributed to variation in injection intervals.

Other side effects attributed to DMPA include weight changes, mood swings, reduced libido, headaches, and decreased bone mineral density. It appears that the decreases in bone mineral density seen in current and recent DMPA users are reversible and are therefore unlikely to have clinical importance. However, many clinicians recommend users take supplemental calcium and vitamin D. Similar side effects are reported in users of MPA/E2C, although there does not appear to be an effect on bone mineral density. DMPA may be used safely by smokers 35 years or older, and by other women at increased risk for arterial or venous events. Use of DMPA has not been associated with clinically significant alterations in hepatic function.

Kaunitz AM: Injectable long-acting contraceptives. Clin Obstet Gynecol 2001;44:73.

Kaunitz AM: Choosing an injectable contraceptive. Contemp OB/GYN 2001;46:29.

IMPLANTS

Subdermal progestin implants are a recent addition to the list of contraceptive choices. The Norplant system was approved for use in the United States in December 1990. Since its introduction, Norplant has been the subject of controversy focusing mainly on its side effects, difficult removal, and coercive application of the method toward low-income and other unempowered groups. It is important to note, however, that the FDA has reaffirmed that Norplant is safe and effective and there is no evidence to the contrary.

Norplant is a subdermal implant consisting of six silastic rods containing 36 mg of crystalline levonorgestrel. The implants release approximately 80 μg of levonorgestrel/24 h during the first year of use, decreasing to 30 μg/day in the latter years of use. It is probably a combination of levonorgestrel's effects on the female reproductive system that results in its high contraceptive efficacy (average of 0.2 pregnancies per 100 woman-years of use). The progestin suppresses the release of gonadotropins, which are responsible for ovulation. In the initial months of use when concentrations of levonorgestrel are the highest, only 10% of women are ovulatory. Toward the fifth year of use, however, more than 50% are ovulatory. Levonorgestrel also exerts a powerful effect on the cervical mucus. The mucus thickens and decreases in quantity, forming a barrier to sperm. Finally, the progestin impairs tubal motility and causes an atrophic endometrium that is inhospitable to implantation. Drugs that accelerate hepatic metabolism, such as phenobarbital, rifampin, phenytoin, and carbamazepine, have been shown to reduce the system's efficacy by accelerating clearance of levonorgestrel.

Individuals adequately trained in the technique should perform insertion of the implants. Proper technique is essential because correctly placed implants usually lead to easy removal, whereas removing poorly placed implants can be very difficult. Ideally the insertion should occur within the first 7 days of the menstrual cycle to diminish the risk of pregnancy and avoid the need for back-up contraception. The implants should be placed in the inner aspect of the upper arm in a fan-like pattern. To facilitate removal, all rods should be placed close to the skin in the same plane. Detailed instructions for insertion and removal are available from the manufacturer. Complications of insertion include ecchymosis, edema, and pain, each of which occurred in 3% or less of recipients by 30 days after insertion. Infection rates are reported to be less than 1%. The most common complications encountered during removal are broken implants (1.7%) and implants imbedded below the subdermal plane (1.2%). Other complications include pain during removal and bleeding.

The most common adverse effects reported during Norplant use are menstrual irregularities, including prolonged bleeding, spotting, irregular onset of bleeding, and amenorrhea. The incidence of bleeding irregularities decreases after the first year of use. Changes in bleeding patterns are reported by most users. If the number of bleeding days or the menstrual flow is excessive, a short course of estrogen can be used. Alternatively, nonsteroidal antiinflammatories have been effective for short-term control of bleeding (eg, ibuprofen 1800–2400 mg/day). Weight gain is a side effect commonly attributed to contraceptives and it is unclear if Norplant is responsible for a small weight gain or if the gain is caused by confounding factors in American society. Other side effects reported by Norplant users include headaches, mood swings, nervousness, dizziness, nausea, facial hair growth, hair loss, acne, mastalgia, galactorrhea, and hyperpigmentation over the implants. Serious complications such as pulmonary embolism, stroke, and myocardial infarction have been reported, but no evidence exists that the incidence of these events is increased, and a causative relationship is not suspected.

Jadelle, a two-rod implant system that releases levonorgestrel, was approved for use in the United States but has not been marketed. Its intended duration of use is 3 years. Pregnancy rates, discontinuation rates, and side effects are similar to that of Norplant. A single-rod contraceptive implant, Implanon, is marketed by NV Organon in many countries outside of the United States. It contains etonorgestrel (the active metabolite of desogestrel) in an ethylene vinylacetate membrane. It is intended for 3 years of use. Implanon had no method failures in over 70,000 cycles of use, and 82% of women continue use for at least 2 years. Women who discontinue Implanon do so mainly because of menstrual irregularity and weight gain. Because the system consists of only one rod, insertion and removal are greatly simplified.

Kovalevsky G, Barnhart K: Norplant and other implantable contraceptives. Clin Obstet Gynecol 2001;44:92.

INTRAUTERINE DEVICES

Throughout the world, the most common form of reversible contraception is the intrauterine device (IUD), used by almost 100 million women. However, relatively few women in the United States use IUDs, although those that do express a high degree of satisfaction. Currently three IUDs are approved for use by the FDA. The most common IUD used in the United States is the copper-T 380A (Paragard), made of polyethylene with fine wire copper wrapped around the stem and copper in the sleeves of each horizontal arm. It is approved for 10 years of use. The progesterone releasing T (Progestasert) is made of an ethylene vinylacetate copolymer containing 38 mg of progesterone. It is approved for 1 year of contraception. The levonorgestrel IUD (Mirena), the newest IUD, has a polyethylene frame that releases 20 μg of levonorgestrel/day for as long as 5 years. All of the IUDs are visible on X-ray.

The contraceptive action of IUDs is probably a result of a combination of factors. The IUD induces an inflammatory, foreign body reaction within the uterus that causes prostaglandin release. This release results in altered uterine activity, inhibited tubal motility, and a direct toxic effect on sperm. The copper present in the Paragard enhances the contraceptive effects by inhibiting transport of ovum and sperm. IUDs containing a progestin produce a similar effect and, in addition, thicken cervical mucus and suppress ovulation. IUDs are not abortifacients; they prevent conception. The IUD is one of the most effective methods of reversible contraception available. Among women who use the IUD perfectly (checking strings regularly to detect expulsion), the probability of pregnancy in the first year of use is 0.6% for Paragard, 1.5% for Progestasert, and 0.1% for Mirena.

The progestational activity of the levonorgestrel IUD results in noncontraceptive benefits. It has therapeutic benefit for menorrhagia, and early investigations indicate it will likely benefit women with endometriosis, adenomyosis, and fibroids. Given its 5-year period of efficacy, the levonorgestrel IUD represents a more practical form of intrauterine progestin delivery than the progesterone IUD, which has a life span of only 1 year.

Screening is critical for identifying women at risk for IUD-associated complications. The main goal of patient selection is to prevent insertion of an IUD in a patient who has an STD or is at high risk for exposure to one. Women who have more than one sexual partner or whose partner has other sexual partners are at high risk for acquiring an STD and are more likely to develop pelvic inflammatory disease (PID) if they use an IUD instead of other barrier or hormonal methods of birth control. The risk of developing PID associated with IUD use is related to insertion of the IUD and subsequent exposure to STDs. The greatest risk of PID occurs during the first few weeks following insertion, possibly because of contamination of the endometrial cavity at the time. The use of prophylactic antibiotics at the time of IUD insertion has not been shown to decrease the risk of PID. Concern about the potential risk of PID and subsequent tubal infertility has led to the recommendation that IUDs not be placed in women who have never been pregnant. However, a case–control study of over 1800 women showed that the IUD can be used safely in appropriately selected nulligravid women with no increased risk of tubal infertility.

The most common side effects reported by IUD users are cramping and bleeding. These symptoms can be minimized with the use of a nonsteroidal antiinflammatory drug (NSAID). However, if symptoms are persistent or severe the patient should be evaluated for infection or perforation. Patients can be reassured that the amount of bleeding and cramping usually decreases with time.

Expulsion occurs in 2–10% of women in the first year of use, with most expulsions occurring in the first 3 months. Nulliparity, an abnormal amount of menstrual flow, and severe dysmenorrhea are risk factors for expulsion. In addition, the expulsion rate may be higher when the IUD is inserted at the time of the menses. Pregnancy may be the first sign of expulsion. Therefore, patients should be taught to check for the IUD strings after each menstrual cycle. If a pregnancy does occur with an IUD in place, the IUD should be removed as soon as possible. In the presence of an IUD 50–60% of pregnancies spontaneously abort. The risk drops to 20% when the IUD is removed. Septic abortion is 26 times more common in women with an IUD. The copper-T IUD protects against ectopic pregnancy, whereas the progesterone IUD increases the risk of ectopic pregnancy almost two-fold.

The treatment of *Actinomyces* discovered on routine Papanicolaou (Pap) smear is one of the most controversial areas in the IUD literature. This finding on cervical cytology is more common in IUD users than in other women. There was concern that *Actinomyces* was associated with IUD-related PID. However, this relationship has been questioned. If *Actinomyces* is detected on Pap smear and the patient has signs or symptoms of PID, the IUD should be removed immediately and the patient should be treated with doxycycline. If the patient is asymptomatic, antibiotic treatment is not recommended and the Pap smear should be repeated in 1 year.

Canavan T: Appropriate use of the intrauterine device. Am Fam Physician 1998;58:2077.

Lee NC, Rubin GL, Borucki R: The intrauterine device and pelvic inflammatory disease revisited: new results from the Women's Health Study. Obstet Gynecol 1988;72:1.

BARRIER CONTRACEPTION

According to the 1995 National Survey of Family Growth, condom use, both at first intercourse and currently, has increased markedly since the 1970s with over 9 million women in the United States reported using condoms for contraception or protection from STDs. Condoms are inexpensive, easy to use, and available without a prescription. Until the late 1990s, most commercially available condoms were manufactured from latex. Now, polyurethane condoms are also available for latex-sensitive individuals. Although polyurethane and latex condoms offer similar protection against pregnancy, breakage and slippage rates appear to be higher with the polyurethane condom. Natural membrane condoms (made from sheep intestine) are also available, but they do not offer the same degree of protection from STDs. Because couples vary widely in their ability to use condoms consistently and correctly, the failure rate also varies. The percentage of women experiencing an unintended pregnancy within the first year of use ranges from 3% with perfect use to 14% with typical use. Women relying on condoms for contraception and protection from STDs should be reminded that oil-based lubricants reduce the integrity of a latex condom and facilitate breakage. Because vaginal medications (eg, for yeast infections) often contain oil-based ingredients, they can damage latex condoms as well.

There are several vaginal barrier contraceptives available that are easy to use, effective, and also reduce the risk on contracting some STDs. The contraceptive efficacy of all barrier methods depends on their consistent and correct use. The percentage of women experiencing an unintended pregnancy within the first year of typical use ranges from 15% to 32%.

The Reality Female Condom is a soft, loose fitting polyurethane sheath with two flexible polyurethane rings at either end. One ring is inserted into the vagina and lies adjacent to the cervix. The other ring remains outside of the vagina, against the perineum. Sperm is captured within the condom. The sheath is coated on the inside with a silicone-based lubricant. It is available without a prescription and is intended for one-time use. Female and male condoms should not be used together because the two condoms can adhere to one another, causing slippage and displacement.

The diaphragm is a dome-shaped rubber cup with a flexible rim. It is inserted, with a spermicide, into the vagina before intercourse. Once in position, the diaphragm provides contraceptive protection for 6 h. If a longer interval has elapsed, insertion of additional spermicide is required. After intercourse the diaphragm must be left in place for 6 h, but no longer than 24 h. Use of the diaphragm has been associated with an increased risk of urinary tract infections (UTIs), the result of exposure to spermicide (which alters vaginal flora) as well as possible mechanical factors in diaphragm use. Use of the diaphragm requires an appointment with a health care provider for education, fitting, and a prescription. Oil-based vaginal products should not be used with the latex diaphragm.

The cervical cap is a soft, deep latex rubber cap that fits snugly over the cervix. Spermicide is placed in the dome of the cap prior to insertion and is held in place against the cervix until the cap is removed. The cap provides continuous contraception for 48 h regardless of how many times intercourse occurs. Additional spermicide is not necessary. The cervical cap must be professionally fitted and requires a prescription. Insertion and removal are somewhat more difficult than with a diaphragm.

The contraceptive sponge is a small, pillow-shaped polyurethane sponge containing a spermicide. The sponge protects for up 12–24 h, no matter how often intercourse occurs. After intercourse, the sponge must be left in place for at least 6 h before it is removed and discarded. The sponge comes in one universal size and does not require a prescription. Although no longer available in the United States, the contraceptive sponge is still manufactured in many other countries including Canada.

The newest barrier device on the market is Lea's Shield. It is a reusable elliptical bowl made of medical-grade silicone rubber. It has an anterior loop to assist with removal and a centrally located valve that allows passage of cervical secretions. Lea's Shield offers several advantages over other vaginal barriers. Because the device is made of silicone, latex allergy and reaction with vaginal medications are not a concern. The device comes in only one size, which simplifies the fitting process. The manufacturer does recommend clinician instruction and the device does require a prescription. The shield can be worn for up to 48 h and, unlike the diaphragm, additional spermicide is not required for each repeated act of intercourse.

Women should be counseled that spermicides are an integral component of barrier contraceptives. Nonoxynol-9, the active chemical agent in spermicides available in the United States, is a surfactant that destroys the sperm cell membrane. It comes in a variety of formulations including gel, foam, creme, film, suppository, and tablet. Spermicide use may lower the chance of becoming infected with a bacterial STD by as much as 25%. However, women at high risk for acquiring human immunodeficiency virus (HIV) should not use products containing nonoxynol-9. Some studies have shown it causes vaginal lesions that could serve as entry points for HIV.

Abma JC et al: Fertility, family planning, and women's health: new data from the 1995 National Survey of Family Growth. Vital Health Statist 1997;(19):1.

Gilliam ML, Derman RJ: Barrier methods of contraception. Obstet Gynecol Clin North Am 2000;27:841.

EMERGENCY CONTRACEPTION

Three million unintended and unwanted pregnancies occur in the United States each year, with 80% occurring in women older than 19 years of age. As many as half of these pregnancies result from condom failure, missed birth control pills, or incorrect or inconsistent use of barrier contraception. Optimal use of emergency contraception could reduce unintended pregnancy in the United States by as much as 50%. Emergency contraception, available as combined oral contraceptives, progestin-only pills, and the copper intrauterine device, are safe and effective. When taken as directed, emergency contraceptive pills (ECPs) can reduce the risk of pregnancy by 75–89% after a single act of unprotected intercourse, whereas a copper IUD inserted within 5 days of intercourse can reduce the risk by 99%.

Emergency contraception is appropriate when no contraception was used or when intercourse was unprotected due to contraceptive accidents. Because pill regimens involve only limited exposure to hormones, ECPs are safe. They have not been shown to increase the risk of venous thromboembolism, stroke, myocardial infarction, or any other cardiovascular event. In addition, ECPs will not disrupt an implanted pregnancy and will not cause birth defects. Although the mechanism of action of ECPs is not fully understood, it is thought to involve inhibition of ovulation and prevention of fertilization and/or implantation. Unfortunately ECPs do not protect against STDs.

Use of combined oral contraceptives for emergency contraception is frequently referred to as the Yuzpe method. It is prepackaged and marketed under the trade name Preven. The initial dose is two tablets, containing a total of 50 μg EE and 250 μg levonorgestrel, taken up to 72 h after unprotected intercourse. The second two-pill dose is taken 12 h later. Commercially available COCs containing EE and levonorgestrel or norgestrel can be used as emergency contraception. Each dose must contain at least 100 μg EE plus 0.5 mg levonorgestrel or 1.0 mg norgestrel (eg, Lo/Ovral four white pills per dose). When used correctly, the Yuzpe method decreases expected pregnancies by 75%. More specifically, eight of every 100 women who have unprotected intercourse once during the second or third week of their cycles will become pregnant; two of 100 will become pregnant if the Yuzpe method is used. The most common adverse effects are nausea (50%) and vomiting (20%). Antiemetics taken 30–60 min before each dose help to minimize these symptoms. Other side effects include delayed or early menstrual bleeding. Some women also experience heavier menses.

When used for emergency contraception, the initial dose of the progestin-only pill is 0.75 mg levonorgestrel taken no more than 72 h after unprotected intercourse and repeated in 12 h. This regimen is marketed under the trade name Plan B. If Plan B is not available the dosage can be formulated from commercially available progestin-only pills. The initial dose of Ovrette, for example, is 20 pills, which is repeated 12 h later. The progestin-only regimen may be somewhat more effective than the Yuzpe method, preventing 85% of expected pregnancies in one study. In addition, nausea occurs in less than 25% of patients and vomiting is reduced to about 5% in women taking the progestin-only regimen.

To prevent pregnancy, a copper-containing IUD can be inserted up to 5 days after unprotected intercourse. The IUD is highly effective and can be used for long-term contraception. An IUD is not recommended for anyone at risk for STDs or an ectopic pregnancy, or if long-term contraception is not desired. The IUD is the most effective method of emergency contraception, with failure rates of less than 1%.

Screening patients for ECP use is based on the time of unprotected intercourse and the date of the last normal menstrual period. There are no preexisting disease contraindications and inadvertent use in pregnancy has not been linked to birth defects. Neither a pregnancy test nor a pelvic examination is required, although these may be done for other reasons (eg, screening for STDs). In contrast, IUD insertion for emergency contraception is an office-based procedure that requires the same counseling and screening as IUD insertion for contraception.

Counseling regarding the availability of emergency contraception can occur whenever contraception or family planning issues are discussed. It is especially appropriate if the patient is relying on barrier methods or does not have a regular form of contraception. The counseling can be reinforced when patients present with contraceptive "mishaps." Information that should be discussed includes the definition of emergency contraception, indications for use, mechanism of action, lack of protection against STDs, instructions on use, and follow-up plans including ongoing contraception.

Glasier A: Emergency postcoital contraception. New Engl J Med 1997;337:1058.

Stone MH, Westley E, Cullins VE: Emergency contraception: America's best kept secret. Contemp OB/GYN 2002;47:106.

Task Force on Postovulatory Methods of Fertility Regulation: Randomised controlled trial of levonorgestrel versus the Yuzpe regimen of combined oral contraceptives for emergency contraception. Lancet 1998;352:428.

SPECIAL POPULATIONS

Adolescents

Adolescent pregnancy continues to be a serious public health problem in the United States. Almost 1 in 10 adolescent females becomes pregnant each year, with half of the pregnancies ending in abortion. The general approach to adolescent contraception should focus on keeping the clinician–patient encounter interactive. Several suggestions include avoiding "yes/no" questions, keeping clinician speaking time short and focused, and avoiding the word "should."

Abstinence deserves emphasis, especially in young teenagers. Counseling should focus not on "just say no" but rather on "know how to say no." COCs and condoms are the most common contraceptive methods chosen by teens. Many clinicians promote using both methods simultaneously as an approach to preventing pregnancy and STDs. The main concern adolescents have regarding COCs is weight gain. They can be reassured that many studies have proven that COCs do not cause weight gain. Another issue that may contribute to the reluctance of adolescents to seek contraception is fear of a pelvic examination. Contrary to popular belief, a pelvic examination is not necessary when contraception is prescribed, especially if it will delay sexually active teens' access to needed pregnancy prevention. Adolescents should be counseled regarding missed pills and given anticipatory guidance about breakthrough bleeding and amenorrhea. The contraceptive patch may be an attractive alternative to some teens who find it difficult to take a daily pill.

Although only a small proportion of adolescents use the long-acting progestin methods of contraception, they have obvious benefits in terms of not requiring daily pill administration or action at the time of coitus. Like COCs they do not protect against STDs. Counseling issues include anticipatory guidance regarding changes in menstrual patterns and, in the case of Depo-Provera, how the patient will access the provider every 12 weeks for her injection.

Vaginal barrier contraceptives are not ideal choices for several reasons. Many adolescents are not prepared to deal so intimately with their own bodies and do not wish to prepare so carefully for each episode of intercourse. However, they can be an effective method for highly motivated, educated adolescents. The IUD is normally not appropriate for adolescents because of the risk of PID in this population.

A discussion of emergency contraception should be part of contraceptive counseling for all adolescents. To increase the availability of emergency contraception, teens may be given a replaceable supply of ECPs to keep at home. Some states allow distribution of emergency contraception by pharmacists without a physician's prescription.

Breast-feeding Women

The lactational amenorrhea method is a highly effective, although temporary method of contraception. However, to maintain effective protection against pregnancy, another method must be used as soon as menstruation resumes, the frequency or duration of breast-feeds is reduced, bottle-feeds or regular food supplements are introduced, or the baby reaches 6 months of age. Other good contraceptive options for lactating women include barrier methods, progestin-only methods, or an IUD. Some experts recommend that breast-feeding women delay using progestin-only contraception until 6 weeks postpartum. This recommendation is based on a theoretical concern that early neonatal exposure to exogenous steroids should be avoided if possible. The combined pill is not a good option for lactating women because estrogen decreases breast milk supply.

Perimenopausal Women

Perimenopause represents a transition period lasting about 5 years before the permanent cessation of periods. Although the likelihood of pregnancy is not high, when it does occur, it is likely to be unintended. Women over the age of 40 have the second highest proportion of unintended pregnancies, 77%, exceeded only by girls 13–14 years old. Although women still need effective contraception during perimenopause, issues including bone loss, menstrual irregularity, and vasomotor instability also need to be addressed. Oral contraceptives offer many benefits for healthy, nonsmoking perimenopausal women. They have been found to decrease the risk of postmenopausal hip fracture, regularize menses in women with dysfunctional uterine bleeding, and decrease vasomotor symptoms.

Progestin-only pills are another good option and can be used by women who have contraindications to estrogen. Long-acting progestin contraceptives can be continued through menopause. However, irregular bleeding patterns sometimes associated with these methods can create problems for perimenopausal women. Abnormal bleeding that is persistent, even if contraceptive hormone exposure is the most likely cause, will need to be evaluated. Other contraceptive options include condoms, vaginal barriers, and IUDs.

Physiologically, menopause is the permanent cessation of menstruation as a consequence of termination of ovarian follicular activity. Determining the exact onset of menopause in a woman using hormonal contraception can be tricky. Many clinicians measure the level of follicle-stimulating hormone (FSH) during the pill-free interval to diagnose menopause. However, because suppression of ovulation can vary from month to month, a single FSH value is unreliable. In addition, in women using COCs, FSH levels can be suppressed even on the seventh pill-free day. Given that many women do not become menopausal until their mid-50s, and considering the limited utility of FSH testing, one approach to managing this transition avoids FSH testing entirely. Women continue to use their COCs until age 55 at which time they can discontinue use.

Davis AJ: Adolescent contraception and the clinician: an emphasis on counseling and communication. Clin Obstet Gynecol 2001;44:114.

Greydanus DE, Patel DR, Rimsza ME: Contraception in the adolescent: an update. Pediatrics 2001;107:562.

Kaunitz AM: Oral contraceptive use in perimenopause. Am J Obstet Gynecol 2001;185:S32.

Adult Sexual Dysfunction

18

T.A. Miller, MD, & Margaret R.H. Nusbaum, DO, MPH

Introduction

Sexual dysfunction is defined as a disturbance in one or more of the aspects of the sexual response cycle or as pain associated with sexual intercourse. The concept of the sexual response cycle is based largely on the work of Masters and Johnson as later revised by Kaplan. The sexual response cycle can be divided into the following four phases:

1. Desire/Interest/Libido: This phase consists of fantasies about sexual activity and interest or motivation to engage in sexual activity. This requires androgens and the sensory system. For men this might be largely visual whereas it is more relationship based for women.
2. Excitement/Arousal: This phase consists of a subjective sense of sexual pleasure and accompanying physiological changes. The major changes in the male consist of penile tumescence and erection. The major changes in the female consist of vasocongestion in the pelvis, vaginal lubrication, and expansion and swelling of the external genitalia. This requires an intact parasympathetic nervous system and vascular system.
3. Orgasm/Ejaculation: This phase consists of a peaking of sexual pleasure, with release of sexual tension and rhythmic contraction of the perineal muscles. In the male, there is a sensation of ejaculatory inevitability, followed by ejaculation of semen. In the female there are contractions of the wall of the outer third of the vagina. In both genders, the anal sphincter rhythmically contracts. This requires an intact sympathetic nervous system.
4. Resolution: This phase consists of a sense of muscular relaxation and general well being. During this phase, males are physiologically refractory to further erection and orgasm for a variable period of time. In contrast, females may be able to respond to additional stimulation almost immediately.

The *Diagnostic and Statistical Manual of Mental Disorders,* 4th edition (*DSM-IV*), categorizes dysfunction by the phase of the cycle most directly impacted. More recently, a modifier has been added—personal distress must be associated with the problem to meet the criteria of a dysfunction.

American Psychiatric Association: *Diagnostic and Statistical Manual of Mental Disorders,* ed 4. R.R. Donnelley, 1994.

Kaplan H: *Disorders of Sexual Desire.* Brunner/Mazel, 1979.

Masters W, Johnson VE: *Human Sexual Inadequacy.* Little, Brown, 1970.

General Considerations

Sexual dysfunctions are extremely common. A survey of young to middle-aged adults found that 31% of men and 43% of women in the general population reported some type and degree of sexual dysfunction. Sexual problems appear to have a higher prevalence in certain clinical populations. The Massachusetts Male Aging Study reported that 50% of men between 40 and 70 years of age experienced erectile dysfunction. As outlined in Table 18–1, recognition of sexual dysfunction is important whether specific treatment is available or desired. Sexual dysfunction may be the initial manifestation of significant underlying disease or provide a marker for disease progression and severity. Sexual dysfunction should be a consideration when managing a number of chronic medical conditions. Provider awareness of the impact that therapeutic management decisions may have on sexual function may improve patient adherence to medical regiments. Sexual dysfunction is positively correlated with low physical and emotional satisfaction in relationships as well as with general happiness.

Despite this, only 10% of men and 20% of women with sexual dysfunctions seek medical care for their sexual difficulties. The key to the identification of sexual function disorders is for the provider to inquire about their presence. Primary care providers are in an ideal position to identify sexual dysfunction. Patients often

Table 18–1. Reasons to inquire about sexual health.

Morbidity and mortality associated with sexual activity: sexually transmitted diseases, including human immunodeficiency virus

Medical disorders can be a cause or effect of sexual problems (eg, diabetes, depression, cardiovascular disease)

Trauma or surgical treatment side effects can adversely affect sexual functioning (eg, transurethral resection of prostate)

Medications used to treat chronic conditions may exacerbate sexual dysfunction (antihypertensive agents, antidepressants)

Past events may explain present problems (eg, history of abuse and lack of sexual desire)

Sexual dysfunctions, difficulties, and concerns are common

Sexual activity is associated with health, happiness, and longevity

Sexual health is integral to general health assessment

It is potentially negligent or unethical to ignore: consider child sexual abuse

---

From Maurice WL: *Sexual Medicine in Primary Care.* Mosby, 1999.

want to talk about sexual dysfunction or concerns related to sexuality but are too embarrassed to raise the topic themselves and want physicians to initiate the discussion. A discussion of sexual health can be initiated in a wide variety of ways. Informing patients of the importance of sexual health can start as soon as a patient arrives in the office. Educational material or self-administered screening forms can be placed in the waiting area or the examination rooms. Doing so sends the message that sexual health is important and is a topic that can be discussed in the physician's office. Table 18–2 lists a number of self-administered screening forms that can be easily incorporated into a busy office practice.

Sexual history can be included as part of the social history or as part of the review of systems under genitourinary systems. Incorporating sexual history into social history acknowledges the social aspect of sexual

Table 18–2. Sexual health screening questionnaires.

Sexual Health Inventory for Men (SHIM)

International Index of Erectile Function (IIEF)

World Health Organization (WHO) Intensity Score

Androgen Deficiency in the Aging Male (ADAM)

Female Sexual Function Index (FSFI)

Sexual Energy Scale

Brief Index of Sexual Function Inventory (BISF-W)

Changes in Sexual Functioning Questionnaire (CSFQ)

---

relations whereas including it under genitourinary systems readily identifies sexual functioning as part of genitourinary health. Including sexual history in routine health screening in whatever manner seems most appropriate to the clinician gives a clear message to the patient that this is an important part of an individual's general health. There are many other opportunities to bring a discussion of sexual health into the clinical encounter as outlined in Table 18–3. Asking patient permission may reduce clinician anxiety about how the patient might react to having a sexual history taken: "Studies show that sexual health is important to one's overall quality of life and that patients prefer that their doctors initiate the topic. Would it be OK if I ask you a few questions about your sex life?"

Once the history confirms the existence of a sexual problem, clarifying which aspect of the sexual response cycle is most affected as well as the course of the problem is essential. Obtain as clear a description as possible regarding the aspect of the sexual response cycle most involved, as well as onset, progression, and associated medical problems (Table 18–4). Clarify terminology that is vague or unclear. Asking patients what they believe to be the cause can help the clinician identify possible relationship, health, and iatrogenic etiologies. Ask patients to identify what they have tried to do to resolve the problems and to clarify their expectations for resolution. Involving the partner in both identification and subsequent management can be very valuable.

Table 18–3. Sexual health inquiry.

Review of systems or social history

    What sexual concerns do you have?

    Has there been any change in your (or partner's) sexual desire or frequency of sexual activity?

    Are you satisfied with your (or partner's) present sexual functioning?

    Is there anything about your sexual activity (as individuals or as a couple) that you (or your partner) would like to change?

When counseling about healthy life-style (smoking or alcohol cessation, exercise program)

When discussing effectiveness and side effects of medications

Inquire before and after medical event on procedures likely to impact sexual function (myocardial infarction, prostate surgery)

Inquire when there is about to be or has been a life cycle change such as pregnancy, new baby, teenager, children leaving the home, retirement, menopause

---

From Nusbaum MRH, Hamilton C: The proactive sexual health inquiry: key to effective sexual health care. Am Fam Physician 2002;66(9):1705 and Nusbaum MRH: *Sexual Health.* American Academy of Family Physicians, 2001.

Table 18–4. The sexual problem history.

Description of the problem:
 As detailed as possible, have the patient describe the problem in his or her own terms, clarifying as necessary. Try to understand what the patient means; try not to label. Determine the frequency of the problem (eg, erectile difficulty—does it occur with the spouse but not in an extramarital affair)?

Development and course of the problem:
 When did it begin and what has been the course of the problem (does it wax and wane)?

Patient's assessment of the cause of the problem:
 The patient may have a good idea about the cause or, perhaps, there is room for sexual information (myth): What do you think the cause of the problem might be? How do you think the problem came to be?

History of attempts to resolve the difficulty:
 Past professional treatment or books read. What has been tried to rectify the problem? What are the outcomes of these attempts?

Patient's expectations and goals:
 What does the patient expect? Whose goal is it?

Medications/associated medical conditions:
 Cause/impact on prescription

From Annon JS: *The Behavioral Treatment of Sexual Problems,* Vol. 1. Enabling Systems Inc., 1974.

Table 18–5. Conditions associated with sexual dysfunction.

Aging
Chronic disease
 Diabetes mellitus
 Heart disease
 Hypertension
 Lipid disorders
 Renal failure
 Vascular disease
Endocrine abnormalities
 Hypogonadism
 Hyperprolactinemia
 Hypo/hyperthyroidism
Life-style
 Cigarette smoking
 Chronic alcohol abuse
Neurogenic causes
 Spinal cord injury
 Multiple sclerosis
 Herniated disc
Penile injury/disease
 Peyronie's plaques
 Priapism
Prescription medications
Psychological issues
 Depression
 Anxiety
 Social stresses
Trauma/injury
 Pelvic trauma/surgery
 Pelvic radiation

Sexual dysfunction is associated with a long list of common medical conditions and medical therapies (Table 18–5). In some instances the underlying medical condition may be the cause of the sexual dysfunction, such as arterial vascular disease causing erectile dysfunction. In other instances the sexual dysfunction contributes to the associated condition (erectile dysfunction leads to loss of self-esteem and depression). It is important to recognize these associations in order to optimally manage patients with chronic disease.

Johannes C et al: Incidence of erectile dysfunction in men 40–69 years old: longitudinal results from the Massachusetts male aging study. J Urol 2000;163:460.

Nusbaum MR et al: The high prevalence of sexual concerns among women seeking routine gynecological care. J Fam Pract 2000; 49(3):229.

Nusbaum MRH, Pathman DE, Gamble G: Seeking medical help for sexual concerns: frequency, barriers, and missed opportunities. J Fam Pract 2002;51(8):706.

DISORDERS OF DESIRE

General Considerations

Concerns about sexual desire are the most common sexual complaint heard by health professionals. Over 33% of women and 16% of men in the general population reported experiencing an extended period of lack of sexual interest. Other investigators have reported prevalence rates as high as 87% in specific populations. Women who were younger, separated, black, less educated, and of lower socioeconomic status reported the highest rates. Among men, the same demographics as well as increasing age were associated with the highest rates.

Classification

Disorders of sexual desire are divided into two major categories: hypoactive sexual desire disorder (HSD) and sexual aversion disorder (SAD). Hypoactive sexual desire disorder is much more common and is likely to be seen in the primary care setting. It is characterized by persistent or recurrently deficient (or absent) sexual fantasies and desire for sexual activity that cause marked distress or interpersonal difficulty. HSD is further classified as life-long (primary) or acquired (secondary) and generalized or situational in occurrence. SAD is characterized by persistent or extreme aversion to, and avoidance of, any genital contact with a sexual partner, causing marked distress or interpersonal difficulty.

Although not considered a sexual dysfunction, a common situation in clinical practice is sexual desire discrepancy, in which partners differ in their level of sexual desire. Although most couples negotiate a workable solution, in some instances it may be significant enough to cause relationship dissatisfaction.

Pathogenesis

Changes in or a loss of sexual desire can be the result of biological, psychological, or social and interpersonal factors (Table 18–6). Numerous medical conditions are directly or indirectly associated with decreased sexual desire. Conditions that impact endocrine function can cause reduced levels of androgens and/or elevated levels of prolactin. Conditions that primarily impact other aspects of the sexual response cycle may indirectly decrease sexual desire—ie, erectile dysfunction due to arterial vascular disease or dyspareunia due to estrogen deficiency-induced atrophic vaginitis. Androgen levels influence sexual desire. The role of androgens is well established in men, although there is an increasing body of evidence for a significant role in women. An estimated 4–5 million men in the United States are affected by hypogonadism.

Table 18–6. Common medical conditions that may decrease sexual desire.

Pituitary/hypothalamic
    Infiltrative diseases/tumors
Endocrine
    Testosterone deficiency
        Castration, adrenal disease, age related bilateral salpingo-
            oophorectomy, adrenal disease
    Thyroid deficiency
    Endocrine-secreting tumors
    Cushing's syndrome
    Adrenal insufficiency
Psychiatric
    Depression and stress
    Substance abuse
Neurological
    Degenerative diseases/trauma of the central nervous
        system
Urological/gynecological (indirect cause)
    Peyronie's, phimosis
    Gynecological pain syndromes
Renal
    End-stage renal disease, renal dialysis
Conditions that cause chronic pain, fatigue, malaise
    Arthritis, cancer, chronic pulmonary, hepatic disease

Decreased sexual desire is a common manifestation of some psychiatric conditions, particularly affective disorders. A number of medications may decrease sexual desire (Table 18–7). The agents most commonly involved are psychoactive drugs, particularly antidepressants, and medications with antiandrogen effects. Many psychosocial issues impact sexual desire. Factors as widely varied as religious beliefs, primary sexual interest in individuals outside of the main relationship, specific sexual phobias or aversions, fear of pregnancy, lack of attraction to the partner, and poor sexual skills in the partner can all diminish sexual desire.

Clinical Findings

A. Symptoms and Signs

The evaluation of the patient concerned with decreased sexual desire should include a detailed sexual problem history. Detailed information should be obtained to categorize the specific type of desire disorder and the association of any predisposing conditions. In addition to loss of desire, other manifestation of androgen deficiency include a diminished sense of well being, depression, lethargy, osteoporosis, loss of muscle mass, and erectile dysfunction.

The physical examination and laboratory testing should be guided by historical findings. The physical examination in patients with an acquired generalized loss of desire should be directed toward the identification of unrecognized conditions such as endocrine abnormalities (hypogonadism, hypothyroidism)

B. Laboratory Findings

In patients with desire complaints, an assessment of hormone status is recommended. The specific hormone studies remain open to debate. In men an assessment of androgen status is indicated. In women an assessment of both androgens and estrogens is indicated. Testosterone levels peak in both men and women in the fourth decade of life and then decrease by 1–2% per year. Testosterone studies should be obtained in the morning as testosterone is secreted in a diurnal manner with the highest levels in the morning. The total plasma testosterone, which measures bioavailable testosterone plus protein-bound testosterone, is the most readily available study. A total testosterone level of <300 ng/dL in a man suggests hypogonadism, particularly when accompanied by clinical signs and symptoms. Because testosterone is highly protein bound with sex hormone-binding globulin (SHBG) and other serum proteins, as men and women age their SHBG levels increase, thereby lowering bioavailable testosterone. Total testosterone may in some instances not reflect the patient's true androgenic status. Free (bioavailable) testosterone

Table 18–7. Drugs most commonly associated with sexual dysfunction.[1]

Medication	Type of Sexual Dysfunction
Antihypertensive medications	
Diuretics	
Thiazides	ED, decreased libido
Spironolactone	ED, decreased libido
Sympatholytics	
Central agents (methyldopa, clonidine)	ED, decreased libido
Peripheral agents (reserpine)	ED, ejaculatory dysfunction
α-Blockers	ED, ejaculatory dysfunction
β-Blockers (particularly nonselective agents)	ED, decreased libido
Psychiatric medications	
Antipsychotics	Multiple phases of sexual function
Antidepressants	
Tricyclic antidepressants	Decreased libido, ED
MAO inhibitors	Multiple phases of sexual function
SSRIs	Ejaculatory dysfunction, ED
Anxiolytics	
Benzodiazepines	Decreased libido
Antiandrogenic agents	
Digoxin	Decreased libido, ED
H-2 receptor blockers	Decreased libido, ED
Others	
Alcohol (long-term heavy use)	Decreased libido, ED
Ketoconazole	Decreased libido, ED
Niacin	Decreased libido
Phenobarbital	Decreased libido, ED
Phenytoin	Decreased libido, ED

[1]ED, erectile dysfunction; MAO, monoamine oxidase; SSRI, selective serotonin reuptake inhibitors.

more accurately reflects androgen status. Free testosterone (<50 pg/mL) suggests hypogonadism. Consensus measurement of other androgenic agents formed earlier in the steroid hormone synthesis pathway has been advocated. If low testosterone is confirmed, further endocrine assessment and imaging are indicated to determine the specific underlying etiology.

Treatment

Treatment is directed at the underlying etiology and consists of both nonspecific and specific therapy. Lifelong decreased desire is unlikely to benefit from therapy, particularly in the primary care setting. Treatment directed toward substantially enhancing the patient's level of sexual desire would likely not be productive. Acquired situational HSD requires psychologically based treatment.

The approach to couples with sexual desire discrepancy should include discussing the epidemiology of decreased sexual desire with patient and partner. Educating couples about the impact of extraneous influences—fatigue, preoccupation with childrearing, work

stress, and interpersonal conflict—can improve awareness of these issues. Encouraging couples to set time aside for themselves and to schedule dates can be very effective. Educating partners, particularly men, about gender generalities can be helpful. The quality of the relationship appears to be a critical component for women's sexual response cycles. An emotionally and physically satisfying relationship enhances sexual desire and arousal and has a positive feedback on the quality of the relationship. The importance of allowing time for sexual relations, incorporating the senses, understanding what is pleasing to one's partner, and incorporating seduction cannot be overemphasized.

Potentially reversible medical conditions or the impact of medications on sexual desire should be addressed. Treating organic etiologies such as depression, hypothyroidism, hyperprolactinemia, and androgen deficiency can often restore sexual interest. Options available when decreased sexual desire is attributed to medical therapy can be challenging. Treatment approaches can include lowering the dosage, suggesting drug holidays, discontinuing potentially offensive medications, and switching to a different agent. In some situations where continuation of therapy is indicated, adding specific agents to address the sexual manifestations can be useful.

In men and women with acquired generalized HSD hormone replacement is a consideration. There is an expanding level of knowledge in this area. Testosterone may be helpful to women who report diminished libido beginning in the perimenopausal time period. Androgen replacement options for both men and women are listed in Table 18–8.

A. ANDROGEN REPLACEMENT

The goal of androgen replacement therapy is to raise the level of androgens to a mid-physiological range. For both genders, oral testosterone is not recommended due to the prominent first pass phenomenon, variable blood levels, and potential for significant liver toxicity. For men, intramuscular injections every 3–4 weeks had been the mainstay of treatment, but this results in dra-

matic fluctuations in blood levels—with supraphysiological levels early and subphysiological levels prior to the next injection. Application of topical preparations offers the advantage of consistently maintaining levels in the normal range. With patches, applied in the evening, local skin reactions are common. Topical gels are applied each morning and have fewer skin side effects.

A diagnosis of androgen insufficiency should be made only in women who are adequately estrogenized, whose free testosterone is at or below the lowest quartile of the normal range for reproductive age (20–40 years), and who present with clinical symptoms. Androgen, testosterone, and dihydroepiandrosterone (DHEAS) supplementation appears to be helpful for women and men. DHEAS is available over the counter and is dosed at 25–75 mg/day based on response. Testosterone is available transdermally, parenterally, and enterally. Transdermal testosterone can be admin-

Table 18–8. Androgens: forms and dosages.

Form	Dosage for Women	Dosage for Men
Oral[1]		
Methyltestosterone	10 mg: 1/4 to 1/2 tablet daily or 10 mg Monday, Wednesday, Friday	10–50 mg/day
Testosterone micronized	2.5 mg daily[2]	
Halotestin (fluoxymesterone)	2 mg: 1/2 tablet daily or 1 tablet every other day	5–20 mg/day
Estratest and Estratest HS	Either 1.25 or 0.625 mg	
Winstrol (Stanozolol)	2 mg: 1/2 tablet every day or 1 tablet every other day	
Dehydroepiandrosterone	25–75 mg 3 times weekly to daily[1]	
Buccal		
Methyltestosterone[3]	5–25 mg daily	5–25 mg/day
	USP tablet, 0.25 mg[2]	
Sublingual		
Methyltestosterone	0.25 mg[2]	
Testosterone micronized		
USP tablet		
Transdermal		
Testosterone patch	2.5–5.0 mg applied every day or every other day	4–6 mg/day
Topical testosterone	1% vaginal cream daily to clitoris and labia	5–10 mg/day (Androderm)
Testosterone micronized	1–2% gel daily to clitoris and labia[2]	
Testosterone proprionate	2% lotion daily to clitoris and labia[2]	
Testosterone micronized	2% lotion daily to clitoris and labia[2]	
Intramuscular		
Testosterone enanthate	200 mg/ml: 0.25–0.5 ml every 3–5 weeks	50–400 mg every 2–4 weeks
Testosterone cypionate	100 mg/ml: 0.25–0.5 ml every 3–4 weeks	50–400 mg every 2–4 weeks

From Nusbaum MRH: *Sexual Health.* American Academy of Family Physicians, 2001 and Wallis L, Kasper AS, Reader GG: Hormone replacement therapy (HRT). In: *Textbook of Women's Health.* Lippincott-Raven, 1998: p 731.
[1]Oral methyltestosterone, aside from the combination estratest, should be used only short term due to the risk of hepatotoxicity.
[2]Must be compounded by a pharmacist.
[3]Guay A: Advances in the management of androgen deficiency in women. Med Aspects Hum Sexuality, 2001.

istered via skin patches (androderm, testoderm) or gels (androgel), and can be compounded as a 1–2% cream, gel, or lotion that can be applied to the labial and clitoral area. Oral methyltestosterone can have varying rates of absorption and is available as Estratest for women. Estratest has been used safely for years. Oral methytestosterone is the less preferred route given its erratic absorption and concern for liver effects. Intramuscular testosterone can be used for both men and women but tends to have a supraphysiological effect in the first week or two after injection. Topical administration has been found to deliver testosterone in a more physiological manner. Although concerns exist for the potential risks of long-term androgen supplementation, no reports of negative consequences on liver function, lipids, or cardiovascular morbidity has been reported to date. Further studies with long-term data are needed.

Exogenous estrogens and progestins in the form of hormone replacement therapy lower physiologically available androgens and can contribute to decreased sexual interest. Addition of androgens, methyltestosterone, or DHEAS can offset this negative impact. If no benefit occurs from this change, the physician should reassess the quality of the sexual relationship and also consider discontinuing the exogenous hormones. All oral contraceptive agents lower bioavailable androgen levels as a result of high SHBG levels. Changing to an oral contraceptive pill (OCP) with greater androgen activity, such as those containing norgestrel, levonorgestrel, and norethrindrone acetate, may be effective (Table 18–9).

Table 18–9. Relative androgenicity of progestational components of oral contraceptive agents.

Least
  Norethindrone (0.4–0.5 mg)[1]
  Norgestimate (0.18–0.25 mg)
  Desogestrel (0.15 mg)
  Ethynodiol diacetate (1.0 mg)
Medium/neutral
  Norethindrone (0.5–1.0 mg)[1]
Greatest
  Levonorgestrel (0.1–0.15 mg)
  Norgestrel (0.075–0.5 mg)
  Norethindrone acetate (1.0–1.5 mg)

From Nusbaum MRH: *Sexual Health.* American Academy of Family Physicians, 2001 and Burham T, Short R (editors): *Drug Facts and Comparisons.* Mosby, 2001.
[1]Norethindrone (0.35 mg) without estrogen, in progestin-only oral contraceptive pills, has medium relative androgenicity.

B. TESTOSTERONE THERAPY

Because testosterone treatment may stimulate tumor growth in androgen, estrogen, and/or progesterone-dependent cancers, it is contraindicated in men with prostate cancer and men and women with a history of breast cancer. Preexisting sleep apnea and hyperviscosity, to include deep venous thrombosis or pulmonary embolism, are relative contraindications to testosterone use.

Certain patient populations such as the elderly and patients with a first-degree relative with prostate cancer may be at increased risk. Serious hepatic and lipid changes have been associated with the use of oral preparations available in the United States. In addition to hepatotoxicity, benign prostatic hyperplasia, lipid changes, gynecomastia, sleep apnea, and increased oiliness of skin acne are reported side effects.

Although it is known that testosterone accelerates the clinical course of prostate cancer and may stimulate the growth of previously undiagnosed prostate tumors, there is no conclusive evidence in short-term studies that testosterone therapy increases the incidence of prostate cancer. In an analysis of eight studies, no correlation was found between increased serum testosterone and subsequent development of prostate cancer. In a four-study analysis, no relationship was documented between bioavailable testosterone levels and the risk of developing prostate cancer several years later. If androgen prescription is initiated for both men and women, close follow-up is recommended to assess androgen levels, lipid profile, hematocrit levels, and liver function. Additionally, periodically checking the prostate-specific antigen should be considered. Until more data regarding long-term use become available, it is probably most prudent to check these levels every 3–6 months.

Bachmann G et al: Female androgen insufficiency: the Princeton consensus statement on definition, classification and assessment. Fertil Steril 2002;77(4):660.

Basson R et al: Report of the International Consensus Development Conference on female sexual dysfunction: definitions and classifications. J Urol 2000;163:888.

Janssens H, Vanderschueren DM: Endocrinological aspects of aging in men: is hormone replacement of benefit? Eur J Obstet Gynecol Reprod Biol 2000;92(1):7.

Johannsson G et al: Low dose dehydroepiandrosterone affects behavior in hypopituitary androgen-deficient women: a placebo-controlled trial. J Clin Endocrinol Metab 2002;87 (5):2046.

Munarriz R et al: Androgen replacement therapy with dehydroepiandrosterone for androgen insufficiency and female sexual dysfunction: androgen and questionnaire results. J Sex Marital Ther 2002;28(Suppl 1):165.

Reiter WJ et al: Dehydroepiandrosterone in the treatment of erectile dysfunction: a prospective, double-blind, randomized, placebo-controlled study. Urology 1999;53(3):590

DISODERS OF EXCITEMENT/AROUSAL

General Considerations

Arousal disorders appear to affect 18.8% of women and 5% of men in the general population. The prevalence of erectile dysfunction (ED) is much higher in certain patient populations, especially men with depression, diabetes, and heart disease. Approximately 75% of women in patient samples have reported difficulty with lubrication.

Pathogenesis

Arousal disorders are divided into two etiological categories: psychogenic and organic. Most arousal disorders were once considered to be of psychogenic origin, but current evidence suggests that up to 80% of cases have an organic etiology. Organic causes are subdivided into vasculogenic, neurogenic, and hormonal etiologies. Vasculogenic represents the largest group with arterial or inflow problems being by far the most common. Regardless of the primary etiology, a psychological component frequently coexists. Although influenced by other systems, arousal is primarily a neurovascular process. Optimal function requires an intact nervous system and a responsive arterial vasculature. Sexual stimulation results in nitric oxide release, which initiates a cascade of events leading to a dramatic increase in blood flow to the penis in men and the vagina and clitoris in women. Nitric oxide enters into vascular smooth muscle cells, causing an increase in the production of cyclic guanosine monophosphate (cGMP). As cGMP concentrations rise, vascular smooth muscle relaxes, allowing increased arterial blood flow. The cGMP build-up is countered by the enzyme phosphodiesterase type 5 (PDE-5). Inhibiting the action of PDE-5 results in higher levels of cGMP, causing increased and sustained vasodilatation. Arousal disorders appear to increase with age, but it is unclear whether age alone versus associated illnesses, medication, or lifestyle factors contributes. DHEAS and testosterone levels decline with age and may have an indirect negative affect on the sexual response cycle (SRC) for men and women by its association with nitric oxide (NO).

Clinical Findings

A. SYMPTOMS AND SIGNS

The history is the most important part of the evaluation. The provider should ensure that arousal problems are the primary problem. Some men may complain of erectile difficulties but on detailed questioning may not be experiencing erections due to lack of desire or many may not be able to sustain the erection due to premature ejaculation. Detailed information on the onset, duration, progression, severity, and association with medical conditions, medications, and psychosocial factors will enable the provider to determine if the etiology is primarily organic or pyschogenic.

The physical examination should be focused and directed by the history. It is necessary to assess overall health, including life-style topics such as exercise, tobacco use, and alcohol use, and, additionally, to screen for manifestations of affective, cardiovascular, neurological, or hormonal etiology.

B. LABORATORY FINDINGS

If not previously done, basic studies, such as a lipid profile and fasting blood sugar, should be considered to identify unrecognized systemic disease that may predispose to vascular disease. Most authorities recommend endocrine assessment with a morning testosterone. Assessing DHEAS levels should be considered, particularly if androgen supplementation is being considered.

Treatment

Chronic medical conditions should be treated or controlled to reverse or slow the progression of associated conditions. If medications such as antihypertensive agents are contributing to arousal problems, the provider should reduce the dose, replace it with an alternative agent less likely to cause arousal problems, or continue with the agent and treat the sexual dysfunction. Potentially reversible causes should be addressed. If there is evidence of hypogonadism, testosterone supplementation should be considered as previously discussed.

Maximizing glucose control in diabetics, encouraging exercise, and smoking cessation are important lifestyle changes necessary to enhance arousal. Nitric oxide appears to be androgen sensitive, so correcting androgens might be critical before PDE-5 inhibitors will be successful. Vaginal lubricants such as astroglide, Replens, and KY jelly can be helpful not only in adding lubrication but also in enhancing sensuality.

A. ORAL AGENTS

Sildenafil is currently the only PDE-5 inhibitor approved for the treatment of male erectile dysfunction. Two additional agents (vardenafil and tadalafil) are soon likely to be approved. PDE-5 inhibitors do not result in spontaneous erection and require physical stimulation to be maximally effective. They have demonstrated effectiveness in both organic and psychogenic causes of erectile dysfunction. PDE-5 inhibitors are contraindicated in any patient taking organic nitrates (nitric oxide donors) of any type. The concomitant use of a PDE-5 inhibitor and a nitrate can result in profound hypotension. PDE-5 inhibitors are also contraindicated in patients with recent cardiovascular events and patients who are clinically hypotensive.

The side effects of PDE-5 inhibitors are related to the presence of PDE-5 in other parts of the body and to cross-reactivity with other PDE enzyme subtypes. A transient disturbance in color vision characterized typically by a greenish-blue hue is due to a slight cross-reactivity with PDE-5 isoenzyme in the retina. Because of this cross-reactivity, sildenafil should not be used in patients with retinitis pigmentosa. The most common side effects of sildenafil include headache, flushing, dyspepsia, and rhinitis. These symptoms are usually mild and transient.

Sildenafil is not approved by the Food and Drug Administration for use in women. Studies evaluating its effectiveness have resulted in mixed findings. Caruso et al reported significant effectiveness in improving arousal and orgasm in a group of young premenopausal women affected with arousal disorder. The frequency of sexual fantasies, sexual intercourse, and enjoyment improved. In postmenopausal women treated with sildenafil there was much less improvement. It is likely that PDE-5 inhibitors will have a role in treating female arousal disorder.

B. VACUUM CONSTRICTION DEVICES

These devices are effective for most causes of erectile dysfunction, are noninvasive, and are a relatively inexpensive treatment option. The device consists of a cylinder, vacuum pump, and constriction band. The flaccid penis is placed in the cylinder. Pressing the cylinder against the skin of the perineum forms an airtight seal. Negative pressure from the pump draws blood into the penis, resulting in increased firmness. When sufficient blood has entered the erectile bodies, a constriction band is placed around the base of the penis, preventing the escape of blood. Following intercourse the band is removed. Side effects include penile pain, bruising, numbness, and impaired ejaculation.

C. INTRACAVERNOSAL INJECTION

With this method, synthetic formulations of prostaglandin E1 (alprostadil alone or in combination with other vasoactive agents) are injected directly into the corpus cavernosum. This results in spontaneous erection. Intracavernosal injection is effective in producing erection in most patients with erectile dysfunction, including some who failed to respond to oral therapy.

D. PENILE PROSTHESIS

In patients not responding to other therapies, a permanent penile prosthesis has proven to be safe and effective. Current models have a 7–10 year life expectancy or longer. Overall patient satisfaction is excellent.

Caruso S et al: Premenopausal women affected by sexual arousal disorder treated with sildenafil: a double blind, cross-over, placebo-controlled study. Br J Gynecol 2001;108:623.

Guay A et al: Efficacy and safety of sildenafil citrate for treatment of erectile dysfunction in a population with associated organic risk factors. J Androl 2001;22(5):793.

Lue T: Erectile dysfunction. New Engl J Med 2000;342(24):1802.

SEXUAL PAIN SYNDROMES

Sexual pain syndromes can negatively affect arousal for both men and women. Sexual pain syndromes are estimated in 14% of women and 3% of men in the general population, and over 70% of samples of female patients. Peyronnie's or other penile deformity, priapism, and lower urinary tract symptoms can be etiologic in male sexual pain syndrome. For women, vaginitis, vestibulitis, pelvic pathology, vaginismus, and inadequate vaginal lubrication are among the etiologies of sexual pain syndromes for women. Sexual pain syndromes negatively feedback for both desire and arousal phases of the SRC.

DISORDERS OF ORGASM & EJACULATION

Premature ejaculation (PE) is the most common sexual dysfunction for men, affecting 29% of men in the general population. The inability to have an orgasm affects 8% of men and 24% of women in the general population. Over 80% of women in patient populations report difficulties with orgasm.

PE results from a shortened plateau phase of the SRC. In addition to heightened sensitivity to erotic stimulation and often learned behavior from rushed sexual encounters, there may be a possible organic etiology to PE. Although in general PE tends to improve with age by the natural lengthening of the plateau phase of the SRC, PE persists well into aging for many men, giving further support to the organic etiology theory. PE, like ED, is often associated with shame and depression.

Difficulty or inability to orgasm affects a greater number of women than men, and is the result of a prolonged arousal phase, typically from inadequate stimulation by self or partner. Medications can also interfere with these phases of the SRC. Selective serotonin reuptake inhibitors (SSRIs) raise the threshold for orgasm, which makes them highly effective treatment options for men with PE, but highly problematic for both genders who have difficulty having orgasm. Medications that lower the threshold for orgasm can be very problematic for the man with PE but can be very effective for treating problems with orgasm. These include periactin, bupropion, and possibly sildenafil. These agents can be helpful for men with delayed ejaculation (DE)—commonly called retarded ejaculation—which affects 8% of men in the general population. Medications, particularly psychotropic agents, and alcohol use can often be etiologic. Medications used as rescue agents to treat sexual side effects of psychotropic agents or to lower the threshold for orgasm in women having difficulty with orgasm are also useful for treating DE (Table 18–10).

In retrograde ejaculation (RE) the seminal fluid is ejaculated from the posterior urethra into the bladder. This can result from an abnormal function of the internal sphincter of the urethra, from an anatomical disruption such as transurethral prostatectomy, from sympathetic nervous system disruptions, such as damage from surgery, lymph node invasion, or diabetes, from interference with sphincter function from medications such as antipsychotics, antidepressants, and antihypertensive agents, as well as from alcohol use. Dextroamphetamine, ephedrine, phenylpropanolamine, and pseudoephedrine have been found to be effective in treating RE.

Evaluation should include a history of sexual problems, medications, and quality of the relationship. Treatment approaches to difficulty with orgasm can include discontinuing, decreasing the dosage of, or drug holidays for offending medications. Small studies show benefit from rescue agents that can be added as a standing or as-needed medication (Table 18–10). SSRIs, the treatment of choice for PE, are also used as a standing or as-needed basis. Additionally, it will be helpful if

Table 18–10. Antidotes for psychotropic-induced sexual dysfunction.

Drug	Dosage
Yohimbine	5.4–16.2 mg, 2–4 h prior to sexual activity
Bupropion	100 mg as needed or 75 mg three times daily
Amantadine	100–400 mg as needed or daily
Cyproheptadine	2–16 mg a few hours before sexual activity
Bethanechol	10–40 mg prior to sex or 30–100 mg daily
Pemoline	18.75 mg daily
Methylphenidate	5–25 mg as needed
Dextroamphetamine	5 mg sublingually 1 h prior to sex
Nefazodone	150 mg 1 h prior to sex
Sildenafil	50–100 mg as needed

From Nusbaum MRH: *Sexual Health.* American Academy of Family Physicians, 2001 and Maurice W: Ejaculation/orgasm disorders. In: *Sexual Medicine in Primary Care.* Mosby, 1999: p 192.

women become familiar with themselves and with what stimulation they require for orgasm and communicate this to their partners. An excellent reference for patients is the book *Becoming Orgasmic.*

The resolution phase is typically not problematic for either gender but misunderstandings of age-related changes can occur. Men need to understand that with increasing age the refractory period—a period of time where no genital response to sexual stimulation is possible—lengthens, sometimes up to 24 h. Additionally, men and their partners need to know that men might require more direct penile stimulation for sexual response as they age.

Heiman JR, LoPicolo J: *Becoming Orgasmic: A Sexual & Personal Growth Program for Women.* Prentice Hall, 1988.

SEXUAL ACTIVITY & CARDIOVASCULAR RISK

Sexual activity and intercourse are associated with physiological changes in heart rate and blood pressure. A patient's ability to meet the physiological demands related to sexual activity should be assessed, particularly if the patient is not accustomed to the level of activity associated with sex or may be at increased risk of a cardiovascular event. Typical sexual intercourse is associated with an oxygen expenditure of 3–4 metabolic equivalents (METS) whereas vigorous sexual intercourse can expend 5–6 METS. Patients unaccustomed to the level of exercise with sexual activity who have risk factors for cardiovascular events present a clinical challenge. An algorithm based on expert opinion has been developed to assist clinicians in determining which patients can be safely advised that sexual activity and treatment can be undertaken without further risk stratification and which need further evaluation. In this algorithm patients are classified as low risk if they have fewer than three risk factors (age, hypertension, diabetes, obesity, cigarette smoking, dyslipidemias, and sedentary lifestyle). Patients in the intermediate risk group should undergo risk stratification into either the low-risk or high-risk group. This assessment may include cardiac stress testing.

Debusk R et al: Management of sexual dysfunction in patients with cardiovascular disease: recommendations of the Princeton consensus panel. Am J Cardiol 2000;86(2):175.

Cardiovascular Disease

19

Stephen A. Wilson, MD[1]

General Considerations

Cardiovascular disease (CVD), synonymous with coronary artery disease (CAD) and coronary heart disease (CHD), is a condition that affects the coronary arteries, which supply oxygenated blood to the heart muscle and enable it continually to perform—resting only between beats—its life-sustaining task of pumping oxygenated, nutrient-rich blood to the entire body. It is the result of multifactorial and complex depository and reactive processes that lead to atheromatous narrowing, inflammation, and subsequent occlusion of the coronary arteries; the inflammatory process involves vascular cell walls, monocytes, T-lymphocytes, proinflammatory cytokines, chemoattractant cytokines (chemokines), and growth factors. Coronary artery occlusion can lead to angina (chest pain or pressure), myocardial ischemia, myocardial infarction, and eventually death if blood flow is not restored in a manner timely and adequate enough to supply the demands of the body upon the heart. This is a treatable, delayable, if not preventable, disease.

The epidemiology of cardiovascular disease is presented in Tables 19–1, 19–2, and 19–3.

Grech ED: Pathophysiology and investigation of coronory artery disease. Br Med J 2003;306:1027.

Saadeddin SM, Habbab MA, Ferns GA: Markers of inflammation and coronary artery disease. Med Sci Monit 2002;8(1):RA5.

Pathogenesis

Atherosclerotic disease is the thickening and hardening (loss of elasticity) of the arterial wall due to the accumulations of lipids, macrophages, T-lymphocytes, smooth muscle cells, extracellular matrix, calcium, and necrotic debris. These multiple components and other circum-

stances (eg, diet, exercise, smoking), each with varying levels of contribution that are different for each person, interact to result in CAD: nature (genetics) meets nurture (environment) and they responsively interrelate (Table 19–4).

A. GENETIC PREDISPOSITION

Animal models and family and twin studies contribute to our understanding of a genetic predisposition to CAD. The best indicator of predisposition to CAD is a family history of CAD. Genes affect the development and progression of disease and its response to risk factor modification and life-style decisions. Inherited cardiovascular risk factors, such as low-density lipoprotein (LDL) cholesterol, homocysteine, and lipoprotein (a), [LP(a)], can be modified. There is currently a lack of information on how to use data on genetic predisposition to prevent clinical events, or if early detection in such individuals leads to improved morbidity and mortality.

B. ATHEROSCLEROSIS PROGRESSION

Foam cells, found within the intima of 45% of infants, are monocyte-derived macrophages that migrate into the arterial intima and ingest lipids. Fatty streaks are accumulated foam cells plus lipid droplets extracellular to and within smooth muscle cells. They have been found in 65% of 12–14 year olds. Microatheromas are fatty streaks with a cap of smooth muscle cells and collagen. They progress at variable rates. A mature plaque is composed of two components: the lipid core and its fibrous capsules, a connective tissue matrix. The lipid core is mainly released from necrotic foam cells. The connective tissue matrix derives from smooth muscle cells, which migrate from the media into the intima, where they proliferate and form a fibrous capsule around the lipid core (Figures 19–1 and 19–2).

Our understanding of the role of immune and inflammatory responses in this process is expanding. Oxygen-free radicals oxidize, bind with, and alter other molecules. This is a normal bodily occurrence. However, some environmental toxins, such as smoke, pro-

[1]Special thanks and appreciation to Amy Haugh, Head of Library Science, UPMC St. Margaret Hospital, and Paula Preisach, UPMC St. Margaret Faculty Development Fellowship. Their assistance was timely, necessary, and indispensable.

Table 19–1. Epidemiology of cardiovascular disease.

Afflicts 7–12 million Americans[1,2]

Leading cause of death and premature disability for both men and women in the United States[1,3]

Of women almost 50% die of CAD or stroke versus ~4% of breast cancer[4]

Prevalence increases with age (Table 19–2) but 8% of cases are diagnosed before age 50[1]

Those of Hispanic origin have a lower death rate from CHD than non-Hispanics[2]

Kills more men than women and more blacks than whites (Table 19–3)

80% of CHD deaths occur in those over 65 years old; CHD is the leading cause of death in this group

Annual mortality rate is 3–4%

Risk factors[5]

  Male sex, in particular, males >45 years old

  Females who are postmenopausal or >55 years old

  Diabetes mellitus

  Hypertension (systolic and diastolic are independent risk factors)

  Smoking; the increased risk abates after 3 years cessation

  Low high-density lipoprotein (HDL) [<35 mg/dL (<0.91 mmol/L)], especially in women

  High low-density lipoprotein (LDL) (>130 mg/dL)

  Left ventricular hypertrophy

  Homocysteine elevation; methylene tetrahydrofolate reductase (MTHFR)

    $677C \rightarrow T$ genotype

  C-reactive protein (CRP) elevation on high-sensitivity CRP test (hs-CRP)

  Obesity

  Lipoprotein—Lp(a)

  Family history of CAD

  Sedentary/physical inactivity

  Excessive alcohol intake

Protective factors[5]

  Exercise

  Moderate alcohol use (two drinks/day for men; one drink/day for women)[6]

  High HDL [>60 mg/dL (>1.55 mmol/L)]

---

[1]http://www.nhlbi.gov/health/public/heart/other/chdfacts.html.

[2]Center for Disease Control: Mortality from coronary heart disease acute myocardial infarction—United States, 1998. MMWR 2001; 50(06):90.

[3]American Heart Association: *2001 Heart and Stroke Statistical Update.* American Heart Association, 2000.

[4]Brown KS: Heart disease: women's unique risks demand attention. Ann Intern Med 1997;127:952.

[5]Link N, Tanner M: Coronary artery disease: Part 1. Epidemiology and diagnosis. West J Med 2001;174:257.

[6]One drink = 0.5 oz or 15 mL ethanol: 12 oz beer, 5 oz wine, or 1.5 oz 80-proof whiskey.

Table 19–2. Age-specific death rates[1] for coronary heart disease[2] and acute myocardial infarction[3]—United States, 1998.

Age Group (Years)	Coronary Heart Disease	
	No.	**Rate**
<25	160	0.2
25–34	936	2.4
35–44	6,535	14.7
45–54	20,165	58.3
55–64	40,968	180.7
65–74	89,625	487.2
75–84	149,668	1,252.2
≥85	151,765	3,743.9

Source: Center for Disease Control: Mortality from coronary heart disease and acute myocardial infarction—United States, 1998. MMMR 2001;50(06):90.

[1]Per 100,000 population.

[2]International Classification of Diseases, Ninth Revision, codes 410.0–414.9.

[3]Code 410.

duce excess amounts. LDLs, which carry cholesterol, are oxidized by free radicals in the arterial linings, resulting in the deposition of mushy atheromatous oxidized cholesterol. As this accumulates the immune system is triggered to relax white blood cells, especially neutrophils and macrophages. This immune response triggers an inflammatory response. Macrophages come and ingest oxidized cholesterol because it is recognized as foreign debris. These become the foam cells described above that eventually attach to the smooth muscle cells and harden into formed plaque (Figures 19–1 and 19–2). The immune system then responds by releasing cytokines, which attract more white blood cells and perpetuate the cycle.

The injured endothelial lining cannot produce enough nitric oxide, a vasodilator critical for helping maintain blood vessel elasticity. This all combines to produce hardened arteries that progressively narrow. When, between plaque accumulation and decreased elasticity, a >50% diameter stenosis, which equals a 75% decrease in cross-sectional area, occurs, CAD often becomes symptomatic with exertion. As demand outstrips supply ability, chest pain (angina) may occur.

Damage to the endothelium is important because the endothelium

1. Provides a high selective permeability barrier that contains LDL receptors.

2. Is a nonthrombogenic surface that (a) secretes prostaglandin I_2, a potent vasodilator and in-

Table 19–3. Age-adjusted death rates[1] for coronary heart disease[2] and acute myocardial infarction[3] for persons ages ≥35 years, by sex and race/ethnicity—United States, 1998.

Sex	Coronary Heart Disease		Acute Myocardial Infarction	
	No.	Rate	No.	Rate
Men				
White	209,457	440.0	95,617	196.7
Black	19,138	421.6	9,185	198.7
Hispanic	8,431	285.4	3,735	121.6
Asian/Pacific Islander	3,247	258.3	1,417	109.1
American Indian/Alaska Native	750	246.7	377	120.9
Women				
White	202,056	263.8	85,248	113.2
Black	21,202	301.9	9,873	140.4
Hispanic	7,602	189.8	3,102	76.7
Asian/Pacific Islander	2,259	148.1	607	62.2
American Indian/Alaska Native	617	160.2	268	69.3

Source: Center for Disease Control: Mortality from coronary heart disease and acute myocardial infarction—United States, 1998. MMMR 2001;50(06):90.
[1]Per 100,000 population. Standardized to the 2000 U.S. Bureau of Census population of persons aged ≥35 years.
[2]International Classification of Disease, Ninth Revision, codes 410.0–414.0.
[3]Code 410.

hibitor of platelet aggregation; (b) secretes plasminogen, which is crucial for fibrinolysis; and is (c) coated with heparan sulfate, a heparin-like substance that binds antithrombin III, an inhibitor of coagulation.

3. Can be procoagulant by secreting von Willebrand factor (vWF), which is necessary for platelet adherence to the vessel wall.

4. Secretes nitric oxide (previously called EDRF—endothelium-derived relaxing factor), a potent vasodilator involved in the homeostasis of arterial dilation and contraction.

5. Interacts with platelets, monocytes, macrophages, T-lymphocytes, and smooth muscle cells via various cytokines and growth factors.

The mechanism of coronary artery thrombosis is depicted in Figure 19–3.

Table 19–4. Genetic and environmental influences on CAD predisposition.[1]

Gene–Environment Interaction	Favorable Genes	Unfavorable Genes
Favorable environment	Low risk	Moderate risk
Unfavorable environment	Moderate risk	High risk

Source: Scheuner MT: Genetic predisposition to coronary artery disease. Curr Opin Cardiol 2001;16:251.
[1]The manifestation of coronary artery disease (CAD) is caused by the interaction of several unfavorable genetic and environmental factors. Those with the greatest number of genetic and environmental risk factors will face the highest risks. Those with favorable genotypes might not develop CAD despite substantial environmental risk factors. Conversely, those with favorable environmental factors might develop CAD given the presence of unfavorable genetic factors.

Chasen CA, Muller JE: Triggers of myocardial infarction. Cardiol Special Ed 1997;3:57.

Grech ED: Pathophysiology and investigation of coronary artery disease. Br Med J 2003;326:1027.

Scheuner MT: Genetic predisposition to coronary artery disease. Curr Opin Cardiol 2001;16:251.

Worthley SG et al: Coronary artery disease: pathogenesis and acute coronary syndromes. Mt. Sinai J Med 2001;68(3):167.

Prevention

CAD is a delayable, if not preventable, condition. Prevention targets risk factors and attempts to positively impact the modifiable. *Primary prevention* is an attempt to prevent disease before it develops (Table 19–5). *Secondary prevention* is an attempt to prevent disease progression by identifying and treating a symptomatic person who already has risk factors or preclinical disease

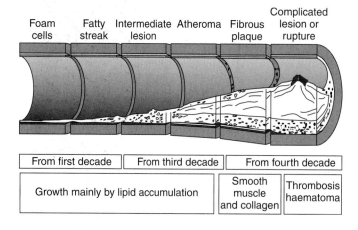

Figure 19–1. Atheromatous plaque progression. (From Grech ED: Pathophysiology and investigation of coronary artery disease. Br Med J 2003;326:1027.)

but not clinically manifested disease. *Tertiary prevention* is treatment of established disease to restore and maintain highest function, minimize negative disease effects, and prevent complications. There are many risk factors for CAD (Table 19–6). The more risk factors present in an individual, the greater the risk of developing and dying of CAD and its sequelae.

Primary prevention of CAD should begin in childhood by discouraging tobacco use and by risk reduction education (ie, diet and exercise), which should be for the whole family. Individual risk factors should be screened and assessed regularly and individuals should be encouraged to pursue a healthy diet, an active exercise regimen, and weight control [body mass index (BMI) = 18.5–25 kg/m^2], and to discontinue use of tobacco.

Secondary and tertiary prevention involves progressively more aggressive management of those with known CAD (Figure 19–4 and Table 19–7). It is important to note that the association between cholesterol

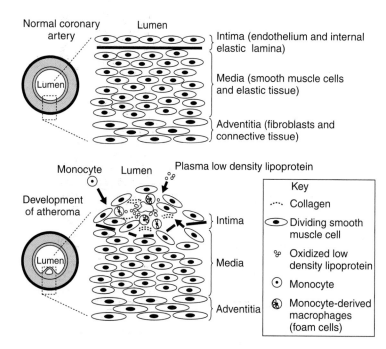

Figure 19–2. Mechanism of plaque development. (From Grech ED: Pathophysiology and investigation of coronary artery disease. Br Med J 2003;326:1027.)

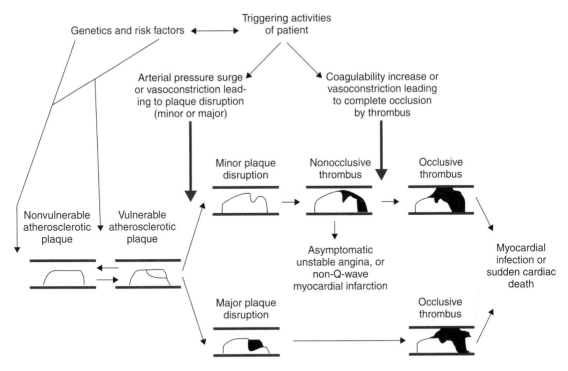

Figure 19–3. Mechanism of coronary artery thrombosis.
Hypothetical methods of possible trigger for coronary thrombosis: (1) physical or mental stress leads to hemodynamic changes leads to plaque rupture; (2) activities causing an increase in coagulability; and (3) stimuli leading to vasoconstriction. The role of coronary thrombosis in unstable angina, MI, and sudden cardiac death has been well described. (From Muller JE et al: Triggers, acute risk factors and vulnerable plaques: the lexicon of a new frontier. J Am Coll Cardiol 1994;23:809. Reprinted with permission from the American College of Cardiology. Chasen CA, Muller JE: Triggers of myocardial infarction. Cardiol Special Ed 1997;3:57.)

and CHD death is weaker in the elderly (>65 years old) than in younger patients. Still, statin treatment, compared to placebo, is beneficial and positively impacts morbidity and mortality.

In contrast to prior observational data, recent prospective, randomized, double-blind, placebo-controlled trials indicate that there is no role for hormone replacement therapy (HRT), which may cause harm, in prevention. Estrogen plus progestin HRT should not be initiated or continued as a form of primary, secondary, or tertiary prevention of CAD. Questions and doubts have been raised concerning the value of the antioxidants vitamins C and E in prevention of CHD.

Grady D et al: Cardiovascular disease outcomes during 6.8 years of hormone therapy. JAMA 2002;288(1):49.

Grech ED: Pathophysiology and investigation of coronary artery disease. Br Med J 2003;326:1027.

Grundy SM et al: Guide to primary prevention of cardiovascular diseases: a statement for healthcare professionals from the task force on risk reduction. Circulation 1997;95(9):2329.

Krantz DS et al: Effects of mental stress in patients with coronary artery disease. JAMA 2000;283(14):1800.

Waters DD et al: Effects of hormone replacement therapy and antioxidant vitamin supplementation on coronary atherosclerosis in postmenopausal women. JAMA 2002;288:2432.

Writing Group for the Women's Health Intitiative Investigators: Risks and benefits of estrogen plus progestin in healthy postmenopausal women. JAMA 2002;288:321.

Clinical Findings

A. Symptoms and Signs

CAD often remains clinically unsuspected until angina occurs. Because one-third of people with CAD progress to myocardial infarction (MI) without experiencing chest pain, it is important to be knowledgeable of other

Table 19–5. Guide to primary prevention of cardiovascular disease.[1]

Risk Intervention	Recommendations	
Smoking Goal Complete cessation	Ask about smoking status as part of routine evaluation. Reinforce nonsmoking status. Strongly encourage patient and family to stop smoking. Provide counseling, bupropion therapy, nicotine replacement, and formal cessation programs as appropriate.	

Blood pressure control
Goal
  ≤140/90 mm Hg
  Optimal: 115/75
	Measure blood pressure in all adults at least every 2½ years. Promote life-style modifications: weight control, physical activity, moderation in alcohol intake, moderate sodium restriction. If blood pressure ≥140/90 mm Hg after 3 months of life habit modification or if initial blood pressure >160/100 mm Hg: add blood pressure medication; individualize therapy to patient's other requirements and characteristics.	

Cholesterol management
Primary goal
  LDL <160 mg/dL if 0–1 risks or
  LDL <130 mg/dL if ≥2 risks
 	
Secondary goals
  HDL >35 mg/dL
  TG <200 mg/dL
	Ask about dietary habits as part of routine evaluation. Measure total and HDL cholesterol in all adults ≥20 years and assess positive and negative risk factors at least every 5 years. Promote AHA Step 1 diet (≤30% fat, <10% saturated fat, <300 mg/day cholesterol), weight control, and physical activity.
	
	Measure LDL if total cholesterol ≥200 mg/dL or ≥200 mg/dL with ≥2 risk factors or if HDL <35 mg/dL.	

	If LDL
	  ≥160 mg/dL with 0–1 risk factors or
	  ≥130 mg/dL on two occasions with ≥2 risk factors; then
	  Start Step II diet (≤30% fat, <7% saturated fat, <200 mg/dL cholesterol) and weight control.
	  Rule out secondary causes of high LDL (LFTs, TFTs, UA).
	
	If LDL
	  ≥160 mg/dL plus 2 risk factors or
	  ≥190 mg/dL; or
	  ≥220 mg/dL in men <35 years; or in premenopausal women; then
	Consider adding drug therapy to diet therapy for LDL levels greater than those listed above that persist despite Step II diet.
		Risk factors: age (men ≥45, years women ≥55 years or postmenopausal), hypertension, diabetes, smoking, HDL <35 mg/dL, family history of CHD in first-degree relatives (in male relatives <55 years, female relatives <65 years), HDL ≥60 mg/dL: Subtract 1 risk factor from the number of positive risk factors.

	Suggested drug therapy for high LDL levels (≥160 mg/dL) (drug selection priority modified according to TG level)	

TG <200 mg/dL	TG 200–400 mg/dL	TG >400 mg/dL	HDL <35 mg/dL
Statin Resin Niacin	Statin Niacin	Consider combined drug therapy (niacin, fibrates, statin)	Emphasize weight management and physical activity, avoidance of cigarette smoking. Niacin raises HDL. Consider niacin if patient has ≥2 risk factors and high LDL (except patients with diabetes).

If LDL goal not achieved, consider combination drug therapy.	

(continued)

Table 19–5. Guide to primary prevention of cardiovascular disease.[1] (Continued)

Risk Intervention	Recommendation

Physical activity
Goal
  Increase amount of exercise
  regularly to 3–4 times
  per week for 30 min
	Ask about physical activity status and exercise habits as part of routine evaluation.
	Encourage 30 min of moderate-intensity dynamic exercise 3 to 4 times per week as well as increased physical activity in daily life habits for persons who are inactive.
	Encourage regular exercise to improve conditioning and optimize fitness level.
	Advise medically supervised programs for those with low functional capacity and/or comorbidities.
	Promote environmental factors conducive to health (ie, golf courses that permit walking).

Weight management
Goal
  Achieve and maintain
  desirable weight (BMI
  18.5–25 kg/m²)
	Measure patient's weight and height, BMI, and waist-to-hip ratio at each visit as part of routine evaluation.
	Start weight management and physical activity as appropriate. Desirable BMI range: 18.5–25 kg/m².
	BMI of 25 kg/m2 corresponds to percentage desirable body weight of 110%; desirable waist-to-hip ratio for men, <0.9: for middle-aged and elderly women, <0.8.

Source: Grundy SM et al: Guide to primary prevention of cardiovascular diseases. A statement for healthcare professionals from the Task Force on Risk Reduction. Circulation 1997;95:2329 (with modifications).
[1]TG, triglycerides; LFTs, liver function tests; TFTs, thyroid function tests; UA, uric acid; CHD, coronary heart disease; BMI, body mass index.

Table 19–6. Risk factors for coronary artery disease.

Nonmodifiable/uncontrollable
  Male sex
  Age
    Men ≥45 years old
    Women ≥55 years old or postmenopausal
  Positive family history of CAD
Modifiable with demonstrated morbidity and mortality benefits
  Hypertension
  Dyslipidemia
  Smoking
  Diabetes mellitus
  Overweight and obesity
  Sedentary/physical inactivity
  Excessive alcohol intake[1]
Potentially modifiable but no demonstrated mortality and morbidity effects of treatment
  Stress
  Depression
  Hypertriglyceridemia
  Renin
  C-reactive protein
  Uric acid
  Lp(a) lipoprotein
  Fibrinogen
  Infection (*Chlamydia pneumoniae*)

[1]Two drinks (ie, 1 oz or 30 mL ethanol: eg, 24 oz beer, 10 oz wine, or 3 oz 80-proof whiskey) per day in most men and no more than one drink per day in women and lighter weight persons.

symptoms of disease. There are a variety of symptom descriptors the patient may relate:

- Dull, heavy pressure in or on the chest.
- Sensation of a heavy object on the chest.
- Pain that radiates to the back, neck, jaw, left arm, or shoulder.
- Accompanying diaphoresis.
- Pain initiated by stress, exercise, large meals, or anything that increases the body's demand upon the heart.
- Shortness of breath. This can be the only sign in the elderly, is more common in black than in white patients, and is more common in women than in men.
- Left-sided chest pain. This is more common in black patients.
- Levine's sign—discomfort described as a clenched fist over the sternum.
- Angor Anami—great fear of impending doom or death.
- Pain high in the abdomen or chest, nausea, extreme fatigue after exercise, back pain, and edema. These are all more common in women.
- Less commonly there is mild, burning chest discomfort, sharp chest pain, pain that radiates to the right arm or back, or an urge to defecate.

B. LABORATORY FINDINGS

Asymptomatic CAD is likely to be absent of laboratory findings. Total cholesterol, LDLc, or triglyceride levels may be elevated and HDLc levels may be reduced. Ta-

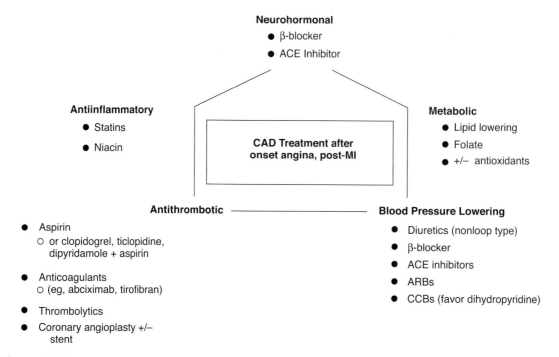

Figure 19–4. Tertiary prevention for CAD. ACE, angiotensin-converting enzyme; ARB, angiotensin receptor blocker; CCB, calcium channel blocker; MI, myocardial infarction.

bles 19–5 and 19–7 address CAD stage-specific approaches to these. Homocysteine and high-sensitivity C-reactive protein (hs-CRP) can be elevated. However, there is no evidence that implementing treatments to lower these leads to improved morbidity and mortality. Currently, markers of inflammation such as Lp(a), fibrinogen, interleukin-1, interleukin-6, tumor necrosis factor-α, chemokines, and serum amyloid A are considered to be nonspecific or without a reproducible diagnostic test assay. Furthermore, it is still undetermined whether markers of inflammation have a causal relationship with CVD, or if they merely reflect the underlying disease. Symptomatic CAD may present with elevations in myocardial-specific creatine kinase or troponin levels.

C. Imaging Studies, Special Tests, and Examinations

Tests for CVD can be classified as noninvasive and invasive.

1. Noninvasive tests—Noninvasive tests include chest radiography (CXR), electrocardiography (ECG), cardiac stress testing, echocardiography (ECHO), radionuclide myocardial perfusion imaging, magnetic resonance imaging (MRI), and electron-beam computed topography (EBCT).

CXR is usually normal in patients without prior heart disease.

ECG may show evidence of prior infarction. When abnormal it increases suspicion of CAD, but a normal ECG does not exclude CAD. Many findings are nonspecific and 25–50% of people with angina or silent ischemia have a normal ECG. The presence of bundle branch block, interventricular conduction delay, or Wolff–Parkinson–White syndrome further reduces the diagnostic reliability of an ECG.

In *cardiac stress testing,* the stress may be achieved through exercise or chemical means. Exercise is the preferred method, but chemicals can be used when the patient is not able to exercise enough to produce a test adequate for interpretation. Dobutamine increases myocardial contraction and heart rate. Dipyrimadole and adenosine dilate coronary arterioles. They are the most common chemicals used and have similar prognostic and diagnostic value. Life-threatening events are rare, ~1/500 for the former and ~1/1000 for the latter.

Exercise electrocardiography is the main test for evaluating those with suspected angina or heart disease. While connected to an ECG patients walk on a treadmill or ride a stationary bicycle until the heart rate is 85% of the maximum rate or there is angina, dysrhythmia, or fatigue. The test is interpreted in terms of

Table 19–7. Guide to comprehensive risk reduction for patients with coronary artery disease.

Risk Intervention	Recommendation

Smoking
  Goal
    complete cessation
	Strongly encourage patient and family to stop smoking.
	Provide counseling, nicotine replacement, and formal cessation programs as appropriate.

Lipids
  Primary goal
    LDL <100 mg/dL
  Secondary goals
    HDL >35 mg/dL
    TG <200 mg/dL
	Start AHA Step II diet in all patients (30% fat, <200 mg/day cholesterol).
	Assess fasting lipid profile. In post-MI patients, lipid profile may take 4–6 weeks to stabilize. Add drug therapy according to the following:

LDL <100 mg/dL No drug therapy	LDL 100–130 mg/dL Consider adding drug therapy to diet, as follows:		LDL >130 mg/dL Add drug therapy to diet, as follows:	HDL <35 mg/dL Emphasize weight management and physical activity. Advise smoking cessation. If needed to achieve LDL goals, consider niacin, statin, fibrates.
	Statins as first-line suggestion drug therapy			
	TG <200 mg/dL	TG 200–400 mg/dL	TG >400 mg/dL	
	Statin Resin Niacin	Statin Niacin	Consider combined drug therapy (niacin, fibrates, statin)	
	If LDL goal not achieved, consider combination therapy.			

Risk Intervention	Recommendation
Physical activity Minimum goal 30 min three to four times per week	Assess risk, preferably with exercise test, to guide prescription. Encourage minimum of 30–60 min of moderate-intensity activity three to four times weekly (walking, jogging, cycling, or other aerobic activity) supplemented by an increase in daily life-style activities (eg, walking breaks at work, using stairs, gardening, household work). Maximum benefit 5–6 h a week. Advise medically supervised programs for moderate- to high-risk patients.
Weight management	Start intensive diet and appropriate physical activity intervention, as outlined above, in patients >120% of ideal weight for height. Particularly emphasize need for weight loss in patients with hypertension, elevated triglycerides, or elevated glucose levels; ideal BMI: 18.5–25 kg/m^2.
Antiplatelet agents/ anticoagulants	Start aspirin 80–325 mg/day if not contraindicated. Manage warfarin to international normalized ratio = 2–3.5 for post-MI patients not able to take or fails aspirin, then consider ticlopidine, clopidogrel, or dipyridamole + aspirin.
ACE inhibitors Post-MI	Start early post-MI in stable patients, especially those with anterior MI, CHF, renal insufficiency, EF <40% (LV dysfunction). Maximize dose as tolerated indefinitely. Use as needed to manage blood pressure or symptoms in all other patients.
β-Blockers	For all patients, especially post-MI, as tolerated.
Estrogens	Limited, if any, role. More evidence of harm than help.

Blood pressure
  Control
  Goal
    ≤140/90 mm Hg
Optimal: 115/75
	Initiate life-style modification: weight control, physical activity, alcohol moderation, and moderate sodium restriction in all patients with blood pressure >140 mm Hg systolic or 90 mm Hg diastolic.
	Add blood pressure medication, individualize to other patient requirements and characteristics (ie, age, race, need for drugs with specific benefits) if blood pressure is not less than 140 mm Hg systolic or 90 mm Hg diastolic in 3 months of if initial blood pressure is >160 mm Hg systolic or 100 mm Hg diastolic.

Source: Smith SC Jr et al: AHA consensus panel statement. Preventing heart attack and death in patients with coronary disease. In: *Therapeutic Options for Effective Management of Coronary Artery Disease.* Dedwania PC, Gheorghiade M (editors). American Heart Association, 1999 (modified).
[1]ACE, angiotensin-converting enzyme; MI, myocardial infarction; TG, triglycerides; LV, left ventricular; CHF, congestive heart failure; BMI, body mass index; EF, ejection fraction.

achieved workload, symptoms, and ECG response. This test is less accurate for women, and has a 10% false-positive rate.

Stress echocardiography has a higher sensitivity and specificity than exercise electrocardiography. Stress-induced impairment of myocardial contraction precedes ECG changes and angina.

Radionuclide myocardial perfusion imaging can be added to improve sensitivity, specificity, and accuracy of exercise stress tests. Thallium-201 or technetium-99m (^{99m}Tc-sestamibi, ^{99m}Tc-tetrofosmin) is given intravenously at peak stress; its myocardial distribution relates to coronary flow. Images, acquired with a gamma camera, can distinguish between reversible and irreversible ischemia (the latter signifying infarcted tissue). It is especially useful in patients with a nondiagnostic exercise test or limited exercise ability. Multi-gated acquisition (MUGA) scans can be used to assess left ventricular function and reveal salvageable myocardium in patients with chronic coronary artery disease. They can be performed with either thallium scintigraphy at rest or metabolic imaging with fluorodeoxyglucose by means of either positron emission tomography (PET) or single-photon emission computed tomography (SPECT).

MRI is a nonradioactive method used to provide information on arterial blood flow, including small vessels not accessible or visible to angiography. Because its sensitivity and specificity for detecting CAD plaque do not eclipse the gold standard, its role in the detection of CAD is limited and it does not yet have a justified clinical role.

EBCT is useful to determine the progression and regression of calcium in coronary arteries, but it does not predict which artery will rupture and when. There is also a large amount of test-to-test variability and suboptimal interrater reliability. The Agency for Health Care Research and Quality, American College of Cardiology, and American Heart Association concur that it is promising, but further testing must be done before it can become a recommended tool that impacts clinical outcomes.

2. Invasive tests—Invasive tests include coronary angiography, intravascular ultrasound (IVUS), and Doppler flow wire and pressure wire.

Coronary angiography, the gold standard and absolute method to evaluate CAD, is usually part of cardiac catheterization, which includes left ventricular angiography and hemodynamic measurements, providing a more complete evaluation of an individual's cardiac status. Angiography is expensive and carries risks of death (1 in 1400), stroke (1 in 1000), coronary artery dissection (1 in 1000), arterial access complications (1 in 500), and other more minor risks (arrhythmias,

hematoma, pseudoaneurysm, vagal reaction during the insertion or withdrawal of the catheter, and dye reaction—anaphylactic or renal impairment). Risk is mediated by patient age, coronary anatomy, impaired left ventricular function, valvular heart disease, clinical setting, and noncardiac disease. Indications for angiography are listed in Table 19–8. Ten percent to 30% of them are normal.

Intravascular ultrasound (IVUS) provides a cross-sectional, three-dimensional image of the full circumference of the artery, thereby allowing precise measurement of plaque length and thickness and minimum lumen diameter. Plaque composition can also be described.

Doppler flow wire and pressure wire provide information on the physiological importance of a diseased coronary artery. They are usually used when angiography shows a stenosis that is of intermediate severity, or to determine the functional severity of a residual stenosis after percutaneous coronary intervention. Intracoronary adenosine is used to dilate the distal coronary vessels to maximize coronary flow.

Grech ED: Pathophysiology and investigation of coronary artery disease. Br Med J 2003;3261027.

Lee TH, Boucher CA: Noninvasive tests in patients with stable coronary artery disease. New Engl J Med 2001;344(24):1840.

Saadeddin SM, Habbab MA, Ferns GA: Markers of inflammation and coronary artery disease. Med Sci Monit 2002;8(1):RA5.

The Writing Group for the ACC/AHA Expert Consensus Document: American College of Cardiology/American Heart Asso-

Table 19–8. Main indications for coronary angiography.

Uncertain diagnosis of angina (coronary artery disease cannot be excluded by noninvasive testing)
Assessment of feasibility and appropriateness of various forms of treatment (percutaneous intervention, bypass surgery, medical)
Class I or U stable angina with positive stress test or class III or W angina without positive stress test
Unstable angina or non-Q-wave myocardial infarction (medium- and high-risk patients)
Angina not controlled by drug treatment
Acute myocardial infarction—especially cardiogenic shock, ineligibility for thrombolytic treatment, failed thrombolytic reperfusion, reinfarction, or positive stress test
Life-threatening ventricular arrhythmia
Angina after bypass surgery or percutaneous intervention
Before valve surgery or corrective heart surgery to assess occult coronary artery disease

Source: Grech ED: Pathophysiology and investigation of coronary artery disease. Br Med J 2003;326:1027.

ciation expert consensus document on electron-beam computed tomography for the diagnosis and prognosis of coronary artery disease. Circulation 2000;102(1):126.

Differential Diagnosis

The differential diagnosis for coronary artery disease is given in Table 19–9.

Complications

Complications of CVD include cardiac disability, in which a person's life-style and activity options are diminished because the coronary arteries are unable to supply the heart muscle and therefore the heart is unable to supply the oxygenated blood the body needs to

Table 19–9. Differential diagnosis of CAD.

Prinzmetal's angina (coronary vasospasm)—more common
   in women
Esophagitis
Esophageal spasm
Gastritis
Hiatal hernia
Gastroesophageal reflux disease (GERD)
Peptic ulcer disease (PUD)
Duodenal ulcer
Cholecystitis
Costochondritis
Pleurisy/pleuritis
Pulmonary hypertension
Pulmonary embolus
Pneumothorax
Diaphragmatic irritation/inflammation due to
   Mass effect from nearby cancer
   Infection
   Pancreatitis
   Hepatitis
   Pulmonary edema/effusion
Aortic aneurysm
Aortic dissection
Cardiomyopathy
Supraventricular tachycardia
Pericardial effusion
Cardiac tamponade
Shoulder arthropathy
Radiculopathy
Generalized anxiety disorder (GAD)
Panic attack
Stress reaction/anxiety
Anemia
Hyperthyroidism
High-altitude exposure
Vasculitis

fulfill its demand. Acute coronary syndrome results in angina, myocardial infarction, and death.

Treatment

CAD is a treatable condition that causes myocardial infarction in either of two ways: (1) plaque build-up increases until the artery is totally occluded or (2) an atheromatous plaque ruptures or tears leading to occlusions via inflammatory response and thrombus formation as platelets adhere to the site to seal off the plaque. The superimposition of thrombus upon a disrupted atherosclerotic plaque is more common in the final potential adverse outcomes of CAD—unstable angina pectoris, acute myocardial infarction, and cardiac death.

The goal of treatment is to reduce myocardial oxygen demand and/or to increase oxygen supply. Therapeutic approaches mainly focus upon reducing plaque build-up or reducing thrombotic sequelae by use of antiplatelet, anticoagulant, and thrombolytic therapies. Because many aspects of treatment are the same as those for prevention (Tables 19–5 and 19–7), this section emphasizes the care of persons with acute coronary syndrome (ACS)—a spectrum of increasingly severe conditions, including unstable angina, non-ST segment elevation acute MI, and persistent ST segment elevation acute MI—and the additional therapeutic regimen that best benefits them if they survive (Figure 19–4).

No treatment is of greater importance than blood pressure (BP) control. Although the minimal goal for BP should be <140/90, the optimal goal should be closer to 115/75, because in 40–70 year olds each increment of 20 mm Hg in systolic BP or 10 mm Hg in diastolic BP doubles the risk of CVD across the entire BP range from 115/75 to 185/115 mm Hg. Other concomitant therapies include increasing cardiac or body efficiency in terms of oxygen demand and supply through diet and exercise therapy. Weight loss helps to decrease the demand (less tissue requires a smaller oxygen supply) and exercise can help to lose weight and create a more efficient supplier. Moderate exercise also causes neurohormonal and neurovascular responses that positively affect mortality and morbidity through effects on plaque (formation, degradation, and stabilization) and endothelium at the cellular and molecular levels.

Indications for referral of patients with CVD to cardiology or admission to the hospital include new onset of symptoms, rapidly progressing symptoms, concerns about possible aortic stenosis, questions of exercise capacity, questions regarding work capacity/capability, severe symptoms such as nocturnal angina, angina with minimal exertion, or angina at rest, angina refractory to medical treatment, and clinician uncertainty or unease with patient management.

Patients with ACS should be hospitalized and medically stabilized and should receive, as appropriate, further cardiac evaluation and treatment: consultation, echocardiography, stress testing, or catheterization. Medical management should start with HOBANA—an achronymic guide in which the dosing of each drug is dynamic and subject to the individual patient:

Heparin (low molecular weight or unfractionated)

Oxygen

β-Blocker

Aspirin (325 mg)

Nitroglycerin (sublingual or drip to pain/blood pressure intolerance)

ACE inhibitor

Morphine may be added for pain and anxiety relief. It also provides some afterload reduction. There is an evolving role for platelet glycoprotein IIB/IIIA (GP IIB/IIIA) receptor inhibitors. GP IIB/IIIA receptors are the final common pathway for platelet aggregation and thrombus formation. If the heart is to survive, blood flow must be restored. Some situations, such as infarctions, will require medical thrombolysis or emergent angioplasty to achieve this. Angioplasty, the opening of a clogged coronary artery via insufflating a balloon over a guidewire, is often accompanied by the deployment of a stent used to help keep the artery open and the clot from reforming. Antiplatelet therapy is required after angioplasty.

Revascularization is achieved by bypassing clogged coronary arteries with healthy veins or arteries autologously transplanted to circumnavigate blood flow around the clot. Revascularization by angioplasty or bypass grafting is generally reserved for patients with symptoms such as unstable angina or with involvement of multiple vessels or the left main coronary artery. There is little evidence that revascularization prolongs life in asymptomatic persons.

Jelinek M: The clinical basis for the management of coronary artery disease. Intern Med J 2002;32;11.

JNC 7 Express: The 7th Report of the Joint National Committee on Prevention, Detection, Evaluation and Treatment of High Blood Pressure. NIH Publication No. 03-5233, 2003.

Salam Am, Suwaid JA: Platelet glycoprotein IIb/IIIa antagonists in clinical trial for the treatment of coronary artery disease. Expert Opin Invest Drugs 2002;11(11):1645.

Worthley SG et al: Coronary artery disease: pathogenesis and acute coronary syndromes. Mt. Sinai J Med 2001;68(3):167.

Prognosis

From 1988 to 1998 the death rate from CHD decreased 26%. However, it still remained the number one cause of death for men and women. Case-fatality rates of myocardial infarction patients who reach the hospital and in-hospital total mortality for patients with suspected myocardial infarction have decreased. This reflects primarily advances in care closer to the final stages—use of thrombolytic agents, anticoagulants, angioplasty, β-blockers, cholesterol-lowering agents [mainly hydroxymethylglutaryl coenzyme A (HMG-CoA) reductase inhibitors], aspirin, and angiotensin-converting enzyme inhibitors. Care for the more acutely sick has improved and is increasingly effective. Also, some posit that there is a link between an individual's capacity for coronary angiogenesis, that is, the development of coronary collaterals that circumvent blocked arteries to some degree. Still, CAD remains the number one disease from which people eventually die.

Prognosis for CHD, especially prior to its acute stages, depends upon the willingness and ability of people to adhere to current primary and secondary prevention recommendations. Recent findings indicate that those with the methylene tetrahydrofolate reductase (MTHFR) 677C→T genotype are at increased risk for CHD. Whether these people will benefit from earlier more aggressive therapies, primarily folic acid, will be determined by clinical investigation. However, such findings indicate that there is potential for the ethical application of the discoveries of genetic science to current paradigms for treatment, prevention, and even pathogenesis of CHD. The future seems to hold improved prognosis for those with or predisposed to CAD.

American Heart Association: *2001 Heart and Stroke Statistical Update.* American Heart Association, 2000.

Bata IR et al: Decreasing mortality from acute myocardial infarction: effects of attack rates and case severity. J Clin Epidemiol 1997;50:787.

Centers for Disease Control: MMWR 1997;46:941.

Koerselman J et al: Coronary collaterals: an important and underexposed aspect of coronary artery disease. Circulation 2003; 107:2507.

Tavazzi L, Volpi A: Remarks about post infarction prognosis in light of the experience with the GISSI trials. Circulation 1997;95:1341.

WEB SITES FOR CARDIOVASCULAR DISEASE

American Academy of Family Physicians
http://familydoctor.org
American College of Cardiology
http://www.acc.org
American Heart Association
http://www.americanheart.org
Aspirin Foundation of America
http://www.aspirin.org

Centers for Disease Control

http://www.cdc.gov

Facts about Coronary Artery Disease

http://home.mdconsult.com/das/patient/body/0/10041/5558.html

http://home.mdconsult.com/das/patient/body/0/10062/8281.html

http://www.pajournalcme.com/pajournal/cme/pa004as6.htm

http://www.nhlbi.nih.gov/health/public/heart/other/chdfacts.htm.

http://www.nhlbi.nih.gov/nhlbi.cardio/other/gp/chdfacts.htm

Healthfinder

http://www.healthatoz.com

Mayo Clinic.Com

http://www.mayoclinic.com/invoke.cfm?id=DSDS00064&

MEDLINE Plus

http://www.nlm.nih.gov/medlineplus/coronarydisease.html.

Medtronic

http://www.medtronic.com/cad

The Merck Manual

http://www.merck.com/pubs/mmanual/section16/chap-ter202/202a.htm

National Institutes of Health—Health Topics

http://health.nih.gov/

National Women's Health Information Center

http://www.4woman.gov/faq/coronary.htm

UPMC Patient Information

http://patienteducation.upmc.com/C.htm#Cardiology

Dyslipidemias

Brian V. Reamy, MD, Col, USAF, MC[1]

General Considerations

The Framingham Heart Study firmly established an epidemiological link between elevated serum cholesterol and an increased risk of morbidity and mortality from atherosclerotic cardiovascular disease (ASCVD). Although the benefits of lowering cholesterol were assumed for many years, not until the past decade has enough evidence accumulated to show unequivocal benefits from using dietary and pharmacological therapy to lower serum cholesterol. Evidence in support of using statin agents is particularly strong and has revolutionized the treatment of dyslipidemias.

The efficacy of lipid reduction for both the secondary prevention of ASCVD (reducing further disease-related morbidity in those with manifest disease) as well as the primary prevention of ASCVD (reducing the risk of disease occurrence in those without overt cardiovascular disease) has been proven in multiple studies. The evidence from these studies led to the release in 2001 of extensively revised treatment guidelines from the National Cholesterol Education Program (NCEP), Adult Treatment Panel (ATP) III. These guidelines emphasize aggressive treatment of dyslipidemias for the prevention of ASCVD.

Pathogenesis

Serum lipids are primarily composed of triglycerides and cholesterol. Serum cholesterol is carried by three major lipoproteins: high-density lipoprotein (HDL), low-density lipoprotein (LDL), and very low-density lipoprotein (VLDL). Most clinical laboratories measure the total cholesterol, the total triglycerides, and the HDL fraction. VLDL cholesterol can be estimated by using the following formula:

$$VLDL\ Cholesterol = Triglycerides/5$$

(This estimation is accurate when the triglyceride level is less than 500 mg/dL.) The LDL level is also estimated, and not directly measured, by using the following formula:

$$LDL\ Cholesterol = Total\ Cholesterol - HDL\ Cholesterol - Triglycerides/5$$

Total serum cholesterol is relatively stable over time and does not depend on whether the patient is fasting. The triglyceride fraction (and to a lesser extent the HDL level), however, varies considerably depending on the fasting status of the patient. Because the evidence regarding the benefits of lowering cholesterol is derived from studies utilizing fasting cholesterol values to determine treatment plans, an accurate estimation of the various cholesterol subfractions represents the key to following the new treatment algorithms from the NCEP/ATP III. It is important that only fasting measurements including total cholesterol, triglycerides, HDL cholesterol, and a calculated LDL cholesterol be used to guide management decisions.

Different populations have different median cholesterol values. For example, Asian populations tend to have total cholesterol values 20–30% lower than populations living in Europe or the United States. It is important to recognize that unlike a serum sodium electrolyte value, there is no normal cholesterol value. Instead, there are cholesterol values that predict higher morbidity and mortality from ASCVD if left untreated, and cholesterol values that correlate with less likelihood of cardiovascular disease if they are below certain levels.

Clinical Trials & Prevention

Basic science studies have established that atherosclerosis is an inflammatory disease. Inflammatory cells and mediators participate at every stage of atherogenesis from the earliest fatty streak to the most advanced fibrous lesion. Elevated glucose, increased blood pressure, and inhaled cigarette byproducts can trigger in-

[1]The opinions contained herein are those of the author. They do not represent the opinions or official policy of the Department of the Air Force, the Department of Defense, or the Uniformed Services University.

flammation. But one of the key factors triggering this inflammation is oxidized LDL. When LDL is taken up by macrophages it triggers the release of inflammatory mediators that can lead to thickening and/or rupture of plaque lining the arterial walls. Ruptured or unstable plaques are responsible for clinical events such as myocardial infarction and stroke. Lipid lowering, whether by diet or medication, can therefore be thought of as an antiinflammatory and plaque-stabilizing therapy. In addition, hydroxymethylglutaryl coenzyme A (HMG-CoA) reductase inhibitor medications (statins) have shown primary antiinflammatory benefits regardless of the degree of LDL reduction achieved.

Older trials, done in the 1980s prior to the advent of statin drugs, provided several insights into the benefits of cholesterol reduction that formed the basis of earlier recommendations from the NCEP. The Lipid Research Clinics Coronary Primary Prevention Cholestyramine trial showed that lowering total cholesterol by 9% resulted in a 19% reduction in coronary artery disease (CAD) morbidity and mortality. The resin agent colestipol was tested in combination with nicotinic acid in the Cholesterol Lowering Atherosclerosis Study (CLAS) and showed a significant reduction in angiographic progression of atherosclerosis versus a control group receiving no medication.

Fibrate agents were also tested in a number of early trials with conflicting results. The Helsinki Heart Study, which tested gemfibrozil, showed reduced CAD mortality, but not all-cause mortality. Troublesome results of trials of clofibrate also showed that its use lowered CAD mortality, but led to an unexplained increase in all-cause mortality from violent death that initially tempered enthusiasm for the use of cholesterol lowering agents.

The statins were introduced against this backdrop of the questionable effects of cholesterol reduction on all-cause mortality. Several large, prospective, randomized double blind trials of statin agents for both the primary and secondary prevention of ASCVD were completed in the 1990s. Five of these trials were especially significant (Tables 20–1 and 20–2).

Two of the trials were primary prevention trials. The West of Scotland Coronary Prevention Study (WOSCOPS—1995) treated 6596 men with markedly elevated cholesterol levels with 40 mg/day of pravastatin. After just 5 years a reduction of relative risk in all end points was observed. Coronary events were reduced by 31%, CAD deaths by 28%, coronary revascularizations by 37%, and all-cause mortality by 22%. The numbers needed to treat (NNT) to reach these goals vary according to the age and risk status of the patient but approach 35:1.

The second primary prevention trial was the Air Force/Texas Coronary Atherosclerosis Prevention Study (AFCAPS/TEXCAPS—1998). This trial treated 6605 patients (15% women) whose cholesterol values were in the average range for the United States population. All were treated with either 20 or 40 mg of lovastatin. Remarkably, even in this **low-risk** group of patients, after 5 years of therapy there was a 25% risk reduction in nonfatal myocardial infarction and CAD deaths, a 40% risk reduction in fatal and nonfatal myocardial infarctions, and a 33% reduction in revascularizations. There was, however, no change in total mortality.

The three remaining landmark trials clearly established the use of statins in secondary prevention. The Scandanavian Simvastatin Survival Study (4S—1994) studied 4444 patients (19% women) for 5.4 years.

Table 20–1. Major trials of statin treatment for coronary heart disease (CHD) primary prevention.

Trial	Number of Patients	% Men/ % Women	RX	Baseline Labs (mg/dL)	Post-treatment	% Risk Reduction
WOSCOPS	6596	100/0	Pravastatin, 40 mg/day	TC = 272	–20%	Nonfatal MI/CHD death –31%
				LDL = 192	–26%	CHD mortality –28%
				HDL = 44	+5%	Total mortality –22%
				TG = 164	–12%	Revascularizations –37%
AFCAPS/TEXCAPS	6605	85/15	Lovastatin, 20 to 40 mg/day	TC = 221	–19%	Nonfatal MI/CHD death –25%
				LDL = 150	–26%	Fatal/nonfatal MI –40%
				HDL = 37	+5%	Total mortality no change
				TG = 158	–13%	Revascularizations –33%

Table 20–2. Major trials of statin treatment for coronary heart disease (CHD) secondary prevention.

Trial	# pts.	% Men/ % Women	RX	Baseline Labs (mg/dL)	Post-treatment	% Risk Reduction
4S	4444	81/19	Simvastatin 20 to 40 mg/day	TC = 261	−26%	Nonfatal MI/CHD death −34%
				LDL = 188	−36%	Fatal/nonfatal MI −42%
				HDL = 46	+7%	Total mortality −30%
				TG = 134	−17%	CHD mortality −42%
LIPID	9014	83/17	Pravastatin 40 mg/day	TC = 218	−18%	Nonfatal MI/CHD death −24%
				LDL = 150	−25%	Fatal/nonfatal MI −29%
				HDL = 36	+5%	Total mortality −22%
				TG = 138	−11%	CHD mortality −24%
CARE	4159	86/14	Pravastatin 40 mg/day	TC = 209	−20%	Nonfatal MI/CHD death −24%
				LDL = 139	−28%	Fatal/nonfatal MI −29%
				HDL = 39	+5%	Total mortality −22%
				TG = 155	−14%	CHD mortality −20%

Treated patients received either 20 or 40 mg of simvastatin. The patients were high risk in terms of both the presence of preexisting disease and markedly unfavorable cholesterol profiles. In this study CAD deaths were reduced by 34%, all myocardial infarcts by 42%, revascularizations by 37%, and all-cause mortality by 30%. For the first time, stroke was included as an end point and its risk was reduced by 30%.

The Long Term Intervention with Pravastatin in Ischemic Disease Study Group (LIPID—1998) followed 9014 patients (17% women) for 6.1 years. All were treated with pravastatin 40 mg/day. Initial lipid values were at the level of population means. Again, a reduction in relative risk across all end points was observed: nonfatal infarcts were reduced by 24%, all infarcts by 29%, revascularizations by 20%, all-cause mortality by 22%, and stroke by 19%.

The last large secondary prevention trial was the Cholesterol and Recurrent Events (CARE—1996). This study enrolled 4519 patients (14% women) with cholesterol values close to ideal. All were placed on 40 mg of pravastatin/day. Relative risk was reduced for all clinical end points, including nonfatal infarcts (24%), all infarcts (25%), revascularizations (27%), and stroke (31%). A conceptual summary of the results of the five large statin trials is outlined in Table 20–3.

Fibrates were retested in a 1999 Veteran's Administration study (VA-HIT) that evaluated secondary prevention in men with a near normal LDL (mean = 111 mg/dL) but HDL less than 40 mg/dL. Gemfibrozil

was used as the trial medication, and as in the statin trials, a 22% reduction in coronary heart disease events was noted in just 5 years.

Clinical Findings

A. SYMPTOMS AND SIGNS

The majority of patients with dyslipidemias have no signs or symptoms of disease. Rarely, patients with fa-

Table 20–3. Statin trials.[1]

200		
High HDL	WOSCOPS	4S
		LIPID
150		
Low LDL	AFCAPS/TEXCAPS	CARE
100		
	No CAD (primary prevention)	CAD (secondary prevention)

[1]WOSCOPS, West of Scotland Coronary Prevention Study; 4S, Scandanavian Simvastatin Survival Study; LIPID, Long Term Intervention with Pravastatin Trial; AFCAPS/TEXCAPS, Air Force/Texas Coronary Atherosclerosis Prevention Study; CARE, Cholesterol and Recurrent Events.

milial forms of hyperlipidemia may present with yellow xanthomas on the skin or in tendon bodies, especially the patellar tendon, achilles tendon, and the extensor tendons of the hands. Dyslipidemia is usually detected by routine laboratory screening in an asymptomatic individual.

There are a few associated conditions that can cause a secondary hyperlipidemia (Table 20–4). These conditions should be considered before lipid-lowering therapy is begun or when the response to therapy is much less than predicted. In particular, poorly controlled diabetes and untreated hypothyroidism can lead to a significant elevation of serum lipids. The control of elevated blood glucose can lead to remarkable improvement in elevated triglyceride levels and depressed serum HDL cholesterol.

B. SCREENING

There is no evidence that establishes a particular age to begin screening, an age at which to stop screening, or the optimum frequency of screening for elevated lipid levels. The U.S. Preventive Services Task Force (USP-STF) recommends periodic screening for high serum cholesterol for all men 35 years of age and older and women 45 years of age and older. They state that screening after age 65 years of age should be undertaken on a case-by-case basis, with a focus on high-risk individuals. Although the USPSTF does not specify the exact interval for screening, they conclude that "an interval of five years has been recommended by experts, but longer intervals may be recommended for low risk subjects." The American College of Physicians (ACP) and the American Academy of Family Physicians (AAFP) recommend screening males between 35 and 65 years of age and females between 45 and 65 years of age. The new NCEP guidelines state that screening should occur in all adults aged 20 years or older with a fasting, complete lipid profile once every 5 years. As stated previously, there are practical reasons in support of always obtaining fasting serum specimens and a complete profile to include subfractions.

Screening children and adolescents is controversial because of a lack of studies proving the benefits of reducing elevated serum cholesterol and the lack of medications indicated for treatment in children. Some expert opinion recommends screening only those children over 2 years of age with significant family histories of hypercholesterolemia or premature ASCVD.

Treatment

The treatment of a high-risk cholesterol profile should be guided by current evidence. The current NCEP/ATP III treatment guidelines released on May 15, 2001, are as rooted in evidence as possible and used expert opinion only when evidence was lacking. It is available in print or online at www.nhlbi.nih.gov. In addition, electronic versions of the guidelines and the Framingham risk calculators can be downloaded from this site to a personal computer or for use in a handheld personal data assistant (PDA).

The new NCEP/ATP III guidelines reviewed below follow a nine-step process. Additional relevant evidence and information from other evidence-based treatment guidelines are incorporated into the discussion (Table 20–5). Although only a few steps may be relevant for patients at low risk, patients with abnormalities in all lipid subfractions may require the application of all nine steps.

The **first step** begins after obtaining fasting lipoprotein levels. The patient's profile is categorized based on the LDL, HDL, and total cholesterol values as follows:

Table 20–4. Secondary causes of lipid abnormalities.

Hypercholesterolemia
  Hypothyroidism
  Nephrotic syndrome
  Obstructive liver disease
  Acute intermittent porphyria
  Diabetes mellitus
  Chronic renal insufficiency
  Cushing's disease
  Drugs (oral contraceptives, diuretics)

Hypertriglyceridemia
  Diabetes mellitus
  Alcohol use
  Obesity
  Chronic renal insufficiency
  Drugs (estrogens, isotretinoin)

Hypocholesterolemia
  Cancer
  Hyperthyroidism
  Cirrhosis

LDL Cholesterol (mg/dL)

<100	Optimal
100–129	Near optimal
130–159	Borderline high
160–189	High
≥190	Very High

HDL Cholesterol (mg/dL)

<40	Low
≥60	High

Table 20–5. Summary of nine steps in NCEP/ATP III guidelines.

Step 1	Determine lipoprotein levels after a 9–12 h fast.
Step 2	Identify the presence of coronary heart disease or equivalents (coronary artery disease, peripheral arterial disease, abdominal aortic aneurysm, diabetes mellitus).
Step 3	Determine the presence of major risk factors, other than LDL (smoking, hypertension, HDL <40 mg/dL, family history of premature coronary disease, men ≥45 years and women ≥55 years).
Step 4	Assess level of risk [use Framingham risk tables if two or more risk factors and no coronary heart disease (or equivalent) is present].
Step 5	Determine risk category, LDL goal, and the threshold for drug treatment.
Step 6	Initiate therapeutic life-style changes (TLC) if LDL is above goal.
Step 7	Initiate drug therapy if LDL remains above goal.
Step 8	Identify the presence of the metabolic syndrome and treat. Determine the triglyceride and HDL goals of therapy.
Step 9	Treat elevated triglycerides and reduced HDL with TLC and drug therapy to achieve goals.

Total Cholesterol (mg/dL)

<200	Desirable
200–239	Borderline high
≥240	High

Step 2 focuses on determining the presence of clinical atherosclerotic disease such as coronary heart disease, carotid artery disease, peripheral arterial disease, an abdominal aortic aneurysm, or diabetes mellitus.

In **Step 3** the clinician should determine the presence of other major CAD risk factor including cigarette smoking, age greater than 45 years in men (55 years in women), hypertension, HDL cholesterol less than 40 mg/dL, a family history of premature CHD in a male first-degree relative less than 55 years of age or a female first-degree relative less than 65 years of age. An HDL cholesterol greater than 60 mg/dL negates one risk factor.

Step 4 classifies the patient into one of three risk categories: *high-risk*, having coronary artery disease or an equivalent; *medium-risk*, having greater than two risk factors or a 10-year risk of coronary heart disease of less than 20% based on the Framingham risk tables; or *low-risk*, having zero to one risk factors. The Framingham risk tables can be printed or downloaded to a personal computer or handheld PDA from the links found at www.nhlbi.nih.gov.

Step 5 is the key step that determines the patient's risk category and suggested LDL cholesterol treatment goals and the methods to reach these goals. Table 20–6 summarizes determination of risk category and treatment goals.

Step 6 reviews the contents of therapeutic life-style changes (TLC). The previously used American Heart Association step diets have been eliminated in favor of a single dietary recommendation modeled after the old step II diet. Saturated fat is limited to less than 7% of total calories and cholesterol intake to less than 200 mg/day. In addition, weight management and increased physical activity are encouraged. TLC also includes advice to increase the consumption of soluble fiber (10–25 g/day) and the intake of plant sterols (sitostanol approximately 2 g/day). Since the advent of several margarines (Benecol, Take Control) containing these plant sterols and evidence that they work in conjunction with all prescribed cholesterol-lowering drugs, the only barrier to their increased utilization is their cost.

Table 20–6. Risk category determination and LDL cholesterol goals.[1]

Risk Category	LDL Goal	LDL Level at Which to Begin Therapeutic Life-style Changes (TLC)	LDL Level at Which to Consider Drug Treatment
CHD or equivalent (10 year risk >20%)	<100 mg/dL	≥100 mg/dL	≥100 mg/dL (minimum goal of <130 mg/dL)
2+ risk factors (10 year risk ≤20%)	<130 mg/dL	≥130 mg/dL	10 year risk 10–20% ≥130 mg/dL 10 year risk <10% ≥160 mg/dL
0 to 1 risk factor	<160 mg/dL	≥160 mg/dL	≥190 mg/dL (160–189 mg/dL drug use optional)

[1]Adapted from NCEP/ATP III Treatment Guidelines.

The cultural background of the patient will impact the choice of dietary recommendations. A skilled nutritional medicine consultant can easily adapt the fat/cholesterol intake recommendations to a variety of culturally normative diets. Indeed, components of some cultures' diets that encourage the consumption of soluble fiber, plant sterols, soy protein, or fish oils can be encouraged to facilitate compliance and enhance the cholesterol-lowering effect of dietary guidance. Dietary advice given without regard to a patient's culturally accepted diet is unsuccessful over the long term and counterproductive to effective cholesterol reduction.

A. MEDICATIONS

Step 7 reviews the options for drug therapy if required (Table 20–7). Of note, NCEP/ATP III now recommends the simultaneous use of TLC and drugs in patients with known coronary heart disease or equivalents. Medications should be added to TLC after 3 months if goal LDL levels are not reached. Given their proven efficacy, ease of administration, and enhanced patient compliance over other classes of medications, statin agents are the drugs of first choice for most patients. In particular, patients with diabetes or those in the highest risk category derive special benefits from

their use due to their innate antiinflammatory and antithrombogenic effects. Myopathy and increased liver enzymes are the main potential side effects from statin agents. An increase of serum aminotransferase levels to more than three times normal occurs in 1% of patients taking high doses of statins. Symptomatic hepatitis is rare. Monitoring of liver function tests at 6 weeks, 12 weeks, 6 months, and annually thereafter can help identify patients with asymptomatic hepatic side effects and facilitate prompt discontinuation of the agents before clinical illness occurs. Rhabdomyolysis occurs in less than 0.1% of cases. It can be prevented by the prompt discontinuation of the agent when muscle pain and elevated muscle enzymes occur. Unexplained pain in large muscle groups should prompt investigation for myopathy; however, routine monitoring of muscle enzymes is not supported by any evidence. Side effects from statins are *not* typically class specific. Therefore, a side effect with one agent should not discourage a trial with another statin agent. In addition, pravastatin has a distinct pathway of metabolism that makes it less likely to cause drug–drug interaction problems compared to other statins. Prior concerns about statins causing cataracts or cancer have been alleviated by the release of two large meta-analyses in 2001 of randomized trials of

Table 20–7. Pharmacologic therapy of elevated cholesterol.

Drug Class	Drugs	Typical Effects[1]	Side Effects
Statins	Lovastatin Pravastatin Simvastatin Fluvastatin Atorvastatin	LDL –20–50% HDL +5–15% TG –10–25%	Myopathy Increased liver enzymes
Bile acid sequestrants	Cholestyramine Colestipol Colesevelam	LDL –15% HDL Minimal TG May increase 10%	Gastrointestinal (GI) distress Constipation Decreased absorption of other drugs
Nicotinic acid	Immediate release Extended release Sustained release	LDL –20% HDL +20–35% TG –20–50%	Flushing GI distress Hyperglycemia Hyperuricemia Hepatotoxicity
Fibrates	Gemfibrozil Fenofibrate Clofibrate	LDL –5–15% HDL +15% TG –20–50%	GI distress Gallstones Myopathy
Absorption blocker	Ezetimibe	LDL –17% HDL +1.3% TG –6%	Gallstones

[1]Lipid effects represent the average seen in most patients. Individual patients may display markedly different effects. This reinforces the need for dosage titration and close monitoring of lipid effects during drug initiation.

cholesterol lowering. These showed that statin agents were not associated with an increase in fatal or nonfatal cancers and that there was no link between long-term statin use and cataracts.

Atorvastatin and simvastatin are the most potent LDL-lowering agents. Atorvastatin also has the greatest effect on lowering triglycerides of the statin agents. Simvastatin, pravastatin, and lovastatin were the only agents used in the five large prevention trials discussed previously.

Statin agents can be combined with fibrates and nicotinic acid, but the potential for side effects is increased. A good rule-of-thumb is to halve the dose of the statin agent when adding a fibrate and then titrate the dosage of the statin upward to reach the therapeutic goal while monitoring for side effects. Fibrate agents have special efficacy in patients with primary low HDL and elevated triglycerides. Dyspepsia, gallstone formation, and a risk of myopathy are the main possible side effects. Nicotinic acid is the most potent HDL-elevating agent and the agent that affects all cholesterol subfractions in a positive fashion. Yet long-term patient compliance is difficult due to flushing, nausea, and abdominal discomfort. Additionally, nicotinic acid can cause an increase in blood glucose, which can limit its use in diabetic patients. The bile acid sequestrants cause a great deal of gastrointestinal side effects and can lead to decreased absorption of other medications. Given their relative decreased potency they are mainly useful as adjunctive agents.

Two new drugs deserve comment: ezetimibe (Zetia) and extended-release niacin plus lovastatin (Advicor). Ezetimibe is the first of a new class of agents that selectively inhibit intestinal absorption of dietary and biliary cholesterol at the brush border of the small intestine. In clinical studies it is remarkably well tolerated in contrast to the bile acid sequestrants. It may predispose to gallbladder disease. A single 10 mg/day dose lowered LDL by 17% and triglycerides by 6% and increased HDL by 1.3%. In addition, it is easily combined with statins and helps to augment their effect without increasing side effects. Advicor combines two older agents, niacin and lovastatin, in several fixed dose combinations that provided potent cholesterol control (LDL decrease of 45%, triglycerides decrease of 42%, and HDL increase of 41%), with a marked reduction in the flushing and hepatotoxicity associated with any of the individual components alone.

B. Complementary and Alternative Therapies

Many other complementary or alternative therapies are also employed for cholesterol reduction. The evidence supporting their use is variable. Several are harmless and some could lead to significant side effects. Oat bran (1/2 cup/day) is a soluble fiber that can reduce TC by 5 mg/dL and TG by 5%. Fish oil (1 g daily of unsaturated omega-3 fatty acids) can reduce triglycerides by up to 30% and raise HDL slightly with long-term use. A study compared users of fish oil supplements to nonusers for secondary prevention after a recent myocardial infarction. After 3 years, clinical events were reduced by 16% in the fish oil users. Fish oil can impair platelet function and potentiate bleeding.

Garlic has minimal side effects but several trials have shown that it is not efficacious. Soy can reduce LDL by up to 15%, but requires the intake of 25 g/day to achieve this effect. This amount is unlikely to be achieved in a western-style diet. Went yeast is the natural source for statin agents. As such, it is effective at lowering lipid values, but carries the same side effect profile as statins. Of concern is that the concentration of active agent in most Went yeast extracts is unpredictable and most patients do not undergo monitoring for potential hepatic or muscle side effects. Red wine can raise HDL and the chemical component responsible for this effect has been identified. However, in amounts greater than two glasses per day, red wine will raise TG and potentially cause hepatic damage and other deleterious health effects. Myrrh is used as a supplement in some countries. It has lipid-lowering effects but there is no trial evidence supporting its effect on clinical end points at present. Several other supplements such as ginseng, chromium, and calcium all have putative cholesterol-lowering effects but no patient-oriented clinical outcome evidence supporting their use.

Step 8 of the NCEP/ATP III guidelines encourages clinicians to look for the "metabolic syndrome" in their patients. The components of this syndrome are abdominal obesity, hypertriglyceridemia, low HDL, hypertension, and glucose intolerance. Aggressive treatment of inactivity, obesity, and hypertension, and the use of low-dose aspirin are encouraged in patients with evidence of the metabolic syndrome. In addition, drug therapy to treat the abnormal TG and HDL level should be utilized after 3 months of TLC.

Step 9 is the final step of the algorithm. Prior to beginning this step the LDL goal should have been reached. This step focuses on how to treat elevated triglycerides and low HDL as secondary end points of cholesterol therapy. Triglycerides are classified as follows:

<150 mg/dL	Normal
150–199 mg/dL	Borderline high
200–499 mg/dL	High
≥500 mg/dL	Very high

The initial steps are to employ TLC (weight reduction, increased physical activity, dietary change) and then to add a drug to reduce TG and raise HDL to reach therapeutic goals after 3–6 months of TLC. There is some indication that elevated triglycerides are a more significant risk factor for women than for men. The results of trials focusing on larger numbers of women may help to better define this risk. If needed to reach goal levels, a fibrate or nicotinic acid can be added to another medication or started primarily. Combination therapy with a statin is frequently needed and caution should be exercised due to the increased potential for side effects.

C. Surgery

Surgical management of the dyslipidemias is a less frequently utilized modality due to concerns about safety, cost, availability, and long-term clinical outcomes. Despite this, there continue to be positive results from the cohort followed in the Program on the Surgical Control of the Hyperlipidemias (POSCH). This study utilized a partial ileal bypass to promote cholesterol reduction as a secondary prevention strategy in 838 patients after a myocardial infarction. At 5-year follow-up, total cholesterol was reduced 27% and LDL by up to 42%, and HDL increased by up to 8%. This procedure can be a possible therapy in patients with genetic hypercholesterolemia resistant to usual pharmacological therapy.

Treatment of Special Groups

The treatment of dyslipidemias in special groups presents additional problems. Data on women, children, the elderly, and adults less than 35 years of age is incomplete.

1. Women—Four of the five major statin trials included women, although they accounted for only about 15–20% of the total enrolled patient population. Subset analysis and meta-analysis reveal that statins reduced coronary events by a similar proportion in women as in men. The reduction of coronary events involved fewer nonfatal events in women than in men. Further information on the benefits of lipid lowering in women will come from the results of the Women's Health Initiative and the PROSPER trial described below.

2. Elderly—Given that ASCVD is more common in the elderly it is expected that the benefits of cholesterol lowering would extend to this subgroup. Indeed, for patients 65–75 years of age subgroup analysis confirms this benefit. Given the increased frequency of ASCVD events in this population the NNT is reduced from approximately 35:1 in patients 40–55 years of age to almost 4:1 in patients 65–75 years of age. The PROSPER study investigated the benefits of lipid lowering with pravastatin 40 mg/day for the primary and secondary prevention of ASCVD in patients 72–84 years of age. More than 50% of the patients were women.

This study demonstrated a 24% relative risk reduction in cardiovascular end points. The medication was tolerated very well, even in patients with multiple prescriptions. PROSPER thus confirms the benefits of statins for older patients.

3. Children—No clinical trials have included children. There are accumulating anecdotal reports on the safety of cholesterol lowering in children. However, given the theoretical concerns of interrupting cholesterol synthesis in the growing body it is unlikely that data on cholesterol lowering in children will be forthcoming. Clearly, therapeutic life-style interventions are safe and can have a profound impact on the long-term health of the child if they are followed. Cholesterol levels should not be checked in children younger than 2 years old because marked elevations are normal for this age group.

4. Patients less than 35 years of age—Numerous studies have shown pathoanatomic evidence of ASCVD at all ages. The PADY study in Louisiana has demonstrated the ability to correlate degrees of arterial intimal narrowing with the risk factors present in a patient at the time of autopsy across all age groups. Given that atherosclerosis can start at very young ages in some patients it seems arbitrary that most programs do not recommend treatment until after 40 years of age.

Cholesterol treatment studies have not enrolled patients younger than 35 years of age because the frequency of clinical end points would be reduced and the duration of the studies would need to increase. The elevation of the NNT in young patients also makes treatment less economically attractive. There is no question that from an economic perspective not treating patients less than 35 years of age makes sense—the issue is whether we are truly aiding the primary prevention of ASCVD to the extent possible. The new NCEP/ATP III guidelines specifically address this issue for patients 20–35 years of age. They state that even though clinical CHD is rare in young adults, coronary atherosclerosis may progress rapidly, and young men who smoke and have an LDL of 160–189 mg/dL may be candidates for drug therapy. In addition, for young men and women with an LDL greater than 190 mg/dL, drug therapy should be considered as in adults of other ages.

E. Indications for Referral

Patients who do not respond to combination therapy or have untoward side effects on therapy should be considered for specialty consultation. Combinations of multiple agents in low doses may sometimes be required in high-risk individuals. Surgical referral for a partial ileal bypass should not be forgotten, but is clearly an option to be considered very carefully. The use of TLC including weight loss, a healthful culturally acceptable diet, soluble fiber intake, and aerobic exercise should be emphasized with all patients regardless of the treatment options chosen.

Ansell BJ, Watson CE, Fogelman AM: An evidence based assessment of the NCEP Adult Treatment Panel II Guidelines. JAMA 1999;282:2051. (A source for an alternative evidence-based algorithm to guide the treatment of dyslipidemias. Much of it was incorporated into the ATP III guidelines—this algorithm is a bit more aggressive.)

Choice of Lipid-Regulating Drugs: Med Lett 2001;43:1105 (also available online at www.medletter.com). (The best unbiased review of drug treatment—updated approximately every 2–3 years.)

Clinical Evidence, ed 5: BMJ Publishing Group, June 2001. (Updates are published every 6 months of this excellent source of patient-oriented evidence.)

Moghadasian MH et al: Surgical management of dyslipidemia: clinical and experimental evidence. J Invest Surg 2001;14 (2):71. (A good review of the state of the art in the surgical treatment of dyslipidemias.)

Ross R: Atherosclerosis—an inflammatory disease. New Engl J Med 1999;340;115. (An excellent review of the basic science supporting the evidence of atherosclerosis as an inflammatory condition and the clinical implications of this evidence for treatment.)

Third Report of the National Cholesterol Education Program (NCEP) Expert Panel on the Detection, Evaluation, and Treatment of High Blood Cholesterol in Adults (Adult Treatment Panel III): NIH/NHLBI, May 2001 (also available at www.nhlbi.nih.gov).

WEB SITE

The Nutritionist's Tool Box (a good web site that reviews nutritional interventions to lower cholesterol).

http://fscn.che.umn.edu/tolls.htm

Urinary Tract Infections

Shersten Killip, MD, MPH

Urinary tract infections (UTIs) are the most common bacterial infection encountered in medicine. Accurately estimating incidence is difficult, as UTIs are not reportable, but estimates range from 650,000 to 7 million office visits per year, with costs ranging as high as 1.6 billion dollars in 1995 alone. For a condition involving so many patients, pathophysiology and knowledge are not as well defined as they could be.

A UTI is defined by urologists as any infection involving the urothelium, which includes urethral, bladder, prostate, and kidney infections. Some of these are diseases that have been clearly characterized, such as cystitis and pyelonephritis, whereas others, such as urethral and prostate infections, are not as well understood or described.

Simple or uncomplicated UTI is a term often used to refer to cystitis; in this chapter UTI will refer to any infection of the urinary tract and cystitis will specify a bladder infection. A complicated UTI is a generic term often used to refer to a cystitis that occurs in a person with preexisting metabolic, immunological, or urological abnormalities, including kidney stones, diabetes, and acquired immune deficiency syndrome (AIDS) or that is caused by multiply-resistant organisms.

This chapter will cover asymptomatic bacteriuria, two urethral syndromes, four prostatitis syndromes, uncomplicated cystitis, complicated cystitis, and pyelonephritis. Some of these syndromes, such as the four prostatitis syndromes, have only recently been defined and therefore there is little research available to answer basic clinical questions related to diagnosis, prevention, treatment, and prognosis. In these cases differentiating between syndromes and deciding treatment(s) may be left very much to the physician.

Antibiotic resistance is a topic that has also been left mostly to the physician. General recommendations about specific antibiotics are inappropriate, given that antibiotic resistance changes from location to location. It is the responsibility of the individual physician to be familiar with local antibiotic resistances, and to determine the best first-line therapies for patients. Always keep in mind that antibiotic use breeds resistance, and

try to keep first-line drugs as simple and narrow spectrum as possible.

Foxman B: Epidemiology of urinary tract infections: incidence, morbidity, and economic costs. Am J Med 2002;113(1A):5.

ASYMPTOMATIC BACTERIURIA

 ESSENTIALS OF DIAGNOSIS

- *Asymptomatic patient.*
- *Urine culture with $>10^5$ organisms, or bacteria in spun urine, or dipstick positive for leukocytes and/or nitrites.*

General Considerations

As this is no longer considered a pathological syndrome, it is not surprising that diagnostic criteria are not well defined. The essential criterion is that the patient be asymptomatic, ie, should not be experiencing dysuria, suprapubic pain, fever, urgency, frequency, or incontinence. Any sign of bacteria in the urine will be sufficient to suspect asymptomatic bacteriuria. Culture does not need to be done, as this syndrome does not need to be treated in young healthy women, elderly healthy or institutionalized women, diabetics, men of any age, or self-catheterizing patients. Hospitalized patients with indwelling catheters are outside the scope of this chapter. Pregnant women are now the only group that should be routinely screened and treated for asymptomatic bacteriuria. Asymptomatic bacteriuria ($>10^5$ organisms on clean-catch mid-stream urine) is present in 2–7% of pregnant women and has been associated with premature birth. Multiple guidelines recommend screening pregnant women for asymptomatic bacteriuria. In the United States this is usually done by urine culture as dipstick screening can miss patients without pyuria or with unusual organisms. A positive dipstick, however, can be taken as evidence of bacteri-uria.

Treatment

Treatment should be guided by local rates of resistance. The usual first-line treatment in the absence of significant resistance or penicillin allergy is 7 days of amoxicillin. Nitrofurantoin or a cephalosporin is suggested for penicillin-allergic pregnant patients, again for 7 days.

Anderson RU: Management of lower urinary tract infections and cystitis. Urol Clin North Am 1999;26(4):729.

Reid G, Nicolle LE: Asymptomatic bacteriuria in spinal cord patients and the elderly. Urol Clin North Am 1999;26(4):789.

Warren JW et al: Guidelines for antimicrobial treatment of uncomplicated acute bacterial cystitis and acute pyelonephritis in women. Clin Infect Dis 1999;29:745.

ACUTE URETHRAL SYNDROME

 ESSENTIALS OF DIAGNOSIS

- Dysuria.
- Frequency and urgency.
- No vaginal discharge.
- Dipstick may be negative or positive.
- Negative culture.

General Considerations

Acute urethral syndrome is a term used by some to describe a young, healthy, sexually active woman who complains of recent-onset symptoms of cystitis but does not meet older, strict guidelines for diagnosis (growth of >10^4 or 10^5 organisms on culture). Some studies indicate that the presence of even 100 colony-forming units on culture of a dysuric woman represents a true UTI. Because most laboratories are equipped to detect only 10^4 organisms or more, these are patients in usual practice found to have "negative" cultures. They may have positive or negative dipsticks and positive or negative spun urine for bacteria, although bacteria and white blood cells in the urine are more convincing for cystitis than a completely negative workup

Clinical Findings

Testing will depend on the physician's assessment of the patient. In a patient at low risk of STD, no testing might be appropriate, or testing only after failure of empirical treatment for cystitis. In patients at higher risk of STD, *Chlamydia* testing, either by cervical swab or urine polymerase chain reaction (PCR) or ligase chain reaction (LCR), might be appropriate.

Differential Diagnosis

This syndrome is clearly not well defined. It is usually taken to represent an early cystitis, but it can also be a sexually transmitted disease (STD). One study found that *C trachomatis* was not uncommonly found in women with the symptoms described above.

Treatment

Depending on the physician's assessment, treatment might involve the use of usual cystitis agents (see the section on "Cystitis") or STD agents (see Chapter 15). Because the prevalence of *C trachomatis* was found to be high in at least one study of women with these symptoms, routine *Chlamydia* testing for patients who do not respond completely to a course of antibiotics would be highly recommended.

Stamm WE et al: Diagnosis of coliform infection in acutely dysuric women. New Engl J Med 1982;307(8):463.

URETHRITIS

 ESSENTIALS OF DIAGNOSIS

- Pain or irritation on urination.
- No frequency or urgency.
- Discharge from the urethra (predominantly males).
- Vaginal discharge possible.

General Considerations

Isolated urethritis in men or women is almost always a sexually transmitted disease, most often caused by *C trachomatis*. This syndrome is differentiated from acute urethral syndrome by the time course of symptoms; symptoms that have a gradual onset and/or persist without evolution into classic cystitis symptoms, including suprapubic symptoms such as pain, urgency, or frequency, are more indicative of urethritis.

Clinical Findings

It can be very difficult to separate a symptomatic *Chlamydia* infection from a bacterial cystitis with coliform organisms, and testing for both may be required.

The new *Chlamydia* urine PCR or LCR tests make ruling out *Chlamydia* much easier than in the past.

Treatment

See Chapter 15 for current diagnosis and treatment of STDs such as *Chlamydia*.

ACUTE BACTERIAL PROSTATITIS

ESSENTIALS OF DIAGNOSIS

- *Dysuria, frequency, urgency.*
- *Tender prostate.*
- *Systemic symptoms such as fever, nausea, vomiting.*
- *Leukocyte esterase or nitrite on dipstick.*
- *Positive urine culture.*

General Considerations

Prostatitis is a very common disease among men with a prevalence and incidence ranging between 5% and 8%. Some 2 million office visits a year are made for prostatitis (1% of all primary care office visits), so it is useful for the primary care practitioner to be able to evaluate men for symptoms of prostatitis.

Until recently, prostatitis could be described as "acute," "chronic," or "nonbacterial." The National Institutes of Health (NIH) revised the categorization of prostatitis in 1995. Prostatitis can now be divided into Category I or acute bacterial prostatitis, Category II or chronic bacterial prostatitis, Category IIIA or inflammatory chronic pelvic pain syndrome, Category IIIB or noninflammatory chronic pelvic pain syndrome, and Category IV or asymptomatic inflammatory prostatitis. That last is a diagnosis made incidentally, while working up other symptoms, and is not believed to require treatment. The other categories will be discussed in separate chapters; this chapter will focus on Category I or acute bacterial prostatitis.

Acute bacterial prostatitis is different from other types of prostatitis in that it is a well-defined entity with a relatively clear-cut etiology, diagnosis, and treatment. It is caused by typical uropathogens and responds well to antibiotic treatment. Unfortunately, despite its clear-cut etiology, there is still no good agreement on how to diagnose this disorder. Acute bacterial prostatitis has been referred to as a "clinical" diagnosis that does not require positive urine cultures, whereas others believe that urinary pathogens are almost always recovered from urine even without prostatic massage.

Prevention

There is no evidence for interventions that will prevent spontaneous prostatitis.

Clinical Findings

A. SYMPTOMS AND SIGNS

Symptoms include dysuria, frequency, and urgency; low back, perineal, penile, and/or rectal pain; tense or "boggy" tender prostate; and fever and chills, which may also be present.

B. LABORATORY FINDINGS

A urine dipstick is positive for leukocyte esterase and/or nitrites and urine culture is positive for a single uropathogen.

C. IMAGING STUDIES

These are generally not done for acute uncomplicated prostatitis.

D. SPECIAL TESTS

Prostatic massage is generally not done for acute bacterial prostatitis as it may lead to acute bacteremia. It can be done carefully if postmassage urine is required, but should be avoided if abscess is suspected.

Differential Diagnosis

Abnormal anatomy may include urethral strictures, polyps, diverticulae, redundancies, or valves anywhere in the system from the penis to the kidneys (Table 21–1).

Complications

Complications of acute bacterial prostatitis may include ascending infection, infection-related stones, abscess, fistula, cysts, and acute urinary retention. In the case of acute urinary retention precipitated by prostatitis, a suprapubic catheter rather than a Foley catheter should be placed to avoid damage to the prostate.

Treatment

The usual treatment is quinolone antibiotics for 28 days. Trimethoprim/sulfamethoxazole or trimethoprim alone is also acceptable, depending on local resistance rates for uropathogens.

Table 21–1. Differential diagnosis of dysuria in men.

If Patient Has	Consider
Acute, colicky flank pain or history of kidney stones	Kidney stone; complicated cystitis
Costovertebral angle tenderness, fevers	Pyelonephritis
Urethral discharge	Sexually transmitted disease
Diabetes/immunosuppression	Complicated cystitis, unusual pathogens
Testicular pain	Torsion; epididymoorchitis
Joint pains	Spondyloarthropathy (ie, Reiter's or Behçet's syndrome)
History of childhood UTI or urological surgery	Abnormal anatomy; complicated cystitis
Recurrent symptoms after treatment	Abnormal anatomy; abscess; stone; chronic prostatitis; resistant organism; inadequate length of treatment; Munchausen's; somatization disorder

Prognosis

The prognosis is very good for acute uncomplicated bacterial prostatitis.

Nickel JC: Prostatitis: evolving management strategies. Urol Clin North Am 1999;26(4):737.

CHRONIC BACTERIAL PROSTATITIS

ESSENTIALS OF DIAGNOSIS

- *Dysuria, frequency, urgency.*
- *Symptoms for more than 3 months.*
- *Urine dipstick positive for leukocyte esterase and/or nitrites.*
- *Pyuria on microscopy.*
- *Positive four-glass or two-glass test for prostatic origin.*

General Considerations

Chronic bacterial prostatitis, or NIH Category II prostatitis, is quite rare, and consequently very few studies have been done on it. Chronic bacterial prostatitis makes up only a small percentage of the cases of chronic prostatitis. It has been estimated that the percentage of both acute and chronic bacterial prostatitis is only between 5% and 10% of all prostatitis diagnoses, and of the bacterial cases the vast majority are acute.

Prevention

Early and sufficient treatment of acute bacterial prostatitis may prevent chronic prostatitis.

Clinical Findings

A. SYMPTOMS AND SIGNS

Symptoms include dysuria, frequency, and urgency; prostatic tenderness on examination; and low back, perineal, penile, and/or rectal pain. Symptoms should be present for more than 3 months.

B. LABORATORY FINDINGS

A urine dipstick is positive for leukocyte esterase and/or nitrites and/or a four-glass or two-glass test for prostatic origin is positive.

C. IMAGING STUDIES

A transrectal prostatic ultrasound should be done if abscess or stones are suspected.

D. SPECIAL TESTS

1. Four-Glass Test—Not used by the majority of practitioners, this is a localization test for chronic prostatitis. The patient should not have been on antibiotics for a month, should not have ejaculated for 2 days, and needs a reasonably full bladder. Signs and symptoms of urethritis and/or cystitis should have been worked up previously and treated. To perform the test, the patient first cleans himself and carefully retracts the foreskin, then urinates the first 5–10 mL into a sterile container (VB_1). He then urinates 100–200 mL into the toilet, and a second 10–20 mL sample into a sterile container (VB_2). Prostatic massage is then done, milking secretions from the periphery to the center, and any expressed prostatic secretions are caught in a third sterile container (EPS). The patient then urinates a final 10–20 mL sample into a fourth container (VB_3).

All urine samples are then examined microscopically and cultured. Expressed prostatic secretions are wet-mounted, examined, and cultured. The test is positive for prostatic localization if white blood cells/high powered filter (WBC/hpf) and colony counts in VB_3 are at least 10 times greater than in VB_1 or VB_2, or if there are ≥10 polymorphonuclear leukocytes (PMNL)/hpf in the ESP wet mount. If there is a significant colony count in both VB_2 and VB_3, treat the patient for 3 days with nitrofurantoin, which does not penetrate the prostate, and repeat the test.

2. Two-Glass Test—This is an experimentally verified modification of the four-glass test. This test requires an initial clean-catch urine, a prostatic massage, and a postmassage urine. It is functionally equivalent to the VB_2 and VB_3 portions of the four-glass test.

Differential Diagnosis

See Table 21–1.

Complications

Complications of chronic bacterial prostatitis may include ascending infection, infection-related stones, abscess, fistula, cysts, and/or acute urinary retention.

Treatment

Treatment of prostatitis with antibiotics such as trimethoprim, trimethoprim/sulfamethoxazole, or quinolones has been suggested for up to 12 weeks in this rare population of patients.

Prognosis

The prognosis for treatment of chronic bacterial prostatitis is not known. A clear differentiation of which patients will respond to antibiotics and which will not has not been made.

Walker P, Wilson J: 2001 national guideline for the management of prostatitis. Clin Effect Group Sex Transm Infect 1999;75 (suppl 1):S46.

CHRONIC ABACTERIAL PROSTATITIS/CHRONIC PELVIC PAIN SYNDROME

 ESSENTIALS OF DIAGNOSIS

- *Not very well characterized; most suggestive symptoms include*
  - *Perineal pain.*
  - *Lower abdominal pain.*
  - *Penile, especially penile tip, pain.*
  - *Testicular pain.*
  - *Ejaculatory discomfort or pain.*
- *STD/bacterial prostatitis tested for and ruled out.*

General Considerations

Chronic abacterial prostatitis was renamed by the NIH in 1995. It is now called chronic pelvic pain syndrome, and can be further subclassified into inflammatory, meaning with inflammatory cells isolated in tests, or noninflammatory. This change was made in an attempt to recognize that the pain syndrome physicians have been referring to as "chronic abacterial prostatitis" or even "prostatodynia" in the absence of inflammatory cells on examination has never been proven to originate in the prostate. This NIH categorization is still quite new, and unfortunately the literature has not to date separated studies of chronic abacterial prostatitis into "inflammatory" and "noninflammatory" categories. In the "inflammatory" case, leukocytes are found in semen, in expressed prostatic secretions, or in a postprostatic massage urine sample. In "noninflammatory" prostatitis no leukocytes are found in secretions. Current research efforts include the Chronic Prostatitis Clinical Research Network, funded in 1997 by the NIH to investigate the chronic pelvic pain syndrome. It is to be hoped that this work will help to separate out etiological factors and useful treatments for chronic pelvic pain syndrome.

We still know very little about chronic abacterial prostatitis. There is no gold standard test for supposed prostatitis; diagnostic trials are of low quality; and treatment trials are few, are methodologically weak, and have small sample sizes.

The etiology of chronic prostatitis remains unknown. Current theories include infection with unusual or fastidious organisms; lower urinary tract obstruction or dysfunctional voiding; intraprostatic ductal reflux and subsequent chemical irritation with urea from urine forced into the gland; immunological or autoimmune processes; or neuromuscular causes, such as reflex sympathetic dystrophy. None of these theories has been proven, but this may be because previous attempts to investigate chronic prostatitis lumped together too many truly disparate syndromes. Continued research will hopefully supply more information.

Prevention

There are no trials of preventive measures for chronic prostatitis or chronic pelvic pain syndrome. Risk factors have not been investigated.

Clinical Findings

A. SYMPTOMS AND SIGNS

Symptoms include dysuria, frequency, urgency, and other irritative voiding symptoms as well as pain in the perineal area for more than 3 months in the last 6 months.

B. LABORATORY FINDINGS

Findings include no current cystitis or demonstrable bacterial infection and for inflammatory-type chronic pelvic pain syndrome, leukocytes in expressed prostatic secretions or postprostatic massage urine.

C. SPECIAL TESTS

If the patient has hematuria, a urine cytology should be done. The two-glass test (first part of a clean-catch urine sample in one bottle; prostatic massage milking from periphery to center; second urine sample into a sterile container) has been shown to be as reliable as the more complicated four-glass test at distinguishing inflammatory or chronic bacterial prostatitis from noninflammatory prostatitis.

Differential Diagnosis

See Table 21–1.

Treatment

There is no clear-cut prescription for the treatment of chronic prostatitis of either the inflammatory or noninflammatory type. Because the reclassification of prostatitis is so new, most published studies to date have not separated the entities. This treatment discussion will therefore group inflammatory and noninflammatory prostatitis into one entity for discussion. More type-specific information should be published soon.

Trials have been done for α blockers [prostatitis from benign prostatic hypertrophy (BPH) or obstructive symptoms], antibiotics (prostatitis from unusual or fastidious organisms), nonsteroidal antiinflammatory drugs (NSAIDs) (prostatitis from inflammation), pentosan polysulfate (prostatitis as a form of interstitial cystitis), allopurinol (irritation from urea in the prostate after reflux), quercitine (a bioflavonoid/herbal treatment), ejaculation three times a week (prostatitis from "congestion" in the gland), balloon dilation (see α blockers), transurethral and/or transrectal thermal treatment, transurethral needle ablation of the prostate, transurethral resection of the prostate, and radical prostatectomy.

The Cochrane Review looked at treatments for chronic prostatitis in August 1999. At that time the conclusion was that no treatments were substantiated, including BPH medications, NSAIDS, antibiotics, miscellaneous medications, and thermotherapy. Ther-

motherapy showed the most promising results and it was noted that further investigations should be done. Table 21–2 is a brief review of controlled trials that have shown possible efficacy of treatments.

Despite the lack of evidence for efficacy, 28- to 42-day courses of antibiotics suitable for bacterial prostatitis continue to be used by practitioners and suggested by panels of experts.

Prognosis

The prognosis for chronic prostatitis/chronic pelvic pain syndrome Category III is not good. A large number of well-designed treatment studies should be published in the next few years, which hopefully will bring some relief to the many men with this condition.

McNaughton Collins M, MacDonald R, Wilt TJ: Diagnosis and treatment of chronic abacterial prostatitis: a systematic review. Ann Intern Med 2000;133:367.

Nickel JC: Prostatitis: evolving management strategies. Urol Clin North Am 1999;26(4):737.

UNCOMPLICATED BACTERIAL CYSTITIS

 ESSENTIALS OF DIAGNOSIS

- *Dysuria.*
- *Frequency and/or urgency.*
- *Dipstick positive for nitrites or leukocyte esterase.*
- *Positive urine culture >10^4 organisms.*
- *No vaginal discharge, fever, or flank pain.*

General Considerations

Acute, uncomplicated cystitis is most common in women. Approximately 33% of all women will have experienced at least one episode of cystitis by the age of 24 years, and 40–50% will experience at least one during their lifetime. Young women's risk factors include sexual activity, use of spermicidal condoms or diaphragm, and genetic factors such as blood type or maternal history of recurrent cystitis.

Healthy, noninstitutionalized older women can also experience recurrent cystitis. Risk factors among these women include changes in the perineal epithelium and vaginal microflora after menopause, incontinence, and a history of cystitis before menopause.

Although men can also suffer from cystitis, it is rare (<0.01% of men 21–50 years old/year) in men with normal urinary anatomy under the age of 35 years.

Table 21–2. Effective therapies for chronic bacterial prostatitis.

Therapy	Dose	Comments
Finasteride	5 mg every day	Symptom score but not pain score dropped in one small, pilot study; placebo group had less pain to start, results may therefore be spurious[1]
Terazosin	1 mg every day for 4 days 2 mg every day for 10 days 5 mg every day for 12 weeks	1.5-fold greater reduction in NIH symptom scores with terazosin than without; responders had lower pain scores to start; moderate benefit only[2]
Quercitine	500 mg twice a day	Small pilot study with good preliminary results; decrease in symptoms from 21 (NIH) to 13 in active drug; 67% of patients on quercitine responded (with a 25% improvement in symptoms) versus 20% of placebo patients. The addition of bromelain and papain (Prosta-Q) in an open-label trial increased the response rate to 82%[3]
Allopurinol		Per the Cochrane Review, on small trial provided some evidence of benefit[4]
Pentosan polysulfate	100 mg three times a day for 6 months	Open-label Phase II trial completed; Phase III trial pending; not a controlled trial, difficult to draw any conclusions yet[5]
Thermotherapy		Not enough data at this time to be considered anything but experimental[6]

[1]Leskinen M, Lukkarinen O, Martilla T: Effects of finasteride in patients with inflammatory chronic pelvic pain syndrome: a double-blind, placebo-controlled pilot study. Urology 1999;53(3):502.
[2]Cheah PY et al: Terazosin therapy for chronic prostatitis/chronic pelvic pain syndrome: a randomized, placebo controlled trial. J Urol 2003;169:592.
[3]Shoskes DA et al: Quercetin in men with category III chronic prostatitis: a preliminary prospective, double-blind, placebo-controlled trial. Urology 1999;54(6):960.
[4]McNaughton Collins M, Wilt T: Allopurinol for chronic prostatitis. (Cochrane Review) In *The Cochrane Library,* Issue 1. Update Software, 2003.
[5]Nickel JC et al: Pentosan polysulfate therapy for chronic nonbacterial prostatitis (chronic pelvic pain syndrome category IIIa): a prospective multicenter clinical trial. Urology 2000;56(3):413.
[6]Zeitlin SI: Heat therapy in the treatment of prostatitis. Urology 2002;60(suppl 6A):38.

Urethritis from sexually transmitted pathogens should always be considered in this age group, and prostatitis should always be ruled out in the older age group by a rectal examination. Any cystitis in a man is complicated, due to the presence of the prostate gland, and should be treated for 7–10 days to prevent a persistent prostatic infection.

Prevention

A. YOUNG WOMEN

Considering the frequency and morbidity of cystitis among young women, it is hardly surprising that the lay press and medical literature contain a host of ideas about how to prevent recurrent cystitis. These range from the old suggestion that cotton underwear is "healthier" to wiping habits, voiding habits, and choice of beverage. Unfortunately, the vast majority of these preventive measures do not hold up to scientific study (Table 21–3).

Recent studies have shown no effect of back-to-front wiping, pre- or postcoital voiding, tampon use, underwear fabric choice, or use of noncotton hose or tights.

Table 21–3. UTI risk in young women.

Factors with No Evidence of Effect on Cystitis	Factors with Evidence for Effect on Cystitis	
	Promote	Prevent
Precoital voiding		
Postcoital voiding	Spermicide[1]	Cranberry juice
Underwear fabric	Diaphragm[1]	Prophylactic
Wiping pattern	Cervical cap[1]	Antibiotics
Douching	Sexual activity	
Hot tub use	Genetic predisposition	

[1]Spermicide on condoms, as contraceptive foam [Hooton TM et al: Escherichia coli bacteriuria and contraceptive method. JAMA 1991;265(1):64.], in diaphragms, and in cervical caps has been shown to adversely affect the vaginal flora, predisposing to *E coli* colonization and UTI.

Behaviors that do appear to impact frequency of cystitis in young women include sexual activity (four or more episodes/month in one study), use of spermicidal condoms (several studies), use of unlubricated condoms (one study), use of diaphragms and/or cervical caps, and intake of cranberry juice.

It can be concluded from Table 21–3 that there is not much to offer young women who suffer from recurrent cystitis in terms of behavior. Recommending a change in contraception to oral contraceptive pills, intrauterine devices, and/or nonspermicidal, lubricated condoms may be helpful.

The cranberry juice question is a bit more complicated. No studies used cranberry juice cocktail; all used pure cranberry juice or cranberry tablets. The optimal dose has not been determined; doses ranged from 200 mL once a day to 250 mL three times a day. Also, there have been studies showing that the cost of daily ingestion of cranberry juice far outweighs that of prophylactic antibiotics. However, for patients who prefer not to use medications or practitioners concerned about antibiotic resistance, suggesting a trial of cranberry juice, one to three glasses daily, or cranberry tablets twice a day (1:30 concentration minimum) is reasonable.

Prophylactic antibiotics, either low-dose daily antibiotics or postcoital antibiotics, remain the mainstay of prevention for young women, and can reduce recurrence rates up to 95%.

B. Postmenopausal Women

Risk factors for cystitis in older women include urological factors such as incontinence, cystocele, and/or postvoid residual; hormonal factors resulting in a lack of protective lactobacillus colonization; and a prior history of cystitis. Among these, estrogen is the most easily administered effective prevention.

There are many possible ways to administer estrogen: traditional oral hormone replacement therapy (HRT), which is still considered indicated (after a thorough discussion with the patient of risks and benefits) for menopausal symptoms, vaginal estrogen rings, or creams.

Estriol is an end-product, low-potency estrogen that preferentially binds to urogenital binding sites, not endometrial sites. It is therefore safe to administer on its own, either as a cream or an oral pill, without adding progesterone. Overall levels of estrogen are lower using a pill than using cream, because of the first-pass effect of the liver on estriol, but endometrial response may be greater to the pill than the cream. Contraindications to estriol include a history of endometrial carcinoma, breast carcinoma, thromboembolic disorders, and liver disease, as with all estrogens. Consideration should be made of a patient's functional and cultural abilities before prescribing vaginal applications.

No studies have been done of older women, cranberry juice, and UTI. It is likely that cranberry juice could help older as well as younger women; however, the cranberry juice will acidify the urine, which could lead to discomfort if the woman has atrophic changes of the vulva.

C. Young Men

There are no studies on prevention of cystitis in young men.

D. Future Trends in Prevention

Some work is being done on probiotics and vaccines for the prevention of UTI. Probiotics are benign living organisms, which in this case are used to bolster the vaginal flora. They then defend against pathological bacteria by competing for adhesion receptors and nutrients. Some species such as lactobacillus even produce antimicrobial substances. At this time, there are oral and vaginal vaccines working their way through clinical trials, but they are not yet commercially available, and whether they will prove to be more efficacious than prophylactic antibiotics is yet to be determined. One study explored intentional colonization of the urothelium with *Escherichia coli* 83972 in spinal patients; there was colonization in 13 of 21 participants, which lasted for a mean of 12.3 years. During that time no colonized patient had a symptomatic UTI.

Clinical Findings

A. Symptoms and Signs

Symptoms include dysuria, ideally felt more internally than externally, and of sudden onset; suprapubic pain; cloudy, smelly urine; frequency; and/or urgency.

Physical examination in the afebrile, otherwise healthy patient with a classic history is done essentially to rule out other diagnoses and to ensure that red flags are not present. The examination might range from checking a temperature and percussing the costovertebral angles to a full pelvic examination, depending on where the history leads. There are no pathognomonic signs on physical examination for cystitis.

B. Laboratory Findings

Findings include a dipstick positive for leukocyte esterase and/or nitrite. There is now support for treatment of simple, uncomplicated UTI in the young, nonpregnant woman on the grounds of clinical history alone, if that history leads to a high suspicion for cystitis (and low suspicion of STD). For women with an equivocal clinical history, urine dipstick may be enough to reassign the women to a high or low suspicion group and treat or not treat accordingly. One study, using 10^4 organisms on culture as its gold standard, came up with a false-positive rate of 11% and a false-negative rate of 31% by sequencing clinical impression and dipstick results for diagnosis. These numbers seem high, but they are in fact comparable to other studies using rapid diagnostic methods. Other results include urinalysis positive for WBC, with no epithelial cells (more expensive than dipstick, but minimally more accurate) and a positive urine culture.

One of the reasons a diagnostic algorithm is difficult to define for cystitis is that there is no agreement on what constitutes the gold standard. Some clinicians are pushing for symptoms of cystitis with as few as 100 (10^2) organisms on culture, whereas others retain the traditional gold standard of 100,000 (10^5). Most laboratories are not equipped to detect fewer than 10^4 organisms. Culture is strongly suggested if a relapsing UTI or pyelonephritis is suspected to be sure of sensitivities and eradication.

In some cases no laboratory tests may be required to diagnose cystitis with high accuracy. This should probably occur only in settings in which follow-up can be easily arranged in case of failure of treatment, which would of course indicate further workup.

C. IMAGING STUDIES

Imaging studies generally are not required for simple uncomplicated UTIs.

D. SPECIAL TESTS

Generally special tests are required only for failures of treatment or symptoms suggesting a diagnosis other than cystitis and/or complicated cystitis (see "Complicated Cystitis" below).

Differential Diagnosis

See Table 21–4.

Complications

There are virtually no complications from repeated uncomplicated cystitis if it is recognized and treated. Delay in treatment may lead to ascending infection and pyelonephritis, but this has not been confirmed. In the case of infection with urea-splitting bacteria, "infection stones" of struvite with bacteria trapped in the interstices may be formed. These stones will lead to persistent bacteriuria and must be completely removed to clear the infection. *Proteus mirabilis, Staphylococcus saprophyticus,* and *Klebsiella* bacteria can all split urea and lead to stones.

Table 21–4. Red flag symptoms and differential diagnoses.

If Patient Has	Consider
Fever	Urosepsis, pyelonephritis, pelvic inflammatory disease (PID)
Vaginal discharge	Sexually transmitted disease (STD), PID
External burning pain	Vulvovaginitis, especially candidal vaginitis
Costovertebral angle tenderness	Pyelonephritis
Nausea/vomiting	Pyelonephritis, urosepsis, inability to tolerate orally
Recent UTI (<2 weeks)	Incompletely treated, resistant pathogen; urological abnormality, including stones and unusual anatomy; interstitial cystitis
Dyspareunia	STD, PID, psychogenic causes
Recent trauma or instrumentation	Complicated UTI
Pregnancy	Antibiotic choice, treatment duration
Severe, colicky flank pain	UTI complicated by stones; preexisting or struvite stone caused by urea-splitting bacteria
Joint pains, sterile urine	Spondyloarthropathy, eg, Reiter's or Behçet's syndrome
History of childhood infections, urological surgery	Abnormal anatomy
History of kidney stones	Complicated UTI; bacterial persistence in stones
Diabetes	Complicated UTI
Immunosuppression	Complicated UTI

Treatment

A. ACUTE CYSTITIS

Current evidence-based guidelines are available from the Infectious Diseases Society of America for the treatment of uncomplicated acute bacterial cystitis in women. The guidelines note that there is evidence from randomized clinical trials to support 3-day antibiotic therapy as superior to 1-day treatment and equivalent to therapy for longer periods of time. Trimethoprim/sulfamethoxazole, in the absence of allergies to sulfa and local resistance rates >10–20%, should be considered first-line therapy. Use of fluoroquinolones as first-line therapy should be discouraged, considering the frequency of cystitis and the consequent potential for antibiotic resistance. β-Lactam antibiotics are not as effective as other classes of drugs against urinary pathogens, and should not be used as a first-line drug except in the case of pregnancy.

B. ACUTE CYSTITIS IN THE PREGNANT WOMAN

Treatment with amoxicillin for 7 days remains the standard, with follow-up cultures to demonstrate bacterial eradication. Asymptomatic bacteriuria, if found on cultures, is treated in the pregnant population (see section on "Asymptomatic Bacteriuria).

C. PROPHYLAXIS FOR RECURRENT CYSTITIS

Low-dose, prophylactic antibiotics have been shown to decrease recurrences by up to 95%. The recommendation is to start prophylaxis after a patient has had more than three documented UTIs in one year. Prophylactic antibiotics are usually administered for 6 months to 1 year, but can be given for longer periods of time. Antibiotics can be taken daily at bedtime or used postcoitally for women whose infections are associated with intercourse. Unfortunately, prophylaxis does not change the propensity of these women for recurrent UTI; when the prophylaxis is stopped, approximately 60% of women will have a UTI within 3–4 months. Prophylaxis should not start until cultures have shown no growth after treatment, to rule out bacterial persistence (Table 21–5).

Prognosis

Long-term prognosis in terms of kidney function is excellent; prognosis of arresting recurrent cystitis without permanent prophylaxis is not as good. Hopefully some of the new preventive treatments currently being explored will prove beneficial.

Engel JD, Schaeffer AJ: Evaluation of and antimicrobial therapy for recurrent urinary tract infections in women. Urol Clin North Am 1998;25(4):685.

Kiel RJ, Nashelsky J: Does cranberry juice prevent or treat urinary tract infection. J Fam Pract 2003;52(3):154.

Naber KG: Treatment options for acute uncomplicated cystitis in adults. J Antimicrob Chemother 2000;46(suppl S1):23.

Table 21–5. Prophylactic antibiotics for recurrent UTI in women.

Regimen	Drug and Dose
Daily	Trimethoprim 100 mg every day
	Nitrofurantoin 50 mg every day
	Nitro. macrocrystals 100 mg every day
	Co-Trimoxazole 240 mg every day
	Cranberry juice 250 mL three times a day
	Cranberry tablets 1:30 twice a day
Postcoital	One dose of any of the above antibiotics after coitus

Orenstein R, Wond ES: Urinary tract infections in adults. Am Fam Phys 1999;59(5):1225.

Raz R: Hormone replacement therapy or prophylaxis in postmenopausal women with recurrent urinary tract infection. J Infect Dis 2001;183(suppl 1):S74.

Schaeffer AJ et al: Overview summary statement. Urology 2002; 60(suppl 6A):1.

Scholes D et al: Risk factors for recurrent urinary tract infection in young women. J Infect Dis 2000;182:1177.

Sultana RV et al: Dipstick urinalysis and the accuracy of the clinical diagnosis of urinary infection. J Emerg Med 2001;20(1):13.

COMPLICATED CYSTITIS & SPECIAL POPULATIONS

ESSENTIALS OF DIAGNOSIS

- Any cystitis not resolved after 3 days of appropriate antibiotic treatment.
- Any cystitis in a special population, such as
  — A diabetic.
  — A man.
  — A patient with an abnormal urinary tract.
  — A patient with stones.
  — A pregnant woman.
- Any cystitis involving multiply resistant bacteria.

General Considerations

These are the infections for which a physician should consider further workup and/or referral to a urologist. These infections should all be cultured to be sure the antibiotics used are appropriate and that the organisms are sensitive to the chosen antibiotic.

Clinical Findings

Special tests should include x-ray or computed tomography (CT) for stones, intravenous pyelogram (IVP) for anatomy and/or stones, and/or cystoscopy and biopsy to rule out interstitial cystitis, cancer, or unusual pathogens.

Treatment

Patients with complicated UTIs should be treated with long-course, appropriate antibiotics. Single-dose or 3-day regimens are not appropriate for this group of patients.

PYELONEPHRITIS

ESSENTIALS OF DIAGNOSIS

- *Fever.*
- *Chills.*
- *Flank pain.*
- *>100,000 colony-forming units (CFU) on urine culture.*

General Considerations

Pyelonephritis is an infection of the kidney parenchyma. It has been estimated to result in more than 100,000 hospitalizations per year. Information on outpatient visits is not easily available, but because many cases of pyelonephritis are now managed on an outpatient basis, it is likely to be seen by most primary care doctors. It usually results from upward spread of cystitis, but can also result from hematogenous seeding of the kidney from another infectious source. Pyelonephritis can be complicated by infection stones or renal scarring if left untreated, but usually resolves without sequelae in young healthy people if treated promptly.

The most common bacteria involved are the same as for uncomplicated cystitis, *E coli, S saprophyticus, Klebsiella* spp, and occasionally *Enterobacter* spp. As with simple cystitis, some women with genetic predispositions are more commonly affected than other women.

Prevention

There are no recent studies on prevention of pyelonephritis. Prompt treatment of cystitis may prevent some cases of pyelonephritis, but this has not been demonstrated.

Clinical Findings

A. SYMPTOMS AND SIGNS

Symptoms include fever, chills, and malaise; dysuria; flank pain; and/or nausea and vomiting.

B. LABORATORY FINDINGS

Findings include a dipstick that is positive for leukocyte esterase or nitrites and a urine culture with >100,000 CFU.

C. IMAGING STUDIES

Imaging studies are generally not required unless the patient is diabetic or stones that may complicate the infection are suspected, in which case a CT scan is the test of choice.

Differential Diagnosis

See Table 21–6.

Complications

Diabetics can experience emphysematous pyelonephritis. This is diagnosed by an x-ray or another imaging study showing gas in the renal collecting system and/or around the kidney. In a diabetic patient, the treatment of choice is emergency nephrectomy, as the mortality rate in diabetics approaches 75%. This condition may rarely occur in nondiabetic patients, and is often related to obstruction. In some of these cases relief of the obstruction and antibiotics may suffice.

Stones can complicate pyelonephritis by causing a partial or complete obstruction. These stones can be spontaneous or "infection" stones of struvite, caused by urea-splitting organisms. Stones complicating pyelonephritis must be removed before the infection will completely resolve.

People with a history of childhood pyelonephritis can have renal scarring and recurrent infections. These scars are unusual in healthy adults with pyelonephritis. Young men with pyelonephritis should be investigated for a cause.

Table 21–6. Differential diagnosis of pyelonephritis.

If Patient Has	Consider
Negative urine dipstick or culture	Pelvic inflammatory disease; stone obstructing ureter; lower-lobe pneumonia; herpes zoster
Guarding/rebound	Acute cholecystitis; acute appendicitis; perforated viscus
Recurrent infection	Kidney stone, spontaneous or infection related; anatomical abnormality; resistant organism; inadequate treatment
Diabetes	Emphysematous pyelonephritis
History of childhood infections, urological surgery	Abnormal anatomy
History of kidney stones	Pyelonephritis complicated by stones

Patients who do not respond to 48 h of appropriate antibiotics should be worked up for occult complicating factors and/or other diagnoses.

Treatment

The best drugs for treatment of pyelonephritis are bactericidal, with a broad spectrum to cover gram-positive and gram-negative bacteria, that concentrate well in urine and renal tissues. Aminogylcosides, aminopenicillins such as amoxicillin with or without clavulinic acid, ticarcillin, or piperacillin, cephalosporins, fluoroquinolones, or, in extreme cases, imipenem are all appropriate. First-line outpatient treatment is usually a fluoroquinolone. There are no recent studies, but cure rates have been reported to approach 90% with a 10-day to 2-week course of antibiotics.

Patients experiencing severe nausea and vomiting who are unable to tolerate oral medications may have to be admitted to the hospital for parenteral therapy. Patients with severe illness, suspected bacteremia, and/or sepsis should also be admitted.

Prognosis

Prognosis after an acute uncomplicated pyelonephritis in a previously healthy adult is excellent.

Roberts, JA: Management of pyelonephritis and upper urinary tract infections. Urol Clin North Am 1999;26(4):753.

Arthritis: Osteoarthritis, Gout, & Rheumatoid Arthritis

22

Bruce E. Johnson, MD

Arthritis is a complaint and a disease afflicting many of our patients and filling our office schedules. Surveys suggest that 10% of appointments to a generalist practice involve a musculoskeletal complaint. Of course, such surveys convey a more monolithic appearance than is actually true. Arthritis is multifaceted and can be categorized in several different fashions. For simplicity, this chapter focuses on conditions afflicting the anatomic joint composed of cartilage, synovium, and bone. Other discussions would include other types of arthritis, localized disorders of the periarticular region (such as tendinitis, bursitis, and bone lesions), and systemic disorders that have arthritic manifestations (such as vasculitides, polymyalgia rheumatica, and fibromyalgia). The chapter includes discussion of three prototypical arthritides: osteoarthritis, as an example of a cartilage disorder; gout, as an example of both a crystal-induced arthritis and an acute arthritis; and rheumatoid arthritis, as an example of an immune-mediated, systemic disease and a chronic deforming arthritis.

OSTEOARTHRITIS

ESSENTIALS OF DIAGNOSIS

- *Degenerative changes in the knee, hip, thumb, ankle, foot, or spine.*
- *Pain with movement that improves with rest.*
- *Synovitis.*
- *Sclerosis, thickening, spur formation, warmth, and effusion in the joints.*

General Considerations

Arthritis is among the oldest identified conditions in humans. Anthropologists examining skeletal remains from antiquity deduce levels of physical activity and work by searching for the presence of osteoarthritis (OA). Such observations have parallels in the present as OA is more prevalent among people in occupations characterized by steady, physically demanding activity such as farming, construction, and production-line work. (Curiously, OA is not found in increased incidence in recreational joggers who apparently practice caution so as not to suffer traumatic or overuse injuries to the joints.) Obesity is a significant risk factor for OA, especially of the knee, although it is unclear whether weight loss prevents further joint damage once begun. Heredity and gender play a role in a person's likelihood of developing OA, regardless of work or recreational activity. For instance, distal interphalangeal OA (Heberden's nodes) is autosomal dominant in women. For reasons currently not well understood, OA of the knee is twice as common in women as men. Estrogen may be somewhat protective for OA, as the incidence of symptomatic disease rises after menopause. However, studies are mixed as to whether hormone replacement lowers the risk of large joint OA.

Pathogenesis

Part of the pathophysiology of OA involves microfracture of cartilage with incomplete healing. The disruption of the otherwise smooth cartilage surface allows differential pressure on the underlying bone resulting in bone abrasion, and a partial source of joint pain. The debris resulting from cartilage breakdown causes a low-level inflammation within the synovial fluid, almost like a crystal-induced arthritis. Such inflammation leads to synovitis, effusion, and, of course, pain with movement.

Prevention

It is difficult with any assurance to advise patients on measures to prevent arthritis. Obese persons should lose weight, but few occupational or recreational precautions can be expected to alter the natural history of OA. Arthritis has multiple etiologies and no consistent preventive steps are available to patients.

Clinical Findings

A. Symptoms and Signs

Symptomatic OA represents the culmination of damage to cartilage, usually over many years. The presentation of OA passes from symptomatic pain to physical findings to loss of function. OA can occur at any joint, but the most commonly involved joints are the knee, hip, thumb (carpometacarpal), ankle, foot, and spine. The strongly inherited spur formation at the distal interphalangeal joint (Heberden's nodes) and proximal interphalangeal joint (Bouchard's nodes) is often classified as OA, yet, although deforming, only infrequently causes pain or disability (Figure 22–1). The pain of OA is at the joint, but can be confusing. Cartilage has no pain fibers, so the pain of OA arises from secondary causes.

Osteoarthritic pain is typically associated with movement, meaning that at rest the patient may be relatively asymptomatic. Recognition that at rest the joint is less painful can be maladaptive. Patients learn to "favor" the involved joint, leading to disuse of supporting muscle groups and contributing to weakness at the joint. Such weakness accounts for the complaint that an involved joint "gives way," resulting in dropped items if at the wrist or falls if at the knee. In joints with mild OA, pain may counterintuitively improve with exercise or activity. This observation is probably explained by a shock-absorber effect well-maintained muscle provides at a joint.

Advanced OA is characterized by bony destruction and alteration of joint architecture. Secondary spur formation with deformity, instability, or restricted motion is a common finding. Fingers, wrist, knees, and ankles appear abnormal with asymmetric growth. Warmth and effusion is seen in joints with advanced OA. At this stage, pain may be frequent and exacerbated by any movement, weight bearing or otherwise. The site of OA involvement also dictates the intensity and persistence of pain with OA of the neck and spine often continuous and OA of the upper and lower extremities more closely associated with volitional movement. Pain associated with neck and spine OA results from the constant movement expected of those mobile joints to maintain posture.

B. Laboratory Findings

There are few laboratory studies of relevance to the diagnosis of OA. Rarely, the erythrocyte sedimentation rate (ESR) will be raised, but only if an inflammatory effusion is present [and even then an elevated ESR or C-reactive protein (CRP) is more likely to be misleading than helpful]. If an effusion is present, arthrocentesis can be helpful in ruling out other conditions (see below, laboratory findings in gout). OA can be a secondary effect of several other conditions and these diseases may have laboratory tests that can confirm a diagnosis and direct specific treatment. Examples include OA secondary to hemochromatosis (elevated iron and ferritin, liver enzyme abnormalities), Wilson's disease (elevated copper), acromegaly (elevated growth hormone), and Paget's disease (elevated alkaline phosphatase). Obviously, the OA may fit into the diagnostic picture if another disease is suspected, but rarely is OA a primary reason to search for other diseases.

C. Imaging Studies

Radiographs are usually not needed for the initial diagnosis of the arthritides. Other means of diagnosing OA are more useful. Radiographs may be misleading in OA by suggesting more advanced disease than consistent with the patient's symptoms.

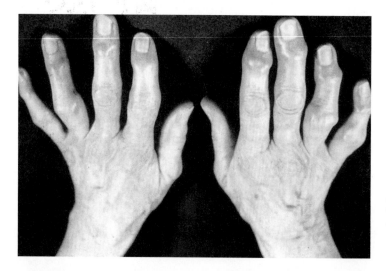

Figure 22–1. Heberden's nodes (distal interphalangeal joint) noted on all fingers and Bouchard's nodes (proximal interphalangeal joint) noted on most fingers.

Plain films of joints afflicted with OA show characteristic changes of sclerosis, thickening, spur formation, loss of cartilage with narrowing of the joint space, and malalignment (Figure 22–2). If effusion is present, this may be seen as bulging or separation of tissue planes. An interesting finding on plain films, especially at the knee or the triangular cartilage at the base of the thumb, is chondrocalcinosis. This finding is often associated with calcium pyrophosphate deposition disease, making the presence of chondrocalcinosis in the setting of acute monoarthritis strongly suggestive of pseudogout.

Most changes in OA described above are relatively late occurrences. Changes do not always correlate with symptoms. Patients may complain of significant pain despite a relatively normal appearance of the joint and, conversely, considerable apparent destruction of a joint may exist with only modest symptoms voiced by the patient. In addition, plain film radiography does not provide good information about cartilage, tendons, ligaments, or any soft tissue. Such findings may be crucial to explaining a patient presentation, especially if there is loss of function of a joint.

To see cartilage, ligaments, and tendon, magnetic resonance imaging (MRI) is important and, in many instances, essential. MRI can detect abnormalities of the meniscus or ligament of the knee, cartilage or femoral head deterioration at the hip, misalignment at the elbow, rupture of muscle and fascia at the shoulder, and a host of other abnormalities. All these findings may be incorrectly attributed to "OA" before MRI scanning.

Computed tomography (CT) and ultrasonography have lesser, more specialized uses in the diagnosis and management of OA. CT, especially with contrast, can detect structural abnormalities of large joints such as the knee or shoulder. Ultrasonography is an inexpensive means of detecting joint or periarticular fluid, or unusual collections of fluid such as a popliteal (Baker's) cyst at the knee.

Differential Diagnosis

In practice, it is should not be difficult to differentiate between the three prototypical arthritides discussed in this chapter. Nonetheless, Table 22–1 suggests some key findings for diagnosis of OA.

A common source of confusion and misdiagnosis occurs when bursitis/tendinitis syndromes mimic the pain of OA. A common example is anserine bursitis. This bursitis, located medially just at the tibial plateau, presents in a fashion similar to OA of the knee, but can be differentiated by a few simple questions and directed physical findings.

Treatment

All three types of arthritis discussed in this chapter have inflammation, making treatment of inflammation a cornerstone of medical management. However, inflammation has a different meaning in each disease. In OA, when treatment of inflammation is necessary, such treatment represents, in part, progression of joint destruction and the failure of conservative therapy.

By the time treatment of OA is considered necessary, a number of significant and probably irreversible steps have occurred. With few exceptions, the early development of OA is silent. When pain occurs, and pain is almost always the presenting complaint, the osteoarthritic process has resulted in joint destruction that

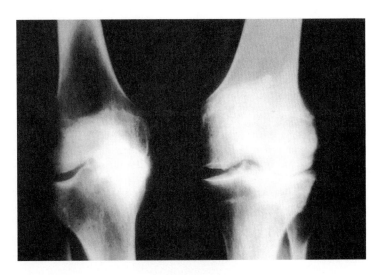

Figure 22–2. Osteoarthritis of the knees showing loss of joint space with marked reactive sclerosis and probable malalignment.

Table 22–1. Essentials of diagnosis.

	Osteoarthritis	Gout	Rheumatoid Arthritis[1]
Key presenting symptoms	Pauciarticular. Pain with movement, improving with rest. Site of old injury (sport, trauma). Obesity. Occupation.	Monoarticular. Abrupt onset. Pain at rest and movement. Precipitating event (meal, physical stress). Family history.	Polyarticular. Gradual, symmetric involvement. Morning stiffness. Hands and feet initially involved more than large joints. Fatigue, poorly restorative sleep.
Key physical findings	Infrequent warmth, effusion. Crepitus. Enlargement/spur formation. Malalignment.	Podagra. Swelling, warmth. Exquisite pain with movement. Single joint (exceptions—plantar fascia, lumbar spine). Tophi.	Symmetric swelling, tenderness. MCP, MTP, wrist, ankle usually before larger, proximal joints. Rheumatoid nodules.
Key laboratory, x-ray findings	Few characteristic (early). Loss of joint space, spur formation, malalignment (late).	Synovial fluid with uric acid crystals. Elevated serum uric acid. 24 h urine uric acid.	Elevated ESR/CRP. Rheumatoid factor. Anemia of chronic disease. Early erosions on x-ray, osteopenia at involved joints.

[1]MCP, metacarpophalangeal; MTP, metatarsophalangeal; ESR, erythrocyte sedimentation rate; CRP, C-reactive protein.

is unlikely changed. Cartilage is damaged, bone reaction is established, and debris mixes with synovial fluid. Consequently, when a diagnosis of OA is established, goals of therapy become control of pain, restoration of function, and reduction of disease progression. Although control of the patient's complaints is possible, and long periods of few or no symptoms may ensue, the patient permanently carries a diagnosis of OA.

Treatment of OA involves multiple modalities and is inadequate if treatment involves only the prescription of antiinflammatory drugs. Patient education, assessment for physical therapy and devices, and consideration of intraarticular injections are essential steps to consider in the total management of the patient. In some patients, preparation for surgical correction may also be relevant, although only after other measures have been exhausted.

A. PATIENT EDUCATION

Patient education is a crucial step. Informing the patient of the likelihood for relief of symptoms, and of the limitations of treatment, is time well spent. The patient also must be made aware of the role he or she plays in successful therapy. Many resources are available to assist the provider in patient education. Patient education pamphlets are widely available from such varied sources as government organizations, physician organizations [eg, American Academy of Family Physicians (AAFP) or American College of Physicians (ACP)], insurance companies, pharmaceutical companies, or patient advocacy groups (eg, The Arthritis Foundation). Many communities have self-help or support groups that are

rich sources of information, advice, and encouragement.

One of the most effective long-term measures to both improve symptoms and slow progression of disease is weight loss. Less weight carried by the hip, knee, ankle, or foot reduces stress on the involved arthritic joint, decreases the pathophysiological processes, and probably slows progression of disease. Unfortunately, in many instances, OA makes weight loss more difficult. Diet and exercise are concurrently advised for effective weight loss, and OA with pain of lower extremity joints limits exercise. Recognizing this limitation in weight management enhances one's credibility; nonetheless, weight loss should be encouraged at each visit.

On the other hand, exercise is a crucial modality that should not be overlooked. Evaluation for appropriate exercise focuses on two issues—overall fitness (with possible weight loss) and correction of any joint-specific disuse atrophy. Flexibility in choices of the type of exercise should be employed. Many persons with significant lower joint pain can still exercise in water. Swimming is an excellent exercise that spares stress on the lower extremities. Although many older persons are reluctant to learn to swim anew, they may be amenable to water aerobic exercises. Water aerobics are now widespread with enlightened programs within relatively easy access at all but the most remote locations. These exercises encourage calorie expenditure, flexibility, and both upper and lower muscle strengthening in a supportive atmosphere. Stationary bicycle exercise is also accessible to most people, is easy to learn, and does not stress the lower extremity joints.

B. PHYSICAL THERAPY AND ASSISTIVE DEVICES

The pain of OA not infrequently results in muscular disuse. The best, and perhaps most frequent, example is quadriceps weakness in OA of the knee. The patient who "favors" the involved joint reduces quadriceps strength. This has two repercussions: the cushioning effect of muscle strength in regular walking is lost, resulting in more weight and pressure directly on the joint; and the stabilizing effect of adequate strength is lost. The latter is usually the cause of the patient complaint of the knee "giving way." Sudden buckling at the knee, often when descending stairs or rapidly changing direction, is not due to destruction of cartilage or bone but rather to inadequate strength in the quadriceps to handle the load required at the joint. Physical therapy with quadriceps strengthening is highly efficacious, resulting in improved mobility, increased patient confidence, and reduction in pain.

The physical therapist or physiatrist should also be consulted for advice regarding assistive devices. Advanced OA of lower extremity joints may cause instability and fear of falls that can be addressed by canes of various types. Altered positioning or alignment can be corrected by orthotics, which has the advantage, when used early, of slowing progression of OA. Braces can protect the truly unstable joint and permit continued ambulation.

C. MEDICATIONS

The patient wants relief of pain. Despite the widespread promotion of nonsteroidal antiinflammatory drugs (NSAIDs) for OA, there is no evidence that NSAIDs alter the course of the disease. That being the case, NSAIDs are being used for their analgesic, rather than antiinflammatory, effects. Although effective as analgesics, NSAIDs have significant side effects and should not always be considered a first-line drug. Regrettably, no pharmacological therapy changes the course of OA and all medication should be considered for symptomatic effect rather than any disease-modifying benefit.

Most recommendations begin with adequate doses of acetaminophen. The patient must understand how acetaminophen is being prescribed. A frequent reason given by the patient for discontinuation of the drug is because it "doesn't work," but on closer questioning the patient has often taken just a few doses, or only used the medicine intermittently, before reaching this conclusion. Acetaminophen should be prescribed in large doses, starting at 3–4 g/day, and continued at this level until pain control is attained. At that point, dosage can be reduced if possible. Maintenance of adequate blood levels is essential and because acetaminophen has a relatively short half-life, frequent dosing is necessary (three or four times a day). High doses of acetaminophen are generally well tolerated, although caution must be employed in patients with liver disease or in whom alcohol ingestion is heavy.

Another relatively common non-NSAID oral treatment for OA is a combination of glucosamine and chondroitin sulfate. These are components of glycosaminoglycans, which make up cartilage, although there is no evidence that orally ingested glucosamine or chondroitin sulfate is actually incorporated into cartilage. Studies, mostly from Europe and of variable quality, suggest these agents are superior to placebo in symptomatic relief of mild OA. The onset of action is somewhat delayed from other oral agents, but the effect seems to be prolonged after treatment is stopped. Glucosamine/chondroitin sulfate combinations are available over the counter and are generally well tolerated by patients.

Capsaicin, a topically applied extract of the chili pepper also available over the counter, relieves pain by depletion of substance P, a neuropeptide involved in pain sensation. Capsaicin is suggested for tendinitis or bursitis, but may be tried for OA of superficial joints such as the fingers. The cream should be applied three or four times a day for 2 weeks or more before concluding any lack of benefit.

NSAIDs come in two main classes largely based on half-life. NSAIDs with shorter half-lives (eg, diclofenac, etodolac, ibuprofen, and indomethacin) need more frequent dosing than longer acting agents. Several of the NSAIDs are available as generics and/or over the counter, which may significantly reduce cost. Despite different pharmacologies of the NSAIDs, there actually is little difference in efficacy, so choice of medication should be made on the basis of individual patient issues such as dosing intervals, tolerance, toxicity, and cost. As with acetaminophen, or for that matter virtually any therapy, adequate doses must be used to attain maximal effectiveness. For example, ibuprofen at doses up to 800 mg three or four times a day should be maintained (if tolerated) before concluding that another agent is necessary. Examples of NSAID dosing are given in Table 22–2.

Prostaglandins are intimately involved in the inflammation process and blockage of prostaglandin synthesis reduces inflammation. Prostaglandins are also important, among many other functions, in maintenance of stomach mucosal protection and glomerular filtration. NSAIDs inhibit production of prostaglandin, explaining their efficacy when inflammation is present but also predicting side effects. Alteration of the gastrointestinal mucosal layer produces symptoms of irritation ("heartburn," "indigestion") and leads to tissue breakdown. NSAIDs are the leading cause of hospital admission for gastrointestinal bleeding. Reduction of renal blood flow

Table 22–2. Selected nonsteroidal antiinflammatory drugs with usual and maximal doses.

Drug	Frequency of Administration	Usual Daily Dose (mg/day)	Maximal Dose (mg/day)
Oxaprozin (eg, Daypro)	Every day	1200	1800
Piroxicam (eg, Feldene)	Every day	10–20	20
Nabumetone (eg, Relafen)	One to two times a day	1000–2000	2000
Sulindac (eg, Clinoril)	Twice a day	300–400	400
Naproxen (eg, Naprosyn)	Twice a day	500–1000	1500
Diclofenac (eg, Voltaren)	Two to four times a day	100–150	200
Ibuprofen (eg, Motrin)	Three to four times a day	600–1800	2400
Etodolac (eg, Lodine)	Three to four times a day	600–1200	1200
Ketoprofen (eg, Orudis)	Three to four times a day	150–300	300

and glomerular filtration is rarely a clinical concern in healthy persons but can cause worsening of renal insufficiency [especially with concurrent use of diuretics or angiotensin-converting enzyme (ACE) inhibitors] in patients with hypertension or congestive heart failure or in patients who are volume depleted, or fluid retention in patients with cirrhosis, nephrosis, or congestive heart failure. Because an age-related decline in renal function is widespread in the elderly, these patients are particularly likely to experience adverse effects of NSAIDs.

The cyclooxygenase system is found in the early steps of synthesis of prostaglandins. The cyclooxygenase system has at least two isoforms: COX-1 helps produce prostaglandin's physiological activities in the gastrointestinal (GI) tract, the kidneys, platelets, and elsewhere; COX-2 is stimulated by cytokines and contributes to prostaglandin production in inflammatory settings. NSAIDs nonselectively block both COX pathways. Selective COX-2 inhibitors are available that successfully block at least one pathway to inflammation without disrupting the beneficial functions of prostaglandins in the GI tract or kidneys. COX-2 inhibitors, eg, celecoxib (Celebrex) and rofecoxib (Vioxx), have antiinflammatory efficacy roughly equivalent to older NSAIDs but with fewer side effects. They may be considered if acetaminophen dosing is inadequate due to the presence of inflammation, or if there have been serious NSAID-related adverse effects. The cost of COX-2 inhibitors is considerably higher than nonselective NSAIDs and many insurance companies that provide drug benefits require a declaration that NSAIDs have been tried and failed before coverage is extended.

D. INTRAARTICULAR INJECTIONS

Hyaluronic acid (Hyalgan, Synvisc) is a constituent of both cartilage and synovial fluid. Injection of hyaluronic acid, usually in a series of three to five weekly intraarticular insertions, has been shown to provide symptomatic improvement for up to 6 months in symptomatic OA. It is unknown why hyaluronic acid

helps; there is no evidence hyaluronic acid is incorporated into cartilage and it does not slow the progression of OA. It is very expensive and the injection process is painful. Use of this agent is usually limited to patients who have failed other forms of OA therapy.

Intraarticular injection of corticosteroids has both been under- and overutilized in the past. There is little question that use of steroids in this manner rapidly reduces inflammation and eases symptoms. Soon after intraarticular injection was first used (actually overused) it was noted that serious degenerative complications ensued, suggesting even a hastening of the need for surgical or other intervention. Combining these observations with the knowledge that oral steroid use was not effective in preventing progression of OA (and had significant side effects) resulted in limited use of intraarticular injection. However, in selected cases, intraarticular steroid use is effective and gives rapid symptomatic relief. The best case is one in which the patient has an exacerbation of pain accompanied by signs of inflammation (warmth, effusion). The knee is most commonly implicated and is most easily approached. Most authorities recommend no more than two injections during one episode and limiting injections to no more than two or three episodes per year. Benefits of injection are often shorter in duration than similar injection for tendinitis or bursitis, but the beneficial outcome is often used to help reestablish therapy with another oral agent.

E. SURGERY

Until recently, orthopedic surgeons have performed arthroscopic surgery on osteoarthritic knees in an effort to remove accumulated debris and to polish or debride frayed cartilage. However, a clinical trial demonstrated that any purported benefit of this practice could be explained by the placebo effect. The procedure was never advocated as a "cure" for OA and it remains to be seen if the numbers of these procedures will decline.

Joint replacement is a rapidly expanding option for treatment of OA, especially of the knee and hip. Pain is reduced or eliminated altogether. Mobility is improved, although infrequently to previous levels. Expenditures for total joint replacement are likely to increase dramatically as the baby-boomer generation reaches the age at which OA of large joints is more common. Indications for joint replacement (which can also be considered for several other joints, including shoulder, elbow, and fingers) include pain poorly controlled with maximal therapy, malalignment, and decreased mobility or ambulation. Improvement in pain relief and quality of life should be seen in about 90% of patients undergoing the procedure. As complications of both the surgery and rehabilitation are increased by obesity, many orthopedic surgeons will not consider hip or knee replacement without at least an attempt by the patient to lose weight. Patients need to be in adequate medical condition to undergo the operation, and even more so to endure the often lengthy rehabilitation process. Some surgeons refer patients for "prehabilitation" or physical training prior to the operation. Counseling of patients should include the fact that there often is a 4–6 month recovery period involving intensive rehabilitation. A good outcome cannot be expected without the enthusiastic participation of the patient in the postoperative program.

American College of Rheumatology Subcommittee on Osteoarthritis Guidelines: Recommendations for the medical management of osteoarthritis of the hip and knee. Arthritis Rheum 2000;43:1905.

Bielak KM, Merket RM: Exercise. Clin Fam Pract 2000;2:407.

Kirwan JR, Rankin E: Intra-articular therapy in osteoarthritis. Baillieres Clin Rheumatol 1997;11:769.

Langman MJ et al: Adverse upper gastrointestinal effects of rofecoxib compared with NSAIDs. JAMA 1999;282:1929.

McAlindron TD et al: Glucosamine and chondroitin for treatment of osteoarthritis: a systemic quality assessment and meta-analysis. JAMA 2000;283:1469.

Moseley JB et al: A controlled trial of arthroscopic surgery for osteoarthritis of the knee. New Engl J Med 2002;347:81.

Slemenda C et al: Quadriceps weakness and osteoarthritis of the knee. Ann Intern Med 1997;127:97.

GOUT

ESSENTIALS OF DIAGNOSIS

- *Podagra (intense inflammation of the first metatarsophalangeal joint).*
- *Inflammation of the overlying skin.*
- *Pain at rest and intense pain with movement.*
- *Swelling, warmth, redness, and effusion.*
- *Tophi.*
- *Elevated serum uric acid level.*

General Considerations

Gout, first described by Hippocrates in the fourth century BCE, has a colorful history, characterized as a disease of excesses, primarily gluttony and sexual. Sydenham, in the seventeenth century, first differentiated gout from other types of arthritis. An association with diet is germane, as gout is less common in countries in which obesity is uncommon and the diet is relatively devoid of alcohol and reliance on meat and abdominal organs (liver, spleen). Gout is strongly hereditary as well, affecting as many as 25% of the men in some families.

Prevention

Despite the associations noted above, it is difficult with any assurance to advise patients on measures to prevent arthritis. Even thin vegetarians develop gout, although at a markedly lower incidence than obese, alcohol-drinking men. Gout has multiple etiologies and no consistent preventive steps are available to patients.

Clinical Findings

A. Symptoms and Signs

Gout classically presents as an acute monoarthritis. Classic podagra—abrupt, intense inflammation of the first metatarsophalangeal joint—remains the most common presentation of gout (Figure 22–3). The first attack often occurs overnight with intense pain awakening the patient. Any pressure, even a bedsheet on the toe, increases the agony. Walking is difficult due to pain. The overlying skin can be intensely inflamed. On questioning, an exacerbating event may be elicited. Common stories include an excess of alcohol, a heavy meal of abdominal organs (liver, spleen), or a recent physiological stress such as surgery or serious medical disease. Alcohol alters renal excretion of uric acid, allowing rapid buildup of serum uric acid levels. Abdominal organs (along with other foods such as anchovies, sardines, asparagus, salmon, and legumes) contain relatively large quantities of purines that, when broken down, become uric acid.

Acute gout is not limited to the great toe; any joint may be affected, although lower extremity joints are more common. In fact, the abruptness of many gouty attacks and the single joint presentation (acute monoarthritis) at any joint other than the great toe may lead to diagnostic confusion (Table 22–3).

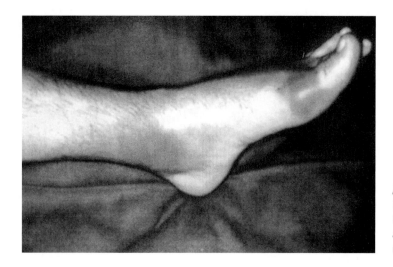

Figure 22–3. Classic podagra involving the first metatarsophalangeal joint. In this photo, the ankle is also involved and the intense erythema could be mistaken for cellulitis.

Gout in joints other than the great toe is frequently missed, occasionally for years. Atypical gout is not uncommon in older women and in men who have already experienced multiple previous episodes of podagra. Foot pain simulating plantar fasciitis is seen in older women. Gout of the ankle (with a positive Homan's sign) can be mistaken for phlebitis. Gout in the lumbar spine, at which synovitis is difficult to imagine much less detect, may go for years before diagnosis.

The intense inflammation at some joints, especially smaller joints such as the ankle, can be impressive. The inflammation may appear to be spreading, encompassing an area greater than what is thought to be the joint. Such cases can be mistaken for cellulitis (Figure 22–3) or superficial phlebitis. The subsequent lack of response to outpatient treatment of cellulitis can cascade to hospital admission and treatment with increasingly strong and expensive antibiotics.

Untreated, attacks of gout slowly resolve with the involved joint becoming progressively less symptomatic over 8–10 days. Long-standing gout with multiple attacks results in destructive changes that both in appearance and symptoms are similar to established OA, although characterized by more inflammatory signs (warmth, redness, effusion). Unlike the other major crystal-induced arthritis, calcium pyrophosphate deposition disease or pseudogout, gout is distinguished by the development of extraarticular manifestations. Tophi are deposits of urate crystals and are found in the ear helix or as nodules elsewhere; atypically placed tophi serve as the source of colorful medical anecdotes. Chronic, untreated gout is a contributor to renal insufficiency (especially in association with heavy metal lead exposure).

Physiological stress is a common precipitating factor. Acute monoarthritis within days of a surgical procedure or a serious medical incident raises concern of infection (which it should!) but is explained by attacks of either gout or pseudogout. In some circumstances, prophylaxis in a person with known gout can prevent these attacks.

About 10% of kidney stones include uric acid. A person with nephrolithiasis due to uric acid stones need

Table 22–3. Inflammatory and noninflammatory causes of monoarthritis.

Inflammatory	Noninflammatory
Crystal-induced	Fracture or meniscal tear
Gout	Other trauma
Pseudogout (calcium pyrophosphate deposition disease)	Osteoarthritis
	Tumors
Apatite (and others)	Osteochondroma
Infectious	Osteoid osteoma
Bacteria	Pigmented villonodular synovitis
Fungi	
Lyme disease or other spirochetes	Cancerous
	Osteonecrosis
TB and other mycobacteria	Hemarthrosis
Viruses (eg, HIV, hepatitis B)	Cancers
Systemic diseases	
Psoriatic or other spondyloarthopathies	
Reactive (eg, inflammatory bowel, Reiter's)	
Systemic lupus erythematosus	

Adapted from Schumacher HR: Signs and symptoms of musculoskeletal disorders. A. Monoarticular joint disease. In Klipper JH (editor). *Primer on the Rheumatic Diseases*, ed 11. Arthritis Foundation, 1997;116.

not have attacks of gout, but patients with gout are at increased risk of developing uric acid stones. A prior history of nephrolithiasis is an important factor in defining therapy in the patient with gout.

Gout is largely a disease of men, with a male:female ratio of 9:1. The first attack of podagra typically occurs in patients in their 30s or 40s although acute gout may present at any age. Interestingly, one attack need not necessarily predict future attacks. In fact, in up to 20% of all men who have one attack of gout, a second episode never follows. Even after a second attack, a sizable percentage (as many as 5%) does not progress to chronic, recurrent gout.

Premenopausal women rarely have gout and then usually in association with other urate metabolic abnormalities. Diagnosis of gout in elderly, postmenopausal women is rare, less because it does not occur than because it is uncommonly suspected.

B. Laboratory Findings

The fundamental abnormality in gout is excess uric acid. In most first attacks of gout, serum uric acid is elevated. In long-standing disease, the uric acid may be normal and symptoms still occur. It is important to note, however, that mild hyperuricemia has a rather high prevalence in the general population. In fact, fewer than 25% of persons with elevated uric acid will ever have gout. Elevation of serum uric acid alone does not confirm a diagnosis of gout, nor does an elevated uric acid predict future attacks.

During acute attacks of gout, the white blood cells (WBC) may be slightly elevated and ESR increased, reflecting acute inflammation. If long-standing gout has caused renal insufficiency, elevations of blood urea nitrogen (BUN) and creatinine are seen along with other electrolyte abnormalities. If gout is indeed suspected as a cause of renal insufficiency, it is well worth measuring the serum lead concentration since "saturnine" gout represents a unique enhancement of the renal destructive characteristics of each component alone.

Gout is generally due to either inappropriately low renal excretion of uric acid (implicated in 90% of patients) or abnormally high endogenous production of uric acid. (The release of huge quantities of urate precursors during chemotherapy for certain hematological cancers is easily predicted and prophylaxis can be instituted.) Collecting a 24-h urine for uric acid and creatinine clearance can be instructive. If the creatinine clearance is greater than 50 mL/min, and the 24-h uric acid excretion is >600 mg, the patient is an overproducer and will respond to specific therapy. Uric acid excretion <600 mg/day, which is the case for most patients with gout, suggests somewhat different therapies.

A strong recommendation must be made to attempt arthrocentesis of the joint in suspected acute gout for several reasons. First episodes of gout present as an acute monoarthritis, for which the differential diagnosis is noted in Table 22–3. Infectious arthritis is a medical emergency, the correct diagnosis of which must be made rapidly and appropriate antibiotic therapy started to avoid destructive changes. Pseudogout is rarely distinguished from gout on the basis of symptoms alone (although pseudogout is a little more likely to occur in larger joints). The settings of both pseudogout and gout can be similar, eg, immediately after surgery. Clinical features of many of the monoarthritides are not characteristic enough to ensure a correct diagnosis. However, crystal examination of synovial fluid is diagnostic of gout. An accurate diagnosis of gout need only be established once, with all subsequent therapeutic decisions confidently made since gout and other crystal-induced arthritides rarely coexist. Characteristics of synovial fluid in selected disease settings is highlighted in Table 22–4.

C. Imaging Studies

Radiographs are usually not needed for the initial diagnosis of the arthritides. Other means of diagnosing gout are more useful.

Phalanges with lateral erosions, distal bone cysts, or the presence of fluffy tophaceous material makes for exciting and characteristic plain film radiographs. However, with our present diagnostic capability, gout should not progress untreated to these late-stage findings. But the changes are characteristic and do not require sophisticated CT or MRI scanning to confirm. Similarly, scintigraphy of gouty joints would be expected to light up but would be a nonspecific means of differentiating monoarthritis due to gout or infection.

Differential Diagnosis

In practice, it is should not be difficult to differentiate between the three prototypical arthritides discussed in this chapter. Nonetheless, Tables 22–1 and 22–3 suggest some key findings for the differential diagnosis of gout.

Treatment

The inflammation of acute gout is easily and effectively managed with antiinflammatory medications, but the major decision is in choice of therapy to prevent attacks.

The often dramatic presentation of gout has a parallel in the often dramatic response to therapy. Once recognized, most cases of gout can be controlled within days, occasionally within hours. Remaining as a challenge is the decision regarding long-term treatment.

Table 22–4. Synovial fluid analysis in selected rheumatic diseases.

	Fluid	White blood cell count	Differential	Glucose	Crystals
Gout	Clear/cloudy	10–100,000	>50% PMNs[1]	Normal	Needle-shaped, negative birefringement
Pseudogout	Clear/cloudy	10–100,000	>50% PMNs	Normal	Rhomboid-shaped, positive birefringement
Infectious	Cloudy	>50,000	Often >95% PMNs	Decreased	None[2]
Osteoarthritis	Clear	2–10,000	<50% PMNs	Normal	None[2]
Rheumatoid arthritis	Clear	10–50,000	>50% PMNs	Normal or decreased	None[2]

[1]PMN, polymorphonuclear leukocytes.
[2]Debris in synovial fluid may be misleading on plain microscopy but only crystals respond to polarizing light.

Standard therapy for acute gout is a short course of NSAIDs at adequate levels. As one of the first NSAIDs developed, indomethacin (50 mg three or four times a day) is occasionally thought to be somehow unique to gout. In fact, all NSAIDs are probably equally effective, although many practitioners feel response is faster with short-acting agents such as naproxen (375–500 mg three times a day) or ibuprofen (800 mg three or four times a day). Response to NSAID therapy is rapid, and treatment is often needed for no more than 3–5 days.

The other standard therapy for acute gout is colchicine. Typically given orally, the instructions to the patient can sound bizarre. The drug is given as a 0.5 or 0.6 mg tablet every 1–2 h "until relief of pain or uncontrollable diarrhea." Most attacks actually respond to the first two or three pills with a maximum of six pills in 24 h a prudent suggestion. Most patients will develop diarrhea well before the sixth pill. In fact, colchicine is well tolerated. At one time, colchicine was believed to be specific to gout and that response to colchicine in essence confirmed the diagnosis. This is not accurate as pseudogout also responds to the drug. As with NSAIDs, colchicine is continued for 3–4 days after the onset of gout at a three times a day dosing interval.

On occasion, corticosteroids are indicated in acute gout. Either oral prednisone (eg, up to 60 mg), methylprednisolone or triamcinolone (eg, 40–80 mg) intramuscularly, or intraarticular agents can be used. Indications include intense overlying skin involvement (mimicking cellulitis), polyarticular presentation of gout, and poor response to NSAID or colchicine therapy. Intraarticular steroid use should be considered for ankle or knee gout, if presenting as a monoarthritis and infection is ruled out. Patients have considerable anxiety and pain with arthrocentesis of the great toe and infrequently allow a second attempt (this assumes the first attempt was to collect synovial fluid for diagnosis).

Decisions regarding long-term treatment of gout must take into account the natural history of attacks. The first attack, especially if the man is young and there is a clear precipitating event (such as an alcohol binge), may not be followed by a second attack for years, even decades. As stated earlier, as many as 20% of men will never have a second gouty attack. Data from the Framingham longitudinal study suggest that intervals of up to 12 years are common between first and second attack. This is not always the case for young women with gout (who tend to have a uric acid metabolic abnormality) or for either men or women who have polyarticular gout. But for many young men, a reasonable recommendation after a first episode is not to treat prophylactically.

The doctor and patient may even decide to withhold prophylactic medication after a second attack, but when episodes of gout become more frequent than one or two a year, both parties are ready to consider long-term medication. The primary medications used at this point are probenecid and allopurinol. Probenecid is a uric acid tubular reuptake inhibitor, resulting in increased excretion of uric acid in the urine. Allopurinol inhibits the uric acid synthesis pathway, blocking the step converting xanthine to uric acid. Xanthine is much more soluble than uric acid and is not implicated in either acute arthritis, nephrolithiasis, or renal insufficiency. The 24-h uric acid excretion can be helpful at this time. The patient with low excretion of uric acid ("underexcretor") should respond to probenecid. A typical dose is 500 mg/day and with infrequent rash the only side effect. Probenecid loses effectiveness when the creatinine clearance falls below 50 mL/min, so alternative therapy is necessary in renal insufficiency. If the patient has uric acid nephrolithiasis, probenecid is contraindicated so as not to increase delivery of uric acid to the stone-forming region.

Some "underexcretors" and virtually all "overproducers" of uric acid will require allopurinol. Typically dosed at 300 mg/day, allopurinol predictably lowers serum uric acid levels and is highly effective at preventing gouty attacks. It is a well-tolerated drug with only infrequent side effects of nausea, diarrhea, or headache. The side effect of concern is rash. Although truly rare, allopurinol-induced rash can progress to a toxic hypersensitivity with fever, leukocytosis, epidermal necrolysis, and renal failure. Patients should be cautioned, but not alarmed, about this complication.

Allopurinol is especially indicated for treatment of tophaceous gout (Figure 22–4) and for uric acid nephrolithiasis. Allopurinol is also the drug of choice for those with uric acid metabolic abnormalities (often young women) and polyarticular gout. Caution must be used, however, when starting allopurinol (and probenecid) for the first time. Rapid lowering of the serum uric acid causes instability of uric acid crystals within the synovial fluid and can actually precipitate an attack of gout. Consequently, prior establishment of either NSAID or colchicine therapy is necessary to prevent this complication.

Patients are occasionally seen on long-term therapy with colchicine. There is a conceptual attraction to this choice. Between attacks of gout, the so-called "intercritical period," examination of synovial fluid continues to show uric acid crystals. These may be free-floating or even ingested by white blood cells. Using colchicine to prevent the spiral to inflammation seems appealing. But this choice is deceptive. Colchicine does nothing to lower uric acid levels. Long-term use allows deposition of uric acid into destructive tophi or contributes to renal disease and kidney stones. Colchicine can be an effective prophylactic agent, for instance, if started prior to a surgical procedure in a patient with known gout but not on allopurinol or probenecid. But use of this drug as a solo agent courts other, significant complications.

Agudelo CA, Wise CM: Crystal-associated arthritis in the elderly. Rheum Dis Clin North Am 2000;26:527.

Roubenoff R et al: Incidence and risk factors for gout in white men. JAMA 1991;266:3004.

Wartmann RL: Gout and hyperuricemia. Curr Opin Rheumatol 2002;14:281.

RHEUMATOID ARTHRITIS

ESSENTIALS OF DIAGNOSIS

- *Arthritis of three or more joint areas.*
- *Arthritis in both hands and/or both feet (bilateral joint involvement).*
- *Morning stiffness.*
- *Fatigue.*
- *Swelling, tenderness, warmth, and loss of function.*
- *Rheumatoid nodules.*
- *Elevated erythrocyte sedimentation rate/C-reactive protein.*
- *Positive test for rheumatoid factor.*

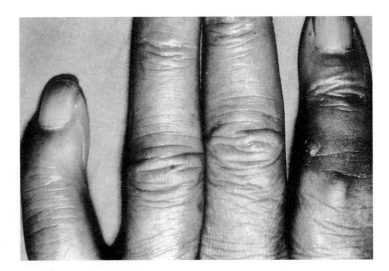

Figure 22–4. Tophaceous gout with subcutaneous nodule almost breaking through the skin.

General Considerations

Bony changes consistent with rheumatoid arthritis (RA) have been found in the body of a Native American who lived 3000 years ago. Differentiation of RA from other arthritides is more recent, having occurred in the late nineteenth century. RA is more frequently seen in women, with the ratio of premenopausal women to age-matched men approximately 4:1; after the age of menopause, the ratio is closer to 1:1. An estrogen:androgen ratio found in premenopausal women (and aging men) may provide a permissive environment for other factors to initiate the processes resulting in RA. Some contend that estrogenic xenobiotics, estrogen-like agents found in products as diverse as plastics and pesticides, account for a purported rise in incidence of RA. Even so, it is unlikely that the estrogen:androgen ratio makes more than a minor contribution to the onset of the disease.

Pathogenesis

Although the etiology of RA is not known, the pathophysiology has been elucidated to a remarkable degree in recent decades. Important knowledge of all inflammatory processes has come from studies in RA. Early, the synovium of joints is targeted by T cells (this is the feature that leads to the "autoimmune" moniker applied to RA). Release of interleukins, lymphokines, cytokines, tissue necrosis factor, and other messengers attracts additional inflammatory cells to the synovium. Intense inflammation ensues, experienced by the patient as pain, warmth, swelling, and loss of function. Reactive cells move into the inflammatory synovium, attempting to repair damaged tissue. Uncontrolled response develops into the pathological tissue called pannus, an exuberant growth of tissue engulfing the joint space and causing destruction itself. The response of cartilage is breakdown of tissue, deterioration, and eventual destruction. Periarticular bone responds to inflammation with resorption, seen as erosions on x-ray. All these changes clearly are maladaptive and responsible for destruction-causing deformity and disability.

Prevention

It is difficult with any assurance to advise patients on measures to prevent arthritis. Changing the estrogen:androgen ratio through oral contraceptives or hormone replacement therapy does little to prevent, or enhance, the likelihood of developing RA. RA has multiple etiologies and no consistent preventive steps are available to patients.

Clinical Findings

A. SYMPTOMS AND SIGNS

RA is a systemic disease, causing fatigue, rash, nodules, depression, and more as joints become progressively stiff and inflamed. RA is a systemic disease with most, but by no means all, symptoms initially in the joints. It is characterized by inflammation, so the presence of swelling, warmth, and loss of function is imperative to the diagnosis. Joints of the hands (Figure 22–5) and feet are typically affected first, although larger joints can be involved at any time. The disease is classically symmetrical with symptoms in both hands and/or both feet. This mirroring of symptoms is almost unique to RA with few other rheumatic diseases characteristically having bilateral, similar joint involvement. Even systemic lupus erythematosus, which is often confused with RA in its early stages, is not so consistently symmetrical.

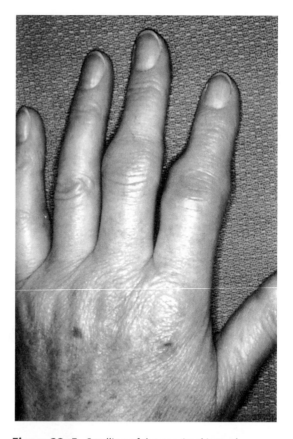

Figure 22–5. Swelling of the proximal interphalangeal joints of the second and third fingers in rheumatoid arthritis. Symmetrical swelling might be expected on the other hand.

Fingers and wrists are stiff and sore in the mornings, requiring heat, rubbing, and movement to be functional ("morning stiffness"). The morning stiffness is in contrast, again, to most other arthritic conditions. Stiffness after prolonged lack of movement ("gelling") is not uncommon in many joint disorders, but the morning stiffness of RA is so prolonged and characteristic that queries regarding this symptom are one of the essentials of diagnosis.

The patient reports fatigue out of proportion to lack of sleep. Daytime naps are almost unavoidable, yet are not fully restorative. Anorexia, weight loss, even low-grade fever can be present. Along with musculoskeletal complaints, these somatic concerns may contribute to mistaken diagnoses of fibromyalgia or even depression.

RA can eventually involve almost any joint in the body. Selected important manifestations of RA in specific joints are listed in Table 22–5. The cause of any one manifestation may be unique to a particular joint, but common features include inflammation-induced stretching of tendons and ligaments resulting in joint laxity, subconscious restriction of movement resulting in "frozen" joints, and consequences of inflammatory synovitis with cartilage destruction and periarticular bone erosion. An objective sign of destruction includes the high-pitched, "crunchy" sound of crepitus. Functional deterioration with loss of grip, strength, gait, or movement represents considerable, usually permanent destruction.

Table 22–5. Manifestations of rheumatoid arthritis in specific joints.

Joint	Complication[1]
Hand	Ulnar deviation (hand points toward ulnar side)
	Swan-neck deformity (extension of PIP joint)
	Boutonniere deformity (flexion at DIP)
Wrist	Swelling causing carpal tunnel syndrome
Elbow	Swelling causing compressive neuropathy
	Deformity preventing complete extension, loss of power
Shoulder	"Frozen shoulder" (loss of abduction, nighttime pain)
Neck	Subluxation of C1–C2 joint with danger of dislocation and spinal cord compression ("hangman's injury")
Foot	"Cock-up" deformity and/or subluxation at MTP
Knee	Effusion leading to Baker's cyst (evagination of synovial lining and fluid into popliteal space)

[1]PIP, proximal interphalangeal; DIP, distal interphalangeal; MTP, metatarsophalangeal.

Extraarticular manifestations of RA can be seen at any stage of disease. Most common are rheumatoid nodules, found at some point in up to 50% of all patients with RA. These occur almost anywhere in the body but usually subcutaneously, especially along pressure points (the typical olecranon site), along tendons, or in bursae. Vasculitis is an uncommon initial presentation of RA, but when present includes either a leukocytoclastic or purpuric skin appearance. Dry eyes and mouth are seen in the RA-associated sicca syndrome. Dyspnea, or cough, or even chest pain may signal respiratory interstitial disease. Cardiac, gastrointestinal, and renal involvement by RA is not common. Peripheral nervous system symptoms usually are seen as compression neuropathies (eg, carpal or tarsal tunnel syndrome) and reflect not so much direct attack on nerves as consequences of squeezing compression as nerves are forced into passages narrowed by nearby inflammation.

B. LABORATORY FINDINGS

In contrast to OA and gout, the laboratory findings in RA can be significant and helpful. The complete blood count (CBC) is not infrequently abnormal with a normocytic anemia common in active disease. This anemia is almost always the so-called anemia of chronic disease. Although sometimes confused with iron deficiency, the anemia of chronic disease represents a suppression of erythrocyte maturation independent of iron stores. Treatment of this disorder is directed at control of the inflammatory process, not at iron supplementation. The white blood cell count is usually normal or even slightly elevated; an exception is the rare Felty's syndrome (splenomegaly and leukopenia in a patient with known RA).

RA does not typically affect electrolytes and renal function. There is no pathophysiological reason why transaminases, bilirubin, alkaline phosphatase, or other liver, pancreatic, or bone enzymes should be altered. Similarly, calcium, magnesium, and other cations, and phosphate should be unchanged. Most hormone measurements are normal, particularly thyroid and the adrenal axis. Chronic inflammatory disease may alter the menstrual cycle but measurement of luteinizing hormone and follicle-stimulating hormone is of little help in active RA.

Elevations of the ESR and the CRP are frequent. An elevated ESR is long established in RA, and in aggressive or explosive disease may even approach 100 mm/h. The CRP is considered by many rheumatologists to be a more sensitive indicator of inflammation, and might be increased in circumstances in which the ESR is either "normal" or minimally elevated. Although quite reliable, there are circumstances in which the ESR is false (Table 22–6). The CRP is more expensive and

Table 22–6. Nondisease factors that influence the ESR.[1]

Increase ESR	Decrease ESR	No Effect on ESR
Aging	Leukocytosis (>25,000)	Obesity
Female	Polycythemia (Hgb >18)	Body tempera-
Pregnancy	Red blood cell changes	ture
Anemia	Sickle cell	Recent meal
Macrocytosis	Anisocytosis	Aspirin
Congenital hyper-	Microcytosis	NSAID
fibrinogenemia	Acanthocytosis	
Technical factors	Protein abnormalities	
Dilutional	Dysproteinemia with	
Elevated	hyperviscosity	
specimen	Hypofibrinogenemia	
temperature	Hypogammaglobulin	
	Technical factors	
	Dilutional	
	Inadequate mixing	
	Vibration during test	
	Clotting of specimen	

Modified from Brigden ML: Clinical utility of the erythrocyte sedimentation rate. Am Fam Physician 1999;60:1443.
[1]ESR, erythrocyte sedimentation rate; Hgb, hemoglobin; NSAID, nonsteroidal antiinflammatory drug.

Table 22–7. Conditions associated with a positive rheumatoid factor.

Normal aging

Chronic bacterial infections
  Subacute bacterial endocarditis
  Tuberculosis
  Lyme disease
  Others

Viral disease
  Cytomegalovirus
  Epstein–Barr virus
  Hepatitis B

Chronic inflammatory diseases
  Sarcoidosis
  Periodontal disease
  Chronic liver disease (especially viral)
  Sjögren's disease
  Systemic lupus erythematosus
  Mixed cryoglobulinemia

somewhat cumbersome to perform, but is increasingly used by specialists in management monitoring.

The test most associated with RA is the rheumatoid factor (RF). This protein actually represents a family of antibodies, the most common of which is an immunoglobulin M (IgM) antibody directed against the Fc portion of immunoglobulin G (IgG). There is no question this antibody is frequently present in RA, with RF-negative RA accounting for only about 5% of all patients with RA. The problem is with the low specificity of the test. Surveys demonstrate that in a young population, 3–5% of "normal" individuals have a positive RF whereas in an older cohort the prevalence of positive RF reaches 25%. With the national prevalence of RA at only 1% (at most), it is clear that many people with a positive RF do not have RA. Some of the conditions that are associated with a positive RF are listed in Table 22–7.

C. Imaging Studies

Radiographs are usually not needed for the initial diagnosis of the arthritides. Other means of diagnosing RA are more useful.

The appearance of characteristic, and prognostically useful, bony changes can be detected relatively earlier in joints damaged by RA than either OA or gout. Because RA is a disease of synovial tissue, and because the synovium lies on and attaches to distal bone, inflammation of this tissue can cause early alterations on plain film radiography. Small erosions, or lucencies, on the lateral portions of phalanges are early indications of significant inflammation (Figure 22–6). Such signs were used, until relatively recently, as an indication to pursue more aggressive treatment of RA. Especially in the current setting of early intervention, the presence of erosions should prompt immediate suppressive treatment.

Plain film radiographs are an accurate and inexpensive means of documenting malalignments and subluxation of joints. These findings, along with a progressive decline in function, serve as milestones for decisions regarding surgical replacement of joints.

CT and MRI have particular value in detecting a major undesired complication of treatment of RA. Changes of marrow infarction, as seen in aseptic necrosis (eg, of the femoral head), have characteristic findings with either of these modalities. Scintigraphy is useful in detecting aseptic necrosis, but, along with MRI, is also employed to differentiate the intense synovitis of RA from infection such as septic arthritis or overlying cellulitis. Osteomyelitis situated close to a joint involved with RA may be diagnosed with either MRI or three-phase bone scan.

Differential Diagnosis

In practice, it is should not be difficult to differentiate between the three prototypical arthritides discussed in

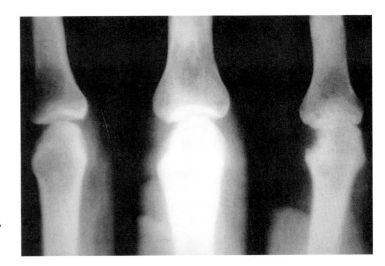

Figure 22–6. Progressive bony changes characteristic of rheumatoid arthritis at a metacarpophalangeal joint. At the left, soft tissue swelling alone is seen. In the middle, early thinning of the cortex is noted. At the right, the thinning has resulted in an erosion with associated loss of joint space.

this chapter. Nonetheless, Table 22–1 suggests some key findings for diagnosis of RA.

Treatment

Therapy of RA has changed from methods of managing inflammation to specific measures directed against the fundamental sources of the inflammation.

In just the past decades, treatment of RA has undergone perhaps the most wholescale shift of any of the rheumatological conditions. From a practice that used to proceed step-wise from conservative (but high-dose) treatment with aspirin or NSAIDs to more toxic agents, RA is now treated almost as a "medical emergency." Therapy is directed at fundamental processes and begins with aggressive, potentially toxic disease-modifying drugs. The outlook can be hopeful, with preservation of joints, activity, and life-style a realistic goal. RA need no longer be the "deforming arthritis" by which it was known just a short time ago.

An early decision by the primary care doctor is whether, and when, to refer the patient with suspected or confirmed RA. Diagnosis can be established, or strongly suspected, by assessment for the criteria developed and confirmed by specialty organizations (Table 22–8). However, relatively recent studies still suggest a considerable lag between onset of symptoms and initiation of disease-modifying treatment. Unfortunately, delay allows inflammation to become established with changes on radiographs already present. For all but mild disease, RA is increasingly being treated with combinations of drugs that target different aspects of the pathophysiology. These drug combinations resemble the chemotherapy regimens used by oncologists, with careful timing of administration and watchful surveillance for toxicities.

A. ASSESSMENT OF PROGNOSTIC FACTORS

One of the early steps in treating RA is to assess prognostic factors in the individual patient. Poor prognosis leads to the decision to start aggressive treatment earlier. Some prognostic features are demographic such as female sex, age greater than 50 years, low socioeconomic status, and a first-degree relative with RA. Clinical features associated with poor prognosis include large

Table 22–8. 1987 American College of Rheumatology diagnostic criteria for rheumatoid arthritis.

The diagnosis of rheumatoid arthritis is confirmed if the patient has had at least four of the seven following criteria, with criteria 1–6 having been present for at least 6 weeks:

1. Morning stiffness (at least 1 h)
2. Arthritis of three or more joint areas (areas are right or left of proximal interphalangeal joints, metacarpophalangeal, wrist, elbow, knee, ankle, and metatarsophalangeal)
3. Arthritis of hand joints (proximal interphalangeal joints or metacarpophalangeal joints)
4. Symmetric arthritis, by area
5. Subcutaneous rheumatoid nodules
6. Positive test for rheumatoid factor
7. Radiographic changes (hand and wrist radiography that show erosion of joints or unequivocal demineralization around joints)

Arnett FC et al: The American Rheumatism Association 1987 revised criteria for the classification of rheumatoid arthritis. Arthritis Rheum 1988;31:315.

number of affected joints, especially involvement of the flexor tendons of the wrist, with persistence of swelling at the fingers; rheumatoid nodules (Figure 22–7); high ESR or CRP and high titers of RF; presence of erosions on radiographs; and evidence of functional disability. Formal functional testing along with disease activity questionnaires is frequently employed, not only in establishing stage of disease but also at many interval visits.

B. Patient Education

Therapy begins with patient education and again there are multiple sources of information from support/advocacy groups, professional organizations, government sources, and pharmaceutical companies. Patients should learn about the natural history of RA and the multiple therapies to interrupt the course. They should learn about joint protection and the likelihood that at least some activities need to be modified or discontinued. RA, especially before disease modification is established, is a fatiguing disorder. Patients should realize that rest is as important as appropriate types of activity. Of vital importance is the patient's acknowledgment that drug regimens about to be started are complex but that compliance is critical to successful outcomes. The patient should frankly be told that the drugs are toxic and are likely to have adverse effects but that the effects can often be treated or substitute medications utilized.

C. Medications

Pain is caused by inflammation and establishment of effective antiinflammatory drugs is the first goal of medication. NSAIDs, at doses recommended earlier (Table 22–2), give the patient an early indication that relief can be achieved. NSAIDs are used throughout the course of treatment; it is not uncommon to switch from one to another as efficacy seems to slide. Desirable qualities of the NSAID chosen are simplicity of dosing, low cost, and lack of side effects.

If the patient is reluctant to start drugs, there are short-term trials of fish oil suggesting symptomatic relief. Both omega-3 and omega-6 fatty acids in fish oil modulate synthesis of highly inflammatory prostaglandin E_2 and leukotriene E_4, favoring production of less inflammatory compounds. The fish oil chosen must contain high concentrations of the relevant fatty acids, a large number of capsules need to be taken, and palatability, diarrhea, and halitosis are frequent accompaniments. γ-Linolenic acid interrupts the pathway of arachidonic acid, another component of the inflammatory cascades. Extracted from the oils of plant seeds such as linseed, sunflower seed, and flaxseed, γ-linolenic acid demonstrates some efficacy in short-term studies using large doses of the extract.

Neither NSAIDs nor "natural" products are disease modifying. Disease-modifying antirheumatic drugs (DMARDs) are drugs that not only control patient symptoms but also suppress the underlying factors that result in synovitis, tissue reactivity (eg, pannus), erosions, ligament/tendon laxity, subluxations, and all the other complications of RA. DMARDs are almost always used in combinations, both to enhance efficacy and to decrease dosage and potential toxicity. Toxicity is a major concern with DMARDs and, in fact, the monitoring for adverse effects may account for almost as much cost and inconvenience as the drugs themselves. For instance, hydroxychloroquine requires baseline and follow-up ophthalmologic visits whereas methotrexate requires baseline and follow-up renal and liver tests and even the occasional liver biopsy.

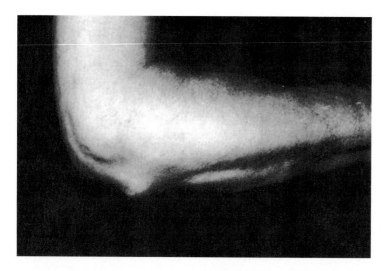

Figure 22–7. Rheumatoid nodule located at the pressure point near the olecranon.

Frequently accompanying NSAID therapy is either sulfasalazine or hydroxychloroquine. Both of these drugs (developed initially for inflammatory bowel disease and malaria, respectively, and coincidentally noted to be effective in RA) have beneficial effects in RA. They are weak DMARDs, with the antimalarial seemingly a more common first choice. Both drugs may allow NSAID therapy at lower doses and clearly are additive. Hydroxychloroquine, as noted above, requires baseline and ophthalmological examinations every 6–12 months to detect color change and/or deposition of drug in the retina. The eye complications of hydroxychloroquine are rare and typically are seen with a higher than recommended dose of 200 mg twice a day. Sulfasalazine is remarkably well tolerated and safe when prescribed at doses up to 2–3 g/day. A few patients experience gastric intolerance; the unlikely occurrence of leukopenia requires hematological monitoring with some regularity (as often as every 2 months). Some patients with mild RA experience control of symptoms and delay or even suppression of disease progression with a combination of NSAID and hydroxychloroquine or sulfasalazine. Gold preparations, either oral (auranofin) or parenteral (thiomalate, aurothioglucose), had been a standard therapy.

These drugs have disease-modifying properties in both short-term and intermediate use. Long-term use of gold is problematic as symptom control can be maintained but disease progression, as measured by appearance of erosions, appears. These are not easy drugs to use. Gastrointestinal side effects are common with oral gold and often result in discontinuation. Mucositis, usually oral ulcers, is an uncomfortable side effect of auranofin. Parenteral administration is cumbersome. Both types of preparations can have significant renal adverse effects and surveillance by urinalysis is required. Thrombocytopenia and leukopenia, although uncommon and seen more often with parenteral gold, may not resolve with discontinuation; treatment with corticosteroids and even granulocyte colony-stimulating factor may be necessary. Gold products are still used, especially in people with mild RA intolerant of other agents, but they have largely been supplanted by different regimens.

Penicillamine is another drug that had been widely, although cautiously, used. It does have DMARD properties and is so effective at low enough doses (eg, 250 mg/day) that adverse effects are not common. But it now is prescribed only in refractory RA cases because the adverse effects, when they do occur, are complex and difficult to treat. Leukopenia responds to discontinuation of drug. Of much more concern are unusual autoimmune disorders such as a myasthenic syndrome, a lupus-like condition, and a disorder that resembles polymyositis. These effects can be treated, and even cured, but they are alarming and produce considerable anxiety.

Minocycline is included in many combination therapies. This antibiotic is not used for its antibacterial effects (although many practitioners believe activity of RA can be diminished if occult infection, particularly sinusitis, is treated). Rather, minocycline is an inhibitor of metalloproteinase, an enzyme involved in the production of pannus within joints. Several well-done studies support the use of minocycline at a dose of 100 mg twice a day in moderate to even severe RA, typically in combination regimens.

The drug that has become a standard in treatment of RA is methotrexate. Especially when used in combination with an antimalarial or sulfasalazine, methotrexate presents all the benefits of a disease-modifying drug. Response is common and relatively rapid with symptom control within weeks. Early fears of liver toxicity and cirrhosis have largely been allayed by longer term studies, but frequent measurement of liver enzymes is required. At doses recommended, no more than 15–20 mg/week, gastrointestinal, mucocutaneous, and hematological adverse effects are not common or intolerable. Methotrexate, along with cyclophosphamide, affects T cells. The pathology of RA is complex, but enhanced activity of T cells, especially with movement into the synovium, is the key to the development of destructive pannus (and other nonarticular manifestations of RA). The ability of methotrexate to reduce this step is the key to disease modification.

Methotrexate is the most commonly used DMARD. But that does not mean it is an easy drug to use. Patients who imbibe large quantities of alcohol must alter this habit as adverse liver effects with methotrexate are considerably heightened. Folic acid is usually prescribed with methotrexate and, in addition to preventing macrocytic anemia, seems to diminish gastrointestinal side effects. Dosing starts low, as little as 5–7.5 mg/week, and only gradually increases to avoid mucositis or other gastrointestinal side effects. As noted, dosing is weekly, which, ironically, actually decreases compliance in some patients who seem to remember daily drugs better. Liver enzymes and blood counts need to be done every 6–8 weeks as long as the patient is on the drug. An early fear that long-term use of methotrexate would result in increased infectious incidents or cancers has not materialized. Nonetheless, awareness of infectious complications, including organisms such as *Pneumocystis carinii*, is necessary. There are a few reports of non-Hodgkin's lymphoma developing in patients on methotrexate. Perhaps of even more concern is the development of a diffuse pulmonary alveolitis. Usually responsive to discontinuation of methotrexate and corticosteroid administration, it appears this complication is more likely to occur in patients with preexisting pulmonary disease. Methotrexate-induced painful nodules, different from rheumatoid nodules, appear on the fingers. These can be progressive, even after discontinuation, but respond to colchicine.

Finally, an ironic side effect of methotrexate use is that disease flare is extremely common (>75%) should methotrexate have to be stopped. The flare, which develops within 2–3 months, proves resistant to reinduction therapy, either with methotrexate or other DMARDs. All that being said, methotrexate is almost universally used in RA, has efficacy in most patients, and counts as one of the most significant advances in disease treatment in the past decades.

Azathioprine and cyclophosphamide are two other chemotherapy drugs not infrequently used in RA drug regimens. These agents do not have either the efficacy or side effect profile of methotrexate, but are turned to in circumstances in which additional drugs are needed to control symptoms or halt disease progression. Azathioprine use is limited to moderate or severe RA unresponsive to other DMARDs. Gastrointestinal and hematological adverse effects are most commonly experienced, with discontinuation of the drug usually all that is required. Azathioprine has been used with success in treatment of serious extraarticular manifestations. There does not appear to be an increased risk of cancer. Cyclophosphamide has such frequent problems with bone marrow suppression, cystitis, bladder hemorrhage, and risk of cancer that its use is infrequent. However, used in combination with high-dose corticosteroids, use of cyclophosphamide is perhaps indicated in life-threatening rheumatoid vasculitis.

Leflunomide is a pyrimidine synthesis inhibitor with efficacy equivalent to methotrexate. Even when used in low doses (10–20 mg/day after a loading dose), there is considerable liver toxicity and surveillance with blood tests for liver enzyme abnormalities is required. Leflunomide is not cleared from the body as rapidly as methotrexate, which is sometimes seen as an advantage (prompting the concept of a "drug holiday"). But similar to other chemotherapy agents, leflunomide is a teratogen, making the prolonged presence in body tissues a deceptive problem. Women of childbearing age must remain on effective contraception for as much as a year after stopping leflunomide. This drug is being investigated for use in moderate to severe RA, occasionally in combination with methotrexate.

Cyclosporine was once promoted for RA treatment as a DMARD with unique beneficial properties. It suppresses immunological processes at steps different than chemotherapy agents. It is effective, as demonstrated in several studies. But the toxicity of cyclosporine is considerable, especially renal effects with development of a particularly resistant type of hypertension and reduc-

tion in renal clearance. The latter effect does not reverse with discontinuation of the drug. Cyclosporine use is currently limited to combinations with methotrexate in severe RA poorly responsive to other therapies.

A different approach to management of RA has followed the development of tumor necrosis factor (TNF) inhibitors. TNF is a messenger attracting other inflammatory cells to a site. In addition, TNF is also involved in production of interferon and interleukines. Blockade of these effects diminishes the inflammatory response, both decreasing patient symptoms and slowing disease progression. Etanercept (Enbrel), infliximab (Remicabe), and adalimumab (Humira) are current examples of TNF inhibitors. These drugs require subcutaneous or intravenous injection, as often as every other week. Despite that, they are relatively well tolerated and associated with hematological toxicity that responds to discontinuation. The TNF inhibitors are indicated for moderate to severe RA, are infrequently given as single agents or first-line drugs, and require regular blood count surveillance. Following in the same physiological idea, an interleukin-1 receptor antagonist (anakinra-Kineret) has recently been introduced. This drug has modest benefit as both a single agent (for which it really is not recommended) and in combination with an agent such as methotrexate. Side effects are relatively common, with leukopenia and sepsis of most concern.

Corticosteroid use in RA goes back to the earliest days of steroid development. It was the dramatic demonstration of symptom reduction in RA that propelled the use of corticosteroids in rheumatic diseases, resulting in a Nobel Prize in Medicine in 1950. But it was the use of high-dose steroids in RA that also led to the recognition of serious complications, and the cautions employed every day in decisions regarding use of steroids. Steroids reduce inflammation and improve symptoms in patients with RA. Finding the correct use is the challenge. Current recommendations suggest use of steroids in limited, but not infrequent, settings.

Corticosteroids can be useful in suppressing activity of RA while establishing other DMARDs, which typically take much longer to have an effect. As initial therapy for a patient with moderate, active disease, steroids (eg, prednisone 40–60 mg/day) can rapidly control symptoms, decrease inflammation, and provide time for DMARDs to begin to have an effect. Similarly, if a patient has flared and the decision is made to change DMARD therapy, steroids can provide "bridging" to the new therapy. If the patient has one or two joints that persist in inflammation and symptoms despite adequate overall control, intraarticular steroids provide an excellent and appreciated intervention. As with use of intraarticular injection in OA (and even gout), this treatment should not be overused; the perceived requirement for frequent intraarticular injection should instead prompt review of the patient's current regimen.

More controversial is the long-term use of corticosteroids, usually at relatively low dose (eg, prednisone 5–10 mg/day). Although most studies note symptom control but disease progression, a few recent studies suggest slowing of joint destruction. The focus of this very low-dose treatment (<5 mg/day) might be metalloproteases more than inflammation. Concern about progressive long-term complications to bone, skin, and other connective tissues has not been allayed with these recent reports.

D. SURGERY

Joint instability and resultant disability are often due to a combination of joint destruction, a primary effect of synovial inflammation, and tendon/ligament laxity, a secondary effect or "innocent bystander." The innocent bystander effect asserts that these connective tissues are stretched, weakened, or malaligned due to inflammation of the joints over which they connect or cross but not due to a direct attack on the tendon/ligament itself. Nonetheless, at some point joint destruction and connecting tissue dysfunction combine to give useless, and frequently painful, joints. At this point, the surgeon has much to offer. Joint stabilization, connecting tissue reinsertion, and joint replacement of both small (interphalangeal) and large (hip, knee) joints provide return of function and reduction of pain. The timing of surgery is still an art and is most effective when close collaboration exists between the medical doctor and surgeon.

Complications

Serious extraarticular manifestations of RA are not infrequent. Some of these are life-threatening and require sophisticated management by doctors experienced in dealing with these crises. The responsibility often remains with the primary care doctor to recognize these conditions and refer appropriately. Table 22–9 lists several of these complications with a brief description of the clinical presentation.

Prognosis

Morbidity and mortality are increased in patients with RA over age-matched persons without RA. Correlated with active disease, there is a well-described increase in stroke and myocardial infarct. These manifestations may be due to a hypercoagulable state induced by the autoimmune process and circulating antibodies. Otherwise, with long-standing RA, even with conscientious treatment, complications from infection, pulmonary and renal disease, and gastrointestinal bleeding occur at rates higher than the general population. Many of these latter diseases are related as much to drugs used to control the disease as to the disease itself.

Table 22–9. Extraarticular manifestations of rheumatoid arthritis.

Complication	Brief Comments
Rheumatoid nodules	Found over pressure points, classically olecranon. Typically fade with disease-modifying antirheumatic drug (DMARD) therapy. Also may be found in internal organs. If causing disability, may attempt intralesional steroids, or surgery.
Popliteal cyst	Usually asymptomatic unless ruptures; then mimics calf thrombophlebitis. Ultrasonography (and high index of suspicion) useful.
Anemia	Usually "chronic disease" and, despite low measured iron, does not respond to oral iron therapy. Improves with control of inflammatory disease.
Scleritis/episcleritis	Inflammatory lesion of conjunctiva. More prolonged, intense, and uncomfortable than "simple" conjunctivitis. Requires ophthalmological management.
Pulmonary disease	Ranges from simple pleuritis and pleural effusion (noted for low glucose) to severe bronchiolitis, interstitial fibrosis, nodulosis, and pulmonary vasculitis. May require high-dose steroid therapy once diagnosis established by bronchoscopy or even open lung biopsy.
Sjögren's syndrome	Often occurring with RA, includes sicca syndrome with thickened respiratory secretions, dysphagia, vaginal atrophy, hyperglobulinemia, and distal renal tubule defects. Treatment of sicca syndrome possible with muscarinic-receptor agonists; other manifestations more difficult.
Felty's syndrome	Constellation of RA, leukopenia, splenomegaly, and often anemia, thrombocytopenia. Control underlying RA with DMARDs; may need granulocyte colony-stimulating factor, especially if infectious complications are frequent.
Rheumatoid vasculitis	Spectrum from digital arteritis (with hemorrhage) to cutaneous ulceration to mononeuritis multiplex to severe, life-threatening multisystem arteritis involving heart, gastrointestinal tract, and other organs. Resembles polyarteritis nodosum.

Bluhm GB et al: Radiographic results from the Minocycline in Rheumatoid Arthritis (MIRA) trial. J Rheumatol 1997;24:1295.

Cutolo M, Wilder RL: Different roles for androgens and estrogens in the susceptibility to autoimmune rheumatic diseases. Rheum Dis Clin North Am 2000;26:825.

Kirwan JR, Lim KK: Low dose corticosteroids in early rheumatoid arthritis. Can these drugs slow disease progression? Drugs Aging 1996;8:157.

Moreland LW, Bridges SL Jr: Early rheumatoid arthritis: a medical emergency? Am J Med 2001;111:498.

O'Dell JR: Combination DMARD therapy for rheumatoid arthritis: a step closer to the goal. Ann Rheum Dis 1996;55:781.

O'Dell JR et al: Treatment of rheumatoid arthritis with methotrexate alone, sulfasalazine and hydroxychloroquine, or a combination of all three medications. New Engl J Med 1996;334:1287.

Sox HC Jr, Liang MH: The erythrocyte sedimentation rate: guidelines for rational use. Ann Intern Med 1986;104:515.

Suarez-Almazor ME et al: Utilization and predictive value of laboratory tests in patients referred to rheumatologists by primary care physicians. J Rheumatol 1998;25:1980.

Tugwell P et al: Combination therapy with cyclosporine and methotrexate in severe rheumatoid arthritis. New Engl J Med 1995;333:137.

Wållberg-Honsson S et al: Extent of inflammation predicts cardiovascular disease and overall mortality in seropositive rheumatoid arthritis. A retrospective cohort study from disease onset. J Rheumatol 1999;26:2562.

WEB SITES

American Academy of Family Physicians. Like the ACP site, of more relevance to member practitioners. Does have a link to www.familydoctor.org, which is an excellent source of general medical information for patients.

www.aafp.org.

American College of Physicians. Free access information helpful but limited for nonmembers. More relevant to member practitioners.

www.acponline.org

American College of Rheumatology. Limited free access information, more relevant to practitioners than patients. www.rheumatology.org

Arthritis Foundation. Helpful and user-friendly information for patients, written without medical jargon. A strong section on advocacy.

www.arthritis.org.

Mayo Clinic. A fine source of patient friendly information.

www.mayoclinic.com

National Guideline Clearinghouse. Supported by the governmental Agency for Health Care Policy and Research. Excellent source for guidelines on all topics from many sources. More relevant to practitioners.

www.guideline.gov

National Institute for Arthritis and Musculoskeletal and Skin Diseases (NIH). A web site with much information for practitioners as well as practical information for patients.

www.niams.nih.gov

National Library of Medicine and NIH. An excellent source of unbiased information for practitioners and patients. Tutorials help patients with numerous topics, starting with the most basic information.

www.medlineplus.gov

The Virtual Hospital. A site supported by the University of Iowa, has many different layers with different relevance to practitioners and patients. Navigating this site is sometimes confusing, but the clinical topics are peer reviewed and updated frequently.

www.vh.org.

Low Back Pain

23

Charles W. Webb, DO, & Francis G. O'Connor, MD, FACSM

General Considerations

Low back pain (LBP) is one of the most frequently encountered conditions in primary care, second only to the common cold. With an annual incidence of 5% and a lifetime prevalence of 60–90%, LBP is the leading cause of disability in the United States for adults under 45 years of age. At any given time 1% of the U.S. population is chronically disabled and another 1% is temporarily disabled as a result of back pain. It is responsible for one-third of workers' compensation costs and accounts for direct medical costs in excess of $25 billion per year. Although numerous studies report a favorable natural history for acute LBP, with 90% of patients recovering within 6–12 weeks with or without physician intervention, back pain is often recurrent and may be chronically disabling.

LBP, as a common clinical problem with high morbidity, has been the focus of a number of evidence-based reviews and clinical practice guidelines. The evidence-based assessment and management discussed in this chapter is from the Veterans Administration/Department of Defense (VA/DoD) Clinical Practice Guideline, which is based on the Agency for Health Care Policy and Research (AHCPR) Clinical Practice Guideline. This guideline uses an algorithmic approach, which is divided into three phases: assessment, initial management of acute LBP, and management of chronic LBP (Figure 23–1).

Anatomy & Biomechanics of the Lumbar Spine

The motion segment of the lumbar spine is a three-joint complex consisting of an intervertebral disc (and its adjacent vertebral bodies) and two zygapophyseal (facet) joints (Figure 23–2). The intervertebral disc consists of an inner nucleus pulposus and the surrounding annulus fibrosis. The nucleus pulposus is primarily composed of a matrix of proteoglycans (PG). As an individual ages, the water-binding capacity of the PG decreases, resulting in degenerative changes (spondylosis)

in the disc. The annulus fibrosis is a fibrocartilage composed of 20 concentric rings of collagenous fibers that interdigitate to accommodate torsional movements. The inner fibers of the annulus envelop the nucleus and are attached to the end plate of the vertebral body.

The facet joints are non-weight-bearing joints located on the vertebral arches. The superior facets face posteromedially and the inferior facets face anterolaterally. These joints are typical synovial joints composed of cartilage, a joint capsule, and a synovial membrane. As disc degeneration (spondylosis) progresses weight bearing is transferred to the facet joints, producing inflammation, arthropathy, and increased force upon adjacent discs leading to herniation.

The intervertebral discs (IVD) are essentially avascular, with only the periphery receiving a blood supply. They also have a limited nerve supply, with only the outer third of the annulus fibrosis containing nerve fibers. The pain-sensitive structures surrounding the disc include the anterior longitudinal ligament, posterior longitudinal ligament, vertebral body, nerve root, and cartilage of the facet joint. Nerve roots exit through intervertebral foramina named for the vertebra above it. Because the L5 and S1 segment bears more weight than any other level, it is the most common site of pathology in the vertebral column.

Two muscular groups support the lumbar spine. The psoas and the abdominal muscles comprise the anterior group and the superficial, middle, and deep layers of the paraspinal muscles comprise the posterior group. The three layers of the posterior musculature are compartmentalized by the thoracolumbar fascia, which communicates with the anterior musculature. The superficial paraspinal layer is composed of the erector spinea (iliocostalis, longissimus, and spinalis). This layer functions as the primary extensor of the vertebral column. The middle layer is composed of the multifidi muscles and the deep layer consists of small intersegmental muscles.

The primary planes of lumbar motion include flexion (40–60°) (forward bending), extension (20–35°) (backward bending), lateral bending (15–20°), and rota-

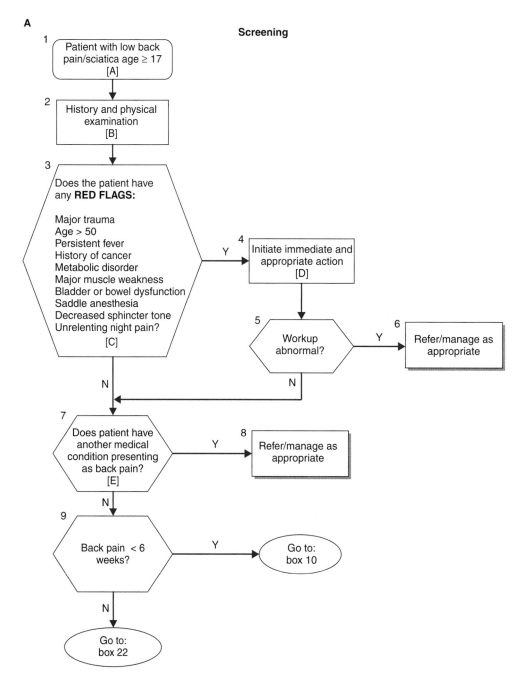

Figure 23–1. **A:** Acute LBP screening algorithm. **B:** Acute phase treatment algorithm. **C:** Chronic phase treatment algorithm.

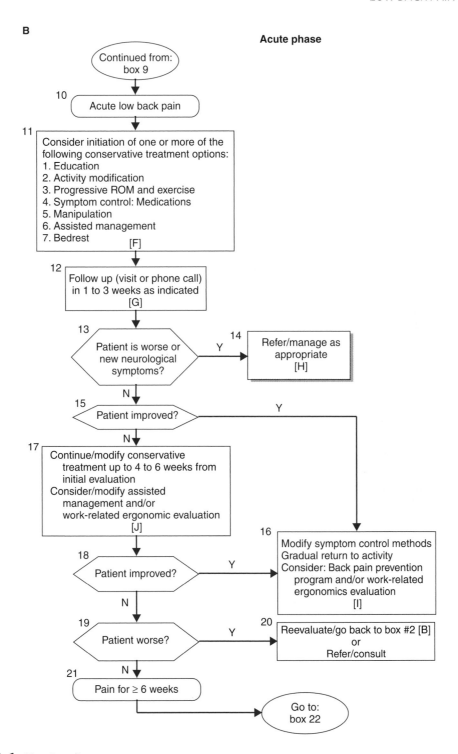

Figure 23–1. (*Continued*)

C

Chronic phase

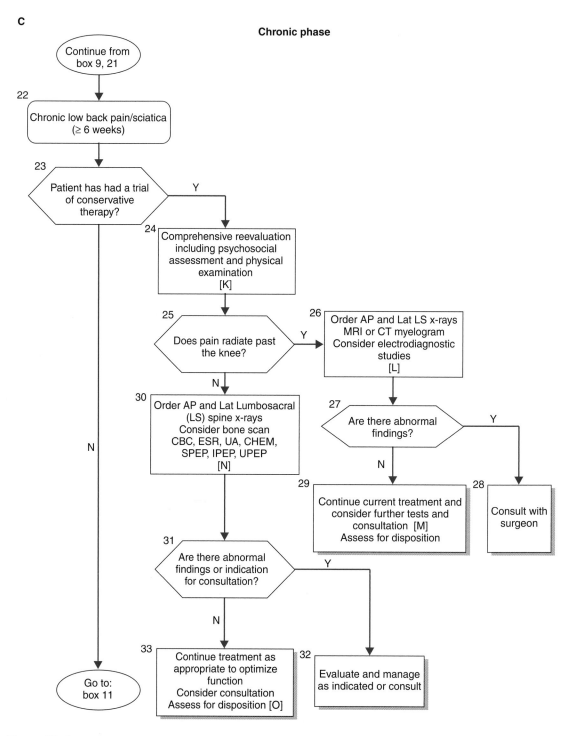

Figure 23-1. (*Continued*)

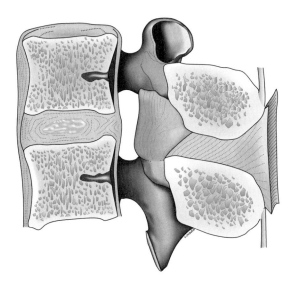

Figure 23–2. Lumbar vertebral segment—anatomy of the spine.

tion (3–18°). Flexion and extension occur mainly at the lower two segments (L4–L5 and L5–S1). Rotation at each lumbar segment is limited to only a few degrees secondary to the position of the facet joints. Because rotation in the lumbar spine involves shearing movement of each lumbar vertebrae, movements that combine flexion and rotation have the highest potential for injury. Another movement of the spine is compression, which although underestimated, may be the most clinically relevant. Although compression load occurs understandably secondary to body weight, up to 90% of total compression load is produced by the lumbar back muscles.

Pathogenesis

LBP, despite its prevalence and morbidity, remains poorly understood in terms of etiology. Many believe that the pain and dysfunction of LBP are the result of a complex interaction between the structural anatomy of the spine and its associated neurophysiology and biochemistry.

A recently proposed functional model that synthesizes the pathophysiology of the lumbar spine with the observed clinical presentations of patients with recurrent LBP is the degenerative cascade model. This model, built upon the work of Kirkaldy-Willis, is based on the concept of the previously described three-joint complex or motion segment. The model reflects the basic concept that injury to one component affects its function as well as the function of the other two components. Trauma and repetitive stress result in an injury cascade that proceeds through three overlapping stages:

stage I (dysfunction), stage II (instability), and stage III (stabilization).

In stage I, trauma and cumulative stress contribute to facet joint synovitis and annular tears of the IVD. At this point pathological changes are minor and may be reversible with proper intervention. The clinical presentation may be quite varied with either an acute or chronic presentation. Stage II follows when persistent stress results in increasing facet joint cartilaginous deterioration, capsular laxity, increased annular tears, and the potential of nuclear and annular disruption. In stage III, the facets demonstrate hypertrophy and spurring, whereas the IVDs show progressive degeneration. End plate abnormalities, loss of disc space height, osteophytes, and nerve root scarring ultimately contribute to patient symptomology.

Clinical Findings

A. SYMPTOMS AND SIGNS

The cornerstone of the assessment of the patient with acute LBP is a careful medical history and physical examination (Figure 23–1A, Box 2), which is critical in determining the presence of more serious conditions. The history should focus on the location of the pain, the mechanism of injury (what the patient was doing when he or she first noticed the pain; whether it was insidious or there was a specific trauma or activity), and the character (mechanical, radicular, caludicant, or nonspecific) and duration (acute is less than 6 weeks and chronic is greater than 6 weeks) of the pain. The provider must identify neurological symptoms (bowel/bladder symptoms, weakness in the extremities, saddle anesthesia) suggestive of cauda equina syndrome (CES), a true neurosurgical emergency. The functional status of the patient should be noted as should any exacerbating or ameliorating factors. The presence of fever, weight loss, and night pain is of particular concern as these could indicate a more serious disease, such as an underlying cancer. The social history should include information about drug use/abuse, intravenous drug use, tobacco use, and the presence of physical demands at work. Past medical and surgical history should also be obtained, particularly a history of previous spinal surgery or immunosuppression (history of cancer, steroid use, human immunodeficiency virus). A thorough history enables the primary care provider to identify any "red flags" that require a more extensive medial workup to rule out more serious disease processes.

The physical examination supplements the information obtained in the history by helping to identify underlying serious medical conditions or possible serious neurological compromise. The primary elements of the physical examination are inspection, palpation, observation (including range of motion testing), and specialized neuromuscular evaluation. The examination should start with an evaluation of the spinal curvature, lumbar range of motion, and amount of pain-free movement. Palpation should include the paraspinal muscles, the spinous processes, and the sacroiliac joints as well as the piriformis muscles and the position of the pelvic bones [anterior and posterior superior iliac spine (ASIS and PSIS)]. Because the lumbar spine is kinetically linked to the pelvis (particularly the sacroiliac area), pain from the pelvis can be referred to the lumbar spine. To address the pelvis the provider must be aware of the location of the ASIS and the PSIS in evaluating any rotational deformity of the pelvis as a cause for the LBP. The hip flexor and hamstring flexibility should also be assessed.

The neurological evaluation should include Achilles (S1) and patellar (L2–L4) reflex testing, ankle and great toe dorsiflexion (L4–L5) and plantarflexion (S1) strength, as well as the location of sensory complaints (dermatomes involved). Light touch testing for sensation in the medial (L4), dorsal (L5), and lateral (S1) aspects of the foot should be performed. In patients presenting with acute LBP and no specific limb complaints, a more elaborate neurological examination is not usually necessary. The straight leg raise (SLR) test should be done in both the seated and supine positions to evaluate for nerve root impingement. This abbreviated neurological evaluation of the lower extremity allows detection of clinically significant nerve root compromise at the L4–L5 and L5–S1 levels. These two sites make up over 90% of all significant radiculopathy secondary to lumbar disc herniation. Because this abbreviated examination may fail to diagnose some of the less common causes of LBP, any patient who has not improved in 4–6 weeks should return for further evaluation.

All patients with acute LBP should be risk stratified with an initial assessment attempting to identify red flags (Figure 23–1A, Box 3). Red flag signs or symptoms are responses or findings in the history and physical examination that indicate a potentially serious underlying condition, such as fracture, tumor, infection, acute abdominal aneurysm, or CES, that can lead to considerable patient morbidity and/or mortality. These clinical clues include a history of major trauma, minor trauma in patients older than 50 years of age, persistent fever, history of cancer, metabolic disorder, major muscle weakness, bladder or bowel dysfunction, saddle anesthesia, decreased sphincter tone, and unrelenting night pain. Red flags risk stratify the patient to an increased risk and should prompt earlier clinical action (Figure 23–1A, Box 4). Table 23–1 lists red flags and their related conditions.

C. LABORATORY FINDINGS

Laboratory testing should be reserved for patients who may have conditions that present as simple LBP or patients with red flags suggesting cancer or infection (Ta-

bles 23–1 and 23–2). Laboratory tests found to be helpful in evaluating these patients include a complete blood count (CBC) with differential and an erythrocyte sedimentation rate (ESR). An ESR over 50 mm/h is suggestive of cancer, infection, or inflammatory disease. Blood urea nitrogen (BUN), creatinine (Cr), and urinalysis (UA) are helpful in identifying underlying renal or urinary tract disease. Serum calcium, phosphorus, and alkaline phosphatase should be tested in patients with osteopenic, osteolytic vertebral lesions or vertebral body collapse. If prostate carcinoma is suspected, prostate-specific antigen and acid phosphatase levels should be checked. If multiple myeloma is suspected a serum immunoelectrophoresis can help guide treatment.

Historical red flags such as fever, intravenous drug abuse, and immunocompromise should raise concern for an underlying infection. Several laboratory studies are helpful in determining the underlying cause. An elevated white blood cell (WBC) count is an indication of an underlying infection, although the count can be within normal limits even in acute infection. The ESR and C-reactive protein (CRP) can be used to monitor the course of treatment in spinal infections. Urinalysis and urine culture should be obtained because urinary tract infection (UTI) often precedes spinal infection. Blood cultures should be obtained as well. Although they are usually negative, positive cultures identify the infecting organism and provide antibiotic sensitivity to guide treatment. Diagnostic imaging plays a central role in diagnosing spinal infections. Plain films should be obtained, although they are often diagnostic only in the advanced stages of the infection. MRI is the imaging modality of choice in evaluating spinal infection. When infection is identified or suspected a spinal surgeon should be consulted.

B. IMAGING STUDIES

Diagnostic imaging (Table 23–3) is rarely indicated in the acute setting of LBP. After the first 4–6 weeks of symptoms, the majority of patients have recovered from their back pain. However, if the patient is still limited by back symptoms diagnostic imaging should be considered to look for other conditions that present as LBP (Figure 23–1C, Boxes 24, 26, and 30). Patients for whom diagnostic imaging should be considered include children, patients over the age of 50 years, trauma patients, and patients for whom back pain fails to improve despite appropriate conservative treatment. Imaging studies must always be interpreted carefully since disc degeneration and protrusion have been noted in 20–25% of asymptomatic individuals. Therefore, abnormal findings on diagnostic imaging may or may not represent the reason for the patient's pain.

Plain films remain the most widely available modality for imaging the lumbar spine. Plain x-rays are rarely

Table 23–1. Red flags and appropriate actions.[1]

Condition	Red Flag	Action
Cancer	History of cancer Unexplained weight loss Age ≥50 Failure to improve with therapy Pain ≥4–6 weeks Night/rest pain	If malignant disease of the spine is suspected, imaging is indicated and CBC and ESR should be considered; identification of possible primary malignancy should be investigated, eg, PSA, mammogram, UPEP/SPEP/IPEP
Infection	Fever History of intravenous drug use Recent bacterial infection: UTI, skin, pneumonia Immunocompromised states (steroid, organ transplants, diabetes, HIV) Rest pain	If infection in the spine is suspected, MRI, CBC, ESR, and/or UA are indicated
Cauda equina syndrome	Urinary retention of incontinence Saddle anesthesia Anal sphincter tone decrease/fecal incontinence Bilateral lower extremity weakness/numbness or progressive neurological deficit	Request immediate surgical consultation
Fracture	Use of corticosteroids Age ≥70 years or history of osteoporosis Recent significant trauma	Appropriate imaging and surgical consultation
Acute abdominal aneurysm	Abdominal pulsating mass Other atherosclerotic vascular disease Rest/night pain Age ≥60 years	Appropriate imaging (ultrasound) and surgical consultation
Significant herniated nucleus pulposus (HNP)	Major muscle weakness	Appropriate imaging and surgical consultation

[1]CBC, complete blood count; ESR, erythrocyte sedimentation rate; PSA, prostate-specific antigen; UPEP, urine protein electrophoresis; SPEP, serum protein electrophoresis; IPEP, immunoprotein electrophoresis; UTI, urinary tract infection; HIV, human immunodeficiency virus; MRI, magnetic resonance imaging; UA, urinalysis.

useful in evaluating or guiding treatment of adults with acute LBP in the absence of red flags. Anteroposterior (AP) and lateral views allow assessment of lumbar alignment, the IVD space, and bone density, and allow a limited evaluation of the soft tissues; oblique views are used to detect spondylolysis; and sacroiliac views are used to evaluate ankylosing spondylitis. The primary objective of x-ray is to identify any bony and/or structural abnormality associated with back pain. Plain lumbar x-rays are helpful in detecting spinal fractures and in evaluating tumor and/or infection.

Plain x-rays of the lumbar spine are recommended for ruling out fractures in patients with acute LBP when the following red flags are present: recent major trauma (any age), age greater than 50 years with a history of mild trauma, history of corticosteroid use, osteoporosis, and age greater than 70 years. Plain x-rays in combination with CBC and ESR may be useful for ruling out tumor or infection in patients with acute LBP when the following red flags are present: prior cancer or recent infection, fever over 100°F, intravenous drug abuse, prolonged steroid use, LBP that is worse with rest, and unexplained weight loss.

When the history or physical examination suggests an anatomic abnormality as a cause for the back pain with neurological deficits four imaging studies are commonly used: plain myelography, computed tomography (CT) scan, magnetic resonance imaging (MRI) scan,

Table 23–2. Masqueraders of LBP.

System	Conditions	System	Conditions
Vascular	Expanding aortic aneurysm	Psychogenic	Affective disorder
Gastrointestinal	Pancreatitis		Conversion disorder
	Peptic ulcers		Somatization disorder
	Cholecystitis		Malingering
	Colonic cancer	Infection	Osteomyelitis
Genitourinary	Endometriosis		Epidural/paraspinal abscess
	Tubal pregnancy		Disc space infection
	Kidney stones		Pyogenic sacroiliitis
	Prostatitis	Neoplastic	Skeletal metastases
	Chronic pelvic inflammatory disease		Spinal cord tumors
	Perinephric abscess		Leukemia
	Pyelonephritis		Lymphoma
Endocrinological/ metabolic	Osteoporosis		Retroperitoneal tumors
	Osteomalacia		Primary lumbosacral tumors
	Hyperparathyroidism		Benign
	Paget's disease		Malignant
	Acromegaly	Miscellaneous	Sarcoidosis
	Cushing's disease		Subacute endocarditis
	Ochronosis		Retroperitoneal fibrosis
Hematological	Hemoglobinopathy		Herpes zoster
	Myelofibrosis		Fat herniation of lumbar space
	Mastocytosis		
Rheumatological	Spondyloarthropathies		
	Ankylosing spondylitis		
	Reiter's syndrome		
	Psoriatic arthritis		
	Enteropathic arthritis		
	Beçhet's syndrome		
	Familial Mediterranean fever		
	Whipple's disease		
	Diffuse idiopathic skeletal hyperostosis		

Adapted from Branch CL et al: *LBP Monograph, Edition No. 185. Home Study Self Assessment Program.* American Academy of Family Physicians, 1994; and Bagduk N: The innervation of the lumbar spine. Spine 1983;8(3):286.

and CT myelography. These four tests are used in similar clinical situations and provide similar information. The objective of these studies is to define a medically or surgically remediable anatomic condition. These tests are not done routinely, and should be used only for patients who present with certain clinical findings, such as radicular symptoms and clinically detectable nerve root compressive symptoms severe enough to consider surgical intervention (major muscle weakness, progressive motor deficit, intractable pain, and persistent radicular pain beyond 6 weeks). Other indications include a history of neurogenic claudication suggesting spinal stenosis or examination findings suggesting CES, spinal fracture, infection, or tumor. For a patient with a neurological deficit, a positive tension sign (straight leg raising), and a correlative imaging study, the clinical accuracy is 95%. MRI is probably the most accurate imaging modality, with CT myelography next.

Other imaging studies, such as bone scan, are recommended to evaluate acute LBP only when spinal tumor, infection, or occult fracture is suspected based on the medical history or physical examination. Thermography and discography are not recommended for assessing patients with acute LBP. Thermography has been shown to be abnormal in a substantial proportion of asymptomatic patients as well as those with myofascial pain syndromes.

Table 23–3. Special tests and indications/recommendations.[1]

Special Test	Indication/Recommendation
Plain x-ray	Not recommended for routine evaluation of acute LBP unless red flags present Recommended for ruling out fractures Obliques are recommended only when findings are suggestive of spondylolisthesis or spondylolysis
Electrophysiological tests (EMG and SEP)	Questionable nerve root dysfunction with leg symptoms ≥6 weeks Not recommended if radiculopathy is obvious
MRI or CT myelography	Back-related leg symptoms and clinically detectable nerve root compromise History of neurogenic claudication suspicious for spinal stenosis Findings suggesting CES, fracture, infection, tumor
ESR	Suspected tumors, infection, inflammatory conditions, metabolic disorders
CBC	Suspected tumors, myelogenous conditions, infections
UA	Suspected UTI, pyelonephritis, myeloma
IPEP	Suspected multiple myeloma
Chemistry profile to include TSH, calcium, and alkaline phosphatase	Suspected electrolyte disorders, thyroid dysfunction, metabolic dysfunction
Bone scan	Suspected occult pars interarticularis fracture or metastatic disease Contraindicated in pregnant patients

LBP, low back pain; EMG, electromyelogram; SEP, serum electrophoresis; MRI, magnetic resonance imaging; CT, computed tomography; CES, cauda equina syndrome; ESR, erythrocyte sedimentation rate; CBC, complete blood count; UA, urinalysis; UTI, urinary tract infection; IPEP, immunoprotein electrophoresis; TSH, thyroid-stimulating hormone.

Differential Diagnosis

After potential red flags have been ruled out, the differential diagnosis for LBP remains extensive. Box 7 in Figure 23–1A directs the provider to consider other medical conditions that can present as LBP. Table 23–2 presents a list of conditions that can masquerade as simple LBP.

Treatment

If the patient has no red flags and the history and physical examination do not suggest an underlying cause, the diagnosis of mechanical LBP can be made, and treatment may be initiated (Figure 23–1B, Box 11). There are multiple treatments available for low back problems. Methods of symptom control should focus on providing comfort and keeping the patient as active as possible while awaiting spontaneous recovery. Evidence for the most common treatments currently used in the primary care setting follows.

A. PATIENT EDUCATION

Patient education is the cornerstone of effective treatment of LBP. Patients who present to the primary care clinic with acute LBP should be educated about expectations for recovery and the potential recurrence of symptoms. They should be informed of safe and rea-

sonable activity modifications and should also be given information on how to limit the recurrence of low back problems through proper lifting techniques, treatment of obesity, and tobacco cessation. If medications are prescribed, patients should be given information on their use and their potential side effects. Patients should be instructed to follow up in 1–3 weeks if they fail to improve with conservative treatment or if they develop bowel or bladder dysfunction or worsening neurological function.

B. ACTIVITY MODIFICATION

Patients with acute LBP may be more comfortable if they are able to temporarily limit or avoid specific activities that are known to increase mechanical stress on the spine. Prolonged unsupported sitting and heavy lifting, especially while bending or twisting, should be avoided. Activity recommendations for the employed patient with acute LBP should consider the patient's age and general health and the physical demands of the job. A recent randomized control trial of an educational program to prevent work-associated low back injury by Daltroy et al found no long-term benefits associated with the training. Weber and colleagues found that focused educational programs can improve self-help in patients with LBP.

C. Bed Rest

A gradual return to normal activities is more effective than prolonged bed rest for the treatment of LBP. Bed rest for longer than 4 days may lead to debilitation and is not recommended. Most patients with acute LBP will not require bed rest. For patients with severe initial symptoms, however, limited bed rest for 2–4 days remains an option.

D. Medications

Oral medications [acetaminophen, nonsteroidal antiinflammatory drugs (NSAIDs), muscle relaxants and opioids] and injection treatments are available for the treatment of LBP. A recent review of clinical trials found that NSAIDs are more effective for short-term symptomatic relief in patients with acute LBP. One NSAID has not been shown to be more effective than another for the treatment of LBP. Muscle relaxants are not as effective as NSAIDs in treating LBP and no additional benefit is noted when muscle relaxants are used in combination with NSAIDs. Muscle relaxants have more potential side effects than NSAIDs, a factor that should be considered when deciding upon treatment. Because opioids are no more effective in relieving low back symptoms than other analgesics (aspirin, acetaminophen) and because of their potential for other complications (dependency), opioid analgesics, if used, should be used only over a time-limited course. Oral steroids are not recommended for the treatment of acute LBP.

Injection therapy for the treatment of low back symptoms includes trigger point, ligamentous, sclerosant, facet joint, and epidural injections. Injections are an invasive treatment option that exposes patients to potentially serious complications. No conclusive studies have proven the efficacy of trigger point, sclerosant, ligamentous, or facet joint injections in the treatment of acute LBP. However, epidural and facet joint injections may benefit patients who fail conservative treatment as a means of avoiding surgery.

Acupuncture and other dry needling techniques have not been found to be beneficial for treating patients with acute LBP. However, recent evidence suggests that traditional Chinese medical acupuncture and therapeutic massage are beneficial for treating chronic LBP.

E. Spinal Manipulation

There is some evidence supporting the use of manipulative therapy in the treatment of acute LBP. Spinal manipulation techniques attempt to restore joint and soft tissue range of motion. Impaired motion of synovial joints has a detrimental effect on joint cartilage leading to degenerative spinal changes. Decreased motion in the spine also has a degenerative effect on vertebral disc metabolism. Manipulation is useful early after symptom onset for patients who have acute LBP without radiculopathy. If the patient's physical findings suggest progressive or severe neurological deficit, manipulation should be postponed pending an appropriate diagnostic assessment. Patients who have symptoms for longer than 4–6 weeks despite manipulation should be reevaluated.

F. Physical Agents and Modalities

There are no well-designed controlled trials to support or discourage the use of physical agents or modalities for acute LBP. Physical agents include ice and moist heat treatments. Self-administered home programs using moist heat and cold are often used. Both ice and moist heat can be applied to the area for 20 min two or three times per day, although moist heat should not be used in the first 72 h after injury.

Transcutaneous electrical nerve stimulation (TENS) is a modality that uses a small battery-operated device worn by the patient to provide a pulse of electricity to the injured area through surface electrodes. TENS is thought to modify pain perception by counterstimulation of the nervous system. There is insufficient evidence on the efficacy of the TENS unit to recommend its routine use.

Shoe insoles (or inserts) can vary from over-the-counter foam, rubber inserts to custom orthotics. These devices aim to reduce back pain due to leg length discrepancies and/or abnormal foot mechanics during gait. There is limited evidence that shoe orthotics (either over the counter or custom) may provide short-term benefit for patients with mild back pain, although there is no evidence supporting long-term use. The role of leg length discrepancies in LBP has not been established and differences of less than 2 cm are unlikely to produce symptoms.

Lumbar support devices for low back problems include corsets, support belts, various types of braces, molded jackets, and back rests for chairs and car seats. Lumbar corsets and support belts may be beneficial in preventing LBP and in reducing time lost from work for individuals whose jobs require frequent lifting. Lumbar corsets have not been proven to be beneficial in the treatment of acute LBP.

G. Exercise

Therapeutic exercises should be started early to control pain, avoid deconditioning, and restore function. No single treatment or exercise program has proven effective for all patients with LBP. Initial exercises should focus on strengthening and stabilizing the spine and stretching the hip flexors. Lower extremity muscle tightness is common with LBP and must be corrected to allow normal range of motion of the lumbar spine. Tight hip flexors (iliopsoas and rectus femoris) cause excessive anterior pelvic rotation and increased lumbar lordosis. Stretching the hip flexors and strengthening the hip extensors will potentially rotate the pelvis back to a neutral position, resulting in a decrease in LBP.

In a similar fashion tight hamstrings place excessive posterior tilt on the pelvis, decreasing lumbar lordosis. This places the erector spinea at a mechanical disadvantage, making the spine less resilient to axial loads and increasing the likelihood of injury. Stretching the hamstrings and strengthening the back extensors restore neutral pelvis positioning and reduce patient pain. For patients with acute LBP, the McKenzie method of physical therapy and chiropractic manipulation are more effective than receiving an education booklet.

H. REEVALUATION

Patients with LBP should be reevaluated as indicated after 1–3 weeks to assess progress (Figure 23–1B, Box 12). This can be accomplished with either a follow-up phone call or office visit. This empowers patients to take the initiative in their disease course. Patients must be advised to follow up sooner if their condition worsens. Any worsening of neurological symptoms warrants a complete reevaluation.

Conservative treatment is warranted for 4–6 weeks from the initial evaluation. The follow-up visit is the appropriate time to consider a work-related ergonomic evaluation. As the patient improves there should be a gradual return to normal activity and a weaning of the medications. Schools for back problems and work-re-lated ergonomic programs might contribute to the prevention of injuries and reinjuries; however, the long-term benefits are inconclusive (Figure 23–1B, Box 16). For patients who have failed to improve, a comprehensive reevaluation is warranted (Figure 23–1C, Box 24).

I. REFERRAL

For patients with pain that radiates below the knee, especially with a positive tension sign, the anatomy must be evaluated with an imaging study (Figure 23–1C, Box 25). If there are abnormal findings then consultation with a neurosurgeon or back surgeon is appropriate (Figure 23–1C, Box 27). If, however, the imaging study does not reveal anatomic pathology then a nonsurgical back specialist may be necessary to help manage the patient (Figure 23–1C, Box 29). Table 23–4 lists these specialists and indications for their referral.

If there are no abnormal findings on a comprehensive reassessment, including selected diagnostic tests, it is crucial to start patients on a program that will enable them to resume their usual activities. The management of the patient without structural pathology should be directed toward a physical conditioning program designed with exercises to progressively build activity tolerance and overcome individual limitations. This may include referral to behavior modification specialists, activity-specific educators, or an organized multidisciplinary back rehabilitation program.

Agency for Health Care Policy and Research: Study compares ways of treating LBP. Press Release, October 7, 1998. http://www.ahrq.gov/news/press/loback.htm.

Table 23–4. Nonsurgical back specialists.

Specialist	Indications
Physiatrist/physical medicine and rehabilitation	Chronic back pain for more than 6 weeks
	Chronic sciatica for more than 6 weeks
	Chronic pain syndrome
	Recurrent back pain
Neurology	Chronic sciatica for more than 6 weeks
	Atypical chronic leg pain (negative straight leg raising)
	New or progressive neuromotor deficit
Occupational medicine	Difficult workers' compensation situations
	Disability/impairment ratings
	Return to work issues
Rheumatology	Rule out inflammatory arthropathy
	Rule out fibrositis/fibromyalgia
	Rule out metabolic bone disease (eg, osteoporosis)
Primary care sports medicine specialist	Chronic back pain for more than 6 weeks
	Chronic sciatica for more than 6 weeks
	Recurrent back pain

Bigos S et al: *Acute Low Back Problems in Adults. Clinical Practice Guideline,* No. 14. AHCPR Publication No. 95-0642.

Agency for Health Care Policy and Research, Public Health Service, U.S. Department of Health and Human Services, 1994.

Bronfort G: Lower back pain: spinal manipulation, current state of research and its indications. Neurol Clin 1999;17(1):91.

Cherkin DC et al: A comparison of physical therapy, chiropractic manipulation, and provision of an educational booklet for the treatment of patients with low back pain. New Engl J Med 1998;339(15):1021.

Cherkin DC et al: Medication use for low back pain in primary care. Spine 1998;23(5):607.

Curatolo M, Bogduk N: Pharmacologic pain treatment of musculoskeletal disorders: current perspectives and future prospects. Clin J Pain 2001;17(1):25.

Daltroy LH et al: A controlled trial of an educational program to prevent low back injuries. New Engl J Med 1997;337(5):322.

Drezner JA, Herring SA: Managing low-back pain: steps to optimize function and hasten return to activity. Physician Sportsmed 2001;29(8):37.

Harwood MI: What is the most effective treatment for acute low back pain. J Fam Pract 2002;51(2):118.

Kirkaldy-Willis WH, Mierau D: The three phases and three joints. In: *Managing LBP,* ed 4. Kirkaldy-Willis WH, Bernard TN (editors). Churchill Livingstone, 1999.

Patel AT, Ogle AA: Diagnosis and management of acute low back pain. Am Fam Physician 2000;61(6):1779.

Ren XS et al: Assessment of functional status, low back disability, and use of diagnostic imaging in patients with LBP and radiating leg pain. J Clin Epidemiol 1999;52(11):1063.

Rosomoff HL, Rosomoff RS: Low back pain: evaluation and management in the primary care setting. Med Clin North Am 1999;83(3):643.

Shiple BJ: Treating low-back pain: exercise knowns and unknowns. Physician Sportsmed 1997. http://www.physsportsmed.com/issues/1997/08aug/shiple.htm.

Van Tulder MW et al: Non-steroidal anti-inflammatory drugs for low back pain. Cochrane Database System Rev 2000.

Veterans Health Administration and Department of Defense Clinical Practice Guideline: *Low Back Pain or Sciatica in the Primary Care Setting.* The Low Back Pain Workgroup, Contract No. V101(93)P-1633, 1999.

Ward RC: *Foundations for Osteopathic Medicine.* Williams & Wilkins, 1997.

Neck Pain

Thomas M. Howard, MD

General Considerations

Neck pain is a common clinical problem. Two-thirds of all people will experience neck pain at some time in their life, with the prevalence being highest in middle-aged adults. In addition to being a common problem, neck pain is quite disabling, and in some countries accounts for nearly as much disability as low back pain. Neck pain is also quite similar to low back pain in that the etiology is poorly understood and the clinical diagnoses are quite vague. Unlike low back pain, however, which has been the subject of numerous clinical practice guidelines, neck pain has received limited study with few randomized controlled studies (RCTs). A review of the National Guidelines Clearinghouse at www.ngc.gov indicates only one published guideline on neck pain, which pertains to the use of imaging in chronic neck pain. This chapter will review the epidemiology and anatomy of neck pain and provide an evidence-based assessment of the evaluation, diagnosis, and management of this challenging disorder.

Neck pain usually resolves in days to weeks, but like low back pain can become recurrent. Almost 85% of neck pain may be attributed to chronic stress and strains or acute or repetitive injuries. Radicular neck pain occurs later in life with an estimated incidence of 10% in the 25–29 year age group, rising to 25–40% in the over 45 year old group. The incidence of chronic neck pain is about 10% and about 5% of people will experience severe disability. Patients who experience symptoms for at least 6 months have a less than 50% chance of recovering even with aggressive therapy. Predictors of chronic neck pain include a prior history of neck pain or injury, female gender, greater number of children, poor self-assessed health, poor psychological status, and a history of low back pain.

Up to 40% of patients with whiplash injuries will report symptoms for up to 15 years postinjury. These patients have a three times higher risk of neck pain in the next 7 years. Initial signs and symptoms that are predictive of slower recovery from whiplash-type injuries include age >60 years, female gender, neck pain on palpation, muscle pain, headache, and pain or numbness radiating to the arms, hands, or shoulders. The single best estimation of handicap due to whiplash injury is return of normal cervical range of motion. The economic impact of whiplash injuries is estimated to be $3.9 billion.

Occupational neck pain is ubiquitous and is not limited to any particular work setting. Predictors for occupational neck pain include little influence on the work situation, work-related psychosocial factors, perceived general tension, and prolonged sitting at work (>95% of the workday), especially with the neck flexed forward 20° or more for more that 70% of the work time.

Functional Anatomy

The cervical spine is a highly mobile column that supports the 6–8 pound head and functions as protection for the cervical spinal cord. The cervical spine consists of 7 vertebrae, 5 intervertebral discs, 14 facet (zagoapophyseal joints or Z-joints), 12 joints of Luschka, and 14 paired anterior, lateral, and posterior muscles. The vertebrae can be grouped into three major groups: C1 or the atlas, C2 or the axis, and the others, C3–C7. The atlas is a ring-shaped vertebra with superior and inferior facets to articulate with the occiput and C2 and an anterior portion of the ring to articulate with the odontoid process of C2. The axis consists of a large vertebral body (the largest in the c-spine) with the anterior odontoid process articulating with C1 and inferior and superior facet joints. The atlantooccipital articulation accounts for 50% of the flexion and extension range of motion of the neck and the atlantoaxial joint accounts for 50% of the rotational range of motion of the neck.

Each of the remaining cervical vertebrae consists of an anterior body with a posterior projecting ring of the transverse and spinous processes that forms the vertebral foramen for the spinal cord. The most prominent spinous processes that can be palpated are C2 and C7. The spinous and transverse processes are the origin and insertion of the multiple interspinous and intervertebral ligaments and muscles. Between each vertebral body are intervertebral discs consisting of a gelatinous center with a multilayered (onion-skin-like) surrounding annulus fibrosis. Each vertebral body from C2–C7 articulates with the others through a bony lip off the lateral margins called joints of Luschka. These are not true joints (no synovium); however, they may develop degenerative spurs limiting motion. The facet joints, which are part of the transverse process and are paired superiorly and inferiorly, have articular cartilage and a synovium that can be involved in degenerative and inflammatory processes. There are multiple interspinous and intervertebral ligaments, but the most important are the anterior and posterior longitudinal ligaments along the vertebral bodies and the ligamentum nuchae along the spinous process. There are eight cervical nerve roots exiting posterolaterally through the neuroforaminae. Given that there are seven vertebrae, each cervical root emerges through a neuroforamen above the vertebrae of its number (ie, the C6 root arises between C5 and C6) with C8 exiting between C7 and T1. The cervical cord gives rise to the nerves that innervate the neck, upper extremity, and diaphragm. To evaluate problems related to the cervical spine, it is necessary to have a basic understanding of the motor and sensory innervations/examination of the upper extremity (Table 24–1).

The musculature of the cervical spine includes flexors, extensors, lateral flexors, and rotators. Major flexors include the sternocleidomastoid, scalenes, and prevertebrals. Extensors include the posterior paravertebral muscles (spleneus, semispinalis, capitis) and trapezius. Lateral flexors include the scalenes and interspinous (between the transverse processes) muscles and the rotators include the sternocleidomastoid and the interspinous muscles. The ability of the cervical spine to absorb the energy from acute injuries is related to its lordotic curvature and the energy absorption of the paraspinal muscles and intervertebral discs.

The combined motion of all the above joints gives a significant range of motion to the neck, allowing the head to scan the environment with the eyes and ears. The normal range of motion includes extension, 70° (chin straight up to the ceiling); flexion, 60° (chin on chest); lateral flexion, approximately 45° (ear to shoulder); and rotation, approximately 80° (looking right and left). The center of motion for flexion is C5–C6 and for extension is C6–C7, hence degeneration and injury often occur at these levels. The range of motion can be reduced by injury to muscles or the vertebrae/disc or by the degenerative process causing spondylosis.

Clinical Findings

A. Symptoms and Signs

The mechanism of injury of the cervical spine like other injuries can be classified in multiple ways: acute injuries including a fall, blow to the head, or the whiplash injury or chronic-repetitive injury associated with recreational or occupational activities. Other classifications can include the direction of the force generating an injury: flexion, extension/hyperextension, axial load, lateral flexion, or rotation. It should be noted that at a forward flexion of 30° the cervical spine is straight and most vulnerable to axial load-type injuries. Most chronic neck pain is associated with poor posture, anxiety/depression, neck strain, or occupational and sport-related injuries.

Table 24–1. Upper extremity motor and sensory innervations.

Spinal Level	Motor	Reflex	Sensory	Peripheral Nerve
C5	Deltoid Biceps	Biceps	Lateral deltoid	Axillary
C6	Biceps Wrist extensors	Brachioradialis	Dorsal first web space	Musculocutaneous
C7	Triceps Wrist flexion Finger extension	Triceps	Dorsal middle finger	
C8	Finger flexors	None	Ring finger Small finger Medial forearm	Medial Antebrachial Cutaneous
T1	Hand intrinsics	None	Medial arm Axilla	Medial brachial Cutaneous

In the evaluation of cervical spine problems the most important first step is to obtain a good history. The mechanism of injury should be identified, which may identify the injury or guide the physical examination. The examiner should identify any history of old injuries or problems with the cervical spine, ie, a history of prior disc surgery or degenerative arthritis. Radicular or radiating symptoms in the upper extremity should be identified. This includes radiating pain, weakness, or paresthesias of the arm or shoulder. Additionally the examiner should ask about any symptoms related to upper motor neuron pathology. This includes bowel or bladder dysfunction or gait disturbance.

Additional history should include the duration of symptoms, aggravating motions or activities, and attempted prior treatments initiated by the patient or by other providers. Comorbid diseases such as inflammatory spondyloarthropathies, cardiac disease, or gastrointestinal problems should be identified as well as a history of tobacco use. A history of current occupational and recreational activities and requirements should be identified as they may contribute to the underlying problem and identify the desired end point for recovery and return to activity.

B. Laboratory Findings

Electromyography (EMG) should be considered in the evaluation of upper extremity neurological disorders to distinguish between peripheral (including brachial plexus) versus nerve root injuries and stable versus an active denervating or recovery process. After an acute nerve injury it may take 3–4 weeks before EMG can be diagnostic, so this study should not be ordered in the acute setting.

Other laboratory studies including complete blood count, sedimentation rate, and rheumatoid factor should be reserved for the evaluation of spondyloarthropathies and play little role in the evaluation of most neck pain.

C. Imaging Studies

Potential imaging studies of the cervical spine can include plain radiographs, magnetic resonance imaging (MRI), computed tomography (CT), bone scan, and myelography. Bone scan does not significantly contribute to the evaluation of neck pain in the acute or chronic settings. Plain films include the basic three-view series (anteroposterior, lateral, open mouth), oblique, and lateral flexion/extension views. Recommendations about the use of imaging studies in the evaluation of neck pain can be divided into recommendations for acute/traumatic or chronic neck pain.

In the acute trauma situation the three-view radiograph is the basic study of choice. In a recent study of 34,000 blunt trauma patients the three-view radiograph was abnormal and diagnostic in 498 of 818 patients, nondiagnostic in 320 of 818 patients, and failed to indicate abnormality in 23 of 818 patients. CT or lateral flexion and extension views can be used to further evaluate nondiagnostic radiographs or cases of high clinical suspicion for injury.

Cervical fractures may be "ruled out" on a clinical basis if the patient **does not** complain of neck pain when asked, **does not** have a history of loss of consciousness, **does not** have mental status change from trauma, drugs, or alcohol, **does not** have symptoms referable to the neck (paralysis or sensory change—present or resolved), and **does not** have other distracting painful injuries.

The American College of Radiology (www.acr.org) published the ACR Appropriateness Criteria for imaging of chronic neck pain in 1998. It concluded that there are no existing guidelines for the evaluation of patients with chronic neck pain. The initial imaging study should be the three-view series. The most common findings include a loss of lordosis (straight c-spine) or disk space narrowing with degenerative change at the C5–C6 and C4–C5 levels. Oblique and flexion/extension views should be ordered at the discretion of the attending physician. Consider lateral flexion/extension views in cases of chronic neck pain after hyperextension or flexion injury with normal radiographs and persistent pain or evidence of neurological injury to rule out instability. Abnormal findings include >3.5 mm horizontal displacement or >11° rotational difference to that of the adjacent vertebrae on resting or flexion/extension lateral radiographs. MRI should be performed on all patients who have chronic neck pain with neurological signs or symptoms or both. If there is a contraindication to MRI (pacemaker, nonavailability, claustrophobia, or interfering hardware in the neck), CT myelography is recommended. Consider oblique radiographs to look for bony encroachment of the neuroforaminae in the evaluation of radicular neck pain.

D. Examination and Tests

The examination of the cervical spine should be organized and systematic. It should include adequate exposure of the neck, upper back, and shoulders for observation, palpation of bony and soft tissues, range of motion (ROM), a Spurling test for nerve root irritation, an upper extremity motor and sensory examination, and evaluation for upper motor neuron symptoms.

Observation should begin as the patient walks into the examination room, looking for the presence or absence of normal fluid motion of the neck and arm swing with walking. After exposure the examiner may note the posture (many patients have a poor head forward/rounded shoulder posture that will contribute to chronic cervical muscular strain), shoulder position (looking for elevation from muscle spasm), and evidence of atrophy. Also observe for head tilt or rotation.

Palpation should be performed of major bony prominences and the soft tissues. The spinous processes and the facet joints (about 1 cm lateral and deep to the spinous process) should be gently palpated, noting pain. Note that if enough pressure is applied to the spinous process pain can be produced in most patients. Palpation of the pre- and paravertebral muscles should be performed noting tension, pain, or the presence of tender or trigger points. Common sites for trigger points include the levator scapulae (off the superior, medial margin of the scapula), upper trapezius, rhomboids, and upper paraspinals near the insertion into the occiput.

Active ROM should be tested first with judicious use of passive motion as pain permits. Motion should be tested in the six prime directions: forward flexion, extension, left and right lateral flexion, and left and right rotation. The ROM can be recorded in degrees from the erect/neutral position or as a percentage of the expected norm of chin on chest, chin to sky, ear to each shoulder, and rotation to each shoulder.

The Spurling test is a test for evidence of nerve root irritation. This irritation can be related to spondolytic compression, discogenic compression, or the Stinger (compression or stretch injury in football). Extend, side bend, and partially rotate the head toward the side being tested. Then gently apply an axial load to the top of the head. A positive test is indicated by radiating pain, generally into the posterior shoulder or arm on the ipsilateral side. Although the Spurling test is felt to be reliable, Tong et al recently published an evaluative study indicating that in normal and symptomatic patients, confirmed by EMG, the Spurling test had a sensitivity of 30% and a specificity of 93%. It is therefore not a definitive screening test, but is useful in helping confirm cervical radiculopathy.

Upper extremity motor evaluation includes muscle testing and deep tendon reflexes (DTRs). A quick pneumonic to keep the upper extremity motor findings in order is *blocker, beggar, kisser, grabber, spock* (Figure 24–1). By assuming these positions the examiner can remember the motor innervation of the cervical roots in the upper extremity. The examiner can quickly check arm abduction (blocking position) for deltoid function, then resisted elbow flexion and extension (biceps and triceps), wrist extension and flexion, grip, and finger abduction (spread fingers). DTRs should be checked for the biceps (C5), triceps (C7), and brachioradialis (C6). Sensory testing should focus on the dermatomes for the cervical roots with emphasis on the lateral deltoid area (C5), dorsal first web space (C6), dorsal middle finger (C7), small finger (C8), and inner arm (T1).

Lower extremity testing for upper motor neuron findings should be checked to include DTRs (looking for hyperreflexia), clonus in the ankle, and the Babinski. If the examiner has not queried about bowel and bladder function, it can be done at this time.

Differential Diagnosis

For the differential diagnosis of neck pain, see Table 24–2.

Treatment

Multiple treatment options are available for the patient and practitioner, although there is limited evidence-based support for the efficacy of most treatment options utilized. Initial management should include avoidance of aggravating factors at work or associated with recreational activities as well as pain management, knowing that most pain is self-limiting. Subsequent management should focus on early return to motion, isometric strengthening, and modification of occupational or recreational aggravating factors with return to activity.

Absolute rest should be limited to a very short period of time, ie, 1–2 days. This includes the use of cervical collars. Early motion should be encouraged as soon as severe pain will allow. Early mobilization after whiplash-type injury is associated with better pain relief and return of motion. Patients should focus on proper posture (neck centered and back over the shoulders) and gentle motion of the neck in the six major motions mentioned above. Each position should be held for 15–20 s. Proprioceptive neuromuscular facilitation (PNF) may be employed in a structured program with physical therapy or a home program with the goal to improve motion. This is done by having patients move their heads in a direction to the point of pain. They then attempt to move in the opposite direction against the resistance of their own hand on the chin for a count of 5, and then to further move in the original direction, usually with improved motion.

Pain management may take the form of ice, medications, or physical modalities. Application of ice (15 min every 2 h) is effective for acute pain after injury or for postactivity pain during the recovery process.

A. MEDICATIONS

Medications used in the management of acute and chronic neck pain include salicylates (aspirin 500 mg four times a day or Disalcid 500 mg three times a day), nonsteroidal antiinflammatory drugs (NSAIDs) (ibuprofen 600 mg four times a day or 800 mg three times a day, naproxen 500 mg twice a day, indomethecin 25–50 mg three times a day, piroxicam 20 mg/day, and COX-

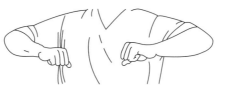

C5: Blocker
    Arm abduction
    Elbow flexion

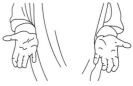

C6: Beggar
    Elbow flexion
    Wrist extension

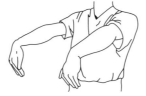

C7: Kisser
    Elbow extension
    Wrist flexion
    Finger extension

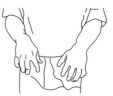

C8: Grabber
    Finger flexion

Figure 24–1. Upper extremity motor evaluation.

T1: Spock
    Finger abduction

Table 24–2. Differential diagnosis of neck pain.

Acute Injury	Noninflammatory Disease	Inflammatory Disease	Infectious Causes	Neoplasm	Referred pain
Cervical sprain/ whiplash	Cervical osteoarthritis (spondylosis)	Rheumatoid arthritis	Meningitis	Primary Myeloma	Temperomandibular joint
Cervical instability	Discogenic neck pain	Spondyloarthropathies	Osteomyelitis	Cord	Cardiac
Fractures	Cervical spinal stenosis	Juvenile rheumatoid	Infectious discitis	tumor	Diaphragmatic irritation
Vertebral body	Fibromyalgia	arthritis		Metastatic	Gastrointestinal
Compression	Myofascial pain	Ankylosing spondylitis			Gastric ulcer
Tear drop	Torticollis				Gallbladder
Spinous process					Pancreas
Transverse process					
Facet					
Hangman's					
Jefferson					

2 inhibitors—rofecoxib 25–50 mg/day and celecoxib 200 mg/day), Tylenol (500-1000 mg four times a day), muscle relaxants (Valium 5 mg three times a day, methocarbamol 1000–1500 mg four times a day, and cyclobenzaprine 10 mg three times a day), narcotic medications (Tylenol with codeine, Percocet, and Demerol), and corticosteroids. For acute radicular symptoms consider a short course of corticosteroids (prednisone 40–60 mg/day for 5–7 days) to reduce inflammation associated with herniated nucleus pulposus (HNP). Although there is no literature to support use of systemic steroids, anecdotal evidence suggests that they may be helpful in the acute setting. For pain that is becoming more chronic (>30 days), tricylic antidepressants (TCAs) (nortriptyline 25–50 mg or amitriptyline 10–50 mg) or selective serotonin reuptake inhibitors (SSRIs)(fluoxetine 10–60 mg or sertraline 25–100 mg at bedtime) may be used at night to manage the pain and to manage the sleep disturbance that often accompanies chronic pain of any source. Side effects of TCAs include excessive drowsiness, dry mouth, urinary retention, and potential cardiac conduction problems. Side effects of SSRIs include insomnia, drowsiness, dry mouth, nausea, headache, and anorexia. Note that the combination of SSRIs and TCAs may result in increased serum levels of the TCA and toxicity. RCTs support the use of simple analgesics and NSAIDs in the management of acute pain but do not support the other treatment options.

B. PHYSICAL MODALITIES

Multiple physical modalities are available for the management of pain and to improve motion, although there is little clinical evidence of their effectiveness. These can include application of heat, ultrasound, cervical traction, acupuncture, and electric stimulation (e-stim and transcutaneous electrical nerve stimulation). Cervical traction can be effective for relief of spasm or in the management of radicular pain from HNP or spondylosis. Traction may be performed in a controlled setting at physical therapy or with the use of home traction units. Typical sessions in physical therapy are 2–3 days/week for 30 min per session. Heat, ultrasound, and electric stimulation may all be effective in local pain management to allow early return to normal motion. There are no RCTs that support the use of physical modalities in the management of acute or chronic neck pain.

C. ACUPUNCTURE

Acupuncture has been shown to be effective in the treatment of acute pain, although its effectiveness beyond five treatments is limited. A home program of ischemic pressure (acupressure) with stretching has also been shown to be effective in the management of myofascial neck pain.

D. MANUAL THERAPY

Manual therapy (chiropractic manipulation) is commonly used in the management of chronic neck and lower back pain. A study on the use of manual therapy in the treatment of neck and low back pain showed an average improvement of 53.8% in acute pain and 48.4% in chronic pain with 12 treatments over a 4-week period of time. A recent case report of a patient with persistent neck and arm pain after failed cervical disk surgery with resolution after a program of manual therapy and rehabilitative exercises further supports the use of manual therapy in the management of both myofascial and radicular neck pain.

E. ISOMETRIC EXERCISE

As patients recover a program of strengthening should be instituted. Simple isometric exercises focusing on resisted forward flexion, extension, and right and left lateral flexion will reduce pain and improve strength to contribute to recovery and long-term resistance to further injury.

F. SPECIALTY REFERRAL

Specialty referral may be considered at multiple points in the recovery process to aid in diagnosis or treatment of acute or chronic neck pain. Physical therapy may be utilized early in the process for use of physical modalities and initiation of a strengthening program. Typical consultations are for two or three sessions per week for 4–6 weeks with follow-up evaluation by the primary provider. Physical medicine and rehabilitation (PM&R) may be considered for comanagement of chronic pain of any source and to obtain EMGs. Neurology may be considered to obtain EMG or for consultation for confusing neurological conditions. Neurosurgery or orthopedic spine surgery should be considered for patients requiring operative management. Early referral should be considered for severe muscle weakness, fractures, and evidence of myelopathy (long-track signs). Success rates for surgery have been reported to be as high as 80–90% for radicular pain and 60–70% for myelopathy. There is insufficient evidence to compare conservative treatment to surgical management of patients with neck pain and radiculopathy. Referral for chronic pain should be considered for chronic radiating pain after failure of 9–12 weeks of conservative management. Anesthesia/pain clinic referral should be considered for comanagement of chronic pain or consideration for epidural steroid (ESI) or facet injections. There are no RCTs on the effects of ESI and insufficient evidence to compare conservative treatment to surgical management of patients with neck pain with radiculopathy.

Prevention strategies for high-risk groups have been employed for both neck and lower back pain. Investigations of educational efforts, exercise, ergonomics, and risk factor modification found that only strengthening exercises were an effective prevention strategy.

Alcantara J et al: Chiropractic care of a patient with vertebral subluxations and unsuccessful surgery of the cervical spine. J Manipulative Physiol Ther 2001;24(7):477.

Aptaker RL: Neck pain, Part II: optimizing treatment and rehabilitation. Phys Sportsmed 1996;24(11):54.

Ariens GA et al: Are neck flexion, neck rotation, and sitting at work risk factors for neck pain? Results of a prospective cohort study. Occup Environ Med 2001;58(3):200.

Ariens GA et al: High quantitative job demands and low coworker support as risk factors for neck pain. Spine 2001;26(17):1896.

Berglund A et al: The association between exposure to rear-end collision and future neck or shoulder pain: a cohort study. J Clin Epidemiol 2000;53:1089.

Binder A: Neck pain. Clin Evid 2001;6:884.

Chronic Neck Pain: ACR Appropriateness Criteria. American College of Radiology, 1998.

Cote P, Cassidy D, Carroll L: The Saskatchewan health and back survey: the prevalence of neck pain and related disability in Saskatchewan adults. Spine 1998;23:1689.

Croft PR et al: Risk factors for neck pain: a longitudinal study in the general population. Pain 2001;93:317.

Eck JC, Hodges SD, Humphreys SC: Whiplash: a review of a commonly misunderstood injury. Am J Med 2001;110:651.

Graber MA, Kathol M: Cervical spine radiographs in the trauma patient. Am Fam Physician 1999;59(2):331.

Hanten WP et al: Effectiveness of a home program of ischemic pressure followed by sustained stretch for treatment of myofascial trigger points. Phys Ther 2001;81:1059.

Irnich D et al: Randomized trial of acupuncture compared with conventional massage and "sham" laser acupuncture for treatment of chronic neck pain. Br Med J 2001;322:1574.

Kasch H, Bach FW, Jensen TS: Handicap after acute whiplash injury: a 1 year prospective study of risk factors. Neurology 2001;56:1637.

Linton SJ, van Tulder MW: Prevention interventions for back and neck pain problems. Spine 2001;26(7):778.

Lu DP, Lu GP, Kleinman L: Acupuncture and clinical hypnosis for facial and head and neck pain: a single crossover comparison. Am J Clin Hypn 2001;44(2):141.

McMorland G, Suter E: Chiropractic management of mechanical neck and low-back pain: a retrospective, outcome-based analysis. J Manipulative Physiol Ther 2000;23(5):307.

Nakano KK: Neck pain. In: Kelley's Textbook of Rheumatology, ed 6. W.B. Saunders, 2001.

Narayan P, Haid R: Neurologic treatment. Neurol Clin 2001;19(1):217.

Suissa S, Harder S, Veilleux M: The relation between initial symptoms and signs and the prognosis of whiplash. Eur Spine J 2001;10(1):44.

Tong HC, Haig AJ, Yamakawa K: The Spurling test and cervical radiculopathy. Spine 2002;27(2):156.

Torg JS, Ramsey-Emrheim JA: Management guidelines for participation in collision activities with congenital, developmental or post injuries involving the cervical spine. Clin J Sport Med 1997;7:273.

Vasseljen O, Holte KA, Westgaard RH: Shoulder and neck omplaints in customer relations: individual risk factors and perceived exposures at work. Ergonomics 2001;44(4):355.

WEB SITES

Useful web sites for patient education on home rehabilitation as well as correction of occupational and postural risk factors:

http://orthoinfo.aaos.org

http://www.nismat.org/ptcor/neck http://famildoctor.org/flowcharts/513.htm

http://www.nismat.org/orthocor/programs/neck/ neckex.html

A useful provider web site:

http://www.spineuniverse.com

Evaluation of Breast Lumps

Jo Ann Rosenfeld, MD

General Considerations

A woman's discovery of a breast lump always brings the specter of breast cancer, disfigurement, and death, even when it is judged benign. The physician who finds a lump or who helps a woman who has discovered a lump must realize that rapid and accurate diagnosis and appropriate treatment are essential. "Triple assessment—clinical examination, imaging and pathology—is now the standard approach to all breast lumps" (Hughes et al, 2000, p. 35).

There are many causes of breast lumps, many of them normal or benign (Table 25–1). "Most benign disorders are related to normal processes of reproductive life" (Hughes et al, 2000, p. 23). Cysts are the most common mass found in patients in a breast clinic.

Age is related to the number of lumps found and the risk that the lump is cancer. The percentage of lumps that are cancer increases with age from less than 1% of all breast lumps in women younger than age 30 years to 70% of breast lumps in women older than age 70 years (Figure 25–1). In young women less than age 20 years, cancer is uncommon and premenarchal breast buds and fibroadenomas are much more common. Localized benign breast masses, cysts, and fibroadenomas are the most common causes in women younger than age 50 years. In women aged 30–35 years, cancer is still uncommon, although its prevalence is not negligible with a rate of 25 per 100,000 women. A new breast lump in a postmenopausal woman is very worrisome.

During pregnancy, mastitis or breast abscesses are the most common cause of a breast mass. Galactocoeles are also found.

Prominent or asymmetric ribs, inflammatory lymph nodes in the axilla, sebaceous cysts, often in the axillae, scars, and accessory breasts may be causes of breast lumps in women at any age.

Fibrocystic breast disease, a cause of multiple or recurrent breast cysts and lumps, occurs in up to 19% of women. The cysts usually start in women in their 20s and 30s and increase with age. The lumps are usually multiple and bilateral and cause cyclic pain, often reduced with use of oral contraceptives. However, there may be just one "lump" at any one time. Fibrocystic disease and its symptoms should decrease with menopause.

Breast lumps may be an incidental finding on a mammogram or may be found by the woman in self-breast examinations or by the physician in a clinical breast examination. Associated symptoms may be pain, discharge, or skin changes.

Clinical Findings

A. Symptoms and Signs

The duration and relation of the lump in size to the menstrual period and whether the lump is tender or painful may help determine the etiology. New breast pain is the presenting complaint for cancer in 6% of women with breast cancer. Figure 25–2 outlines the evaluation of breast lumps.

Because lumps or cysts may be related to the menstrual cycle, evaluating the woman twice—once immediately and once 2 weeks later—may be advisable, especially in a young woman who is nearing her menses. If any associated symptoms are more worrisome or the woman is postmenopausal, waiting 2 weeks before proceeding to radiological studies and pathology may not be sensible.

Although radiological tests may be definitive, the clinical breast examination can contribute to the diagnosis and delineation of the cause of a lump. Both breasts should be examined in detail, from the axillae to the areolae, visually and by palpation.

Skin changes are important; dimpling, thickening of the skin of the breast (peau d'orange—"orange skin"), or nipple inversion is worrisome for cancer. Nipple retraction is often, but not always, a sign of cancer. Two benign lumps, skin fixation, or a chronic abscess can cause nipple retraction or skin attachment.

Noting whether the lump is soft, cyst-like, hard, or firm and noting its size and mobility (whether it is at-

Table 25–1. Causes of breast lumps.

Normal nodularity
    Fat lobules, prominent ribs, etc
Inflammatory
    Abscess; fat necrosis
Common benign changes
    Fibroadenomas, cysts, galactocoeles
Benign tumors
    Duct papillomas, lipomas,
Malignant
    Carcinoma *in situ*, primary or secondary cancers
Skin lesions
    Sebaceous cysts, hidroadenitis, malignant or benign skin
    tumors

Data from Hughes LE, Mansel RE, Webster DJT: *Benign Disorders and Diseases of the Breast,* ed 2. Saunders, 2000: 94–121.

tached to the chest wall, other breast tissue, or freely moving) are important. Fibroadenomas are usually rubbery, smooth, and mobile. Cysts can be soft or hard, depending on the pressure of the contents, and are usually less mobile than fibroadenomas. Abscesses are often tender, fluctuant, and warm, with the surrounding tissue often erythematous and warm, if not hot.

Lymph node enlargement, tenderness, or thickenings should be noted. The presence and placement of other lumps or breast tissue should be observed. Draw-

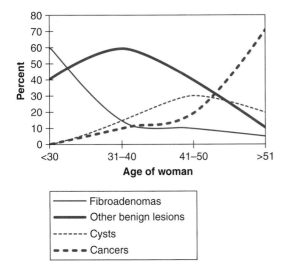

Figure 25–1. Types of breast lumps by age. (Data from Dixon JM, Mansel RE: ABC of breast diseases: symptoms assessment and guidelines for referral. Br Med J 1994;309:722.)

ing pictures of the breast with placement and sizing of the lump(s) in the medical record is also useful.

The woman whose lump is not felt by the physician should nonetheless be subject to the same complete evaluation.

B. Laboratory Findings

No laboratory tests will help define the breast lump. A white blood count and other tests may be useful if an abscess, cellulitis, or cancer is suspected, but the information only adds to the data.

C. Imaging Studies

The primary way to image the breast is with mammography. Despite current controversy over the relative benefits of prevention or detection of cancer by mass screening, every woman over age 35 years with a lump needs a mammogram, even if a screening mammogram has recently been done. Mammography is the imaging technique of first choice in women 35 years of age or older. In women younger than age 35 years, breasts are usually denser and more glandular, cancer occurs less often, and, thus, ultrasonography becomes the primary radiological study.

1. Mammography—Mammography is safe and reliable and often is sufficient to make the diagnosis of a breast lump. Benign breast lesions are usually rounded or ovoid with smooth margins. Benign lesions, such as cysts or fibroadenomas, may show "halos" of compressed fat that suggest there has been no infiltration. Cysts may also show eggshell-like rims of calcifications whereas fibroadenomas often show popcorn-like calcifications. Calcifications in benign lesions are often smooth or follow the ducts.

Additional specific mammographic views and ultrasonography may often be needed to delineate the cause of a breast lump.

2. Ultrasonography—Ultrasound is used, often in conjunction with mammography, to determine whether a lump is cystic or solid or whether the lump is discrete or is associated with other nodularity, and to assist in localization and targeting for needle and other biopsy

3. Fine needle aspiration—Use of fine needle aspiration (FNA) has become almost mandatory in the diagnosis of breast lumps. FNA will assess the consistency of a mass, aspirate fluid, "cure" the lump if it is a cyst, and even provide a specimen for cytology, if possible. Usually it is performed under mammographic or ultrasound direction.

Cytology from an FNA has an accuracy of up to 99%, with as few as 0.4% false positives.

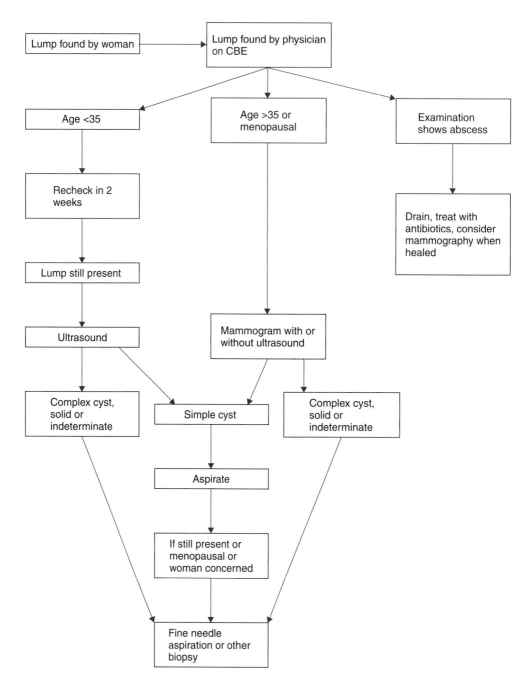

Figure 25–2. Evaluation of breast lumps.

Treatment

Treatment depends on diagnosis. If there is uncertainty after FNA, a wide needle or open biopsy is indicated. Abscesses should be drained; consultation with a surgeon may be necessary, especially if they are large, deep, or involved.

Skin abscesses such as those from sebaceous cysts and those in the axillae can often be drained in the office. Antibiotics, oral or parenteral, are indicated. If the woman is not breast-feeding and surgical drainage is performed, the excised tissue should be sent for cytology or the woman should have another mammogram after the abscess heals to evaluate for inflammatory cancers.

Physicians comfortable with the procedure can drain cysts. If the examination, mammogram, and ultrasound show the lump is a cyst, an aspiration can be diagnostic and therapeutic. If after anesthesia, the needle encounters fluid, and when aspirated, the lump disappears, the lump was definitely a cyst and further evaluation may not be needed. The fluid can be sent for cytology. Larger cysts may need to be aspirated or drained surgically. However, women with breast cysts have a moderately higher risk of breast cancer.

Lumps definitely diagnosed by mammography as fibroadenomas can be watched or excised. Recent research suggests that for younger women conservative watching may be acceptable psychologically and a reasonable risk. Repeat mammography in 6 months may be an adequate evaluation and no other treatment is necessary.

The treatment of fibrocystic breast disease has not been extensively studied. Dietary additions and avoidance of caffeine, chocolate, and alcohol have been suggested by observational studies without proof of efficacy in case-controlled studies. Diuretics have not been shown to be useful. Use of oral contraceptives for 12–24 months has shown some reduction in cysts and pain. In severe cases, danazol and gonadotropin-releasing hormone analogs have been used, but they are not approved for use in fibrocystic disease.

Women whose lumps show pathology that indicates cancer or *in situ* cancer should be immediately referred to an oncologist, preferably one specializing in breast cancers.

Bundred NJ et al: Is there an increased risk of breast cancer in women who have had a breast cyst aspirated? Br J Cancer 1991;64:935.

Dixon JM, Mansel RE: ABC of breast diseases: symptoms assessment and guidelines for referral Br Med J 1994;309:722.

Geller BM et al: Use of the American College of Radiology BI-RADS to report on the mammographic evaluation of women with signs and symptoms of breast disease. Radiology 2002; 222(2):536.

Greenberg R, Skornick Y, Kaplan O: Management of breast fibroadenomas. J Gen Intern Med 1998;13(9):640.

Hughes LE, Mansel RE, Webster DJT: *Benign Disorders and Diseases of the Breast,* ed 2. Saunders, 2000.

Jatoi I, Trott PA: False positive reporting in breast fine-needle aspiration cytology. Incidence and causes. Breast 1996;5:270.

Lubin F et al: A case control study of caffeine and methyl xanthines in benign breast diseases. JAMA 1985;253:2388.

Marchant DJ: Controversies in benign breast disease. Surg Oncol Clin North Am 1998;7:285.

Preece PE et al: Importance of mastalgia in operable breast cancer. Br Med J 1982;284:1299.

Seltzer MH: The significance of breast complaints as correlated with age and breast cancer. Am Surg 1992;58.

Stone AM, Shenker RI, McCarthy K: Adolescent breast masses. Am J Surg 1977;134:275.

Walls JB: Breast lumps in young women. Letter. Br Med J 1998; 317:209.

Respiratory Problems

William J. Hueston, MD

Respiratory infections and chronic lung diseases are among the most common reasons that patients consult primary care physicians. Most of the respiratory problems encountered by primary care physicians are acute, with the majority involving respiratory infections, exacerbations of asthma, chronic obstructive pulmonary diseases, and pulmonary embolism. This chapter will examine some of the more common respiratory conditions encountered in primary care.

■ UPPER RESPIRATORY TRACT INFECTIONS

COMMON COLDS/UPPER RESPIRATORY TRACT INFECTIONS

ESSENTIALS OF DIAGNOSIS

- Sore throat, congestion, low-grade fever, mild myalgias, and fatigue.
- Symptoms last 12–14 days.

General Considerations

The common cold is a very common infectious condition. Adults typically have two to four colds each year and children in day care have as many as six or seven. Although colds are mild, tend to get better on their own, and are of short duration, they are a leading cause of sickness and of industrial and school absenteeism. Each year, colds account for 170 million days of restricted activity, 23 million days of school absence, and 18 million days of work absence.

Colds have a seasonal variation with an increased prevalence in the United States between September and

March. It is unclear why this variation exists, although it may be related to increased crowding of indoor populations in the colder months. Temperature is not the key to seasonal variation. Evidence from Antarctica showed that spacious well-ventilated rooms reduced transmission of colds compared to crowded poorly ventilated rooms regardless of temperature.

The majority of colds are caused by viruses. Rhinoviruses are the most common type of virus and are found in slightly more than half of all patients. Coronaviruses are the second most common cause. In rare instances (0.05% of all cases), bacteria can be cultured from individuals with cold symptoms. It is not clear if these bacteria cause the cold, are secondary infectious agents, or are simply colonizers. Bacterial pathogens that have been identified include *Chlamydia pneumoniae, Haemophilus influenzae, Streptococcus pneumoniae,* and *Mycoplasma pneumoniae.*

Prevention

The mechanisms of transmission suggest that colds can be spread through contact with inanimate surfaces, but the primary transmission appears to be via hand-to-hand contact. The beneficial effects of removing viruses from the hands are supported by observations that absences due to colds among children in day care or school settings have been reduced through the use of antiseptic hand wipes throughout the day.

Clinical Findings

Colds generally last 12–14 days. Telling patients that colds last no longer than a week underestimates the actual natural history of an uncomplicated viral respiratory tract infection and leads patients to believe that symptoms that persist beyond a week are not normal. When the symptoms of congestion persist longer than 2 weeks, consideration should be given to other causes of chronic congestion (Table 26–1).

Symptoms of colds include sore throat, congestion, low-grade fever, and mild myalgias and fatigue. In general, early in the development of a cold the discharge is

Table 26–1. Differential diagnosis for congestion and rhinorrhea.

Common cold
Sinusitis
    Viral
    Allergic
    Bacterial
    Fungal
Seasonal allergic rhinitis
Vasomotor rhinitis
Rhinitis secondary to α-agonist withdrawl
Drug-induced rhinitis (eg, cocaine)
Nasal foreign body

---

clear. As more inflammation develops, the discharge takes on some coloration. Yellow, green, or brown-tinted nasal discharges are indicators of inflammation, not secondary bacterial infection. Discolored nasal discharge does raise the likelihood of sinusitis, but only if other predictors of sinusitis are present. In addition, a number of studies have shown that patients with discolored discharge respond to antibiotics no better than they respond to placebos.

Differential Diagnosis

The differential diagnosis of colds includes complications of the cold such as sinusitis or otitis media, acute bronchitis, and noninfectious rhinitis. Influenza shares many of the symptoms of a common cold, but generally the patient will have a much higher fever, myalgias, and more intense fatigue.

Differentiating sinusitis from upper respiratory infections (URIs) can be difficult. About half of all patients with URIs do have sinus inflammation present on computed tomography (CT) scan, but these patients do not have any additional symptoms suggestive of sinusitis and their cold resolves with no antibiotic therapy. Therefore, sinus tenderness or a sensation of "fullness" in the sinuses is not necessarily indicative of a more serious infection.

Treatment

Despite the widespread recognition that viruses cause common colds, several studies have shown that the majority of cases of the common cold seen in physicians' offices are treated with antibiotics. This practice continues despite convincing evidence that antibiotic treatment of colds has no benefit. The overprescribing of antibiotics for self-limited viral illness is believed to contribute significantly to the growing multidrug resistance being observed in respiratory pathogens. In areas in which prescribing antibiotics for respiratory infections has been curtailed, reversals in antibiotic drug resistance have been observed.

A variety of alternatives to antibiotics for colds have been investigated and have their advocates, if not strong evidence of effectiveness. Currently, the most effective symptomatic treatments are over-the-counter decongestants, the most popular of which include pseudoephedrine hydrochloride and topically applied vasoconstrictors. These agents produce short-term symptomatic relief. However, patients must be warned to use topical agents cautiously because prolonged use is associated with rebound edema of the nasal mucosa (rhinitis medicamentosa).

Antihistamines, with a few exceptions, have not been shown to be effective treatments. Therefore, the use of over-the-counter antihistamines such as diphenhydramine and chlorpheniramine is not recommended. A number of over-the-counter medications have a mix of decongestants, cough suppressants, and pain relievers. Again, the use of these preparations will not cure the common cold, but will provide symptomatic relief.

Vitamins and minerals have also been suggested as a remedy for the common cold. Vitamin C has many advocates, although systematic reviews of the literature provide only weak support for its effectiveness. However, many people (including the late Nobel laureate Linus Pauling) advocated the use of vitamin C as a stimulant for the immune system. As for minerals, zinc gluconate lozenges are available without a prescription, but a meta-analysis of 15 previous studies on zinc concluded that zinc lozenges were not effective in reducing the duration of cold symptoms.

Some herbal medicines are also useful for treatment of the common cold. Echinacea, also known as the American ConeFlower, has been purported to reduce the duration of the common cold by stimulating the immune system. However, evidence for its efficacy is mixed. Echinacea should be used only for 2–3 weeks to avoid liver damage and other possible side effects that have been reported during long-term use of this herb.

Another herbal remedy that is useful in treating the symptoms of the common cold is ephedra, also known as Ma Huang. This herb has decongestant properties that make it similar to pseudoephedrine. Ephedra is more likely than pseudoephedrine to cause increased blood pressure tachyarrhythmia. This is especially true if used in conjunction with caffeine. Other herbal remedies for the common cold include goldenseal, yarrow, eyebright, and elderflower. However, no systematic evidence supports the use of these herbs for treating the common cold.

Some homeopathic remedies can be used to reduce the duration and severity of the common cold, the most common being *zincum gluconicum*. Preliminary studies suggest that patients who used this preparation had their symptoms resolve faster than patients on a placebo.

A commonly used nutritional therapy for the common cold that has been the focus of discussions in both scientific communities and around dinner tables is chicken soup. Chicken soup has been shown to inhibit neutrophil chemotaxis *in vivo* in a dose–response fashion. The beneficial effects appear to lie in the liquid component of the soup; further investigation showed that the liquid portion inhibits chemotaxis while the chicken showed no cytotoxic activity.

Recently, attention has turned to antiviral agents in hopes of developing drugs that will cure colds or at least reduce their symptomatic duration. Studies with tremacamra, a molecule that blocks viral binding, showed some reduction in cold symptoms. One antiviral agent currently in clinical trial may be approved soon.

Complications

Primary complications from upper respiratory tract infection are otitis media and sinusitis. These complications develop from obstruction of the Eustachian tube or sinus ostea from nasal passage edema. Although treatment of these infections with antibiotics is common, the vast majority of infections clear without antibiotic therapy.

One misconception is that using antibiotics during the acute phase of a cold can prevent these complications. Evidence shows that taking antibiotics during a cold does not reduce the incidence of sinusitis or otitis media.

Gonzales R, Steiner JF, Sande MA: Antibiotic prescribing for adults with colds, upper respiratory tract infections, and bronchitis by ambulatory care physicians. JAMA 1997;278: 901.

Mainous AG III, Hueston WJ, Clark JR: Antibiotics and upper respiratory infection: do some folks think there is a cure for the common cold? J Fam Pract 1996;42:357.

Makela MJ et al: Viruses and bacteria in the etiology of the common cold. J Clin Microbiol 1998;36:539.

Williams JW, Simel DL: Does this patient have sinusitis: diagnosing acute sinusitis by history and physical examination. JAMA 1993;270:1242.

SINUSITIS

ESSENTIALS OF DIAGNOSIS

- *"Double-sickening" phenomenon.*
- *Maxillary toothache and purulent nasal discharge.*
- *Poor response to decongestants.*
- *History of discolored nasal discharge.*

General Considerations

Because sinusitis is most often a complication of upper respiratory viral infections, the incidence peaks in the winter. Among children, sinusitis is frequently found as a comorbidity with otitis media. Children are also more likely to have posterior ethmoidal and sphenoid inflammation whereas among adults maxillary and anterior ethmoidal sinusitis are more common. Medical conditions that may increase the risk for sinusitis include cystic fibrosis, asthma, immunosuppression, and allergic rhinitis. Cigarette smoking may also increase the risk of bacterial sinusitis during a cold because of reduced mucociliary clearance.

Viral, fungal, and bacterial infections as well as allergies can cause sinus inflammation. The majority of acute sinusitis is caused by viral infection. The inflammation associated with viral infection clears without additional therapy. Bacterial superinfection of URIs is rare and occurs in only 0.5–1% of colds.

Cultures of material obtained from patients with sinusitis show that the most prevalent organisms are *S pneumoniae* and, especially in smokers, *H influenzae*. These two organisms are present in 70% of cases of bacterial acute sinusitis. Antibiotics used for the treatment of bacterial sinusitis, should include sufficient coverage of these two organisms. Fungal sinusitis is very rare and usually occurs in immunosuppressed individuals or those with diabetes mellitus.

Clinical Findings

Acute sinusitis has considerable overlap in its constellation of signs and symptoms with URIs. One-half to two-thirds of patients with sinus symptoms seen in primary care are unlikely to have sinusitis. In 300 patients who presented with a URI, 19% had radiographic evidence of maxillary sinusitis, but had no symptoms of sinus infection. URIs are often precursors of sinusitis and at some point symptoms from each condition may overlap. Sinus inflammation from a URI without bacterial infection is also common. In a series of 60 children undergoing CT for non-sinus-related diagnoses, 47% had evidence of sinus inflammation with no clinical signs of sinusitis and with complete resolution following their viral illness.

Acute sinusitis tends to start with a URI that leads to sinus ostial obstruction. The signs and symptoms that increase the likelihood that the patient has acute sinusitis are a "double sickening" phenomenon whereby the patient seems to improve following the URI and then deteriorates, maxillary toothache, purulent nasal discharge, poor response to decongestants, and a history of discolored nasal discharge.

Treatment

Antibiotics are commonly prescribed for adult patients who present with complaints consistent with acute sinusitis. The effectiveness of antibiotics is unclear. Some evidence supports their use, some evidence has yielded mixed results, and other evidence showed no beneficial effect. Trials demonstrating effects suggested that patients with more severe signs and symptoms, as well as radiographic or CT confirmation, may benefit from an antibiotic. A meta-analysis of 32 randomized trials of antibiotics versus placebo and antibiotics of different classes cited in computerized databases such as MEDLINE and studies from pharmaceutical companies indicated that acute maxillary sinusitis may benefit from penicillin or amoxicillin for 7–14 days. If an antibiotic is used, evidence with trimethoprim/sulfamethoxazole suggests that short duration treatment (eg, 3 days) is as effective as longer treatment. Further, a meta-analysis indicates that narrow spectrum agents are as effective as broad spectrum agents.

De Bock GH et al: Antimicrobial treatment in acute maxillary sinusitis: a meta-analysis. J Clin Epidemiol 1997;50:881.

Evans KL: Diagnosis and management of sinusitis. Lancet 1994;309:1415.

Lindbaek M, Hjortdahl P, Johnsen UL-F: Use of symptoms, signs, and blood tests to diagnose acute sinus infections in primary care: comparison with computer tomography. Fam Med 1996;28:183.

Williams JW Jr et al: Antibiotics for acute maxillary sinusitis. Cochrane Database Syst Rev 2000;(2):CD000243.

OTITIS MEDIA

ESSENTIALS OF DIAGNOSIS

- *Decreased hearing, pain, fever, malaise.*
- *Visualization of the tympanic membrane reveals purulent-appearing fluid and reduced movement of the eardrum with pneumatic insufflation.*

General Considerations

Decreased hearing, pain, and systemic signs of infections such as fever or malaise characterize middle ear infections. The peak onset of middle ear infections is in the first 6 years of life. About one-third of children have their first episode of otitis media in the first year of life and often have repetitive episodes throughout their childhood, another one-third have only a small number of ear infections (fewer than three), and the remaining one-third have no ear infections.

Dysfunction of the Eustachian tube disrupts proper ventilation of the middle ear and can result in a negative pressure that pulls fluid into the middle ear space. Stasis of this fluid combined with colonization with nasopharyngeal organisms can result in otitis media. Conditions that are associated with poor Eustachian tube function or occlusion of the lower Eustachian tube such as allergic rhinitis or upper respiratory tract infections increase the risk of otitis media. Additionally, poor function of the tensor veli palatini muscle, which is seen in some families as well as in patients with trisomy 21 (Down's syndrome), also increases the risk of otitis media. Finally, patients with craniofacial abnormalities that may involve the Eustachian tube also have higher incidences of otitis media.

Clinical Findings

In most cases of otitis media, the diagnosis can be made based on physical examination. Visualization of the tympanic membrane reveals purulent-appearing fluid with reduced movement of the eardrum with pneumatic insufflation. However, physical examination alone has poor accuracy compared with other modalities.

Tympanometry improves the sensitivity and specificity of the diagnosis of middle ear effusion. Tympanometry testing measures the amount of a test sound that transverses the tympanic membrane at given positive and negative auditory canal pressures. The tympanometer forms an airtight seal around the auditory canal and a sound wave is introduced by pushing a button on the instrument. The machine monitors the amount of the sound reflected back from the tympanic membrane. This procedure is repeated at various positive and negative pressures and the results are plotted based on the amount of sound transmitted. In a series of studies evaluating this test, the sensitivity of tympanometry compared to myringotomy was 79–95% with a corresponding specificity of 57–93%. However, the reliability of the test is influenced by the level of cooperation by the patient. In poorly cooperative children, the predictive value drops substantially.

Acoustic reflectometry is another adjunctive test that measures sound reflected off the tympanic membrane. The amount of sound reflected is measured in decibels with the most appropriate cut-off value for a positive test still controversial. Studies of acoustic reflectometry have used either tympanometry or clinical examination as the gold standards, which limits their application. Even with these weak gold standards, positive and negative predictive values are in the 80% range.

Treatment

Despite many debates, there is no consensus regarding which antibiotics are most appropriate for initial or recurrent therapy, the optimal duration of therapy, or even whether antibiotics should be used. Although internationally there is great variation in the percentage of cases treated with antibiotics, in the United States, routine use of antibiotics for otitis media has been the tradition. Data from two meta-analyses showed that routine use of amoxicillin is associated with a 12.3–13.7% lower failure rate than observation (or placebo). This translates into a number needed to treat (NNT) of 6 to prevent one case of failure in a patient not treated with antibiotics.

When the effectiveness of multiple antibiotics was compared, there appeared to be no difference among drugs as first-line therapy. Additionally, a shorter duration of antibiotic use (5 days) appears to be equally effective as a longer duration. In addition to short-duration therapy compared to long-duration therapy with oral antibiotics, a single intramuscular dose of ceftriaxone was just as effective as a longer duration of other antibiotics.

Because of the emergence of multiple drug-resistant strains of *S pneumoniae,* there has been some concern that standard doses of medications might not be sufficient to cover strains that are intermediately resistant. However, two controlled studies of high-dose amoxicillin-clavulanate have shown no greater effectiveness than standard dosing regimens.

The treatment of recurrent otitis media after a previous resistant episode is another area of controversy. Some physicians treat recurrent infection failure with a second-line drug to avoid a second treatment failure. However, recurrences several weeks after an initial episode are usually produced by a new organism and do not necessarily have the same resistance pattern as previous infections. One nonrandomized study that investigated the effectiveness of a second-line drug versus a first-line agent (amoxicillin or trimethoprim-sulfamethoxazole) showed no benefit of the broader spectrum second-line agent in a recurrent infection following a previously resistant episode. To reduce the development of resistance, new episodes should be treated with narrower spectrum agents.

In children with multiple episodes of otitis media, prevention of recurrent infections may be necessary. Recurrent otitis is defined as three or more episodes in a 6-month period or four episodes in a year with a normal examination documented between each infection. The first approach in preventing recurrences is to identify conditions that predispose children to Eustachian tube dysfunction. Most commonly, this is an upper respiratory infection that cannot be prevented. However, in some children this is a chronic allergic rhinitis. Treatment of these children with antihistamines or nasal steroids may reduce their risk of a recurrent infection.

For children with no evidence of allergy, options include chronic antibiotic prophylaxis and surgical ventilation of the inner ear through the placement of tubes. Tympanostomy tubes and antibiotic prophylaxis have nearly equal effectiveness for the prevention of recurrence, but medication use is associated with fewer side effects. Antibiotic prophylaxis can be achieved with either amoxicillin or sulfamethoxazole given as a single dose at bedtime. The usual dose is one-half of the total daily treatment dose. If antibiotic prophylaxis fails, it is most likely to fail in the first 6 months, so a short trial of antibiotic suppression is probably indicated in most patients. For children who continue to have episodes of otitis media despite antibiotic prophylaxis, the insertion of tympanostomy tubes is indicated. Children who already have language delay and recurrent infections complicated by persistent serous otitis media may benefit from tympanostomy tubes as initial therapy. However, a recent controlled trial showed no benefit for early insertion of tubes.

Koryrskyj AL et al: Treatment of acute otitis media with a shortened course of antibiotics: a meta-analysis. JAMA 1998;279: 1736.

Stewart MH, Siff JE, Cydulka RK: Evaluation of the patient with sore throat, earache, and sinusitis: an evidence based approach. Emerg Med Clin North Am 1999;17:153.

PHARYNGITIS

 ESSENTIALS OF DIAGNOSIS

- *Fever and cervical lymphadenopathy accompany the sore throat.*
- *Rhinorrhea and cough.*
- *Positive throat culture or rapid streptococcal antigen test.*

General Considerations:

The most common causes of pharyngitis are respiratory viruses. Adenovirus and the rhinoviruses account for about 80% of cases of sore throat in children who are seen by a physician. Coxsackievirus, herpesvirus, and Epstein–Barr virus (EBV) can cause tonsillitis, but are less common that adenovirus.

Group A β-hemolytic streptococcus can cause an acute tonsillopharyngitis, but may colonize the oropharynx without symptoms. The asymptomatic carrier rate of group A streptococcus is usually reported to be less than 10%. However, positive cultures can result from colonization rather than true infection. In contrast to group A streptococcal tonsillopharyngitis, treatment of the carrier state is not necessary and does not reduce symptoms or reduce complications. The peak occurrence of both viral and group A streptococcal pharyngitis is winter and early spring. Streptococcal infection, in particular, can be recognized in epidemic patterns frequently affecting groups that spend considerable time together in close quarters, such as day cares, schools, and places of employment. Strep throat also is related to patient age. Streptococcal pharyngitis is rare in the very young (<1 year old), but increases in early childhood with a peak occurrence for strep throat between 3 and 10 years of age. The risk of strep throat decreases in those over the age of 20.

Chlamydia and *Mycoplasma* species also have been identified in patients with acute pharyngitis. However, there have been few treatment trials that demonstrate any benefit of treating these agents; patients who received placebo had the same speed of symptom resolution as those treated with active antibiotics.

Another cause of acute pharyngitis, especially in preteen and early teen children, is mononucleosis. Infectious mononucleosis is spread through salivary excretion of the EBV. Clinical characteristics of infectious mononucleosis include an exudative tonsillitis/pharyngitis, cervical lymph node enlargement, fever, malaise, and hepatosplenomegaly. Fever and lymphadenopathy are the most common symptoms of infectious mononucleosis and occur in over 90% of children with this infection. Tonsillitis occurs in 70–80% of children with mononucleosis. Because of the similarities in presenting symptoms with streptococcal pharyngitis, infectious mononucleosis can be mistaken for strep throat early in the course of illness.

In addition to the common causes, several other conditions can cause pharyngitis. These include infections with Coxsackie viruses (herpangina), *Candida*, other bacteria (diphtheria, *Neisseria gonorrhea*), and spriochetes (leptospirosis). Retropharyngeal or peritonsillar abscesses also can present as sore throats. A complete history including exposure to common infectious agents, risks for immunosuppression, history of smoking and alcohol use, and duration of symptoms can be useful in distinguishing situations in which atypical causes for pharyngitis are more likely.

Clinical Findings

Table 26–2 shows some of the causes of sore throat that should be considered in the primary care setting. The findings of other symptoms suggestive of a URI such as rhinorrhea or cough are useful in suggesting a viral cause for a sore throat. Although exudative tonsillitis is thought to signal streptococcal infection, adenovirus,

Table 26–2. Differential diagnosis for sore throat.

Pharyngeal infection
  Bacterial infection
    Group A streptococcus
    Chlaymdia
    Mycoplasma
    Diphtheria
    Mycobacterium tuberculosis
    Neisseria gonorrhea
  Viral infection
    Adenovirus
    Respiratory syncytial virus
    Influenza virus
    Parainfluenza virus
    Epstein–Barr virus (mononucleosis)
    Coxsackie virus (herpangina)
  Fungal infections
    Candidiasis
Noninfectious causes
  Trauma
  Smoke inhalation

coxsackievirus, and EBV also cause exudative pharyngitis that can mimic the appearance of streptococcal infection. Consequently, the use of exudate alone is a poor indicator of a bacterial pharyngitis.

Streptococcal pharyngitis is more likely when signs of URI are not present and when a fever and cervical lymphadenopathy accompany the sore throat. Several clinical decision rules have been developed that help clinicians determine the risk of a strep throat based on these clinical criteria, but none has been accurate enough to replace microbiological testing in identifying a strep throat. A positive throat culture or rapid streptococcal antigen test usually confirms streptococcal pharyngitis. One dilemma in testing children for group A streptococcus is that the sensitivity of first-generation rapid group A antibody kits was not very high when compared to a throat culture. Early versions of rapid antigen detection kits showed sensitivities in the range of only 30–50%. Recently developed optical immunoassays (OIA) that use a polymerase chain reaction (PCR) technique to amplify certain streptococcal antigens show a sensitivity of 80–82% and a specificity of 87–97% compared to cultures for group A streptococcus. When compared to other reference criteria, the PCR test was equally sensitive and specific to blood agar cultures. OIA has been found to be superior to previous "first-generation" strep tests. Because these tests now have suitable sensitivity, follow-up throat culture is not cost effective.

Mononucleosis should be suspected when extensive adenopathy is present along with hepato- or splenomegaly or when symptoms of pharyngitis persist longer than 10–14 days. The typical incubation period between exposure to EBV and the development of symptoms of infectious mononucleosis is 5–7 weeks. However, studies in families with one child who contacts infectious mononucleosis have shown that the delay between exposure and symptoms can sometimes exceed 6 months. The diagnosis of EBV mononucleosis is usually made through the identification of immunoglobulin M (IgM) antibodies to the Epstein–Barr virus. A rapid test for the presence of these heterophil antibodies is positive in about 80% of children above the age of 4 years who have infectious mononucleosis, but is much less sensitive under this age. The IgM response can usually be detected within 3–4 weeks after the onset of symptoms. So, early in the course of the illness testing for mononucleosis is not helpful and can be confusing since a negative heterophil antibody can be misinterpreted as excluding the diagnosis of infectious mononucleosis. Additionally, there may be some confusion in patients who have an unconfirmed history of a prior mononucleosis infection. In this case, complete EBV serology for IgM, IgG, and antinuclear antibody can be useful.

Treatment

If group A streptococcus is identified, antibiotic treatment is indicated. The selection of an appropriate antibiotic and duration of therapy are important considerations in treating strep pharyngitis. Penicillin V resistance in group A streptococcus as well as erythromycin resistance has led to investigations of other drugs for management of strep throat. Single-dose therapy with amoxicillin at 40 mg/kg/day for 10 days appears to be very successful, resulting in excellent clinical responses and low (5–10%) posttreatment carrier rates. Treatment with other agents such as azithromycin and clarithromycin produces results no better than treatment with amoxicillin or penicillin V, but at much greater expense.

Attempts at "short-course" therapy have been studied with azithromycin. Both short-course treatment with azithromycin and 10 days of cefaclor have exactly the same clinical cure rates (86%) by Day 3 of therapy. However, patients treated with cefaclor were less likely to become recolonized with group A streptococcus over the next 45 days than those treated with the short course of azithromycin (20% versus 55%). Because the significance of rapid recolonization is still unclear, short course therapy with azithromycin or other antibiotics still requires additional investigation.

Although the carrier state does not require treatment, some clinicians attempt to treat those colonized by group A streptococcus to prevent spread to other family members and close contacts. A regimen of intramuscular penicillin V plus oral rifampin has been shown to reverse the carrier status in 93% of patients treated. No studies indicate whether this regimen remains effective with increased group A streptococcus resistance to penicillin.

EBV-associated infectious mononucleosis is a self-limited condition that usually resolves over several weeks. Fever, often the earliest manifestation of illness, abates usually after 1 or 2 weeks, but malaise and hepatosplenomegaly may take 4–6 weeks to resolve. During this time activities that could result in splenic trauma, such as contact sports, should be avoided. Although the exact time to return to full activities is predicated on the degree of splenic rupture and absence of other complications, a minimum of 1 month to recuperate is suggested.

Some patients with infectious mononucleosis experience severe tonsillitis with potential compromise of their airways. In these patients, administration of corticosteroids should be considered. If airway obstruction is severe and life-threatening, an artificial airway should be provided. Installation of an airway is preferable to emergency tonsillectomy.

Finally, some investigation has focused on antiviral therapy with acyclovir for infectious mononucleosis. However, acyclovir in doses of 600 mg for 10 days did not appear to reduce clinical symptoms, although it did reduce viral shedding. Combining acyclovir with steroids did not appear to produce any clinical benefit either.

Treatment of nonbacterial sore throats should focus on alleviation of symptoms. Routine use of antibiotics in this group has not been shown to offer any benefit. Symptomatic care includes pain relief with acetominophen, ibuprofen, or other nonsteroidal antiinflammatory agents plus topical treatment with local anesthetics such as those found in over-the-counter throat lozenges. Gargling with salt water is commonly used as well, although there is little evidence that this is beneficial.

Complications

The complications of pharyngitis of most concern are rheumatic fever, peritonsillar abscess, and poststreptococcal glomerulonephritis.

Poststreptococcal rheumatic fever was once a common problem in industrialized countries. Until the 1960s, rheumatic fever ranked as the most common cause of cardiac valvular disease in adults. However, rheumatic fever has been declining in industrialized countries since the 1950s. Treatment with antibiotics reduces the likelihood that rheumatic fever will develop even when strains carrying the M antigen are responsible for the infection. Currently, the annual incidence of rheumatic fever is now 0.5 cases per 100,000 children in industrialized nations.

Peritonsillar abscess is a more common complication of streptococcal pharyngitis. Abscess development is most common in adolescents and young adults. Patients present with increased sore throat, fever, and difficulty swallowing and speaking. The affected tonsils are large and usually displace the palate. Visualization of the uvula deviated to the contralateral side is a useful indicator of peritonsillar abscess. Treatment focuses on draining the infection usually with an 18-gauge needle inserted into the tonsil along with antibiotic therapy. Single aspiration with antibiotics has been shown to result in cure rates of 92%, which compared favorably with more aggressive surgical management. Without therapy, peritonsillar abscesses may invade into the head and neck with fatal consequences.

Like rheumatic fever, several subtypes of group A streptococcus can cause acute poststreptococcal glomerulonephritis (APSGN). Unlike rheumatic fever that develops after a throat infection, APSGN can result from both pharyngeal and skin infections. APSGN occurs most often in young school-aged children and is rare in those under the age of 3. Overall, the prognosis of APSGN is excellent, with 98% of children eventually recovering full renal function.

Olivier C: Rheumatic fever—is it still a problem? J Antimicrob Chemother 2000;45(Suppl);13.

Peter J, Ray CG: Infectious mononucleosis. Pediatr Rev 1998; 19:276.

Tynell E et al: Acyclovir and prednisolone treatment of acute infectious mononucleosis: a multicenter, double-blind, placebo-controlled study. J Infect Dis 1996;174:324.

■ LOWER RESPIRATORY TRACT INFECTIONS

ACUTE BRONCHITIS

ESSENTIALS OF DIAGNOSIS

- Cough lasting more than 3 weeks.
- Fever, constitutional symptoms, and a productive cough.

General Considerations

Acute bronchitis in the otherwise healthy adult is one of the most common medical problems encountered in primary care. The prevalence of acute bronchitis peaks in the winter and is much less common in the summer.

Viral infection is the primary cause of most episodes of acute bronchitis. A wide variety of viruses have been shown to cause acute bronchitis, including influenza, rhinovirus, adenovirus, coronavirus, parainfluenza, and respiratory syncytial virus. Nonviral pathogens including *M pneumoniae* and *C pneumoniae* (TWAR) have also been identified as causes.

The etiological role of bacteria such as *H influenzae* and *S pneumoniae* in acute bronchitis is unclear because these bacteria are common upper respiratory tract flora. Sputum cultures for acute bronchitis are therefore difficult to evaluate because it is unclear whether the sputum has been contaminated by pathogens colonizing the nasopharynx.

Clinical Findings

Patients with acute bronchitis may have a cough for a significant time. Although the duration of the condition is variable, one study showed that 50% of patients had a cough for more than 3 weeks and 25% had a cough for more than 4 weeks. Other causes of chronic cough are shown in Table 26–3.

Both acute bronchitis and pneumonia can present with fever, constitutional symptoms, and a productive cough. Although patients with pneumonia often have rales, this finding is neither sensitive nor specific for the illness. When pneumonia is suspected on the basis of the presence of a high fever, constitutional symptoms, severe dyspnea, and certain physical findings or risk factors, a chest radiograph should be obtained to confirm the diagnosis.

Differential Diagnosis

Asthma and allergic bronchospastic disorders can mimic the productive cough of acute bronchitis. When obstructive symptoms are not obvious, mild asthma may be diagnosed as acute bronchitis. Further, because respiratory infections can trigger bronchospasm in asthma, patients with asthma that occurs only in the presence of respiratory infections resemble patients with acute bronchitis.

Finally, nonpulmonary causes of cough should enter the differential diagnosis. In older patients, congestive heart failure may cause cough, shortness of breath, and wheezing. Reflux esophagitis with chronic aspiration can cause bronchial inflammation with cough and wheezing. Bronchogenic tumors may produce a cough and obstructive symptoms.

Treatment

Antibiotic treatment for acute bronchitis is quite common with evidence indicating that 60–75% of adults

Table 26–3. Causes of chronic cough.

Pulmonary causes
  Infectious
    Postobstructive pneumonia
    Tuberculosis
    Pneumocystis carinii
    Bronchiectasis
    Lung abscess
  Noninfectious
    Asthma
    Chronic bronchitis
    Allergic aspergillosis
    Bronchogenic neoplasms
    Sarcoidosis
    Pulmonary fibrosis
    Chemical or smoke inhalation

Cardiovascular causes
  Congestive heart failure/pulmonary edema
  Enlargement of left atrium

Gastrointestinal tract
  Reflux esophagitis

Other causes
  Medications, especially angiotensin converting enzyme
    (ACE) inhibitors
  Psychogenic cough
  Foreign body aspiration

visiting a doctor for acute bronchitis receive an antibiotic. Clinical trials of the effectiveness of antibiotics in treating acute bronchitis have had mixed results. Meta-analyses indicated that the benefits of antibiotics in a general population are marginal and should be weighed against the impact of excessive use of antibiotics on the development of antibiotic resistance.

Data from clinical trials suggest that bronchodilators may provide effective symptomatic relief to patients with acute bronchitis. Treatment with bronchodilators demonstrated significant relief of symptoms including faster resolution of cough, as well as return to work. The effect of albuterol in a population of patients with undifferentiated cough was evaluated and no beneficial effect was found. Because a variety of conditions present with cough, there may have been some misclassification in generalizing this to acute bronchitis.

Bent S et al: Antibiotics in acute bronchitis: a meta-analysis. Am J Med 1999;107:62.

Nyquist AC et al: Antibiotic prescribing for children with colds, upper respiratory tract infections, and bronchitis. JAMA 1998;279:875.

Smucny JJ et al: Are antibiotics effective treatment for acute bronchitis? A meta-analysis. J Fam Pract 1998;47:453.

COMMUNITY-ACQUIRED PNEUMONIA

 ESSENTIALS OF DIAGNOSIS

- *Fever and cough (productive or nonproductive).*
- *Tachypnea.*
- *Rales or crackles.*
- *Positive chest radiograph.*

General Considerations

Pneumonia is the cause of over 10 million visits to physicians annually and in the United States accounts for 3% of all hospitalizations and is the sixth leading cause of death. Pneumonia occurs in about 12 people/1000 per year, but is much higher in the elderly population (estimated at about 30 cases/1000 per year).

In addition to age, other risk factors for pneumonia should be noted. Among the elderly, institutionalization and debilitation increase the risk for acquiring pneumonia. Of patients aged 55 years or older, smokers and patients with chronic respiratory diseases are more likely to require hospitalization for pneumonia. Those with congestive heart failure, cerebrovascular diseases, cancer, diabetes mellitus, and poor nutritional status are more likely to die. Thus, age and comorbidities are important factors to consider when deciding whether to hospitalize a patient with pneumonia. These risk factors are summarized in Table 26–4.

In the past, over 80% of confirmed cases of pneumonia were caused by *S pneumoniae* with mortality rates between 20% and 40%. Although pneumococcal disease still represents the largest single cause of pneumonia, other bacterial causes and nonbacterial pathogens now represent the majority of cases. Prevalence data from a number of North American studies estimate that pneumococcal pneumonia now represents about 20–60% of documented cases with atypical agents such as *Legionella* and *Mycoplasma* species responsible for another 10–20%, viruses causing 2–15%, and other bacterial agents such as *H influenzae* (3–10%), *Staphylococcus aureus* (3–5%), and gram-negative organisms (3–10%) less common.

Primary care physicians must be cautious when interpreting the data on the prevalence of causative agents for pneumonia. These data are generally derived from a few academic medical centers and may include only cases in which a causative agent was identified. The increase in

Table 26–4. Risk factors associated with mortality in community-acquired pneumonia.

Category	Characteristics	Mortality	Location of Care
Very low risk	Age <60, no comorbidities	<1%	Outpatient
Low risk	Age >60, but healthy	3%	80% can be cared for as outpatient (depending on comorbidity)
	Age <60, mild comorbidity		
Moderate risk	Age >60 with comorbidity	13–25%	Hospitalization
High risk	Serious compromise present on presentation (hypotension, respiratory distress, etc) regardless of age	50%	Intensive care unit

the number of patients who are immunosuppressed from drug therapy or human immunodeficiency virus (HIV) disease and the trend toward treating less severely ill individuals as outpatients has skewed the spectrum of illness cared for in the hospital setting. An example of this are data from Johns Hopkins Hospital in 1991 where pneumococcus was the most common cause of pneumonia, but was followed in frequency by *Pneumocystic carinii,* which accounted for 13% of all cases.

Prevention

Pneumococcal pneumonia may be prevented through immunization with multivalent pneumococcal vaccine. Pneumococcal vaccination is indicated for individuals over age 65, and for those 2 years of age or older with diabetes mellitus, chronic pulmonary or cardiac disease, or without a spleen. Additionally, people in certain high-risk populations such as Native Americans, Alaska Native populations, and those people over age 50 living in chronic care facilities should be vaccinated. Immunosuppressed patients including those with HIV, alcoholism, cirrhosis, chronic renal failure, sickle cell disease, or multiple myeloma may benefit from immunization, but the evidence is less convincing.

In addition to initial vaccination, clinicians should advise patients that the duration of protection is uncertain. For those at particularly high risk of mortality from pneumococcal pneumonia, such as patients over age 75 and those with chronic pulmonary disease or lacking a spleen, revaccination every 5 years is a worthwhile precaution.

A conjugated pneumococcal vaccination is effective for children under the age of 2. Current recommendations are to immunize all children under the age of 2 and high-risk children under age 7.

Clinical Findings

The most common presenting complaints for patients with pneumonia are fever and a cough that may be either productive or nonproductive. As an example, in one study, 80% of patients with pneumonia had a fever. Other symptoms that may be suggestive of pneumonia include dyspnea and pleuritic chest pain. However, none of these symptoms is specific for pneumonia.

Symptoms of pneumonia may be nonspecific in older patients. Elderly individuals who suffer a general decline in their function, who become confused or have worsening dementia, or experience more frequent falls should receive a chest x-ray even if no pulmonary symptoms or physical findings are present. Elderly patients who have preexisting cognitive impairment or depend on someone else for support of their daily activities are at highest risk for not exhibiting typical symptoms of pneumonia.

The most consistent sign of pneumonia is tachypnea. In one study of elderly patients, tachypnea was observed to be present 3 to 4 days before the appearance of other physical findings of pneumonia. Rales or crackles are often considered the hallmark for pneumonia, but these may be heard in only 75–80% of patients. Other signs of pneumonia such as dullness to percussion or egophony, which are usually believed to be indicative of consolidation, occur in less than a third of patients with pneumonia.

Chest radiography is the standard for diagnosing pneumonia. In rare cases, the chest x-ray may be false negative. These generally occur in patients exhibiting profound dehydration, early pneumonia (first 24 h), infection with *Pneumocystis,* and severe neutropenia.

Microbiological testing for pneumonia is not very useful in relatively well patients with nonsevere pneumonia. Blood and sputum cultures are most likely to be beneficial in patients with risk factors for unusual organisms or who are very ill.

Differential Diagnosis

Every infiltrate is not a pneumonia. Other conditions such as postobstructive pneumonitis, pulmonary infarct from an embolism, radiation pneumonitis, and interstitial edema from congestive heart failure all may produce infiltrates that are indistinguishable from an infectious process.

Treatment

With the emergence of other pathogens causing pneumonia and the development of resistance penicillin and other drugs in *S pneumoniae,* treatment decisions have become more complex. A Centers for Disease Control and Prevention (CDC) working group on drug-resistant *S pneumoniae* released recommendations on management of community-acquired pneumonia (CAP) (Table 26–5). For outpatient treatment of CAP, suitable empirical oral antimicrobial agents include a macrolide (eg, erythromycin, clarithromycin, azithromycin), doxycycline (or tetracycline) for children aged 8 years or older, or an oral β-lactam with good activity against pneumococci (eg, cefuroxime axetil, amoxicillin, or a combination of amoxicillin and clavulanate potassium).

Suitable empirical antimicrobial regimens for inpatient pneumonia include an intravenous β-lactam, such as cefuroxime, ceftriaxone sodium, cefotaxime sodium, or a combination of ampicillin sodium and sulbactam sodium plus a macrolide. New fluoroquinolones with improved activity against *S pneumoniae* can also be used to treat adults with CAP. To limit the emergence of fluoroquinolone-resistant strains, the new fluoroquinolones should be limited to adults (1) for whom one of the above regimens has already failed, (2) who are allergic to alternative agents, or (3) who have a documented infection with highly drug-resistant pneumococci (eg, penicillin MIC 4 μg/mL). Vancomycin hy-

drochloride is not routinely indicated for the treatment of CAP or pneumonia caused by drug-resistant *S pneumoniae.*

Bartlett JG, Mundy LM: Community-acquired pneumonia. New Engl J Med 1995;333:1618.

Houston MS, Silverstein MC, Suman, VJ: Community-acquired lower respiratory tract infection in the elderly: a community-based study of incidence and outcome. J Am Bd Fam Pract 1995;8:247.

■ NONINFECTIOUS RESPIRATORY PROBLEMS

ASTHMA

ESSENTIALS OF DIAGNOSIS

- *Recurrent wheezing, shortness of breath, or cough.*
- *Histories of allergies in children.*
- *Increase in airway secretions.*
- *Airway constriction and/or obstruction.*
- *Bronchospasm documented on spirometry.*
- *Dyspnea.*

Table 26–5. Recommendations for empiric treatment of community-acquired pneumonia.

Treatment of patients not requiring hospitalization
  Preferred (in no special order): Macrolide, fluoroquinolone with enhanced pneumococcal activity,[1] doxycycline
  Alternatives not active against atypical agents: Amoxicillin/clavulinic acid, selected second-generation cephalosporins (cefuroxime, cefpodoxime, or cefprozil)

Treatment of hospitalized patients not critically ill
  Preferred (in no special order): β-Lactam with or without a macrolide or fluoroquinolone with enhanced pneumococcal activity[1]
  Alternatives: Cefuroxime with or without a macrolide or azithromycin alone

Treatment of critically ill hospitalized patients
  Preferred (in no special order): Erythromycin, azithromycin, or fluoroquinolone with enhanced pneumococcal activity,[1] *plus* cefuroxime, ceftriaxone, or a β-lactam with β-lactamase inhibitor

Other situations
  Treatment of patients with penicillin allergy: Fluoroquinolone with enhanced pneumococcal activity[1]
  Suspected aspiration: Fluoroquinolone with enhanced pneumococcal activity[1] *plus* clindamycin or a β-lactam with β-lactamase inhibitor

From Bartlett JG et al: ISDA Guidelines for CAP in Adults. *Clin Infect Dis* 31:347–382.
[1]Includes levofloxacin, sparfloxicin, grepafloxicin, and trovofloxicin.

General Considerations

Asthma is one of the most common illnesses in childhood. Up to 25% of all children will experience an asthma attack with 3–5% continuing to have asthma symptoms into adulthood. Both asthma and the number of deaths from this disease have been steadily increasing in the United States over the past two decades. It is estimated that approximately 5000 individuals die from asthma in the United States annually.

Risk factors for the development of asthma include living in poverty and being in a nonwhite racial group. Part of the difference in asthma rates in different races may be increased exposure to allergens and other irritants such as air pollution, cigarette smoke, dust mites, and cockroaches in less affluent families, but racial differences persist even after adjusting for socioeconomic status.

Asthma results from inflammation in the airways, which is caused by allergies, environmental insults, or unknown causes. The inflammation causes an increase in airway secretions and contraction of the bronchial musculature, both of which result in airway constriction. Acute inflammation produces the asthma "attacks" that patients suffer, but even during periods of symptomatic quiescence, the inflammatory process continues and can produce long-term remodeling of the airways. Chronic changes in the bronchial wall musculature can result in long-term airway narrowing and resistance to bronchodilating agents.

Allergy is an important factor in asthma development in children, but does not appear to be as significant a factor in adults. Although as many as 80% of children with asthma also are atopic, 70% of adults under 30 and less than half of all adults over the age of 30 have any evidence of allergy. So, although an allergic component should be sought in adults it is less commonly found than in children with asthma.

Clinical Findings

In most cases, asthma is diagnosed based on symptoms of recurrent wheezing, shortness of breath, or cough. Children with recurrent cases of "bronchitis" who experience night cough or have difficulty with exercise tolerance should be suspected of having asthma. An additional history of allergies is useful since 80% of childhood asthma is associated with atopy.

Formal spirometry testing can usually be accomplished in children as young as 5 years of age and can confirm the diagnosis of asthma. Both the forced expiratory volume in 1 s (FEV_1) and FEV_1 to forced vital capacity (FVC) ratio are useful in documenting obstruction to airway flow. Further confirmation is provided by improvement of the FEV_1 by 12% or more following the use of a short-acting bronchodilator. For a valid test, though, children should avoid using a long-acting β-agonist in the previous 24 h or a short-acting β-agonist in the previous 6 h.

In some patients with asthma, spirometry may be normal. When there is a high index of suspicion that asthma may still be present, provocative testing with methacholine may be necessary to make the diagnosis. Bronchospasm documented on spirometry after inhalation of a challenge dose of metacholine is evidence of abnormal bronchial hyperreactivity. Methacholine challenge testing can result in severe bronchospasm and should be used judiciously. In most cases, this test is rarely necessary.

It also is useful to stratify patients with asthma by the severity of their illness. The severity of illness is thought to be related to the risks of long-term respiratory problems related to airway remodeling and also guides the treatment. Severity categorization should not be construed to mean that distinct differences exist in the patient population nor should it be interpreted to mean that patients remain in one category continuously. Instead, severity is a continuum that refers to a patient's current disease state and patients may move between severity stages throughout the course of their illness.

The severity of asthma is based on the frequency, intensity, and duration of baseline symptoms, level of airflow obstruction, and the extent to which asthma interferes with daily activities. Stages of severity range from severe persistent (step 4), where symptoms are chronic and limit activity, to mild intermittent (step 1), where symptoms are present no more than twice a week and pulmonary function studies are normal between exacerbations (Table 26–6). Patients are classified as to severity based upon their worst symptom and frequency, not upon having met all or the majority of the criteria in any category.

Finally, patients with asthma may benefit from allergy testing. The identification of specific allergens usually does not help in making the diagnosis of asthma, but may be useful in assisting families in avoiding provoking allergens or in providing immunotherapy when allergies persist despite avoidance measures.

Treatment

The approach to managing asthma relies on acute management of exacerbations, treatment of chronic airway inflammation, monitoring of respiratory function, and control of the factors that precipitate wheezing episodes. For all of these, patient and family education is vital.

Treatment of persistent asthma requires daily medication to prevent long-term airway remodeling. Mild, intermittent asthma may require therapy only during wheezing episodes. Guidelines for the management of

Table 26–6. Classification of asthma severity.

Step	Symptoms	Nighttime Symptoms	Lung Function

Step 4
Severe
    persistent
	Continual symptoms
	Limited physical activity
	Frequent exacerbations
		Frequent	FEV_1 or peak expiratory flow (PEF)
			    ≤60% predicted
			PEF variability >30%

Step 3 Moderate persistent	Daily symptoms Daily use of inhaled short-acting β_2-agonist Exacerbations affect activity Exacerbations ≥2 times a week; may last days	>1 time a week	FEV_1 or PEF >60%–<80% predicted PEF variability >30%
Step 2 Mild persistent	Symptoms >2 times a week but <1 time a day Exacerbations may affect activity	>2 times a month	FEV_1 or PEF ≥80% predicted PEF variability 20–30%

Step 1
Mild
    intermittent
	Symptoms <2 times a week
	Asymptomatic and normal PEF between exacer-
	    bations
	Exacerbations are brief; variable intensity
		≤2 times a month	FEV_1 or PEF ≥ 80% predicted
			PEF variability <20%

asthma are based on the child's age (6 years of age or younger) and are stratified by severity of illness. Guidelines for older children, adults, and younger children are provided in Table 26–7.

The treatment of exacerbations of asthma relies on fast-acting bronchodilators to produce rapid changes in airway resistance along with management of the late-phase changes that occur several hours after the initial symptoms are manifested. The failure to recognize the late-phase component of an acute exacerbation may lead to a rebound of symptoms several hours after the patient has left the office or emergency room. Corticosteroids are the mainstay for preventing the late-phase response.

For patients with persistent symptoms (step 2 and higher), chronic therapy is required. The management of persistent asthma may include long-acting bronchodilators to control intermittent symptoms and nighttime cough, but also should provide chronic antiinflammatory therapy to prevent long-term remodeling. Both inhaled steroids and nonsteroidal antiinflammatory medications (ie, cromoglycates) can provide antiinflammatory therapy. When symptoms are recurrent or large doses of antiinflammatory agents are required, treatment with a leukotriene inhibitor can provide additional antiinflammatory therapy and may allow a reduction in the dose of other antiinflammatory agents such as steroids.

When drugs are selected for the treatment of asthma, the potential side effects of each agent need to be weighed against the potential benefits. For children, chronic use of inhaled steroids has been associated with a small decrease in total height attained. Although the difference in height attainment is small (up to 1 inch), it might be preferable to use nonsteroidal antiinflammatory agents such as cromolyn and nedocromil in children.

In addition to pharmacological management, patients with asthma should avoid known and possible airway irritants. These include cigarette smoke (including second-hand inhalation of smoke), environmental pollutants, suspected or known allergens, and cold air. Children who have difficulty participating in sports may benefit from the use of a short-acting β-agonist such as albuterol before participating in exertion to prevent wheezing or cough.

The monitoring of pulmonary function is an important component of asthma management for all patients with persistent disease. Children and adults should be provided with a peak flow meter and instructed on how to use the device reliably. The use of a peak flow meter can determine subtle changes in respiratory function that may not cause symptoms for several days. To use a peak flow meter, patients must establish a "personal best," which represents the best reading that they can obtain when they are as asymptomatic as possible. Daily or periodic recordings of peak flows are compared to this personal best to gauge the current pulmonary function. Readings between 80% and 100% of the personal best indicate that the patient is doing well. Peak flows between 50% and 80% of an individual's person best are cause for concern even if symptoms are mild. Patients should be instructed beforehand how to respond in these instances. If a repeat of the peak flow later in the day after appropriate measures have been taken does not show improvement, patients should seek further medical attention. Patients should be told that severe decreases in peak flow to less than 50% are cause for immediate medical attention.

Table 26–7. Asthma drug therapy based on severity.

	Ages 6 Years Through Adulthood	
Step	**Daily Medications**	**Quick Relief**

Step 4
Severe
  persistent
	Choose all needed
	  High-dose inhaled corticosteroid
	  Long-acting bronchodilator
	  A leukotriene modifier
	  Oral corticosteroid
		Short-acting bronchodilator
		Daily or increasing use of short-acting
		  inhaled β_2-agonist indicates need for additional long-term
		  control therapy

Step 3
Moderate
  persistent
	Usually need 2
	  Either low- to medium-dose inhaled
	    corticosteroid
	  Long-acting bronchodilator
		Short-acting bronchodilator
		Daily or increasing use of short-acting inhaled β_2-agonist indicates
		  need for additional long-term control therapy

Step 2
Mild
  persistent
	Choose one
	  Low-dose inhaled corticosteroid
	  Cromolyn
	  Sustained-release theophylline (to
	    serum concentration of 5–15 µg/mL)
	  A leukotriene modifier
		Short-acting bronchodilator
		Daily or increasing use of short-acting inhaled β_2-agonist
		  indicates need for additional long-term control therapy

Step 1 Intermittent	No daily medication needed	Short-acting bronchodilator Use of short-acting inhaled β_2-agonist >2 times per week indicates need for additional long-term control therapy

	Step Down
	Review treatment every 1–6 months; a gradual stepwise
	  reduction in treatment may be possible
		Step Up
		If control is not maintained, consider step up; first, review patient
		  medication technique, adherence, and environmental control
		  (avoidance of allergens and/or other factors that contribute to
		  asthma severity)

Step	**Daily Antiinflammatory Medications**	**Quick Relief**

Step 4
Severe
  persistent
	High-dose inhaled corticosteroid with
	  space/holding chamber and facemask
	  and if needed, add systemic corticos-
	  teroids 2 mg/kg/day and reduce to
	  lowest daily or alternate-day dose that
	  stabilizes symptoms
		Short-acting bronchodilator as needed for symptoms
		By nebulizer or metered dose inhaler (MDI) with spacer/holding
		  chamber and facemask **or** oral β_2-agonist
		Daily or increasing use of short-acting inhaled β_2-agonist indi-
		  cates need for additional long-term control therapy

Step 3
Moderate
  persistent
	Either medium-dose inhaled cortico-
	  steroid with spacer/holding chamber
	  and facemask **or** low- to medium-dose
	  inhaled corticosteroid and long-acting
	  bronchodilator (theophylline)
		Short-acting bronchodilator as needed for symptoms
		By nebulizer or MDI with spacer/holding chamber and facemask
		  or oral β_2-agonist
		Daily or increasing use of short-acting inhaled β_2-agonist indicates
		  need for additional long-term control therapy

Step 2
Mild
	Young children usually begin
	  with a trial of cromolyn **or** low-dose
	  inhaled corticosteroid with spacer/
	  holding chamber and facemask
		Short-acting bronchodilator as needed for symptoms
		By nebulizer or MDI with spacer/holding chamber and facemask
		  or oral β_2-agonist
		Daily or increasing use of short-acting inhaled β_2-agonist indicates
		  need for additional long-term control therapy

Step 1
Intermittent
	No daily medication	Short-acting bronchodilator as needed for symptoms <2 times a
		  week
		By nebulizer or MDI with spacer/holding chamber and facemask
		  or oral β_2-agonist
		Two times weekly or increasing use of short-acting inhaled
		  β_2-agonist indicates need for additional long-term control
		  therapy

	Step Down
	Review treatment every 1–6 months; a gradual stepwise
	  reduction in treatment may be possible
		Step Up
		If control is not maintained, consider step up; first, review patient
		  medication technique, adherence, and environmental control
		  (avoidance of allergens and/or other factors that contribute to
		  asthma severity)

For patients with allergic symptoms, the use of immunotherapy should be considered. However, although immunotherapy usually results in improvements in symptoms of allergic rhinitis, it often does not improve asthma symptoms.

NIH Publication: *Guidelines for the Diagnosis and Management of Asthma.* Expert Panel Report 2. U.S. Department of Health and Human Services, 1997, No. 97-4051.

CHRONIC OBSTRUCTIVE PULMONARY DISEASE

 ESSENTIALS OF DIAGNOSIS

- *Productive cough featuring sputum production for at least 3 months for two consecutive years.*
- *Chronic dyspnea.*
- *FEV$_1$ below 80% predicted.*

General Considerations

Chronic obstructive pulmonary diseases cause about 80,000 deaths in the United States each year. In addition to mortality, chronic airway disease is the second leading cause of disability in the United States after coronary artery disease. Symptoms of chronic bronchitis first develop when patients are between 30 and 40 years of age and progressively become more common as patients reach their 50s and 60s. The development of chronic bronchitis is associated with heavier cigarette use; those smoking over 25 cigarettes per day have a risk of chronic bronchitis that is 30 times higher than nonsmokers. Although chronic bronchitis affects both genders and all socioeconomic strata, it is more commonly observed in men and in those of lower socioeconomic classes. It is presumed that these populations may be at higher risk due to higher consumption of cigarettes observed in these groups.

In addition to smoking, air pollution may play a role in the development and exacerbation of symptoms in patients with chronic bronchitis. Evidence shows that exposure to heavy doses of pollutants in ambient air is associated with increases in cardiopulmonary mortality as well as lung cancer. Patients with chronic obstructive pulmonary diseases who live in industrialized areas with heavy levels of particulate air pollution may be at increased risk of recurrent disease and death.

Patients with emphysema experience progressive destruction of the lung paryenchema resulting in the loss of interstitial lung tissue, enlarged alveolar air spaces, and damaged alveolar walls. These changes result in increased lung compliance and decreased elasticity. In contrast to patients with chronic bronchitis who have difficulty getting air in and clearing their mucus, patients with emphysema have greater difficulty exhaling and must use their accessory muscles to compress the lung to move air. This increased work results in dyspnea, the hallmark of emphysema.

Only 10–15% of smokers will develop chronic obstructive pulmonary disease (COPD), so other factors must also play a role in the progression from acute to chronic lung damage. The development of chronic bronchitis is thought to include both a predisposition to inflammatory damage plus exposure to the proper stimuli that cause inflammation, such as cigarette smoke or pollutants. Genetic factors, prolonged heavy exposure to other inflammatory mediators such as environmental pollutants, preexisting lung impairment from other inflammatory processes such as recurrent infection or childhood passive smoke exposure, and other mechanisms may all predispose individuals to the development of chronic bronchitis from smoking.

α_1-Antitrypsin deficiency is a rare genetic abnormality that causes panlobular emphysema in adults, and is responsible for approximately 1% of cases of COPD. This trait is inherited in an autosomal recessive pattern. Nonsmokers with this genetic defect develop emphysema at young ages. Those with this trait who smoke develop progressive emphysema at very early ages.

Clinical Findings

COPD includes both chronic bronchitis and emphysema. Chronic bronchitis is characterized by a productive cough featuring sputum production for at least 3 months for two consecutive years. Emphysema causes chronic dyspnea due to destruction of lung tissue, resulting in enlargement of air space and reduced compliance. In most cases, chronic bronchitis and emphysema can be differentiated based on whether the predominant symptom is a chronic cough or dyspnea. In contrast to asthma, changes in COPD are relatively fixed and only partially reversible with bronchodilator use.

When suspected clinically, COPD can be confirmed with chest radiography and spirometry. Chest radiographs in emphysema have several findings such as flattening of the diaphragm, irregularity in the lucency of the lung fields, enlargement of the retrosternal space, and blunting of the costophrenic angle. Although chest radiographic findings occur much later in the course of the disease than alterations in pulmonary function testing, a chest x-ray may be useful in patients suspected of having COPD because it can detect a number of other clinical conditions often found in these patients.

Spirometry is usually used to diagnose COPD because it can detect small changes in lung function and is easy to quantify. Changes in the FEV_1 and the FVC can provide an estimate of the degree of airway obstruction in these patients. Symptoms of COPD usually develop when FEV_1 falls below 80% of the predicted rate. In addition, a peak expiratory flow rate (PEFR) under 350 L/min in adults is a sign that COPD is likely to be present.

Spirometry also is useful in gauging the severity of COPD. Although there is some disagreement between the American Thoracic Society and the British Thoracic Society over the precise values that indicate severity of illness, decreases in FEV_1 over time are associated with overall mortality and with the frequency of exacerbations. A number of studies have shown that FEV_1 along with the patient's age is one of the best predictors of survival in patients with COPD. Decreases in FEV_1 on serial testing are associated with increased mortality rates; ie, patients with a faster decline in FEV_1 have a higher rate of death. The major risk factor associated with an accelerated rate of decline of FEV_1 is continued cigarette smoking. Smoking cessation in patients with early COPD improves lung function initially and slows the annual loss of FEV_1. Once FEV_1 falls below 1 L, 5-year survival is approximately 50%. FEV_1 less than 750 mL or less than 50% predicted on spirometric testing is associated with worsening disease and poorer prognosis.

Treatment

A. Nonpharmacological Therapy

The first step in treating the patient with chronic bronchitis/COPD is promoting a healthy life-style. Regular exercise and weight control should be started and smoking stopped to maximize the patient's therapeutic options.

Smoking cessation is the first and most important treatment option in the management of chronic bronchitis or COPD. A number of interventions to assist patients in smoking cessation are available. These include behavioral modification techniques as well as pharmacological treatments (see below). A combination of behavioral and pharmacological approaches such as nicotine replacement appears to yield the best results. Even minimal counseling from the provider improves the effectiveness of the nicotine patch.

Once patients have stopped smoking, those who are hypoxemic with a PaO_2 less than or equal to 55 mm Hg or an O_2 saturation of 88% or less while sleeping should receive supplemental oxygen. Along with smoking cessation, home oxygen is the only therapy shown to reduce mortality in COPD. Continuous long-term oxygen therapy (LTOT) should be considered in those patients with stable chronic pulmonary disease with PaO_2 <55 mm Hg on room air, at rest and awake. The presence of polycythemia, pulmonary hypertension, right heart failure, and/or hypercapnia (PaO_2 >45 mm Hg) is also an indication for use of continuous LTOT.

Exercise and pulmonary rehabilitation may also be beneficial as adjunct therapies for patients whose symptoms are not adequately controlled with appropriate pharmacotherapy. Exercise and pulmonary rehabilitation are most useful for patients who are restricted in their activities and have decreased quality of life. Rehabilitation that includes arm exercise reduces metabolic and ventilatory requirements for simple arm elevation. Specific ventilatory exercises, breathing retraining, and breathing education also can allow patient self-monitoring, which can be useful in the long-term management of chronic bronchitis.

B. Pharmacological Therapy

1. Smoking cessation pharmacotherapy—Multiple medications are available to assist with smoking cessation. Nicotine can be substituted 1 mg (1 cigarette) per milligram with the use of the patch, gum, or inhaler to help with symptoms of nicotine withdrawal. Patches and gum are both available over the counter as well as by prescription. Nicotine gum comes in two strengths (2 mg and 4 mg) so that the dosage can be titrated to the smoking level of the patient. Nicotine patches are available from four different manufacturers; two of these are over the counter. Doses range from 7 mg to 22 mg. Some evidence suggests that use of the patch and gum simultaneously enhances quit rates, but use of both is not approved by the Food and Drug Administration. Although all these products state that patients must not smoke while using nicotine replacement because of early case reports of myocardial infarction, more recent studies show that smoking is relatively safe when using nicotine replacement and may help reduce smoking before a patient actually quits. However, even at best, the cessation rate is only about 20–30% at one year.

Bupropion also is approved for smoking cessation as an adjunct to behavior modification. The main effect of buproprion is to reduce symptoms of nicotine withdrawal. Bupropion should be instituted for 2 weeks before the quitting target date. Then a nicotine substitute can be utilized in combination to maximize alleviation of symptoms of nicotine withdrawal. Because many patients with chronic bronchitis are already taking multiple medications, potential drug interactions and adverse effects must be taken into consideration before instituting therapy with buproprion.

Other agents are currently being developed and evaluated for smoking cessation. Vigabatrin, an antiepileptic medication used primarily for refractory seizure disorders, has shown promise, in preliminary studies, in blocking nicotine-induced dopamine production, which is a key player in the pleasure centers of the brain. Other agents such as clonidine, lobeline (a chemical derived from the *Lobelia* plant and the active agent in *CigArrest*), and silver acetate lozenges (which create an unpleasant taste when combined with cigarette smoke) have been shown to be of little benefit. Two potential nicotine receptor blockers, mecamylamine and naltrexone, actually appear to increase the number of cigarettes smoked.

2. Bronchodilators—The anticholinergic agent ipratropium bromide is the drug of choice for patients with persistent symptoms of chronic bronchitis. Ipratropium bromide has fewer side effects and a better response than intermittent β-agonists. Although ipratropium has a delayed onset of action compared to short-acting β-agonists, the beneficial effects are prolonged.

For patients with mild to moderately severe symptoms, intermittent use of a β-agonist inhaler such as albuterol is sometimes beneficial even without significant changes in their FEV_1. Adverse effects of β-agonist agents include tachycardia, nervousness, and tremor. Short-acting β-agonists may not last through the night; when nighttime symptoms develop, long-acting β-agonists such as salmeterol may be more useful. Levabuterol, the active agent of racemic albuterol, has recently been studied and appears to have greater efficacy than albuterol with fewer side effects.

Combination inhalers of ipratropium bromide and albuterol have also been utilized for chronic bronchitis patients, but have demonstrated only minimal changes in outcomes compared to single agents.

3. Antibiotics—Patients with acute exacerbations of chronic bronchitis pose a more difficult therapeutic dilemma. Many of these exacerbations are probably due to viral infections. However, a meta-analysis of studies using a wide range of antibiotics (ampicillin, sulfamethoxasole/trimethoprim, and tetracyclines) did demonstrate some benefit from empiric use of antibiotics for exacerbations of chronic bronchitis. For patients with moderately severe symptoms of chronic bronchitis, any change in cough that produces either increased sputum volume or purulent appearance is an indication for antibiotics. For patients with severe chronic bronchitis (defined as FEV_1 <50%, advanced age, four or more exacerbations/year, or a significant comorbidity such as cardiac disease or diabetes), a quinolone, penicillin plus β-lactamase inhibitor, a second- or third-generation cephalosporin, or a broad spectrum macrolide might be considered.

4. Other agents—As symptoms increase, addition of inhaled β-agonists, theophylline, and corticosteroids may provide symptomatic relief of symptoms of chronic bronchitis. In a multicenter randomized placebo-controlled trial, patients who used inhaled fluticasone had improved peak expiratory flows, FEV_1, FVC, and mid-expiratory flow. At the end of treatment patients also showed increased exercise tolerance compared to the placebo group. Corticosteroids at a therapeutic dose of 60 mg/day for 5 days have been shown to provide some symptomatic relief for severe exacerbations.

Mucolytics have not been shown to be beneficial. Iodinated glycerol has not been shown to improve any objective outcome measurements.

Newer agents such as aerosolized surfactant also have been utilized to treat stable chronic bronchitis. A prospective randomized controlled trial showed a minimal but statistically significant improvement in spirometry and sputum clearance. However, the cost of such a treatment regime is high and may not add any advantage to the underlying treatment.

For the treatment of cough, agents that may be of benefit for patients with chronic bronchitis include ipratropium bromide, guaimeseal, dextromethorphan, and viminol.

Anabolic steroids have recently been utilized for patients who have severe malnutrition and in those in whom weight loss is a concern. These agents show some beneficial effects.

Bach PB et al: Management of acute exacerbations of chronic obstructive pulmonary disease: a summary and appraisal of published evidence. Ann Intern Med 2001;134:600.

Celli BR: Standards for the optimal management of COPD. Chest 1998;113:283.

Dewey SL, Brodie JD, Gerasimov M: A pharmacologic strategy for the treatment of nicotine addiction. Synapse 1999;31:76.

Lynn J EE et al: Living and dying with chronic obstructive pulmonary disease. J Am Geriatr Soc 2000;48:S91.

Snow V, Lascher S, Mottur-Pilson C, for the Joint Expert Panel on Chronic Obstructive Pulmonary Disease of the American College of Chest Physicians and the American College of Physicians-American Society of Internal Medicine: Evidence base for management of acute exacerbations of chronic obstructive pulmonary disease. Ann Intern Med 2001;134:595.

EMBOLIC DISEASE

 ESSENTIALS OF DIAGNOSIS

- *Dyspnea.*
- *Hypoxia.*
- *Pleuritic pain.*

General Considerations

Pulmonary embolism usually results from the mobilization of blood clots from thromboses in the lower extremities or pelvis. However, embolization of other materials including air, fat, and amniotic fluid also can obstruct the pulmonary vasculature. The symptoms of pulmonary embolism range from mild, intermittent shortness of breath or pleuritic chest pain to complete circulatory collapse and death.

Amniotic fluid, fat, and air emboli are uncommon and generally associated with clear risk factors or precipitating events. Amniotic fluid embolism results from entry of amniotic fluid into the venous circulation usually in the second stage of labor. Deposition of amniotic fluid in the lungs results in fibrin deposition in the vasculature with resulting abrupt occlusion of blood flow and circulatory collapse. Dramatic falls in blood pressure and oxygenation are the hallmarks of this syndrome that carries a high mortality rate even if recognized and treated promptly.

Fat emboli usually occur in the setting of a lower limb, long bone fracture. Embolism occurs usually in the first 24–72 h after trauma. In addition to dyspnea and hypoxia, patients with fat emboli are usually agitated and confused.

Air emboli are uncommon and result from entry of air into the venous circulation usually from trauma or, more commonly, from insertion of an external catheter into a large intrathoracic vein. During inspiration, the negative thoracic pressure can pull air through an unsecured catheter into the venous system. Symptoms can range from dyspnea and chest pain to profound hypotension and hypoxia.

The most common source of embolism, though, is the disruption of thrombi formed in the deep veins. The estimated annual incidence of pulmonary embolism in the United States is estimated at 0.5 per 1000, resulting in about 250,000 new cases a year. Mortality in untreated cases in 30%, but can be reduced to 2% with prompt recognition and appropriate management. Recurrent pulmonary embolism carries a very high mortality in the range of 45–50%.

Risk factors for pulmonary embolism include venous stasis, trauma, abnormalities in the deep veins, and hypercoagulable states. Hypercoagulability occurs with some cancers as well as with inherited conditions such as Factor V Leiden mutation that results in resistance to the anticoagulant effects of protein C. Other congenital hypercoagulation disorders include protein C deficiency, protein S deficiency, and antithrombin III deficiency.

Hypercoagulation states also exist with the use of certain medications. Use of estrogens either as part of hormone replacement therapy or for contraception increases the risk by a factor of three. The effects of these drugs are compounded in patients with Factor V Leiden mutation. The risk of deep venous thrombosis with estrogen use appears to be related to the length of use.

In addition, smoking appears to an independent risk factor for deep vein thrombosis and pulmonary embolism.

Prevention

Because pulmonary emboli usually arise from lower extremity thromboses, prophylactic anticoagulation can be used to reduce the incidence of these thrombi in high-risk individuals. Both low-molecular-weight heparin products and unfractionated heparin are effective in preventing deep venous thrombosis. Selection of the agent and the dose is based on the risk factor and other characteristics of the patient as shown in Table 26–8.

In addition to preventing initial thrombi, the pulmonary embolism can be reduced through the use of a vena-caval filter in patients with known thrombi and contraindications to long-term anticoagulation. The long-term impact of intravenacaval (IVC) filters has not been studied extensively. One study showed a complication rate, such as thrombi trapped in the filter or the filter tilting, malpositioning, or migrating, in nearly 50% of those who survived 3 years. However, given the high mortality rates from recurrent pulmonary embolism, the complication rates from long-term IVC filter insertion appear to be a worthwhile trade-off in high-risk patients.

Clinical Findings

Patients with pulmonary emboli usually exhibit dyspnea and hypoxia, and often have pleuritic chest pain. However, other than hypoxia, most routine studies including chest radiographs may be normal. Suspicious signs of embolism on a chest radiograph include a wedge-shaped infiltrate resulting from lobar infarction and/or a new pleural effusion.

Confirmation of a pulmonary embolism is based on either demonstrating obstruction of vascular flow through pulmonary angiography, finding a mismatch of perfusion and ventilation, or visualization of a clot on spiral (helical) CT scanning. Although pulmonary angiography is considered the gold standard, because of its invasiveness spiral CT and ventilation/perfusion scan are usually employed to make the diagnosis. Of the noninvasive tests available, spiral CT has the best sensitivity for detecting pulmonary artery thrombi (95–100%), although it is not as useful in identifying subsegmental emboli.

Table 26–8. Strategies to prevent venous thromboembolism.

Condition or Procedure	Prophylaxis
General surgery	Unfractionated heparin, 5000 U two or three times a day
	Enoxaparin, 40 mg/day subcutaneously
	Dalteparin, 2500 or 5000 U/day subcutaneously
	Nadroparin, 3100 U/day subcutaneously
	Tinzaparin, 3500 U/day subcutaneously, with or without graduated-compression stockings
Total hip replacement	Warfarin (target INR, 2.5)
	Intermittent pneumatic compression
	Enoxaparin, 30 mg subcutaneously twice daily
	Danaparoid, 750 U subcutaneously twice daily
Total knee replacement	Enoxaparin, 30 mg subcutaneously twice daily
	Ardeparin, 50 U/kg subcutaneously twice daily
General medical condition requiring hospitalization	Graduated-compression stockings, intermittent pneumatic compression, or unfractionated heparin, 5000 U two or three times daily
Condition requiring hospitalization in the intensive care unit	Graduated-compression stockings and intermittent pneumatic compression, with or without unfractionated heparin, 5000 U two or three times daily
Pregnancy in high-risk patient[1]	Dalteparin, 5000 U/day subcutaneously
	Enoxaparin, 40 mg/day subcutaneously

From Goldhaber SZ: Pulmonary embolism. New Engl J Med 1998;339:93.
[1]High risk includes patients with previous pulmonary embolism or deep venous thrombosis.

D-dimer testing has been evaluated as a serum marker for pulmonary embolism or deep vein thrombosis. D-dimer is a product of the degradation of fibrin during fibrinolysis. During episodes of thrombosis, D-dimer is elevated. The presence of D-dimer is not specific for thrombotic disease since D-dimer also rises in other conditions such as recent surgery, congestive heart failure, myocardial infarction, and pneumonia. Although the presence of D-dimer is not useful in diagnosing thombosis/embolism, the negative predictive value of the absence of D-dimer is very high (97–99%), so this test can be useful in ruling out embolism.

Treatment

Options for management of the patients with an acute pulmonary embolism include anticoagulation to prevent further embolism from occurring, clot lysis with thrombolytic agents, or surgical removal of the clot.

Most patients without life-threatening embolism are managed with acute anticoagulation with heparin followed by long-term maintenance on warfarin. Unfractionated heparin is administered intravenously and titrated to produce a suitable anticoagulation state. The use of a weight-based nomogram for loading and maintenance dosing can improve the time to achieve adequate anticoagulation and reduce the risks of bleeding. The drawbacks of unfractionated heparin include the need for hospitalization to monitor coagulation status and administer the intravenous drug plus the possibility

of thrombocytopenia associated with the use of this agent.

An alternative to unfractionated heparin is low-molecular-weight heparin that can be administered as a daily intramuscular dose. The decreased risk of bleeding with the use of low-molecular-weight heparin also means that laboratory monitoring of the patient's coagulation status is not necessary. The result of this is that therapy can be provided in the patient's home. Currently, enoxaparin sodium is the only low-molecular-weight heparin product approved for use in the United States. In a study using doses of 1 mg/kg and 1.5 mg/kg once a day, both doses were equivalent to unfractionated heparin in patients with deep venous thrombosis (DVT) or pulmonary embolism (PE).

Warfarin should be started promptly at a dose of 5 mg/day. Starting with a higher dose of warfarin does not appear to achieve oral anticoagulation any faster or reduce the days that heparin is needed. Heparin can be discontinued when a prothrombin time indicates that the international normalized ratio (INR) has reached 2.0–3.0.

The duration of anticoagulation for PE depends on whether the precipitating event is known and reversible or whether the cause is unknown. In situations in which the thrombosis and embolism are the result of an acute event such as an injury or surgery, treatment for 6 months is recommended. If the risk factor associated with the embolic event is not reversible such as cancer or coagulation disorder, then lifetime anticoagulation is advisable. When a risk factor or event causing the embolism is not known, so-called idiopathic embolism, treatment with anticoagulants for 6 months is indicated.

The use of thrombolytic agents for PE is usually reserved for patients with extensive embolism who show hemodynamic instability. Thrombolytic agents available for use in this situation include urokinase, streptokinase, tissue plasminogen activator (tPA), and reteplase. When used for the treatment of a pulmonary embolism, tPA is administered in a 100 mg infusion over 2 h whereas streptokinase is given as a 250,000 IU loading dose followed by 100,000 IU/h for 24 h. Once the infusion is completed intravenous heparin therapy can be continued as long as the activated partial thromboplastin time (aPTT) is less than twice normal. Although thrombolytic agents can cause rapid hemodynamic improvement in patients presenting with shock, the use of these agents does not significantly improve overall mortality.

Embolectomy is rarely performed and is reserved for patients in whom embolism is rapidly diagnosed and a very large embolism is suspected that completely occludes the pulmonary arteries. In most situations, this is treated as a "last ditch" effort to save the patient.

Becker DM et al: D-dimer testing and acute venous thromboembolism: a short-cut to accurate diagnosis? Arch Intern Med 1996;156:939.

Gould MK et al: Low molecular weight heparins compared with unfractionated heparin for the treatment of acute deep vein thrombosis: a meta-analysis of randomized controlled trials. Ann Intern Med 1999;130:800.

Remy-Jardin MJ et al: Diagnosis of acute pulmonary embolism with spiral CT: comparison with pulmonary angiography and scintigraphy. Radiology 1996;200:699.

Evaluation & Management of Headache

C. Randall Clinch, DO

ESSENTIALS OF DIAGNOSIS

- *Migraine.*
  - *Headache lasts 4–72 h.*
  - *Unilateral location.*
  - *Pulsating quality and moderate or severe intensity of pain.*
  - *Aggravated by physical activity.*
  - *Nausea and photophobia.*
  - *Presence of an aura.*
- *Cluster headache.*
  - *Unilateral orbital, supraorbital, and/or temporal pain lasting 15–180 min.*
  - *Explosive excruciating pain.*
  - *One attack every other day to eight attacks per day.*
- *Tension-type headache.*
  - *Pericranial muscle tenderness.*
  - *Bilateral band-like distribution of pain.*
  - *Headache more than 180 days/year.*

General Considerations

Headache is among the most common pain syndromes presenting in primary care. Each year over 10 million patients visit their primary care provider's office or the emergency department with a complaint of headache. Up to 17 billion dollars is spent annually on the direct medical and indirect costs of migraine headache alone; the cost of lost work days and medical benefits is over 50 billion dollars annually in the United States. The main task before the primary care provider is to determine if the patient has a potentially life-threatening headache disorder and, if not, to provide appropriate management to limit disability from headache.

Although a classification system for a variety of head, neck, and facial pain has been provided by the International Headache Society, such a detailed system has limited utility in daily clinical practice. A distinc-

tion between primary headaches (benign, recurrent headaches having no organic disease as their cause) and secondary headaches (those caused by an underlying, organic disease) is more practical. Over 90% of patients presenting to primary care providers have a primary headache disorder (Table 27–1). These disorders include migraine (with and without aura), tension-type headache, and cluster headache. Secondary headache disorders comprise the minority of presentations; however, given that their underlying etiology may range from sinusitis to subarachnoid hemorrhage, these headache disorders often present the greatest diagnostic challenge to the practicing clinician (Table 27–2).

Solomon GD et al: National Headache Foundation: Standards of care for treating headache in primary care practice. Clev Clin J Med 1997;64(7):373.

Solomon S: Diagnosis of primary headache disorders: validity of the International Headache Society Criteria in clinical practice. Neurol Clin 1997;15(1):15.

Clinical Findings

A. SYMPTOMS AND SIGNS

1. **History**—Because the majority of patients presenting with headache have a normal neurological and general physical examination, the headache history is of utmost importance (Table 27–3). Key issues in the headache history include identifying which patients present with red flags, prompting greater concern for the presence of a secondary headache disorder and a greater potential need for additional laboratory evaluation and neuroimaging (Table 27–4).

The onset of primary headache disorders is usually between 20 and 40 years of age; however, they may occur at any age. Patients without a history of headaches presenting with a new onset headache outside of this age range should be considered at higher risk for a secondary headache disorder. Serious consideration should be given to performing additional testing and/or neuroimaging in these patients or those complaining of their "first or worst" headache. Temporal (giant cell) arteritis should be a consideration in any patient 50 years of age or older with a new complaint of head, facial, or

Table 27–1. Primary headache disorders.

More Common	Less Common
Migraine with or without aura	Paroxysmal hemicrania
Tension-type	Idiopathic stabbing headache
Cluster	Cold stimulus headache
	Benign cough headache
	Benign exertional headache
	Headache associated with sexual activity

Adapted from Classification and diagnostic criteria for headache disorders, cranial neuralgias and facial pain. Headache Classification Committee of the International Headache Society. Cephalalgia 1988;8(suppl 7):1.

Table 27–2. Secondary headache disorders.

Headache associated with head trauma
    Acute posttraumatic headache
Headaches associated with vascular disorders
    Subarachnoid hemorrhages
    Acute ischemic cerebrovascular disorder
    Unruptured vascular malformation
    Arteritis (eg, temporal arteritis)
    Carotid or vertebral artery pain
    Venous thrombosis
    Arterial hypertension
Headaches associated with nonvascular intracranial disorder
    Benign intracranial hypertension (pseudotumor cerebri)
    Intracranial infection
    Low cerebrospinal fluid pressure (eg, lumbar puncture headache)
Headaches associated with substances or their withdrawal
    Acute substance use or exposure
    Withdrawal headache (acute use)
    Withdrawal headache (chronic use)
Headaches associated with noncephalic infection
    Viral infection
    Bacterial infection
Headache associated with metabolic disorder
    Hypoxia
    Hypercapnia
    Mixed hypoxia and hypercapnia
    Hypoglycemia
    Dialysis
    Headache related to other metabolic abnormality
Headache or facial pain associated with disorder of cranium, neck, eyes, ears, nose, sinuses, teeth, mouth, or other facial or cranial structures
Cranial neuralgias, nerve trunk pain, and deafferentation pain

Adapted from Classification and diagnostic criteria for headache disorders, cranial neuralgias and facial pain. Headache Classification Committee of the International Headache Society. Cephalalgia 1988;8(suppl 7):1.

Table 27–3. Questions to ask in obtaining a headache history.

Is this your first or worst headache? How bad is your pain on a scale of 1 to 10 (1 means not too bad, and 10 means very bad)? Do you have headaches on a regular basis? Is this headache like the ones you usually have?
What symptoms do you have before the headache starts?
What symptoms do you have during the headache? What symptoms do you have right now?
When did this headache begin? How did it start (gradually, suddenly, other)?
Where is your pain? Does the pain seem to spread to any other area? If so, where?
What kind of pain do you have (throbbing, stabbing, dull, other)?
Do you have other medical problems? If so, what?
Do you take any medicines? If so, what?
Have you recently hurt your head or had a medical or dental procedure?

From Clinch CR: Evaluation of acute headaches in adults. Am Fam Physician 2001;63:685.

scalp pain, diplopia, and/or jaw claudication. An erythrocyte sedimentation rate (ESR) should be included in the evaluation of these patients; a normal ESR makes this diagnosis very unlikely.

Symptoms suggesting a recurring, transient neurological event, typically lasting 30–60 min and preceding headache onset, strongly suggest the presence of an aura and an associated migraine headache disorder (Table 27–5). Migraine without aura, the most common form of migraine (formerly called common migraine), may present with unilateral pain in the head (cephalgia) with subsequent generalization of pain to the entire head. Bilateral cephalgia is present in a small percentage of migraneurs at the onset of their headache. Nausea accompanying a migraine may be debilitating and warrant specific treatment.

Cluster headaches are strictly unilateral in location and are typically described as an explosive, deep, excruciating pain. They are associated with ipsilateral autonomic signs and symptoms, and have a much greater prevalence in men (Table 27–6). Compared to migraine headache sufferers who often desire sleep and a quiet, dark environment during their headache, individuals with cluster headache pace the floor unable to find a position of comfort. Tension-type headaches, the most prevalent form of primary headache disorder, typically present with pericranial muscle tenderness and a description of a bilateral band-like distribution of the pain (Table 27–7).

Patients with chronic medical conditions have a greater possibility of having an organic cause of their

Table 27–4. Red flags in the evaluation of acute headaches in adults.

Red Flag	Differential Diagnosis	Possible Work-Up
Headache beginning after 50 years of age	Temporal arteritis, mass lesion	Erythrocyte sedimentation rate, neuroimaging
Sudden onset of headache	Subarachnoid hemorrhage, pituitary apoplexy, hemorrhage into a mass lesion or vascular malformation, mass lesion (especially posterior fossa mass)	Neuroimaging, lumbar puncture, if neuroimaging is negative[1]
Headaches increasing in frequency and severity	Mass lesion, subdural hematoma, medication overuse	Neuroimaging, drug screen
New-onset headache in patient with risk factors for HIV[2] infection or cancer	Meningitis (chronic or carcinomatous), brain abscess (including toxoplasmosis), metastasis	Neuroimaging, lumbar puncture, if neuroimaging is negative[1]
Headache with signs of systemic illness (fever, stiff neck, rash)	Meningitis, encephalitis, Lyme disease, systemic infection, collagen vascular disease	Neuroimaging, lumbar puncture,[3] serology
Focal neurological signs or symptoms of disease (other than typical aura)	Mass lesion, vascular malformation, stroke, collagen vascular disease	Neuroimaging, collagen vascular evaluation (including antiphospholipid antibodies)
Papilledema	Mass lesion, pseudotumor cerebri, meningitis	Nauroimaging, lumbar puncture[3]
Headaches subsequent to head trauma	Intracranial hemorrhage, subdural hematoma, epidural hematoma, posttraumatic headache	Neuroimaging of brain, skull, and, possibly, cervical spine

From Clinch CR: Evaluation of acute headaches in adults. Am Fam Physician 2001;63:685.
[1]Lumbar puncture may follow a negative neuroimaging procedure if suspicion of hemorrhage, infection, or cancer remains high.
[2]HIV, human immunodeficiency virus.
[3]Suspicion of specific central nervous system infections (Lyme disease, syphilis, etc) or intracranial hypertension (pseudotumor cerebri) warrants lumbar puncture with cerebrospinal fluid analysis and pressure measurement.

headache (Table 27–4). Patients with cancer, hypertension (with diastolic pressures higher than 110 mm Hg), or human immunodeficiency virus (HIV) infection may present with central nervous system metastases, lymphoma, toxoplasmosis, or meningitis as the etiology of their headache. Numerous medications have headache as a reported adverse event and medication overuse headache (formerly drug-induced headache) may occur following frequent use of analgesics or any antiheadache medication, including the triptans. The duration and severity of withdrawal headache following discontinuation of the medication vary depending upon the medication itself; withdrawal is shortest for triptans (4.1 days) compared to ergots (6.7 days) or analgesics (9.5 days), respectively. Medical or dental procedures (lumbar punctures, rhinoscopy, tooth extraction, etc) may be associated with postprocedure headaches. Any history of head trauma or loss of consciousness should prompt concern for an intracranial hemorrhage in addition to a postconcussive disorder.

2. Physical examination—Physical examination is performed to attempt to identify a secondary, organic cause for the patient's headache. Additionally, special attention should be paid to any red flags identified during the headache history (Table 27–4). A general physical examination should be performed including vital signs, general appearance, and examinations of the head, eyes (including a funduscopic examination), ears, nose, throat, teeth, neck, and cardiovascular regions. Particular attention should be given to palpation of the head, face, and neck.

A detailed neurological examination should be performed and the findings well documented. Assessment includes mental status testing, level of consciousness, pupillary responses, gait, coordination and cerebellar function, motor strength, sensory, deep tendon, and pathological reflex testing, in addition to cranial nerve tests. The presence or absence of meningeal irritation should be sought. Examinations such as Kernig's (the patient is supine with hips and knees flexed to 90°;

Table 27–5. Diagnostic criteria for migraine headaches.

Migraine without aura
  A. At least five attacks fulfilling B–D
  B. Headache attacks lasting 4–72 h (untreated or unsuccessfully treated)
  C. Headache has at least two of the following characteristics
    1. Unilateral location
    2. Pulsating quality
    3. Moderate or severe intensity
    4. Aggravation by walking stairs or similar physical activity
  D. During headache at least one of the following
    1. Nausea and/or vomiting
    2. Photophobia and phonophobia

Migraine with aura
  A. At least two attacks fulfilling B
  B. At least three of the following four characteristics
    1. One or more fully reversible aura symptoms indicating focal cerebral cortical and/or brain stem dysfunction
    2. At least one aura symptom develops gradually over more than 4 min or two or more symptoms occur in succession
    3. No aura symptom lasts more than 60 min; if more than one aura symptom is present, accepted duration is proportionally increased
    4. Headache follows aura with a free interval of less than 60 min (it may also begin before or simultaneously with the aura)

Adapted from Classification and diagnostic criteria for headache disorders, cranial neuralgias and facial pain. Headache Classification Committee of the International Headache Society. Cephalalgia 1988;8(suppl 7):1.

Table 27–6. Diagnostic criteria for cluster headache.

A. At least five attacks fulfilling criteria B through D
B. Severe unilateral orbital, supraorbital, and/or temporal pain lasting 15–180 min (untreated)
C. Headache associated with at least one of the following signs on the pain side:
    1. Conjunctival injection
    2. Lacrimation
    3. Nasal congestion
    4. Rhinorrhea
    5. Forehead and facial sweating
    6. Miosis
    7. Ptosis
    8. Eyelid edema
D. Frequency of attacks: one attack every other day to eight attacks per day

---

Adapted from Classification and diagnostic criteria for headache disorders, cranial neuralgias and facial pain. Headache Classification Committee of the International Headache Society. Cephalalgia 1988;8 (suppl 7):1.

Table 27–7. Diagnostic criteria for tension-type headache.

I. Episodic tension-type headache
  A. At least 10 previous headache episodes fulfilling criteria B–D. Number of days with such headache <180/year
  B. Headache lasting from 30 min to 7 days
  C. At least two of the following pain characteristics
    1. Pressing/tightening (nonpulsating) quality
    2. Mild or moderate intensity
    3. Bilateral location
    4. No aggravation by walking stairs or similar routine physical activity
  D. Both of the following
    1. No nausea or vomiting (anorexia may occur)
    2. Photophobia and phonophobia are absent or one but not the other is present
II. Chronic tension-type headache
  A. All of the above criteria except number of days with such headache >180 days per year

---

Adapted from Classification and diagnostic criteria for headache disorders, cranial neuralgias and facial pain. Headache Classification Committee of the International Headache Society. Cephalalgia 1988;8 (suppl 7) : 1.

there is pain in the hamstring muscles and low back when the examiner attempts to extend the knee) and Brudzinski's signs (the patient is supine; passive neck flexion produces pain in the neck and flexion of the hips) should be documented; both signs may be absent, however, even in the presence of subarachnoid hemorrhage.

B. LABORATORY FINDINGS AND IMAGING STUDIES

Additional laboratory investigations should be driven by the history and by any red flags that have been identified (Table 27–4). The routine use of electroencephalography (EEG) is not warranted in the evaluation of the patient with headache. In the primary care setting, computed tomographic (CT) scanning was shown to have been ordered on approximately 3% of patients with headache, the majority because of a suspected intracranial tumor (49%); however, only 8.2% of patients with intracranial tumor present with isolated headache as their first and only symptom. Interestingly, patients with a primary or metastatic brain tumor may exhibit headache symptoms that are similar to migraine, tension-type, or other primary headache disorders; however, the "classic" early morning brain tumor headache is uncommon. Although there are different characteristics that may lead to choosing either CT or magnetic resonance imaging (MRI) (Table 27–8), routine use of neuroimaging is not cost effective.

The U.S. Headache Consortium has provided evidence-based guidelines on neuroimaging in the patient with nonacute headache. They revealed the prevalence of patients with a normal neurological examination and migraine having a significant abnormality (acute cerebral infarct, neoplastic disease, hydrocephalus, or vascular abnormalities, eg, aneurysm or arteriovenous malformation) on a neuroimaging test is 0.2%. Their recommendations are as follows:

- Neuroimaging should be considered in patients with nonacute headache and an unexplained abnormal finding on neurological examination.
- Evidence is insufficient to make specific recommendations in the presence or absence of neurological symptoms.
- Neuroimaging is not usually warranted for patients with migraine and normal neurological examination. For patients with atypical headache features or patients who do not fulfill the strict definition of migraine (or have some additional risk factor), a lower threshold for neuroimaging may be applied.

Table 27–8. Computerized tomographic (CT) scans versus magnetic resonance imaging (MRI) in patients with headaches.

CT Scan	MRI
Need to identify an acute hemorrhage	Need to evaluate the posterior fossa
Generally more readily available at most medical centers	More sensitive at identifying pathological intracranial processes[1]
Generally less expensive at most medical centers	

[1]Increased sensitivity may not correlate with an improved health outcome and may be associated with identifying more clinically insignificant findings.

- Data were insufficient to make an evidence-based recommendation regarding the use of neuroimaging for tension-type headache.
- Data were insufficient to make any evidence-based recommendations regarding the relative sensitivity of MRI compared with CT in the evaluation of migraine or other nonacute headache.

Although the U.S. Headache Consortium based the above recommendations on a review of the best available evidence, clinicians must individualize management plans to meet a variety of needs including addressing patient fears and medicolegal concerns.

Within the first 48 h of acute headache, CT scanning without contrast medium followed, if negative, by lumbar puncture and cerebrospinal fluid (CSF) analysis is the preferred approach to attempt to diagnose subarachnoid hemorrhage. Xanthochromia, a yellow discoloration detectable on spectrophotometry, may aid in diagnosis if the CT scan and CSF analysis are normal but suspicion of subarachnoid hemorrhage remains high. Xanthochromia may persist for up to a week following a subarachnoid hemorrhage.

In addition to CSF analysis, lumbar puncture is useful for documenting abnormalities of CSF pressure in the setting of headache. Headaches are associated with low CSF pressure (less than 90 mm H_2O as measured by a manometer) and elevated CSF pressure (greater than 200–250 mm H_2O). Headaches related to CSF hypotension include those caused by posttraumatic leakage of CSF [ie, after lumbar puncture or central nervous system (CNS) trauma]. Headaches related to CSF hypertension include those associated with idiopathic intracranial hypertension and CNS space-occupying lesions (ie, tumor, infectious, mass, hemorrhage).

Becker LA et al: Use of CT scans for the investigation of headache: a report from ASPN, Part 1. J Fam Pract 1993;37(2):129.

Clinch CR: Evaluation of acute headaches in adults. Am Fam Physician 2001;63(4):685.

Consortium U.S. Headache: Evidence-based guidelines in the primary care setting: neuroimaging in patients with nonacute headache, 2000.

Ekbom K, Hardebo JE: Cluster headache: aetiology, diagnosis and management. Drugs 2002;62(1):61.

Katsarava Z, Diener HC, Limmroth V: Medication overuse headache: a focus on analgesics, ergot alkaloids and triptans. Drug Safety 2001;24(12):921.

Katsarava Z et al: Clinical features of withdrawal headache following overuse of triptans and other headache drugs. Neurology 2001;57(9):1694.

Schulman EA: Overview of tension-type headache. Curr Pain Headache Rep 2001;5(5):454.

Sturmann K: The neurologic examination. Emerg Med Clin North Am 1997;15(3):491.

Vazques-Barqureo A et al: Isolated headache as the presenting clinical manifestation of intracranial tumors: a prospective study. Cephalalgia 1994;14(4):270.

Zakrzewska JM: Cluster headache: review of the literature. Br J Oral Maxillofac Surg 2001;39(2):103.

Differential Diagnosis

The differential diagnosis for acute headaches in adults is presented in Table 27–4.

Treatment

Treatment of headache is best individualized based upon a thorough history, physical examination, and the interpretation of appropriate ancillary testing. Secondary headaches require accurate diagnosis and therapy directed at the underlying etiology (Tables 27–2 and 27–4). Nonpharmacological measures and cognitive–behavioral therapy (CBT) are worth consideration in most patients with primary headache disorders. CBT may have a prophylactic effect in migraine similar to propranolol (an approximate 50% reduction). Cluster headache, chronic daily headache, and medication overuse headache respond poorly to CBT as monotherapy. A critical analysis of 27 clinical trials of acupuncture in headache suggests a possible benefit. However, methodological inadequacies in many of the trials leave the evidence about the efficacy and indication for acupuncture in question. A systematic review of nine randomized clinical trials involving 683 patients with chronic headache showed there was moderate evidence that spinal manipulative therapy has short-term efficacy in prophylactic treatment of chronic tension-type headache and migraine; it is also more efficacious than massage for cervicogenic headache. Caution should be used, however, in applying the results of this review, given the small number of studies available for analysis. One randomized controlled trial of spinal manipulation in episodic tension-type headache showed that participants receiving manipulation alone did not obtain any significant positive effects versus control subjects with respect to daily hours of headache, pain intensity per episode, or daily analgesic use.

A. MIGRAINE

The U.S. Headache Consortium lists the following general management guidelines for treatment of migraine patients:

- Educate migraine sufferers about their condition and its treatment, and encourage them to participate in their own management.
- Use migraine-specific agents [triptans, dihydroergotamine (DHE), ergotamine, etc] in patients with more severe migraine and in those whose headaches respond poorly to nonsteroidal antiinflammatory drugs (NSAIDs) or combination analgesics such as aspirin plus acetaminophen plus caffeine.
- Select a nonoral route of administration for patients whose migraines present early with nausea or vomiting as a significant component of the symptom complex.
- Consider a self-administered rescue medication for patients with severe migraine who do not respond well to (or fail) other treatments.
- Guard against medication-overuse headache (the terms "rebound headache" and "drug-induced headache" are sometime used interchangeably with "medication-overuse headache").

Pharmacological treatment options are numerous in the management of migraine headache. Table 27–9 details a hierarchy of evidence-based treatment options during acute migraine episodes. Of those therapies supported by the best evidence (Table 27–9, Group 1), DHE and the triptans are migraine specific. Of note, meperidine (Demerol) intravenously or intramuscularly has not been shown to be superior to other effective therapies, such as chlorpromazine (Thorazine) IV, for acute migraine. Studies comparing DHE IV or Ketorolac IV with meperidine were inconclusive. Despite this evidence, meperidine remains a commonly used (and abused) abortive therapy for acute migraine headache.

The goal of therapy in migraine prophylaxis is a reduction in the severity and frequency of headache by 50% or more. Table 27–10 details pharmacological management options for prevention of migraine. The strongest evidence surrounds the use of amitriptyline (10 mg at bedtime, titrate slowly over 2–3 weeks; maximum 150 mg daily), propranolol (begin at 80 mg divided three to four times daily; maximum 240 mg daily), timolol (10 mg orally twice daily), and divalproex sodium (200–500 mg orally twice daily with food) for migraine prevention.

B. TENSION-TYPE HEADACHE

Initial medical therapy of episodic tension-type headache often includes aspirin, acetaminophen, or NSAIDs. Avoidance of habituating, caffeine-containing over-the-counter or prescription drugs as well as butalbital-, codeine-, or ergotamine-containing preparations (including combination products) is recommended given the significant risk of developing drug dependency or medication-overuse headache.

Similar general management principles for treatment of migraine headaches can be applied to the treatment of chronic tension-type headaches. In a randomized placebo-controlled trial of tricyclic antidepressant use (amitriptyline hydrochloride, up to 100 mg/day, or

Table 27-9. Acute therapies for migraine.[1]

Group 1: Proven Pronounced Statistical and Clinical Benefit (at least two double-blind, placebo-controlled clinical studies + clinical impression of effect)	Group 2: Moderate Statistical and Clinical Benefit (one double-blind, placebo-controlled study + clinical impression of effect)	Group 3: Statistically But Not Proven Clinically or Clinically But Not Proven Statistically Effective (conflicting or inconsistent evidence)	Group 4: Proven to Be Statistically or Clinically Ineffective (failed efficacy versus placebo)	Group 5: Clinical and Statistical Benefits Unknown (insufficient evidence available)
Acetaminophen plus aspirin plus caffeine PO	Acetaminophen plus codeine PO	Butalbital, aspirin, plus caffeine PO	Acetaminophen PO	Dexamethasone IV
Aspirin PO	Butalbital plus aspirin plus caffeine, plus codeine PO	Ergotamine PO	Chlorpromazine IM	Hydrocortisone IV
Butorphanol IN		Ergotamine plus caffeine PO	Granisetron IV	
DHE SC, IM, IV	Butorphanol IM		Lidocaine IV	
DHE IV plus antiemetic	Chlorpromazine IM, IV	Metoclopramide IM, PR		
DHE IN	Diclofenac K, PO			
Ibuprofen PO	Ergotamine plus caffeine plus pentobarbital plus Belafolline PO			
Naproxen sodium PO				
Prochlorperazine IV				
Rizatriptan PO	Flurbiprofen, PO			
Sumatriptan SC, IN, PO	Isometheptine compound, PO			
Zolmitriptan PO	Ketorolac IM			
	Lidocaine IN			
	Meperidine IM, IV			
	Methadone IM			
	Metoclopramide IV			
	Naproxen PO			
	Prochlorperazine IM, PR			

From U.S. Headache Consortium, Evidence-based guidelines for migraine headache in the primary care setting: pharmacological management of acute attacks. http://www.aan.com/public/practiceguidelines/03.pdf, 2000. Access date 9/5/2001.
[1]PO, orally; IN, intranasally; SC, subcutaneously; IM, intramuscularly; IV, intravenously; PR, rectally; DHE, dihydroergotamine.

nortriptyline hydrochloride up to 75 mg/day) and stress management (eg, relaxation, cognitive coping) therapy, combined therapy produced a statistically and clinically greater reduction (≥50%) in headache activity. A meta-analysis of antidepressant treatment (eg, tricyclic antidepressants, serotonin antagonists, and selective serotonin reuptake inhibitors) of chronic headache (eg, migraine, tension-type, or both) revealed treated study participants were twice as likely to report headache improvement and consumed less analgesic medication than nontreated patients. Other considerations for prophylaxis of chronic tension-type headaches include calcium channel blockers and β-blockers.

C. CLUSTER HEADACHE

Acute management of cluster headache involves 100% oxygen at 6 L/min, DHE, and the triptans. Verapamil,

lithium, divalproex sodium, methysergide, and prednisone may be considered for prophylaxis. Due to side effects related to chronic use, methysergide and prednisone should be used with caution.

D. REFERRAL

Referral to a headache specialist should be considered in cases that are difficult to classify into a primary or secondary headache disorder. Additionally, referral is often warranted in cases of daily or intractable headache, drug-rebound, habituation, or medication-overuse headache, or in any scenario in which the primary care provider feels uncomfortable in making a diagnosis or offering appropriate treatment. Patients who request referral, who do not respond to treatment, or whose condition continues to worsen should be considered for referral.

Table 27–10. Preventive therapies for migraine.

Group 1: Medium to High Efficacy, Good Strength of Evidence, and a Range of Severity (Mild to Moderate) and Frequency (Infrequent to Frequent) of Side Effects	Group 2: Lower Efficacy Than Those Listed in Group 1, or Limited Strength of Evidence, and Mild to Moderate Side Effects	Group 3: Clinically Efficacious Based on Consensus and Clinical Experience, But No Scientific Evidence of Efficacy	Group 4: Medium to High Efficacy, Good Strength of Evidence, But with Side Effect Concerns	Group 5: Evidence Indicating No Efficacy over Placebo
Amitriptyline	Aspirin[1]	**Mild to moderate side effects**	Methysergide	Acebutolol
Divalproex sodium	Atenolol	Cyproheptadine	Flunarizine[2]	Alprenolol[2]
Lisuride[2]	Cyclandelate[2]	Bupropion	Pizotifen[2]	Carbamazepine
Timolol	Fenoprofen	Diltiazem	TR-DHE[2]	Clomipramine
	Feverfew	Doxepin		Clonazepam
	Flurbiprofen	Fluvoxamine		Clonidine DEK[2]
	Fluoxetine (racemic)	Ibuprofen		Femoxitine[2]
	Gabapentin	Imipramine		Flumedroxone[2]
	Guanfacine	Mirtazepine		Indomethacine
	Indobufen[2]	Nortriptyline		Iprazochrome[2]
	Ketoprofen	Paroxetine		Lamotrigine
	Lornoxicam[2]	Protriptyline		Mianserine[2]
	Magnesium	Sertraline		Nabumetone
	Mefenamic acid	Tiagibine		Nicardipine
	Metoprolol	Topiramate		Nifedipine
	Nadolol	Trazadone		Oxprenolol[2]
	Naproxen	Venlafaxine		Pindolol
	Naproxen sodium			Tropisetron[2]
	Nimodipine	**Side effect concerns**		Vigabatrin[2]
	Tolfenamic acid[2]	Methylergonovine (methylergometrine)		
	Verapamil	Phenelzine		
	Vitamin B_2			

From U.S. Headache Consortium, Evidence-based guidelines for migraine headache in the primary care setting: pharmacological management for prevention of migraine. http://www.aan.com/public/practiceguidelines/04.pdf, 2000. Access date 9/5/2001.
[1]Does not include combination products.
[2]Currently not available in the United States.

Bronfort G et al: Efficacy of spinal manipulation for chronic headache: a systematic review. J Manipulative Physiol Ther 2001;24(7):457.

Consortium, U.S. Headache: Evidence-based guidelines for migraine headache in the primary care setting: pharmacological management of acute attacks, 2000.

Consortium, U.S. Headache: Evidence-based guidelines for migraine headache in the primary care setting: pharmacological management for prevention of migraine, 2000.

Dalessio DJ: Relief of cluster headache and cranial neuralgias. Promising prophylactic and symptomatic treatments. Postgrad Med 2001;109(1):69.

Dodick DW, Capobianco DJ: Treatment and management of cluster headache. Curr Pain Headache Rep 2001;5(1):83.

Holroyd KA et al: Management of chronic tension-type headache with tricyclic antidepressant medication, stress management therapy, and their combination: a randomized controlled trial. JAMA 2001;285(17):2208.

Lake AE 3rd: Behavioral and nonpharmacologic treatments of headache. Med Clin North Am 2001;85(4):1055.

Manias P, Tagaris G, Karageorgiou K: Acupuncture in headache: a critical review. Clin J Pain 2000;16(4):334.

Tomkins GE et al: Treatment of chronic headache with antidepressants: a meta-analysis. Am J Med 2001;111(1):54.

Osteoporosis

28

Jeannette E. South-Paul, MD

General Considerations

Osteoporosis is a public health problem affecting more than 40 million people, one-third of postmenopausal women and a substantial portion of the elderly in the United States, and almost as many in Europe and Japan. An additional 54% of postmenopausal women have low bone density measured at the hip, spine, or wrist. Osteoporosis results in more than 1,500,000 fractures annually in the United States alone. At least 90% of all hip and spine fractures among elderly women are a consequence of osteoporosis. The direct expenditures for osteoporotic fractures have increased during the past decade from $5 billion to almost $15 billion per year. Thus, family physicians and other primary care providers will (1) frequently care for patients with subclinical osteoporosis, (2) recognize the implications of those who present with osteoporosis-related fractures, and (3) determine when to implement prevention for younger people.

Of the 25 million women in the United States thought to have osteoporosis, 8 million have a documented fracture. The female-to-male fracture ratios are reported to be 7:1 for vertebral fractures, 1.5:1 for distal forearm fractures, and 2:1 for hip fractures. Approximately 30% of hip fractures in persons over 65 years of age occur in men. Osteoporosis-related fractures in older men are associated with lower femoral neck bone mineral density (BMD), quadriceps weakness, higher body sway, lower body weight, and decreased stature. Osteoporotic fractures are more common in whites and Asians than in African-Americans and Hispanics, and more common in women than in men. Little is known regarding the influence of ethnicity on bone turnover as a possible cause of the variance in bone density and fracture rates among different ethnic groups. Significant differences in bone turnover in premenopausal and early perimenopausal women can be documented. The bone turnover differences do not appear to parallel the patterns of BMD. Other factors, such as differences in bone accretion, are likely responsible for much of the ethnic variation in adult BMD.

Finkelstein JS et al: Ethnic variation in bone turnover in pre- and early perimenopausal women: effects of anthropometric and lifestyle factors. J Clin Endocrinol Metab 2002;87:3051.

Finkelstein JS et al: Ethnic variation in bone density in premenopausal and early perimenopausal women: effects of anthropometric and lifestyle factors. J Clin Endocrinol Metab 2002;87:3057.

National Osteoporotic Foundation: 1996 and 2015 osteoporosis prevalence figures: state-by-state report. January 1997. Women's Health Matters 1998;2(3):1.

Taxel P: Osteoporosis: detection, prevention, and treatment in primary care. Geriatrics 1998;53(8):22.

Pathogenesis

Osteoporosis is characterized by microarchitectural deterioration of bone tissue that leads to decreased bone mass and bone fragility. The major processes responsible for osteoporosis are (1) poor bone mass acquisition during adolescence and (2) accelerated bone loss during the perimenopausal period (mid-50s—the sixth decade in women and the seventh decade in men) and beyond. Both processes are regulated by genetic and environmental factors. Reduced bone mass, in turn, is the result of varying combinations of hormone deficiencies, inadequate nutrition, decreased physical activity, comorbidity, and the effects of drugs used to treat various medical conditions.

Primary osteoporosis, deterioration of bone mass not associated with other chronic illness, is related to increasing age and decreasing gonadal function. Therefore, early menopause or premenopausal estrogen deficiency states may hasten its development. Prolonged periods of inadequate calcium intake, a sedentary lifestyle, and tobacco and alcohol abuse also contribute to primary osteoporosis.

Secondary osteoporosis results from chronic conditions that contribute significantly to accelerated bone loss. These include endogenous and exogenous thyroxine excess, hyperparathyroidism, cancer, gastrointestinal diseases, medications, renal failure, and connective tissue diseases. Secondary forms of osteoporosis are listed in Table 28–1. If secondary osteoporosis is suspected,

Table 28–1. Secondary forms of osteoporosis.

Endocrine or metabolic causes	Drugs
Acromegaly	Cyclosporine
Anorexia nervosa	Excess thyroid
Athletic amenorrhea	medication
Type 1 diabetes mellitus	Glucocorticoids
Hemochromatosis	Prolonged heparin Rx
Hyperadrenocorticism	Phenytoin
Hyperparathyroidism	Methotrexate
Hyperprolactinemia	Phenobarbital
Thyrotoxicosis	Gonadotropin-releasing
	hormone agonists
	Phenothiazines
Collagen/genetic disorders	**Nutritional**
Ehlers–Danlos syndrome	Alcoholism
Glycogen storage disease	Calcium deficiency
Marfan syndrome	Chronic liver disease
Osteogenesis imperfecta	Gastric operations
Homocystinuria	Malabsorptive
Hypophosphatasia	syndromes
	Vitamin D deficiency

appropriate diagnostic workup may identify a different management course.

Harper KD, Weber TJ: Secondary osteoporosis. Diagnostic considerations. Endocrinol Metab Clin North Am 1998;27(2):325.

Heaney RP: Pathophysiology of osteoporosis. Endocrinol Metab Clin North Am 1998;27(2):255.

Prevention

A. NUTRITION

Bone mineralization is dependent on adequate nutritional status in childhood and adolescence. Therefore, measures to prevent osteoporosis should begin with increasing the milk intake of adolescents to improve bone mineralization. Nutrients other than calcium are also essential for bone health. Adolescents must, therefore, maintain a balance in calcium intake, protein intake, other calorie sources, and phosphorus. Substituting phosphorus-laden soft drinks for calcium-rich dairy products and juices compromises calcium uptake by bone and promotes decreased bone mass.

Eating disorders are nutritional conditions that affect BMD. Inability to maintain normal body mass promotes bone loss. The body weight history of women with anorexia nervosa has been found to be the most important predictor of the presence of osteoporosis as well as the likelihood of recovery. The BMD of these patients does not increase to a normal range, even several years after recovery from the disorder, and all persons with a history of an eating disorder remain at high risk for osteoporosis in the future.

Major demands for calcium are placed on the mother by the fetus during pregnancy and lactation. The axial spine and hip show losses of BMD during the first 6 months of lactation, but this bone mineral loss appears to be completely restored 6–12 months after weaning. Risk factors for osteoporosis are summarized in Table 28–2.

B. LIFE-STYLE

Sedentary life-style and/or immobility (being confined to bed or a wheelchair) increase the incidence of osteoporosis. Low body weight and cigarette smoking negatively influence bone mass. Excessive alcohol consumption has been shown to depress osteoblast function and, thus, to decrease bone formation. Those at risk for low BMD should avoid drugs that negatively affect BMD (Table 28–1).

C. BEHAVIORAL MEASURES

Behavioral measures that decrease the risk of bone loss include eliminating tobacco use and excessive consumption of alcohol and caffeine. A balanced diet with adequate calcium and vitamin D intake and a regular exercise program (see below) retard bone loss. Medications, such as glucocorticoids, that decrease bone mass should be avoided if possible. The importance of maintaining estrogen levels in women should be emphasized. Measurement of bone density should be considered in the patient who presents with risk factors, but additional evidence is needed before instituting preventive measures.

D. EXERCISE

Regular physical exercise can reduce the risk of osteoporosis and delay the physiological decrease of BMD.

Table 28–2. Risk factors for osteoporosis.

Female gender
Petite body frame
White or Asian race
Sedentary life-style/immobilization
Nulliparity
Increasing age
High caffeine intake
Renal disease
Lifelong low calcium intake
Smoking
Excessive alcohol use
Long-term use of certain drugs
Postmenopausal status
Low body weight
Impaired calcium absorption

Short-term and long-term exercise training (measured up to 12 months; eg, walking, jogging, stair climbing) in healthy, sedentary, postmenopausal women results in improved bone mineral content. Bone mineral content increases more than 5% above baseline after short-term, weight-bearing exercise training. With reduced weight-bearing exercise, bone mass reverts to baseline levels. Similar increases in BMD have been seen in women who participate in strength training. In the elderly, progressive strength training has been demonstrated to be a safe and effective form of exercise that reduces risk factors for falling and may also enhance BMD.

Estrogen deficiency results in diminished bone density in younger women as well as in older women. Athletes who exercise much more intensely and consistently than the average person usually have above average bone mass. However, the positive effect of exercise on the bones of young women is dependent upon normal levels of endogenous estrogen. The low estrogen state of exercise-induced amenorrhea outweighs the positive effects of exercise and results in diminished bone density. When mechanical stress or gravitational force on the skeleton is removed as in bed rest, space flight, immobilization of limbs, or paralysis, bone loss is rapid and extensive. Weight-bearing exercise can significantly increase the BMD of menopausal women. Furthermore, weight-bearing exercise and estrogen replacement therapy have independent and additive effects on the BMD of the limb, spine, and Ward's triangle (hip).

There have been no randomized prospective studies systematically comparing the effect of various activities on bone mass. Recommended activities include walking and jogging, weight training, aerobics, stair climbing, field sports, racquet sports, court sports, and dancing. Swimming is of questionable value to bone density (as it is not a weight-bearing activity) and there are no data on cycling, skating, or skiing. It should be kept in mind that any increase in physical activity may have a positive effect on bone mass for women who have been very sedentary. To be beneficial, the duration of exercise should be between 30 and 60 min and the frequency should be three times per week.

Cadogen J et al: Milk intake and bone mineral acquisition in adolescent girls: randomised, controlled intervention trial. Br Med J 1997;315:1255.

Ernst E. Exercise for female osteoporosis. A systematic review of randomised clinical trials. Sports Med (NZ) 1998;25(6):359.

Clinical Findings

A. SYMPTOMS AND SIGNS

The history and physical examination are neither sensitive enough nor sufficient for diagnosing primary osteoporosis. However, they are important in screening for secondary forms of osteoporosis and directing the eval-

uation. A medical history provides valuable clues to the presence of chronic conditions, behaviors, physical fitness, and/or the use of long-term medications that could influence bone density. Those already affected by complications of osteoporosis may complain of upper or mid-thoracic back pain associated with activity, aggravated by long periods of sitting or standing, and easily relieved by rest in a recumbent position. The history should also assess the likelihood of fracture. Low bone density, a propensity to fall, greater height, and the presence of prior fractures are indications of increased fracture risk.

The physical examination should be thorough for the same reasons. For example, lid lag and/or enlargement or nodularity of the thyroid suggest hyperthyroidism. Moon facies, thin skin, and a buffalo hump suggest hypercortisolism. Cachexia mandates screening for an eating disorder or cancer. A pelvic examination is one aspect of the total evaluation of hormonal status in women and a necessary part of the physical examination in women. Osteoporotic fractures are a late physical manifestation. Common fracture sites are the vertebrae, forearm, femoral neck, and proximal humerus. The presence of a "Dowager's hump" in elderly patients indicates multiple vertebral fractures and decreased bone volume.

B. LABORATORY FINDINGS

Basic chemical analysis of serum is indicated when the history suggests other clinical conditions influencing bone density. The tests presented in Tables 28–3 and 28–4 are appropriate for excluding secondary causes of osteoporosis. These tests provide clues to serious illnesses that may otherwise have gone undetected and that, if treated, could result in resolution or modification of the bone loss. Specific biochemical markers (human osteocalcin, bone alkaline phosphatase, immunoassays for pyridinoline cross-links and type 1 collagen-related peptides in urine) that reflect the overall rate of bone formation and bone resorption are now available. These markers are primarily of research interest and are not recommended as part of the basic workup for osteoporosis. They suffer from a high degree of biological variability and diurnal variation and do not differentiate causes of altered bone metabolism. For example, measures of bone turnover increase and remain elevated after menopause but do not necessarily provide information that can direct management.

C. IMAGING STUDIES

Plain radiographs are not sensitive enough to diagnose osteoporosis until total bone density has decreased by 50%, but bone densitometry is useful for measuring bone density and monitoring the course of therapy (Table 28–5). Single or dual photon absorptiometry

Table 28–3. Abnormalities in routine laboratory studies and suggested pathology.[1]

Abnormal Study	Suggested Pathology
↑Creatinine	Renal disease
↑Hepatic transaminases	Hepatic disease
↑Calcium	Primary HPT or malignancy
↓Calcium	Malabsorption, vitamin D deficiency
↓Phosphorus	Osteomalacia
↑Alkaline phosphatase	Liver disease, Paget's disease, fracture, other bone pathology
↓Albumin	Malnutrition
↓TSH	Hyperthyroidism
↑ESR	Myeloma
Anemia	Myeloma
↓24 h calcium excretion	Malabsorption, vitamin D deficiency

Source: Harper KD, Weber TJ: Secondary osteoporosis. Diagnostic considerations. Endocrinol Metab Clin North Am 1998;27(2):325.
[1] HPT, hyperparathyroidism; TSH, thyroid-stimulating hormone; ESR, erythrocyte sedimentation rate; ↑, increased; ↓, decreased.

(SPA, DPA) has been used in the past but provides poorer resolution, less accurate analysis, and more radiation exposure than x-ray absorptiometry. The most widely used techniques for assessing bone mineral density are dual-energy x-ray absorptiometry (DXA) and quantitative computerized tomography (CT). These methods have errors in precision of 0.5 –2%. Quantitative CT is the most sensitive, but results in substantially greater radiation exposure than DXA.

D. SPECIAL TESTS

Of these methods, DXA is the most precise and the diagnostic measure of choice. Smaller, less expensive systems for assessing the peripheral skeleton are now available. These include DXA scans of the distal forearm and the middle phalanx of the nondominant hand and a variety of devices for performing quantitative ultrasound (QUS) measurements on bone. The predictive value of these peripheral measures to assess fracture risk at the hip or vertebra is not clear. Ideally, therefore, measurements should be taken at both a central and a peripheral site for baseline. If follow-up BMD measurements are needed to monitor therapy, the peripheral scans can be compared to the original measurements. Follow-up measures must be done using the same instruments to ensure reliability of data.

Bone densitometry reports provide a T score (the number of standard deviations above or below the

Table 28–4. Directed laboratory assessment for secondary osteoporosis.[1]

Hypogonadism	↓Testosterone in men
	↓Estrogen in women
	↑Gonadotropins (LH and FSH)
Hyperthyroidism	↓TSH
	↑T$_4$
Hyperparathyroidism	↑PTH
	↑Serum calcium
	↑1,25(OH)D
Vitamin D deficiency	↓25-Hydroxycalciferol
Hemochromatosis	Serum iron
	Ferritin
Cushing's syndrome	24 h urine free cortisol excretion
	Overnight dexamethasone suppression test
Multiple myeloma	Serum protein electrophoresis—M spike and Bence–Jones proteinuria
	↑ESR
	Anemia
	Hypercalcemia
	↓PTH

Modified from Harper KD, Weber TJ: Secondary osteoporosis. Diagnostic considerations. Endocrinol Metab Clin North Am 1998;27(2):325.
[1] LH, luteinizing hormone; FSH, follicle-stimulating hormone; TSH, thyroid-stimulating hormone; T$_4$, thyroxine; PTH, parathyroid hormone; 1,25(OH)D, 1,25-hydroxyvitamin D; ESR, erythrocyte sedimentation rate; ↑, increased; ↓, decreased.

Table 28–5. Indications for measuring bone density.

Concerned perimenopausal women willing to start therapy
Radiographic evidence of bone loss
Patient on long-term glucocorticoid therapy (more than 1 month at ≥ 7.5 mg of prednisone/day)
Asymptomatic hyperparathyroidism where osteoporosis would suggest parathyroidectomy
Monitoring therapeutic response in women undergoing treatment for osteoporosis if the result of the test would affect the clinical decision

mean BMD for sex and race matched to young controls) or Z score (comparing the patient with a population adjusted for age as well as for sex and race). The BMD result enables the classification of patients into three categories: normal, osteopenic, and osteoporotic. Normal patients receive no further therapy; osteopenic patients are counseled, treated, and followed so that no further bone loss develops; osteoporotic patients receive active therapy aimed at increasing bone density and decreasing fracture risk. Osteoporosis is indicated by a T score of more than 2.5 standard deviations below the sex-adjusted mean for normal young adults at peak bone mass. Z scores are of little value to the practicing clinician.

There is little evidence from controlled trials that women who receive bone density screening have better outcomes (improved bone density or fewer falls) than women who are not screened. The U.S. Preventive Services Task Force suggests the primary argument for screening is that postmenopausal women with low bone density are at increased risk for subsequent fractures of the hip, vertebrae, and wrist, and that interventions can slow the decline in bone density after menopause. The presence of multiple risk factors (age over 80 years, poor health, limited physical activity, poor vision, prior postmenopausal fracture, psychotropic drug use, and others) seems to be a stronger predictor of hip fracture than low bone density. The patient who is not asymptomatic but may have only one or two risk factors can benefit from BMD screening. Indications for BMD screening are outlined in Table 28–5.

Blake GM, Fogelman I: Applications of bone densitometry for osteoporosis. Endocrinol Metab Clin North Am 1998;27(2): 267.

Kroger H, Reeve J: Diagnosis of osteoporosis in clinical practice. Ann Med 1998;30:278.

U.S. Preventive Services Task Force: *Guide to Clinical Preventive Services.* Williams & Wilkins, 1996.

Differential Diagnosis & Screening

The approach to the patient is governed by the presentation. The greatest challenge for clinicians is to know which asymptomatic patients would benefit from screening for osteoporosis, rather than determining a treatment regimen for those with known disease (Table 28–2). All women and girls should be counseled as to appropriate calcium intake and physical activity. Assessment of osteoporosis risk is also important when following a patient for a chronic disease known to cause secondary osteoporosis (Table 28–1). An algorithm is presented to assist in the evaluation. Preventive measures (Figure 28–1) are always the first step in therapy.

Should there be a suspicion of osteoporosis in a man or evidence of a pathological fracture in a man or a woman, assessment of risk via medical history and determination of BMD should be completed. BMD measurement and laboratory evaluation are necessary to document the extent of bone loss and to rule out secondary causes of osteoporosis. Should there be clinical evidence of a particular condition, the evaluation can focus on the suspected condition once the basic laboratory work has been completed as described in Table 28–3 and Figure 28–1.

Recognizing the variety of conditions conferring risk of osteoporosis, the National Osteoporosis Foundation makes the following recommendations to physicians:

1. Counsel all women on the risk factors for osteoporosis. Osteoporosis is a "silent" risk factor for fracture just as hypertension is for stroke; one of two white women will experience an osteoporotic fracture at some point in her lifetime.

2. Perform evaluation for osteoporosis on all postmenopausal women who present with fractures, using bone BMD testing to confirm the diagnosis and determine the disease severity.

3. Recommend BMD testing to postmenopausal women under age 65 years who have one or more additional risk factors for osteoporosis in addition to menopause.

4. Recommend BMD testing to all women aged 65 years and older regardless of additional risk factors.

5. Advise all patients to obtain an adequate intake of dietary calcium (at least 1200 mg/day, including supplements if necessary).

6. Recommend regular weight-bearing and muscle-strengthening exercise to reduce the risk of falls and fractures.

7. Advise patients to avoid tobacco smoking and to keep alcohol intake moderate.

8. Consider all postmenopausal women who present with vertebral or hip fractures candidates for treatment of osteoporosis.

9. Initiate therapy to reduce fracture risk in women with BMD T scores below −2 in the absence of risk factors and in women with T scores below −1.5 if other risk factors are present.

10. Pharmacological options for prevention and/or treatment of osteoporosis include hormone replacement therapy, alendronate, raloxifene (prevention), and calcitonin (treatment).

Treatment

Decisions to intervene when osteoporosis is diagnosed reflect a desire to prevent early or continuing bone loss, a belief that there can be an immediate impact on the

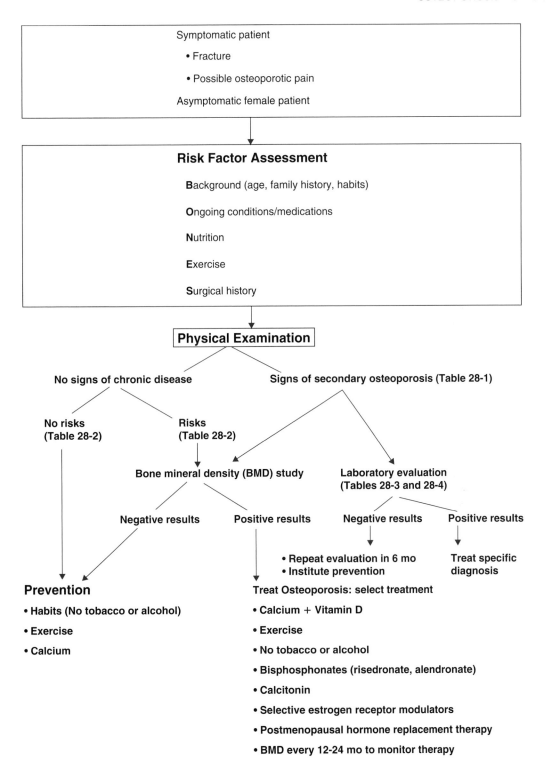

Figure 28–1. Approaching osteoporosis.

patient's well-being, and a willingness to comply with the patient's desires. Bone densitometry can assist in the decision-making process if the patient's age confers risk, there are no manifestations of disease, and the decision point is prevention rather than treatment. BMD measurements can also assist in therapy when there are relative contraindications to a specific agent and demonstrating efficacy could encourage continuation of therapy. Medicare currently reimburses costs of bone densitometry according to the conditions outlined in Table 28–6. The decision to intervene with pharmacological therapy involves clinical judgment based upon a global assessment, rather than BMD measurement alone. All currently approved therapeutic agents for the prevention and treatment of osteoporosis work by inhibiting or decreasing bone resorption.

A. ESTROGEN

Adequate estrogen levels remain the single most important therapy for maintaining adequate bone density in women. Prior to 2003, estrogen replacement therapy (ERT) was considered for all women with decreased bone density, absent contraindications. However, in July 2002, the Women's Health Initiative (WHI) randomized controlled primary prevention trial was stopped at a mean 5.2 years of follow-up by the data and safety monitoring board because the test statistic for invasive breast cancer exceeded the stopping boundary for the adverse effect of estrogen and progesterone versus placebo. Estimated hazard ratios were excessive for coronary heart disease, breast cancer, and strokes, but were less than 1.0 for colorectal cancer, endometrial cancer, and hip fracture. Therefore, careful risk assessment is needed for each patient to determine whether the improvement of risk for hip fracture (0.66) balances the risk for cardiovascular and breast disease. Contraindications to estrogen replacement therapy are listed in Table 28–7.

Studies have been done to determine the effect of the timing of initiation and the duration of postmenopausal estrogen therapy on BMD. Current users who started at menopause had the highest BMD levels,

Table 28–6. Conditions qualifying for Medicare coverage of densitometry.

Estrogen-deficient woman at clinical risk for osteoporosis
Individual with vertebral abnormalities (eg, osteopenia, vertebral fractures, osteoporosis)
Individual receiving long-term (more than 3 months) glucocorticoid therapy
Primary hyperparathyroidism
Individual being monitored to assess response to osteoporosis drug therapy

Table 28–7. Contraindications to estrogen replacement therapy.

Absolute
History of breast cancer
Estrogen-dependent neoplasia
Undiagnosed or abnormal genital bleeding
History of or active thromboembolic disorder
Relative
Migraine
History of thromboembolism
Familial hypertriglyceridemia
Uterine leiomyomas
Uterine cancer
Gallbladder disease
Strong family history of breast cancer
Chronic hepatic dysfunction
Endometriosis

Source: Scientific Advisory Board, Osteoporosis Society of Canada: Clinical practice guidelines for the diagnosis and management of osteoporosis. Can Med Assoc J 1996;155:1113.

which were significantly higher than never users or past users who started at menopause (with a duration of use of at least 10 years). BMD was similar for women using unopposed estrogen or estrogen plus progestin, for women younger or older than 75 years, and for current smokers or nonsmokers. Current users who started estrogen within 5 years of menopause had a decreased risk of hip, wrist, and all nonspinal fractures compared with those who never used estrogen. Long-term users who initiated therapy 5 years after menopause had no significant reduction in risk for all nonspinal fractures, despite an average duration of use of 16 years. Therefore, early initiation of estrogen with respect to menopause may be more important than the total duration of use. Estrogen initiated early in the menopausal period and continued into late life appears to be associated with the highest bone density.

As more and more women utilize estrogen therapy, there has been increasing concern regarding its impact on breast cancer risk. The relation between the use of hormones and the risk of breast cancer in postmenopausal women was assessed in a follow-up survey of participants in the Nurses' Health Study in 1992. The risk of breast cancer was significantly increased among women who were currently using estrogen alone or estrogen plus progestin, as compared with postmenopausal women who had never used hormones. Women currently taking hormones who had used such therapy for 5–9 years had an adjusted relative risk of breast cancer of 1.46, as did those currently using hormones who had done so for a total of 10 or more years

(RR = 1.46). The addition of progestins to estrogen therapy does not reduce the risk of breast cancer among postmenopausal women.

The only randomized trial of estrogen–progesterone therapy describes secondary prevention of coronary heart disease in postmenopausal women (HERS) and included only women who had a prior history of cardiovascular disease. Women received either estrogen or estrogen and progesterone. There was an excess of deaths from coronary heart disease and a three-fold excess risk of venous thrombosis during the first year of the trial for women on estrogen and a small risk of stroke in women on estrogen and progesterone. Recommendations at the conclusion of the trial included not starting women who already have clinical cardiovascular disease on estrogen and progesterone therapy (ie, secondary prevention).

B. CALCIUM AND VITAMIN D

Calcium supplementation produces small beneficial effects on bone mass throughout postmenopausal life and may reduce fracture rates by more than the change in BMD would predict—possibly as much as 50%. Postmenopausal women receiving supplemental calcium over a 3-year period in a placebo-controlled, randomized clinical trial had stable total body calcium and BMD in the lumbar spine, femoral neck, and trochanter compared with the placebo group.

Vitamin D increases calcium absorption in the gastrointestinal tract, so that more calcium is available in the circulation and is subsequently reabsorbed in the renal proximal tubules. There is now evidence of significant reductions in nonvertebral fracture rates from physiological replacement of vitamin D in the elderly. Vitamin D supplementation is important in those of all ages with limited exposure to sunlight.

Dietary calcium augmentation should be recommended to maintain lifetime calcium levels and to help prevent early postmenopausal bone loss (Table 28–8). Adults should ingest 1000 mg of elemental calcium per

Table 28–8. Calcium-rich foods.[1]

Milk (skim, lowfat, or whole), 8 oz
Plain yogurt, 8 oz
Frozen yogurt, fruit, 8 oz
Swiss cheese, 1 oz
Ricotta cheese, part skim, 4 oz
Sardines, canned, 3 oz
Cooked greens, collards, or mustard, 8 oz
Firm cheeses (Edam, Brick, Cheddar, Gouda, Colby, Mozzarella), 1 oz
Calcium-fortified orange juice, 8 oz

[1]Approximately 300 mg.

day for optimal bone health. Teenagers, pregnant/lactating women, women greater than 50 years of age taking ERT, and everyone greater than 65 years of age should ingest 1500 mg of elemental calcium per day for optimal bone health. If this cannot be achieved by diet alone, calcium supplementation is recommended. Calcium preparations should be compared relative to elemental calcium content. Therefore, attention to which form the patient is ingesting is important.

C. CALCITONIN

Calcitonin, a hormone directly inhibiting osteoclastic bone resorption, is an alternative for patients with established osteoporosis in whom estrogen replacement therapy is not recommended. A unique characteristic of calcitonin is that it produces an analgesic effect with respect to bone pain and, thus, is often prescribed for patients who have suffered an acute osteoporotic fracture. The American College of Rheumatology recommends treatment until the pain is controlled, followed by tapering of medication over 4–6 weeks. Calcitonin decreases further bone loss at vertebral and femoral sites in patients with documented osteoporosis, but has a questionable effect on fracture frequency. Calcitonin has been shown to prevent trabecular bone loss during the first few years of menopause, but it is unclear whether it has any impact on cortical bone. Calcitonin is also thought to be effective in decreasing the fracture rate of vertebrae and peripheral bones.

The PROOF (Prevent Recurrence of Osteoporotic Fractures)—a 5-year double-blind study that randomized 1255 postmenopausal women with osteoporosis to receive placebo or one of three dosages of intranasal calcitonin (100, 200, or 400 IU/day)—demonstrated a 36% reduction in the relative risk of new vertebral fractures compared with placebo. There was no effect with 100 IU/day and no significant change in the reduction seen with 400 IU/day.

For reasons poorly understood, the increase in BMD associated with administration of calcitonin may be transient or there may be the development of resistance. Calcitonin can be provided in two forms. Nasal congestion and rhinitis are the most significant side effects of the nasal form. The injectable formulation has gastrointestinal side effects and is less convenient than the nasal preparation. The increase in bone density observed by this therapy is significantly less than that achieved by bisphosphonates or estrogen and may be limited to the spine, but it still has recognized value in reducing risk of fracture.

D. BISPHOSPHONATES

Bisphosphonates are effective for preventing bone loss associated with estrogen deficiency, glucocorticoid treatment, and immobilization. All bisphosphonates act similarly on bone in binding permanently to mineralized bone surfaces and inhibiting osteoclastic activity. Thus, less bone is degraded during the remodeling cycle. First-, second-, and third-generation bisphosphonates are now available (etidronate, alendronate, and residronate). The Fracture Intervention Trial investigated the effect of alendronate on the risk of fractures (both inapparent as well as clinically evident) in postmenopausal women with low bone mass. The risk of any clinical fracture was half that of the placebo group in those taking alendronate. Because food and liquids can reduce the absorption of alendronate, it should be given with a glass of plain water 30 min before the first meal or beverage of the day. Patients should not lie down for at least 30 min to lessen the chance of esophageal irritation. In addition, patients should consider taking supplemental calcium and vitamin D if their dietary intake is inadequate.

Bisphosphonates are of comparable efficacy to hormone replacement therapy (HRT) in preventing bone loss and have a demonstrated positive effect on symptomatic and asymptomatic vertebral fracture rate as well as on nonvertebral fracture rate (forearm and hip). More than 4 years of treatment would be needed in women with low bone density (T score >-2.0), but without preexisting fractures, to substantially reduce the risk of clinical fracture.

In clinical trials, alendronate was generally well tolerated and no significant clinical or biological adverse experiences were observed. Alendronate appears to be effective at doses of 5 mg daily in preventing osteoporosis induced by long-term glucocorticoid therapy. In placebo-controlled studies of men and women (ages 17–83) who were receiving glucocorticoid therapy, femoral neck bone density and the bone density of the trochanter and total body increased significantly in patients treated with alendronate.

Alendronate appears to be a safe and well-tolerated agent for the treatment of osteoporosis. Some small studies do suggest an additional benefit of adding alendronate to HRT and ongoing studies should provide additional information. However, all of the bisphosphonates accumulate over time in bone, and further research is needed to determine their long-term impact as well as their potential for use in premenopausal women and men.

Risedronate is a pyridinyl bisphosphonate approved as treatment for several metabolic bone diseases in 2000. In doses of 5 mg daily, risedronate reduces the incidence of vertebral fractures in women with two or more fractures by rapidly increasing BMD at sites of cortical and trabecular bone. In a randomized trial of 2458 postmenopausal women with diagnosed osteoporosis participants were treated with either 2.5 mg or 5 mg of risedronate or placebo as well as calcium supplementation and cholecalciferol if they had low baseline 25-hydroxyvitamin D levels. The 2.5 mg dose was found to be ineffective in other trials and was discontinued. After 3 years of treatment, the 5 mg residronate group showed a 41% reduction in risk of new vertebral fractures and a 39% reduction in incidence of nonvertebral fractures.

In a large, prospective, hip fracture prevention trial of elderly women, residronate was shown to significantly reduce the risk of hip fracture in women with osteoporosis. Bisphosphonates should be prescribed for 3–4 years in women with osteoporosis and low bone density.

E. Selective Estrogen Receptor Modulators

Raloxifene is the first drug to be studied from a new class of drugs termed selective estrogen receptor modulators. This drug has a mixed agonist/antagonist action on estrogen receptors—estrogen agonist effects on bone and antagonist effects on breast and endometrium. Its discovery evolved from a structural rearrangement of the antiestrogen tamoxifen, although it is structurally very different. It is thought to block estrogen in a manner similar to tamoxifen, while also binding and stimulating other tissue receptors to act like estrogen. Raloxifene inhibits trabecular and vertebral bone loss in a manner similar, but not identical, to estrogen—ie, by blocking the activity of cytokines that stimulate bone resorption.

Raloxifene therapy results in decreased serum total and low-density lipoprotein (LDL) cholesterol without any beneficial effects on serum total high-density lipoprotein (HDL) cholesterol or triglycerides. Reported side effects of raloxifene are vaginitis and hot flashes. Investigators in the Multiple Outcomes of Raloxifene (MORE) trial of over 7000 postmenopausal, osteoporotic women over 3 years showed a decreased risk of breast cancer in those already at low risk for the disease. The study results were analyzed separately for women presenting with preexisting fracture. Although treatment effectiveness was similar in both groups, the absolute risk of fractures in the group with preexisting fractures was 4.5 times greater than in the group with osteoporosis, but no preexisting fracture (21% versus 4.5%). Thus, it is important to identify and treat patients at higher risk. Studies of women at higher risk for breast cancer are currently underway.

A summary of overall treatment strategies is given in Table 28–9 and guidelines for dosing the pharmacological agents are given in Table 28–10. Table 28–11 summarizes the risks and benefits of osteoporosis therapy.

F. Other Modalities

Fluoride increases bone formation by stimulating osteoblasts and increasing cancellous bone formation in

Table 28–9. Treatment strategies.

Overall
Calcium-rich diet ± vitamin D supplements
Weight-bearing exercise
Avoidance of alcohol, tobacco products, excess caffeine, and drugs
Estrogen replacement within 5 years of menopause, and used for 10+ years
Alendronate
Raloxifene
Calcitonin

For patients on glucocorticoids
Lowest dose of a short-acting glucocorticoid or topical preparations whenever possible
Maintain a well-balanced, 2- to 3-g sodium diet
Weight-bearing and isometric exercise to prevent proximal muscle weakness
Calcium intake of 1500 mg/day and vitamin D intake of 400–800 IU/day after hypercalciuria is controlled
Gonadal hormones in all postmenopausal women, premenopausal women with low levels of estradiol, and men who have low levels of testosterone (unless contraindicated)
Thiazide diuretic to control hypercalciuria
Measure bone mineral density at baseline and every 6–12 months during the first 2 years of therapy to assess treatment efficacy
If bone loss occurs during treatment or hormone replacement therapy is contraindicated, treat with calcitonin or bisphosphonate

Source: Lane NE, Lukert B: The science and therapy of glucocorticoid induced bone loss. Endocrinol Metab Clin North Am 1998; 27(2):465.

patients with osteoporosis. However, the bone is formed only in the spine and is abnormal—irregularly fibrous and woven with lacunae of low mineral density. Cessation of therapy resulted in rapid loss of much of the bone formed during treatment. The major side effect of fluoride therapy is gastric distress, thought to be related to the direct effect of hydrofluoric acid on the gastric mucosa. Fluoride is also associated with joint pain and swelling. For these reasons, sodium fluoride is not routinely used for treatment of osteoporosis and does not have Food and Drug Administration (FDA)-approved labeling for this indication.

A variety of other drugs have been studied for the treatment of osteoporosis, but are not accepted therapies for various reasons. Anabolic steroids produce some increased bone mass. Despite these benefits, these drugs are seldom used for osteoporosis in the United States because of the long-term effects on multiple organ systems—significant hepatotoxicity, reduced HDL, and elevated LDL cholesterol. Testosterone replacement is acceptable therapy for many of the causes of hypogonadism in men [eg, Klinefelter's syndrome, isolated gonadotropin deficiency (Kallman's syndrome)].

G. Complementary and Alternative Therapies

Evidence from animal studies suggests a beneficial effect of phytoestrogens on bone, but long-term human studies are lacking. Epidemiological evidence that Asian women have a lower fracture rate than white women even though the bone density of Asian women is less than that of African-American women promotes consideration of the impact of nutrition. It is possible that high soy intake contributes to improved bone quality in Asian women. A comparison study of a soy protein and high isoflavone diet versus a milk protein diet or medium isoflavone and soy protein diet demonstrated

Table 28–10. Pharmacological doses.

Medication	Dosage	Route
Estradiol patch	0.05 mg every week	Topical
Elemental calcium	1000–1500 mg/day	Oral
Calcitonin	200 IU/day or 50–100 IU/day	Intranasal or subcutaneous/intramuscular
Vitamin D	400 IU/day (800 IU/day in winter in northern latitudes)	Oral
Alendronate	10 mg/day (treatment) or 70 mg once weekly	Oral
Raloxifene	60 mg/day	Oral
Risedronate	5 mg/day or 35 mg once weekly	Oral
Conjugated estrogens[1]	0.625–1.25 mg/day	Oral

[1]Patients should discuss risks carefully with a physician.

Table 28–11. Risks and benefits of osteoporosis therapy.[1]

	Estrogen	Raloxifene	Calcitonin	Alendronate	Risedronate
Reduction of vertebral fracture	Yes	Yes	Yes	Yes	Yes
Reduction of non-vertebral fracture	Yes	No	No	Yes	Yes
Experience with long-term use	Large epidemiological studies over decades	RCT 3 years in length	RCT 5 years in length	RCT 4 years in length	RCT 3 years in length
Administration	Orally: once daily any time	Orally: once daily any time	Intranasally: once daily any time	Once daily in morning, 30 min before eating, with water while upright; or weekly	Once daily (or weekly) in morning, 30–60 min before eating, with water, while upright
Adverse effects	Breast tenderness, vaginal bleeding, thromboembolic disorders	Increased risk of venous thrombo-sis, hot flashes, leg cramps	Nasal irritation	Dyspepsia; esophagitis; avoid in patients with esophagheal disorders	Dyspepsia
Effect on CV mortality	Increased in those with preexisting CV disease	No final outcome data	None	None	None
Breast cancer	Increased	Possibly decreased risk of estrogen receptor-positive breast cancer	None	None	None
Endometrial cancer	Increased if unopposed estrogen used	None	None	None	None

Modified from *Managing Osteoporosis—Part 3: Prevention and Treatment of Postmenopausal Osteoporosis.* AMA CME Program, 2000.
[1]RCT, randomized clinical trial; CV, cardiovascular.

that only those receiving the higher isoflavone preparation were protected against trabecular (vertebral) bone loss.

A topical form of natural progesterone derived from diosgenin in either soybeans or Mexican wild yam has been promoted as a treatment for osteoporosis, hot flashes, and premenstrual syndrome, and a prophylactic against breast cancer. However, eating or applying wild yam extract or diosgenin does not produce increased progesterone levels in humans because humans cannot convert diosgenin to progesterone.

H. GLUCOCORTICOID-INDUCED OSTEOPOROSIS

Glucocorticoids are widely used in the treatment of many chronic diseases, particularly asthma, chronic lung disease, and inflammatory and rheumatological disorders, and in those who have undergone organ transplantation. The risk oral steroid therapy poses to bone mineral density, among other side effects, has been known for some time. As a result clinicians have eagerly substituted inhaled steroids in an endeavor to protect the patient from unwanted negative steroid effects. Recent evaluations of the effects of inhaled glucocorticoids on bone density in premenopausal women demonstrated a dose-related decline in bone density at both the total hip and the trochanter. Women with asthma were enrolled and were divided into three groups: those using no inhaled steroids, those using four to eight puffs per day, and those using more than eight puffs per day at 100 μg per puff. No dose-related effect was noted at the femoral neck or the spine. Serum and urinary markers of bone turnover or adrenal function did not predict the degree of bone loss. To achieve the best possible outcome for the patient, given the potentially devastating effects of systemic steroids, therapy to combat the steroids should begin as soon as the steroids are begun. See Table 28–9 for specific guidelines.

Col NF et al: Patient-specific decisions about hormone replacement therapy in postmenopausal women. JAMA 1997;277:1140.

Colditz GA et al: The use of estrogens and progestins and the risk of breast cancer in postmenopausal women. New Engl J Med 1995;332:1589.

Ettinger B et al: Reduction of vertebral fracture risk in post-menopausal women with osteoporosis treated with raloxifene. Results from a 3 year randomized clinical trial. JAMA 1999; 282:637.

Harris ST et al: Effects of residronate treatment on vertebral and nonvertebral fractures in women with postmenopausal osteo-porosis. A randomized controlled trial. JAMA 1999;282: 1344.

Israel E et al: Effects of inhaled glucocorticoids on bone density in premenopausal women. New Engl J Med 2001;345:941.

Potter SM et al: Soy protein and isoflavones: their effects on lipids and bone density in postmenopausal women. Am J Clin Nutr 1998;68:(6, Suppl):1375S.

Reid IR: The role of calcium and vitamin D in the prevention of osteoporosis. Endocrinol Metab Clin North Am 1998;27(2): 389.

Roussouw JE et al: Risks and benefits of estrogen plus progestin in healthy postmenopausal women. JAMA 2002;288:321.

Saag KG et al: Alendronate for the prevention and treatment of glucocorticoid-induced osteoporosis. New Engl J Med 1998; 339(5):292.

Watts NB: Treatment of osteoporosis with bisphosphonates. En-docrinol Metab Clin North Am 1998;27(2):419.

WEB SITE

The National Osteoporosis Foundation
http:/www.nof.org

Abdominal Pain

29

Cindy Barter, MD, & Laura Dunne, MD

General Considerations

Abdominal pain is the chief complaint for 5–10% of patients presenting to the emergency room and is one of the top 10 outpatient complaints. Accurately diagnosing abdominal pain is difficult due to the enormously varied group of causes. Because the array of possible problems associated with abdominal pain is wide, it is necessary to focus upon a detailed history and a thorough physical examination, including laboratory and radiological evaluations.

Clinical Findings

A. HISTORY

When evaluating a patient with abdominal pain the history is one of the most important factors and can help direct the subsequent workup. The first priority is to determine whether the pain is acute or chronic in nature. The sudden and/or severe onset of abdominal pain, particularly pain associated with hemodynamic changes, leads toward an emergent evaluation and intervention.

A thorough and accurate history requires good communication skills on the part of the clinician. Physicians are more likely to collect the full history when implementing the "engage, empathize, educate, and enlist" method. Patients should be allowed to tell their story, which usually takes 1 or 2 min, and often answers the questions regarding the onset, intensity, location, and frequency of the problem.

Sudden and severe onset of abdominal pain is often seen in appendicitis, leaking or ruptured abdominal aortic aneurysm (AAA), a perforated ulcer, pancreatitis, obstruction, and nongastrointestinal sources of pain—ectopic pregnancy, myocardial infarction, sickle cell crisis, and kidney stones. Gastroesophageal reflux disease (GERD), chronic pancreatitis, functional bowel disease (irritable bowel syndrome), abdominal wall pain, celiac disease, constipation, chronic diarrhea, and nongastrointestinal sources—prostatitis, ovarian cyst, and pelvic inflammatory disease—can all be characterized by a more gradual onset of abdominal pain and by abdominal pain that is chronic in nature (Table 29–1).

The patient's description of the quality of the pain provides clues to the etiology of the problem. For example, "burning" is often used to describe GERD. A pressure-like description ("there's an elephant sitting on me") suggests cardiac ischemia. Patients suffering from peptic ulcer disease (PUD) often describe their pain as a gnawing or hunger-like sensation.

The location of the pain coupled with any radiation can be helpful. For example, pain from an acute appendicitis may start as epigastric or periumbilical pain prior to settling in the right lower quadrant of the abdomen. Pain that starts in the midepigastric region and then radiates to the back suggests pancreatitis. Gallbladder pain typically radiates to the scapula. Pain from the lower esophagus may be referred higher in the chest and is often confused with pain associated with cardiac conditions, such as an acute myocardial infarction (MI).

The frequency and pattern of the pain are particularly useful in identifying abdominal pain that is gradual in onset. Pain that worsens nocturnally upon lying down suggests GERD. Pain occurring after the consumption of high-fat meals increases the probability of gallbladder disease. Pain that is relieved after a bowel movement is indicative of functional bowel symptoms.

Physicians need to determine if other associated symptoms are present. Fever and chills suggest an infectious etiology. Nausea and vomiting are associated with pancreatitis. Hematemesis can indicate a Mallory–Weiss tear or PUD. Feculent emesis is correlated with bowel obstruction. The presence of blood or melena in the stool requires further evaluation due to the possibility of gastrointestinal bleeding. Emotional stress can exacerbate functional bowel disease. However, it should not be used as a primary diagnostic discriminator between functional and organic disease as many organic diseases can be accentuated by emotional stress.

Past medical history can provide important clues to the etiology of abdominal pain. A history of previous episodes can help direct further evaluation. Previous ab-

Table 29–1. Common causes of abdominal pain by location.[1]

Localized
  Midepigastric
    Dyspepsia
    GERD
    Pancreatitis
    PUD
  RUQ
    Gallbladder diseases
    Hepatitis
    Hepatomegaly
  RLQ
    Appendicitis
    Crohn's disease
    GYN-related diseases
      Ruptured ovarian cyst
      Ectopic pregnancy
      PID
      Pregnancy
    Meckel's diverticulitis
  LUQ
    MI
    Pneumonia
    Sickle cell crisis
    Lymphoma
    Splenomegaly—EBV
    Gastritis
  LLQ
    Diverticulitis
    Bowel obstruction
    Ischemic colitis
    Ulcerative colitis
    Urinary calculi
  Suprapubic
    Cystitis
    Prostatitis
    Urinary retention
Generalized
  Abdominal wall pain—multiple causes
  Celiac disease
  Constipation
  Chronic diarrhea
  IBS
  Gastroenteritis/infectious diarrhea
  Mesenteric lymphadenitis
  Perforated colon
  Ruptured aortic aneurysm
  Trauma

[1]GERD, gastroesophageal reflux disease; PUD, peptic ulcer disease; GYN, gynecological; PID, pelvic inflammatory disease; MI, myocardial infarction; EBV, Epstein–Barr virus; IBS, inflammatory bowel disease; RUQ, right upper quadrant; RLQ, right lower quadrant; LUQ, left upper quadrant; LLQ, left lower quadrant.

dominal surgery increases the risk for bowel obstruction secondary to adhesions, strangulation, or hernia. Patients with a history of cardiovascular disease are at greater risk for bowel infarction. A history of tobacco or alcohol use is associated with an increased incidence of GERD and PUD. Alcohol abuse is also a common cause of pancreatitis. Multiparity, obesity, and diabetes mellitus all increase the risk of gallbladder disease. Tubal ligation or a history of pelvic inflammatory disease (PID) indicates a greater risk for an ectopic pregnancy.

No medical history is complete without a medication history that also includes both over-the-counter drugs and herbal supplements. Aspirin, nonsteroidal antiinflammatories, and warfarin increase the risk of gastrointestinal bleeding. Alendronate sodium (Fosamax) increases the probability that the patient's symptoms of abdominal pain include epigastric pain, which further indicates erosive esophagitis. Antibiotics can be associated with nausea and/or diarrhea.

Advancing age can change the patient's presentation and perception of abdominal pain. There is a 10–20% reduction in intensity of pain per decade of age over 60 years old. In one study it was found that only 22% of the elderly with appendicitis presented with the classic symptom pattern. Young patients are twice as likely to present with epigastric pain with PUD than are elderly patients. Obtaining a detailed history including the onset, intensity, location, and frequency of the pain can often help focus the physical examination.

B. THE PHYSICAL EXAMINATION

The physical examination must be thorough, but the history obtained dictates the focus of the abdominal examination. In addition to the abdominal examination, a pelvic examination is frequently indicated in females presenting with abdominal pain.

An effective physical examination of the abdomen has many steps that flow intuitively. The physician should begin by positioning the patient supine with the knees slightly bent. From this position many different aspects of the abdomen can be assessed. An inspection for distention, discoloration, scars, and striae should then be conducted. Distention suggests ascites, obstruction, or other masses increasing the abdominal contents. Discoloration may include bruising as in the case of hemoperitoneum, found in the central portion of the abdomen, especially following abdominal trauma. The presence and location of scars help clarify and confirm the history previously obtained. Striae suggest rapid growth of the abdomen. Old striae tend to be white, whereas new striae or those related to endocrine abnormalities tend to be purplish or dark pink. The abdomen should also be inspected when the patient is upright, as many hernias resolve when the patient is in a supine position.

Auscultation should be performed prior to palpation. The physician should listen for the quality of bowel sounds: normal, hypoactive, hyperactive, or high pitched. Hypoactive and hyperactive bowel sounds can both be present in the case of total or partial bowel obstruction, or ileus. It is also necessary to listen for bruits over the aorta, renal arteries, and femoral arteries when auscultating. Bruits may be suggestive of aneurysms in those areas. Palpating gently while auscultating decreases the likelihood of guarding, embellishment, or symptom magnification on the part of the patient.

Palpation of the abdomen should be done in several steps, beginning with the lightest of touches and beginning away from the area of greatest pain, moving closer to the tender area as the examination progresses. There are several aspects to palpation, including consistency, tenderness, masses, and organ size. The consistency can range from soft to rigid. Increased rigidity is indicative of an acute abdomen needing more emergent intervention.

Tenderness can be separated by location, radiation, and associated rebound or guarding. The specific site of tenderness is classic in many sources of abdominal pain. For example, rebound tenderness and sharp pain upon palpation of McBurney's point are indicative of appendicitis. McBurney's point is located 2 inches from the anterior superior iliac spine on a line drawn from this process through the umbilicus. However, the actual site of the appendix (and therefore the location of pain with palpation) is often found some distance from the classic McBurney's point. Additionally, Murphy's sign, sudden cessation of the patient's inspiratory effort during deep palpation of the right upper quadrant (RUQ), is suggestive of acute cholecystitis.

Pain stemming from visceral organs may appear to radiate secondary to other areas being inervated by the same nerve. For example, the pain caused by pancreatitis often radiates to the back. Kehr's sign, abdominal pain radiating to the left shoulder, is indicative of splenic rupture, renal calculi, or ectopic pregnancy. Radiation of pain can also be caused by inflammation of surrounding tissues.

It is difficult to palpate the deep muscles of the abdomen, but the same effect can be obtained by examining pain with motion of muscles. For example, the iliopsoas muscle test can test for inflammation within the psoas muscle or inflammation of overlying structures such as the appendix. The test is performed by having the patient lie supine, then lift the right leg, flexing at the hip. Resistance is applied to the leg. Pain with this maneuver is suggestive of appendicitis or retroperitoneal dissection.

Rebound tenderness indicates peritoneal irritation, which can come from perforation along the gastrointestinal (GI) tract or from non-GI sources such as a ruptured ovarian cyst or PID. When there is peritoneal irritation the patient will often demonstrate guarding. Guarding can be voluntary or involuntary. Voluntary guarding can occur when the patient anticipates the pain. The "closed eye" sign has been shown to help differentiate the etiology of the pain. Patients whose pain has an organic etiology will keep their eyes open and watch as the examiner approaches the abdomen. Patients who close their eyes (the closed eye sign) are more likely to have psychosocial factors contributing to their abdominal pain.

Involuntary guarding is caused by flexion of the abdominal wall muscle as the body attempts to protect the internal organs. This protective reflex can be used to differentiate visceral pain from abdominal wall or psychogenic pain, demonstrated with Carnett's test. The test is performed by finding the area of greatest tenderness. The patient then flexes the abdominal wall and the point is palpated again. Pain that is less severe with palpation of the flexed abdomen wall has a high probability of being visceral. Pain that remains the same or is worsened with this maneuver likely stems from the abdominal wall or nonorganic causes.

Palpation of the abdomen of a ticklish patient can be difficult. There are two ways to palpate these patients more thoroughly. One method is to first use the stethoscope for light palpation and then curl the fingers past the edge of the stethoscope to create a less sensitive touch. In an alternative technique the patient places his or her hands on the abdomen and the examiner palpates through the patient's hands and just over the edge of the patient's fingers. This permits deep palpation without contraction of the abdominal muscles from laughing.

In addition to feeling for tenderness with palpation, the physician should examine the abdomen for masses and organ size. Palpable masses include colon cancer masses, kidney abnormalities, non-GI tumors, aneurysms, or other organ abnormalities. Most are found on deep palpation. This palpation can be facilitated by having the patient in the supine position with the knees slightly bent, to allow for relaxation of the abdominal muscles. If a mass is palpated, it should be examined for location, size, shape, consistency, pulsations, mobility, and movement with respiration.

When palpating for organ size, the liver and spleen should be examined. It can be helpful to have the patient take a deep breath prior to trying to palpate the lower border of the liver or spleen and to have the patient exhale while palpating deeper to appreciate the lower border of the liver or tip of the spleen. The normal liver span at the mid-clavicular line is 6–12 cm. The liver of males and taller individuals tends to be larger than the liver of females and shorter individuals. Additionally, the liver span in the mid-sternal line can be helpful. This span is normally 4–8 cm. Anything larger than 8 cm should be considered enlarged. The size of the liver may better be appreciated by percussion along the mid-clavicular line. The examiner should start in an area of tympany, and progress to an area of dullness, both from above the liver and below the liver. The upper border generally sits at the fifth to seventh intercostal space. Being inferiorly displaced is suggestive of emphysema or other pulmonary disease.

The spleen may not be palpable or just a tip of the spleen may be palpable. Both of these findings are normal. The actual span of the spleen can be determined by percussion. The area of dullness related to the spleen is generally from the sixth to tenth rib. It should be percussed in the left mid-axillary line.

Percussion can be helpful to determine both the size of the organs as well as other information about the abdomen. Percussion over the liver or spleen should be slightly dull. A change in the character of the sound can indicate that the edge of the organ is reached. This can also be determined by the scratch test, a gentle form of percussion. The scratch test is very useful in determining the size of the liver. It is performed by placing the stethoscope over the liver, then gently scratching the surface of the skin beginning above the upper border of the liver and progressing down below the lower border of the liver. The quality of the sound changes as the examiner's scratch travels from the lung field to the liver and then to the abdomen. These changes in sound help to identify the borders of the liver.

After determining the size of organs, the rest of the abdomen can be examined for other abnormalities. Tympany should be present over the stomach bubble because of the air present. Tympany related to the stomach should be found in the area of the left lower border of the rib cage and the left epigastrum. However, any increased tympany throughout the rest of the abdomen suggests dilation or perforation of the bowel. Dullness can be stationary, as with solid masses, or shifting, as with mobile fluid. Shifting dullness is generally present with significant ascites.

C. LABORATORY FINDINGS

As a general rule, the laboratory tests ordered are determined by the history obtained and the results of the physical examination of the patient. Specific tests are indicated when specific processes are suspected.

Frequently indicated tests include, but are not limited to, complete blood count (CBC), liver function tests (LFTs), electrolytes, blood urea nitrogen (BUN), creatinine, erythrocyte sedimentation rate (ESR), C-reactive protein (CRP), stool studies, pregnancy test, urinalysis (UA), amylase, and lipase. Specifically, the hemoglobin and hematacrit should be examined for evidence of blood loss, to go along with other warning signs. The CBC is helpful in identifying infection as in appendicitis, diverticulitis, peritonitis, and PID. Amylase is a test often used to try to identify pancreatitis, but it can be elevated in many abdominal processes. Lipase and trypsin are both more specific to pancreatitis and can be helpful in clarifying the etiology of pain. Electolytes, BUN, and creatinine can help identify dehydration, kidney failure, and acidotic or alkolotic states. Patients with inflammatory bowel disease tend to have elevated ESR and CRP, especially during times of exacerbation of the disease. The UA can indicate confusing results. Evidence of red or white blood cells in the urine may suggest a kidney stone or a urinary tract infection. However, these findings can be present in any inflammatory process in proximity to the bladder, such as prostatitis, appendicitis, PID, and diverticulitis. A pregnancy test should be performed upon any female patient of childbearing age. If a patient has abdominal pain, a prior history that includes a tubal ligation does not rule out the possibility of pregnancy and increases the risk of ectopic pregnancy. In summary, there are many helpful laboratory studies, but they must be examined with careful clinical correlation.

D. IMAGING STUDIES

There are several tests available to visualize the abdomen that help to delineate the source of abdominal pain. Radiological examination is a rapidly evolving field and therefore "the single best test" may change as technology advances.

Computerized tomography (CT) scan of the abdomen and pelvis with and without contrast is usually the most helpful. CT scans provide an adequate view of many of the causes of abdominal pain and are most useful due to the wide range of problems that can be revealed. Vascular lesions such as abdominal aortic aneurysms or aortic ruptures are well visualized using CT scans, as are diverticulitis, pancreatitis, appendicitis, and bowel obstructions. A CT scan is superior to simple radiographs in detecting pneumoperitoneum specifically and perforated viscus generally. A spiral (or helical) CT of the urinary tract is comparable to intravenous pyelography (IVP) for imaging kidney stones and urinary obstructions. With certain exceptions, a CT scan is the single most effective way to confirm a diagnosis or, upon its failure to confirm a suspected diagnosis, to dictate the need for additional further testing.

Ultrasound or sonography is another highly useful diagnostic tool. It involves the formation of a two-dimensional image used for the examination and measurement of internal body structures and the detection of bodily abnormalities. The advantages of ultrasound include low cost, low risk (due to the absence of contrast materials), reliable imaging of biliary systems, and more reliable imaging of the female pelvic organs. Ultrasound is the most reliable method to diagnose biliary disease. Because as many as 25% of biliary stones are isodense to bile, these stones cannot be visualized via CT scan. Exceptions to the general rule exist in the cases of obese individuals, where the study can be technically difficult, and those instances in which the skill and experience of the operator are substandard. Ultrasound has been used for focused study of the appendix, but spiral CT scans have been shown to be more accurate for diagnosing appendicitis. An exception to this general rule is pregnant women, for whom ultrasound is the test of choice. Ultrasound can also be helpful in children who are unable to remain still for the duration of a CT scan.

Magnetic resonance imaging (MRI) is a useful test in certain situations. The magnetic resonance cholangiopancreatography (MRCP) is a noninvasive way to obtain high-quality images of the biliary tree and the liver paranchyma. MRCP is uniquely effective for patients who are unable to tolerate the administration of contrast or who are obese and patients for whom CT or ultrasound has shown lesions that need further characterization or for whom endoscopic retrograde cholangiopancreatography (ERCP) poses a significant risk. MRI has recently been used to visualize pancreatic cancer, but it has not proven to be any more useful than CT scans in this regard.

In some cases endoscopy, colonoscopy, or angiography may be indicated. Further discussion of these tests can be found in the individual sections later in this chapter.

The systematic approach to abdominal pain will be grouped by general region of symptoms. Conditions that are more likely to be managed primarily by family physicians will be discussed in greatest detail while conditions requiring referral are focused on the primary care physician's initial diagnosis.

Seidel HM et al: Abdomen. In: *Mosby's Guide to Physical Examination*, ed 3. Mosby-Year Book, 1995.

Thompson WG et al: Functional bowel disorders and functional abdominal pain. In: *The Functional Gastrointestinal Disorders*, ed 2. Drossman DA et al (editors). Degnon Associates, 2000.

DYSPEPSIA

General Considerations

The word "dyspepsia" first appeared in the early eighteenth century to describe a person's ill humor, indigestion, or disgruntlement. The modern family practitioner uses the term to describe a set of symptoms that can encompass several different diseases and the etiology associated with them. Chronic or recurrent discomfort centered in the upper abdomen is the description most commonly used by clinicians for dyspepsia. Dyspepsia can be associated with heartburn, belching, bloating, nausea, or vomiting. Common etiologies include PUD and GERD. Rare causes include gastric and pancreatic cancers.

Dyspepsia is reported to affect 40% of the world's adult population and accounts for 2–3% percent of all visits to primary care providers. Only a small portion (about 10%) of the vast number of adults suffering from the condition seek medical advice for dyspepsia. Approximately 15–25% of dyspepsia is caused by PUD and 5–15% is caused by GERD.

No specific etiology is found for approximately 50–60% of patients who present with epigastric pain. When a patient has suffered at least 3 months of dyspepsia without a definitive structural or biochemical explanation, the clinical term applied is nonulcer dyspepsia and, less commonly, functional dyspepsia. Other etiologies that occur infrequently include gastric or esophageal cancer, biliary tract disease, gastroparesis, pancreatitis, carbohydrate malabsorption, medication-induced symptoms, non-GI diseases affecting the stomach (sarcoidosis, diabetes, and thyroid and parathyroid diseases), metabolic disturbances (hypercalcemia and hyperkalemia), hepatoma, intestinal parasites, and other cancers, particularly pancreatic cancer.

The history is often similar, whether the symptoms are from PUD, GERD, or nonulcer dyspepsia. Studies have shown that the symptoms and the degree of symptoms do not correlate with the findings on endoscopy.

The physical examination is also similar. There may be tenderness in the midepigastric area. Unless an ulcer has perforated, causing signs of peritonitis, the rest of the abdominal examination is unremarkable.

The treatment for dyspepsia depends on the etiology and will be discussed in the different sections on PUD, GERD, and nonulcer dyspepsia.

Bazaldua OV, Schneider FD: Evaluation and management of dyspepsia. Am Fam Physician 1999;60:1773.

McNamara DA, Buckley M, O'Morain CA: Nonulcer dyspepsia: current concepts and management. Gastroenterol Clin North Am 2000;29(4):807.

1. Peptic Ulcer Disease

General Considerations

The four major causes of ulcers include *Helicobacter pylori*-induced ulcers, nonsteroidal antiinflammatory drugs (NSAIDs), acid hypersecretory conditions, and idiopathic ulcers.

There is clear evidence to support the eradication of *H pylori* in patients who have documented ulcers. In the 1980s *H pylori* was associated with 90% of peptic ulcers. In the late 1990s *H pylori* was associated with 60–70% of all peptic ulcers. This decrease is related to increased treatment of *H pylori* infections. *H pylori* infections have been commonly associated with low income, low educational levels, and overcrowded living conditions. African-Americans and Hispanics have about a one-third higher rate of infection than white Americans. In the United States, 40% of all adults are infected with *H pylori* by the time they reach 50 years of age, compared to only 5% of all children aged 6–12 years. In developing countries, children are more commonly infected at a younger age and there is a higher incidence of infection throughout the entire population.

Pathogenesis

Infection with *H pylori* is the leading cause of peptic ulcers and use of NSAIDs is the second leading cause. In the United States, one in seven individuals uses NSAIDs. Of long-term NSAID users 5–20% have an ulcer when an upper endoscopy is performed. Risk factors for developing an ulcer due to NSAID use are a personal history of ulcer, age over 65 years, current steroid use, use of anticoagulants and/or a history of cardiovascular disease, or the impairment of another major organ. NSAIDs are prescribed to nearly 40% of all persons over the age of 65. Elderly patients who commence a course of treatment with NSAIDs have a 1–8% chance of being hospitalized within the first year of therapy for GI complications caused by NSAIDs. Patients who are *H pylori* positive and who are taking NSAIDs have a higher risk of complications.

Prevention

Eradication of *H pylori* infection prior to starting a course of treatment with NSAIDs reduced the risk of developing an ulcer early in the treatment.

Clinical Findings

As with most diagnosis of abdominal pain, the history obtained provides the majority of information used to focus the differential diagnosis. Factors pointing toward PUD include a gnawing pain with the sensation of hunger, a prior personal or family history of ulcers, tobacco use, and/or a report of melena.

The diagnostic test of choice is esophagogastroduodenoscopy (EGD), which allows both visualization and biopsy of the ulcer as well as testing for *H pylori*.

Complications

In the elderly (over 80 years old) who have ulcers the incidence of complications is much higher in patients who are taking aspirin and are *H pylori* infected. The eradication of *H pylori*, if present, should be considered prior to beginning long-term aspirin therapy. A hypersecretory condition, such as Zollinger–Ellison syndrome, is suspected in patients who have multiple ulcers and is caused by a gastrin-producing tumor. To complicate matters further, there is an increasing incidence of idiopathic ulcers in the U.S. population at large.

Treatment

Treatment of peptic ulcers requires the initial eradication of *H pylori* if present, stopping or reducing the dose of NSAIDs, and treatment with an H_2 blocker or a proton pump inhibitor (PPI) (see Table 29–2 for evaluation for *H pylori*-related disease). Many Food and Drug Administration (FDA)-approved treatment regimens exist to eradicate *H pylori*. They usually include two or three antibiotics plus a PPI or an H_2 blocker for 10–14 days. Because antibiotic resistance changes and subsequently recommended treatment options change it is necessary to refer to current guidelines either locally or from the Centers for Disease Control and Prevention (CDC). Treatment of the *H pylori* infection facilitates the healing of the ulcer and decreases the rate of recurrence in the first year from 75% to only 10%. Medical treatment of peptic ulcer has become very effective and surgical intervention needs to occur less frequently. When surgery is performed it is more commonly done with a laparoscopic repair.

Chan FK et al: Randomised trial of eradication of *Helicobactor pylori* before non-steroidal anti-inflammatory drug therapy to prevent peptic ulcers. Lancet 1997;350:97.

Megraud F, Marshall BJ: How to treat *Helicobacter pylori*: first-line, second-line, and future therapies. Gastoenterol Clin North Am 2000;29(4):759.

Meurer LN, Bower DJ: Management of *Helicobacter pylori* infection. Am Fam Physician 2002;65:1327.

Smoot DT, Go MF, Cryer B: Peptic ulcer disease. Prim Care 2001; 28(3):487.

2. Gastroesophageal Reflux Disease

Clinical Findings

Heartburn is the single most common symptom of GERD. Ten percent of the U.S. population experiences heartburn at least once per day and almost 50% experience symptoms at least once per month. Other common symptoms include regurgitation, belching, and dysphagia. GERD can also be associated with multiple

Table 29–2. Evaluation for *Helicobacter pylori*-related disease.[1]

Clinical Scenario	Recommended Test	Levels of Evidence[2] and Comments
Dyspepsia[3] in patient with alarm symptoms for cancer or complicated ulcer (eg, bleeding, perforation)	Promptly refer to a gastroenterologist for endoscopy	A
Known PUD, uncomplicated	Serology antibody test; treat if result is positive	A—Best evidence for eradication in presence of documented gastric or duodenal ulcer
Dyspepsia in patient with previous history of PUD not previously treated with eradication therapy	Serology antibody test; treat if result is positive	A
Dyspepsia in patient with PUD previously treated for *H pylori* results	Stool antigen or urea breath test; if positive, treat with regimen different from the one previously used; retest to confirm eradication; consider endoscopy	B—Urea breath test should be delayed for 4 weeks following treatment, as acid suppression can lead to false-positive results
Undifferentiated dyspepsia (without endoscopy)	Serology antibody test; treat if result is positive	B—Supported by cost–benefit analyses and recent small RCTs
Documented nonulcer dyspepsia (after endoscopy)	Unnecessary	B—RCTs and meta-analyses on this topic are mixed but indicate that few patients benefit from treatment
GERD	Unnecessary	B—GERD is not associated with *H pylori* infection
Asymptomatic with history of documented PUD not previously treated with eradication therapy	Serology antibody test; treat if result is positive	C
Asymptomatic	Screening unnecessary	C

[1]PUD, peptic ulcer disease; GERD, gastroesophageal reflux disease; RCT, randomized controlled clinical trial.
[2]Levels of evidence: A, strong evidence, based on good-quality RCTs or meta-analysis of RCTs; B, moderate evidence, based on high-quality cohort studies, case-control studies, or systematic reviews of observational studies or lower-quality RCT; C, based on consensus or expert opinion.
[3]Defined as pain or discomfort centered in the upper abdomen and persisting or recurring for more than 4 weeks.

extraesophageal symptoms and conditions. Pulmonary conditions that can be caused by GERD include asthma, chronic bronchitis, aspiration pneumonia, sleep apnea, atelectasis, and interstitial pulmonary fibrosis. Ear, nose, and throat manifestations of GERD include chronic cough, sore throat, hoarseness, halitosis, enamel erosion, subglottic stenosis, vocal cord inflammation, granuloma, and possibly cancer. Noncardiac chest pain, chronic hiccups, and nausea are also associated with GERD.

Changes in body position tend to exacerbate the symptoms of GERD, particularly lying down or bending forward. Complications include Barrett's esophagus, esophageal strictures, ulceration, hemorrhage, and, rarely, perforation. Of all patients who undergo an upper endoscopy for GERD, 8–20% are found to have Barrett's esophagus.

The esophagus has three mechanisms in place to try to prevent mucosal injury. The lower esophageal sphincter creates a barrier to acid reflux. Peristalsis, gravity, and saliva provide acid clearance mechanisms. The third defense mechanism is epithelial resistance.

Diagnosis is made using the medical history and treatment with H_2 receptor antagonists, prokinetic agents, or PPIs. Symptomatic improvement following treatment can be indicative of GERD. Upper endoscopy fails to reveal 36–50% of all patients who have been diagnosed via esophageal pH monitoring. Endoscopy should always be performed if alarming symptoms are present such as bleeding, weight loss, or dysphagia, especially if the alarm symptoms occur in an elderly patient.

Treatment

Treatment of GERD involves life-style modification and medication. Life-style modifications that have the greatest impact in reducing symptoms of GERD and that also provide positive health benefits include cessation of smoking, temperance in the consumption of alcohol, weight loss in the case of overweight patients, and reduction of dietary fat intake. Certain foods that decrease lower esophageal sphincter (LES) pressure (chocolate), stimulate acid secretion (coffee, tea, and cola beverages), or produce symptoms by their acidity (orange or tomato juice) should be avoided. Medicines that can irritate the mucosa (aspirin and NSAIDS) should be avoided or used only sparingly. Other medicines to avoid if possible include α-adrenergic antagonists, anticholinergics, β-adrenergic agonists, calcium channel blockers, diazepam, narcotics, progesterone, and theophylline.

Medication treatment options are designed to decrease the acid or increase the defense mechanisms. Commonly used over-the-counter medications include antacids, gaviscon, and H_2 blockers. Prescription medicines include prescription strength H_2 blockers, PPIs, prokinetic agents (Reglan), bethanechol, and sucralfate.

In addition, elevating the head of the bed by 6 inches, avoiding bedtime snacks, and reducing meal size, particularly the evening meal, can all help ameliorate symptoms of GERD.

If the patient's symptoms have resolved or significantly improved with the above treatment then no further evaluation is needed. If the symptoms have not improved, usually within 1–2 weeks, then endoscopy would be the next step. Symptoms do not always correlate with the pathology seen at the time of endoscopy. Even as symptoms improve over time there still may be a risk of developing long-term complications. Patients who have developed Barrett's esophagus need closer follow-up and monitoring as they have a 50- to 100-fold increased risk of developing esophageal cancer.

Isolauri J et al: Natural course of gastroesophageal reflux disease: 17-22 year follow-up of 60 patients. Am J Gastroenterol 1997;92(1):37.

Richter JE: Extraesophageal manifestations of gastroesophageal reflux disease. Clin Perspect 1998;1:28.

3. Nonulcer Dyspepsia

General Considerations

Nonulcer dyspepsia (NUD), also referred to as idiopathic or functional dyspepsia, is defined as a minimum of 12 consecutive or nonconsecutive weeks of persistent or recurrent dyspepsia without evidence of organic disease, not relieved by defecation, and not associated with the onset of change in stool frequency or form (which would indicate irritable bowel syndrome). NUD is divided into four groups based on their symptoms: ulcer-like dyspepsia, reflux-like dyspepsia, dysmotility-like dyspepsia, and nonspecific dyspepsia.

There is overlap between the four different groups and with irritable bowel syndrome (IBS). It has been suggested that separating the functional GI symptoms of dyspepsia and IBS may be inappropriate.

Pathogenesis

The pathophysiology of nonulcer dyspepsia is not entirely clear and is probably multifactorial. Suggested causes include changes in gastric physiology, nociception, motor dysfunction, central nervous system dysfunction, and pyschological and environmental factors (see the section on IBS). *H pylori* and its effects on NUD are highly controversial. A percentage of patients with NUD and *H pylori* have significant improvement in their symptoms after using eradication therapy, yet improvement cannot be guaranteed. Approximately 50% of patients with NUD are *H pylori* positive.

Clinical Findings

NUD is diagnosed by excluding other causes of dyspepsia. The "gold standard" is the esophagogastroduodenoscopy (EGD). Cost effectiveness data indicate that testing for *H pylori* and treating the patient if it is found decrease the amount of EGDs performed by approximately one-third.

Treatment

Management of NUD is multifactorial and includes making a diagnosis early and explaining as much physiology as possible to the patient. It is important for the physician neither to investigate excessively nor to investigate the presenting symptoms alone. New investigation in a patient who has been previously diagnosed with NUD should be done whenever alarm symptoms present (weight loss, vomiting, or blood in the stool) or if there is a new objective symptom. It is important for the physician to determine why the patient with chronic symptoms presented at this particular time.

Psychosocial factors can exacerbate symptoms, so it is important for physicians to address these issues and offer counseling. A mainstay of management is postevaluation reassurance of the patient concerning the diagnosis and the absence of alarm symptoms. Patients should avoid any food or substance that tends to exacerbate symptoms (NSAIDS, alcohol, tobacco, and certain foods). Not all patients want or need to take prescription medicine. For these patients other treatment options should be explored. If symptoms of bloating or postprandial fullness are present, the patient should eat six small meals per day, which may help ameliorate symptoms.

A remarkable number of different medicines have been used in studies of NUD. Confounding the results is the fact that the studies do not use the same definition for NUD and do not differentiate between the different symptom types. For example, PPIs appear to have some benefit in ulcer-like dyspepsia whereas patients with dysmotility-like dyspepsia do not respond. Medicines that have been used include antacids, H_2 blockers, PPIs, bismuth, and sucralfate. Prokinetic agents such as metoclopramide have been poorly studed. Cisapride, which was taken off the market, showed a two-fold decrease in symptoms over placebo. Domperodone, which is not available in the United States, has been shown to be superior to placebo and does not produce central nervous system side effects as it does not cross the blood–brain barrier. Peppermint oil and caraway oil have been compared to cisapride with similar results. Motilin agonists such as erythromycin increase the rate of gastric emptying. Visceral analgesics such as fedotozine reduce gastric hypersensitivity. Buspirone and 5-HT_1 agonists such as sumatriptan are promising in tests that have been done. Antispasmodics such as dicyclomine have not been shown to be more effective than placebo in patients with dyspepsia. Antinausea agents such as ondansetron and perchlorperazine have been shown to provide modest symptom improvement with the second agent having more side effects. Antihistamines such as dimenhydrinate and cyclizine decrease gastric dysrhythmias. Promethazine has been used to treat mild nausea. Of the antidepressants only tricyclic antidepressants have been studied in functional dyspepsia. Selective serotonin reuptake inhibitors have had some promising results with other functional bowel diseases (IBS).

Other approaches that are being used include acupuncture, acupressure, and gastric electrical stimulation. However, there are no randomized, double-blind controlled trials to evaluate their effectiveness. After discussing if medications are needed and writing a prescription if necessary, physicians should schedule a follow-up appointment to assess the patient's function and to determine if there are any responses to the treatment.

Smucny J: Symptomatic treatment and *H. pylori* eradication therapy for nonulcer dyspepsia. Am Fam Physician 2001;64(9): 1605.

Talley NJ: Therapeutic options in nonulcer dyspepsia. J Clin Gastroenterol 2001;32(4):286.

DISEASES OF THE GALLBLADDER

General Considerations

The three main causes of abdominal pain related to the gallbladder are biliary colic, gallstones, and cholecystitis.

Approximately 10% of the U.S. population have gallstones and are at greater risk of developing complications related to diseases of the gallbladder. Cholecystectomy, removal of the gallbladder, is the most com-

monly performed abdominal surgical procedure. Risk factors for gallstones and other diseases of the gallbladder can be easily remembered by the mnemonic **ABCDEFGHI:**

A—Older age: 80% of men and women in their 90s have gallstones.

B—Body habitus: obesity or rapid weight loss.

C—Childbearing.

D—Drugs: contraceptive steroids, hormone replacement therapy (HRT) estrogen and progesterone, and ceftriaxone (Rocephin).

E—Ethnicity: Pima Indians, Scandinavians, and African-Americans are hospitalized at approximately 40% the rate of white Americans.

F—Family: a family history of gallstones in a first-degree relative increases the likelihood of developing gallstones by 4.5 times.

G—Gender: women have double the prevalence of gallstones than men in each age group except the very elderly.

H—Hyperalimentation or fasting.

I—Ileal and other metabolic diseases [Crohn's disease, alcoholic cirrhosis, hypertriglyceridemia, diabetes, low high-density lipoprotein (HDL) cholesterol, and hyperparathyroidism].

Biliary Colic

The pain associated with biliary colic is actually not colicky in nature. It tends to be fairly constant in its intensity. Pain from biliary colic comes on suddenly and usually last less than 3 h. It is caused by a spasm of the cystic duct, usually when obstructed by a stone. Biliary colic is not associated with fat intolerance. As compared to acute cholecystitis, the body temperature is normal. Any pain associated with the gallbladder may radiate to the right shoulder, right scapula, right clavicular area, or back.

Biliary colic lacks specific laboratory abnormalities. The white blood cell count might be slightly elevated, but LFTs are usually within normal limits.

The physical examination reveals midepigastric or RUQ pain. If there are peritoneal signs then the examination is not consistent with uncomplicated biliary colic and other diagnoses need to be included in the differential.

Gallstones

Cholelithiasis, stones located in the gallbladder, and choledocholithiasis stones located in the extrahepatic bile ducts (common bile duct), both present with similar types of pain in the RUQ. Multiple factors contribute to the formation of gallstones. Hypersecretion of cholesterol accelerates crystallization of the cholesterol. Gallbladder hypomotility and decreased contractility lead to bile stasis. Of gallstones 70–80% contain more than 50% cholesterol and are referred to as cholesterol stones. Black stones contain 20–30% cholesterol and are related to increased production of conjugated bilirubin. Brown stones contain less than 20% cholesterol and are related to bacterial invasion with the stone matrix coming from bacterial synthetic products.

Of patients with gallstones 66% are not aware that they have them. There is a 1–4% per year risk of developing symptoms in patients who have asymptomatic gallstones. Patients presenting with symptoms most commonly present with biliary colic without complications. Once patients present with symptoms they are very likely to have recurrent symptoms. One study found that 50% of patients had recurrent symptoms within 1 year. Up to 30% of patients will not have a recurrent episode and will never need to have a cholecystectomy.

Cholecystitis

Acute cholecystitis is the most frequent complication of gallstones. Inflammation of the gallbladder occurs after impaction of the cystic dust by a gallstone 90% of the time. Ten percent of the time acute cholecystitis occurs without a stone being present (acalculus cholecystitis). Frail elderly men more commonly have acalculus cholecystitis as opposed to stone-related acute cholecystitis, which occurs more frequently in young otherwise healthy women. Recurrent episodes of acute cholecystitis lead to thickening of the gallbladder walls with loss of contractility and concentrating functions.

Another complication of gallstones is pancreatitis, which will be discussed in the next section.

The physical examination is similar to that of biliary colic. However, in acute cholecystitis the pain may last longer than 3 h, there is usually a fever, and one in five patients have mild jaundice. One-third of patients have a palpable gallbladder, particularly on the first attack. As stated earlier, Murphy's sign—the cessation of inspiration during palpation of the RUQ when the patient takes a deep breath—is often positive.

Laboratory findings include leukocytosis with a left shift, mild elevations in serum transaminase and alkaline phosphatase, mild elevation of bilirubin (2–4 mg/dL), and nonspecific elevations of amylase and lipase.

The principal imaging study of the gallbladder is ultrasound. A distended bile-filled gallbladder improves imaging of gallstones, so a patient should have an ultrasound done after 8 h of fasting. Ultrasound is a less sensitive imaging study for choledocholithiasis and gallstone complications such as abscess, perforation, and

pancreatitis. A CT or MRI is noninvasive and can provide the same information. An ERCP is the gold standard for diagnosis of choledocholithiasis. It is usually performed in the setting of acute cholecystitis with elevated LFTs or amylase and lipase. Another test occasionally utilized is cholescintigraphy (HIDA, DISIDA), used when acute cholecystitis is suspected and on an emergent basis in a nonfasting patient. A normal scan virtually rules out acute cholecystitis.

Treatment

Treatment of patients with biliary colic and asymptomatic gallstones usually involves observation. If no further episodes of pain occur then no further treatment is needed. Symptomatic gallstones and/or recurrent episodes of cholecystitis are usually treated with a cholecystectomy, most commonly performed laproscopically. Patients with acute cholecystitis should be admitted to the hospital for hydration and bowel rest. If the patient appears toxic or if a complication is suspected such as perforation, antibiotics that cover gram-negative enteric bacteria should be given. Patients with choledocholithiasis need endoscopic intervention. Emergent ERCP is indicated if obstructive jaundice or cholangitis is present.

Ahmed A, Cheung RC, Keeffe EB: Management of gallstones and their complications. Am Fam Physician 2000;61:1673.

Kalloo AN, Kantsevoy SV: Gallstones and biliary diseases. Prim Care 2001;28(3):591.

PANCREATITIS
General Considerations

Pancreatitis can vary from a very mild, self-limited disease to fulminate pancreatitis with subsequent hypovolemia, shock, acute respiratory distress syndrome (ARDS), and multisystem organ failure. Acute pancreatitis is an acute inflammatory process that occurs after activated digestive enzymes are released into the interstitium resulting in autodigestion. Chronic pancreatitis occurs when there is progressive loss of structure and function of the pancreas and can be associated with steatorrhea and diabetes mellitus.

Acute pancreatitis was the reason for hospitalization in approximately 215,000 cases in 1993, with 33% of the patients being over the age of 65 years. The incidence of pancreatitis increased 10-fold from 1960 to 1980. The mortality rate is 5–10% overall and 20–25% in the elderly.

Pathogenesis

The etiology of pancreatitis is varied with the most common causes being related to gallstones or alcohol intake. Between 10% and 30% of cases of pancreatitis are still idiopathic. Other miscellaneous causes include genetic (cystic fibrosis), developmental abnormalities, hyperlipidemia, metabolic abnormalities, neoplasms, vascular disease, medications, infections, trauma, and autoimmune disorders.

Gallstones are the cause of approximately 50% of the cases of pancreatitis and may be a factor in many idiopathic cases. Gallstones are frequently found in the feces of pancreatitis patients even if they are not observed on ultrasound or CT. Alcohol is responsible for at least 30% of cases of pancreatitis in the United States.

Clinical Findings

A. Symptoms and Signs

Abdominal pain caused by pancreatitis tends to be diffuse throughout the entire upper abdomen with frequent radiation to the back. Pain is usually moderate to very severe and can last for hours with little relief from parenteral narcotics. Nausea and vomiting are often present at the time of presentation and may persist for hours.

On physical examination the patient may appear to be in mild distress or can appear toxic with hypotension, tachycardia, fever, and tachypnea. In more severe cases mental status may be altered. If gallstones are present in the common bile duct the patient may appear jaundiced. Auscultation reveals decreased bowel sounds secondary to ileus and possible decreased breath sounds in the left lung base secondary to pleural effusion. Palpation of the abdomen shows tenderness in the upper abdomen with guarding. Diffuse peritoneal signs with rigidity are not usually present. Ecchymosis in the flanks (Gray Turner sign) or of the periumbilical region (Cullen sign) can be a result of extravasation of pancreatic exudates.

B. Laboratory Findings

Laboratory tests including amylase, lipase, white blood cell count (WBC), and LFTs can be helpful. Amylase is widely available and quite sensitive but is not specific for pancreatitis. Lipase has similar sensitivity yet has higher specificity as almost all lipase originates from the pancreas. Lipase can be elevated in association with renal insufficiency and other intraabdominal conditions similar to acute pancreatitis, although it is usually less than three times normal. A greater than three times normal lipase is very sensitive and specific for acute pancreatitis. WBCs, glucose, and transaminase can also be elevated; however these tests are better used to assess severity and prognosis.

Ranson's criteria are used to assess severity and prognosis. Eleven factors are evaluated: five on admission and the remaining six during the initial 48 h of admission. Poor prognosis is indicated by age >55 years, WBC >16,000/mm^3, glucose >200 mg/dL, lactate dehydrogenase >350 IU/L, and aspartate aminotransferase >250 U/L in the initial tests at admission. The remaining six criteria that reflect the development of systemic complications include hematocrit decrease of >10 mg/dL, BUN increase of >5 mg/dL, calcium <8 mg/dL, PaO$_2$ <60 mm Hg, base deficit >4 mEq/L, and fluid sequestration >6 L. Other criteria have been developed to identify early prognostic indicators.

A commonly used scoring system is the Acute Physiology and Chronic Health Evaluation (APACHE-II), which uses 12 items: temperature, mean arterial pressure, heart rate, respiratory rate, oxygenation, arterial pH, sodium, potassium, creatinine, hematocrit, WBC, and the Glasgow coma score. The patient's age and severity of other chronic health problems are added to the previous 12 items.

C. Imaging Studies

Several imaging techniques can be used to evaluate for pancreatitis. Plain radiographs of the abdomen may show anterior displacement of the stomach with separation of the contour from the transverse colon secondary to pancreatic exudate. An ileus, calcified gallstones, and the colon cutoff sign may be seen. The colon cutoff sign occurs when exudate from the pancreas inflames the colon, with the inflammation producing colonic spasm that results in dilatation of the proximal colon.

CT is the study of choice for imaging the pancreas, assessing pancreatitis and its possible complications, and helping to differentiate pancreatitis from other diseases with a similar presentation. A CT scan may not be necessary in patients with mild acute pancreatitis. It is necessary in patients with a Ranson score greater than 3, an APACHE-II score greater than 8, no response to conservative management in 48–72 h, or who are deteriorating. A CT scan may show fluid collections, pseudocysts, or pancreatic necrosis.

Ultrasound may be used, particularly if biliary causes are suspected. ERCP is mainly used to remove a common bile duct stone that has caused obstruction in severe gallstone pancreatitis. The role of the MRI in evaluation of acute pancreatitis remains to be defined.

Treatment

Determining the severity of pancreatitis helps predict the course and define the management plan. Clinical monitoring detects about 39% of severe cases. Because clinical monitoring is not adequate to monitor disease progression it is important to use severity classification systems such as Ranson or APACHE-II. A five-point increase in the APACHE-II score has been associated with an increase in intensive care unit (ICU) deaths.

Mild acute pancreatitis is usually managed with supportive therapy including fluid replacement and pain management. Demerol is often used secondary to the risk that morphine may cause the sphincter of Oddi tone to increase. There is no clear evidence that morphine exacerbates the disease process. A nasogastric tube may be useful if there is an ileus or if there is intractable nausea and vomiting. It is otherwise not needed for the treatment of pancreatitis. Antibiotics are generally not needed for mild pancreatitis. There is no clear evidence as to when to refeed patients who have mild acute pancreatitis. General practice is to restart small meals after abdominal pain has decreased, bowel sounds have returned, and the patient has an appetite. H_2 blockers and PPIs have not been shown to decrease or prevent recurrence of pain.

Severe pancreatitis usually necessitates intensive care with a multidisciplinary approach. Severe systemic complications that can occur include cardiovascular collapse, renal failure, hypovolemia, shock, respiratory failure, ARDS, metabolic disturbance, congestive heart failure (CHF), MI, acute fluid collections, diffuse intravascular coagulation (DIC), and/or GI bleeding. Purtscher's angiopathic retinopathy can occur; it presents with a sudden onset of blindness, does not relate to the severity of the disease, and its pathogenesis is unknown. Encephalopathy with mental status changes can occur; fortunately this is a rare complication of severe pancreatitis. Necrotizing pancreatitis often involves infection and can lead to sepsis, which accounts for more than 80% of deaths from acute pancreatitis. Late complications that can occur include pseudocysts and abscesses. Although a multitude of different medical treatment options have been studied, none has been proven to be of benefit. Surgical intervention may be necessary including debridement, particularly if infected necrosis of the pancreas occurs.

Trying to prevent a recurrence of pancreatitis by avoiding any known offending agent (alcohol, cholecystectomy if related to gallstones) is the goal after the first episode.

Munoz A, Katerndahl DA: Diagnosis and management of acute pancreatitis. Am Fam Physician 2000;62:164.

IRRITABLE BOWEL SYNDROME

General Considerations

Estimates indicate that symptoms consistent with a diagnosis of IBS are present in from 3% to 20% of adult Westerners. Although IBS occurs worldwide, cultural and social factors affect its presentation. In Western countries, women have a higher incidence of the condition and are more likely to consult a physician. In India and Sri Lanka men have a higher incidence of IBS. In black South Africans, IBS symptoms are common in people who live in urban zones and are unusual in people who live in rural areas. In the United States, prevalence is similar between blacks and whites and some studies show a lower prevalence in Hispanics from Texas and Asians from California.

There are between 2.4 and 3.5 million physician visits a year for IBS in the United States, for which 2.2 million prescriptions are written. IBS accounts for up to 40% of gastroenterology referrals, often perceived by GI specialists as very difficult. Primary care providers see a larger percentage of patients suffering from IBS than GI specialists. Primary care physicians also find patients with symptoms of IBS less difficult to manage than patients with pelvic pain, headache, and backache, especially with regard to difficulty in distinguishing functional IBS from organic disease, satisfying the patient, and time consumption. Primary care providers in Canada estimated that they referred approximately 14% of their patients with symptoms of IBS to specialists. In the United Kingdom, 29% of patients were referred to specialists. Follow-up evaluation showed that of all patients diagnosed with IBS by their primary care provider, 91% actually had a functional bowel disease (IBS), indicating that the majority of the time the primary care providers accurately diagnosed the condition.

A large percentage of individuals (up to 50%) with symptoms consistent with a diagnosis of IBS never seek a doctor's care. Those who do have often had a major life event such as a death in the family or loss of their job before presenting with GI complaints.

Pathogenesis

The physiology contributing to symptoms of IBS has not been elucidated. Many theories exist, including disturbance in motility, altered perception either locally in the GI tract or in the central nervous system, visceral hypersensitivity, mucosal inflammation, autonomic nerve dysfunction, and/or psychological disturbance, but no theory works for every patient who has symptoms of IBS. In one study a positron emission tomography (PET) scan was used to examine the activity of the brain when GI symptoms were induced. Patients with IBS did not activate the anterior cingulate cortex that is associated with opiate binding but did activate the prefrontal cortex that is associated with hypervigilance and anxiety. Studies of whether patients with IBS have a lower threshold of pain with colonic distention are inconclusive. All that can be stated with reasonable certainty is that studies have not clarified whether symptoms of IBS are a normal perception of an abnormal function or an abnormal perception of a normal function.

Clinical Findings

A. SYMPTOMS AND SIGNS

IBS belongs to a group of functional bowel disorders (ie, no organic cause can be identified) in which abdominal discomfort or pain is associated with defecation or a change in bowel habits and with features of disordered defecation. Diagnostic criteria developed by the Rome Consensus Committee for IBS are at least 12 or more weeks, not necessarily consecutive, in the preceding 12 months of abdominal discomfort or pain that is characterized by two of the following three features: (1) it is relieved with defecation, (2) its onset is associated with a change in frequency of stool, and/or (3) its onset is associated with a change in the form and/or appearance of the stool.

The Bristol Stool Form Scale (Figure 29–1 and Table 29–3) is used as a standard description for seven types of stool forms. Other symptoms that support the diagnosis of IBS include abnormal stool frequency (more than three/day or less than three/week), abnormal stool form (lumpy/hard or loose/watery), abnormal stool passage (straining, urgency, or feeling of incomplete evacuation), passage of mucus, and a sensation of bloating or feeling of abdominal distention.

Table 29–3. The Bristol Stool Form Scale.

Type	Description
1	Separate hard lumps like nuts (difficult to pass)
2	Sausage shaped but lumpy
3	Like a sausage but with cracks on its surface
4	Like a sausage or snake, smooth and soft
5	Soft blobs with clear-cut edges (passed easily)
6	Fluffy pieces with ragged edges, a mushy stool
7	Watery, no solid pieces, entirely liquid

Stool form has been demonstrated to be reflective of GI transit time. Using the Bristal Stool Form Scale and frequency of bowel movements is more diagnostically precise and useful than using the imprecise terms diarrhea and constipation, which can have different meanings to different patients. Patients may complain of feeling constipated, attributable to a feeling of incomplete evacuation despite having just passed soft or watery stool.

B. HISTORY

The patient history is the single most useful tool in diagnosing IBS. Continuity of care and a well-established rapport contribute significantly to obtaining an accurate and exhaustive history. Allowing patients the first 1–2 min to "tell their story" not only contributes to a high level of patient satisfaction, but also improves information gathering and diagnosis with a decrease in time spent in consultation. When physicians missed clues that where being offered by their patients, the appointment took longer. A positive physician–patient interaction, including a psychosocial history, precipitating factors, and a discussion of diagnosis and treatment with patients, results in fewer return visits for IBS and lower utilization of health care resources. Chronic/recurrent abdominal pain indicates a need to assess quality of life. In one study undergraduate students with IBS had quality of life scores that were similar to patients with CHF, indicating a significant impact by IBS symptoms.

A history of abuse should be sought in patients with chronic abdominal pain. A study at a tertiary care gastroenterology clinic reported that 60% of the overall study population, all female, reported a history of physical or sexual abuse. The self-reported history of abuse was highest for those with functional bowel disease (up to 84%) and lowest for those with organic bowel disease, such as ulcerative colitis (38%). Of course not all patients with IBS have a history of abuse, but it is worthwhile to overtly assess a patient's psychosocial stressors as they can affect the success of the course of treatment. A physician should always assess for abuse when considering referral to a gastroenterologist. Family physicians, due to the continuous nature of their

Type 1	
Type 2	
Type 3	
Type 4	
Type 5	
Type 6	
Type 7	Entirely liquid

Figure 29–1. Bristol Stool Form Scale. See Table 29–3 for standard description for each of the seven types.

contact with patients and their biopsychosocial training, are uniquely positioned to assess and address issues associated with abuse.

Patients with IBS have not been demonstrated to have a higher incidence of psychiatric diagnosis such as depression, anxiety, somatization, stress, lack of social support, or abnormal illness behavior compared to other patients presenting with abdominal pain of organic origin. However, patients presenting with abdominal pain do have more psychosocial abnormalities than control subjects without abdominal pain. Psychosocial factors have not been shown to be helpful in differentiating between organic and functional abdominal disease, but they have been helpful in understanding some of the health-seeking behavior.

Stressful life events such as the death of a family member or loss of a job often precede the onset of symptoms of IBS. Although such stressful life events may not be the cause of IBS, they might factor into the decision by patients to seek care for their symptoms. In women who have symptoms of IBS, the decision to seek care has been shown to have a significant and positive correlation between daily stress levels and daily symptoms of IBS.

In gathering the history of a patient with IBS, signs or symptoms of an anatomic disease should be absent. These might include the fever, GI bleeding, unintentional weight loss, anemia, and abdominal mass. Physicians should assess for laxative use as laxatives could be a significant cause of IBS-like symptoms.

Patients with IBS may have had surgery, particularly appendectomy, or women may have had a hysterectomy or ovarian surgery. The most common discharge diagnosis of patients admitted to the hospital for abdominal pain is "nonspecific abdominal pain." A study of patients discharged with the diagnosis of "nonspecific abdominal pain" showed that 37% of women and 19% of men met the criteria for IBS 1–2 years after discharge. Of such patients 70% had other prior attacks of abdominal pain and at the initial admission only 6% of the charts had IBS listed in the differential diagnosis. Of patients presenting with acute pain of less than 1 week in duration 50% had symptoms of IBS at the time of admission. It appears that assessing for diagnostic criteria of IBS symptoms can reduce the length of hospitalization and reduce the extent of testing and thus decrease the cost of treatment of patients presenting with acute abdominal pain who do not need immediate surgical intervention.

C. Physical Examination

The physical examination is usually fairly unremarkable, except for some abdominal tenderness and an increased likelihood of abdominal scars.

D. Special Tests

No specific testing is required for diagnosis of IBS, although some physicians would be reassured by a normal CBC and ESR. Patients who meet the criteria to screen for colon cancer (older than 50 or a family history of colon cancer) should be examined by either flexible sigmoidoscopy or colonoscopy. A colonoscopy should always be performed if there is a family history of colon cancer. Other tests to consider are *Clostridium difficile* toxin if the patient has been on antibiotics recently, stool evaluation for giardiasis in areas in which giardiasis is common (Rocky Mountains), and serology or gluten elimination diet for evaluation for celiac disease.

Treatment

A. Therapeutic Relationship

Treatment options are varied. A therapeutic relationship is critical to the management of IBS. The therapeutic relationship is achieved by obtaining the history through a nondirective, patient-centered interview, being nonjudgmental, eliciting the patient's understanding of the illness and his or her concerns, identifying and responding realistically to the patient's expectation for improvement, setting consistent limits, and involving the patient in the treatment approach. The most effective treatment option is explanation and reassurance. A confident diagnosis based on the above clinical criteria helps explain that the symptoms are not associated with a higher risk of other diseases such as cancer or GI bleeding and helps the patient to understand that IBS symptoms are chronic in nature, are very likely to wax and wane over time, and may not ever completely go away. Patients' reasons for seeking care at the time they did and whether any psychosocial issues are contributing to the symptoms should be assessed. Counseling regarding psychosocial stressors in patients' lives may not resolve all the symptoms of IBS, but may help patients to better cope with the symptoms.

B. Diet

Many different dietary approaches have been tried. Patients in whom gas-forming vegetables, lactose, caffeine, or alcohol exacerbate symptoms should be counseled to minimize their exposure to the offending substance. Food intolerance and elimination diets have not been proven to be effective. Dietary fiber has been shown to improve symptoms of constipation, hard stools, and straining, particularly if 30 g of fiber is consumed each day. Patients often need to gradually increase the amount of fiber to improve adherence, as a sudden increase can lead to increased symptoms of bloating and gas. The most common reason for failure of a high-fiber diet is insufficient dose. Fiber is very safe and inexpensive and should be routinely recommended, particularly to patients for whom constipation is a component of their IBS symptoms.

C. HERBAL MEDICATIONS

A meta-analysis of five double-blind, placebo-controlled randomized trials suggested a significant (p <0.001) positive effect of peppermint oil compared to placebo. Peppermint oil was given as a monopreparation in a dosage range of 0.2–0.4 mL. A randomized controlled trial of Chinese herbal medicine indicated that both a standardized herbal formulation as well as individualized Chinese herbal medicine treatment improved symptoms of IBS compared to placebo.

D. HYPNOTHERAPY AND PSYCHOTHERAPY

Hypnotherapy has been studied regarding its effectiveness in treating patients with symptoms of IBS. Dramatic improvements in a high proportion of patients with poorly controlled IBS symptoms were seen for both individual and group hypnotherapy. Therapeutic audiotapes are easy to use and low cost, although somewhat inferior to hypnotherapy.

Psychotherapies rely on the relationship between the therapist and the patient and can vary according to that relationship, which makes them difficult to evaluate in a randomized, controlled way.

E. DRUGS

Drugs have been used for the treatment of IBS without proven benefit and with some troublesome side effects. A meta-analysis that concluded that smooth muscle relaxants and anticholinergics were better than placebo has been criticized for methodological inadequacies. The most frequently used drugs and most common complaints that they are used to treat include the following:

> **Constipation:** psyllium, methylcellulose, calcium polycarbophil, lactulose; 70% sorbitol and polyethylene glycol (PEG) solution
> **Diarrhea:** loperamide, cholestyramine
> **Gas, bloating, or flatus:** simethicone, β-D-galactosidase (Beano)
> **Abdominal pain:** anticholinergics/antispasmodics
> **Chronic pain:** tricyclic antidepressants, selective seratonin reuptake inhibitors

Patients seeing their family physician on a consistent and regular basis with the purpose of reassurance, reinforcement, and explanation combined with communication in a positive therapeutic relationship can prevent the continual quest by patients for a "miracle" cure for IBS.

Levy RL et al: The relationship between daily life stress and gastrointestinal symptoms in women with irritable bowel syndrome. J Behav Med 1997;20(2):177.

Lewis SJ, Heaton KW: Stool Form Scale as a useful guide to intestinal transit time. Scand J Gastroenterol 1997;32:920.

Owens DM, Nelson DK, Talley NJ: The irritable bowel syndrome: long-term prognosis and the physician-patient interaction. Ann Intern Med 1995;122:107.

Thompson WG et al: Irritable bowel syndrome in general practice: prevalence, characteristics, and referral. Gut 2000;46:78.

APPENDICITIS

General Considerations

Appendicitis can occur in people of any age, but is most common in older children to young adults. When appendicitis occurs in young children or in the elderly, the presentation is often not classic. There does not seem to be any race or gender predilection, although diagnosis in females can be more difficult.

Pathogenesis

The appendix is a long diverticuli extending from the cecum. It has a long lumen. When this lumen is occluded, appendicitis results. The most common cause of obstruction of the lumen is proliferation of lymphoid tissue, often associated with viral infections, Epstein–Barr virus (EBV), upper respiratory infection (URI), or gastroenteritis. Lymphoid tissue proliferation is the most common cause of appendicitis in the young adult. Other causes of occlusion include tumors, foreign bodies, fecolith, parasites, or complications of Crohn's disease.

Clinical Findings

A. SYMPTOMS AND SIGNS

The most important indicator in the diagnosis of appendicitis is history. It is crucial because missing the diagnosis of appendicitis can cause severe complications. There are six historical indicators that should be examined. In close to 100% of patients there is abdominal pain, usually right lower quadrant (RLQ) pain, often preceded by periumbilical pain. Also in nearly 100% of patients there is anorexia. Ninety percent of patients have nausea, with vomiting in around 75% of patients. The progression of abdominal pain from periumbilical to RLQ is present around 50% of the time as is the classic progression of appendicitis from vague abdominal pain to anorexia/nausea/vomiting to RLQ pain to low-grade fever.

B. Physical Examination

Careful examination of the abdomen is very helpful in diagnosing appendicitis. Inspection then palpation then percussion of the abdomen can often identify the cause of abdominal pain. Other helpful signs on physical examination include the peritoneal signs, rigidity, rebound tenderness, guarding, and low-grade fever (100.4°F, 38°C).

It is important to perform a pelvic examination on all women who present with RLQ pain to rule out multiple gynecological causes. A thorough respiratory and genitourinary examination is often helpful as well. A rectal examination is useful only when the diagnosis remains unclear, and thus should not be used unless necessary.

There is some debate about the use of analgesics during the evaluation of possible appendicitis. Traditional practice suggested that pain medication may mask important signs or symptoms, although a recent study showed that the use of analgesic, specifically tramadol, did not compromise the ability to identify acute appendicitis. In fact, although pain was decreased in many patients, specific signs related to appendicitis were more clearly evident with the use of analgesic. Additional studies suggest that informed consent is compromised by not using adequate pain medication. The use of an observational unit can be helpful as well to examine the progression of signs and symptoms.

C. Laboratory Findings

There are many laboratory studies performed routinely on patients with abdominal pain. However, very few if any are truly helpful in the diagnosis and management of the patient with possible appendicitis. In fact, laboratory studies can often be misleading and delay diagnosis in cases of appendicitis. The WBC has classically been used, but studies suggest that there are few times when this is helpful diagnostically. If the WBC is less than 7000, it is unlikely that the patient has appendicitis. If the WBC count is greater than 19,000, the patient has a greater than 80% chance of having appendicitis. The presence of neutrophilia makes the diagnosis of appendicitis more likely, but is not diagnostic. The presence of increased WBC with neutropenia is generally accompanied by increased C-reactive protein levels. The presence of all three is not diagnostic, but the absence of all three does rule out appendicitis.

The routine use of a chemistry examination is helpful only to determine the level of dehydration. UA commonly shows some leukocytosis and some increased red blood cells (RBCs). Despite these common findings, it is more often misleading than helpful. The most important use of UA is as a screening test for urinary tract infection (UTI). All women of childbearing age should have a pregnancy test.

D. Imaging Studies

The CT scan is the single best test for diagnosing appendicitis. US can be useful in situations in which a CT is not possible. Plain radiographs can be misleading and are not diagnostic in most cases. The cost of a complete abdominal series is about the same as that of a CT. US is very helpful, is less invasive, and is cost efficient. It can be considered normal only if a normal appendix is seen. If the appendix is retoperitoneal or pelvic, it can be difficult to visualize. US is most helpful in women in whom other pathologies can be identified. It is also a good choice in children because of the lack of contrast and easier patient compliance with the test. US can be used in pregnant patients to evaluate the appendix. CT is more sensitive and more specific and provides access to visualization or many other possible problems. If the diagnosis of appendicitis is suspected, a focused helical CT without contrast can be performed in less than an hour and can be very specific for appendicitis.

Treatment

Treatment has not changed in several hundred years. The treatment is surgical removal of the inflamed appendix. The methods for removal have changed slightly. There are two choices: laparotomy or laparoscopic assisted. Laparotomy is a faster, simpler procedure. Laparoscopy allows visualization of other possible causes. Laparoscopy is more expensive and has a higher rate of complications.

Hardin DM: Acute appendicitis: review and update. Am Fam Physician 1999;60:2027.

Schrock TR: Appendicitis. In: *Gastrointestinal and Liver Disease: Pathophysiology/Diagnosis/Management,* ed 6. Feldman M et al (editors). W.B. Saunders, 1998.

INFLAMMATORY BOWEL DISEASE

General Considerations

A careful study of the epidemiology of inflammatory bowel disease (IBD) demonstrates that it is currently in a state of flux. In spite of the confusion, environmental factors appear to contribute to the occurrence of the condition. IBD is most common in northern regions of northern countries, occurs most frequently in whites, especially those who are Jewish, and has been found to be more common in higher socioeconomic populations.

Environmental factors may make IBD more prevalent in people who work indoors and less prevalent in manual laborers who work outdoors. There is a 20–50% increase in the prevalence of IBD in first-degree relatives, and a 50-to 100-fold increase in the offspring of patients afflicted with IBD.

Risk factors seem to include work environment and diet. There is a difference among the subtypes of IBD with regard to risk factors. Smoking appears to decrease the risk of ulcerative colitis (UC) but to increase the risk of Crohn's disease (CD). Birth control pills seem to increase the risk of CD. There is some evidence in support of these findings, but further studies are needed.

Pathogenesis

The etiology of these diseases is unknown. There are many theories related to infection, autoimmune disorders, as well as environmental factors. There appear to be genetic factors as well.

Clinical Findings

A. SYMPTOMS AND SIGNS

IBD has several subtypes, the most common being UC and CD. Both can present with abdominal pain. UC can have associated abdominal pain, but almost always presents with perirectal pain and bloody diarrhea. On the other hand, CD more commonly causes abdominal pain, and can be more difficult to differentiate from other diseases based on history and physical examination alone. The pain with CD is most often RLQ. This is due to the fact that the terminal ileum is involved in 85% of cases.

B. PHYSICAL EXAMINATION

Unfortunately the physical examination is not very specific. Evaluation of the rectum for evidence of fissures, ulceration, or abscess can be helpful. Fullness or a palpable mass can suggest associated abscess. But generally, the examination reveals nonspecific generalized tenderness, with focal findings depending on the extent and activity of the disease. Skin examination may be useful as CD is associated with erythema nodosa, whereas UC is associated with pyoderma gangrenosa.

C. LABORATORY FINDINGS

Recommended laboratory tests include ESR, CBC, LFTs, albumen, electrolytes, B_{12} level, folate level, and stool studies. The ESR is elevated in 80% of patients

with CD and 40% of patients with UC. Anemia is often related to the disease as a result of iron deficiency and blood loss. There is often leukocytosis with increased eosinophilia. LFTs are needed because there can be liver involvement with CD. Albumen is an indicator of malnutrition associated with malabsorption. Stool studies are important to rule out infectious etiologies of colitis.

D. IMAGING STUDIES

There are many imaging options for IBD. The most accurate test is the colonoscopy, as this allows direct visualization of the mucosa and biopsy. Use of colonoscopy is not recommended in the setting of acute active disease. Plain films can be most helpful when looking for toxic megacolon, or if "thumbprinting" is seen, as with bowel wall edema. The classic string sign can be seen on barium enema. Abdominal CT can be useful for diagnosis and management of IBD. CT is most helpful in identifying abscesses, fistulas, bowel wall thickening, and fat stranding.

Treatment

Management of IBD includes immunosuppressive therapy, nutritional support, psychological support, and surveillance for cancer. The risk of colon cancer related to UC is higher than that of CD. Current recommendations involve colonoscopy with biopsy annually for UC. There are no set guidelines for cancer screening in CD because of the variations in areas of disease involvement and unclear risk. However, the risk of other types of cancer, such as adenocarcinoma of the jejunum and ileum (when involved in disease), lymphoma, and squamous cell carcinoma of the vulva and rectum, is increased in CD.

Familial counseling is also important to help family members cope with the many exacerbations of the disease. Genetic counseling is needed because of the strong inheritance factor in this disease.

Chutkan RK: Gastroenterology: inflammatory bowel disease. Prim Care 2001;128(3):539.

Hyams J: Inflammatory bowel disease. Pediatr Rev 2000;l21(9): 291.

DIVERTICULITIS

General Considerations

The epidemiology of diverticulitis has been changing over the past hundred years. It is directly related to the increase in diverticulosis. Diverticulitis occurs in 10–25% of patients with diverticulosis. In the twentieth century, the incidence of diverticulosis increased as fiber intake decreased. In addition to insufficient fiber, age is the single greatest risk factor contributing to diverticulosis. Typically, diverticulosis is seen in patients 60 years of age and older. It is uncommon before age 40, and is present in 50% of people over the age of 90 years. There is an increased prevalence of left-sided diverticuli in patients of Western descent and an increased prevalence of right-sided diverticuli in people of Asian descent.

Pathogenesis

The pathology of diverticulitis is directly related to the anatomy of the bowel wall. A true diverticuli consists of outpouching of all three layers: mucosa, submucosa, and muscular layer. However, in most cases of diverticulitis, there are only pseudodiverticulae. These consist of a herniation of the mucosa and submucosa through the muscular layer. The diverticulae tend to form in rows between the mesenteric and lateral teniae. The area of penetration of the vasa recta has the greatest muscular weakness. This area is therefore the most common site of herniation. Lack of dietary fiber contributes to development of diverticuli. As fiber content of the stool decreases, the colonic pressure increases and the transit time decreases. These changes result in high pressure in the colon, which essentially blows out areas of weakness in the colon wall.

Diverticulitis occurs when there is infection associated with one or more of these diverticuli. There can be micro- or macroperforations of the diverticuli, resulting in bowel contents contacting the peritoneum and infecting the pericolonis fat, mesentery, and associated organs. This process can be localized and can result in the development of an abscess or peritonitis or in the formation of a fistula. The most common fistula is a colovesical fistula.

Clinical Findings

A. Symptoms and Signs

Diverticulitis commonly presents with left lower quadrant (LLQ) pain, which is seen in 93–100% of cases. However, pain can be right sided, especially in patients of Asian descent. Commonly, patients have nausea, vomiting, constipation, or diarrhea. Dysuria and urinary frequency can also be present. Complicated diverticulitis, as with a colovesical fistula, can present with recurrent urinary tract infections. If there is macroperforation, diffuse abdominal pain is present. Although LLQ pain is the most common, diverticulitis can occur with right lower quadrant (RLQ) pain. When this is the case, a duration of 3 or more days is suggestive of diverticulitis rather than appendicitis.

Examining the vital signs gives some evidence supportive of the diagnosis of diverticulitis. The presence of temperature at or greater than 100.7°F and the presence of tachycardia are consistent with diverticulitis. Fever is present in 57–100% of cases.

B. Physical Examination

The examination should include a complete abdominal examination. Signs suggestive of diverticulitis include tender LLQ (or RLQ in more infrequent right-sided cases), signs of peritoneal irritation such as guarding or tenderness to percussion, and occasionally the presence of a tender mass, which is suggestive of abscess. The rectal examination may demonstrate rectal tenderness or occasionally a tender rectal mass.

C. Imaging Studies

Patients suspected of having diverticulitis should have a CBC and UA. Flat and upright abdominal films, or CT of the abdomen and pelvis if the diagnosis is less clear, should be obtained. There is frequently an increased WBC count with a high prevalence of polymorphonuclear leukocytes. Leukocytosis is present in 69–83% of cases. There can be anemia if there is associated diverticular bleeding. UA can show evidence of inflammation if there is irritation of the peritoneum surrounding the bladder or evidence of infection if a fistula is present.

The abdominal films can show evidence of free air, ileus, or mass. If the diagnosis is in doubt, a CT of the abdomen and pelvis can help clarify the cause of pain. In cases of diverticulitis, CT shows a thickened colonic wall and can show an abscess if present. These same findings can be seen on US, but CT best confirms diverticulitis because it reveals the presence and location of an abscess more easily. Ureteral obstruction, fistula, or air in the bladder can also be seen. The CT will show and allow for percutaneous drainage of an abscess. The US can also be used to identify inflammation in the colon and allow for percutaneous drainage of an abcess.

Treatment

Treatment depends on the severity of the disease and the health of the patient. Outpatient treatment includes a clear liquid diet and oral broad-spectrum antibiotics. Current recommendations include ciprofloxacin and metronidazole for 7–10 days. Due to the ever-changing nature of antibiotic treatment and variations of resistance in different areas, the CDC guidelines or Sanford antibiotic recommendations should be followed. Pain medications such as morphine should be avoided as they increase colonic pressure and contribute to the problem.

If there are signs and symptoms of inflammation such as fever and leukocytosis, hospitalization is needed.

Patients should have complete bowel rest, intravenous fluids, and intravenous broad-spectrum antibiotics such as cefoxitin. Meperidine can be used if needed, as it decreases intraluminal pressure. A nasogastric tube is not needed unless there is significant ileus or obstruction. Most patients should improve in 48–72 h, at which time they can resume diet, change to oral antibiotics, and be discharged home with close follow-up. If needed, invasive studies, such as colonoscopy, should be delayed 4–6 weeks. A high-fiber diet is recommended for all patients. Surgical resection is recommended for some.

Surgery is not recommended after the first attack because the recurrence rate is only 20–30%. The incidence of recurrence increases with each subsequent attack and therefore surgery should be considered after the second or third attack. An exception to this is patients under 40 years of age. Younger patients tend to have more aggressive disease and more complications, and thus should consider surgery after the first attack.

Additionally, there is a specific type of diverticulum, called Meckel's diverticulum, that can present with abdominal pain, nausea, vomiting, or intestinal bleeding. The pathology of this is different. This diverticulum is a congenital anomaly of the GI tract that can cause pain and bleeding. This tissue often contains gastric or pancreatic tissue. It can cause complications including diverticulitis, intussusception, perforation, and obstruction. The best test for diagnosis is the technetium-99m pertechnetate scan. Treatment is surgical.

Marinella MA, Mustafa M: Acute diverticulitis in patients 40 years of age and younger. Am J Emerg Med 2000;18(2):140.

ABDOMINAL WALL PAIN

There are many presentations of abdominal wall pain because there are many different causes of abdominal wall pain. Several examination findings might suggest the abdominal wall as the source of pain. The lack of evidence for an intraabdominal process is a good first indicator. When visceral problems have been ruled out, the physician should look for abdominal wall abnormalities. The pain is usually not related to meals or bowel function, but is related to posture. Often a trigger point can be found. Most of the time there is a positive Carnett's sign.

Carnett's sign is elicited by having the patient tense the abdominal muscles and then examining the patient's abdomen. Places that are tender prior to tensing the abdomen and that are still tender afterward are considered positive and are suggestive of the abdominal wall as the source of pain. Most visceral pain will decrease with this maneuver. Causes of abdominal wall pain include hernias, herpes zoster, neuromas, hematomas of the ab-

dominal wall or rectus sheath, desmoid tumor, endometriosis, myofascial tears, intraabdominal adhesions, neuropathies, slipping rib syndrome, and general myofascial pain.

Hernias

Types of hernias include inguinal, femoral, umbilical, epigastric, spigelian, and Richter's hernia. These are more commonly found on examination rather than from the history. The history can be suggestive of many types of hernias, although it can be confusing if there is herniation of the bowel wall or omentum. Bowel herniation will cause visceral pain and obstruction, whereas omentum herniation will cause visceral pain with no signs of obstruction. A history of prior surgery, especially laparoscopic surgery, increases the likelihood of the presence of a hernia.

Certain hernias are more common in certain patients. Males more typically develop inguinal hernias, whereas women tend to develop femoral hernias. Umbilical and epigastic hernias are more common in obese or gravid patients. The spigelian hernia, a hernia along the border of the arcuate ligament, is most common in athletes.

Richter's hernia is defined by the pathology rather than the location of the hernia. The side of the bowel wall herniates rather than the entire bowel segment. Because this type of hernia results in subtle findings there is often a delay in diagnosis and therefore a higher fatality rate. The epidemiology of patients with Richter's hernia has changed over the years. It is generally found in women over 50 years old, but is increasing in frequency in young men, primarily due to an increase in laparoscopic procedures. Because the size of the instruments used for laparoscopy is small, the abdominal wall defect left after surgery can allow only a portion of the bowel wall to herniate. It is a tight hernia, resulting in strangulation of the tissue that passes through. On examination, prior surgical sites must be examined. Erythema at these sites is a bad sign. There is often a slight bulge that is confused with adenopathy or fat tissue.

A CT scan can be used to identify hernias. However, these are often overlooked by the radiologist unless the radiologist is focused on more thoroughly examining the abdominal wall.

Hernias are best treated surgically. If surgery is contraindicated, hernias that cause pain or pose a risk of bowel obstruction can be treated with a truss or other restrictive garment.

Rectus Sheath Hematoma

Rectus sheath hematoma can be equally difficult to diagnose. They tend to occur more commonly in elderly or pregnant patients. The epigastric vessels are sheared, resulting in intramuscular bleeding. The shearing can occur from trauma or twisting motions. Again, the history is the most important factor in helping to direct the clinician. A history of unilateral mid-abdominal pain, use of anticoagulants such as aspirin or coumadin, and abdominal trauma are all important risk factors for hematoma. On examination, the pain is worse when patients tense their abdominal muscles. The pain is unilateral. There is often a palpable mass within the rectus sheath.

Coagulation studies and blood count are the most useful laboratory studies. Helpful imaging studies include CT, US, and MRI. Ultrasound is the cheapest and most useful study if the diagnosis is highly suspected. CT is more useful for identifying other possible causes. MRI is sometimes helpful if the diagnosis remains unclear. Treatment is generally expectant, but severe cases may warrant reversal of coagulation abnormalities, administration of fluids, or even surgical evacuation and ligation or coagulation of vessels.

Herpes Zoster

Any time there is an abrupt onset of severe abdominal wall pain, herpes zoster should be suspected. The pain associated with zoster can precede the rash by more than 1 week, although commonly it is only 2–4 days. Zoster occurs most frequently in patients over the age of 50 years. There can be postherpetic neuralgia (PHN) causing similar pain in patients with a history of zoster. PHN increases in frequency in patients as they get older, with most patients over 60 years. A good history and close follow-up are the best way to establish this diagnosis. Prophylactic treatment includes the varicella vaccine. Treatment of acute herpes zoster with acyclovir, valacyclovir, or famciclovir in combination with a prednisone taper seems to decrease the incidence and severity of PHN. Treatment of PHN has proven difficult. Many modalities have been tried with only minor success. Treatments include analgesics, narcotics, nerve stimulation, antidepressants, capsaicin, biofeedback, and nerve blocks.

Other Causes of Abdominal Wall Pain

Surgical scars are the location of many causes of abdominal wall pain. Hernias are frequently present at the site of scars as previously discussed. Endometriosis can recur at the site of surgical scars and neuromas often form at the border of scars. Other unusual causes include desmoid tumors, myofascial tears, and intraabdominal adhesions. The desmoid tumor is a dysplastic tumor of the connective tissue that tends to form in young adults and can be identified only after surgical removal. Myofascial tears and intraabdominal adhesions occur most frequently in athletes.

Treatment

Most abdominal wall pain has a trigger point that reproduces the pain. Finding this point can help in both diagnosis and treatment. These trigger points are often found along the lateral border of the rectus abdominis muscle where nerve roots can become stretched, compressed, and irritated. These points are also found at areas of tight fitting clothing or at insertion points of muscles. The Carnett's sign is useful for diagnosis of trigger points.

Management of this type of pain can be difficult. Patient education and reassurance are both very important. Preventing further unnecessary testing can be helpful to patients by decreasing their concerns about the pain. Explaining the nature of the pain and its origins helps patients deal with the pain. Tricyclic antidepressants can be useful at low doses.

Treatment of many etiologies of abdominal wall pain can be achieved by injection. This treatment can be both diagnostic and therapeutic. It is necessary to find the point of greatest tenderness, usually an area less than 2 cm. Insertion of the needle into the correct point should elicit intense pain, but the pain should improve dramatically with injection. Lidocaine or an equivalent should be used. For areas that require more than one injection, a small amount of steroid can be used as well. Steroids should be avoided in areas near hernias or into fascia, as they can cause hernia formation. Dry needling has been shown to be as useful, but the initial treatment is followed by more pain at first. For patients with severe needle aversion, a therapeutic trial of a transcutaneous lidocaine patch can be considered. Pain clinics can help patients with more difficult cases.

Edlow JA et al: Rectus sheath hematoma. Ann Emerg Med 1999; 34(5):671.

Suleiman S, Johnston DE: The abdominal wall: an overlooked source of pain. Am Fam Physician 2001;64(3):431.

WEB SITES

American Academy of Pain Management
www.aapainmanage.org
American Pain Society
www.ampainsoc.org

GYNECOLOGICAL CAUSES OF ABDOMINAL PAIN

Gynecological causes of abdominal pain can be separated into three categories: acute causes in the nonpregnant patient, chronic problems in the nonpregnant patient, and acute causes in the pregnant patient. Acute causes include PID, adnexal torsion, ruptured ovarian cyst, hemorrhagic corpus luteum cyst, endometriosis, and tuboovarian abscess. Chronic causes in the non-pregnant patient include dysmenorrhea, mittelschmerz, endometriosis, obstructive müllerian duct abnormalities, leiomyomas, cancer, and pelvic congestion syndrome. In the pregnant patient causes include ectopic pregnancy, retained products of conception, septic abortion, and ovarian torsion. Psychological factors can greatly contribute to pain related to the abdomen and pelvis. Patients can present with acute pain after a sexual assault.

Because of the wide differential, a careful history and a pregnancy test are both very important when evaluating females with abdominal pain. The history should include the last menstrual period, a detailed menstrual history, a sexual history including possible assault, and a family history. The physical examination should include careful abdominal, pelvic, and recto-vaginal examinations. Laboratory evaluation is based on specific findings from the physical examination. In evaluating PID LFTs can identify possible Fitz–Hughes–Curtis syndrome, especially in the presence of RUQ pain.

The incidence of PID is 11% in American women of reproductive years, although it is rare in pregnancy. Numerous biological factors contribute to a higher incidence of PID in adolescents. There is a lower prevalence of protective chlamydial antibodies. The cervical mucus is more penetrable. The larger zones of cervical ectopy with more columnar cells are more vulnerable to bacterial and viral agents. Other risk factors that increase the likelihood of PID include early age at first sexual intercourse, a higher number of lifetime partners, or a new partner within the last 30–60 days. Diagnosis of PID requires the presence of abdominal pain, adnexal pain, cervical motion tenderness, and at least one of the following: temperature >101°F, vaginal discharge, leukocytosis >10,500/mm^3, positive cervical cultures, intracellular diplococci, or white blood cells on vaginal smear. Treatment varies depending on whether the patient requires inpatient or outpatient treatment. Inpatient treatment is required if there is a surgical emergency, pregnancy, no response to outpatient therapy in 72 h, nausea and vomiting, or immunodeficiency.

Endometriosis is found in 15–32% of women undergoing laparoscopy for evaluation of abdominopelvic pain. This type of pain is generally cyclical but can present acutely with rupture of an ovarian endometrioma. On physical examination, a retroverted, fixed uterus with ash spots on the cervix suggests endometriosis. Conservative treatment includes the use of NSAIDs and oral contraceptive pills.

Most gynecological causes of abdominal pain are best evaluated with pelvic ultrasound. Sometimes laparoscopy is needed, which is often therapeutic as well, as in the case of ovarian torsion. CT can help delineate unclear findings from US. Consultation or follow-up with a gynecologist is often warranted.

Baines PA, Allen GM: Genitourinary emergencies: pelvic pain and menstrual related illnesses. Emerg Med Clin North Am 2001;19(3):763.

Anemia

30

Brian A. Primack, MD, EdM, & Kiame J. Mahaniah, MD

General Considerations

A. ADULTS

Anemia is defined as an abnormally low circulating red blood cell (RBC) mass, reflected by low serum hemoglobin (HGB). However, the normal range of HGB varies among different populations. For menstruating women, anemia is present if the HGB level is at or below 12 g/dL. In men and postmenopausal women, anemia is present if the HGB level is at or below 13–14 g/dL. Other factors, such as age, race, altitude, and exposure to tobacco smoke, can also alter HGB levels.

Anemia is usually classified by cell size (Table 30–1). Microcytic anemias, or those with mean corpuscular volume (MCV) <80 fL, are usually due to iron deficiency, chronic inflammation, or thalassemia. Macrocytic anemias, those with MCV >100 fL, are classified as megaloblastic or nonmegaloblastic. Megaloblasts, which are large, immature, nucleated precursors to RBCs, are seen with vitamin B_{12} deficiency and folic acid deficiency. Nonmegaloblastic causes of macrocytosis include alcoholism, hypothyroidism, and chronic liver disease. Normocytic anemia (MCV between 80 and 100 fL) can be due to hemolytic or nonhemolytic causes. Hemolysis can result from hereditary abnormalities of the cell contents or cell membrane. Hemolysis can also result from acquired insults caused by autoantibodies, alloantibodies (in, for instance, transfusion reactions), or a nonimmune process such as malaria or hypersplenism. Important nonhemolytic causes of normocytic anemia include poor production of RBCs due to aplastic anemia, renal insufficiency, and bone marrow infiltration.

B. CHILDREN

Normal HGB levels vary significantly with age. At birth, mean HGB is about 16.5 g/dL. This level increases to 18.5 g/dL during the first week of life, followed by a drop to 11.5 g/dL by 1–2 months of age. This physiological anemia of infancy is mediated by changes in erythropoietin levels. By 1–2 years of age the HGB level begins to rise, however, to 14 g/dL in adolescent girls and 15 g/dL in adolescent boys. Other relevant laboratory values also vary in children. The median MCV, for example, can be as high as 120 fL in premature infants and as low as 78 fL in 1-year-old infants. Thus, laboratory values in children should always be compared with age-appropriate norms.

Many inherited causes of anemia are discovered in infancy and childhood. It is therefore important to obtain a careful family history in an anemic child, especially if the episodes of anemia are intermittent. Sickle cell anemia, thalassemia, glucose-6-phosphate dehydrogenase deficiency, and spherocytosis are examples of inherited forms of anemia. When only males in a family are affected, glucose-6-phosphate dehydrogenase deficiency, which is X-linked, should be particularly considered.

Other elements of the history are also important when evaluating a child for anemia. Because infants with anemia can exhibit poor feeding, irritability, and tachycardia rather than classic adult symptoms and signs, these atypical features should be explored with the family. Nutrition should be evaluated carefully, with attention to dietary sources of vitamin B_{12}, folic acid, and iron. Potential sources of lead poisoning must also be considered. Finally, adolescents often require additional support and explanation. For instance, adolescent girls may not know what constitutes a normal menstrual period, so the specific number of tampons and pads used should be obtained.

Bomgaars L. Approach to the child with anemia. UpToDate Online 2000;11.

Brill JR, Baumgardner DJ: Normocytic anemia. Am Fam Physician 2000;62:2255.

Davenport J: Macrocytic anemia. Am Fam Physician 1996;53:155.

Huffstutler SY: Adult anemia. Adv Nurse Pract 2000;8:89.8.

Schrier SL: Approach to the patient with anemia. UpToDate Online 2002;11.

Table 30–1. Anemia classification by cell size.

Microcytic	Macrocytic
Iron deficiency	Megaloblastic
Anemia of chronic disease	Vitamin B_{12} deficiency
Thalassemias	Folic acid deficiency
Sideroblastic anemia	Drug related
	Nonmegaloblastic
	Hypothyroidism
	Liver disease
	Alcoholism
	Myelodysplastic syndromes

Normocytic	
Hemolytic	**Nonhemolytic**
Intrinsic	Acute blood loss
Membrane defects (spherocytosis)	Aplastic anemia
Enzyme deficiencies (G6PD deficiency)	Anemia of chronic disease
Hemoglobinopathies (sickle cell disease)	Chronic renal insufficiency
Extrinsic	Myelophthisis
Autoimmune	
Warm antibody mediated (chronic lymphocytic leukemia, systemic lupus erythematosus, idiopathic)	
Cold antibody mediated (*Mycoplasma*, idiopathic)	
Alloimmune	
Nonimmune	
Splenomegaly	
Physical trauma (thrombotic thrombocytopenic purpura, disseminated intravascular coagulation, burns)	
Infections (malaria)	

■ MICROCYTIC ANEMIA

IRON DEFICIENCY ANEMIA

ESSENTIALS OF DIAGNOSIS

- *Low iron levels, low serum ferritin, and elevated total iron-binding capacity.*
- *Response to therapeutic trial of iron.*
- *In adults, nearly always due to blood loss.*
- *Can also be due to poor iron intake or poor absorption.*

General Considerations

Iron deficiency is the most common cause of anemia. Up to 11% of women and 4% of men have iron deficiency. Only about 2% of women and 1% of men develop anemia due to the deficiency, however.

The average adult has 2–4 g of stored iron. About 65% of this reserve is located in the red blood cells, with the remainder in the bone marrow, liver, spleen, and other body tissues. Iron deficiency results from a net imbalance resulting from either excessive loss or poor intake.

Extracorporeal blood loss is the most common cause of iron deficiency anemia. When red cells are destroyed within the body, on the other hand, the reticuloendothelial system usually adequately recycles iron into the next generation of red blood cells. Poor iron uptake, due either to poor nutrition or inadequate absorption, is a less common cause of iron deficiency anemia.

Women develop iron deficiency more readily than men because of increased potential for iron loss. On average, women lose an additional 1 mg of iron each day due to menstruation. Pregnancy, lactation, and delivery additionally cost a woman an average of 1000 mg of iron each.

Clinical Findings

A. SYMPTOMS AND SIGNS

Iron deficiency can be asymptomatic, especially in the early stages. However, patients can present with varying degrees of any of the common symptoms associated with anemia, such as weakness, fatigue, dizziness, headaches, exercise intolerance, or palpitations. Possible signs on physical examination include tachycardia, tachypnea, and pallor, especially of the palpebral conjunctivae.

One symptom associated with iron deficiency in particular is pica—the craving for ice, clay, or other unusual substances that may or may not contain iron. Rare symptoms include koilonychia (spoon nails), blue sclerae, and atrophic glossitis. Esophageal webs, dysphagia, and iron deficiency characterize the Plummer–Vinson syndrome, a disease of unknown pathophysiology that can increase the risk of squamous cell carcinoma of the pharynx and esophagus.

B. LABORATORY FINDINGS

Hemoglobin levels can be normal in early iron deficiency. Mild deficiency yields HGB levels of 9–11 g/dL, whereas in severe deficiency levels can fall as low as 5 g/dL.

Serum iron levels below 60 µg/dL indicate iron deficiency. As iron stores are depleted, serum ferritin falls below 30 ng/dL. Total iron-binding capacity (TIBC) therefore rises above 400 µg/dL. Percent iron saturation, which is inversely proportional to TIBC, falls below about 15%.

Although serum ferritin levels are often useful in differentiating iron deficiency from other forms of microcytic anemia, it should be noted that ferritin is an acute phase reactant that can be elevated during acute illnesses, chronic inflammatory states, or cancer.

The peripheral blood smear is also a useful test. Iron-deficient red cells manifest varying degrees of hypochromia and microcytosis. However, the gold standard of iron deficiency is bone marrow examination, which shows absent iron reserves in affected patients. A Prussian blue stain is used to examine marrow iron stores.

Another method of diagnosis involves measuring a patient's response to oral iron therapy. Increased reticulocytosis several days after institution of oral iron treatment can be diagnostic.

Treatment

Iron can be increased in the diet. Foods particularly rich in iron include meats (especially liver) and fish. Whole grains, green leafy vegetables, nuts, seeds, and dried fruit also contain iron. Cooking with iron pots and pans also increases iron intake.

Oral iron therapy is available in the form of iron salts. One 300-mg tablet of iron sulfate, for example, delivers 60 mg of elemental iron. One 300-mg tablet of iron gluconate delivers 34 mg of elemental iron and may be better tolerated by some patients. Up to 180 mg of elemental iron can be given each day depending on the degree of deficiency. Absorption of oral iron is dependent on many environmental factors. An acidic environment increases absorption; thus iron tablets are often given with ascorbic acid. For this same reason, antacids should be avoided within several hours of iron ingestion. Other substances that impair the absorption of iron include calcium, soy protein, tannins (found in tea), and phytate (found in bran). Side effects of oral iron therapy include gastrointestinal distress and constipation. For this reason, some physicians routinely prescribe an as-necessary stool softener along with each iron prescription.

Iron can be given intramuscularly or intravenously to patients who cannot tolerate oral iron due to gastrointestinal upset. This route may also be convenient for patients who have concurrent gastrointestinal mal-absorption or ongoing blood loss, such as those with severe inflammatory bowel disease. Phlebitis, muscle breakdown, anaphylaxis, and fever are possible side effects of parenteral iron.

Brittenham GM et al: Clinical consequences of new insights in the pathophysiology of disorders of iron and heme metabolism. Hematology (Am Soc Hematol Educ Program) 2000;39.

Leung AK, Chan KW: Iron deficiency anemia. Adv Pediatr 2001; 48:385.

Massey AC: Microcytic anemia. Differential diagnosis and management of iron deficiency anemia. Med Clin North Am 1992; 76:549.

Rasul I, Kandel GP: An approach to iron-deficiency anemia. Can J Gastroenterol 2001;15:739.

ANEMIA OF CHRONIC DISEASE

 ESSENTIALS OF DIAGNOSIS

- *Presence of a chronic disease or chronic inflammation.*
- *Shortened RBC survival but poor compensatory erythropoiesis.*
- *High or normal serum ferritin and low TIBC.*

General Considerations

Many chronic diseases—such as cancer, collagen vascular disease, chronic infections, diabetes mellitus, and coronary artery disease—can be associated with anemia (Table 30–2). In spite of shortened RBC survival, bone marrow RBC production is low. This is thought to be

Table 30–2. Selected causes of anemia of chronic disease.

Chronic infections
  Abscesses
  Subacute bacterial endocarditis
  Tuberculosis
Collagen vascular disease
  Rheumatoid arthritis
  Systemic lupus erythematosus
  Temporal arteritis
Neoplasia
  Hodgkin's and non-Hodgkin's lymphoma
  Adenocarcinoma
  Squamous cell carcinoma

due to (1) trapping of iron stores in the reticuloendothelial system, (2) a mild decrease in erythropoietin production, and (3) impaired response of the bone marrow to erythropoietin.

Clinical Findings

A. SYMPTOMS AND SIGNS

The anemia of chronic disease (ACD) is often mild and therefore general anemic symptoms, such as fatigue, dizziness, and palpitations, can be low grade or nonexistent. Signs such as pallor of the palpebral conjunctivae are only sometimes present. The condition must therefore be suspected and investigated in patients known to have underlying conditions such as collagen vascular diseases, cancers, or chronic infections.

B. LABORATORY FINDINGS

Hemoglobin levels are generally mildly decreased (10–11 g/dL), but levels can occasionally be below 8 g/dL. RBCs are often hypochromic. MCV can be either normal (80–100 fL) or low (<80 fL). Because RBC production is poor, the absolute reticulocyte count is often low (<25,000/μL). Acute phase reactants such as erythrocyte sedimentation rate (ESR), platelets, and fibrinogen can be elevated.

Because ACD is associated with decreased production of transferrin, serum iron and TIBC are often both low. Calculated percent saturation (iron × 100/TIBC), however, remains normal. This is to be distinguished from iron deficiency anemia, in which TIBC is often high, resulting in low percent saturation. Serum ferritin is high or normal in ACD but low in iron deficiency anemia.

Treatment

Treatment of ACD should be aimed at the underlying condition. Symptomatic patients or heart patients often require packed red blood cell transfusions, especially if the hemoglobin count is <10 mg/dL.

Schrier SL: Anemia of chronic disease. UpToDate Online 2003;11.

Spivak JL: Iron and the anemia of chronic disease. Oncology (Huntingt) 2002;16:25.

Weiss G: Iron and anemia of chronic disease. Kidney Int Suppl 1999;69:S12.

THALASSEMIAS

 ESSENTIALS OF DIAGNOSIS

- *Elevated RBC count in spite of decreased HGB.*
- *Exaggerated microcytosis.*
- *Positive family history.*
- *Mediterranean or African heritage.*
- *Pattern of inheritance.*

General Considerations

One normal adult hemoglobin molecule, also known as hemoglobin A, consists of a heme moiety, two α hemoglobin chains, and two β hemoglobin chains. The thalassemias are the diverse group of genetic diseases resulting from abnormal hemoglobin due to defective α or β chains.

Other hemoglobin chains exist, such as γ and δ chains. Fetal hemoglobin consists of two α chains and two γ chains ($\alpha_2\gamma_2$), and hemoglobin A2 consists of two α chains and two δ chains ($\alpha_2\delta_2$). Although ordinarily these lesser types of hemoglobin comprise no more than 5% of the total amount of hemoglobin, the thalassemias are characterized by increased proportions of non-A hemoglobin because of defective α or β chains. These disorders are classified as α-thalassemias or β-thalassemias, based upon the abnormal gene.

Thalassemia traits are more common in those with Mediterranean, African, and South Asian ancestry. This is at least in part because these parts of the world are inhabited by *Plasmodium* species, and heterozygous thalassemic traits confer survival advantage to those afflicted with malaria.

Because there are four α hemoglobin genes per individual (two on each copy of chromosome 16), there are four major types of α-thalassemia. If only one α hemoglobin gene is damaged, the result is called α-thalassemia minima, an essentially asymptomatic condition. Damage to two different α hemoglobin genes results in α-thalassemia minor, which has only mild clinical significance. Three damaged α hemoglobin genes can lead to a relative abundance of β hemoglobin, causing an abundance of hemoglobin β4, also known as hemoglobin H. This disorder, also called hemoglobin H disease, is characterized by severe clinical manifestations of chronic hemolysis, hospitalizations, and decreased lifespan. Absence of normal α hemoglobin chains causes hemoglobin Barts disease and is fatal *in utero.*

The two β hemoglobin genes are found on chromosome 11. If one is damaged, β-thalassemia minor results, with few clinical effects. Infants with two damaged copies of β hemoglobin will be phenotypically normal at birth due to the predominance of fetal hemoglobin ($\alpha_2\gamma_2$). Affected infants become severely symptomatic in the first year of life, however, and usually die before age 5.

Clinical Findings

A. SYMPTOMS AND SIGNS

α-Thalassemia minima is almost always asymptomatic. α-Thalassemia minor can be accompanied by occasional mild symptoms of anemia, including headaches, fatigue, and dizziness. Patients with hemoglobin H disease, however, can exhibit severe clinical manifestations of chronic hemolytic anemia, including hepatosplenomegaly and cholelithiasis (due to bilirubin gallstones). These patients often require chronic transfusions, usually beginning in late childhood and adolescence. Patients with no normal α hemoglobin develop tetramers of γ hemoglobin *in utero,* known as hemoglobin Barts, which are inefficient at delivering oxygen to the tissues. The accompanying hypoxia results in high output congestive heart failure, severe edema, and hydrops fetalis.

The clinical appearance of β-thalassemia minor often mimics that of mild or moderate iron deficiency, and often laboratory findings are necessary to distinguish the two. β-Thalassemia major, however, results in a severe phenotype. Widespread hemolysis in these patients causes pallor, irritability, jaundice, and hepatosplenomegaly. Eighty percent of patients die in the first 5 years of life due to severe anemia, high-output congestive heart failure, or infection.

B. LABORATORY FINDINGS

As with iron deficiency, hemoglobin levels and MCV are often low with the thalassemias. In contrast to iron deficiency, however, thalassemias are usually characterized by an elevated RBC count. Furthermore, the decrease in MCV is often more exaggerated in the thalassemias; levels as low as 50–60 fL are not unusual. The red cell distribution width (RDW) can also be used to distinguish the two conditions. With iron deficiency, the RDW is elevated due to a variety of cell sizes, whereas the RDW is usually normal in thalassemic patients as RBCs are uniformly small.

Hemoglobin electrophoresis should be ordered for any patient with suspected thalassemia. Although some patients with α-thalassemia minima or media can have normal electrophoresis patterns, abnormalities are often seen in other thalassemic patients. In β-thalassemia minor, for example, relative proportions of fetal hemoglobin and hemoglobin A2 are increased.

Treatment

Patients with β-thalassemia minor, α-thalassemia minima, and α-thalassemia minor are generally asymptomatic and should be treated only if necessary. These patients may require blood transfusions under certain conditions, such as after vaginal delivery or surgery.

Patients with β-thalassemia major and hemoglobin H disease, however, require the care of a hematologist. These patients may require frequent transfusions and/or splenectomy. Iron overload is a frequent complication in these patients, both those with and without transfusion therapy. Chelation therapy is often required to avoid end-organ damage in the heart, endocrine organs, and liver.

Those with a personal or family history of thalassemia should be offered genetic counseling when planning a family.

Benz EJ: Clinical manifestations of the thalassemias. UpToDate Online 2002;11.

Schrier SL: Pathophysiology of thalassemia. Curr Opin Hematol 2002;9:123.

■ MACROCYTIC ANEMIA

VITAMIN B$_{12}$ DEFICIENCY

ESSENTIALS OF DIAGNOSIS

- *Macrocytosis.*
- *Serum vitamin B$_{12}$ <100 pg/mL.*
- *Hypersegmented neutrophils.*

General Considerations

Vitamin B$_{12}$ (cobalamin) is involved in two important enzymatic reactions: the conversion of methylmalonyl-coenzyme A (CoA) to succinyl-CoA and the methylation of homocysteine to methionine. This latter reaction is required for synthesis of thymidine, a component of DNA.

Since vitamin B$_{12}$ is present in all animal products, only people with unusual diets (vegans, fad dieters) receive inadequate intake. Some special populations, such as pregnant women, require increased levels of vitamin B$_{12}$.

Most of the time, however, vitamin B$_{12}$ deficiency reflects a defect in the B$_{12}$ absorption and transport chain. Vitamin B$_{12}$ is transported from the stomach to the jejunum by intrinsic factor (IF), a protein produced in gastric parietal cells. Pernicious anemia occurs when autoantibodies against parietal cells are produced, resulting in a lack of IF and inadequate uptake of vitamin B$_{12}$.

Clinical Findings

A. SYMPTOMS AND SIGNS

Many clinical features are common to all megaloblastic anemias: anemia, pallor, weight loss, fatigue, glossitis, lightheadedness, jaundice, and abdominal symptoms. Neurological symptoms are specific to vitamin B_{12} deficiency, however, beginning with paresthesias in the hands and feet. Disturbances in vision, taste, smell, proprioception, and vibratory sense can also occur. Untreated, vitamin B_{12} deficiency can lead to posterior spinal column demyelination, resulting in spastic ataxia and dementia mimicking that of Alzheimer's disease. These changes are often irreversible. Vitamin B_{12} deficiency can also lead to psychotic depression and paranoid schizophrenia.

B. LABORATORY FINDINGS

The MCV is usually above 100 fL, and vitamin B_{12} levels are usually below 100 pg/mL. Lactate dehydrogenase (LDH) and indirect bilirubin can be modestly elevated because of increased RBC destruction. The reticulocyte count can be depressed. Because DNA synthesis affects all cell lines, pancytopenia can occur. Peripheral blood smear can show markedly abnormal RBCs along with hypersegmented neutrophils, which are pathognomonic for megaloblastic anemia. There is evidence suggesting that early vitamin B_{12} deficiency can be diagnosed by elevated levels of homocysteine or methylmalonic acid.

Examination of the bone marrow shows erythroid hyperplasia and marked asynchrony in maturation between cytoplasmic components and nuclear material.

Although not as frequently used today, the Schilling test has historically been used to confirm the diagnosis of pernicious anemia. In the first stage, a large dose of intramuscular vitamin B_{12} is given, followed by oral ingestion of radiolabeled vitamin B_{12}. Patients with intact vitamin B_{12} absorption will have at least 7% of the oral dose present in urine. In the second stage, radiolabeled vitamin B_{12} is administered with IF. If pernicious anemia is the cause of vitamin B_{12} deficiency, a poor absorption rate in the first stage will be corrected by the combination of vitamin B_{12} and IF in the second stage.

Treatment

Treatment requires monthly parenteral treatment of 100 μg vitamin B_{12} along with concurrent administration of folate, 1–5 mg each day. Many advocate weekly vitamin B_{12} for the first month. Once vitamin B_{12} levels have been reestablished, oral therapy (1 mg/day) can then be substituted. Oral therapy alone may be sufficient.

Oh RC, Brown DL: Vitamin B12 deficiency. Am Fam Physician 2003;67:979.

Savage DG et al: Etiology and diagnostic evaluation of macrocytosis. Am J Med Sci 2000;319:343.

FOLIC ACID DEFICIENCY

 ESSENTIALS OF DIAGNOSIS

- *Reduced RBC or serum folate levels.*
- *Macrocytic anemia.*
- *Normal vitamin B_{12} levels.*
- *Hypersegmented neutrophils.*

General Considerations

In contrast to vitamin B_{12} reserves, which can last 3–5 years, folate reserves last only 4–5 months. The human body requires about 75–100 μg/day of folic acid, which is present in leafy green vegetables, fruits, nuts, beans, wheat germ, and liver. Like vitamin B_{12}, folate is involved in the synthesis of thymidine.

Folic acid deficiency can occur as a result of decreased intake. In spite of supplementation of U.S. wheat products with folate, nutritional deficiencies still occur, especially in alcoholics and patients with atypical diets. Malabsorption can also affect intake of folate. Because small intestine (SI) microvilli convert the ingested complex folic acid molecule into an absorbable one, SI diseases such as gluten enteropathy and Crohn's disease can cause deficiency. Certain drugs, such as anticonvulsants and oral contraceptives, also predispose to folate malabsorption. Other medications—such as antineoplastic agents, trimethoprim, and certain antimalarial drugs—inhibit the enzyme necessary for the replenishment of intracellular folate and can affect folate levels.

Folate deficiency can also result if increased requirements are not met. Pregnancy, for instance, increases folate requirements 5- to 10-fold by the third trimester. Patients with hemolytic anemia and exfoliative skin diseases also have increased requirements and should receive supplementation. Because folate is dialyzable, patients on dialysis can suffer from folate deficiency if they do not receive supplementation.

Folate deficiency is common among alcoholics for several reasons. First, although some folic acid is present in beer, alcoholics tend to consume less of other foods rich in folic acid, such as leafy green vegetables. Alcohol can also adversely affect intracellular processing of folate. Finally, alcohol may suppress bone marrow function. Although alcoholics commonly present with macrocytosis, only those who are folate or vitamin B_{12} deficient will have accompanying megaloblastic anemia with its associated clinical features.

Clinical Findings

A. SYMPTOMS AND SIGNS

Patients with mild folate deficiency often present with anemia on a routine blood screen. Those with more severe disease can present with pallor, weight loss, fatigue, glossitis, lightheadedness, jaundice, or abdominal symptoms, as in vitamin B_{12} deficiency. As opposed to vitamin B_{12} deficiency, however, neurological symptoms are absent.

B. LABORATORY FINDINGS

Many laboratory findings are similar to those of vitamin B_{12} deficiency: HGB levels can be variably depressed, pancytopenia can occur, and hypersegmented neutrophils can be seen on the peripheral blood smear. Also as with vitamin B_{12} deficiency, examination of the bone marrow can show erythroid hyperplasia and marked asynchrony in maturation between cytoplasmic components and nuclear material.

With folate deficiency, however, serum and RBC folate levels are low, whereas vitamin B_{12} levels are normal. RBC folate—which is low at less than 150 pg/L—is thought to be a more precise indicator of chronic folate deficiency than serum folate. The latter is thought to reflect more recent dietary intake.

Treatment

Foods rich in folic acid should be consumed, which include leafy green vegetables, fruits, nuts, beans, wheat germ, and liver. Supplementation with oral folic acid—from 1 to 5 mg daily—is used to treat deficiency. Total correction occurs within 6–8 weeks. Patients with increased folate requirements, such as pregnant women, should receive supplementation.

Barney-Stallings RA, Heslop SD: What is the clinical utility of obtaining a folate level in patients with macrocytosis or anemia? J Fam Pract 2001;50:544.

■ NORMOCYTIC ANEMIA

HEREDITARY SPHEROCYTOSIS

ESSENTIALS OF DIAGNOSIS

- Autosomal dominant inheritance pattern (in most cases).

- Spherocytes on peripheral blood smear.
- Hemolysis.

General Considerations

Hereditary spherocytosis (HS) is the most common inherited defect of the RBC membrane. Patients with this condition inherit one of a series of mutations of the structural proteins of the RBC membrane, such as spectrin and ankyrin. The resulting decreased membrane elasticity causes loss of the normal biconcave shape of the RBC. These deformed, spherical RBCs are then detained and phagocytosed in the narrow fenestrations of the splenic cords.

Less common related defects also exist, including hereditary elliptocytosis and hereditary stomatocytosis.

Clinical Findings

A. SYMPTOMS AND SIGNS

HS can be classified as mild, moderate, or severe. Individuals with mild disease rarely manifest symptoms and signs. Increased erythropoietin levels compensate for early destruction of RBCs. These patients often present as adolescents or adults on routine blood screenings. Individuals with moderate disease comprise 60–75% of HS patients and can develop intermittent episodes of jaundice, dark urine, abdominal pain, and splenomegaly in infancy or early childhood. Individuals with severe disease have more marked jaundice and splenomegaly.

If bilirubin levels are chronically elevated, bilirubin gallstones can form, leading to right upper quadrant abdominal pain and tenderness, nausea, and a positive Murphy's sign.

B. LABORATORY FINDINGS

Patients with mild disease may or may not be anemic. Patients with moderate and severe disease often have low hemoglobin, reticulocyte counts between 5% and 20%, and elevated serum bilirubin.

The mean corpuscular hemoglobin concentration (MCHC) is a useful test in diagnosing HS. It is generally elevated to 36 g/dL in patients with HS, reflecting decreased membrane surface area and increased hemoglobin concentration in the RBC.

The peripheral blood smear of a patient with HS shows characteristic spherocytes—small RBCs that have lost their central pallor. Although a patient with mild disease may have only a few spherocytes, patients with moderate or severe disease can have 30 or more spherocytes per high power field.

Special tests can also be used to evaluate patients for HS. The osmotic fragility test involves suspending a patient's RBCs in increasingly dilute salt solutions and observing for cell lysis. RBCs from patients with HS will be more sensitive to hypotonic solutions because of membrane instability. The newer "acidified glycerol lysis test" is also used.

Treatment

Individuals with mild disease rarely require treatment. For patients with moderate disease blood transfusions may be necessary, and for patients with severe disease regular transfusions are required. Folic acid supplementation is useful for patients with this and other hemolytic diseases.

The definitive treatment is splenectomy, which leads to significantly increased RBC life span. Patients postsplenectomy are at risk for overwhelming sepsis with encapsulated organisms, however, and immunization against *Pneumococcus* and *Meningococcus* is recommended for these patients. Cholecystectomy may be necessary for patients with bilirubin gallstones.

Mentzer WC, Lubin BH: Hereditary spherocytosis: clinical features; diagnosis; and treatment. UpToDate Online 2001;11.

GLUCOSE-6-PHOSPHATE DEHYDROGENASE DEFICIENCY

ESSENTIALS OF DIAGNOSIS

- X-Linked inheritance pattern.
- African or Mediterranean heritage.
- Recent exposure to oxidizing substances such as primaquine, sulfa drugs, naphthalene, or fava beans.

General Considerations

Glucose-6-phosphate dehydrogenase (G6PD) is a cytoplasmic enzyme that prevents oxidative damage to RBCs by reducing NADP to NADPH. Individuals who are deficient in this enzyme are more susceptible to damage from oxidative substances such as superoxide anion (O_2^-) and hydrogen peroxide. In addition to being normal by-products of cell metabolism, these substances are produced by certain drugs, household chemicals, and foods.

The World Health Organization classifies G6PD deficiency into five variants, from class I (the most severe enzyme deficiency) to class V (no clinical significance). The deficiency is most common in people of African and Mediterranean heritage. The disorder is thought to protect against malaria. Although it is primarily seen in men, as are most X-linked disorders, women who carry the defective gene can also manifest symptoms due to inactivation of their normal X chromosomes.

Overall, G6PD deficiency is the most common enzymatic disorder of red blood cells in humans and affects 200–400 million people. Less common enzymatic deficiencies also exist. Pyruvate kinase deficiency, for example, has a similar clinical presentation.

Clinical Findings

Persons affected with G6PD deficiency are often asymptomatic. However, a spectrum of clinical manifestations can occur, from infrequent mild episodic hemolysis to severe chronic hemolysis.

A. SYMPTOMS AND SIGNS

The most common clinical manifestations are jaundice, dark urine, pallor, abdominal pain, and back pain. These symptoms usually occur hours to days after an oxidative insult. Chemicals that can cause such an insult include primaquine, sulfa drugs, dapsone, nitrofurantoin, and naphthalene (found in moth balls). Aspirin and acetaminophen can precipitate hemolysis in certain individuals as well. Attacks can also be associated with infections (such as pneumonia, viral hepatitis, and *Salmonella*), and diabetic ketoacidosis. Finally, foods such as fava beans have been implicated. These beans are common in the Mediterranean and are harvested in late spring (Table 30–3).

Infants with G6PD deficiency can also present with jaundice. Again a spectrum of disease exists, from mild transient jaundice to severe jaundice, kernicterus, and death. Those with class I G6PD deficiency can have life-long, life-threatening chronic hemolysis.

Table 30–3. Selected sources of oxidative damage.

Medications
Aspirin, nonsteroidal antiinflammatory drugs
Antimalarial agents
Nitrofurantoin, sulfonamides
Quinidine
Infections
Naphthalene
Fava beans

B. Laboratory Findings

Hemoglobin levels mirror the severity of disease. During acute attacks in highly susceptible individuals, hemoglobin levels can be as low as 3–4 g/dL. Many asymptomatic individuals, however, have only mildly depressed levels at 11–12 g/dL.

During periods of active hemolysis, other laboratory measures can be abnormal. To compensate for the loss of RBCs, reticulocytosis occurs and the absolute reticulocyte count is elevated above 2–3%, and sometimes above 10–15%. Haptoglobin levels are often depressed below 50 mg/dL, as this plasma protein binds hemoglobin released from fragmented RBCs.

The peripheral blood smear in G6PD deficiency shows characteristic Heinz bodies, which represent masses of denatured, damaged hemoglobin. "Bite cells," which appear as RBCs with a small semicircular defect, can also be seen. The definitive test for G6PD deficiency is an enzymatic assay that measures *in vitro* production of NADPH.

Treatment

Individuals with mild disease require no treatment except for avoidance, whenever possible, of oxidative triggers. Individuals with class I disease may require inpatient treatment of acute exacerbations with transfusion, intravenous fluid support, and monitoring of renal function. Although vitamin E and splenectomy have been advocated as possible treatments in more severe cases, neither has provided consistent benefit.

Glader BE: Glucose-6-phosphate dehydrogenase deficiency and related disorders of hexose monophosphate shunt and glutathione metabolism. In: *Wintrobe's Clinical Hematology.* Lee GR, Foerster J, Lukens J (editors). Williams & Wilkins, 1999.

Glader BE: Diagnosis and treatment of glucose-6-phosphate dehydrogenase deficiency. UpToDate Online 2001;11.

SICKLE CELL ANEMIA

ESSENTIALS OF DIAGNOSIS

- *African, Mediterranean, or Asian heritage.*
- *Family history.*
- *Autosomal recessive inheritance.*
- *Characteristic pattern on hemoglobin electrophoresis.*

General Considerations

Patients with sickle cell anemia are homozygous for a mutation in the β hemoglobin chain; the sixth amino acid is valine instead of glutamate. The resulting hemoglobin S, which consists of two normal α hemoglobin chains and two abnormal β hemoglobin chains, is poorly soluble when deoxygenated. The polymerization of hemoglobin S within the RBC leads to the characteristic "sickle" shape. These abnormal RBCs occlude capillary beds and lead to the many clinical manifestations of sickle cell disease.

A spectrum of other sickle cell syndromes exists. Hemoglobin C results from a different mutation in the β hemoglobin chain. Patients with hemoglobin SC disease have one of each mutation and generally experience a milder phenotype than patients with homozygous sickle cell anemia (hemoglobin SS). Other permutations of abnormal hemoglobin genes can cause similar syndromes. Patients with one sickle cell gene and one β-thalassemia gene, for example, can have significant clinical manifestations of hemoglobinopathy.

Traits that lead to sickle cell anemia are common in those with African and South Asian heritage, as these traits confer resistance to malaria. The gene frequency for sickle cell anemia in African-Americans is about 4%.

Clinical Findings

A. Symptoms and Signs

Patients with homozygous sickle cell anemia manifest disease early. About 30% of patients are discovered by 1 year of age and over 90% by 6 years of age. Acute pain episodes are the most common presentations; they can occur in the extremities, abdomen, back, or chest. Many patients have several hospitalizations each year for acute episodes of pain. Although generally no inciting factor is found, stresses such as cold, infection, and dehydration can precipitate attacks. Fever, joint swelling, vomiting, and tachypnea can accompany pain episodes.

Most patients experience autoinfarction of the spleen by early childhood due to occlusion of splenic capillary beds. For this and other reasons, patients with sickle cell anemia are significantly vulnerable to infection, especially from encapsulated pathogens such as *Streptococcus pneumoniae* and *Hemophilus influenzae.* Pneumonia, meningitis, osteomyelitis, and bacteremia are causes of significant morbidity and mortality in these patients.

Pulmonary complications are the most common causes of death in patients with sickle cell disease. RBCs in the pulmonary system are particularly vulnerable to sickling because of its low PO_2 and relatively low blood pressure. "Acute chest syndrome" refers to the clinical triad of chest pain, pulmonary infiltrate on x-ray, and fever, which can be due to pulmonary infarction, pneumonia, or both.

Sickled RBCs can occlude vasculature and infarct nearly any tissue in the body. Other serious manifestations of sickle cell disease therefore include stroke, myocardial infarction, bone infarction, retinopathy, leg ulcers, and priapism. Depression, low self-esteem, and social withdrawal are common, especially when adequate coping mechanisms are not in place.

B. LABORATORY FINDINGS

Laboratory findings often reflect the chronic hemolysis that accompanies sickle cell anemia. The classic patient will have a reticulocyte count increased to 3–15%, hemoglobin mildly or moderately decreased to 7–11 g/dL, elevated direct bilirubin and LDH, and a depressed haptoglobin level.

The peripheral blood smear will show up to half of the RBCs as sickled. Howell–Jolly bodies and target cells are also present on the smear, indicating hyposplenism. The white blood cell (WBC) count can be elevated at 12–15,000/μL, even in the absence of infection.

Treatment

Several prophylactic measures can reduce the likelihood of pain crises and other manifestations of disease in patients with sickle cell anemia. First, adequate hydration and oxygenation are required at all times to reduce the risk of hemoglobin polymerization and subsequent vasoocclusive crises. Folic acid should be supplemented, 1 mg orally every day. Some physicians recommend hydroxyurea, which seems to reduce the likelihood of RBC sickling by stimulating production of fetal hemoglobin. Infectious complications can be reduced by immunization against *Streptococcus pneumoniae, Hemophilus influenzae* type B, hepatitis B, and influenza. Daily oral penicillin prophylaxis should be given until age 5 years.

Despite these measures, most patients with sickle cell anemia require frequent hospitalization for acute vasoocclusive crises or infectious complications. During acute exacerbations, patients often require hydration and oxygenation, analgesia with nonnarcotic or narcotic medications, antibiotics if appropriate, and/or blood transfusions.

Ballas SK: Complications of sickle cell anemia in adults: guidelines for effective management. Cleve Clin J Med 1999;66:48.

Embury SH, Vichinsky EP: Overview of the management of sickle cell disease. UpToDate Online 2002;11.

AUTOIMMUNE HEMOLYTIC ANEMIA

 ESSENTIALS OF DIAGNOSIS

- *Positive direct Coombs' test.*
- *Elevated indirect bilirubin and decreased serum haptoglobin.*
- *Inciting factor such as medication or illness.*

General Considerations

Autoimmune hemolytic anemia (AIHA) results when a patient produces antibodies directed against self RBCs. AIHA can be classified by the temperature at which the antibodies are most reactive. "Warm" autoantibodies bind most strongly near 37°C, whereas "cold" autoantibodies bind RBCs near 0–4°C. Occasionally, a mixture of both types of autoantibodies is present.

Although in nearly 50% of cases the production of autoantibodies is idiopathic, other times an inciting factor can be found. Lymphoproliferative disorders such as chronic lymphoblastic leukemia and autoimmune disorders such as rheumatoid arthritis, for example, can induce production of either warm or cold autoantibodies. Infections such as *Mycoplasma* and syphilis have been implicated primarily in cold autoimmune hemolytic anemia.

Medications can induce a warm antibody autoimmune reaction. Some drugs, such as methyldopa, alter RBC antigens so that they become targets of the host immune system. Other drugs bind with RBC antigens to form immunogenic complexes. This "hapten" reaction can occur with penicillin as well as a variety of other drugs (Table 30–4).

Table 30–4. Causes of immune hemolytic anemia.

Idiopathic
Transfusion reaction
Drugs (methyldopa, penicillin, quinidine)
Connective tissue disorders
Hematological malignancies (chronic lymphocytic leukemia, non-Hodgkin's lymphoma)
Infections (*Mycoplasma*, syphilis)

Clinical Findings

A. Symptoms and Signs

Overall, a wide spectrum of possible manifestations exists. A typical patient with autoimmune hemolytic anemia presents with pallor, fatigue, or headaches due to loss of circulating RBCs. Jaundice may also be present, due to elevation of indirect bilirubin resulting from the release and breakdown of RBC heme. A patient may also have splenomegaly due to increased sequestration of damaged RBCs within the splenic cords of Billroth. In some cases, hemoglobinuria can lead to renal failure. The rate of disease progression depends on the underlying cause of hemolysis. Although in some patients clinical manifestations progress slowly, in others severe symptoms can develop in a matter of hours.

B. Laboratory Findings

A positive direct Coombs' test helps diagnose AIHA. Direct Coombs' tests involve washing RBCs and then immersing them in a solution containing antibodies against immunoglobulin G (IgG) and/or C3d, a fragment of complement. RBCs with adherent autoantibodies and/or complement will tend to agglutinate or burst.

Other laboratory findings reflect the general hemolytic process. Bilirubin and LDH levels are increased, haptoglobin levels tend to decrease, and the corrected reticulocyte count is increased. Other appropriate laboratory investigations specific to underlying causes—such as collagen vascular diseases, cancer, and infections—may be warranted.

Treatment

Although further hemolysis can result, blood transfusion should be given when the hemoglobin level is significantly low (5–7 g/dL). Corticosteroids are often considered the treatment of choice, especially when autoantibodies are warm. Those who need long-term treatment and cannot take steroids can use other immunomodulating agents such as azathioprine, cyclosporine, and rituximab. Intravenous immunoglobulin is advocated for the acute treatment of adults with AIHA, but it is not as effective in children. Exchange transfusion, which not only delivers new RBCs but also removes destructive autoantibodies and complement, can also be useful. Splenectomy should be considered in refractory cases; any patient who receives a splenectomy should also receive immunizations against *Pneumococcus, Hemophilus,* and *Meningococcus.* Finally, underlying disorders should be treated as appropriate.

Gehrs BC, Friedberg RC: Autoimmune hemolytic anemia. Am J Hematol 2002;69:258.

Rosse WF, Schrier SL: Clinical features and treatment of autoimmune hemolytic anemia: warm agglutinins. UpToDate Online 2002;11.

EXTRINSIC NONIMMUNE HEMOLYTIC ANEMIA

 ESSENTIALS OF DIAGNOSIS

- *Negative Coombs' test.*
- *Negative family history.*
- *Known mechanical trauma to RBCs, hemolytic infection, or drug/toxin exposure.*

General Considerations

There are many causes of extrinsic hemolysis not related to immunity. The first group of conditions results from mechanical damage to RBCs. Any process that enlarges the spleen, for instance, can lead to an acquired hemolytic process as the spleen is the major organ recycling RBCs. Mechanical damage can also occur as RBCs rush past a prosthetic valve or other internal machinery. Disseminated intravascular coagulation (DIC) and thrombotic thrombocytopenic purpura (TTP) can result in hemolysis of RBCs that flow through areas of intravascular coagulation. Mechanical destruction of RBCs can also be due to exposure to heat, burns, or even repeated trauma such as that encountered in the feet while marching long distances.

Infectious diseases such as malaria, babesiosis, and leishmaniasis can also cause an acquired hemolysis. This is due both to direct parasitic action and to increased activity of macrophages within the spleen.

Finally, drugs and toxins can lead to hemolysis. Medications such as primaquine, dapsone, nitrites, and even topical anesthesia can induce oxidative stress, damaging RBCs. This can occur even in patients without G6PD deficiency. Toxins such as lead, copper, and arsine gas, as well as venom from snakes, insects, and spiders, can also cause hemolysis (Table 30–5).

Symptoms and signs, laboratory findings, and treatments will be based upon the specific diagnosis made. Rather than a specific disorder, extrinsic nonimmune hemolytic anemia is a general categorization of heterogeneous disease processes.

Schrier SL: Extrinsic nonautoimmune hemolytic anemia due to drugs and toxins. UpToDate Online 2001;11.

Table 30–5. Nonimmune causes of hemolysis.

Hypersplenism
Microangiopathy
   Disseminated intravascular coagulation
   Thrombotic thrombocytopenic purpura - hemolytic uremic
     syndrome
Physical destruction
   Prosthetic valve
   March hemoglobinuria
   Burns
Infection
   Malaria, babesiosis
   Leishmaniasis
Medications
   Primaquine
   Dapsone
   Nitrates
Toxins
   Lead, copper
   Arsine gas
   Snake, spider venom

APLASTIC ANEMIA

ESSENTIALS OF DIAGNOSIS

- *Pancytopenia.*
- *Hypocellular bone marrow.*
- *Normal hematopoietic cells.*

General Considerations

Aplastic anemia represents the suppression of all bone marrow lines—erythroid, granulocytic, and megakaryocytic—leading to pancytopenia. Most commonly the disorder is idiopathic. However, drugs, toxins, radiation, infections, and pregnancy can all induce aplastic anemia (Table 30–6).

The etiology is unclear. Although some causative agents have been shown to be directly toxic to the bone

Table 30–6. Selected causes of aplastic anemia.

Idiopathic (most common)
Drug induced
Iatrogenic (radiation, chemotherapy)
Infections (hepatitis, parvovirus)
Pregnancy

marrow, others seem to induce an autoimmune process. The prognosis depends on many factors. The specific etiology plays a role: drug-induced aplastic anemia carries a more favorable prognosis than idiopathic aplastic anemia. The more severe the pancytopenia, the worse the prognosis. Age and gender do not seem to play a role.

Clinical Findings

A. Symptoms and Signs

Anemia leads to pallor, fatigue, and weakness. Neutropenia increases susceptibility to bacterial infections. Thrombocytopenia can present as mucosal bleeding, easy bruising, or petechiae. Splenomegaly is common in advanced disease.

B. Laboratory Findings

Pancytopenia is the hallmark of aplastic anemia. The associated anemia can be severe and is generally normocytic. The reticulocyte count is often low. The white count can be lower than 1500/μL and the platelet count is generally less than 150,000/mL. The peripheral blood smear shows RBCs, neutrophils, and platelets that are normal in morphology but decreased in number. Bone marrow aspirate, which reveals marrow hypocellularity, is essential to the diagnosis of aplastic anemia and important in distinguishing it from other causes of pancytopenia.

Treatment

Patients with aplastic anemia should avoid sick contacts and razors. Other means of decreasing risk of infection include the use of stool softeners and antiseptic soaps. Fever or other signs of infection should be aggressively investigated. Often, empiric broad-spectrum antibiotics should be used. Menstrual blood loss can be suppressed with oral contraceptive pills. Although replacement of blood products is often necessary, it should be used as little as possible to avoid sensitizing potential bone marrow transplant candidates. Hematopoietic growth factors (erythropoietin and granulocyte colony-stimulating factor) are not routinely used due to transient or nil effect.

In a patient under 50 years of age with an HLA-matched sibling, immediate bone marrow transplantation is the treatment of choice. The toxicity associated with treatment increases with age, along with the risk of graft-versus-host disease (GVHD). If successful, transplant is curative. Five-year survival rate is approximately 70%.

In those lacking matched siblings or those over 50 years, treatment consists of immunosuppression with antithymocyte globulin (ATG), augmented with high-dose cyclosporine. Most patients relapse, but remission rates with additional ATG treatments are encouraging. Survival at 5 years is about 75%.

Young NS, Maciejewski J: The pathophysiology of acquired aplastic anemia. New Engl J Med 1997;336:1365.

ANEMIA OF CHRONIC RENAL INSUFFICIENCY

ESSENTIALS OF DIAGNOSIS

- *Elevated serum creatinine.*
- *Low HGB.*

General Considerations

Although anemia of chronic renal insufficiency (CRI) commonly occurs in patients with a creatinine clearance of 30 mL/min/1.73 m^2 or less, it can appear in patients with serum creatinine as low as 2 mg/dL. It is caused in part by a decrease in renal production of erythropoietin. The milieu of CRI also adversely affects RBC function. Studies show that RBCs from healthy patients die prematurely when injected into patients with CRI, but RBCs from CRI patients have a normal life span when injected into healthy individuals. Platelets are also affected. Platelet count is decreased and function is impaired.

Clinical Findings

A. SYMPTOMS AND SIGNS

Patients may exhibit bleeding or bruising due to thrombocytopenia and platelet dysfunction. Pallor and fatigue are also common. Early symptoms of uremia include nausea, vomiting, weight loss, malaise, and headache. As the blood urea nitrogen (BUN) level rises, paresthesias, decreased urine output, and waning level of consciousness can be seen. Other signs and symptoms depend on the etiology of the patient's renal insufficiency.

B. LABORATORY FINDINGS

BUN and serum creatinine are generally both elevated, above 30 and 3.0 mg/dL, respectively. The anemia tends to be normocytic, but in some cases it can be microcytic. Hyperphosphatemia, hypocalcemia, and hyperkalemia can occur, as can metabolic acidosis. Reticulocyte count tends to be normal or decreased. The blood smear in the uremic patient can reveal acanthocytes, which are grossly deformed RBCs. Bone marrow is inappropriately normal for the degree of anemia.

Treatment

Erythropoietin or darbopoietin is indicated when the hemoglobin is 11 g/dL or less. Both are recombinant products. Darbopoietin has a longer half-life and more predictable bioavailability. Prior to initiation of therapy, the patient should be screened for deficiency of iron, folate, and vitamin B$_{12}$. Erythropoietin is given at 80–120 units/kg/week. The most common side effect of erythropoietin therapy is hypertension. Intravenous or oral iron replacement may be necessary as well.

There is growing evidence that treatment with erythropoietin has a favorable effect on the progression of renal disease, underscoring the importance of early diagnosis and treatment.

Macdougall IC: Role of uremic toxins in exacerbating anemia in renal failure. Kidney Int Suppl 2001;78:S67.

ANEMIA ASSOCIATED WITH MARROW INFILTRATION

ESSENTIALS OF DIAGNOSIS

- *Anemia with abnormally shaped RBCs on peripheral smear.*
- *Bone marrow study showing infiltration or a "dry tap."*
- *Underlying neoplastic, inflammatory, or metabolic disease.*

General Considerations

The bone marrow can tolerate fairly extensive infiltration. When marrow infiltration causes anemia or pancytopenia, however, it is referred to as myelophthisic anemia. The most common cause of myelophthisis is metastatic carcinoma. Other causes include hematological malignancies, infections, and metabolic diseases (Table 30–7).

Table 30–7. Selected causes of marrow infiltration.

Metastatic malignancy (lung, breast, prostate)
Hematological malignancy (leukemia, lymphoma)
Infection (tuberculosis, fungi)
Metabolic disease (Gaucher's disease, Niemann–Pick disease)

As the marrow is infiltrated by one of these disease processes, hematopoietic precursor cells are unable to mature and differentiate. Eventually, the normal marrow becomes replaced by collagen, reticulin, and other fibrotic cells. The severity of the resulting pancytopenia reflects the degree of infiltration.

Myelophthisis occurs in less than 10% of patients with metastatic disease. The prognosis in patients with marrow metastases is generally poor.

Clinical Findings

A. SYMPTOMS AND SIGNS

Anemia can be manifested by pallor or fatigue. Thrombocytopenia can cause petechiae, bleeding, or bruising. Neutropenia can lead to frequent or atypical infections. Fractures, bony pain, and bony tenderness may occur. Other presenting signs and symptoms are usually related to the underlying cause of marrow infiltration.

B. LABORATORY FINDINGS

The anemia tends to be normocytic and mild to moderate. White cells and platelets may also be decreased.

The peripheral blood smear is characterized by abnormal cells, particularly tear-shaped red cells. The smear may also show poikilocytes and anisocytes. "Leukoerythroblastosis" refers to the presence of immature nucleated red blood cells, immature white cells, and megakaryocyte fragments on the peripheral blood smear—findings that are highly suggestive of infiltration. Because of the hypocellular marrow, aspirate often yields few cells ("dry tap").

Treatment

Treatment targets the underlying disease. Successful treatment of the malignancy, through radiation, chemotherapy, or bone marrow transplant, can resolve the anemia. Erythropoietin or blood transfusion may be used to augment the RBC count. Platelet transfusions may be needed.

Shpall EJ et al: Bone marrow metastases. Hematol Oncol Clin North Am 1996;10:321.

Diseases of the Biliary Tract & Liver

31

Rodrick McKinlay, MD, & Samuel C. Matheny, MD, MPH

■ BILIARY TRACT DISEASES

Rodrick McKinlay, MD

RIGHT UPPER QUADRANT PAIN

General Considerations

Patients complaining of right upper quadrant (RUQ) or epigastric abdominal pain usually have a disorder of the hepatobiliary or upper gastrointestinal system. The first priority is to rule out life-threatening conditions requiring emergent attention. A history and physical examination should be sufficient to make such a determination. Pain that is acute in onset, persists longer than 6 h, and is associated with significant abdominal tenderness often signals a condition requiring surgical (or interventional endoscopic) attention. Such conditions include acute cholecystitis, perforated duodenal or gastric ulcer, pyogenic liver abscess, choledocholithiasis with or without cholangitis, perforated diverticulitis, perforated appendicitis leaking into the right upper quadrant, and severe acute pancreatitis. Other nonsurgical conditions to consider include mild to moderate pancreatitis, perihepatitis from pelvic inflammatory disease (Fitz–Hugh–Curtis syndrome), right lower lobe pneumonia, right-sided pyelonephritis, nephroureterolithiasis, and myocardial infarction.

Clinical Findings

Cost-effective laboratory tests in working up acute right upper quadrant pain stem from the history and physical examination, but in general, they should include a complete blood count, liver function tests, and amylase and lipase. A right upper quadrant ultrasound should be the first imaging study to rule out gallstones and related conditions. If a perforated viscus is suspected, an abdominal series should be ordered to rule out free air. Such a finding necessitates operation. Computed tomography (CT) scans should be reserved for patients whose diagnosis is unclear following laboratory, ultrasound, and plain abdominal radiographs.

An ultrasound is cost effective in confirming the presence of gallstones and biliary-related pathology. A complete blood count, liver function tests, amylase and lipase, thyroid-stimulating hormone (TSH), and a sedimentation rate are advocated as cost-effective tests in the workup of chronic abdominal pain. For patients without gallstones, endoscopy and nuclear medicine studies [eg, hepatic 2,6-dimethyliminodiacetic acid (HIDA) scan] may be beneficial. Endoscopic retrograde cholangiopancreatography (ERCP) should be reserved for patients with ultrasound evidence of bile duct dilatation in whom an obstructing stone, stricture, or neoplasm is suspected, or to enable diagnosis in refractory cases.

Differential Diagnosis

The differential diagnosis for patients with subacute or chronic right upper quadrant pain is rather extensive and consists of symptomatic cholelithiasis (biliary colic), peptic ulcer disease, gastroesophageal reflux, pancreatitis, hepatitis, inflammatory bowel disease, porphyria, intestinal angina, pancreatic cancer, large and small bowel cancer, endometriosis, and right-sided diverticulitis.

Silen W: *Cope's Early Diagnosis of the Acute Abdomen,* ed 20. Oxford University Press, 2000. (Overview of abdominal conditions that require urgent attention.)

CHOLELITHIASIS

General Considerations

Between 16 and 25 million (about 1 in 13) Americans harbor gallstones. The prevalence of gallstones is related to many factors, including gender, age, and ethnic background. Gallstones are more common in women than men and increase in both sexes with age. By age 70 about 25% of women and 10% of men in the United States have gallstones. Gallstones are more prevalent in Native Americans and whites and less prevalent in African-Americans. Gallstones affect greater than 70% of Pima

Indians over 30 years of age. Other risk factors for gallstones include obesity, high estrogen levels, cholesterol-lowering drugs, diabetes, rapid weight loss, fasting, prolonged parenteral nutrition, and conditions of the terminal ileum, such as Crohn's disease. Avoidance or control of these conditions helps to prevent gallstones and their sequelae.

Pathogenesis

Gallstones may be divided pathologically into cholesterol stones and pigment stones. Cholesterol stones develop when the balance of cholesterol, bile salts, and lecithin within the gallbladder bile tips in favor of cholesterol supersaturation. This state allows the formation of solid cholesterol crystals, which then grow into stones by further deposition of cholesterol and calcium salts. Pigment stones are classified into black and brown stones. Black pigment stones are associated with hemolytic states in which the concentration of unconjugated bilirubin increases and precipates with calcium. Brown stones are often formed in the setting of infection, in which bacteria secrete enzymes that hydrolyze bilirubin glucuronide to free bilirubin, which then precipitates with calcium.

Clinical Findings

Asymptomatic gallstones may be found incidentally on plain abdominal radiography, but most gallstones are composed largely of cholesterol, rendering them radiolucent. Ultrasound is the most sensitive and cost-effective test to detect gallstones (>90% sensitivity).

Treatment

Most people with gallstones remain asymptomatic. The risk of developing biliary colic or other complications is about 1–2% per year. Therefore, the incidental finding of asymptomatic gallstones should generally not prompt surgical referral, except in cases in which an elevated risk for gallbladder carcinoma exists (gallstones associated with a calcified, or "porcelain," gallbladder, and possibly those with stones greater than 3 cm). Patients with diabetes, although more likely to have complications from symptomatic disease, still do not require prophylactic cholecystectomy for asymptomatic gallstones. The longer a patient's gallstones remain clinically silent, the less likely the stones will ultimately become symptomatic.

Kalloo AN, Kantsevoy SV: Gallstones and biliary disease. Prim Care 2001;28:591. [PMID: 11483446].

Sheth S, Bedford A, Chopra S: Primary gallbladder cancer: recognition of risk factors and the role of prophylactic cholecystectomy. Am J Gastroenterol 2000;95:1402. [PMID: 10894571]. (A review of the literature regarding risk factors for the development of gallbladder cancer and when prophylactic cholecystectomy may be offered.)

SYMPTOMATIC CHOLELITHIASIS (BILIARY COLIC)

 ESSENTIALS OF DIAGNOSIS

- *Episodic RUQ pain.*
- *Nausea.*
- *Ultrasound evidence of gallstones.*

Pathogenesis

Biliary colic develops when a gallstone or biliary sludge transiently obstructs the gallbladder neck, creating gallbladder distention and pain through visceral afferent fibers.

Clinical Findings

A. SYMPTOMS AND SIGNS

Patients typically complain of RUQ pain after eating a fatty meal. The pain often radiates to the back or to the right scapula and lasts between 30 min and several hours. Nausea may accompany symptoms of pain, but vomiting is uncommon in uncomplicated biliary colic. On physical examination, mild RUQ tenderness may be present.

B. LABORATORY FINDINGS

Laboratory values are normal.

C. IMAGING STUDIES

An ultrasound demonstrates gallstones, with or without gallbladder wall thickening or pericholecystic fluid.

Differential Diagnosis

Other painful disorders of the RUQ include peptic ulcer disease, pancreatitis, hepatitis, gastritis, duodenitis, right-sided diverticulitis, pneumonia of the right lower lobe, and myocardial infarction.

Treatment

Elective laparoscopic cholecystectomy is the gold standard for treatment of symptomatic cholelithiasis. Patients who are young (under 60 years of age) and otherwise healthy can generally expect outpatient treatment with a rapid recovery, returning to work within 1–2 weeks. Older patients also do well after laparoscopic cholecystectomy but usually take longer to recover. Conversion rates to open surgery are rare for elective laparoscopic cholecystectomy (<5%), but are more likely to occur in obese, elderly, and diabetic patients. In the case of conversion, a 2- to 4-day hospital stay is customary. Contraindications for laparoscopic surgery include severe comorbid disease precluding general anesthesia and uncontrolled coagulopathy.

Cheno- and ursodeoxycholic acids may be used to treat symptomatic gallstones in patients who are not candidates for or refuse cholecystectomy, but biliary colic is more likely to recur in these patients compared to those treated with cholecystectomy.

Extracorporeal shock wave lithotripsy has a relatively high rate of stone recurrence and is not approved by the Food and Drug Administration (FDA) in the United States.

Prognosis

Greater than 95% of patients treated with laparoscopic cholecystectomy have no further symptoms related to gallstones. The most feared complication of laparoscopic cholecystectomy is injury to the common bile duct (0.1–0.6%), which may require endoscopic intervention (eg, stent placement) or further surgery to correct. Retained common duct stones and cystic duct leaks occur 2–3% of the time and are usually amenable to endoscopic therapy.

Pregnancy is a risk factor for gallstones. Pregnant patients should generally be treated conservatively as most attacks will abate after the birth of the baby. However, in severe attacks or in acute cholecystitis, laparoscopic cholecystectomy is safe. The best time to perform surgery is during the second trimester.

Gadacz TR: An update on laparoscopic cholecystectomy, including a clinical pathway. Surg Clin North Am 2000;80:1127. [PMID: 10987028]. (A review of the indications, technique, and outcomes of laparoscopic cholecystectomy.)

Kalloo AN, Kantsevoy SV: Gallstones and biliary disease. Prim Care 2001;28:591. [PMID: 11483446].

CHOLECYSTITIS

1. Acute

ESSENTIALS OF DIAGNOSIS

- Persistent severe RUQ pain (>4-6 h).
- RUQ tenderness.
- Fever, leukocytosis.
- Ultrasound evidence of gallstones.

Pathogenesis

Persistent gallbladder outlet obstruction by a stone or sludge causes distention of the gallbladder with resultant significant pain. Engorgement of the gallbladder leads to further inflammation and possible gangrene.

Clinical Findings

A. SYMPTOMS AND SIGNS

Patients with acute cholecystitis complain of persistent RUQ pain, typically lasting more than 4–6 h, which may radiate to the back and right shoulder. Nausea and vomiting are frequently associated with the pain. RUQ tenderness is present on physical examination. The classically described Murphy's sign (arrest of inspiration with RUQ palpation) is not always present, but if it can be elicited, the diagnosis of acute cholecystitis is confirmed.

B. LABORATORY FINDINGS

Laboratory values include elevated white blood cell count and frequently an elevated alkaline phosphatase. The total bilirubin and liver transaminases [alanine aminotransferase (ALT), aspartate aminotransferase (AST)] may also be elevated. A total bilirubin >3 mg/dL or significantly elevated alkaline phosphatase or γ-glutamyltransferase (GGT) should prompt a search for a common duct stone (see the section on "Choledocholithiasis"). Elevation of amylase and lipase should lead to suspicion of gallstone pancreatitis. A significantly elevated white blood cell count (>17K) is associated with an increased likelihood of gallbladder gangrene.

C. IMAGING STUDIES

Right upper quadrant ultrasound typically shows gallstones, a thickened gallbladder wall, and pericholecystic fluid, although the latter two findings may not be present in all cases. If the diagnosis of acute cholecystitis is strongly suspected in the absence of gallstones, an HIDA scan should be performed. Failure to visualize the gallbladder (secondary to obstruction) is indicative of acute cholecystitis.

Differential Diagnosis

Perforated peptic ulcer disease, acute pancreatitis, acute hepatitis, appendicitis, and right-sided diverticulitis may mimic acute cholecystitis.

Treatment

Patients diagnosed with acute cholecystitis should be admitted to the hospital for intravenous antibiotics, analgesics, and bowel rest followed closely by laparoscopic cholecystectomy, which is the definitive treatment of choice for acute cholecystitis. Most studies favor performing surgery during the same hospitalization rather than several weeks after the resolution of the acute episode. Conversion to open surgery for acute cholecystitis occurs more frequently than for biliary colic, but still occurs in only 5–10% of cases.

For patients who are not candidates or refuse cholecystectomy, percutaneous cholecystostomy under radiological guidance is indicated to drain potentially infected bile from the gallbladder. Antibiotic coverage is essential before and after the procedure.

Prognosis

Cholecystectomy alleviates patients of gallstone-related pain and complications in 90% of cases of acute cholecystitis, although complications are slightly more frequent when surgery is performed urgently for acute disease than electively for chronic disease. Postcholecystectomy syndrome—persistent RUQ pain following cholecystectomy—occurs in a small percentage of patients and usually is due to a faulty diagnosis. A small subset of patients may have disordered functioning of the ampulla of Vater requiring further workup and treatment.

2. Chronic

When patients endure multiple episodes of biliary colic or acute cholecystitis without intervention, they may present later with chronic cholecystitis. Keys to diagnosis include a history of multiple episodes of RUQ pain, the absence of RUQ tenderness, and gallstones on ultrasound. Treatment is with laparoscopic cholecystectomy. The gallbladder may be contracted and partially intrahepatic secondary to scarring from previous inflammatory episodes.

Wang CH et al: Rapid diagnosis of choledocholithiasis using biochemical tests in patients undergoing laparoscopic cholecystectomy. Hepatogastroenterology 2001;48:619. [PMID: 11462888]. (A large retrospective series of patients with symptomatic gallstones is analyzed for predictive factors for common bile duct stones.)

GALLSTONE PANCREATITIS

ESSENTIALS OF DIAGNOSIS

- *RUQ pain.*
- *Elevated amylase, lipase.*
- *Ultrasound evidence of gallstones.*

General Considerations

Gallstones are the most frequent cause of pancreatitis in the United States, accounting for more than 50% of cases of acute pancreatitis. Transient or persistent occlusion by a gallstone of the common channel between the common and pancreatic ducts results in pancreatitis.

Clinical Findings

A. SYMPTOMS AND SIGNS

Patients present with RUQ and epigastric pain, which often radiates to the back. Nausea and vomiting often accompany the pain. Physical examination reveals epigastric tenderness.

B. LABORATORY FINDINGS

Depending on the degree of pancreatitis, the WBC count may be significantly elevated. Amylase and lipase are high. Total bilirubin, alkaline phosphatase, AST, and ALT may be elevated as well.

C. IMAGING STUDIES

Ultrasound demonstrates gallstones, with or without gallbladder wall thickening and pericholecystic fluid. Ultrasound is not sensitive for detecting stones in the common bile duct (CBD) (30–50%). For patients with severe pancreatitis, CT is a helpful adjunct to determine the degree of pancreatic necrosis, if present. CT is also more sensitive than ultrasound in detecting CBD stones (greater than 50%). Magnetic resonance cholangiography (MRC) is >90% sensitive for common duct stones but is very expensive and is not cost effective for typical cases of gallstone pancreatitis. In cases in which the bilirubin is elevated (>3–4 mg/dL), consideration should be given to preoperative ERCP to clear the pancreatic duct of stones.

Treatment

To cure a patient of gallstone pancreatitis, cholecystectomy is necessary. The timing of cholecystectomy depends on the severity of the pancreatitis. In cases of mild to moderate pancreatitis, current recommendations are to perform laparoscopic cholecystectomy early in the initial hospitalization, provided evidence exists that pancreatitis is resolving; ie, amylase and lipase are falling toward normal levels. This resolution of pancreatitis typically occurs within 1–2 days of admission with the patient on bowel rest. Intravenous analgesics should be administered. Antibiotics are not always necessary but may be given where there is concomitant evidence of acute cholecystitis (fever, persistent leukocytosis). Many surgeons perform intraoperative cholangiography (IOC) for patients who present with acute cholecystitis to ensure that the common bile duct is cleared of stones. In cases of severe pancreatitis (ie, necrotizing), ensdoscopic clearance of a common duct stone is usually required preoperatively. Laparoscopic or open cholecystectomy should then be performed toward the end of the patient's hospital stay, when pancreatitis is nearly resolved.

Evidence-based management supports early ERCP (within 24–72 h of hospital admission) to extract the stone(s) responsible for pancreatic duct obstruction in patients who are predicted to have a severe attack of pancreatitis. Any time ERCP is performed, a small risk (1–5%) of post-ERCP pancreatitis exists.

Complications of pancreatitis may occur before or after cholecystectomy, including necrotizing pancreatitis, infected pancreatic necrosis, or hemorrhagic pancreatitis. Supportive care in the intensive care unit may be necessary in these cases.

Barkun AN: Early endoscopic management of acute gallstone pancreatitis—an evidence-based review. J Gastrointest Surg 2001;5:243. [PMID: 11419450]. (A review of the evidence to support early ERCP for common duct clearance in patients with a predicted severe attack of pancreatitis, but not to perform ERCP in patients with a predicted mild attack.)

Schirmer B: Timing and indications for biliary tract surgery in acute necrotizing pancreatitis. J Gastrointest Surg 2001;5: 229. [PMID: 11419446]. (Early cholecystectomy is indicated during the initial hospitalization for those with mild-to-moderate gallstone pancreatitis; delayed (but within the same hospitalization) laparoscopic cholecystectomy is indicated for those with more severe forms of pancreatitis.)

CHOLANGITIS/CHOLEDOCHOLITHIASIS

ESSENTIALS OF DIAGNOSIS

- Persistent RUQ pain.
- Jaundice.
- Fever.
- Hypotension, mental status changes (acute suppurative cholangitis).

General Considerations

Common bile duct stones (choledocholithiasis) are present in 10–15% of patients with gallstones. Common duct stones may be symptomatic or asymptomatic. Symptomatic stones cause obstruction of the biliary tract leading to jaundice, pancreatitis, or cholangitis. Biliary stasis predisposes to infection of bile and cholangitis. Pus under pressure in the biliary tract is known as acute suppurative cholangitis and requires emergent decompression of the biliary tree.

Common duct stones are classified into primary stones and secondary stones. Primary stones arise in the common duct *de novo* and are rare (5%). Secondary stones pass into the common duct from the gallbladder and are the most common type of stone (95%).

Clinical Findings

A. SYMPTOMS AND SIGNS

Patients with cholangitis classically present with Charcot's triad: a history of jaundice; acute, severe RUQ pain; and fever. If pus is under pressure in the biliary tree, patients exhibit the additional signs of hypotension and mental status changes (creating the so-called Reynauld's pentad).

B. LABORATORY FINDINGS

Laboratory studies indicate elevated WBC count, hyperbilirubinemia, and elevated alkaline phosphatase. Liver transaminases may also be high.

C. IMAGING STUDIES

Although ultrasound has poor sensitivity for detecting a common duct stone, it may provide convincing indirect evidence of a choledocholithiasis, such as common bile duct dilatation and stones in the gallbladder. To confirm the diagnosis, a CT scan, ERCP, or MRCP may be necessary.

Differential Diagnosis

The differential diagnosis includes periampullary cancer (pancreas, bile duct, or duodenum), liver metastases, cholestatic liver diseases, and hepatocellular jaundice.

Treatment

Priorities in treating cholangitis are resuscitation and decompression of the biliary system. Patients should be aggressively hydrated and given broad-spectrum antibiotics upon presentation. ERCP is effective in extracting the causative stone in the majority of cases and is preferable to surgery on initial presentation. If ERCP fails, the biliary system may be decompressed with a percutaneous transhepatic drain. Failing that, surgery should be undertaken to extract the stone and drain the biliary system. If ERCP or transhepatic cholangiogram (THC) is successful, patients should undergo cholecystectomy within several weeks as tolerated to eliminate the source of stones. This may be performed laparoscopically or open. If surgery is needed to explore the common bile duct, a T tube draining bile from the duct to a skin level bag is left in place for 2–6 weeks. Prior to removing the T tube, a cholangiogram is performed through the T tube to ensure that the duct is clear of stones.

Prognosis

Cholangitis is a serious illness that carries significantly more morbidity and mortality than acute cholecystitis, with mortality rates ranging from 13% to 88%. Poor prognostic indicators include old age, female sex, acute renal failure, concomitant medical illnesses, pH <7.4, preexisting cirrhosis, hepatic abscess, and malignant obstruction.

Lillemoe KD: Surgical treatment of biliary tract infections. Am Surg 2000;66:138. [PMID: 10695743]. (Resusitative measures, antibiotics, and decompression of the biliary system are the mainstay of treatment in acute cholangitis.)

Raraty MG, Finch M, Neoptolemos JP: Acute cholangitis and pancreatitis secondary to common duct stones: management update. World J Surg 1998;22:1155. [PMID: 9828724].

Soetikno RM, Montes H, Carr-Locke DL: Endoscopic management of choledocholithiasis. J Clin Gastroenterol 1998;27:296. [PMID: 9955257].

ACUTE ACALCULOUS CHOLECYSTITIS

ESSENTIALS OF DIAGNOSIS

- *RUQ tenderness.*
- *Critically ill patients.*
- *Diagnosis of exclusion.*

General Considerations

Patients may develop cholecystitis without gallstones. So-called acute acalculous cholecystitis (AAC) represents 5–10% of all episodes of cholecystitis and typically takes a more fulminant course than calculous cholecystitis. The underlying etiology in this instance is ischemia and bile stasis as opposed to stones. AAC generally develops in patients who are critically ill, such as those who have sustained major burns, multiple trauma, or major nonbiliary operations, including cardiopulmonary bypass; however, outpatient cases have been documented, especially among elderly males with vascular disease.

Clinical Findings

A. SYMPTOMS AND SIGNS

RUQ pain and tenderness may be present but difficult to detect secondary to the patient's critically ill state.

B. LABORATORY FINDINGS

Laboratory results show leukocytosis with or without elevation of liver function tests.

C. IMAGING STUDIES

Utrasound reveals a distended gallbladder, often with wall thickening or emphysematous changes. Cholescintigraphy (HIDA scan) shows nonfilling of the gallbladder, but the false-positive rate may be as high as 40% because of the common underlying finding of biliary stasis.

Differential Diagnosis

Perforated peptic ulcer disease, acute/necrotizing pancreatitis, ischemic bowel, and any perforated viscus may mimic AAC.

Treatment

Treatment consists of cholecystectomy, which is usually performed open but may be performed laparoscopically in selected cases. If a patient is unable to tolerate a general anesthetic or is coagulopathic, percutaneous cholecystostomy may be necessary, with interval cholecystectomy after systemic improvement.

Kalliafas S et al: Acute acalculous cholecystitis: incidence, risk factors, diagnosis, and outcome. Am Surg 1998;64:471. [PMID: 9585788]. (Review of 27 patients undergoing open cholecystectomy for acute acalculous cholecystitis.)

Lillemoe KD: Surgical treatment of biliary tract infections. Am Surg 2000;66:138. [PMID: 10695743]. (Acute acalculous cholecystitis is generally found in critically ill patients and requires aggressive management.)

BILIARY DYSKINESIA

ESSENTIALS OF DIAGNOSIS

- *Chronic, intermittent RUQ pain.*
- *Absence of gallstones on ultrasound.*
- *HIDA scan demonstrates gallbladder ejection fraction <35%.*

General Considerations

Biliary dyskinesia may also be referred to as chronic acalculous cholecystitis, which follows a much less fulminant course than acute acalculous cholecystitis. Patients often undergo esophagogastroduodenoscopy (EGD), upper gastrointestinal studies, or even ERCP by the time they reach HIDA scanning in an attempt to diagnose their RUQ pain. Most patients with this disorder are young (under 50 years of age) females.

Clinical Findings

A. SYMPTOMS AND SIGNS

Patients typically present with episodic RUQ pain, intolerance to fatty meals, and mild nausea.

B. LABORATORY FINDINGS

Labarotory values are generally normal.

C. IMAGING STUDIES

Ultrasound studies generally are normal. An HIDA scan performed with cholecystokinin showing <35% gallbladder ejection fraction at 20 min is diagnostic of biliary dyskinesia.

Treatment

Laparoscopic cholecystectomy effectively cures 80–90% of patients with biliary dyskinesia demonstrated by an abnormally low gallbladder ejection fraction. In most cases the pathology report shows evidence of chronic cholecystitis.

Canfield AJ et al: Biliary dyskinesia: a study of more than 200 patients and review of the literature. J Gastrointest Surg 1998;2:443. [PMID: 9843604]. (Reviews a series of 295 patients with 18-month follow-up after cholecystectomy for biliary dyskinesia showing a success rate of 94.5% of those with <50% gallbladder ejection fraction.)

Jones-Monahan K, Gruenberg JC: Chronic acalculous cholecystitis: changes in patient demographics and evaluation since the advent of laparoscopy. JSLS 1999;3:221. [PMID: 10527335]. [Reviews a large series of patients with chronic acalculous cholecystitis, showing that most affected patients (70%) are young females with long-term success after laparoscopic cholecystectomy reaching about 80%.]

BILIARY TRACT NEOPLASIA

ESSENTIALS OF DIAGNOSIS

- RUQ pain.
- Jaundice.
- Weight loss.

General Considerations

Cancer of the gallbladder is relatively uncommon, with 5000 new cases diagnosed each year in the United States. Women are affected two to three times more frequently than men. More than 75% of affected individuals are over 65 years of age. The incidence of gallbladder cancer is higher among Native Americans and is particularly high in Chile.

Cholangiocarcinoma, or cancer of the bile ducts, is even less common than gallbladder cancer, with 2500 to 3000 new cases per year in the Unites States. Men and women are affected equally. The incidence rises with increasing age.

Clinical Findings

A. SYMPTOMS AND SIGNS

Patients with gallbladder cancer most commonly present with biliary colic, complaining chiefly of chronic RUQ pain and mild nausea. However, they also can present with malignant biliary obstruction (jaundice, weight loss) or simply with weight loss and vague abdominal pain. A small subset of patients with gallbladder cancer presents with acute cholecystitis (acute RUQ pain, fever, and leukocytosis).

Patients with bile duct cancer most commonly present with painless jaundice. Other symptoms may include pruritis, fever, vague abdominal pain, anorexia, and weight loss. Except for jaundice, the physical examination is usually unremarkable.

B. LABORATORY FINDINGS

For patients with bile duct cancer total bilirubin may exceed 10 mg/dL and alkaline phosphatase is substantially elevated. CA 19-9 may also be high, helping to distinguish malignant from benign biliary obstruction.

C. IMAGING STUDIES

For patients with gallbladder cancer ultrasound demonstrates a mass replacing the gallbladder or an irregular gallbladder wall. CT is an effective diagnostic tool for those patients in whom ultrasound is not helpful. For patients with bile duct cancer ultrasound and CT are the initial diagnostic studies, with cholangiography following to evaluate for resectability.

Treatment

Patients with gallbladder cancer frequently present at a late stage and often are not candidates for surgical resection. For the small number of patients who present with early gallbladder cancer (Stage T1a—mucosal involvement only), cholecystectomy is curative and survival approaches 100%. For others (Stages T1b and

II–IV—extension into gallbladder muscularis and beyond), extended cholecystectomy is the treatment of choice for resectable tumors, and prognosis is poor. For unresectable tumors, palliative treatment for pain and obstruction is indicated.

Tumors of the bile duct may be curatively resected in a limited number of cases. Like gallbladder cancer, presentation is usually late and palliative therapy is in order.

Rumalla A, Petersen BT: Diagnosis and therapy of biliary tract malignancy. Semin Gastrointest Dis 2000;11:168. [PMID: 10950465].

Sheth S, Bedford A, Chopra S: Primary gallbladder cancer: recognition of risk factors and the role of prophylactic cholecystectomy. Am J Gastroenterol 2000;95:1402. [PMID: 10894571]. (A review of the literature regarding risk factors for the development of gallbladder cancer and when prophylactic cholecystectomy may be offered.)

PRIMARY SCLEROSING CHOLANGITIS

 ESSENTIALS OF DIAGNOSIS

- *Jaundice.*
- *Pruritis.*
- *Abnormal liver function tests.*
- *Association with inflammatory bowel disease (IBD).*

General Considerations

An uncommon disorder, primary sclerosing cholangitis (PSC) is a cholestatic liver disease characterized by fibrotic strictures in the intra- and extrahepatic biliary trees in the absence of a known underlying cause. Men are more commonly affected than women, and the usual presenting age is between 40 and 45 years. Approximately two-thirds of patients with PSC have ulcerative colitis.

Clinical Findings

A. SYMPTOMS AND SIGNS

Patients typically present with jaundice, pruritis, and fatigue, but they may be initially detected by abnormal liver function tests without symptoms.

B. IMAGING STUDIES

The imaging study of choice to confirm the diagnosis and determine the extent of disease is ERCP.

Treatment

Medical management should be directed at control of symptoms and bile cholestasis. Treatment with ursodeoxycholic acid lowers serum bilirubin and liver transaminases but generally does not control symptoms effectively. Percutaneous dilatation of strictured segments may relieve symptoms in the short term. Liver transplantation is the only effective long-term treatment; patients with end-stage liver disease, symptomatic portal hypertension, liver failure, and recurrent cholangitis are candidates.

Lee YM, Kaplan MM: Management of primary sclerosing cholangitis. Am J Gastroenterol 2002;97:528. [PMID: 11922543].

WEB SITES FOR BILIARY TRACT DISEASES

http://www.aafp.org/afp/20000701/tips/16.html (Gallstone pancreatitis.)

http://www.brighamrad.harvard.edu/Cases/bwh/hcache/95/full.html (Acute acalculous cholecystitis.)

http://www.cancer.gov/cancerinfo/pdq/treatment/gallbladder/healthprofessional/ (Gallbladder cancer.)

http://www.emedicine.com/EMERG/topic97.htm (Cholelithiasis and choledocholithiasis.)

http://home.mdconsult.com/das/stat/view/24748043/ctt (For those with access to mdconsult.com, a clinical topic tour updated December 11, 2002, with an overview of gallstone diseases and links to related texts and recent journal articles.)

http://www.ssat.com/guidelines/chole7.htm (Treatment guidelines for cholelithiasis and related diseases.)

http://www.umanitoba.ca/colleges/cps/Guidelines_and_Statements/1011.html (Cholelithiasis.)

■ LIVER DISEASE

Samuel C. Matheny, MD, MPH

VIRAL HEPATITIS

Acute viral hepatitis is a worldwide problem, and in the United States there are probably between 200,000 and 700,000 cases per year according to the Centers for Disease Control and Prevention. Over 32% of cases are caused by hepatitis A, 43% by hepatitis B, 21% by hepatitis C, and the remainder are not identified. Although few deaths are reported yearly from acute hepatitis (around 250 cases per year), considerable morbidity can result from chronic infection of hepatitis B and C, and mortality from complications can be pronounced for years to come.

1. Hepatitis A

General Considerations

Hepatitis A virus (HAV), first identified in 1973, is the prototype for the old term of infectious hepatitis. Over the past several decades, the incidence of hepatitis A has varied considerably, with a significantly high level of cases that are unreported. The virus is a very small viral particle that is its own unique genus (hepatovirus).

The majority of individuals infected worldwide are children. In general, there are four patterns of HAV (high, moderate, low, and very low), which roughly correspond to differing socioeconomic and hygienic conditions. Countries with poor sanitation have the highest rates of infection. Most children under the age of 9 years in these countries have evidence of HAV infection. Countries with moderate rates of infection have the highest incidence in later childhood; food and waterborne outbreaks are more common. Countries with low endemicity are more likely to have the peak age of infection at early adulthood, and in very low endemic countries, outbreaks are uncommon.

HAV is usually transmitted by ingestion of contaminated fecal material of an infected person by a susceptible individual. Contaminated food or water can be the source of infection, but occasionally infection can occur by contamination of different types of raw shellfish from areas contaminated by sewage. The virus can survive from 3 to 10 months in water. Other cases of infection by blood exposures have been reported, but are less common. The incubation period for hepatitis A averages 30 days, with a range of 15–50 days.

In countries of low endemicity, persons at greatest risk for infection include travelers to intermediate and high HAV-endemic countries, men who have sex with men (MSM), intravenous drug users, and persons with chronic liver disease, including those who have received transplants. In areas of high endemicity, all young children are at increased risk.

Prevention

At the present time in the United States, the Centers for Disease Control has recommended that certain populations at increased risk be considered for preexposure vaccination. These include the groups listed above. The immunization schedule consists of three doses for children and adolescents and two doses for adults (Table 31–1). In groups with the potential for high risk of exposure, including any adult over the age of 40 years, prevaccination testing for prior exposure may be cost effective. The appropriate test should be the total anti-HAV. Currently, the routine immunization of all children awaits additional information concerning the duration of protection in children and immugenicity in infants. Travelers who receive the vaccine may assume they are protected 4 weeks after receiving the first dose, although the second dose is needed for long-term protection. If travel is anticipated in less than 4 weeks, immunoglobulin may be given in a different site for additional protection. A combination vaccine with hepatitis B is available for persons over 18 years of age, and is used on the same three-dose schedule as hepatitis B.

Immunoglobulin may also be given for postexposure prophylaxis within 14 days, and would most normally be used for household or intimate contacts of a case, in some institutional settings, or if a common source is identified.

Clinical Findings

A. SYMPTOMS AND SIGNS

The symptoms and signs of acute viral hepatitis are quite similar regardless of type and are difficult to distinguish based on clinical findings. The prodrome for viral hepatitis is variable, and may be manifested by anorexia, including changes in olfaction and taste, as

Table 31–1. Recommended doses and schedules of hepatitis A vaccine.

Group	Age (Years)	Number of Doses	HAVRIX[1] Doses EL.U. (mL)	Schedule (Months)
Children and adolescents	2–18	3	360 (0.5)	0, 1, 6–12
Adults	>18	2	1440 (1.0)	0, 6–12

[1]The dose and schedule of administration for HAVRIX vary according to age. For adults (>18 years of age), 1440 ELISA units (EL.U.) per dose is given in a two-dose schedule 6–12 months apart. For children and adolescents (2–18 years of age), 360 EL.U. per dose is given in a three-dose schedule at 0, 1, and 6–12 months. The vaccine should be given by intramuscular injection into the deltoid muscle.

well as nausea and vomiting, fatigue, malaise, myalgias, headache, photophobia, pharyngitis, cough, coryza, and fever. Dark urine and clay-colored stools may be noticed 1–5 days before jaundice.

Clinical jaundice varies considerably, and may range from an anicteric state to rare hepatic coma. In acute HAV infection, jaundice is usually greater in the older age groups (greater than 14 years—70–80%) and rare in children under 6 years (<10%). Weight loss may also be present, as well as an enlarged liver (70% of cases) and splenomegaly (20% of cases). Spider angiomatas may be manifest without acute liver failure. There may also be a loss of desire for smoking and/or alcohol.

B. Laboratory Findings

Laboratory tests are nonspecific. Usually, the onset of symptoms coincides with the beginning of abnormal laboratory values. Acute elevations of ALT (SGPT) and AST (SGOT) are seen, with levels as high as 4000 units or more in some cases. The ALT is usually higher than the AST. When the bilirubin level is greater than 2.5, jaundice may be obvious. Bilirubin levels may go from 5 to 20, usually with an equal elevation of conjugated and unconjugated. The prothrombin time is usually normal. If it is significantly elevated, it may signal a poor prognosis. The complete blood count (CBC) may demonstrate a relative neutropenia, lymphopenia, or atypical lymphocytosis. Urobilinogen may be present in urine in the late preicteric stage.

Serum IgM antibody (anti-HAV) is present in the acute phase and disappears in 3 months, although it may persist longer in some cases. IgG anti-HAV is used to detect past exposure and persists for the lifetime of the patient. The more commonly available test for IgG anti-HAV is the total anti-HAV (Figure 31–1).

Treatment

Treatment for the most part is symptomatic, with many clinicians prohibiting only alcohol during the acute illness phase. Most patients can be treated at home.

Prognosis

The vast majority of cases of hepatitis A resolve uneventfully within 3–6 months. Rarely, fulminant hepatitis may occur with acute liver failure, and high rates of mortality. There are rare cases of cholestatic hepatitis with persistent bilirubin elevations. Also, relapsing hepatitis may occur, with HAV being reactivated and shed in the stool, and liver function test abnormalities appearing. Virtually all patients recover completely from the relapsing hepatitis as well. HAV does not progress to chronic hepatitis.

2. Hepatitis B

General Considerations

Hepatitis B virus (HBV) is a double-shelled DNA virus. The outer shell contains the hepatitis B surface antigen (HBsAg). The inner core contains several other particles, including a hepatitis B core antigen (HBcAg) and a hepatitis B e antigen (HBeAg). These antigens and their subsequent antibodies are described in more detail in Table 31–2.

In the United States, hepatitis B is normally a disease of young adults. The largest numbers of cases are

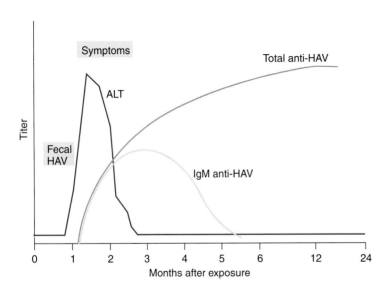

Figure 31–1. Hepatitis A virus infection: typical serological course.

Table 31–2. Interpretation of the hepatitis B panel.

Tests	Results	Interpretation
HBsAg	Negative	Susceptible
Anti-HBc	Negative	
Anti-HBs	Negative	
HBsAg	Negative	Immune due to natural factors
Anti-HBc	Positive	
Anti-HBs	Positive	
HBsAg	Negative	Immune due to hepatitis B vaccination
Anti-HBc	Negative	
Anti-HBs	Positive	
HBsAg	Positive	Acutely infected
Anti-HBc	Positive	
IgM anti-HBc	Positive	
Anti-HBs	Negative	
HBsAg	Positive	Chronically infected
Anti-HBc	Positive	
IgM anti-HBc	Negative	
Anti-HBs	Negative	
HBsAg	Negative	Four interpretations possible[1]
Anti-HBc	Positive	
Anti-HBs	Negative	

[1](1) May be recovering from acute HBV infection. (2) May be distantly immune and the test is not sensitive enough to detect very low levels of anti-HBs in serum. (3) May be susceptible with a false-positive anti-HBc. (4) May be an undetectable level of HBsAg present in the serum and the person is actually a carrier.

reported in people between the ages of 20 and 39 years, although many cases in younger age groups may be asymptomatic and go unreported. Worldwide, the distribution of HBV is quite varied, and is divided into areas of high incidence (>8% of the population), which includes 45% of the global population. Here, the lifetime risk of infection is over 60%, and early childhood infections are very common. Intermediate-risk areas (2–7% of the population) cover 43% of the global population. Here the lifetime risk is between 20% and 60%, and infections occur in various age groups. The low-risk areas (infections <2%) represent around 12% of the global population, and the lifetime risk is <20%. The risk of infections is usually limited here to specific adult risk groups.

Of the specific risk groups in the United States, over 50% in recent studies involve sexual risk factors (more than one sex partner in the past 6 months, sexual relations with an infected person, or MSM transmission). Over 15% had a history of injecting drug use, and 4% had other risk factors such as household contact with HBV or a health care exposure. The mode of transmission can thus be sexual, parenteral, or perinatal, by contact of the infant's mucous membranes with maternal infected blood at delivery. Body fluids with the highest degree of concentration of HBV are blood, serum, and wound exudates. Moderate concentrations are found in semen, vaginal fluid, and saliva, and low or nondetectable amounts are found in urine, feces, sweat, tears, and breast milk. Saliva can be implicated in transmission through bites, but not by kissing.

The average incubation period for hepatitis B is between 60 and 90 days, with a range of 45–180 days. Although the incidence of jaundice increases with age (less than 10% of children under 5 years demonstrate icterus as opposed to 30–50% over 35 years), the likelihood of chronic infection with hepatitis B is greater when contracted at a younger age. Between 30% and 90% of all children under 5 years of age who contract hepatitis B develop chronic disease, compared to 2–10% of people over 35 years of age.

Prevention

Current recommendations in the United States call for routine immunization of all infants, children, adolescents, and adults in high-risk groups. These recommendations include immunizing all children at birth and at 1 and 6 months. Additionally, all high-risk groups should be screened, as well as all pregnant women. Prevaccination testing of patients in low-risk areas is probably not necessary, but in high-risk groups, this may be cost effective. The vaccine contains components of the HBsAg. Pretesting with anti-HB core antibody (anti-HBc) is probably the single best test, as it would identify those who are infected and those who have been exposed. Posttesting for vaccine is not usually recommended in most patients, except for those who may have difficulty mounting an immune response, as in the case of immunocompromised patients. In this case, the HB surface antibody (anti-HBs) would be the appropriate test. Some authorities recommend revaccinating high-risk individuals if titer levels have fallen below 10 IU/L after 5–10 years.

Children born to women of unknown hepatitis B status should also receive their first dose of hepatitis B vaccine at birth, and hepatitis B immune globulin (HBIG) within 7 days of birth if maternal blood is positive. Repeat testing of all infants born to hepatitis B-infected mothers should be repeated at 9–15 months with HBsAg and anti-HBs. Infants born to hepatitis B-infected mothers should receive the first dose of hepatitis B vaccine at birth as well as 0.5 mL of HBIG in separate sites within 12 h after birth. Recommendations for postexposure prophylaxis of hepatitis B can be reviewed in the current recommendations of the CDC.

Clinical Findings

Acute infection may range from an asymptomatic infection to cholestatic hepatitis to fulminant hepatic failure. Usually, HBsAg and other markers should become positive around 6 weeks after infection, and remain positive into the clinical signs of illness. Other biochemical abnormalities will begin to show in the prodromal phase, and may persist several months even with a resolving disease process. Anti-HB core IgM becomes positive early with onset of symptoms, and both anti-HB core IgM and anti-HB core IgG may persist for many months or years. Anti-HBs is the last antibody to appear, and may indicate resolving infection. The presence of HBeAg indicates active viral replication and increased infectivity (Figure 31–2). Liver function tests should be performed early in the course of hepatitis, and evidence of a prolonged prothrombin time (>1.5 INR) should cause concern for hepatic failure. Patients who continue to remain chronically infected may demonstrate HBsAg and HBeAg for at least 6 months, with a usual trend in liver function tests toward normal levels, although they may remain persistently elevated (Figure 31–3).

Complications

Extrahepatic manifestations of disease with hepatitis B are not uncommon, such as serum sickness, polyarteritis nodosa, and membranoproliferative glomerulonephritis. Complications of chronic infection may include progression to cirrhosis and hepatocellular carcinoma. Patients with active viral replication are at highest risk of disease, with 15–20% developing progressive disease over a 5-year period. Continued positivity for HBeAg is associated with an increased risk of hepatocellular carcinoma (HCC). Most patients who are chronically infected remain HBsAg positive for their lifetime.

Screening

There is no general agreement concerning the appropriate screening for patients with chronic infection for HCC. Some experts would not screen carriers if all laboratory tests are normal, but would screen with ultrasound and α-fetoprotein for evidence of chronic active hepatitis every 2–3 years, and more frequently for patients with cirrhosis. However, it appears that the incidence of progression of disease is greater in countries with high endemicity, and clinicians in these countries screen as frequently as every 6 months.

Treatment

Treatment for chronic disease depends on evidence of viral activity, histological evidence of liver injury, and elevated liver function tests. Currently approved treatment modalities include interferon-α, lamivudine, and, most recently, adefovir. Other new antivirals are currently being tested. Sensitive tests for determination of response to therapy, such as covalently closed circuit (ccc) DNA and others, may be more readily available in the future.

3. Hepatitis C

General Considerations

Hepatitis C virus (HCV) has become the most common blood-borne infection and the leading cause of chronic liver disease and liver transplantation in the United

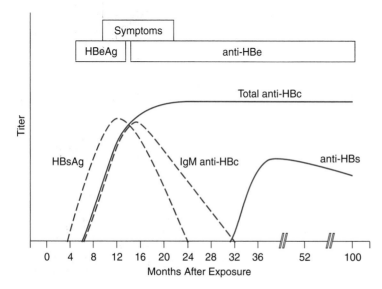

Figure 31–2. Acute hepatitis B virus infection with recovery.

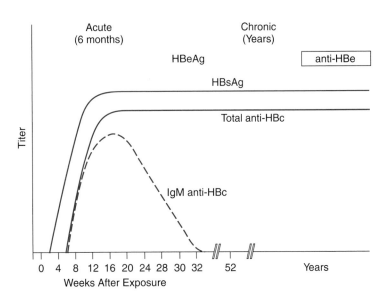

Figure 31–3. Progression to chronic hepatitis B virus infection.

States. Worldwide, there are over 170 million people infected, but the infection rates vary considerably. In the United States, it is estimated that around 3.8% of the population may be infected. The responsible virus is an RNA virus of the Flaviviridae family. Six major genotypes, numbering 1 through 6, are known, with additional subtypes. There are varying distributions of these genotypes. They may also affect the progression of disease and the response to treatment regimens.

HCV is spread primarily through percutaneous exposure to blood. Since 1992, all donated blood has been screened for HCV. Intravenous drug use is responsible for over 50% of new cases. Within 1–3 months after the first incident of needle sharing, 50–60% of intravenous drug users are infected. Other risk factors include use of intranasal cocaine, hemodialysis, tattooing (debatable), and vertical transmission, which is rare. Breast-feeding is low risk. Sexual transmission is uncertain, but is probably 1–3% over the lifetime of a monogamous couple. Health care workers are at particular risk following a percutaneous exposure (1.8% average incidence).

Prevention

No immunizations are currently available for HCV infections. Prevention consists mainly of reduction of risk factors, including screening of blood and blood products, caution to prevent percutaneous injuries, and reduction in intravenous drug use. It is also important to immunize patients with chronic hepatitis C for hepatitis A, as the incidence of fulminant hepatitis A has been shown to be significantly increased in this population. Patients infected with hepatitis C should also abstain from alcohol.

Clinical Findings

A. SYMPTOMS AND SIGNS

1. Acute hepatitis—The incubation period for HCV varies between 2 and 26 weeks, but most commonly is 6–7 weeks. Most cases of HCV are asymptomatic at the time of infection. However, over 20% of all recognized cases of acute hepatitis in the United States are HCV. As many as 30% of adults who are infected may present with jaundice (Figure 31–4).

2. Chronic hepatitis—As opposed to hepatitis A and B, most people infected with HCV (85%) develop a chronic infection, but rarely develop fulminant acute hepatic failure (Figure 31–5). The incidence of significant liver disease is 20–30% for cirrhosis and 4% for liver failure; over 1–4% of patients with chronic infection develop HCC annually, or 11–19% over 4–11 years in one study. Risk factors that increase the likelihood of progression to serious disease include increased alcohol intake, age greater than 40 years, HIV coinfection, and possibly male gender and other liver coinfections.

Extrahepatic manifestations of chronic infection are fairly common and are similar to those of hepatitis B, including autoimmune conditions and renal conditions such as membranous glomerulonephritis.

B. LABORATORY FINDINGS

Tests used in the diagnosis and assessment of hepatitis C are listed in Table 31–3. Asymptomatic patients should first be tested with the enzyme immunoassay (EIA) for HCV. A positive test should be confirmed by a recombinant strip immunoblot assay (RIBA) test for anti-HCV

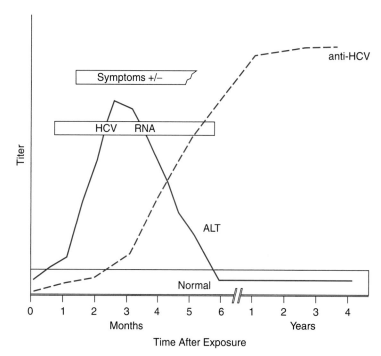

Figure 31–4. Serological pattern of acute hepatitis C virus infection with recovery.

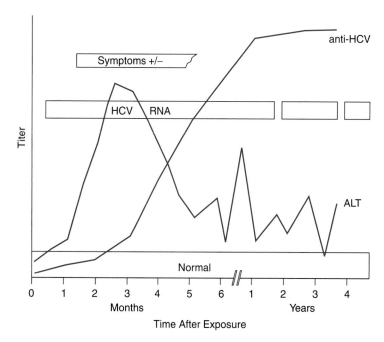

Figure 31–5. Serological pattern of acute hepatitis C virus infection with progression to chronic infection.

or a reverse transcriptase polymerase chain reaction (RT-PCR) for HCV RNA (Figure 31–6). Diagnosis of acute infection may require the use of the RT-PCR, as the anti-HCV may not be positive for several weeks.

Treatment

Treatment for both acute and chronic hepatitis has undergone significant strides in the past few years. A recent study documents the conversion of a significant number of patients to negative serology when treated in the acute phase of infection. Treatment of chronic hepatitis with a combination of pegylated interferon-2b (PEG-IFN) and ribavirin is the current standard of care in the United States, although poorer responses are seen with genotype 1, which is the most common in this country. Newer treatments with PEG-IFN-α-2a are being considered for approval with ribavirin, usually for at least 48 weeks.

4. Other Types of Infectious Hepatitis

Over 97% of the viral hepatitis in the United States is either A, B, or C. Other types of viral hepatitis occur much less frequently, although worldwide, they may be more important.

Hepatitis D

Hepatitis D virus (HDV) is a virus that can replicate only in the presence of HBV infection. This can either occur as a coinfection with the HBV or as a superinfection in a chronically infected individual with HBV. Although coinfection can produce more severe acute disease, a superinfection poses the risk of more significant chronic disease, with 70–80% of patients developing cirrhosis. The mode of transmission is most commonly percutaneous. The only tests commercially available in the United States are IgG-anti-HDV. Prevention of HDV depends on prevention for HBV. There are no products currently available to prevent HDV infection in those patients infected with HBV.

Table 31–3. Diagnostic testing for hepatitis C.

Test[1]	Indication
Anti-HCV antibody (EIA)	Initial screen or diagnosis
RIBA	Confirm EIA
Qualitative PCR for HCV RNA	Confirm EIA
Quantitative PCR or bDNA for HCV RNA	Measure level of serum HCV RNA (not used for diagnosis)

[1]EIA, enzyme immunoassay; RIBA, recombinant immunoblot assay; bDNA, branched DNA; PCR, polymerase chain reaction.

Hepatitis E

Hepatitis E virus (HEV) is the most common cause of enterically transmitted non-A, non-B hepatitis. Acute hepatitis is similar to other forms of viral hepatitis; no chronic form is known. Severity of illness increases with age, and for reasons that are unclear, case fatality rates are particularly high in pregnant women. Most of the cases of HEV reported in the United States have occurred in travelers returning from high endemic areas. In certain areas of the world (North Africa, the Middle East, and Asia) epidemics of hepatitis E may be common. Prevention includes avoiding water and other beverages of unknown purity, uncooked shellfish, and uncooked vegetables and fruits. No vaccines are currently available, and pooled γ-globulin does not appear to be effective.

Hepatitis F and G

The existence of a hepatitis F virus has been debated, and very rare cases of another newly identified virus have been reported labeled hepatitis G. Very little is currently known of transmission, or patterns of illness, although the infectivity level in the United States may be significant.

5. Acute Hepatitis: A Cost-Effective Approach

Because the vast majority of cases of viral hepatitis are caused by HAV, HBV, or HCV, tests to determine the precise etiology are necessary for appropriate primary and secondary prevention for the patient, as well as potential for therapy. Figure 31–7 outlines one cost-effective approach. If these tests fail to indicate a diagnosis, the etiology may be due to less frequent causes of viral hepatitis such as Epstein–Barr virus, in which jaundice can rarely accompany infectious mononucleosis; cytomegalovirus or herpes virus in immunocompromised patients; or other nonviral etiologies, such as alcoholic hepatitis, drug toxicity, Wilson's disease, or an autoimmune hepatitis.

Ahmed A, Keefe E: Cost-effective evaluation of acute viral hepatitis. West J Med 2000;(179):29. [PMID: 10695442]. (Good overview of workup for acute hepatitis.)

U.S. Public Health Service: Prevention of hepatitis A through active or passive immunization: recommendations of the Advisory Committee on Immunization Practices (ACIP). MMWR 1999;48(RR-12):1. [PMID: 10543657].

U.S. Public Health Service: Updated U.S. Public Health Service guidelines for the management of occupational exposures to HBV, HCV, and HIV and recommendations for postexposure prophylaxis. MMWR 2001;50(RR-11):1. [PMID: 11442229].

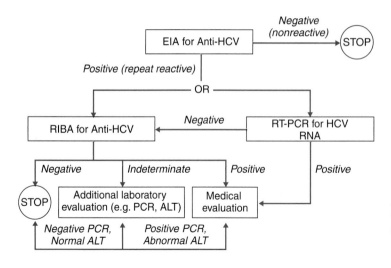

Figure 31–6. Hepatitis C virus infection testing algorithm for diagnosis of chronic illness. [From MMWR 1998;47(RR-19).]

WEB SITES

American Liver Foundation: Liver update: function and disease. (Excellent survey of issues around hepatitis.)

www.liverfoundation.org

Centers for Disease Control: National Center for Infectious Diseases. Hepatitis information. (References for immunization and testing, as well as patient information in several languages.)

www.cdc.gov/ncidod/diseases/hepatitis

National Institutes of Health: Consensus statement: management of hepatitis C.

http://consensus.nih.gov/cons/116/116cdc_intro.htm

ALCOHOLIC LIVER DISEASE

General Considerations

Alcoholic liver disease includes a number of different disease entities, which span a large clinical spectrum. These range from the syndrome of acute fatty liver to severe liver damage as manifested by cirrhosis. **Fatty liver** is usually asymptomatic, and is the histological result of excessive use of alcohol over several days. In this stage, most patients are symptomatic, having occasional evidence of hepatomegaly. **Perivenular fibrosis** usually refers to the deposit of fibrous tissue in the central areas of the liver, particularly the central veins, and is an indication that the individual may then rapidly progress to more severe forms of liver disease. Patients can progress from this stage directly to cirrhosis. **Alcoholic hepatitis** is described as a condition with necrosis of hepatic cells with an inflammatory response, which includes polymorphonuclear cells, along with evidence of fibrosis. **Cirrhosis** may result from continued progression of disease from alcoholic hepatitis, or may occur without prior evidence of alcoholic hepatitis. Cirrhosis is characterized by distortion of the liver structure, with bands of connective tissue forming between portal and central zones. Changes in hepatic blood circulation may also occur, resulting in portal hypertension. Additionally,

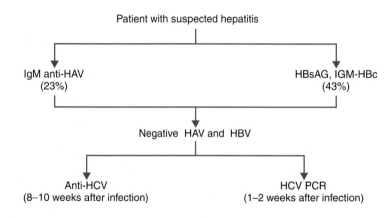

Figure 31–7. Cost-effective workup for acute viral hepatitis. (From Ahmed A, Keefe E: Cost-effective evaluation of acute viral hepatitis. West J Med 2000;172:29.)

evidence of abnormal fat metabolism, inflammation, and cholestasis may also be seen. Progression to **hepatocellular carcinoma (HCC)** may also occur, although it is still unclear exactly what risk cirrhosis poses in the progression to HCC.

It is known that women are more likely to develop alcoholic liver disease than men, although the reasons for this phenomenon are only now being clarified. There may be additional genetic factors, most notably in specific enzyme systems, such as the metabolism of tumor necrosis factor (TNF) and alcohol-metabolizing systems that affect the development of disease. Concomitant disease, such as hepatitis C, is also a risk factor. Other factors such as obesity may play a role in the progression of disease.

Clinical Findings

A. SYMPTOMS AND SIGNS

A history of drinking alcohol in excess of 80 g/day (six to eight drinks) is seen with the development of more advanced forms of the disease, although there is considerable individual variation. Numerous questionnaires have been designed for detection of excessive drinking, but the CAGE questionnaire is probably the most useful.

Clinical findings may be limited at this stage to occasional hepatomegaly, but no other changes may be evident. Alcoholic hepatitis may present with classic signs and/or symptoms of acute hepatitis (see above), including weight loss, anorexia, fatigue, nausea, and vomiting. Hepatomegaly may be evident, as well as other signs of more advanced disease, such as cirrhosis, as the development of cirrhosis may occur concomitant with a new episode of alcoholic hepatitis. These signs include jaundice, splenomegaly, ascites, spider angiomas, and signs of other organ damage secondary to alcoholism such as dementia, cardiomyopathy, and peripheral neuropathy.

B. LABORATORY FINDINGS

In early stages, various commercially available laboratory tests have been used in the detection of excessive alcohol intake. The sensitivity and specificity of these tests vary. Elevated AST, ALT, and GGT are liver function tests frequently used. In addition, elevated MCV has been noted.

Transaminase levels are usually only mildly elevated in pure alcoholic hepatitis unless other disease processes are present, such as concomitant viral hepatitis or acetaminophen ingestion (Figure 31–8). AST is usually greater than ALT. Elevated prothrombin time and bilirubin levels have a significant negative prognostic indication. The *presence of jaundice* may have special significance in any actively drinking person and needs to be carefully evaluated. Several instruments have been used for evaluation of severity, but the most common is the Maddrey discriminant function (DF) [DF = 4.6 × (prothrombin time in seconds − control) + serum bilirubin (mg/dL)]. A score greater than 32 is indicative of high risk of death.

Treatment

Treatment involves avoiding diuretics and ensuring adequate volume replacement, with concern for the ability to handle normal saline. Adequate nutrition should be given, parenterally if necessary. There is no indication that avoidance of protein is helpful in encephalopathy.

Consider broad-spectrum antibiotics early. Many cases will develop spontaneous peritonitis, pneumonia, or cellulitis, and should be treated aggressively.

Abstaining from alcohol is essential. Recovery from the acute episode is associated with an 80% 7-year survival as opposed to a 50% survival in those continuing to drink.

Corticosteroids have been suggested as beneficial, but considerable debate still ensures. A subgroup of patients with hepatic encephalopathy may benefit.

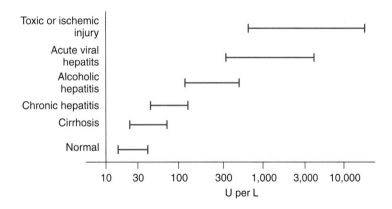

Figure 31–8. Typical AST or ALT values in disease. (From Johnson D: Am Fam Pract 1999.)

Liver transplantation may be an option. Alcoholic liver disease is currently the second most common reason for liver transplantation in the United States. Patients accepted for liver transplantation should not have active alcoholic hepatitis, should have remained sober for over 6 months, and should have had treatment for addiction. The prognosis is excellent if relapse from drinking can be avoided. Relapse occurs in 15–30% of patients.

Other treatment methodologies are in various stages of testing, such as modification of TNF with pentoxifylline; antioxidant therapy with agents such as S-adenosyl-L-methionine (SAMe), silymarin, or vitamin E; or anti-fibrotics such as polyenylphosphatidylcholine (PPC), but more studies are needed to recommend these therapies.

Maher J: Advances in liver disease: alcoholic hepatitis, non-cirrhotic portal fibrosis, and complications of cirrhosis. Treatment of alcoholic hepatitis. J Gastroenterol Hepatol 2002; 17(4):448. [PMID: 11987726]. (Excellent overview of issues of treatment and review of treatment options under consideration.)

Yeung E, Wong FS: The management of cirrhotic ascites. Medscape General Medicine 2002;4(4). http://www.medscape.com/viewarticle/442364. (Overview of the issues concerning appropriate treatment of cirrhosis.)

OTHER LIVER DISEASES

1. Nonalcoholic Fatty Liver Disease (NAFLD) and Nonalcoholic Steatohepatitis (NASH)

A condition first described around 1980, NAFLD encompasses a wide clinical spectrum of patients whose liver histology is similar to patients with alcoholic-induced hepatitis, but without the requisite history. Women are affected more frequently than men. Over 20% of these patients progress to cirrhosis. These are now the most common liver diseases in the United States, occurring in 2–3% of the population. This condition is found very commonly in obese patients as well as in patients with type 2 diabetes mellitus. It may be a part of the "syndrome X," which includes obesity, diabetes mellitus, dyslipidemia, and hypertension. Clinical features include hepatomegaly (75%) and splenomegaly (25%), but no pathognomonic laboratory markers. Elevations of ALT and AST may be up to five times normal, with the AST/ALT ratio <1. Treatment includes weight reduction, treatment of diabetes and lipid disorders, and, possibly, ursodeoxycholic acid and/or vitamin E.

2. Wilson's Disease

Wilson's disease, which is a hepatolenticular degeneration, is caused by the abnormal metabolism of copper, the result of an autosomal recessive inheritance. The prevalence in the general population is about 1:30,000. Patients in asymptomatic stages may manifest only a transaminasemia, or demonstrate the Kayser–Fleisher rings, which are golden-greenish granular deposits in the limbus. Hepatomegaly or splenomegaly may already be present. In most symptomatic patients, serum ceruloplasmin will be <20 mg/dL (96% of patients). In more advanced disease, the patient may manifest symptoms of acute hepatitis or cirrhosis. Neurological signs include dysarthria, tremors, abnormal movements, and/or psychological disturbances. HCC can also be seen in advanced cases. Treatment includes penicillamine, trientine, or zinc salts.

3. Hemochromatosis

Hemochromatosis (HC), an inborn error of iron metabolism leading to increased absorption of iron from the diet, is associated with diabetes, bronze skin pigmentation, hepatomegaly, loss of libido, and arthropathy. Patients may also show signs of cardiac or endocrine disorders. Symptoms usually first manifest themselves between 40 and 60 years of age. Men are 10 times more likely to be affected. This is the most common inherited liver disease found in people of European extraction. Physical signs include hepatomegaly (95% of symptomatic patients), which precedes abnormal liver function tests. Cardiac involvement includes congestive heart failure and arrhythmias. Many patients will have cirrhosis by the time they are symptomatic (50–70%), 20% will have fibrosis, and 10–20% will have neither. HCC is very frequent in patients with cirrhosis (30%) and is now the most common cause of death. Laboratory diagnosis includes an elevated serum iron concentration, increased serum ferritin, and increased transferrin saturation. Treatment involves treating the complications of HCC, removing excess iron by phlebotomy, and, in patients with cirrhosis, surveillance for HCC and treatment of hepatic and cardiac failure.

4. Autoimmune Hepatitis

Autoimmune hepatitis is a hepatocellular inflammatory disease of unknown etiology, with the diagnosis based on histological examination, hypergammaglobulinemia, and the presence of serum autoantibodies. The condition may be difficult to discern from other causes of chronic liver disease, which need to be excluded in making the diagnosis. Immunoserological tests essential for diagnosis are assays for antinuclear antibodies (ANA), smooth muscle antibodies (SMA), and antibodies to liver/kidney microsome type 1 (anti-LKM1), as well as perinuclear antineutrophil cytoplasmic antibodies (aANCAs).

5. Drug-Induced Liver Disease

More than 600 drugs or other medicinals have been implicated in liver disease. Worldwide, drug-induced liver disease represents about 3% of all adverse drug reactions, with over 20% of cases of jaundice due to drugs in the United States occurring in a geriatric population. Acetaminophen and other drugs account for 25–40% of fulminant hepatic failure. Diagnosis is either by discovering abnormalities in hepatic enzymes or by the development of a hepatitis-like syndrome or jaundice. Most cases occur within 1 week to 3 months of exposure, with symptoms rapidly subsiding after cessation of the drug and returning to normal within 4 weeks of acute hepatocellular injury. Hepatic damage may manifest itself as acute hepatocellular injury (isoniazid, acetaminophen), cholestatic injury (contraceptive steroids, chlorpromazine), granulomatous hepatitis (allopurinol, phenylbutazone), chronic hepatitis (methotrexate), vascular injury (herbal tea preparations with toxic plant alkaloids), or neoplastic lesions (oral contraceptive steroids).

6. Primary Biliary Cirrhosis

Primary biliary cirrhosis is an autoimmune disease of uncertain etiology that is manifested by inflammation and destruction of interlobular and septal bile ducts, which can cause chronic cholestasis and biliary cirrhosis. It is predominantly a disease of middle-aged women (the female:male ratio is 9:1), with a particularly high prevalence in northern Europe. The condition may be diagnosed on routine testing, or be suspected in women with symptoms of fatigue or pruritus, or in susceptible individuals with elevated serum alkaline phosphatase, cholesterol, and immunoglobulin M (IgM) levels. Antimitochondrial antibodies (AMA) are frequently found. Ursodeoxycholic acid is the only therapy currently available, although some patients may benefit from liver transplantation.

7. Hepatic Tumors and Cysts

Hepatocellular carcinoma (HCC) is the most common malignant tumor of the liver; it is the fifth most common cancer in men and the eighth most common cancer in women. Incidence increases with age, but the mean age in ethnic Chinese and black African populations is lower. Signs of worsening cirrhosis may alert the clinician to consideration of HCC, but in many cases the onset is subtle. There are no specific hepatic function tests to detect HCC, but elevated serum tumor markers, most notably α-fetoprotein (AFP), are useful. Ultrasound can detect the majority of cases of HCC, but may not distinguish HCC from other solid lesions. CT and MRI are also helpful in making the diagnosis. Risk factors for HCC include hepatitis B, hepatitis C, all etiological forms of cirrhosis, ingestion of foods with aflatoxin B_1, and smoking. High-risk patients for HCC include those with early-onset HBV infection, HCV infection, and HC. In these patients, ultrasound (US) and AFP measurements every 4–6 months are recommended, and in moderate-risk patients (later onset HBV) measurement of AFP every 6 months with US annually is suggested.

8. Benign Tumors

Benign tumors include hepatocellular adenomas, which have become more common with the use of oral contraceptive steroids (OCS), and cavernous hemangiomas, which may occur with pregnancy or use of OCS and are the most common benign tumor of the liver.

9. Liver Abscesses

Liver abscesses can be the result of infections of the biliary tract or can have an extrahepatic source such as diverticulitis or inflammatory bowel disease. In about 40% of cases, no source of infection is found. The most common causative organisms are *Escherichia coli, Klebsiella, Proteus, Pseudomonas,* and *Streptococcus* species. Amebic liver abscesses are the most common extraintestinal manifestation of amebiasis, which occurs in over 10% of the world's population, and is most prevalent in the United States in young Hispanic adults. Amebic abscesses may have an acute presentation, with symptoms present for several weeks; a few patients report typical intestinal symptoms such as diarrhea. US or CT scans with serological tests such as enzyme-linked immunosorbent assay (ELISA) or indirect fluorescent antibody tests help confirm the diagnosis.

Alvarez F et al: International Autoimmune Hepatitis Group report: review of criteria for diagnosis of autoimmune hepatitis. J Hepatol 1999;31:929. [PMID: 10580593]. (Overview of criteria for diagnosis of autoimmune hepatitis.)

Lewis JH: Drug-induced liver disease. Med Clin North Am 2000;84(5):1275. [PMID: 11026929]. (Extensive review of drugs causing liver disease.)

Powell LW, Yapp TR: Hemochromatosis. Clin Liver Dis 2000; 4(1):211. [PMID: 11232185].

Yu AS, Keeffe EB: Nonalcoholic fatty liver disease. Rev Gastroenterol Disord 2002;2(1):11. [PMID: 12122975]. (Overview of the subject.)

Vaginal Bleeding

Patricia Evans, MD

General Considerations

Abnormal bleeding affects up to 30% of women at some time during their lives. Evaluating vaginal bleeding involves an examination of the patient's menstrual cycle. The normal menstrual cycle is generally 21–35 days in length with a menstrual flow lasting 2–7 days and a total menstrual blood loss of 20–60 mL. During the normal menstrual cycle the endometrium is exposed initially to estrogen, followed by ovulation and production of progesterone as well as estrogen, and finally the withdrawal of estrogen and progesterone causing menstruation.

Different diseases are associated with certain patterns of vaginal bleeding, although there is a wide variation in presentation within each. Common terminology used to discuss vaginal bleeding includes menorrhagia, metrorrhagia, menometrorrhagia, hypermenorrhea, polymenorrhea, and oligomenorrhea. The bleeding patterns associated with each term are listed in Table 32–1.

Throughout their lifetimes there are normal changes in most women's menstrual patterns. Just as anovulation is common during the years following menarche, the perimenopausal patient usually experiences changes in her menstrual cycle related to decreasing, irregular anovulation. Although age plays an important role in constructing a differential diagnosis in a patient presenting with vaginal bleeding, many of the causes can occur in any adult woman.

Kjerulff KH, Erickson BA, Langenberg PW: Chronic gynecological conditions reported by U.S. women: findings from the National Health Interview Survey, 1984–1992. Am J Public Health 1996;86:195.

Clinical Findings

A. SYMPTOMS AND SIGNS

1. History—Taking a history of a patient presenting with vaginal bleeding should begin with an exploration of the patient's usual bleeding pattern. The physician should try to establish whether the patient's pattern is cyclic or anovulatory. If the patient menstruates every 21–35 days her cycle is consistent with an ovulatory pattern of bleeding. To confirm ovulation patients can check their basal body temperature, cervical mucus, and luteinizing hormone (LH) levels. Basal body temperature can be checked using a basal body temperature thermometer, which allows for a precise measurement of the patient's temperature within a narrower range than a standard thermometer. The patient takes her temperature orally as soon as she awakens in the morning and records it on a chart. After ovulation the ovary secretes an increased amount of progesterone, causing an increase in temperature of approximately 0.5°F over the baseline temperature in the follicular phase. The luteal phase is often accompanied by an elevation of temperature that lasts 10 days. In addition, patients can be taught to check the consistency of their cervical mucus, watching for a change from the sticky, whitish cervical mucus of the follicular phase to the clear, stretching mucus of ovulation. Finally, the patient can use an enzyme-linked immunosorbent assay (ELISA) available as a home testing kit to check for the elevation of LH over baseline that occurs with ovulation.

The patient should then be asked by the physician to describe the current vaginal bleeding in terms of onset, frequency, duration, and severity. This history will help the physician to focus the differential diagnosis. For example, if the patient reports a longstanding history of anovulatory bleeding the workup can focus on causes for chronic hyperandrogenicity such as polycystic ovarian syndrome and congenital adrenal hyperplasia. Age, parity, sexual history, previous gynecological disease, and obstetrical history will further assist the physician in focusing the evaluation of the women with vaginal bleeding. These questions will help in evaluating the likelihood of pregnancy-related causes of vaginal bleeding, infectious disease, and cancer.

The physician should ask about medications, including contraceptives, prescription medications, and over-the-counter medications and supplements. Contraception is a common cause of vaginal bleeding in women. Specifically, the patient should be asked about any over-the-counter preparations she may be taking.

Table 32–1. Patterns of vaginal bleeding.

Descriptive Term	Bleeding Pattern
Menorrhagia	Regular cycles, prolonged duration, excessive flow
Metrorrhagia	Irregular cycles
Menometrorrhagia	Irregular cycles, prolonged duration, and excessive flow
Hypermenorrhea	Regular cycles, normal duration, and excessive flow
Polymenorrhea	Frequent cycles
Oligomenorrhea	Infrequent cycles

Patients may not be aware that herbal preparations may contribute to vaginal bleeding. Ginseng, which has estrogenic properties, can cause vaginal bleeding and St. John's Wort can interact with oral contraceptives to cause breakthrough bleeding. A review of symptoms should include questions regarding fever, fatigue, abdominal pain, hirsutism, galactorrhea, changes in bowel movements, and heat/cold intolerance. A careful family history will aid in identifying patients with a predisposition to polycystic ovarian syndrome, congenital adrenal hyperplasia, thyroid disease, premature ovarian failure, and cancer. Physicians should also keep in mind that women usually present complaining of vaginal bleeding when symptoms deviate from the patient's normal bleeding pattern. Patients with chronic anovulatory bleeding patterns or lifelong heavy menses secondary to von Willebrand's disease may not perceive their underlying menses pattern as abnormal. Therefore, the physician should avoid asking the patient if her periods been "normal" and instead should ask for specific details regarding the patient's bleeding pattern.

2. Physical examination—The physical examination for women complaining of vaginal bleeding should begin with an evaluation of the patient's vital signs. Does the patient present with a fever (indicating possible infection), increased pulse, low blood pressure, or significant orthostatic changes in her blood pressure (indicating significant acute blood loss)? Has she had a significant weight change and an enlarged or tender thyroid gland indicating thyroid disease? The physician should also evaluate the patient's weight for obesity and hair distribution for hirsutism. These can indicate possible chronic anovulation syndromes. The pelvic examination will aid in identifying other causes of bleeding including anatomic abnormalities such as cervical polyps; signs of infections such as cervical discharge, cervical motion tenderness, and uterine or adnexal tenderness; signs of pregnancy such as changes in the cervix and a symmetrically enlarged uterus; and signs of fibroids such as an enlarged but irregular uterus.

B. EVALUATION

The evaluation of patients presenting with vaginal bleeding includes a combination of laboratory testing, imaging studies, and sampling techniques. The evaluation is directed both by patient presentation and a risk evaluation for endometrial cancer. For example, a patient who presents with a history and physical examination consistent with pelvic inflammatory disease will obviously be tested for gonorrhea and chlamydia. If the physician feels an enlarged uterus on physical examination the initial evaluation will include a pregnancy test followed by a pelvic ultrasound. If the results are inconclusive a sonohysterogram can aid in detecting a focal versus a diffuse lesion. This in turn can lead to a hysteroscopy for further evaluation of a focal lesion or an endometrial biopsy for a diffuse lesion.

The choice of evaluation is also based on the risk of endometrial cancer. For a patient who is at risk, an endometrial biopsy should be included in the evaluation. Patients having prolonged exposure to unopposed estrogen (either iatrogenically or because of chronic anovulation) for more than a year, regardless of age, should also have an endometrial biopsy. In addition, because the incidence of endometrial cancer begins to increase after the age of 35, any patient older than this should also have an endometrial biopsy during an evaluation for unexplained vaginal bleeding.

C. LABORATORY STUDIES

Most patients presenting with vaginal bleeding should be evaluated with a complete blood count. In addition, every woman of reproductive age should have a urine or serum pregnancy test. A thyroid-stimulating hormone (TSH) should be drawn on women presenting with symptoms consistent with hypo- or hyperthyroidism or in women presenting with a change from a normal menstrual pattern.

Adolescents presenting with menorrhagia at menarche should have an evaluation for coagulopathies including a prothrombin time (PT), partial thromboplastin time (PTT), and bleeding time.

There is no general agreement on the diagnostic criteria for polycystic ovarian syndrome (PCOS). In patients with symptoms suggestive of PCOS it is reasonable to check for elevated luteinizing hormone, testosterone, and androstenedione. These may be elevated in patients with PCOS, but due to the large variation among individual women these tests are not definitive. Therefore, the physician needs to interpret test results in conjunction with the clinical picture to make a diagnosis of PCOS.

Overall, the incidence of adult-onset congenital adrenal hyperplasia (CAH) is about 2% in women with hyperandrogenic symptoms. The incidence is higher in individuals of Italian, Ashkenazi, and Yugoslav heritage. Deciding on screening for adult-onset CAH should be based on both the patient's clinical presentation and the patient's ethnic background. A basal 17-hydroxyprogesterone (17-HP) should be drawn in the early morning to screen for adult-onset CAH. Patients with an abnormal result can have another 17-HP level drawn after receiving a dose of ACTH.

D. IMAGING STUDIES

1. Pelvic ultrasound—A pelvic ultrasound can be used to evaluate the ovaries, uterus, and endometrial lining for abnormalities. An evaluation of the ovaries can assist in the diagnosis of PCOS as many women with PCOS will have enlarged ovaries with multiple, small follicles. As with the laboratory testing, this study will not provide a definitive diagnosis.

A pelvic ultrasound is also useful for evaluating an enlarged uterus for the presence of fibroids. Fibroids will appear as hypoechoic, solid masses seen within the borders of the uterus. Subserosal fibroids can be pedunculated and therefore can be seen outside the borders of the uterus.

An endovaginal ultrasound can be used to evaluate the thickness of the endometrial stripe. The results need to be interpreted based on the whether a patient is pre- or postmenopausal. For all women the thicker the endometrial stripe, the more likely the patient has an endometrial abnormality.

An endovaginal ultrasound is a sensitive test for patients with postmenopausal bleeding whether or not they are using hormone replacement therapy. Therefore, postmenopausal patients with an endometrial stripe thicker than 4–5 mm should have a histological biopsy. Hormone replacement therapy can cause proliferation of a patient's endometrium, making an endovaginal evaluation less specific.

An endovaginal ultrasound is also useful in evaluating the endometrial stripe in premenopausal patients. Whereas the normal endometrial stripe is thicker in the premenopausal patient than in the postmenopausal patient, the median thickness of an abnormal endometrium is similar for both. The endovaginal ultrasound examination is less likely to detect myomas and polyps.

2. Sonohysterography—Sonohysterography (SHG) involves performing a transvaginal ultrasound following installation of saline into the uterus. Done after an abnormal vaginal ultrasound, the study is most useful in differentiating focal from diffuse endometrial abnormalities. Detection of a focal abnormality indicates evaluation by hysteroscopy and detection of an endometrial abnormality indicates the need to perform an endometrial biopsy or dilatation and curettage.

3. Magnetic resonance imaging—Magnetic resonance imaging (MRI) can be used to evaluate the uterine structure. The endometrium can be evaluated with an MRI, but the endometrial area seen on MRI does not correspond exactly to the endometrial stripe measured with ultrasound. In most situations, a transvaginal ultrasound is the preferred imaging modality, but if the patient cannot tolerate the procedure MRI does provide an option for evaluation. MRI is better than ultrasound in distinguishing adenomyosis from fibroids, so if the history and examination suggest either of these, an MRI may be the best first choice. MRI is also sometimes used to evaluate fibroids prior to uterine artery embolization.

E. ENDOMETRIAL SAMPLING

The workup for endometrial cancer should be pursued most aggressively with patients at greatest risk for the disease, such as postmenopausal patients who present with vaginal bleeding. In patients younger than 40, endometrial cancer is usually seen in obese patients and/or patients who are chronically anovulatory. Therefore, a patient who presents with an anovulatory pattern of bleeding for greater than a year should be evaluated for hyperplasia and neoplasm with an endometrial sample. In addition, the evaluation of women older than 35–40 years presenting with a new onset of menorrhagia should include endometrial sampling since the incidence of endometrial cancer increases after the age of 35.

Findings from the initial work-up and response to treatment will determine the need for additional studies including sonohysterography, diagnostic hysterography, and MRI.

1. Dilatation and curretage—Dilatation and curretage (D&C) provides a blind sampling of the endometrium. The D&C generally will provide sampling of less than half of the uterine cavity. Because an endometrial biopsy can be completed in the office setting, it has generally replaced the D&C as the initial method of obtaining an endometrial sample. The D&C is useful in patients with cervical stenosis or other anatomic factors that prevent an adequate endometrial biopsy. The D&C is not effective as the sole treatment for menorrhagia.

2. Endometrial biopsy—An endometrial biopsy is an adequate method of sampling the endometrial lining to identify histological abnormalities. A number of devices can be used. Early devices were hooked to an external suction source. More commonly clinicians will use one of the clear, flexible endometrial curettes with an inner plunger or piston that generate suction during the procedure. The different devices available (eg, Pipelle, Explora, Z-Sampler, and Endosampler) provide similar biopsy results. The rates of obtaining an adequate endometrial sample depend on the age of the patient. Because many postmenopausal women will have an atrophic endometrium, sampling in this group will more often result in an inadequate endometrial specimen for examination. In this situation, the clinician must use additional diagnostic studies to fully evaluate the cause of the vaginal bleeding.

3. Diagnostic hysteroscopy—Hysteroscopes come in a variety of forms including rigid, semirigid, and flexible. Diameters range from less than 3 mm to 6 mm. All hysteroscopes uses a light source, camera, and dilating medium to visualize the uterine cavity. The direct exploration of the uterus is useful in identifying structural abnormalities such as fibroids and endometrial polyps. Small-caliber hysteroscopes allow the endometrium to be evaluated without the need for cervical dilatation. Currently these instruments are limited by the fact that they cannot be passed through the endoscope and have a limited field of view. Larger-diameter hysteroscopes allow specific biopsy of lesions. In general, the diagnostic hysteroscopy is combined with a D&C or endometrial biopsy to maximize identification of abnormalities.

Apgar BS, Newkirk GR: Endometrial biopsy. Prim Care Clin Office Pract 1997;24:303.

Bradley LD, Falcone T, Magen AB: Radiographic imaging techniques for the diagnosis of abnormal uterine bleeding. Obstet Gynecol Clin North Am 2000;27:245.

Burkman RT et al: Current perspectives on oral contraceptive use. Am J Obstet Gynecol 2001;185:4.

Klein A, Schwartz ML: Uterine artery embolization for the treatment of uterine fibroids: an outpatient procedure. Am J Obstet Gynecol 2001;184:1556 .

Laing FC, Brown DL, DiSalvo DN: Update on ultrasonography. Radiol Clin North Am 2001;39:523.

Reisman H, Martin D, Gast MJ: A multicenter randomized comparison of cycle control and laboratory findings with oral contraceptive agents containing 100 mcg levonorgestrel with 20 mcg ethinyl estradiol or triphasic norethindrone with ethinyl estradiol. Am J Obstet Gynecol 1999;181:45.

Differential Diagnosis

The differential diagnosis of vaginal bleeding encompasses a wide range of possible etiologies. The patient's history and physical examination will determine the direction of the workup. Age and ovulatory status play important roles in determining the direction of the workup once relatively straightforward causes of vaginal bleeding such as pregnancy and infection have been eliminated.

The history and physical examination will often lead to a narrowing of the differential diagnosis (Table 32–2). The physician should not narrow the differential diagnosis too quickly, as a patient can have more than one possible cause of vaginal bleeding. For example, a patient on oral contraceptives could also present with pelvic inflammatory disease or hypothyroidism. Generating the differential diagnosis will aid the physician in deciding how to further evaluate and treat the patient.

A. PREGNANCY-RELATED BLEEDING

The initial evaluation of any patient presenting with vaginal bleeding should include testing for pregnancy. In recent years urinary assays for β-human chorionic gonadotropin (hCG) have become so sensitive that they are a viable alternative to serum testing. The differential diagnosis for vaginal bleeding for pregnancy varies depending on the estimated gestational age. Early in pregnancy it includes spontaneous miscarriage, ectopic pregnancy, and trophoblastic disease. Later in pregnancy the appearance of bleeding should lead the physician to investigate the possibilities of placenta previa and placental abruption.

B. BLEEDING SECONDARY TO HORMONE MEDICATIONS

1. Contraception—Vaginal bleeding is a common side effect of many forms of contraception. Many women starting oral contraceptive pills (OCPs) experience breakthrough bleeding in the initial months. Lower dose oral contraceptive pills have higher rates of spotting and breakthrough bleeding. Possible causes of vaginal bleeding in patients taking OCPs include inadequate estrogenic or progestogenic stimulation of the endometrium, skipped pills, or altered absorption and metabolism of the pills.

Vaginal bleeding is also frequent with Depo Provera, and is the most commonly cited reason women discontinue taking it as well as OCPs. For this reason, when initiating either form of contraception the expected course of possible bleeding should be discussed with the patient. After the initial dose of Depo Provera 50% of women will experience irregular bleeding or spotting. After a year this decreases to 25%. Norplant users also experience high rates of irregular bleeding. One-third of women continue to have regular cycles after Norplant placement, increasing to two-thirds by the fifth year of use.

2. Hormone replacement therapy—Bleeding is common with hormone replacement therapy, and can occur with both the sequential and continuous regimens. With sequential administration of estrogen and progesterone, most women will experience bleeding near the end or right after taking the progesterone therapy. Although most women taking sequential therapy will

Table 32–2. Differential diagnosis.[1]

Diagnosis	Clinical Presentation	Most Commonly Associated Bleeding Pattern
Contraception	Known OCP/Depo use	OCP: spotting Depo: irregular or continuous bleeding
HRT	Known HRT use	Sequential: menorrhagia or spotting Continuous: irregular spotting
Fibroids	Asymptomatic, pelvic pain, and/or dysmenorrhea	Menorrhagia
Adenomyosis	Dysmenorrhea	Menorrhagia
Endometrial polyps	Asymptomatic	Intermenstrual spotting, metrorrhagia and/or menorrhagia
Cervical polyps	Asymptomatic	Intermenstrual and/or postcoital bleeding
PID	High-risk sexual behavior, fever, pelvic pain, tenderness	Menorrhagia and/or metrorrhagia
PCOS Adult-onset CAH	Hirsutism, acne, central obesity, or asymptomatic	Oligomenorrhea menometrorrhagia
Hyperthyroidism	Nervousness, heat intolerance, diarrhea, palpitations, weight loss	Oligomenorrhea, amenorrhea, polymenorrhea, or menorrhagia
Hypothyroidism	Fatigue, cold intolerance, dry skin, hair loss, constipation, weight gain	Menorrhagia, polymenorrhea, oligomenorrhea, amenorrhea
Bleeding disorder	Asymptomatic mucocutaneous bleeding, easy bruising	Menorrhagia
Endometrial hyperplasia	Asymptomatic	Menorrhagia and/or metrorrhagia
Endometrial cancer	Asymptomatic	Postmenopausal: irregular spotting Perimenopausal: menometrorrhagia
Cervical cancer	Asymptomatic	Irregular spotting, postcoital bleeding

[1]OCP, oral contraceptive pills; HRT, hormone replacement therapy; PID, pelvic inflammatory disease; PCOS, polycystic ovarian syndrome; CAH, congenital adrenal hyperplasia.

continue to bleed every month, women can experience abnormal bleeding patterns including heavy or prolonged bleeding during the regular cycle or bleeding between cycles.

Theoretically patients taking continuous estrogen and progesterone therapy should not experience any bleeding, as the therapy is meant to result in an atrophic endometrium. In reality about 40% of women starting continuous regimens will experience bleeding in the first 4–6 months after starting treatment. To avoid higher rates of irregular bleeding many physicians will use sequential hormonal therapy for 12 months after the start of menopause to avoid the effects of endogenous ovarian function.

C. ANATOMIC CAUSES

1. Fibroids—Fibroids or leiomyomas are benign uterine tumors that are often asymptomatic. The most common symptoms associated with fibroid tumors are pelvic discomfort and abnormal uterine bleeding. Fibroids can be subserosal, intramural, or submucosal. Fibroids located subserosally may be felt on the physical examination as an irregular enlargement of the surface. Depending on the size of the fibroid, intramural and subserosal fibroids can be more difficult to palpate on examination and are more likely to cause abnormal bleeding. Most commonly, women with symptomatic fibroids experience either heavy or prolonged periods. In the past theories about possible mechanisms of uterine bleeding included increased vascularity, interference with uterine contractility, endometrial ulceration, and increased endometrial surface area. More recently, there is evidence to suggest that fibroids involve abnormalities of growth factors that in turn have direct effects on vascular function and angiogenesis.

2. Adenomyosis—Adenomyosis is defined as the presence of endometrial glands within the myometrium.

This is usually asymptomatic, but women can present with heavy or prolonged menstrual bleeding as well as dysmenorrhea. The dysmenorrhea can be severe and begin up to 1 week prior to menstruation. The appearance of symptoms usually occurs after the age of 40.

3. Endometrial and cervical polyps—Endometrial polyps can cause intermenstrual spotting, irregular bleeding, and/or menorrhagia. In contrast, cervical polyps usually cause intermenstrual spotting or postcoital bleeding. Other cervical lesions such as condyloma and herpes simplex virus (HSV) ulcerations can present with similar abnormal bleeding patterns

D. Infectious Causes

Microorganisms including sexually transmitted microorganisms, respiratory pathogens, and endogenous vaginal bacteria can ascend into the endometrium and fallopian tubes, causing pelvic inflammatory disease (PID). Factors that increase endocervical accessibility increase a patient's risk for PID. This occurs during menstruation, and with alterations in the cervical mucus secondary to alterations in the vaginal flora due to bacterial vaginosis. PID in its classic form presents with fever, pelvic discomfort, cervical motion tenderness, and adnexal tenderness. Patients can present atypically with nothing but a change in their bleeding pattern. PID can cause menorrhagia or metrorrhagia, so the patient presenting with abnormal vaginal bleeding should be fully evaluated for PID.

The squamous epithelium of the ectocervix is a continuation of the vaginal epithelium. Therefore, cervical inflammation occurs in the ectocervix when invaded by microrganisms causing vaginitis. The physician will see a bright red cervix (the "strawberry" cervix) in patients with severe cases of trichomonas. The pathogens causing mucopurulent endocervicitis (*Neisseria gonorrhoeae* and *Chlamydia trachomatis*) invade the glandular epithelium of the endocervix. Both kinds of cervical inflammation can cause intermenstrual spotting and postcoital bleeding.

E. Anovulatory Bleeding

When a woman does not ovulate she does not produce a corpus luteum, and then does not produce any progesterone. As a result, the endometrium of the uterus continues to proliferate. Eventually the growth of the endometrium cannot be sustained, resulting in irregular sloughing of the uterine lining. This irregular sloughing causes the bleeding pattern associated with anovulatory bleeding: irregular, heavy periods.

There are multiple causes of anovulation including physiological and pathological etiologies. During the first year following menarche, anovulation is a normal result of an immature hypothalamic–pituitary–gonadal axis. Irregular ovulation also is a normal physiological result of declining ovarian function during the perimenopausal years, and the hormonal changes associated with lactation.

Hyperandrogenic causes of anovulation include PCOS, adult-onset CAH, and androgen-producing tumors. The etiology of PCOS is uncertain, and its clinical features vary. Most recently research has focused on the underlying disorder of insulin resistance in these patients, and the possibility that hyperinsulinemia stimulates excess ovarian androgen production. Making the diagnosis of PCOS involves the evaluation of clinical features and endocrine abnormalities, and the exclusion of other etiologies. Women with PCOS can present with oligomenorrhea or dysfunctional uterine bleeding from prolonged anovulation. In addition, these women can have hirsutism, acne, and central obesity. Endocrinologically they can have increased testosterone activity, elevated luteinizing hormone concentration with a normal follicle-stimulating hormone level, and hyperinsulinemia due to insulin resistance. PCOS usually has its onset during puberty, and so these women often report a long history of irregular periods.

Adult-onset CAH results from an enzyme defect in the adrenal gland, most commonly a deficiency of 21-hydroxylase. There are three hypothesized allelic variants of the 21-hydroxylase deficiency gene: a normal variant, a mild variant, and a severe variant. Patients with adult-onset CAH are either homozygous for the mild allele or have one mild and one severe allele. The genetic defect causes an abnormality in steroid synthesis of glucocorticoids. The hypothalamic–pituitary axis compensates by increasing secretion of ACTH. This in turn causes a hyperplastic adrenal cortex, which produces increased androgens as well as corticoid precursors. Phenotypically women can present in a variety of ways: with PCOS symptoms, with hirsutism alone, or with hyperandrogenic laboratory work but no hyperandrogenic symptoms. Typically patients will present at or after puberty. As a result, these women will also report a long history of irregular periods.

Other causes of anovulation, including androgen-producing tumors, hypothalamic dysfunction, hyperprolactinemia, pituitary disease, and premature ovarian failure, are more likely to present as amenorrhea than vaginal bleeding.

F. Endocrine Abnormalities

Both hyper- and hypothyroidism can cause changes in a woman's menstrual cycle. Hyperthyroidism can cause amenorrhea, oligomenorrhea, hypermenorrhea, or polymenorrhea. Of all the menstrual abnormalities, oligomenorrhea is the most common in patients with hyperthyroidism. Patients who smoke and have higher total thyroxine (T_4) levels tend to have more menstrual disturbances.

A patient with hypothyroidism may experience changes in her menstrual cycle including amenorrhea, oligomenorrhea, polymenorrhea, or menorrhagia. Menstrual abnormalities occur more frequently with severe than with mild hypothyroidism. Hypothyroidism most likely causes menorrhagia through a combination of anovulation and subsequent breakthrough bleeding as well as decreased levels of coagulation factors.

G. BLEEDING DISORDERS

Formation of a platelet plug is the first step of homeostasis during menstruation. Patients with disorders that interfere with the formation of a normal platelet plug can experience menorrhagia. The two most common disorders are von Willebrand's disease and thrombocytopenia. Bleeding can be particularly severe at menarche, due to the dominant estrogen stimulation causing increased vascularity. Patients with von Willebrand's disease will usually present with a long history of heavy periods. Patients with thrombocytopenia can present with menorrhagia with the onset of their disease.

Bleeding disorders resulting from coagulation deficiencies cause impaired formation of fibrin from fibrinogen. These deficiencies are more common in men. They more often cause bleeding in soft tissues and mucocutaneous tissues. Cases of menorrhagia in women with coagulation deficiencies have been reported.

H. ENDOMETRIAL HYPERPLASIA

Endometrial hyperplasia is an overgrowth of the glandular epithelium of the endometrial lining. This usually occurs when a patient is exposed to unopposed estrogen, either estrogenically or because of anovulation. Retrospectively, we know that the rate of neoplasms found with simple hyperplasia is 1% and that the rate with complex hyperplasia is much higher, reaching almost 30% when atypia is present. We do not know if the different types of hyperplasia reflect a spectrum, what percentage progress to invasive cancer, and over what time period this occurs. Most patients without atypia will respond to progestin therapy. Patients having hyperplasia with atypia should have a hysterectomy due to the high incidence of subsequent endometrial cancer.

I. NEOPLASMS

Uterine cancer is the fourth most common cancer in women. Risk factors for endometrial cancer include nulliparity, late menopause (after age 52), obesity, diabetes, unopposed estrogen therapy, tamoxifen, and a history of atypical endometrial hyperplasia. Endometrial cancer most often presents as postmenopausal bleeding in the sixth and seventh decade, although when investigated only 10% of patients with postmenopausal bleeding will have endometrial cancer. In the perimenopausal period endometrial cancer can present as menometrorrhagia.

Vaginal bleeding is the most common symptom in patients with cervical cancer. The increased cervical friability associated with cervical cancer usually results in postcoital bleeding, but also can appear as irregular or postmenopausal bleeding.

Burke TW et al: Endometrial hyperplasia and endometrial cancer. Obstet Gynecol Clin 1996;23:411.

Ewenstein BM: The pathophysiology of bleeding disorders presenting as abnormal bleeding. Am J Obstet Gynecol 1996;175:770.

Hatcher RA et al: *Contraceptive Technology.* Ardent Media, 1998.

Hopkinson ZE et al: Polycystic ovarian syndrome: the metabolic syndrome comes to gynaecology. Br Med J 1998;317:329.

Kaunitz AM: Injectable long-acting contraceptive. Clin Obstet Gynecol 2001;44:73.

Lurain JR: Uterine cancer. In: *Novak's Gynecology.* Berek JS, Adashi EY, Hillard PA (editors). Williams & Wilkins, 1996.

Rapkin AJ: Pelvic pain and dysmenorrhea. In: *Novak's Gynecology.* Berek JS, Adashi EY, Hillard PA (editors). Williams & Wilkins, 1996.

Spencer CP, Cooper AJ, Whitehead MI: Management of abnormal bleeding in women receiving hormone replacement therapy. Br Med J 1997;315:37.

Stovall DW: Clinical symptomatology of uterine leiomyomas. Clin Obstet Gynecol 2001;44:364.

Treatment

The treatment for vaginal bleeding depends on the underlying cause. When the vaginal bleeding is found to have a specific cause, such as an infectious agent or thyroid disease, the treatment should obviously be directed at the specific underlying disease. The primary care physician can also initiate many other treatments for vaginal bleeding. When initial treatment fails, patients can be referred for treatment with surgical options.

A. BLEEDING FROM CONTRACEPTION

Physicians often change formulations of OCPs to try to decrease the incidence of intermenstrual bleeding, although conflicting study results make it difficult to determine whether different formulations actually make a difference. All formulations share the characteristic of a higher incidence of intermenstrual bleeding during the first cycle of use. Therefore, one of the most important things physicians can do is to reassure the patient and encourage continued use. The physician can try adding exogenous estrogen daily for 7–10 days to control prolonged intermenstrual bleeding, but no clinical trials support this strategy. Physiologically, this approach makes sense, as OCPs cause endometrial atrophy.

Similarly, bleeding is common with Depo Provera, especially early during the treatment. Reassurance and patience should be the initial treatment of any bleeding. With continued bleeding physicians can consider the unstudied practice of adding low-dose estrogen supplementation for 1–3 months.

B. FIBROIDS

Administration of a gonadotropin-releasing hormone (GnRH) agonist can greatly reduce the volume of a patient's fibroids. Unfortunately this effect is temporary. As a result, this treatment is largely reserved for preoperative therapy to facilitate the removal of the uterus or fibroid. Pretreatment can also improve the patient's hematological parameters by decreasing vaginal bleeding prior to surgery. The exception to these restrictions is the perimenopausal patient. If a woman is close to menopause, treatment with a GnRH agonist is reasonable. To achieve success, this approach depends on the woman beginning menopause during treatment. This reduces the chance that myomas will increase in size after the cessation of treatment. Because it is impossible to predict the start of menopause, the number of patients benefiting from this approach is limited.

Treatment with nonsteroidal antiinflammatory drugs or oral contraceptives may be effective in decreasing abnormal uterine bleeding, but there is a lack of randomized trials examining these treatments. Ibuprofen at doses of 1200 mg daily effectively reduces bleeding in patients with primary menorrhagia, but this may not be as effective in women with fibroids. Oral contraceptives may reduce the perceived amount of blood loss. Despite this, they can occasionally stimulate the growth of the fibroids causing other bulk-induced symptoms such as pelvic discomfort to increase.

If patients fail these ambulatory approaches surgical options include a myomectomy, hysterectomy, or uterine embolization. Although the primary care physician will refer the patient out for these procedures, patients will often want to discuss possible treatment options with their physicians. Myomectomy is a good option for the patient who does not want her uterus removed or desires future childbearing. The risk exists for the growth of new fibroids and the growth of fibroids too small for removal at the time of surgery. Women having hysterectomies may have the option of an abdominal or vaginal hysterectomy. Vaginal hysterectomies involve fewer complications and shorter hospital stays. The size of the uterus at the time of surgery determines the feasibility of this approach, as the surgeon must be able to remove the uterus completely through a vaginal incision.

Women wanting to avoid hysterectomy now have the option of uterine fibroid embolization. In this procedure an interventional radiologist injects tiny polyvinyl alcohol particles into the uterine arteries. Because the hypervascular fibroids have no collateral vascular supply, they undergo ischemic necrosis. Women with pedunculated or subserosal fibroids are not considered ideal candidates for this procedure. In addition, because the effects of uterine artery embolization on childbearing are not well known, the procedure is generally not done on women desiring future fertility. Menorrhagia is improved in over 90% of women undergoing uterine artery embolization.

C. ANOVULATORY BLEEDING

In general, medical management is the preferred treatment for anovulatory bleeding. Treatment goals should include alleviation of any acute bleeding, prevention of future noncyclic bleeding, a decrease in the patient's future risk of long-term health problems secondary to anovulation, and improvement in the patient's quality of life. Treatment options include prostaglandin synthetase inhibitors, estrogen, oral contraceptives, and cyclic progesterones. Those failing medical management have surgical options including hysterectomy and endometrial ablation.

Blood loss can be reduced by 50% in women treated with prostaglandin synthetase inhibitors including mefenamic acid, ibuprofen, and naproxen. Because many of the studies evaluating the role of prostaglandin synthetase inhibitors were completed in women with ovulatory cycles, the results cannot be directly applied to women with anovulatory bleeding; women with anovulatory bleeding may not find this approach as effective. In addition, this treatment does not address the issues of future noncyclic bleeding and decreasing future health risks due to anovulation.

Estrogen alone is usually used to treat an acute episode of heavy uterine bleeding. Premarin used intravenously will temporarily stop most uterine bleeding, regardless of the cause. The dose commonly used is 25 mg of conjugated estrogen every 4 h. Nausea limits using high doses of estrogen orally, but lower doses can be used in a patient with acute heavy bleeding who is hemodynamically stable. One suggested regimen is 2.5 mg conjugated estrogen every 4–6 h.

After acute bleeding is controlled, the physician should add a progestin to the treatment regimen to induce withdrawal bleeding. A combination of estrogen and progesterone is given for 7–10 days and then stopped, inducing a withdrawal bleed. To decrease the risk of future hyperplasia and/or endometrial cancer, a progestin is continued for 10–14 days each cycle. Traditionally, treatment has been with medroxyprogesterone acetate (Provera) 10 mg. Other progestational agents include norethindrone acetate (Aygestin), norethindrone (Micronor), norgestrel (Ovrette), and micronized progesterone (Prometrium, Crinone). The micronized progesterones are natural progesterones modified to have a prolonged half-life and less destruction in the gastrointestinal tract. Women having problems with mood changes from synthetic progestins may better tolerate treatment with a micronized progesterone.

OCPs provide an option for treatment of both the acute episode of bleeding and future episodes of bleeding as well as prevention of long-term health problems from anovulation. Acutely, one option to control bleeding is to use a 50-μg estrogen OCP four times a day until bleeding ceases, then continue the OCP for a week. This may not be as effective as estrogen alone for quick stoppage of bleeding, but is very convenient and easy. Long term, OCPs are effective in treating all patterns of dysfunctional uterine bleeding. Although the triphasil norgestimate/ethinyl estradiol combination has been studied in a double-blind, placebo-controlled study, various oral contraceptives have been used for decades to control uterine bleeding. Patients with a history of thromboembolism, cerebrovascular disease, coronary artery disease, estrogen-dependent neoplasias, or liver disease should not be started on an oral contraceptive. Relative contraindications include migraine headaches, hypertension, diabetes, age greater than 35 in a smoking patient, and active gallbladder disease.

When evaluating various treatment regimens for dysfunctional uterine bleeding the clinician should realize that there are few studies evaluating the most effective type, dose, regimen, and administrative route. This contributes to a wide range of suggested treatment options, none of which has been proven to be more superior than another.

Patients who are unable to tolerate hormonal management can consider endometrial ablation. Using electrocautery, laser, cryoablation, or thermoablation, these techniques all result in destruction of the endometrial lining. Initially used exclusively in patients with menorrhagia, these treatments are now also used in women with anovulatory bleeding, although outcomes are not well studied for this indication. Because endometrial glands often persist after ablative treatment, most women will not experience long-term amenorrhea after treatment. Also, because endometrial glands do persist, the risk of endometrial cancer is not eliminated after treatment. Women at risk for endometrial cancer from long-term unopposed estrogen exposure still need preventive treatment. This procedure should be used only in women who choose not to preserve future fertility. As pregnancies have occurred after endometrial ablation, some form of contraception may be needed after the procedure.

D. ALTERNATIVE THERAPIES

Although no controlled studies have been completed, small studies suggest that acupuncture may be an option for young women with dysfunctional bleeding and for women with PCOS.

The nomenclature used in traditional Chinese medicine differs from western medicine, so making a direct comparison of treatments is difficult. Again, no controlled studies have been completed, but smaller studies suggest a possible role in certain situations for patients interested in pursuing alternative therapies. Keishibukuryo-gan (KBG) is a traditional herbal remedy that may act as a luteinizing hormone-releasing hormone antagonist and a weak antiestrogen. It has been used successfully in the treatment of uterine fibroids. A smaller number of patients have been treated for acute bleeding and then induction of ovulation.

Agency for Healthcare Research and Quality: Management of uterine fibroids. Summary, evidence report/technology assessment: number 34. Publication no. 01-E051, January 2001. AHRQ, Rockville, MD.

American College of Obstetricians and Gynecologists: Management of anovulatory bleeding. ACOG Pract Bull 2000;14;1.

Apgar BS, Greenberg GG: Using progestins in clinical practice. AFP 2000;8:1839.

Chavez NF, Stewart EA: Medical treatment of uterine fibroids. Clin Obstet Gynecol 2001;44:372.

Guarnaccia MM, Rein MS: Traditional surgical approaches to uterine fibroids: abdominal myomectomy and hysterectomy. Clin Obstet Gynecol 2001;44:385.

Hickey M, Higham J, Fraser IS: Progestogens versus oestrogens and progestogens for irregular uterine bleeding associated with anovulation. Cochrane Database Syst Rev 2000; CD001895.

Kammerer-Doak DN, Rogers RG: Endometrial ablation: electrocautery and laser techniques. Clin Obstet Gynecol 2000;43:561.

Smith SJ: Uterine fibroid embolization. Am Fam Phys 2000;61:3601.

Hypertension

Maureen O'Hara Padden, MD

General Considerations

At least 50 million Americans have hypertension, defined as systolic blood pressure greater than or equal to 140 mm Hg and/or diastolic blood pressure greater than or equal to 90 mm Hg. This translates to one in four adults and one in five Americans. High blood pressure resulted in the death of 44,435 Americans in 1998 and contributed to the death of about 210,000. Of persons with high blood pressure roughly one-third are not aware of their diagnosis. The incidence of hypertension increases with age and is demonstrated by the fact that over 75% of women aged 75 and over and 64% of men aged 75 and over are affected. Hypertension is most prevalent among the black population, affecting one of every three African-Americans. Non-Hispanic blacks and Mexican-Americans are also more likely to suffer from high blood pressure than non-Hispanic whites.

The National High Blood Pressure Education Program (NHBPEP), which is coordinated by the National Heart, Lung, and Blood Institute (NHBLI) of the National Institutes of Health, was established in 1972. The program was designed to increase awareness, prevention, treatment, and control of hypertension. Data from the National Health and Nutrition Examination Survey (NHANES), conducted between 1976 and 1991, revealed that the number of patients aware of their high blood pressure, under treatment for high blood pressure, and achieving control of high blood pressure had increased. Coincident with these positive changes was a dramatic reduction in morbidity and mortality (40–60%) including stroke and myocardial infarction secondary to hypertension. However, the most recent NHANES III survey, conducted in 1991–1994, showed that a leveling off in improvement has occurred in these areas. In addition, the incidence of end-stage renal disease and the prevalence of heart failure continue to increase. Both diagnoses have been linked to uncontrolled hypertension in many cases.

High blood pressure is easily detected and usually controlled with appropriate intervention. However, among persons with high blood pressure, 14.8% are not on diet or medical therapy, 26.2% are receiving inadequate therapy, and only 27.4% are on adequate therapy. Clearly room exists for improvement.

Pathogenesis

A. PRIMARY OR ESSENTIAL HYPERTENSION

In 90–95% of cases of hypertension, no cause can be identified. Genetics clearly plays a role in the development of high blood pressure, although it appears that environment and life-style factors are important cofactors. It has been hypothesized that among other things, alterations in the renin–angiotensin and sympathomimetic systems play a contributory role in the development of hypertension.

B. SECONDARY HYPERTENSION

In only 5% of cases can a cause for hypertension be found. It is reasonable to look for an underlying cause in patients diagnosed with hypertension. History or physical examination may suggest an underlying etiology, or the first clue may come later when patients fail to respond appropriately to standard drug therapy. In addition, secondary hypertension should be considered in those with sudden onset of hypertension, in those with suddenly uncontrolled blood pressure that had previously been well controlled, and in those with Stage 3 hypertension.

Causes of secondary hypertension that must be considered in appropriate patients include use of certain medications such as oral contraceptives, sympathomimetics, decongestants, nonsteroidal antiinflammatory drugs, appetite suppressants, antidepressants, adrenal steroids, cyclosporine, and erythropoietin, all of which can contribute to an elevation in blood pressure. Hypertension can also be related to excessive use of caffeine, ingestion of licorice, or use of illicit drugs such as cocaine or amphetamines.

Hypertension can also occur secondary to any form of intrinsic renal disease including, among others, polycystic kidney disease or diabetic nephropathy, which might be suggested by a flank mass, an elevated creatinine, or abnormal findings such as proteinuria, hematuria, or casts on routine urinalysis. Rarely, hypertension may be related to renal artery stenosis, particularly if onset is before the age of 20 or after the age of 50 years. Abdominal bruits with radiation to the renal area are sometimes heard. Other causes to consider include hypothyroidism, hyperthyroidism, primary hyperaldosteronism, Cushing's syndrome, coarctation of the aorta, and pheochromocytoma in the appropriate clinical presentation. When such causes are entertained, appropriate evaluation should be undertaken.

Prevention

Life-style modifications including maintaining optimal weight and a regular aerobic exercise program can help prevent or delay the onset of hypertension. Patients should be encouraged to follow a diet rich in fruits and vegetables and low in saturated and total fats. Alcohol intake should be in moderation. Life-style modification is discussed in greater detail later.

Clinical Findings

Before patients with hypertension can be offered adequate treatment, they must be properly diagnosed. Because patients are often asymptomatic, the risk factors for hypertension must be understood and appropriate patients must be screened.

Modifiable risk factors include obesity [body mass index (BMI) >30], excessive salt ingestion, heavy alcohol consumption, and lack of exercise. Other significant risk factors that are not modifiable include African-American race, family history of hypertension, and increasing age.

A. Symptoms and Signs

There are usually no physical findings early in the course of hypertension with which to make the diagnosis. In some patients, the presence of hypertension may be signaled by early morning headaches or patients with onset of severe hypertension may experience signs or symptoms associated with target organ damage. Such symptoms might include nausea, vomiting, visual disturbance, chest pain, or confusion. More typically, the first indication is an elevated blood pressure taken, using a sphygmomanometer, at a routine visit or after the patient has had a stroke or myocardial infarction.

Proper measurement of blood pressure should occur with patients seated in a chair with their back supported and their arms bared and supported at heart level. Caffeine and tobacco should be avoided in the 30 min preceding measurement and measurement should begin after 5 min of rest. The cuff size should be appropriate for the patient's arm as evidenced by the bladder encircling 80% of the arm. It is important that the diagnosis be made after the elevation in blood pressure is documented with three separate readings, on three different occasions, unless the elevation is severe or is associated with symptoms requiring immediate attention (hypertensive urgency or emergency). Transient elevation of blood pressure secondary to pain or anxiety, as experienced by some patients when they enter the doctor's office ("White Coat Syndrome"), does not require treatment. In cases in which the diagnosis is in question, 24-h ambulatory blood pressure monitoring can sometimes be useful in clarifying whether the patient has high blood pressure.

1. Classification of blood pressure—The Sixth Report of the Joint National Committee on Prevention, Detection and Treatment of High Blood Pressure (JNC VI) was released in November 1997. It proposed a classification system now well accepted as the standard for adults aged 18 and older (Table 33–1).

This classification assumes that patients are not already taking antihypertensive medication and are not acutely ill. Optimal blood pressure when considering risk for cardiovascular disease is below 120/80 mm Hg. Diagnosis of high blood pressure should be based on the average of two or more readings taken at each of two or more visits after initial screening. When systolic and diastolic blood pressures fall into two different categories, the higher category should be used to classify the patient. For example, a patient whose blood pressure is 165/94 should be classified with Stage 2 hypertension. In the case of a patient with isolated systolic hypertension whose blood pressure reading is 184/76, correct categorization would be Stage 3 hypertension.

Table 33–1. Classification of blood pressure for adults age 18 and older.

Category	Systolic (mm Hg)		Diastolic (mm Hg)
Optimal	< 120	and	< 80
Normal	< 130	and	< 85
High-normal	130–139	or	85–89
Hypertension			
Stage 1	140–159	or	90–99
Stage 2	160–179	or	100–109
Stage 3	≥180	or	≥110

Source: JNC VI Report.

2. Self-monitoring—Patients should be encouraged to do self-monitoring of their blood pressure at home. Many easy-to-use blood pressure monitors are commercially available at reasonable cost for use at home. Validated electronic devices are recommended and independent reviews of available devices, such as that published by Consumer Reports, are periodically published. Self-measurement can be extremely helpful in ensuring that the diagnosis of hypertension is correct, in assessing response to medical therapy, and in encouraging patient compliance with therapy by providing regular feedback on therapy response.

3. Recommendations for follow-up—JNC VI made specific recommendations concerning follow-up for initial blood pressure measurements in adults (Table 33–2). Once again, when systolic and diastolic blood pressures fall into different categories, follow-up should be conservative and a shorter time to follow-up should be recommended. For example, for a patient with a blood pressure of 150/88, recommended follow-up should be within 2 months. Patients whose blood pressure is categorized as high normal (130–139/85–89), in addition to follow-up blood pressure evaluation in 1 year, should be provided with counseling on life-style modifications.

B. Evaluation

Patients with documented hypertension must undergo a thorough evaluation to identify known causes of high blood pressure, to establish whether the patient already manifests evidence of target end-organ disease, and, finally, to identify any cardiovascular risk factors or comorbidities that would necessarily guide therapy.

Table 33–2. Recommendations for follow-up based on initial blood pressure measurement in adults.

Initial Blood Pressure (mm Hg)		Follow-Up Recommended
Systolic	**Diastolic**	
< 130	< 85	Recheck in 2 years
130–139	85–89	Recheck in 1 year
140–159	90–99	Confirm within 2 months
160–179	100–109	Evaluate or refer to source of care within 1 month
≥180	≥110	Evaluate or refer to source of care immediately or within 1 week depending on the clinic schedule

Source: JNC VI Report.

1. Medical history—A thorough history should be taken from the patient diagnosed with hypertension. Any prior history of hypertension should be elicited from the patient as well as response and side effects to any previous hypertension therapy. It is important to inquire as to whether there is any history or symptoms suggestive of coronary artery disease and other significant comorbidities including diabetes, heart failure, dyslipidemia, renal disease, and peripheral vascular disease. The family history should also be reviewed with special attention to the presence of hypertension, premature coronary artery disease, diabetes, renal disease, dyslipidemia, or stroke. Use of tobacco, alcohol, or illicit drugs should be documented as well as dietary intake of sodium, saturated fat, and caffeine. Recent changes in weight and exercise level should be queried. Current medications used by the patient should be reviewed including over-the-counter medications and herbal formulations.

2. Physical examination—The initial physical examination should be comprehensive and should pay careful attention to the following areas.

a. General—Baseline height, weight, and waist circumference should be documented. Upper and lower extremity blood pressures should be taken to assess for coarctation of the aorta. Note any features of Cushing's syndrome.

b. Eyes—Funduscopic examination should be performed looking for any signs of hypertensive retinopathy including arteriolar narrowing, focal arteriolar constriction, atrioventricular nicking, hemorrhages, or exudates.

c. Neck—The neck should be auscultated for carotid bruits and examined for neck vein distention or thyroid gland enlargement.

d. Heart—Cardiac auscultation should assess for abnormalities in rate or rhythm, murmurs, or extra heart sounds.

e. Lungs—Pulmonary auscultation should be used to assess for rales, rhonchi, or wheezes.

f. Abdomen—Auscultation for abdominal bruits suggestive of renal artery stenosis and examination for enlargement of the kidneys (mass) or aortic pulsation suggesting aneurysm should be done.

g. Extremities—Examination and documentation of diminished or absent peripheral arterial pulsations, any edema, or signs of vascular compromise should be performed.

h. Neurological—Examination should be performed to assess for any deficits.

C. Laboratory and Diagnostic Tests

Routine tests should include urinalysis looking for hematuria, proteinuria, or casts suggestive of intrinsic renal disease. Complete blood count rules out anemia or polycythemia. Potassium levels help assess for hyperaldosteronism. Creatinine levels reflect renal function. Fasting glucose is used to assess for diabetes. Other tests include serum sodium level, lipid profile as an indicator of cardiovascular risk, and a 12-lead electrocardiogram. Tests that may be considered if the history or physical examination suggests utility include hemoglobin A1C, calcium, thyroid-stimulating hormone, microalbuminuria, creatinine clearance, and 24-h urine for protein. Echocardiogram and chest x-ray are not routinely recommended for evaluation of the hypertensive patient. In certain cases, however, an echocardiogram may prove useful in guiding therapy when baseline abnormalities are found on the electrocardiogram such as left ventricular hypertrophy or signs of previous silent myocardial infarction. A chest x-ray may be useful if there are abnormal findings on physical examination. Tests that evaluate for rare causes such as renal artery stenosis (renal ultrasound) or pheochromocytoma (24-h urine for catecholamines) should be ordered only for patients whose history and physical examination raise suspicion.

Treatment

A. Cardiovascular Risk Stratification

There is a strong association between hypertension and cardiovascular disease with 50% of patients with known coronary artery disease having coincident high blood pressure. Hypertension is clearly an important, but not the only risk factor for heart disease. JNC VI defines specific components of cardiovascular risk that are used not only in risk stratification but in recommendations for therapy (Table 33–3).

JNC VI recommends that a specific stratification system be used when considering initial therapy for patients with hypertension (Table 33–4). Risk group A has no risk factors, no target organ damage, and no evidence of cardiovascular disease. Life-style modification may be used initially depending on blood pressure level. Risk group B is characterized by at least one risk factor, not including diabetes mellitus, without evidence of target organ damage or cardiovascular disease. Similarly, life-style modification may be used initially depending on blood pressure level. When life-style modification is used as initial therapy for the specified period of time without successful control of blood pressure, drug therapy should then be initiated. Risk group C, which is an indication for drug therapy at all levels of high blood pressure including high-normal blood pressure, is defined by the presence of target organ damage, evidence of cardiovascular disease, and/or diabetes mellitus with or without risk factors. It is important to remember that even when pharmacological therapy is indicated, life-style modification is an important aspect of therapy for *all* patients.

Table 33–3. Components of cardiovascular risk stratification in patients with hypertension.

Major risk factors (RF)
  Smoking
  Dyslipidemia
  Diabetes mellitus
  Age older than 60 years
  Sex (men and postmenopausal women)
  Family history of cardiovascular disease (women under age 65 and men under age 55)

Target organ damage/clinical cardiovascular disease (TOD/CCD)
  Heart disease
    Left ventricular hypertrophy
    Angina pectoris/prior myocardial infarction
    Prior coronary revascularization
    Heart failure
  Stroke
  Nephropathy
  Peripheral artery disease
  Retinopathy

Source: JNC VI Report.

B. Life-style Modification

Life-style modifications can be effective in reducing blood pressure in motivated patients. Overweight patients should be encouraged to lose weight. Even small amounts of weight loss (10 pounds) can improve blood pressure control and reduce cardiovascular risk. Weight loss can be facilitated through dietary changes and increased exercise. Patients should be encouraged to set their exercise goal for 30–45 min of aerobic activity most days of the week. Any use of tobacco should be discouraged and patients currently using tobacco should be counseled to quit as this may help lower blood pressure.

Patients should be encouraged to show moderation in their intake of alcoholic beverages. Alcohol intake should be limited to no more than 1 oz of ethanol, 24 oz of beer, 10 oz of wine, or 2 oz of 100 proof whiskey per day. Women and individuals who are thin should limit daily ethanol intake to 0.5 oz. Sodium intake should be reduced to no more than 100 mmol/day based on available evidence. African-Americans, diabetics, and elderly patients are more likely to show a blood pressure response to reduction in salt intake than others. Adequate intake of potassium should be encour-

Table 33–4. Risk stratification and treatment.[1]

Blood Pressure Stages (mm Hg)	Risk Group A (No RF, No TOD/CCD)	Risk Group B (at Least One RF, Not DM, No TOD/CCD)	Risk Group C (TOD/CCD and/or DM, with or without RF)
High normal (130–139/85–89)	Life-style modification	Life-style modification	Drug therapy[2]
Stage 1 (140–159/90–99)	Life-style modification (up to 12 months)	Life-style modification (up to 6 months)[3]	Drug therapy
Stage 2 and 3 (≥160/≥100)	Drug therapy	Drug therapy	Drug therapy

Source: JNC VI Report.
[1] RF, risk factor; TOD/CCD, target organ damage/clinical cardiovascular disease; DM, diabetes mellitus.
[2] Drug therapy is indicated in patients with diabetes, heart failure, or renal insufficiency.
[3] If more than one risk factor is present consider drug therapy.

aged (90 mmol/day) as blood pressure control may improve. However, patients taking angiotensin-converting enzyme (ACE) inhibitors or angiotensin receptor blockers should be cautioned regarding potassium intake as these medications can result in potassium retention.

C. PHARMACOLOGICAL TREATMENT

Many medications are available to treat hypertension. Medication should be initiated at a low dose and titrated slowly to achieve desired blood pressure control. When available, formulations available in once daily dosing are preferred due to increased patient compliance. Also useful are the many combination formulations now available that incorporate two different classes of drugs. When selecting a medication, side effect profile and patient comorbidities should help guide choice. The recommendations that follow are based on JNC VI. In addition, evidence from trials released since JNC VI was published are discussed. JNC VI recommends initially treating uncomplicated hypertension with diuretics or β-blockers in the absence of a compelling reason to use another agent. This strong recommendation is based on the many randomized controlled trials that have demonstrated a reduction in morbidity, including stroke, coronary artery disease, and congestive heart failure, as well as total mortality.

1. Diuretics—Compared with β-blockers, diuretics are an excellent first choice for therapy in most patients, particularly African-Americans with uncomplicated hypertension. Diuretics should be used cautiously in patients with gout as worsening hyperuricemia can result. They may also cause muscle cramps or impotence in some individuals. Diuretics may be effective at lower doses in patients with dyslipidemia and diabetes mellitus, but patients placed on higher doses must be observed closely for worsening hyperglycemia or hyperlipidemia. The thiazide diuretics are most commonly used in the treatment of hypertension as the loop diuretics are more likely to lead to electrolyte abnormalities such as hypokalemia and to have a shorter duration of action. However, loop diuretics can sometimes be useful in the treatment of hypertension in patients with chronic renal disease and a serum creatinine of greater than 2.5 mg/dL. The loop diuretics have found most utility in the treatment of congestive heart failure. Commonly used diuretics are listed in Table 33–5.

2. β-Blockers—β-Blockers are also an excellent choice for treatment of uncomplicated hypertension, particularly in patients with comorbidities that will benefit from their use, such as angina, a history of myocardial infarction, migraine headache, hyperthyroidism, and anxiety. Patients should be informed that β-blockers may cause sexual dysfunction. β-Blockers should be used with caution, if at all, in patients with a history of depression, asthma or reactive airway disease, second- or third-degree heart block, or peripheral vascular disease. In patients with mild to moderate reactive airway disease, the benefits of cardioselective β-blockers probably outweigh the small risk and warrant a trial of therapy. Studies have suggested that they have little effect on respiratory function in patients with less severe airway disease. The United Kingdom Prospective Diabetes Study (UKPDS) demonstrated that β-blockers can be used safely and effectively for type 2 diabetes mellitus, although there is concern that hypoglycemic episodes might be masked. Any patient with diabetes mellitus placed on a β-blocker should, therefore, be carefully monitored. Although previously not recommended, patients with congestive heart failure are now being successfully treated with β-blockers lacking intrinsic sympathomimetic activity including two of the most studied, carvedilol and metoprolol. Careful use of these agents has shown promise in reducing mortality and improving ejection fraction in patients with NYHA Class II or III congestive heart failure. Commonly used β-blockers are listed in Table 33–6.

Table 33–5. Diuretics.[1]

Drug	Initial Dose	Typical Dose Range	30-Day Cost	Comments
Thiazides				
Hydrochlorothiazide (Esidrix, Hydrodiuril, Microzide, Oretic)	12.5 mg po qd	12.5–50 mg/day	25 mg qd (30) $2.40	G[2]
Chlorathalidone (Hygroton)	12.5 mg po qd	12.5–50 mg/day	25 mg qd 50 mg tabs (15) $2.81	G
Indapamide (Lozol)	1.25 mg po qam	1.25–5.0 mg/day	2.5 mg qd (30) $7.98	G
Metolazone (Zaroxolyn)	1.25–2.5 mg po qd	1.25–10.0 mg/day	2.5 mg qd (30) $24.78	
Loop diuretics				
Furosemide (Lasix)	20 mg po bid	20–120 mg po bid	20 mg bid (60) $8.00	G, short duration
Bumetanide (Bumex)	0.5 mg po qd	0.5–4.0 mg/day (total split in two or three doses)	0.5 mg bid 1 mg tabs (60) $16.04	G, short duration
Other				
Hydrochlorothiazide/ triamterene (Maxide, Diazide)	25/37.5 mg po qd	1–2 tabs once daily	1 tab qd (30) $14.33	G, limit use to patients needing potassium-sparing agent
Hydrochlorothiazide/ amiloride (Moduretic)	½ tab po qd	1–2 tabs once daily	1 tab qd (30) $18.34	
Hydrochlorothiazide/ spirinolactone (Aldactazide)	1 tab po qd	1–2 tabs once daily	1 tab qd (30) $16.69	

[1]po, orally; qd, daily; qam, every morning; tabs, tablets; bid, twice a day.
[2]G, generic available.

3. Calcium channel blockers—There are two classes of calcium channel blockers: the dihydropyridine calcium channel blockers, which vasodilate (nifedipine, amlodipine, felodipine), and the rate-lowering calcium channel blockers (verapamil, diltiazem). They have relatively few side effects but may cause headache, nausea, rash, or flushing in some patients. Calcium channel blockers were not recommended as first-line therapy by JNC VI, although it did suggest that long-acting dihydropyridine calcium channel blockers could have limited use in treating isolated systolic hypertension in elderly patients. This recommendation was based on the lack of evidence in the literature at that time regarding any improvement in morbidity and mortality for calcium channel blockers when compared with diuretics and β-blockers. The Systolic Hypertension in Europe

(SYSEUR) trial released in 1997, however, randomized 5000 elderly patients with isolated systolic hypertension to treatment with either placebo or the long-acting dihydropyridine calcium channel blocker nitrendipine. In 2 years of follow-up there was significant reduction in stroke and cardiovascular events, thus the recommendation for targeted use of dihydropyridine calcium channel blockers for treating isolated systolic hypertension. JNC VI also recommended use of calcium channel blockers to control hypertension in patients with co-morbidities likely to benefit from their use: coincident angina, migraine headaches, and in the case of rate-lowering calcium channel blockers, atrial tacchycardia and atrial fibrillation.

Calcium channel blockers have also been recommended as second-line therapy after diuretics in African-

Table 33–6. β-Blockers.[1]

Drug	Initial Dose	Typical Dose Range	30-Day Cost[2]	Comments[3]
Acebutolol (Sectral)	200 mg po qd	200–800 mg (can split into two doses)	400 mg tabs (30) $21.11	1,2,3,H,R
Atenolol (Tenormin)	25–50 mg po qd	25–100 mg po qd	50 mg tabs (30) $2.40	1,3,R
Betaxolol (Kerlone)	10 mg po qd Renal disease: 5 mg	10–20 mg po qd Renal disease max 20 mg	20 mg tabs (30) $31.95	1,3,H,R
Bisoprolol fumarate (Zebeta)	2.5 mg po qd	2.5–10 mg po qd	10 mg tabs (30) $33.56	1,3,H
Carteolol hydrochloride (Cartrol)	2.5 mg po qd	2.5–10 mg po qd	5 mg tabs (30) $39.57	2,H,R
Metoprolol tartrate (Lopressor)	50 mg po qd–bid	50–300 mg/day (total) split in two doses	50 mg bid (60) $9.56	1,3,H
Metoprolol succinate (TorprolXL)	50 mg po qd	50–300 mg/day	100 mg (30) $27.86	1,H
Nadolol (Corgard)	20–40 mg po qd	20–320 mg/day	40 mg (30) $12.93	3,R
Penbutolol sulfate (Levatol)	10 mg po qd	10–80 mg/day	20 mg tabs (30) $45.93	2,H,R
Pindolol (Visken)	5 mg po bid	10–60 mg/day (total) split in two doses	5 mg bid (60) $13.76	2,3,H,R
Propanolol hydrochloride (Inderal) (Inderal LA)	20–40 mg po bid 60–80 mg po qd	40–480 mg/day (total) split in two doses 60–320 mg po qd	40 mg bid (60) $7.99 80 mg (30) $41.24	3,H
Timolol (Bocadren)	5–10 mg po bid	10–60 mg/day (total) split in two doses	10 mg bid (60) $15.10	3,H,R
Combined α- and β-blocker				
Carvedilol (Coreg)	6.25 bid with food, titrate after 2 weeks	12.5–50 mg/day (total) split in two doses	12.5 mg bid (60) $90.67	H
Labetolol hydrochloride (Normodyne, Trandate)	100 mg po bid	200–1200 mg/day (total) split in two doses	200 mg bid (60) $28.60	3,H

[1]po, orally; qd, daily; tabs, tablets; bid, twice a day.
[2]Average retail cost www.drugstore.com as per Epocrates Rx; generic cost when available.
[3]1, cardioselective; 2, intrinsic sympathomimetic activity; 3, generic available; R, renal metabolism; H, hepatic metabolism.

Americans with hypertension. Diltiazem has been shown to be extremely effective in lowering diastolic blood pressure in African-American males when compared with other agents. Since the release of JNC VI, several studies have involved calcium channel blockers. The Hypertension Outcomes Trial (HOT) revealed that use of the long-acting dihydropyridine calcium channel blocker felodipine led to a reduction in cardiovascular events, especially in the diabetic subpopulation. Meanwhile, the Appropriate Blood Pressure Control in Diabetes (ABCD) trial compared the calcium channel blocker nisoldipine to the ACE inhibitor enalapril. Although the group treated with the ACE inhibitor had significantly fewer fatal and nonfatal myocardial infarctions, there was no comparative placebo control. The evidence is still incomplete as to whether calcium channel blockers are as useful in improving outcomes as the traditionally used β-blockers and diuretics. A large number of trials currently underway comparing calcium channel blockers with other agents should help to clarify this issue. Table 33–7 lists commonly used calcium channel blockers.

Table 33–7. Calcium channel blockers.[1]

Drug	Initial Dose	Typical Dose Range	30-Day Cost[2]	Comments[3]
Dihydropyridine class				
Amlodipine (Norvasc)	5 mg po qd	5–10 mg po qd	5 mg qd (30) $37.62	H
Felodipine (Plendil)	5 mg po qd	5–20 mg po qd	5 mg qd (30) $33.02	H
Isradapine (Dynacirc)	2.5 mg po bid	2.5–10.0 mg bid	2.5 mg bid (60) $56.32	H
Isradapine (Dynacirc CR)	5 mg po qd	5–20 mg po qd	5 mg qd (30) $42.80	H
Nicardipine (Cardene)	20 mg po tid	20–40 mg po tid	30 mg po tid (90) $28.56	G,H
Nifedipine (Procardia XL)	30 mg po qd	30–120 mg po qd	60 mg po qd (30) $49.87	G,H
Nisoldipine (Sular)	10 mg po qd	10–60 mg po qd	30 mg po qd (30) $31.52	H
Nondihydropyridine class				
Diltiazem (Cardizem SR)	60 mg po bid	60–180 mg po bid		
Diltiazem (Cardizem CD)	180 mg po qd	180–360 mg po qd	180 mg qd (30) $49.22	
Verapamil (Calan SR)	180 mg po q am	180–480 mg po qd (if > 240 mg/day split to two doses)	180 mg qd (30) $45.32	

Source: JNC VI Report.
[1]po, orally; qd, daily; bid, twice a day; tid, three times a day; q am, each morning.
[2]Average retail cost www.drugstore.com as per Epocrates Rx; generic cost when available.
[3]G, generic available; H, hepatic metabolism.

4. ACE inhibitors—The ACE inhibitors stimulate vasodilation by blocking the renin–angiotensin–aldosterone system and inhibiting degradation of bradykinin. ACE inhibitors have relatively few side effects, the most significant being a dry cough in some individuals and hyperkalemia. JNC VI recommends that ACE inhibitors be considered first-line treatment of hypertension for diabetics (type I and II) with proteinuria, for patients with congestive heart failure, and for patients who have had a myocardial infarction with systolic dysfunction. ACE inhibitors have also been shown to be more effective in promoting regression of left ventricular hypertrophy (LVH) than diuretics, β-blockers, or calcium channel blockers. LVH is considered one of the best predictors of cardiovascular events in patients with hypertension. However, ACE inhibitors must be used cautiously in patients with known renovascular disease and, when used, may need dose adjustment due to reduced drug clearance. These agents should be used with extreme caution, if at all, in patients whose serum creatinine exceeds 3.0 mg/mL. ACE inhibitors should not be used in patients with bilateral renal artery stenosis.

Since JNC VI was released, several randomized controlled clinical trials have suggested that ACE inhibitors may be as effective in reducing morbidity and mortality as β-blockers and diuretics. In the Captopril Prevention Project (CAPPP) trial released in 1999, patients were randomized to treatment of hypertension with either captopril or conventional therapy (diuretics and β-blockers). In 5 years of follow-up, there was no statistically significant difference in primary end points between the groups including myocardial infaction, stroke, and deaths due to other cardiovascular events. In the Fosinopril Versus Amlodipine Cardiovascular Events Trial (FACET), hypertensive type II diabetics were randomized to treatment with either fosinopril or amlodipine, with the addition of the other drug allowed if blood pressure was not controlled. The ACE inhibitor group had significantly fewer cardiovascular events, but, perhaps most interesting, the group taking both the ACE inhibitor and the calcium channel blocker had the least number of events.

The results of the FACET trial were affirmed in the Appropriate Blood Pressure Control in Diabetes (ABCD) trial, which randomized diabetics to treatment with enalapril or nisoldipine. The ACE inhibitor group again showed a reduction in cardiovascular events. The United Kingdom Prospective Diabetes Study (UKPDS) compared treatment of hypertension in diabetics using either a β-blocker (atenolol) or an ACE inhibitor (captopril). Captopril and atenolol were equally effective in reducing both microvascular and macrovascular events. The Heart Outcomes Prevention Evaluation (HOPE) Study evaluated the effects of ramipril on cardiovascular events in patients considered to be at high risk. The study randomized patients to treatment with either ramipril or placebo. Patients treated with ramipril not only showed a reduction in cardiovascular events, but

showed a measurable reduction in other important outcomes including development of diabetes, progression of diabetic nephropathy, and prevention/remission of LVH.

The CAPPP, FACET, ABCD, UKPDS, and HOPE trials suggest that ACE inhibitors may be as effective as β-blockers and diuretics in reducing morbidity and mortality and that they may be the hypertensive drug of choice in diabetics even when proteinuria is not yet present. The HOPE study was even more interesting in that ACE inhibitors appeared to delay or prevent the onset of diabetes, although this landmark finding needs further study. Table 33–8 lists commonly used ACE inhibitors.

5. Angiotensin II receptor blockers (ARBs)—ARBs selectively block angiotensin II activation of AT1 receptors, which are responsible for mediating vasoconstriction, salt and water retention, and central and sympathetic activation among others. Angiotensin II is still able to activate AT2 blockers, facilitating vasodilation

Table 33–8. ACE inhibitors.[1]

Drug	Initial Dose	Typical Dose Range	30-Day Cost[2]	Comments[3]
Benzapril (Lotensin)	10 mg po qd	10–40 mg po qd	20 mg qd (30) $27.82	
Captopril (Capoten)	25 mg po tid	25–50 mg po tid	25 mg po tid (90) $8.93	G
Enalapril (Vasotec)	5 mg po qd	5–40 mg po qd	10 mg po qd (30) $17.67	
Fosinopril (Monopril)	10 mg po qd	10–40 mg po qd	20 mg po qd (30) $25.16	
Lisinopril (Prinivit®, Zestril®)	10 mg po qd	10–40 mg po qd	20 mg po qd (30) $27.41	
Moexipril (Univasc)	7.5 mg po qd	7.5–15 mg po qd	15 mg po qd (30) $21.96	
Quinapril (Accupril)	10 mg po qd	10–80 mg po qd	20 mg po qd (30) $29.90	
Ramipril (Altace)	2.5 mg po qd	2.5–20 mg po qd		
Trandolapril (Mavik)	1–2 mg po qd	1–4 mg po qd	4 mg po qd (30) $25.76	
Perindopril (Aceon)	4 mg po qd	4–16 mg po qd	4 mg po qd (30) $29.91	

Source: JNC VI Report.
[1]po, orally; qd, daily; tid, three times a day.
[2]Average retail cost www.drugstore.com as per Epocrates Rx; generic cost when available.
[3]G, generic available.

Table 33–9. Angiotensin II receptor blockers.[1]

Drug	Initial Dose	Typical Dose Range	30-Day Cost[2]
Losartan (Cozaar)	25 mg po qd	25–100 mg po qd	50 mg qd (30) $38.86
Valsartan (Diovan)	80 mg po qd	80–320 mg po qd	160 mg qd (30) $43.29
Irbesartan (Avapro)	75–150 mg po qd	75–300 mg po qd	150 mg po qd (30) $42.28
Telmisartan (Micardis)	20 mg po qd	20–80 mg po qd	40 mg po qd (30) $38.18
Eprosartan (Teveten)	400 mg po qd	400–800 mg po qd	400 mg qd (30) $30.94
Candasartan (Atacand)	4 mg po qd	4–32 mg po qd	8 mg po qd (30) $40.23

Source: JNC VI Report.
[1]po, orally; qd, daily.
[2]Average retail cost www.drugstore.com as per Epocrates Rx; generic cost when available.

Table 33–10. Other drugs.[1]

Drug	Initial Dose	Typical Dose Range	30-Day Cost[2]	Comments[3]
Central α-blockers				
Clonidine HCl (Catapres)	0.1 mg po bid	0.1–0.6 mg po bid	0.3 mg po bid (60) $11.73	G, withdrawal rebound
Methyldopa (Aldomet)	250 mg po bid	250–500 mg po bid	500 mg po bid (60) $12.85	G
Guanabenzacetate (Wytensin)	2 mg po bid	2–16 mg po bid	8 mg po bid (60) $48.70	G
Guanfacine HCl (Tenex)	1 mg po qhs	1–3 mg po qhs	2 mg po qhs (30) $25.96	G
α-Blockers				
Doxazosin mesylate (Cardura)	1 mg po qd	1–4 mg po qd; max: 16 mg/day	4 mg po qd (30) $21.70	G
Prazosin HCl (Minipress)	1 mg po bid/tid	3–7 mg po bid	5 mg po bid (60) $10.31	G
Terazosin HCl (Hytrin)	1 mg po qhs	1–5 mg po qhs; max: 20 mg/day	5 mg po qhs (30) $15.88	G
Direct vasodilators				
Hydralazine HCl (Apresoline)	10 mg po qid	10–50 mg po qid	25 mg po qid (120) $21.96	G
Minoxidil (Loniten)	5 mg po qd	10–40 mg po qd	20 mg po qd (30) $16.29	G

Source: JNC VI Report.
[1]po, orally; bid, twice a day; qhs, every night; qd, daily; qid, four times a day.
[2]Average retail cost www.drugstore.com as per Epocrates Rx; generic cost when available.
[3]G, generic available.

and production of bradykinin, which aids in reduction of blood pressure. JNC VI did not recommend that ARBs be used for initial therapy in treatment of hypertension. This was secondary to the lack of randomized controlled clinical trials providing evidence that they are comparable to the β-blockers and diuretics in improving cardiovascular and other outcomes. They have been an attractive option for patients and physicians alike secondary to a side-effect profile that is similar to placebo.

Since JNC VI, ELITE II, released in 2000, compared an ARB (losartan) with an ACE inhibitor (captopril) for use in patients with NY class II–IV congestive heart failure. No differences were found in cardiovascular end points between the two groups. Another study released in 2001 compared an ARB (losartan) with placebo in patients with diabetes and nephropathy to assess for prevention of progression of renal disease. Losartan significantly reduced progression compared with placebo.

Therefore, limited evidence exists for beneficial effects of ARBs used in diabetics with known nephropathy and in patients with class II–IV congestive heart failure. However, ACE inhibitors should still be considered first-line therapy in such patients until more compelling evidence is available, with ARBs used in patients who are unable to tolerate ACE inhibitors. Table 33–9 lists commonly used ARBs.

6. Other drugs —Other drugs, including α-blockers and direct vasodilators, are used to treat hypertension, although less commonly than the other classes of drugs. They are typically used as second- or third-line therapy agents because of increased side effects. JNC VI recommends that the α-blockers be considered for use in treatment of hypertension in patients who also suffer from benign prostatic hypertrophy (BPH) and hyperlipidemia, as they may have beneficial effects on both conditions in addition to lowering blood pressure. Table 33–10 lists other medications used to treat hypertension, although they are typically not first-line agents.

D. Treatment Goals and Follow-Up

Patients initiating medication for treatment of hypertension should be started on an appropriate single agent after consideration of the patient's history and comorbidities. Table 33–11 presents an evidence-based quick reference for medication choice in specific types of patients. A low starting dose as outlined in Tables 33–6 to 33–10 should be begun with titration over subsequent visits to achieve appropriate control (Table 33–12).

Life-style modifications should be initiated with drug therapy. If single-agent therapy is ineffective, a second agent should be added from a different class. It is not uncommon for patients to require a second or even third agent for control of more severe and chronic

Table 33–11. Quick reference list of indications for consideration of specific antihypertensive medications.[1]

Special Situation/ Indication	Antihypertensive
Uncomplicated hypertension	β-Blockers; diuretics; CCB
Myocardial infarction	β-Blockers (non-ISA); ACE-I (with systolic dysfunction)
Diabetes mellitus with proteinuria	ACE-I; ARB if ACE-I not tolerated
Congestive heart failure	ACE-I; diuretics; β-blockers; ARB if ACE-I not tolerated
Angina	β-Blockers; CCB
Atrial tachycardia/ fibrillation	β-Blockers, CCB (rate lowering)
Dyslipidemia	α-Blockers
Hyperthyroidism	β-Blockers
Migraine headaches	β-Blockers (noncardioselective); CCB (rate lowering)
Preoperative hypertension	β-Blockers
Prostatism (BPH)	α-Blockers
Renal insufficiency	ACE-I; loop diuretic if Cr>2.5
Elderly	Diuretics; dihydropyridine CCB; titrate any drugs slowly
African-Americans	Diuretics; CCB; ACE-I

[1]CCB, calcium channel blocker; ISA, intrinsic sympathomimetic activity; ACE, angiotensin-converting enzyme; ARB, angiotensin II receptor blocker; BPH, benign prostatic hyperplasia; Cr, creatinine.

Table 33–12. Goals for antihypertensive therapy.

Uncomplicated hypertension	<140/90
Diabetes	<130/80[1]
Renal insufficiency	<130/85 <125/75 (if proteinuria >1 g/day)

[1] American Diabetes Association.

Table 33–13. Oral agents in hypertensive urgency.

Drug	Dosage	Onset	Duration	Precautions
Nifedipine	10 mg initially; repeat after 30 min	15 min	2–6 h	Sublingual contraindicated
Clonidine	0.1–0.2 mg initially; 0.1 mg every hour to 0.8 mg	30–60 min	6–8 h	Hypotension; rebound
Captopril	25 mg	15–30 min	4–6 h	

hypertension. If triple drug therapy with appropriate drugs from different classes (including a diuretic) does not control blood pressure, investigation must ensue regarding possible etiologies of poor response. These include patient compliance with therapy, secondary causes of hypertension not previously considered, excessive salt intake, and drug-related hypertension (prescription, over the counter, and illicit). Poor response also warrants consideration of referral to a specialist in hypertension for evaluation and recommendations concerning therapy.

E. HYPERTENSIVE URGENCY AND EMERGENCY

Hypertensive urgencies are situations in which the blood pressure must be lowered within several hours either due to an asymptomatic severely elevated blood pressure (>240/130 mm Hg) or a moderately elevated blood pressure (>200/120 mm Hg) with associated symptoms including angina, headache, and congestive heart failure. When such symptoms are present, even lower blood pressures may warrant more urgent treatment. Oral therapy can often be utilized with good response (Table 33–13).

Hypertensive emergencies require treatment of elevated blood pressures within 1 h to avoid significant morbidity and mortality. Symptomatology with which the patient presents warrants the immediate attention, not the actual blood pressure value itself. Such patients show evidence of end organ damage from the elevated blood pressure including encephalopathy (headache, irritability, confusion, coma), renal failure, pulmonary edema, unstable angina, myocardial infarction, aortic dissection, and intracranial hemorrhage. Hypertensive emergency is an indication for hospital admission and such patients typically require intravenous therapy with antihypertensives. The goal of therapy is reduction of systolic pressure by 20–40 mm Hg and diastolic pressure by 10–20 mm Hg. Initial blood pressure target is a

Table 33–14. Drug therapy in hypertensive emergency.

Drug	Dosage	Onset	Duration	Precautions
Nitroprusside (Nipride)	0.25–10 µg/kg/min	Seconds	3–5 min	Risk of cyanide toxicity especially in renal insufficiency
Nitroglycerin	0.25–5 µg/kg/min	2–5 min	3–5 min	Headache, hypotension
Labetalol (Normodyne)	20–40 mg every 10 min; max 300 mg	5–10 min	3–6 h	Hypotension, heart block, heart failure, bronchospasm
Esmolol (Breviblock)	Loading dose 500 µg/kg over 1 min; maintenance 25–200 µg/kg/min	1–2 min	10–30 min	Hypotension, heart block, bronchospasm, heart failure
Hydralazine (Apresoline)	5–20 mg intravenously; may repeat after 20 min	10–30 min	2–6 h	Hypotension, headache, nausea, vomiting
Enalaprilat (Vasotec)	1.25 mg every 6 h	15 min	6 h or more	Hypotension
Furosemide (Lasix)	10–80 mg	15 min	4 h	
Nicardipine (Cardene)	5 mg/h; increase by 1–2.5 mg/h every 15 min to max 15 mg/h	1–5 min	3–6 h	Hypotension, headache, nausea, vomiting

systolic blood pressure in the range of 180–200 mm Hg and a diastolic blood pressure in the range of 110–120 mm Hg. Blood pressure should not be lowered too quickly as doing so can result in hypoperfusion of the brain and myocardium. Once initial treatment goals are achieved, blood pressure can subsequently be reduced gradually to more appropriate levels.

Nitroprusside is the preferred agent in emergencies such as hypertensive encephalopathy, as the infusion can be titrated easily to effect. When myocardial ischemia is present, intravenous nitroglycerin or intravenous β-blockers such as labetolol or esmolol are preferred. Agents commonly used are listed in Table 33–14.

Once blood pressure has been brought under control using intravenous therapy, oral agents should be initiated slowly as intravenous therapy is gradually withdrawn. Whether a patient is being treated for hypertensive urgency, emergency, or benign hypertension, long-term therapy and life-style modification are essential. Patients must receive regular follow-up and meet the treatment goals established by JNC VI to prevent unnecessary morbidity and mortality.

Appel L et al: A clinical trial of the effects of dietary patterns on blood pressure. New Engl J Med 1997;336:1117.

Brenner B et al: Effects of losartan on renal and cardiovascular outcomes in patients with type 2 diabetes and nephropathy. New Engl J Med 2001;345(12):861.

Brown D, Giles W, Croft J: Left ventricular hypertrophy as a predictor of coronary heart disease mortality and the effect of hypertension. Am Heart J 2000;140(6):848.

Burnier M, Brunner H: Angiotensin II receptor antagonists. Lancet 2000;355:637.

Cohn J et al: Safety and efficacy of carvedilol in severe heart failure. The U.S. Carvedilol Heart Failure Study Group. J Cardiac Failure 1997;3(3):173.

Cutler J et al: Effect of reduced dietary sodium on blood pressure: a meta analysis of randomized controlled trials. Am J Clin Nutr 1997;65(suppl):643S.

Database of Abstracts of Reviews of Effectiveness: *Ejection Fraction Improvement by Beta-Blocker Treatment in Patients with Heart Failure: An Analysis of Studies Published in the Literature.* University of York, 2001.

Database of Abstracts of Reviews of Effectiveness: *Effect of Beta-Blockade on Mortality in Patients with Heart Failure: A Meta-Analysis of Randomized Clinical Trials.* University of York, 2001.

ENBbuNational Institutes of Health, National Heart, Lung and Blood Institute: *The Sixth Report of the Joint National Committee on Prevention, Detection, Evaluation and Treatment of High Blood Pressure,* 1997.

Estacio R, Schrier R: Antihypertensive therapy in type 2 diabetes: implications of the Appropriate Blood Pressure Control in Diabetes (ABCD) trial. Am J Cardiol 1998;82:9R-14R.

Heart Outcomes Prevention Evaluation Study Investigators: Effects of ramipril on cardiovascular and microvascular outcomes in people with diabetes mellitus: results of the HOPE study and MICRO-HOPE substudy. Lancet 2000;355:253.

Hilleman D: Role of angiotensin-converting-enzyme inhibitors in the treatment of hypertension. Am J Health-System Pharm 2000;57(19):S8.

Matthew J et al: Reduction of cardiovascular risk by regression of electrocardiographic markers of left ventricular hypertrophy by the angiotensin-converting enzyme inhibitor ramipril. Circulation 2001;104(14):1615.

National Institutes of Health, National Heart, Lung and Blood Institute: *The Sixth Report of the Joint National Committee on Prevention, Detection, Evaluation and Treatment of High Blood Pressure.* NIH, 1997.

Physicians Desktop Reference. Medical Economics Company, 2000.

Psaty B et al: Health outcomes associated with antihypertensive therapies used as first line agents: a systematic review and meta-analysis. JAMA 1997;277:739.

Salpeter S, Ormiston T, Salpeter E: Cardioselective beta-blocker use in patients with reversible airway disease. Cochrane Database Syst Rev 2001;2(CD002992).

Singh V, Christiana J, Frishman W: How to use calcium antagonists in hypertension: putting the JNC-VI guidelines into practice. Drugs 1999;58(4):579.

Staessen J et al: Ramdomized double-blind comparison of placebo and active treatment for older adults with isolated systolic hypertension: the Systolic Hypertension in Europe (SYSEUR) trial. Lancet 1997;350:757.

Stamler J, Caggiula A, Grandits G: Relation of body mass and alcohol, nutrient, fiber and caffeine intakes to blood pressure in the special intervention and usual care groups in the Multiple Risk Factor Intervention Trial. Am J Clin Nutr 1997;65(suppl):338S.

Tatti P et al: Outome results of the Fosinopril versus Amlodipine Cardiovascular Events Trial (FACET). Diabetes Care 1998;21:597.

Trials of Hypertension Prevention Collaborative Research Group: Effects of weight loss and sodium reduction intervention on blood pressure and hypertension incidence in overweight people with high-normal blood pressure. Arch Intern Med 1997;157:657.

United Kingdom Prospective Diabetes Study Group: Efficacy of atenolol and captopril in reducing macrovascular and microvascular complications in type 2 diabetes: UKPDS 39. Br Med J 1998;317:713.

Whelton P et al: Effects of oral potassium on blood pressure: meta analysis of randomized controlled clinical trials. JAMA 1997;277:1624.

Yusuf S et al: Ramipril and the development of diabetes. JAMA 2001;286(15):1882.

WEB SITES

American Heart Association
www.americanheart.org
Centers for Disease Control and Prevention
www.cdc.gov

Diabetes Mellitus

34

Belinda Vail, MD

ESSENTIALS OF DIAGNOSIS

- *Two separate measurements of plasma glucose ≥200 mg/dL.*
- *Polydipsia, polyuria, polyphagia, and/or weight loss.*
- *Fasting plasma glucose ≥126 mg/dL.*
- *Two-hour oral glucose tolerance test ≥200 mg/dL after a 75-g glucose load.*

General Considerations

As the world becomes closer, more populated, and more developed, we are witnessing a dramatic increase in the prevalence of diabetes mellitus. The estimated 150 million people around the world afflicted with diabetes appear to have in common the adoption of a more sedentary, western life-style. With increasing industrialization and an aging population, by 2025 there are expected to be 300 million people with diabetes.

There are an estimated 17 million people in the United States with diabetes comprising about 6.5% of the population. In 1990 only 4.9% of the population was afflicted, and 40 years ago there were only 1.6 million diabetics in the United States. The age-adjusted prevalence of diabetes rose 33% from 1990 to 1998. About 7 million Americans over age 65 are afflicted, or one in five in this population. The fastest rate of increase is in individuals 30–39 years of age; in this group the prevalence rose 70% over the past decade. Thirteen percent of African-Americans, 10% of Hispanic Americans, and 15% of Native Americans have diabetes. One million people over the age of 20 years are diagnosed every year. Diabetes in adolescents has reached epidemic proportions. Due to the rapid rise in obesity and inactivity in youth, type 2 diabetes in individuals under the age of 20 years has risen from 5% to 30% of the newly diagnosed cases in the past 8 years.

Diabetes is now the seventh leading cause of death, and one of every seven health care dollars spent in this country goes to treat diabetes and its complications. Nearly $100 billion is currently spent on the direct and indirect costs of diabetes, with 63% of that on inpatient care. Diabetes is a major cause of blindness, renal failure, lower extremity amputations, cardiovascular and peripheral vascular disease, and congenital malformations. It is the epitome of a chronic disease requiring a multidisciplinary management approach. Treatment of this disease requires commitment from the patient and physician, and a willingness of both to work with other health care professionals. Ninety percent of patients with diabetes receive their care from a primary care physician, not an endocrinologist or diabetologist. Most of these physicians have had little or no specialized training in the care of diabetes. All physicians, regardless of specialty, will care for patients with diabetes and its complications. It is, therefore, imperative that all physicians stay abreast of the rapid developments in diabetes care.

In 1993 the Diabetes Control and Complications Trial (DCCT) Research Group established what had long been hypothesized, that control of hyperglycemia in insulin-dependent diabetics significantly reduced their complication rate. The Kumamato study in Japan found similar results in type 2 diabetic patients, but was a relatively small study. In 1995 information from the large United Kingdom Prospective Diabetes Study (UKPDS) began to emerge showing reduction in complications with tight control of type 2 diabetes and concomitant hypertension. Recently, it has been shown that a sustained reduction in hemoglobin A_{1c} (HgbA$_{1c}$) is associated with significant cost savings within 1–2 years.

Diabetes Control and Complications Trial Research Group: The effect of intensive treatment of diabetes on the development and progression of long-term complications in insulin-dependent diabetes mellitus. New Engl J Med 1993;329:977.

Narayan KMV et al: Diabetes a common, serious, costly, and potentially preventable public health problem. Diabetes Res Clin Pract 2000;50:77.

UKPDS Group: UK Prospective Diabetes Study 17: a nine-year update of a randomized, controlled trial on the effect of improved metabolic control on complications in non-insulin-dependent diabetes mellitus. Ann Intern Med 1996;124:136.

Wagner EH et al: Effect of improved glycemic control on health care costs and utilization. JAMA 2001;285:182.

Pathogenesis

Theory now indicates that both types 1 and 2 diabetes are caused by a complex interaction of environmental and genetic factors. Two chromosomal regions are associated with both types of diabetes (the HLA region on 6p21 and the insulin gene region on 11p15). These two sites contribute to inheritance in about 42% of type 1 and 10% of type 2 diabetics. The autoimmune regulator gene (AIRE gene on chromosome 21q22.3) is responsible for a rare form of autoimmune type 1 diabetes. Even in genetically susceptible individuals, an environmental trigger may be necessary for development of the disease. In type 1 diabetics this trigger may be the coxsackie virus. There are single gene mutations found in type 2 diabetes, but most forms are caused by more than one mutation causing beta cell dysfunction and insulin resistance.

The exact mechanism by which insulin regulates transport of glucose into the cell is not clearly understood. Insulin binds to receptors on the surface of insulin-sensitive cells, particularly in muscle and adipose tissue. This activates the receptors, initiating a series of phosphorylation reactions including insulin receptor substrate 1 (IRS-1), ultimately moving glucose transporter proteins to the cell surface, where they transport glucose through the cell membrane. Even in normal individuals there is great variability in the number of insulin receptors on the cell surface and a variety of defects that may occur throughout this system that lead to insulin resistance. The first compensation for this increased insulin resistance is an increase in insulin production by the pancreatic beta cells. This increased circulating insulin leads to the deposition of greater fat stores and may produce deleterious vascular changes. This resistance becomes progressively greater over time and when a defect in insulin secretion develops, diabetes is the end product. As plasma glucose levels rise, the ability of the pancreatic beta cell to secrete insulin is reduced. In the initial stages, the beta cell response is adequate to maintain glucose control. With aging, the beta cell response decreases and cannot keep up with the demand. Increasing body weight also increases insulin resistance. Decreasing insulin resistance by weight loss or medications will delay the onset of diabetes.

As the availability of food increases, and the work required for obtaining food decreases, there is a corresponding increase in obesity in the population. Although this phenomenon is seen worldwide, it is particularly prevalent in the United States, where over 50% of the population is now overweight. Obesity increased from 12% of the population in 1991 to almost 18% in 1998. This combination of increasing obesity and an increasing percentage of the population surviving into old age accounts for much of the increasing diabetes epidemic.

Recently more evidence is pointing to an inflammatory process that may be active in the development of diabetes. A number of markers for inflammation have been postulated as predictors for the development of diabetes, but the most promising to date is C-reactive protein (CRP). Pradhan et al found CRP to be a "powerful independent predictor" for the development of diabetes in middle-aged women even after controlling for obesity and other risk factors.

Pietropaolo M, LeRoith D: Pathogenesis of diabetes: our current understanding. Clin Cornerstone 2001;4:1.

Pradhan AD et al: C-reactive protein, interleukin 6, and risk of developing type 2 diabetes mellitus. JAMA 2001;286:327.

Prevention

It has been firmly established that life-style changes impact upon the acquisition of type 2 diabetes. It is unknown if significant life-style change can prevent diabetes, but it does delay its development. In a small but randomized controlled trial in Finland of 522 overweight, middle-aged patients with impaired glucose tolerance life-style intervention over a 4-year period reduced the risk of progression to diabetes by 58%. Patients received individualized weight loss and nutritional counseling. They reduced intake of total and saturated fats, increased dietary fiber, and increased physical activity. Weight loss over 2 years was 3.5 kg compared with 0.8 kg in the control group. After 4 years 11% of the interventional group had developed diabetes whereas 23% of the control group progressed to diabetes. Prior studies have shown similar results but were not randomized and controlled.

Preliminary data from the Diabetes Prevention Program, a large randomized, controlled study, show that in patients with impaired glucose tolerance life-style intervention reduced the risk of acquiring type 2 diabetes by 58% and using metformin reduced development of diabetes by 31%.

Motivating and influencing individuals to make life-style changes may be difficult, but it is inexpensive, cost effective, and safe. These changes can reverse or improve the risk factors for developing diabetes. Alteration of life-style can reduce obesity (including central obesity) and hypertension and improve lipid profiles. Low-fat, high-fiber diet, modest exercise, and smoking cessation are modalities vastly superior to the complexities of the care of patients with diabetes and its complications.

National Institute of Diabetes and Digestive and Kidney Disease: Diet and exercise dramatically delay type 2 diabetes: diabetes medication metformin also effective. http://www.niddk.nih.gov/welcome/releases. Accessed June 11, 2002.

Screening

Screening for type 2 diabetes is a controversial topic that has experts divided. Although there is good evidence that treating patients with known disease decreases microvascular complications and reduces cardiovascular risk, there are few data that show similar results for patients at risk for or prior to detection of diabetes. At the time of diagnosis over 50% of patients have evidence of cardiovascular disease and/or microvascular complications. This suggests that the actual disease process begins several years prior to our ability to detect it. The lack of tests that are both sensitive and specific early in the disease process may limit the effectiveness of the screen. The best treatment available for early or developing disease is life-style modification. Therefore, the most cost-effective method for reducing complications of diabetes is primary prevention. For these reasons the U.S. Preventative Services Task Force does not recommend for or against universal screening. It does recommend screening of high-risk individuals. The American Diabetes Association recommends screening all persons 45 years of age and over every 3 years and suggests earlier or more frequent screening when the following risk factors are considered:

1. Family history of diabetes in a first-degree relative.
2. Hypertension (blood pressure >140/90).
3. Obesity.
4. High-risk ethnic group (African-American, Hispanic, Native American).
5. Previous history of impaired glucose tolerance.
6. Abnormal lipid levels [especially high triglycerides and low high-density lipoproteins (HDLs)].
7. History of gestational diabetes or birth of a child >9 pounds.

The American College of Endocrinology and the American Association of Clinical Endocrinologists have recommended screening anyone over 30 years of age who is at risk. They include the above risk factors plus sedentary life-style, cardiovascular disease, and polycystic ovarian disease.

Screening of overweight children with additional risk factors is now recommended by the consensus panel of the National Institute of Diabetes and Digestive and Kidney Diseases (NIDDKD), the Centers for Disease Control (CDC), and the American Academy of Pediatrics (AAP). Overweight is defined as a body mass index (BMI) or weight for height >85th percentile or weight >120% of ideal. Screening should start at age 10 years or at the onset of puberty and should continue every 2 years in children with the following risk factors:

1. Family history of diabetes in first- and second-degree relatives.
2. High-risk racial or ethnic group (Native Americans, African-Americans, Hispanics, or Pacific Islanders).
3. Signs of insulin resistance or conditions associated with insulin resistance (eg, acanthosis nigricans, hypertension, dyslipidemia, and polycystic ovarian syndrome).

Multiple screening tests are available, and the choice of test is probably less important than knowing which patients to screen. Random serum glucose is easy and inexpensive, but specificity is limited. Fasting glucose is more accurate, and is generally accepted as the screening test of choice. It often requires a return trip, so in patients with compliance or transportation problems, a random glucose may be the best option. A glucose tolerance test is more specific, but is also more costly and time consuming. Screening the urine for glycosuria has a high specificity but a low sensitivity, and is not recommended. Community screens often use finger stick methods, but serum glucose is significantly more accurate. The use of glycosylated hemoglobin measurements has not been adequately evaluated as a diagnostic tool to recommend it for screening at the present time. There are questions concerning its accuracy in healthy adults, in patients with impaired glucose tolerance, or in patients with hemolytic anemias or other diseases that affect the red blood cells. Until 1996 there was no standardization of this test, and values fluctuated significantly between laboratories. There is even confusion in terminology and in the actual test ordered. Standardization of this test is being attempted, but about 25% of laboratories remain unstandardized.

Screening for gestational diabetes is also controversial and the U.S. Preventive Services Task Force does not recommend universal screening. The American College of Obstetricians and Gynecologists (ACOG) recommends screening unless a woman meets all of the following criteria:

1. Less than 25 years of age.
2. Not a member of a high-risk racial or ethnic group (Hispanic, African-American, Native American, South or East Asian, Pacific Islander).
3. Body mass index ≤25.
4. No history of abnormal glucose tolerance.
5. No previous history of adverse pregnancy outcomes usually associated with gestational diabetes.
6. No known diabetes in a first-degree relative.

Screening is done with a 1-h glucose tolerance test (GTT), nonfasting, with a 50-g glucose load usually between 24 and 28 weeks of gestation. It may be done as early as 12 weeks in women who are at significant risk. One-hour values ≥135–140 mg/dL indicate the need for a 3-h GTT for confirmation. Three-hour GTT is done following a 10-h fast and with a 100-g glucose load. Two of the following must be abnormal for diagnosis:

1. Fasting ≥95 mg/dL.
2. One hour ≥190 mg/dL.
3. Two hour ≥165 mg/dL.
4. Three hour ≥140 mg/dL.

Women with one abnormal value are considered to have glucose intolerance and many physicians will institute life-style intervention. If one abnormal value is found early in the pregnancy, the test should be repeated later in the pregnancy. Pregnant women with glucose intolerance, as well as gestational diabetes, should be on an exercise program and if obese should have carbohydrates restricted to 35–40% of calories.

American Association of Clinical Endocrinologists and the American College of Endocrinology: AACE guidelines for the management of diabetes mellitus. Endocrine Pract 1995;1(2):151.

Expert Committee on the Diagnosis and Classification of Diabetes Mellitus: Report of the Expert Committee on the Diagnosis and Classification of Diabetes Mellitus. Diabetes Care 1994; 20:1183.

Wareham NJ, Griffin SJ: Should we screen for type 2 diabetes? Evaluation against national screening committee criteria. Br Med J 2001;322:986.

Clinical Findings

A. SYMPTOMS AND SIGNS

The diagnosis of diabetes in all ages may be made by two separate measurements of plasma glucose ≥200 mg/dL with classic signs of diabetes (polydipsia, polyuria, polyphagia, and weight loss), fasting plasma glucose ≥126 mg/dL, or 2-h oral glucose tolerance test ≥200 mg/dL after a 75-g glucose load.

Impaired glucose tolerance is defined as a fasting plasma glucose ≤110–125 mg/dL or 2-h oral glucose tolerance test of 140–190 mg/dL following a 75-g load. Impaired fasting glucose is diagnosed if the fasting glucose is between 110 and 125 mg/dL. Again two abnormal results are recommended for diagnosis.

B. HISTORY AND PHYSICAL EXAMINATION

The initial assessment for new patients with diabetes or patients with a new diagnosis of diabetes is extensive. The use of written checklists or questionnaires or the assistance of a trained nurse or assistant can decrease physician time while still obtaining necessary information. The initial history should include the following:

1. Current symptoms and prior symptoms consistent with diabetes.
2. Weight changes.
3. Eating patterns, nutritional status (growth and development in children).
4. Exercise history and ability to exercise.
5. Details of previous treatment and prior HgbA$_{1c}$ records and monitoring.
6. Current regimen of treatment including medications and diet.
7. Prior acute or severe complications (ie, ketoacidosis or hypoglycemia).
8. Prior and current infections particularly involving the skin, feet, and genitourinary systems.
9. History of hypertension, hyperlipidemia, coronary artery disease, and insulin resistance.
10. Chronic complications including retinopathy, nephropathy, neuropathy, gastrointestinal problems, vascular problems, sexual dysfunction, and foot problems.
11. Medications and allergies.
12. Family history of diabetes, other endocrine disorders, or heart disease.
13. History of gestational diabetes, large-for-gestational-age infants, or miscarriages.
14. Tobacco, alcohol, and drug use.
15. Lipid disorders or hypertension.
16. Life-style, cultural, psychosocial, education, and economic factors influencing control.

Patients who have positive responses in multiple areas may require two or three closely spaced visits to gather all the necessary information unless physician extenders are available.

The initial physical examination should also be detailed, covering all the organ systems as diabetes has a truly systemic effect. Height and weight should be obtained and BMI calculated. Blood pressure including orthostatic measurements should also be recorded. Other points of particular interest include the following:

1. Ophthalmoscopic examination.
2. Oral examination.
3. Thyroid palpation.
4. Cardiac examination.
5. Abdominal examination.
6. Skin examination (including injection sites in patients using insulin).
7. Sexual maturity in children and adolescents.

8. Evaluation of pulses.
9. Neurological examination with particular attention to reflexes, vibratory senses, light touch (monofilament examination of both feet), and proprioception.
10. Pap test and pelvic examination if appropriate.
11. Digital rectal examination if indicated.

Again, a physical examination record tailored to patients with diabetes may help the provider to include all necessary parts of the examination.

Interim visits require a less extensive history, but special attention should be placed on compliance and patients' special issues with their management. Any history of hypoglycemia or hyperglycemia, results of self-monitoring, and adjustments by patients in their therapeutic regimen are of particular importance. A brief history of complications, medications, psychosocial issues, and life-style changes should also be taken. Patients' goals and their motivation for achieving them should be assessed. Nursing personnel may be given additional responsibilities, and standing orders are an excellent way to make physician time more efficient (Table 34–1).

There is also information in the literature concerning novel approaches to patient visits. These include visits in which multiple providers are seen, one after another, keeping physician time low; or group visits in which multiple patients are seen by the provider at the same time, sharing ideas and information among the group.

Interval visits should include determination of weight and blood pressure and ophthalmoscopic, cardiac, and brief skin examinations. Shoes and socks should always be removed to allow visualization of the skin, palpation of pulses, and a monofilament examination of the feet. This examination utilizes a standardized length of 10-gauge nylon monofilament. When the line is touched to the bottom of the foot and bends, the patient should be able to detect its presence. An assessment should be made concerning the status of yearly ophthalmology visits, semiannual dental examinations, and any other required specialist visits. Diabetics are at increased risk for periodontal disease, and should be followed closely by a dentist. Visit frequency should be based on control of diabetes and the patient's understanding and comfort. Patients initiating insulin therapy may require daily contact, by phone or e-mail. Brittle diabetics or patients making multiple management changes might be seen weekly until stable. Uncontrolled type II diabetics may need monthly visits for medication changes. Well-controlled diabetics usually need visits only quarterly, and those in excellent control can be followed with twice yearly visits.

Table 34–1. Standing nursing orders for patients with diabetes.

---

1. Place the flowsheet in the patient's record and update with information from the patient and his or her chart
2. Administer services for **every visit** according to the orders below:
   a. Monitor and record blood pressure in the same arm every visit
   b. Measure and record the patient's weight every visit
   c. If **HgbA$_{1c}$** has not been done in the past 6 months, complete a requisition and attach to the patient's chart for physician approval
   d. If a **urinalysis** and **microalbumin** have not been done in the past year
      i. Perform a urine dipstick and record the results in the chart on the flowsheet
      ii. Complete a requisition for urine microalbumin and attach it to the patient's chart for physician approval
   e. If a **lipid profile** has not been done in the past year, complete a requisition and attach it to the patient's chart for physician approval
   f. If a **dilated eye examination** has not been done in the past year, complete a referral for an ophthalmology examination and attach it to the patient's chart
   g. At every visit ask the patient to remove his or her shoes and socks:
      i. Palpate dorsalis pedis and posterior tibial pulses
      ii. Inspect the skin for any skin breakdown
      iii. Record the findings on the patient's flowsheet

Physician Signature: _____ Date: _____

Vaccination status should be checked, and any missing vaccines given. All patients need assessment of diphtheria/tetanus status and younger patients need assessment of measles/mumps/rubella and hepatitis B status. All patients with diabetes should be encouraged to receive a yearly influenza vaccine. The use of the pneumococcal pneumonia vaccine prior to age 65 years has been somewhat controversial. The position of the U.S. Preventive Services Task Force (USPTF) is that there is insufficient evidence to recommend it for universal use in patients younger than 65 years with chronic diseases. Diabetic patients are more likely to die from pneumonia or influenza than nondiabetic patients, and so the vaccine has been routinely recommended in patients with diabetes.

C. LABORATORY FINDINGS

The frequency of laboratory evaluation and the use of other tests are also not entirely clear. Initially and yearly patients should have a fasting glucose, fasting lipid profile, serum electrolytes and blood urea nitrogen (BUN)/creatinine, urinalysis, microalbumin, thyroid-stimulating hormone, and other routinely recommended screening tests (ie, Pap smear, mammograms, fecal occult blood testing, prostate-specific antigen, etc). Depending on age and length of disease an electrocardiogram (ECG) should be performed, but as microalbuminuria is a marker for cardiovascular disease, an ECG should be performed at onset of microalbuminuria. Generally glycosylated hemoglobin or HgbA$_{1c}$ is measured every 3 months unless patients maintain very tight control without hypoglycemia. In this case levels may be obtained every 6 months. HgbA$_{1c}$ is one of several types of glycosylated hemoglobins. The A$_{1c}$ component comprises about 80% of glycosylated hemoglobin. In the past different laboratories assayed for one or the other, and there was a lack of control and standardization of these levels at various laboratories. Since 1996 the National Glycohemoglobin Standardization Program has influenced most laboratories to pass certification tests for accuracy and precision of HgbA$_{1c}$ levels, improving the validity of this test. Random microalbumin levels may be used for screening and/or monitoring, but patients may require a 24-h urine for protein and creatinine clearance when there are significant changes. A C-terminal peptide can help to distinguish type 2 diabetes from type 1, particularly in young adults. This peptide is cleaved from the end of native insulin during its production. Patients with type 1 diabetes make little insulin and should have low values for this peptide. Patients with type 2 diabetes make an abundance of insulin and the values will be high. In older patients, as the beta cells cease to function, the C-terminal peptide levels will fall, indicating the need for insulin supplementation.

Complications

A. KETOACIDOSIS

Ketoacidosis occurs when there is insufficient insulin to meet the body's needs. This may be due to a deficiency of insulin or an increase in the body's needs (ie, illness, stress, increased glucagon concentrations, or increased epinephrine levels). When this occurs gluconeogenesis and fatty acid oxidation increase, osmotic diuresis occurs, and the patient develops dehydration. This is accompanied by ketogenesis from fatty acid oxidation, resulting in a metabolic acidosis. Ketoacidosis is one of the leading causes of death in children with diabetes. The incidence of ketoacidosis in children is about 8 per 100 person-years. It increases with age in girls, and is highest for children with higher HgbA$_{1c}$ levels, those who are underinsured, and those with psychiatric disorders.

Initial treatment is immediate rehydration with normal saline at 20 mL/kg intravenously over 90 min. The fluid deficit is then replaced with half normal saline. The first half of the replacement should take 12 h, and the second half should be replaced over the next 24 h. Fluid deficit is usually about 10%. In a 20-kg child, that is equal to 2000 mL. Replacement fluid should be added to maintenance fluid and should include 20 mEq of KCl per liter. When the blood glucose falls below 300 mg/dL, 5% dextrose should be added to the fluids. An insulin drip should be initiated immediately with regular insulin at a rate of 0.1 U/kg/h. When the serum glucose falls below 500 mg/dL the insulin drip may be reduced to 0.075 U/kg/h. If only small ketones are present, doses as low as 0.05 U/kg/h may be used.

Patients should have continuous ECG monitoring. Fingerstick glucose and vital signs should be checked hourly with an evaluation of pupils and sensorium. After 12 h if the patient is responding appropriately, these may be extended to every 2 h. Plasma glucose, serum electrolytes, and serum ketones should be checked every 4 h. The insulin drip should be continued and blood glucose maintained between 100 and 200 mg/dL until all ketones have been cleared. It is necessary to watch for signs of increased intracranial pressure and use of sodium bicarbonate, rapid rehydration, or rapid glucose correction should be avoided.

B. INFECTIONS

Patients with diabetes are at greater risk for many infections, common, as well as uncommon. Diabetics have a higher incidence of community-acquired pneumonia, particularly pneumococcal pneumonia; therefore, the pneumococcal vaccine is usually recommended. Diabetic patients also have an increased risk of influenza and should receive the flu shot yearly. Pyelonephritis, perinephric renal abscess, and cholecystitis are more common in diabetic patients. Fungal infections should be considered in diabetic patients. Besides vaginal candidiasis, these patients may develop mucormycosis and fungal eye and skin infections. Foot infections are common including cellulitis, osteomyelitis, plantar abscesses, and necrotizing fasciitis.

C. NEPHROPATHY

Diabetic nephropathy is the most common cause of end-stage renal disease (ESRD), accounting for about 100,000 of the 300,000 patients with ESRD in the United States. The rate of ESRD among African-Americans is four times that of whites, and it is more common in Native Americans, Asians, and Mexican Americans. The rate is much higher in type 1 diabetes, but more type 2 diabetics are afflicted because the percentage of type 1 diabetics is so small. Other risk factors include poor glycemic control, smoking, hypertension, family history, and glomerular hyperfiltration. Diabetic nephropathy is a result of mesangial cell growth within the glomerulus. Hyperglycemia, increased angiotensin II (hypertension), LDL lipids, and tobacco all contribute to this increased cell growth. The first indication of renal compromise is an increase in the glomerular filtration rate; renal lesions then develop, followed by microalbuminuria. All patients with diabetes should have a yearly microalbumin. If microalbuminuria develops, a 24-h urine will better quantify the actual amount of leakage. Once macroalbuminuria develops, the utility of continued screens is questionable. The following values may vary slightly depending on laboratory normals, but these are the general categories for albuminuria:

Normal albuminuria, <30 mg/24 h

Microalbuminuria, 30–300 mg/24 h

Macroalbuminuria, >300 mg/24 h (definition of diabetic nephropathy)

In the DCCT trial intensive therapy reduced the incidence of microalbuminuria by 39% and clinical albuminuria by 56%. The risk of microalbuminuria increased by 25% for each 10% rise in $HgbA_{1c}$. Also, these differences seem to be important early and will continue to show a significant difference even if the control group later achieves tight glycemic control.

The most important treatment is early glycemic control, aggressive blood pressure control to <130/80 mm Hg, and smoking cessation to prevent progression of the microvascular disease. Angiotensin-converting enzyme (ACE) inhibitors are the drug of choice with the appearance of microalbuminuria. Experts disagree, but because renal damage is occurring even before the detection of microalbuminuria, there is some evidence to support using ACE inhibitors prophylactically in diabetics. In a head-to-head trial with amlodipine, ramipril reduced ESRD and death by 41% and proteinuria by 20%, whereas patients on amlodipine saw a 58% increase in proteinuria. Angiotensin II receptor blockers (ARBs) are not proven to have the same effect as ACE inhibitors, but as they block the renin–angiotensin system they are believed to be comparable in efficacy. There is some emerging evidence that because these drugs act on the renin–angiotensin system at two separate points, a combination of the two may be highly effective. Referral to a nephrologist is indicated in the presence of rising creatinine, macroalbuminuria, and increasing microalbuminuria. Restriction of dietary protein (0.8 g/kg/d) is indicated in nephropathy. There is some evidence that plant proteins may not be as destructive as animal proteins. As renal failure progresses, oral hypoglycemic drugs may have delayed

clearance, resulting in improved glycemic control but also in increased episodes of hypoglycemia.

Diabetics are more susceptible to urinary tract infections, pyelonephritis, and perinephric abscess. Persistent fever and flank pain for more than 3–4 days despite appropriate antibiotic treatment should elicit an evaluation (preferably by computed tomography) for a perinephric infection.

D. RETINOPATHY

Retinopathy is the leading cause of blindness in the United States in persons over 60 years of age. The prevalence of retinopathy increases with the duration of the diabetes, but the initial changes may occur even before the disease is diagnosed, with about 20% of diabetics showing signs of retinopathy at the time of their diagnosis. It has been suggested that microvascular disease may put patients at risk for developing diabetes as retinal arteriolar narrowing has been found to be an independent risk factor for development of diabetes. Progression of retinopathy is usually orderly with mild background abnormalities followed by increased vascular permeability and preproliferative retinopathy characterized by vascular closure. Eventually proliferative retinopathy occurs with growth of new vessels on the retina and into the vitreous culminating in vision loss from contraction of fibrous tissue and tractional retinal detachment, hemorrhage, or macular edema. The risk of retinopathy increases with increasing $HgbA_{1c}$ similar to the rate seen in nephropathy. The risk is also increased with duration of the disease, so improving glycemic control means extending the time before onset of retinopathy.

Every office visit by the patient should include an ophthalmoscopic evaluation. The earliest signs of developing retinopathy are small hemorrhages in the retina. Patients with type 1 diabetes may begin yearly ophthalmology visits 5 years after diagnosis. Because type 2 diabetics often have signs of retinopathy at diagnosis, these patients should begin yearly office visits as soon as the diagnosis is made. Glaucoma screening is usually accomplished during the ophthalmology visit.

Treatment options are limited. Tight glycemic and blood pressure control are most important. Laser photocoagulation therapy is currently the only treatment option once the disease progresses. Aspirin has no effect on development of retinopathy or other complications in the eye.

E. NEUROPATHY

Peripheral neuropathy is the major cause of foot problems in diabetics. Twenty-five percent of hospital admissions for diabetes are foot related. Diabetes is the leading cause of lower-extremity amputations, with about 86,000 amputation per year. The incidence is twice as high in African-Americans and up to five times as high in some tribes of Native Americans. In the DCCT trial, the risk of neuropathy at 5 years was reduced by 69% in those patients who entered the study without neuropathy. Screening should include cranial nerves, reflexes, and vibratory, light, and sharp touch. A Semmes Weinstein monofilament can be used at each visit to quickly assess sensation on the soles of the feet. This is a standardized length of 10-gauge monofilament line that can be easily used by the patient as well as the physician. The line is placed against the skin to be tested, and the patient should feel its presence when it is pushed hard enough to bend. Patients should take their shoes and socks off at each office visit and the provider should assess for any skin breaks and the presence of sensation.

Treatment of peripheral neuropathy remains symptomatic. Recombinant human nerve growth factor has been studied as a possible treatment of neuropathy, but phase 3 clinical trials were not promising. Treatment options that have been shown to be effective include nonsteroidal antiinflammatory drugs (NSAIDs), tricyclic antidepressants (particularly amitriptyline 10–150 mg/day), anticonvulsants (particularly gabapentin 900–3600 mg/day and carbamazepine 200 mg twice a day), and topical capsaicin cream.

Autonomic nervous system function affects a large number of organ systems and requires some vigilance in diabetes care. Intermittently patients should be asked about symptoms of autonomic neuropathy, such as orthostatic hypotension, diarrhea and/or constipation, incontinence, impotence, and heat intolerance. Patients should be checked for resting tachycardia, dependent edema to assess impaired venoarteriolar reflex, and decreased diameter of dark-adapted pupil. Orthostatic blood pressures should be checked in symptomatic patients. Gastrointestinal motility may be improved with metoclopramide or erythromycin.

F. CARDIOVASCULAR DISEASE

Heart disease is the leading cause of death in patients with diabetes. The prevalence of fatal and nonfatal coronary heart disease events is 2 to 20 times higher in diabetic patients. Fifty percent of patients diagnosed with diabetes already have coronary artery disease at the time of diagnosis. Although an overall decline in the incidence of cardiovascular disease has been seen in the United States, there has been no decrease in cardiovascular mortality in patients with diabetes. Blood pressure levels in 73% of diabetics are above 130/80 or are controlled with the use of medications. In diabetics, the female protective effect is lost. There is a higher incidence of diffuse, multivessel disease, plaque rupture, and superimposed thrombosis. In diabetics, in-hospital mortality is double that of nondiabetics. Five-year survival

following angioplasty or coronary artery bypass graft (CABG) is lower in patients with diabetes; however, survival rates are significantly higher with CABG than with angioplasty for these patients.

The presence of diabetes, even without known cardiovascular disease, is a risk factor equivalent to known cardiovascular disease in a nondiabetic patient. Tight control of blood pressure is the most important element in preventing the vascular complications of diabetes. Cardiovascular disease, however, is the result of a complex interaction of multiple variables. A growing collection of studies has shown that many of these variables are mediated through angiotensin II–aldosterone mechanisms. The interaction of these substances causes a thickening and loss of compliance of the arterial wall and the left ventricle. This process is counteracted by nitric acid. Secreted from healthy endothelium, nitric acid promotes vascular dilation and inhibits vascular hypertrophy. A combination of genetics and life-style appears to shift the system to angiotensin II–aldosterone dominance. Because this system is so important, the use of ACE inhibitors appears to exert a cardioprotective influence far beyond blood pressure control. ACE inhibitors have produced a significant decrease in myocardial infarction (MI), stroke, and cardiac death in patients with diabetes. They reduce post-MI mortality and dramatically reduce ischemic events following revascularization procedures. They have been shown to reduce left ventricular mass by as much as 40%, thereby reducing the risk of sudden death, CHF, and ventricular dysrhythmias.

Hypertension and insulin resistance also cause hypertrophy and hyperplasia of the arterial walls, leading to a decrease in arterial compliance and endothelial dysfunction. Insulin resistance is significantly decreased with ACE inhibitors. In the Heart Outcomes Prevention Evaluation (HOPE) trial the use of ACE inhibitors correlated with a 34% reduction in the onset of new cases of diabetes. ACE inhibitors also result in a mild improvement in the lipid profile, especially when compared to β-blockers and diuretics.

There have been no definitive head-to-head studies to determine which of the 10 ACE inhibitors on the market is most effective at preventing cardiovascular disease (Table 34–2). Certainly ramipril has the most impressive data from the HOPE trial with a cost per year of life saved of $3100. Trandolapril has the longest half-life, but all except captopril may be dosed daily. Quinapril has a short half-life but has an active metabolite that remains in the circulation for about 24 h. Benazepril and fosinopril have level pricing and are therefore least expensive at maximal dosage. There have been some studies suggesting that aspirin may reduce the beneficial effects of ACE inhibitors. This was not found to be the case in the HOPE study, but the nonsynergis-

Table 34–2. Angiotensin-converting enzyme inhibitors.

	Dosage Range
Benazepril (Lotensin)[1]	5–80 mg/day
Captopril (Capoten)[1]	12.5–150 mg three times a day
Enalapril (Vasotec)[1]	2.5–40 mg/day[2]
Fosinopril (Monopril)	10–80 mg/day
Lisinopril (Prinivil, Zestril)[1]	2.5–40 mg/day
Moexipril (Univasc)[1]	7.5–30 mg/day
Perindopril (Aceon)	2–16 mg/day
Quinapril (Accupril)[1]	10–80 mg/day[2]
Ramipril (Altace)	2.5–20 mg/day
Trandolapril (Mavik)	1–8 mg/day

[1]Available in combination with hydrochlorothiazide.
[2]May also be given in two divided doses.

tic effect may be reduced by limiting aspirin to 81 mg and/or giving the two medications 12 h apart.

Because of the renal and cardiac protection they afford, ACE inhibitors remain the first-line choice for treatment of hypertension in diabetic patients. They should also be used for hypertension in patients with signs of insulin resistance even prior to the development of diabetes. Because of the HOPE trial, the potential decrease in the development of diabetes, and the cardiovascular protection conferred by these medications, it has been recommended that ACE inhibitors be used in all diabetic patients whose systolic blood pressure is >100 mm Hg. Although compelling, the body of data is still insufficient to recommend prophylactic ACE inhibitor therapy for all diabetics.

Microvascular and macrovascular disease appear to be interrelated as microalbuminuria has been shown to be an independent risk factor for cardiovascular disease. Patients with microalbuminuria or even an elevated albumin–creatinine ratio greater than 0.65 mg/mmol had over twice the risk of a cardiovascular event. Microalbuminuria indicates increased risk for MI, hospitalization for CHF, and for all-cause mortality. Albuminuria is an indicator for renal endothelial permeability and may be a marker for diffuse endothelial disfunction.

Reducing systemic hypertension and glomerular capillary pressure is critical in diabetic patients to prevent renal damage as well as cardiovascular disease. In the United Kingdom study reductions in blood pressure with ACE inhibitors or β-blockers were found to be equivalent in preventing microvascular disease. It was postulated that the most important aspect was tight control of hypertension regardless of agent used. β-Blockers and diuretics were underutilized in diabetics in the past because of a potentially mildly deleterious

effect on glycemic control. Following the UKPDS the emphasis has shifted to control of hypertension with all agents having a potential place in management. The National Kidney Foundation recommends blood pressure be maintained below 130/80 mm Hg, and most major groups are following suit. As with all aspects of diabetes, patients should be encouraged to alter their life-style to improve control of their blood pressure. In light of the considerable evidence for using ACE inhibitors and their relative safety profile, they should be readily used without allowing a long period for a trial of diet and exercise.

ACE inhibitors are clearly the first choice for control of hypertension in diabetes. They should be used in the presence of coronary artery disease, CHF, and microalbuminuria. They preferentially dilate the efferent glomerular arteriole, lowering glomerular capillary pressure. Although rising creatinine will eventually necessitate their cessation, current recommendations allow their use up to a creatinine level of ≤3.0 mg/mmol. Potassium levels should be monitored as renal failure develops, but they can be helpful in reversing renal loss of potassium when used in combination with diuretics. ACE inhibitors are contraindicated in pregnancy, so diabetic women attempting pregnancy should be maintained on another agent. All women of childbearing age should be counseled to immediately stop ACE inhibitors and to be tested for pregnancy if they miss their period. The most troublesome side effect is a bradykinin-induced dry cough, which sometimes limits the use of these agents.

ARBs have not been as thoroughly studied as ACE inhibitors, but do reduce the likelihood of developing ESRD. They do not appear to change cardiovascular risk or overall mortality, but are still recommended for use if ACE inhibitors cannot be used.

Thiazide diuretics are effective in lowering blood pressure and have been shown to reduce cardiovascular morbidity and mortality. They may cause short-term dyslipidemia, may interfere slightly with carbohydrate metabolism, and may cause mild hyperinsulinemia, hypokalemia, hypomagnesemia, and hyperuricemia. They therefore should be introduced cautiously at low doses. Studies, however, continue to confirm their usefulness as they appear to have a systemic vasodilatory effect that is independent of their diuretic effect. Loop diuretics should replace thiazide diuretics only when serum creatinine is >2.0. Potassium-sparing diuretics should be avoided because of the greater potential for hyperkalemia.

Calcium antagonists are effective treatment for hypertension but should not be used alone in patients with diabetes. They have no effect on lipids and may reduce proteinuria slightly, but they have not been shown to reduce cardiovascular events. They cause constipation, peripheral edema, and impotence that may be exacerbated by the diabetes.

β-Blockers reduce cardiovascular morbidity and mortality and prevent recurrent myocardial infarction and sudden death. They have a small but adverse effect on glycemic and lipid control. Their presence may interfere with awareness of and recovery from hypoglycemia. Regarding microvascular complications, however, they had the same long-term outcomes as ACE inhibitors in the U.K. study. It has been postulated that this was due to tight control of hypertension in both groups. Despite the small chance of complications resulting from the use of β-blockers in diabetic patients, the reduction in cardiovascular complications that results makes them a reasonable choice.

α_1-Receptor blockers have a beneficial effect on lipids and may improve insulin sensitivity, but they may also cause orthostatic hypotension. These medications may increase the risk of cardiovascular events when used alone. Centrally acting α_2-agonists may worsen orthostatic hypotension and are generally used only in combination with several other medications for severe hypertension.

In a small subset of diabetic patients with severe hypertension, it may be extremely difficult to optimally control blood sugars and blood pressure at the same time. When blood glucose is high, the vascular volume is increased, and the kidney sees a larger blood volume, thereby reducing vasoconstriction. However, when glycemic control improves and blood volume decreases, the kidney responds by vasoconstricting and increasing blood pressure. These patients usually require five to six antihypertensive medications and oral medications plus insulin to obtain reasonable control.

Hormone replacement therapy is currently not recommended for cardiovascular protection in postmenopausal women. However, in type 1 diabetes low-dose oral contraceptives should be considered in girls over 16 years of age who are amenorrheic to protect against skeletal demineralization.

Aspirin therapy in diabetic women with hypertension has been shown to reduce cardiovascular morbidity and mortality. However, it may lessen the beneficial effects of ACE inhibitors in patients with established cardiovascular disease, so alternative antiplatelet agents might be considered.

Smoking cessation is imperative!

G. HYPERLIPIDEMIAS

Patients with type 2 diabetes often have a distinct triad of dyslipidemia. Each of these abnormalities has been shown to be an independent factor in atherogenesis. Elevated triglyceride and LDL levels are accompanied by decreased levels of HDL. Most outcome studies on lipid management have excluded patients with diabetes, but there is subgroup analysis data that show a reduction in cardiovascular events of 25–37% with the use of statins to improve the lipid profile. As with all other aspects, life-style changes with a reduction of saturated fats to <7% of daily calories should be encouraged. But in the absence of significant improvement with life-style change or attempt, management of lipid levels should be aggressive. The following goals are recommended:

Total cholesterol, <200 mg/dL

LDL, <100 mg/dL

Triglycerides, <150 mg/dL

Hydroxymethylglutaryl coenzyme A (HMG-CoA) reductase inhibitors (statins) are the drugs of choice in treating hyperlipidemia in diabetics. They decrease the risk of coronary events, specifically inhibiting the regular enzyme for cholesterol biosynthesis, and are excellent for lowering LDL cholesterol. Their effect on lowering triglycerides is less pronounced, but they are sufficient in many patients. They are contraindicated in pregnancy and so must be used with extreme caution in adolescents.

Niacin increases fatty acid reesterification to triglycerides; it reduces triglycerides by as much as 23%, reduces VLDL secretion, increases HDL by 29%, decreases LDL by 8%, and may increase insulin resistance slightly, so has not been used extensively in diabetics. The ADMIT study showed good efficacy without serious side effects. At doses up to 3000 mg/day there was no significant change in HgbA$_{1c}$ levels.

The fibric acid derivatives gemfibrozil and clofibrate activate lipoprotein lipase, reduce triglycerides, and increase HDL, but have minimal effect on LDL. Bile acid-binding resins (colestipol and cholestyramine) are insoluble ion-exchange resins that bind and sequester bile acids in the GI tract, can elevate triglycerides, and are not frequently used in diabetics

H. DIABETIC FEET

Diabetes is the leading nontraumatic cause of foot amputation in the United States. It is also the leading cause of Charcot foot, caused by a combination of neuropathy, altered foot structure, and vasculopathy. Of diabetics 15% will have a foot ulcer at some time and 20% of these will lead to amputation. Feet should be examined at every office visit and patients should be instructed in foot care. Prevention of skin breakdown and infections is the best treatment. Medicare will pay for special shoes and the fitting of these shoes by a podiatrist or orthotist. However, careful attention to foot care by primary providers was found to be more effective at preventing ulcers than special shoes or inserts.

Treatment of diabetic foot ulcers requires removing pressure or unloading the ulcer. Good wound care with deep debridement and appropriate dressing is the basis of treatment. Betadine is not appropriate for cleaning as it kills normal tissue. Antibiotics should be used only if infection is clearly present, and have been shown to retard healing in the noninfected foot. Wound cultures almost always yield multiple organisms, and usually are helpful only if taken from the bone in cases of osteomyelitis. Becaplermin (Regranex) aids in healing, but is expensive and is usually not necessary. The tool of choice for diagnosis of osteomyelitis is the magnetic resonance imaging (MRI) scan, although bone scans are a good alternative. Treatment efficacy can be followed by monitoring the sedimentation rate.

Evans TC, Capell P: Diabetic nephropathy. Clin Diabetes 2000; 18:7.

Gamel JW: Diabetic retinopathy: an update. Hosp Med 1998; June:51.

Gerstein HC et al: Albuminuria and risk of cardiovascular events, death, and heart failure in diabetic and nondiabetic individuals. JAMA 2001;286:421.

Gleckman RA, Mehrnoosh S: Infection in the diabetic patient: what to look for and how to treat. Consultant 1997;September:2396.

O'Keefe JH et al: Improving the adverse cardiovascular prognosis of type 2 diabetes. Mayo Clin Proc 1999;74:171.

Simmons Z, Feldman EL: The pharmacological treatment of painful diabetic neuropathy. Clin Diabetes 2000;18:116.

Yusuf S et al: Effects of an angiotensin-converting-enzyme inhibitor, ramipril, on death from cardiovascular causes, myocardial infarction, and stroke in high-risk patients. The Heart Outcomes Prevention Evaluation Study Investigators. New Engl J Med 2000;342:145.

Treatment

A. MANAGEMENT

In the DCCT trial, a reduction of HgbA$_{1c}$ to 7.2% in type 1 diabetics produced a 50–70% reduction in risk for microvascular disease. More recent studies in type 2 diabetes have confirmed these findings. Microvascular complications are preventable with good glycemic control in type 1 and 2 diabetics. From both an individual and a societal perspective, glycemic control is cost effective in minimizing microvascular complications. Blood pressure appears to independently affect the progression of microvascular and macrovascular complications, and tight control of blood pressure is as important as tight glycemic control. There is good clinical evidence to support aggressive management of hyperglycemia, hypertension, and hyperlipidemia to reduce nephropathy, retinopathy, neuropathy, and cardiovascular events.

The management goal of the clinician is to maintain fasting glucose levels of 80–100 mg/dL and bedtime levels of 100–140 mg/dL with HgbA$_{1c}$ levels <7; the American College of Endocrinology and the American Association of Clinical Endocrinologists have set a goal for HgbA$_{1c}$ at <6.5% and others may follow suit. As more evidence concerning the importance of tight blood pressure control accumulates the recommended blood pressure level continues to drop. The American Kidney Association now recommends that blood pressure be maintained below 130/80 mm Hg.

Less stringent treatment goals may be appropriate for patients with limited life expectancies, in the very young, in older adults at risk for hypoglycemia, or in patients with comorbid conditions. Diabetes is a disease managed best by the motivated patient. Clinician goals are not always compatible with those of the patient. Patients are most likely to achieve goals if they, not the physician, establish them.

B. EDUCATION

Education is the cornerstone of diabetes management. Because the most important management tool is lifestyle alteration, it is imperative that the patient take ownership of the disease and develop skills for managing it. Clinicians, nurse practitioners, nurses, diabetes educators, dietitians, and others can all contribute to the educational process. Other modalities such as reading materials, Internet sites, and self-tests may also be employed. Patients need to have a basic concept of diabetes and understand the complications of both the disease and the treatments. They should understand the interrelationship of life-style changes, smoking cessation, home monitoring, management of blood pressure and lipids, and foot and skin care. Additionally they need to know and understand their medication and/or insulin regimens and how to recognize problems with medications. Some patients will need instruction in special situations that may involve work or travel. Time should also be devoted to the psychological aspects of the disease including family and other outside support, self-image, and relationships. Finally, as they gain a better understanding of their disease patients will be able to make treatment goals in conjunction with the care team.

Knowledge is ongoing and always changing. A patient's knowledge base will change over time, so periodic assessments will need to be made. There are instruments available to help measure the patient's understanding and motivation, or practices can develop their own. It is preferable to have separate questions for patients with type 1 diabetes as they will need more training in insulin management. Whatever instrument is used, it can provide feedback to the patient and reward increased knowledge acquisition.

C. NUTRITION

The goal of nutritional therapy in diabetes is to maintain a near normal blood glucose level and optimal serum lipid levels. Weight loss in an obese individual of 10–15% will significantly improve glucose control. In a prospective 12-year study of nearly 5000 type 2 diabetic patients, it was found that interventional weight loss reduced mortality by 25%. Improved nutrition should improve overall health and well-being. The shift in nutrition is toward more individualization and achievement of goals, health, and well-being rather than a one-size-fits-all percentage of nutrients approach. Structured programs designed to promote life-style changes that include education, decreased fat and overall calorie intake, regular exercise, and regular follow-up have been shown to produce long-term weight loss of about 5–7%. In insulin-resistant individuals reduced intake and modest weight loss improve insulin sensitivity and hyperglycemia. A reduction of 300–400 kcal/day will induce a modest weight loss in most individuals. Exercise has been shown to be the most important factor in long-term maintenance after weight loss. Programs that do not concentrate on life-style changes and rely on diet alone are unlikely to produce long-term results.

Whether maintaining or losing weight, patients with diabetes should attempt to eat a balanced diet. Older adults have lower energy requirements, and this should be taken into account when suggesting total daily caloric intake. The greatest percentage of carbohydrates should come from whole grains, vegetables, fruits, and low-fat milk or dairy products. Several studies have looked at milk, dairy products, and/or calcium consumption and the risk of developing diabetes. As part of the Coronary Artery Risk Development in Young Adults (CARDIA) study, increased dairy consumption was found to have an inverse relationship to the development of insulin-resistance syndrome (IRS) in overweight, young adults. The implication of this study is that a greater percentage of fat calories should be obtained through dairy products, but the mechanisms or implications for management based on these data are unknown.

Glycemic control is dependent on total caloric intake, not on the type of carbohydrate used. Sucrose does not increase glycemia more than carbohydrates, although the increase may occur more rapidly. Diabetic individuals do not need to give up sucrose-containing foods, but they should be substituted for other carbohydrate sources. Nonnutritive sweeteners are safe when used within the acceptable intake levels recommended by the Food and Drug Administration (FDA). A high-fiber diet (particularly soluble type) improves glycemic control, decreases hyperinsulinemia, and lowers plasma lipid concentrations in type 2 diabetes.

Less than 10% of energy intake should be derived from saturated fats and dietary cholesterol should be less than 300 mg/day. In obese individuals or those with low-density lipoprotein (LDL) cholesterol levels greater than 100 mg/dL, saturated fats should be restricted to less than 7% and cholesterol intake to less than 200 mg/day. Long-term maintenance of low-fat diets contributes to modest weight loss and improvement of dyslipidemia.

Ingested protein stimulates insulin secretion just as carbohydrate ingestion does, but does not increase plasma glucose to the same extent. There is no evidence to support protein restriction in diabetic patients with normal renal function. However, the American diet usually contains much more than the recommended amount of protein, so patients should be encouraged to eat appropriate amounts. There is also no evidence that high-protein diets are harmful to diabetic patients with normal kidney function. These diets may induce fairly rapid weight loss; however, in most cases individuals using these diets do not maintain their weight loss. Questions remain about the effect of these diets on plasma LDL cholesterol levels. In patients with microalbuminuria, there is limited evidence to suggest that restricting daily dietary protein to 0.8–1.0 g/kg body weight may slow the progression of nephropathy.

Patients with hypertension should restrict sodium intake to <2400 mg/day. Alcohol has a high caloric value and should be consumed only in small quantities. There is no clear evidence to recommend vitamin or mineral supplementation for patients with diabetes. Like normal individuals, folate should be used in pregnancy and calcium may be recommended to prevent bone loss. There in some evidence concerning the use of magnesium and chromium and these will be discussed in the section on alternative therapy.

Individuals receiving fixed daily doses of insulin should try to maintain a consistent daily caloric intake. Those on intensive insulin therapy should adjust their insulin based on the carbohydrate content of their meals. With the new rapid acting insulins, some individuals may prefer to eat first, count carbohydrates, and then give the appropriate dose of insulin based on carbohydrate intake immediately following the meal.

D. EXERCISE

Exercise improves self-esteem, reduces stress, lowers heart rate and blood pressure, improves circulation, lowers lipid levels, improves digestion, controls appetite, lowers blood sugar, increases strength and endurance, reduces risk of cardiovascular disease, improves sleep and energy level, may increase HDL cholesterol and insulin sensitivity, and can contribute to weight loss. When combined with dietary therapy, a daily walking program has been shown to decrease weight and improve insulin sensitivity. Exercise programs alone decrease $HgbA_{1c}$ levels by 0.66% with no significant changes in body mass. Benefit seems greatest prior to or early in disease as exercise may help delay or even prevent the onset of type 2 diabetes. It was found that as women increase their regular level of activity, their risk for developing type 2 diabetes decreases. The Diabetes Prevention Program (DPP) was a major clinical trial comparing life-style change with metformin in preventing type 2 diabetes in 3234 individuals with impaired glucose tolerance (IGT). It found that individuals who participated in moderate physical exercise (30 min/day) and lost 5–7 pounds decreased their risk of developing diabetes by 58%

A regular exercise program adapted to complications should be prescribed for all patients. An exercise physiologist, if available, can help create a successful exercise program by helping patients understand the need for exercise, their own limitations, and how to most effectively use their assets to optimize exercise. A basic exercise plan would include moderate aerobic or physical activity for 20–60 min three to five times per week. Heart rate should reach 65–80% of maximum, and energy expenditure should be targeted at 700–2000 calories per week. Patients at increased risk of coronary artery disease should have an exercise stress test performed prior to beginning or significantly advancing an exercise program. Older patients with complications of diabetes should undergo a careful physical examination prior to beginning an exercise program and should avoid sudden, strenuous exercise. Athletes with diabetes may not participate in strenuous exercise when the blood glucose is >300 mg/dL. If glucose levels are >250 mg/dL the urine should be checked for ketones. The presence of ketones precludes exercise. Patients who are ketotic need more insulin. Increasing exercise does not supply more insulin, and so forces the body into more ketosis. Treatment is insulin and careful monitoring without increasing exercise.

E. Home Glucose Monitoring

The consensus panel of the American Diabetes Association (ADA) has recommended that all patients with diabetes should perform home glucose monitoring. This is imperative in patients using insulin and has been shown to be effective in noninsulin users. However, there are few studies that show the accuracy of home glucose monitoring. Only about 50% of patients who regularly monitored their blood sugars were found to be within 10% of the control values recommended by the ADA; however, 84% were within 20% of controls. Patients need adequate instruction and follow-up to assess continued compliance. Monitors should be checked when home values do not correspond to office values.

At least eight companies manufacture blood glucose meters and most make several different models. Newer models are smaller, require less blood, and calculate serum glucose more rapidly. They also have the ability to store previous readings and many have systems that can download the memory onto a personal computer. Home monitors usually provide readings between 50 and 500 mg/dL blood glucose. Sample volume required for the test ranges from 0.3 to 12 µL. Machines usually store 100–250 values but some have no storage capacity and some can store up to 1000 readings. Most machines now can download the data as well. Test time ranges from 5 to 50 s.

Four meters have been approved for testing on the arm or leg (alternative site testing). These are all newer machines, requiring small samples, with memories ranging from 100 to 250 readings and with download capabilities. These machines are the AtLast by Amira Medical, Fast Take and One Touch Ultra by Life Scan Inc., and Free Style by TheraSense Inc. When recommending meters consider the patient's needs for ease of operation, memory, and cost. Many companies provide rebates making the machine very economical but ensuring the long-term use of expensive test strips. Medicare and some insurance companies cover the cost of monitoring so choice of machine may be influenced by insurance coverage.

A wristwatch style device and a soon-to-be marketed continuous monitoring system continuously sample interstitial fluid. This measurement lags about 5–15 min behind blood glucose. A currently available continuous glucose monitoring system provides 3 days of continuous readings that can be downloaded in a graph for later analysis but is not available at the time of measurement.

Type 1 diabetics should monitor blood glucose at least four times a day. Patients with type 2 diabetes will monitor more irregularly based on their degree of control. Adjustments are made based on fasting, bedtime, and pre- and postprandial readings. Patients on intermediate-acting insulin (neutral protamine Hagedorn) may also need some readings at 2:00 to 3:00 AM. Patients will need to vary the times each day until they have several readings in each of the necessary categories. In general, fasting and 2-h postprandial values are the most helpful and predictive of long-term control and minimization of complications.

F. Alternative Therapies

Because the best "alternative" and traditional therapy for diabetes is life-style change, most alternative therapies are in the form of nutritional supplementation. At least two studies have looked specifically at the use of chromium in the treatment of diabetes. It has been studied both in type 2 and in gestational diabetes. It appears to potentiate the action of insulin. It also seems to have beneficial effects on mild glucose intolerance. Chromium picolinate is available over the counter and is usually used in doses of 100–500 μg twice daily. These doses have previously been shown to be safe, but recently questions have been raised concerning possible chromosomal damage with long-term, high-dose therapy. The greatest problem with chromium supplementation is that it seems to be most efficacious in patients with low chromium due to poor dietary intake. There is no readily available assay to detect these patients, so it is difficult to determine which patients to treat. There are no large, randomized, controlled trials showing its efficacy.

Magnesium supplementation has also surfaced as a possible adjunct to treatment. Observations have been made that patients with well-controlled diabetes have magnesium levels in the normal range, and those with poorly controlled diabetes have low levels. If there is a causal effect, it is not known if magnesium influences glucose levels or if elevated glucose levels cause magnesium levels to fall. There are no significant studies that show an improvement in hyperglycemia with magnesium supplementation.

Recently cinnamon has been reported to lower glucose levels, but little information is yet available on this spice as a supplement.

G. Pharmacological Therapy

Until the 1990s the only choice for oral diabetes medication was a sulfonylurea. There are now five categories of oral medications (Table 34–3), and increasing choices for insulin. In most cases, therapy is begun with one medication and dosage is increased before adding a second medication. A second medication may be added before the first reaches maximum strength as two medications are sometimes synergistic. When patients with type 2 diabetes present with extremely high serum glucose levels (>400 mg/dL), insulin can be used initially in combination with an oral medication to lower glucose levels to a manageable number. The CDC Diabetes Cost-Effectiveness Group found that intensive control of diabetes and hypertension and reduction of lipids were all cost effective and led to improved health outcomes.

1. Biguanides—Metformin (Glucophage) has become one of the most important medications in the treatment of type 2 diabetes. It is a biguanide that acts primarily on the liver to decrease glucose output via gluconeogenesis. It also improves insulin sensitivity in the liver and in muscle tissue and may decrease intestinal glucose absorption. It has several other advantages as it does not cause hypoglycemia, lowers insulin levels, and may contribute to some weight loss by decreasing ap-

Table 34–3. Oral medications for diabetes.

	Available Dosage (mg)	Dosage Range (mg/day)
Biguanides		
Metformin (Glucophage)	500, 850, 1000	500–2500
Metformin XR (Glucophage XR)	500	500–2000
Sulfonylureas (second generation)		
Glyburide (DiaBeta, Micronase)	1.25, 2.5, 5	1.25–20
Glyburide, micronized (Glynase)	1.5, 3, 6	1.5–12
Glipizide (Glucatrol)	5, 10	5–40
Glipizide XL (Glucotrol XL)	2.5, 5, 10	2.5–20
Glimepiride (Amaryl)	1, 2, 4	1–8
Meglitinides		
Repaglinide (Prandin)	0.5, 1, 2	0.5–4 (2–4 times/day)
Nateglinide (Starlix)	60–120	60–120 (3 times/day)
Thiazolidinediones		
Rosiglitazone (Avandia)	2, 4, 8	2–8
Pioglitazone (Actos)	15, 30, 45	15–45
α-Glucosidase inhibitors		
Acarbose (Precose)	25, 50, 100	25–100 (3 times/day)
Miglitol (Glyset)	25, 50, 100	25–100 (3 times/day)
Combination		
Glyburide/metformin (Glucovance)	1.25/250, 2.5/500, 5/500	1.25/250–20/2000

petite. It has a beneficial effect on the lipid profile by decreasing serum triglycerides and LDL levels. It has been shown to promote improved endothelial function. Metformin is one of the more potent oral antihyperglycemics, lowering $HgbA_{1c}$ levels by 1.5–2.0%. In the UKPDS it was also shown to decrease cardiovascular events, to reduce diabetes end points by 32%, to decrease diabetes-related deaths by 42%, and to reduce all-cause mortality by 36%.

Gastrointestinal (GI) side effects, particularly nausea and diarrhea, are common, but are reduced by starting at a low dose. The recommended starting dose is 500 mg twice a day, but some patients will have fewer side effects with a single daily dose to start. The maximum dose is 2500 mg/day. The sustained release formulation is now available with a maximum dose of 2000 mg/day, but appears to be of equal efficacy. Both forms may be taken as a single dose with the largest meal, but as the dosage increases the shorter acting form is usually split into two or three doses with meals. The side effect profile may also be somewhat improved with the sustained release formulation. Metformin may not be used in patients with congestive heart failure requiring medication or with renal insufficiency (creatinine >1.5 mg/dL), due to the slight possibility of lactic acidosis. Although rare, lactic acidosis has a 50% mortality rate. Metformin should be used with caution in the elderly or in patients with hepatic dysfunction. It must be stopped when giving intravenous contrast dye and is restarted 48 h after the procedure. A category B drug, it may be used in pregnancy but not during lactation. It is, however, the drug of choice in children with type 2 diabetes. It has been used successfully in children 10 years of age and older, but there is no evidence for its safety in younger children. Metformin is currently being used in patients with impaired glucose tolerance to prolong or prevent the onset of diabetes.

2. Sulfonylureas—Sulfonylureas are the oldest oral medications used for the treatment of diabetes. They are insulin secretagogues that stimulate the pancreatic beta cells to increase insulin production. Hypoglycemia is the most common side effect and is most worrisome in patients with tight control and/or the elderly. Glyburide (DiaBeta, Micronase, Glynase) is the most commonly used, but also has the greatest propensity for hypoglycemia. Glipizide (Glucotrol) is available in an extended release form, the least expensive formulation. The newest addition to this category is glimepiride (Amaryl), which may also be the most efficacious.

The sulfonylureas primarily stimulate pancreatic beta cells to release more insulin but may also have some peripheral effect. They block ATP-sensitive potassium channels leading to insulin exocytosis. Glimepiride has a more rapid onset and longer duration of action but induces less hypoglycemia, and may be the best choice of a sulfonylurea in patients with known coronary disease. The sulfonylureas are efficacious, lowering $HgbA_{1c}$ levels up to 2.0%, but about 20% of patients who start on them will not respond. They tend to lose efficacy over time, and doses must be increased or other medications added.

Sulfonylureas should be taken 1 h before meals to induce insulin secretion or at bedtime where they limit hepatic glucose production. The most common side effects are weight gain and hypoglycemia. Glyburide has now been shown to be safe and efficacious in the treatment of gestational diabetes. Although sulfonylureas have the propensity to cause hypoglycemia, they appear to be safe even in the elderly. In one study, elderly patients on sulfonylureas who fasted for 24 h had increased epinephrine levels but no severe hypoglycemia.

3. Meglitinides—The meglitinides, repaglinide (Prandin) and nateglinide (Starlix), are short-acting insulin secretagogues that bind to ATP-sensitive potassium channels on pancreatic beta cells and increase insulin secretion. They have a rapid onset of action, and their half-life is less than 1 h, so they may be taken immediately before meals. If a meal is skipped, the dose should be skipped as well. Nateglinide has a more rapid onset and shorter duration of action than repaglinide and is indicated for combination therapy with metformin. The meglitinides have been reported to reduce $HgbA_{1c}$ levels from 0.5% to 2.0%, but are significantly more expensive than sulfonylureas. They are particularly useful in patients whose fasting glucose levels are well controlled but who have high postprandial values. They also work well for patients who eat few or irregular meals as the dose is not taken if the meal is skipped.

These medications should be used with caution in patients with hepatic dysfunction and their long-term safety is still unknown. They can, however, be used in patients with renal failure as they are excreted through the liver.

4. Thiazolidinediones—The thiazolidinediones (TZDs), rosiglitazone (Avandia) and pioglitazone (Actos), work primarily by improving target cell response to insulin in muscle and adipose tissue, thereby decreasing insulin resistance. They also decrease hepatic gluconeogenesis and increase peripheral glucose disposal. Pioglitazone has been shown to decrease triglyceride levels by 33% and increase HDL cholesterol levels, but the TZDs may cause a slight increase in LDL cholesterol levels. Because they increase the efficacy of insulin, they also promote weight gain. They are metabolized by the liver, so they may be used in patients with renal failure. Troglitazone was removed from the market following several cases of associated liver failure, and now liver function tests must be monitored every other month for the first year that these medications are used. They do not induce cytochrome P-450 3A4, so do not react with nifedipine, oral contraceptives, metformin, digoxin, ranitidine, or acarbose. Initiating therapy with TZDs requires patience. It may take 12 weeks for the medication to reach its maximum potential. Increases in dosage should be made slowly and only after several weeks on the same dosage.

TZDs cause water retention and peripheral edema and must be used with caution in patients with congestive heart failure (CHF), prompting the FDA to strengthen its precautions and warnings for these medications. They are not currently recommended for children. They may be a good first-line choice in some newly diagnosed diabetics with marked insulin sensitivity. The long-term effect on macrovascular disease is unknown. TZDs are FDA approved for use with insulin, but they should be used with caution in this combination unless other more cardioprotective medications are used as well. They may increase ovulation and, therefore, increase the chance of pregnancy in obese diabetic women.

5. α-Glucosidase inhibitors—The α-glucosidase inhibitors, acarbose (Precose) and miglitol (Glyset), interfere with disaccharide metabolism and delay carbohydrate absorption in the gut by inhibiting α-glucosidase in the brush border of the small intestine. The delayed absorption blunts postprandial hyperglycemia. This mechanism produces a modest reduction in $HgbA_{1c}$ of 0.7–1.0%. The α-glucosidase inhibitors are relatively expensive for the moderate reduction in serum glucose achieved. They work only when taken with food, so they do not cause hypoglycemia when used alone. They can be particularly useful in patients with erratic eating habits as they are taken only with meals and can also be helpful in patients who remain noncompliant with diet. They may be useful in elderly patients who need only mild improvement in control if they can tolerate the side effects.

Therapy should be initiated at a low dose and increased slowly to minimize side effects. If they are used with a sulfonylurea or insulin, and hypoglycemia occurs, the patient must be treated with simple sugars (glucose or lactose), not sucrose.

Gastrointestinal side effects are frequent and objectionable. Flatulence is caused by continued disaccharide decomposition in the large intestine. They should not be used in patients with inflammatory bowel disease or other chronic intestinal disorders. These medications are contraindicated in ketoacidosis, cirrhosis, or GI disorders. Efficacy is altered with digestive enzymes, antacids, or cholestyramine. They are not recommended when serum creatinine >2.0 mg/dL. Serum transaminase levels must be followed every 3 months for the first year.

6. Combination therapy—Insulin, sulfonylureas, and meglitinides all increase insulin levels. They can be used together but are more efficiently used with metformin, and TZD, or an α-glucosidase inhibitor. Combining drugs with different mechanisms of action is most efficacious. Caution must be exercised in combining drugs with similar side effects.

The best results in the UKPDS trial were achieved with the combination of insulin and metformin. Sulfonylurea and metformin combinations also work well, and metformin and glyburide are now available as a combination drug (Glucovance). Combining metformin with the TZDs has been shown to be more effective in a once daily dose than metformin alone, but this combination can be very expensive and requires careful monitoring. Sulfonylureas, the meglitinides, and insulin are commonly combined with metformin or the TZDs. α-Glucosidase inhibitors should be used with caution with the TZDs because both can be hepatotoxic. They also must be carefully monitored with sulfonylureas, meglitinides, and insulin because treatment of hypoglycemia can be difficult. Also, the similar target of postprandial hyperglycemia and the three times daily dosing of the meglitinides and α-glucosidase inhibitors make them a poor combination.

Combinations of three or more classes of oral medication can be used, but are currently not approved. If three medications are needed consider adding insulin. Patients with long-standing diabetes may require the addition of insulin as they age and beta cell function is depleted.

7. Insulin—Despite the rapid growth of pharmacological choices for type 2 diabetes, the use of insulin in type 2 diabetes is on the rise. The UKPDS trial did not show any increase in cardiovascular disease due to the use of insulin and significant improvement in all complications of diabetes with tight control has made insulin again a popular choice in type 2 diabetes. Due to its propensity to cause weight gain and the lingering questions about the safety of the hyperinsulinemic state, insulin is usually used only after life-style changes and combinations of oral agents have been tried. It may be particularly useful, however, in patients with newly diagnosed diabetes and high blood glucose levels. These patients may benefit from short-term insulin use to control blood glucose while initiating oral therapy. Patients with type 1 diabetes and some patients with type 2 diabetes require the use of short- and long-acting insulin. A long-acting insulin provides a basal rate that minimizes hepatic glucose production. A short-acting insulin is used with meals to minimize the postprandial insulin peak. In normal patients circulating insulin returns to the basal level as soon as postprandial blood glucose levels normalize.

With the advent of synthetic insulin analogs, the choice of insulin has increased significantly (Table 34–4). These new designer insulins more closely mimic

Table 34–4. Current insulins.

	Onset of Action	Peak (h)	Duration (h)
Rapid—lispro (Humalog)	5–15 min	1–2	4–5
Rapid—aspart (Novolog)	5–15 min	1–3	3–5
Short—regular	30–60 min	2–4	6–8
Intermediate—NPH or N	1–3 h	5–7	13–18
Intermediate—lente or L	1–3 h	4–8	13–20
Long—ultralente or U	2–4 h	8–14	18–20
Sustained—glargine (Lantus)[1]	2–4 h	None	>24

[1]Glargine insulin cannot be mixed.

the pharmacokinetics of human insulin *in vivo*. Until recently, neutral protamine Hagedorn (NPH), lente, or ultralente insulins were utilized to supply basal metabolic needs. These long-acting insulins have variable absorption rates depending on dose and injection site, making them somewhat unpredictable in efficacy. NPH and lente have an onset of action of about 2 h and a duration of 12–16 h. They are usually given twice a day with peaks occurring in the afternoon and early morning, although they are occasionally given once a day in type 2 diabetics. The variable absorption and peak times expose patients to significant risk of hypoglycemia. Dosage changes are made based on fingersticks taken about 8 h following the dose. Ultralente is a peakless, long-acting insulin designed for once daily use. Its onset of action is 12 h and its duration is 18–24 h. Because it does not always have 24-h duration, it may not meet basal needs, allowing blood glucose to rise until the next dose.

The long-acting insulin analog glargine (Lantus) is a truly peakless insulin with a consistent 24-h duration. This insulin is less soluble in subcutaneous tissue, thereby prolonging absorption. It can be used with any of the short-acting insulins and may be used with oral medications for type 2 diabetics. Glargine, approved in April 2000, is a clear insulin and cannot be mixed with other insulins. It is usually taken in the evening around 8:00 PM. When converting to this insulin, total all insulin that it is replacing and multiply by 0.8. If there are no episodes of severe hypoglycemia after monitoring for two consecutive days, the dose may be increased two units for every 20 mg/dL rise in glucose above 100 mg/dL (ie, glucose 100–120, increase by two units; glucose 120–140, increase by four units, etc, with a maximum increase of eight units).

Until recently short-acting regular insulin was the only insulin used to control postprandial blood glucose primarily in type 1 diabetics. Regular insulin has an onset of action in about 30 min with peak levels in 1–2 h, but its duration of action is 4–6 h, usually long after blood glucose should return to normal. This long duration leads to a blood glucose nadir several hours after meals, often necessitating the use of a snack to maintain blood glucose levels. It is also given about 30 min prior to meals, making any delay in eating a hazard. The synthetic insulin analogs, lispro (Humalog) and aspart (Novolog), have a similar onset and peak, but they have a duration of only 2–4 h, corresponding to a normal fall in postprandial blood glucose. These insulins are given immediately prior to the meal and disappear with the normalization of blood glucose, decreasing postprandial hypoglycemia. They are excellent for motivated patients, but should be used with caution in patients who do not use regular fingerstick monitoring. The names of these insulins reflect the amino acid changes made to human insulin. Switching a lysine and proline makes lispro. Aspart is derived by replacing a proline with an aspartic acid.

Mixtures of short-acting and intermediate-acting insulin are often used and will work if a patient is on a steady regimen. Lente insulin should not be mixed with NPH or short-acting forms. It is very difficult to achieve tight control with mixtures, although regular, lispro, or aspart could still be given between doses if necessary. Humulin 70/30 is a mixture of 70% NPH and 30% regular. Humalog mix 75/25 is a mixture of 75% lispro protamine suspension and 25% lispro (it has the same onset and peak as lispro but has a longer duration of action).

Bioavailability with insulin changes with the site of injection. Abdominal injection (especially above the umbilicus) is the quickest; using the arm is slower, but is faster than using the hip or thigh. The American Diabetes Association now recommends rotating injections within the same area instead of rotating between areas.

When initiating insulin therapy in type 1 diabetics, their total insulin requirement for 24 h (from insulin infusion or sliding scale regular) should be estimated. Half of this amount will be given as an intermediate or long-acting insulin and the other half as a short-acting insulin. If using a long-acting form, 50% of the total insulin will be given as a single dose. If using an intermediate form, its portion is divided with two-thirds given in the morning and one-third in the evening. The short-acting portion is divided with 40% given before breakfast, 40% before supper, and the remaining 20% prior to lunch.

8. Insulin pump—Continuous subcutaneous insulin infusion (CSII) was first reported in the 1970s. These "insulin pumps" have become smaller and easier to use with more safety features. Current pumps weigh about 4 ounces and are about the size of a beeper. CSII allows for continuous use of short-acting insulin with a more consistent absorption rate as the site of injection is not rotated. The newer short-acting insulin analogs (lispro and aspart) appear to be more beneficial in the CSII system. Similar to standard insulin therapy, results with the insulin pump are improved when patients monitor and record their blood glucose three or more times a day and count carbohydrates at meals. When compliant, patients can achieve tighter control with the pump while gaining more flexibility in eating habits and a more normal life-style. Used correctly there are fewer episodes of severe hypoglycemia, a reduction of total insulin usage, and less weight gain. Particularly good candidates for insulin pump therapy are patients who are difficult to control or have wide glucose swings, have erratic schedules, or have a significant dawn phenomenon, pregnant women, and teenagers with poor control and/or frequent episodes of ketoacidosis.

When initiating pump therapy in adults the total dose of insulin may be reduced by 25–30%. In children the total dose usually remains the same. In general, the average adult will require about 0.7 U/kg/day. Older individuals may require only 0.5 U/kg/day, whereas adolescents may need 1.0 U/kg/day. In both groups, all insulin, both short and long acting, is replaced with a short-acting insulin. This insulin is divided in half with 50% given continuously to supply basal needs and the other 50% divided between meals. Individuals vary, but a usual distribution is 20% of total insulin for breakfast, 10% for lunch, and 20% for dinner boluses. Total basal dose is divided by 24 to give the rate per hour. Both dose rates must be adjusted based on blood glucose monitoring before and 2 h after meals and at bedtime, midnight, and 3 AM. Another advantage to the pump is that the basal rate can be changed during the night. Daytime basal rates may be adjusted by delaying a meal and monitoring every 2 h to determine the magnitude of change needed. Mealtime bolus rates are based on carbohydrate intake with the average rate of 1 unit of insulin for every 1–15 g of carbohydrate. Boluses can be divided before and after the meal to more accurately assess actual consumption. When plasma glucose is high, a bolus dose may be calculated by dividing 1500 by the total daily dose of insulin (TDD). This will determine the mg/dL drop that will be produced by one additional unit of insulin (Table 34–5). The newer pumps also allow customization of the bolus rate to allow for a high-fat or small meal.

Because exercise decreases blood glucose levels, the target glucose level prior to exercise should be 120–180 mg/dL. As for all diabetics exercise should not be initiated if the blood glucose is ≥250 mg/dL. Patients may discontinue the pump for exercise, participation in water sports, and contact sports. The pump will need to be reinitiated after 4 h if using regular insulin or after 2 h if using aspart or lispro. As with other forms

Table 34–5. Sample calculation of insulin for pump therapy.

Calculation of insulin for pump therapy for a 70-kg individual:
70 kg × 0.7 = 49 U regular or lispro/aspart insulin
49 ÷ 2 = 24.5
24 U as basal dose ÷ 24 = 1 U/h basal dose
30 U may be used for bolus dosing (12 U prior to breakfast, 6 U prior to lunch, and 12 U prior to dinner)
1500 ÷ 49 = ~30 mg/dL drop per 1.0 U of insulin (if blood sugar is 200 mg/dL, 3 U of insulin should decrease blood glucose to 110 mg/dL)

of therapy, best results are achieved in motivated and educated patients.

9. Transplant—During the 1990s over 250 brittle, insulin-dependent diabetics received islet cell transplants, but only 12% remained insulin independent for over a week. A new method of islet cell injection that also uses an immunosuppressive combination that does not include steroids looks promising. Seven patients who received these transplants remained insulin independent for 4–15 months. Each transplant requires two cadaver donors. The limited supply of donated organs will continue to make this an option only for those diabetics who are most difficult to control.

American Diabetes Association: Clinical practice recommendations. Diabetes Care 2001;24(suppl):594.

Bode BW, Steed RD, Davidson PC: Reduction in severe hypoglycemia with long-term continuous subcutaneous insulin infusion in type 1 diabetes. Diabetes Care 1996;19:324.

Bode BW, Sabbah H, Davidson PC: What's ahead in glucose monitoring? New techniques hold promise for improved ease and accuracy. Postgrad Med 2001;109:41.

Inzucchi SE: Oral antihyperglycemic therapy for type 2 diabetes. JAMA 2002;287:360.

Mayer-Davis EJ et al: Intensity and amount of physical activity in relation to insulin sensitivity. JAMA 1998;279:669.

Pereira MA et al: Dairy consumption, obesity, and the insulin resistance syndrome in young adults: the CARDIA study. JAMA 2002;287:2081.

Ratner RE: Glycemic control in the prevention of diabetic complications. Clin Cornerstone 2001;4:24.

UK Prospective Diabetes Study (UKPDS) Group: Effect of intensive blood-glucose control with metformin on complications in overweight patients with type 2 diabetes (UKPDS 34). Lancet 1998;352:854.

Coding & Reimbursement

In most cases International Classification of Diseases (ICD) 9 coding is fairly simple. The basic code for diabetes is 250. The fourth digit concerns complications. These are listed in Table 34–6. The fourth digit codes of 4–8 are most often used in the office. The fifth digit is for type and control and is also listed in Table 34–6. Therefore, patients with poorly controlled diabetes who return for follow-up of their osteomyelitis would be coded as 250.82. Medicare reimburses at a higher rate when the visit is more complex; therefore, appropriate coding of the complications of diabetes will allow for a higher level office visit if those issues are addressed. Medicare now also reimburses for glucometers, strips, and lancets if these are prescribed. Patients will need a prescription with the type of diabetes and frequency of monitoring. As noted earlier, Medicare does reimburse for special shoes. They also will pay for dietetic and educational counseling. As most insurance companies follow Medicare guidelines to some extent, these services are also often covered by private insurance. This varies by company, and patients will need to check their policy or call their insurance company to ascertain what benefits are covered.

Systems Approach

Numerous studies have looked at the health care system and the delivery of health care for diabetes. A number of approaches have been shown to dramatically improve glycemic control. Development of guidelines helps practitioners to cover all areas of diabetes care in an efficient manner. Diabetes improvement models that target education and quality review of providers have been shown to improve provider compliance. Use of electronic medical records or computerized registry systems can provide recurrent review for all aspects of diabetes care, and can be used for call-back and reminder systems, so fewer patients are lost to care. Most importantly, the patients must become empowered. They need to take ownership of their disease and see the health care team as a resource for assisting them in the care of their disease. Diabetes is a complicated, chronic disease with a complex management requiring a multidisciplinary team approach.

Most importantly, the health care team must continue to educate the public about life-style changes that prevent the onset of diabetes. Prevention of this disease, which has reached pandemic proportions, is clearly far superior to trying to treat the diabetes and its complications. In the native Aborigines of Australia diabetes was an unknown disease prior to adoption of a western diet and life-style. Diabetic Aborigines who return to their native diet see resolution of their diabetes. The evidence is clear that life-style change is the most efficacious and cost-effective therapy for this deadly disease.

Table 34–6. ICD 9 fourth and fifth digit classifications.

Fourth Digit	Organ System Involved
0	No complications
1	Hyperosmolarity
2	Ketoacidosis
3	Coma (with either of the above)
4	Renal
5	Eye
6	Neuro
7	Cardiovascular
8	Bone
9	Unspecified
Fifth digit	**Classification**
0	Type 2 well controlled
1	Type 1 well controlled
2	Type 2 uncontrolled
3	Type 1 uncontrolled

WEB SITES

American Association of Diabetes Educators
http://www.aadenet. org
American Diabetes Association (ADA)
http://www/diabetes.org
Centers for Disease Control and Prevention (CDC), Division of Diabetes
http://www.cdc.gov.diabetes
Joslin Diabetes Center
http://www.joslin.harvard.edu
National Diabetes Education Program
http://ndep.nih.gov
National Institute of Diabetes and Digestive and Kidney Diseases
http://www.niddk.nih.gov

Endocrine Disorders

35

William J. Hueston, MD, & Peter J. Carek, MD, MS

◼ THYROID DISORDERS

Thyroid disorders involve a number of problems that alter the normal function of the thyroid gland. These conditions can be grouped into several large categories that include inflammatory diseases of the thyroid (ie, thyroiditis), autoimmune stimulation of the thyroid (Graves' disease), benign thyroid nodular diseases, and thyroid cancers. Thyroid disorders affect 1 out of 200 adults, but are more common in women and with advancing age. By the time individuals reach "old age," about 1 out of 20 people will have a thyroid abnormality. Hypothyroidism is much more common than hyperthyroidism, nodular disease, or thyroid cancer. Thyroid nodules occur in between 4% and 8% of all individuals and, like other thyroid problems, increase in incidence with age. Although nodules are more common in women, thyroid carcinoma is more common in men.

INFLAMMATORY THYROID DISORDERS (THYROIDITIS)

Symptoms & Signs

Thyroiditis encompasses a number of unrelated clinical conditions that involve either autoimmune, infectious, or unknown insult to the thyroid. Symptoms range from painless or mildly tender enlargement of the thyroid to a frankly swollen, very tender gland with accompanying fever and other stigmata of invasive bacterial infections. Patients with thyroiditis may exhibit hyper- or hypothyroid symptoms or be euthyroid.

Pathogenesis

The most common cause of thyroiditis is chronic lymphocytic or Hashimoto's thyroiditis. Hashimoto's thyroiditis is the most common of the inflammatory thyroid disorders and the most common cause of goiter in the United States. The prevalence of Hashimoto's thyroiditis has been increasing dramatically in the past 50 years in the United States. The cause for this rise is unknown. Hashimoto's thyroiditis is seen most often in middle-aged women and presents with enlargement of the thyroid. The thyroid may be slightly tender on palpation, but also can be pain free. About 20% of patients presenting with Hashimoto's thyroiditis will already be hypothyroid either clinically or on measurement of thyroid-stimulating hormone (TSH). Hashimoto's thyroiditis is caused by an autoimmune disease; 95% of patients will have antithyroid perixodase (formerly known as antimicrosomal) antibodies in their serum.

Subacute lymphocytic thyroiditis, also known as painless or silent thyroiditis, is less common. Subacute lymphocytic thyroiditis is also autoimmune mediated, but the immune insult is usually only transient. Patients with subacute lymphocytic thyroiditis often have fairly acute enlargement of the thyroid without tenderness (hence, the label "painless"). Insult to the thyroid may result in the release of preformed thyroid hormone, resulting in a period of hyperthyroidism. Following this hyperthyroid phase, patients may become hypothyroid as the injured thyroid undergoes repair. Fewer than 10% of patients will remain hypothyroid indefinitely.

Subacute granulomatous thyroiditis, also known as giant cell thyroiditis or deQuervain's thyroiditis, is similar to subacute lymphocytic thyroiditis except it is usually associated with a recent viral illness and does not appear to be autoimmune mediated. In subacute granulomatous thyroiditis, the thyroid enlargement is mildly painful. Acute inflammation in the thyroid may be treated with aspirin or other nonsteroid antiinflammatory agents or, in severe cases, with prednisone. However, it should be noted that a rebound in thyroid swelling and tenderness may occur after prednisone withdrawal. The clinical presentation of subacute granulomatous thyroiditis is similar to subacute lymphocytic thyroiditis with a hyperthyroid stage followed by euthyroid or hypothyroid periods. In most cases, the thyroid damage is minor, but a small number (10%) of patients will suffer enough thyroid dysfunction to require permanent thyroid replacement.

Suppurative thyroiditis is a very rare condition in which there is an acute bacterial infection of the thyroid gland usually with *Staphylococcus aureus, Streptococcus pyogenes* (Group A strep), or *Streptococcus pneumoniae.* Patients have a tender, swollen thyroid, fever, elevated white blood cell count, and other manifestations of an acute bacterial illness.

Finally, invasive fibrous thyroiditis, or Reidel's thyroiditis, presents with a gradually enlarging, firm but nontender thyroid. In this condition, thyroid tissue is infiltrated with dense fibrous tissue that causes a hard, woody goiter. Patients are usually euthyroid, although a small minority can develop hypothyroidism over time.

Laboratory & Imaging Evaluation

In most cases, very few laboratory or imaging tests are necessary for patients with acute thyroiditis. For patients with nonsuppurative thyroiditis, evaluation of the goiter with thyroid function tests is the initial step. If these tests reveal hypothyroidism, then the evaluation is complete. Generally, antithyroid antibody testing does not add any value to further evaluation or long-term management.

For patients with hyperthyroidism on initial testing, thyroid scanning and uptake may be useful to differentiate thyroiditis from Grave's disease. In Grave's disease, hyperthyroidism develops from antithyroid antibodies that stimulate thyroid activity and overproduction of thyroid hormone. In contrast, hyperthyroidism associated with thyroiditis results from abnormal release of large amounts of preformed thyroid hormone. Production of thyroid hormone is actually decreased. Thus, thyroid scanning shows increased uptake and a diffuse "hot" thyroid with Grave's disease whereas in thyroiditis uptake is decreased and the gland may be "cool."

Treatment

Patients with subacute granulomatous thyroiditis may benefit from administration of antiinflammatory medications such as aspirin. These provide symptomatic benefit, but there is little evidence that antiinflammatory treatment reduces the duration of symptoms or changes the long-term likelihood of hypothyroidism. For hyperthyroid states seen in subacute lymphocytic and subacute granulomatous thyroiditis, β-blockers can be effective at reducing symptoms. Most patients can be started on a low dose of a β-blocker with the dosage titrated up to provide maximal symptom relief with the fewest side effects. Because thyroid production is not increased with thyroiditis, the use of propylthiouricil or methimazole is not effective for decreasing hyperthyroid symptoms.

Thyroid replacement is warranted for hypothyroidism associated with Hashimoto's thyroiditis or for the minority of patients with persistent hypothyroidism from subacute lymphocytic or subacute granulomatous thyroiditis. Replacement should start with low doses (25 µg/day) in patients at high risk for ischemic heart disease and advanced slowly to a target between 100 and 150 µg/day. TSH levels may be used every 6–8 weeks to monitor initial changes in thyroid dose and yearly to ensure adequate replacement.

For suppurative thyroiditis, parenteral administration of antibiotics to cover the likely organisms (*Staphylococcus aureus* and streptococcal species) is indicated. Treatment should include parenteral antistaphylococcal drugs such as first-generation cephalosporins. Rarely, aspiration or drainage of an abscess may be required. Unless extensive damage to the thyroid has occurred, patients usually have normal thyroid function following clearance of the acute infection.

Lastly, invasive fibrous thyroiditis generally requires no therapy. Occasionally, because the large, firm thyroid may be uncomfortable or compress nearby structures, surgical removal of the thyroid is warranted. Otherwise, monitoring for symptoms of hypothyroidism is all that is needed.

Farwell AP, Braverman LE: Inflammatory thyroid disorders. Otolaryngol Clin North Am 1997;29:541.

HYPOTHYROIDISM

Symptoms & Signs

Patients with hypothyroidism generally present with a constellation of symptoms that includes lethargy, weight gain, hair loss, dry skin, slowed mentation or forgetfulness, and a depressed affect (Table 35–1). Because of the range of symptoms seen in hypothyroidism, clinicians must have a high index of suspicion, especially in high-risk populations. In older patients, hypothyroidism can be confused with Alzheimer's disease or other conditions that cause dementia. In women, hypothyroidism is often confused with depression.

Physical findings that can occur with hypothyroidism include a low blood pressure and bradycardia, nonpitting edema, generalized hair thinning along with hair loss in the outer third of the eyebrows, skin drying, and a diminished relaxation phase of reflexes.

Pathogenesis

Several conditions can lead to hypothyroidism (Table 35–2). The most common non-iatrogenic condition causing hypothyroidism in the United States is Hashimoto's thyroiditis. Other common causes of hypothyroidism are post-Graves' disease thyroid irradiation and surgical removal of the thyroid.

Table 35–1. Signs and symptoms that occur in 60% or more of patients with hypothyroidism.

Sign or Symptom	Patients in Whom This Occurs (%)
Weakness	99
Skin changes (dry or coarse skin)	97
Lethargy	91
Slow speech	91
Eyelid edema	90
Cold sensation	89
Decreased sweating	89
Cold skin	83
Thick tongue	82
Facial edema	79
Coarse hair	76
Skin pallor	67
Forgetfulness	66
Constipation	61

From Wilson JD et al: *Williams Textbook of Endocrinology*, ed 9. W.B. Saunders, 1998, p. 461.

Another cause of hypothyroidism is secondary hypothyroidism related to hypothalamic or pituitary dysfunction. These conditions are seen primarily in patients who have received intracranial irradiation or surgical removal of a pituitary adenoma.

Laboratory & Imaging Evaluation

The evaluation of a patient with new onset hypothyroidism is quite limited. In primary hypothyroidism the TSH is elevated, indicating insufficient thyroid hormone production to meet metabolic demands. Free

Table 35–2. Causes of hypothyroidism.

Primary hypothyroidism (95% of cases)
Idiopathic hypothyroidism (probably old Hashimoto's thyroiditis)
Hashimoto's thyroiditis
Postthyroid irradiation
Postsurgical
Late stage invasive fibrous thyroiditis
Iodine deficiency
Drugs (lithium, interferon)
Infiltrative diseases (sarcoidosis, amyloid, scleroderma, hemochromatosis)
Secondary hypothyroidism (5% of cases)
Pituitary or hypothalamic neoplasms
Congenital hypopituitarism
Pituitary necrosis (Sheehan's syndrome)

Adapted from Hueston WJ: Thyroid disease. In: *Women's Health in Primary Care* (Rosenfeld JA, editor). Williams & Wilkins, 1997.

thyroid levels will be depressed. In contrast, patients with secondary hypothyroidism will have low or nondetectable TSH levels. A guide to the laboratory diagnosis of hypothyroidism and interpretation of TSH, tetraiodothyronine (T_4), and triiodothyronine (T_3) levels is shown in Table 35–3.

Once the diagnosis of primary hypothyroidism is made, further imaging or serological testing is not necessary if the thyroid is normal on examination. In cases of secondary hypothyroidism, further investigation with provocative testing of the pituitary can be performed to determine if the cause is a hypothalamic or pituitary problem. If pituitary dysfunction is suspected, further evaluation of the anterior pituitary function can be performed using a thyroid-releasing hormone (TRH)-stimulation test. In this test, TSH levels are determined before and after administration of intravenous TRH. In normal circumstances, infusion of TRH results in a modest rise in TSH. With pituitary dysfunction, the TSH response is absent or blunted. If an exaggerated rise in TSH is noted, this indicates that the pituitary is normal and that the lack of production of TSH reflects an abnormality in TRH production in the hypothalamus.

In cases of pituitary dysfunction, imaging of the pituitary to detect microadenomas is indicated along with testing of other hormones that are dependent on pituitary stimulation. In general, evidence of decreased production of more than one pituitary hormone is indicative of panhypopituitary problems.

Treatment

Most healthy adult patients with hypothyroidism require about 1.7 µg/kg of thyroid replacement with requirements falling to 1 µg/kg for the elderly. This usually amounts to between 0.10 and 0.15 mg/day of L-thyroxine. Children may require higher doses of up to 4 µg/kg for full replacement.

In young patients without risks for cardiovascular disease, replacement can start close to the estimated daily requirement. Most individuals start therapy at 0.075 mg/day and increase the dose slowly as indicated by continued elevations in the TSH levels. Older patients or those with risks for cardiovascular compromise that could occur with a rapid increase in resting heart rate and blood pressure should be started on low doses of L-thyroxine with gradual increases over time. The usual starting dose for patients for whom gradual increases in thyroid replacement is preferable is 0.025 mg/day of thyroxine. Doses can be increased in increments of 0.025–0.050 mg every 4–6 weeks until TSH levels return to normal. Thyroxine is usually given once a day, although some evidence suggests that weekly dosing may be effective as well.

Table 35–3. Laboratory changes in hypothyroidism.

TSH Level	Free T$_4$ Level	Free T$_3$ Level	Likely Diagnosis
High	Low	Low	Primary hypothyroidism
High (>10)	Normal	Normal	"Subclinical hypothyroidism" with high risk for future development of overt hypothyroidism
High (6–10)	Normal	Normal	"Subclinical hypothyroidism" with low risk for future development of overt hypothyroidism
High	High	Low	Congenital absence of T$_4$–T$_3$-converting enzyme or amiodarone effect
High	High	High	Peripheral thyroid hormone resistance
Low	Low	Low	Pituitary thyroid deficiency or recent withdrawal of thyroid replacement after excessive replacement

In addition to replacement with thyroxine, some evidence suggests that providing low doses of T$_3$ may be beneficial for some elderly patients with hypothyroidism. An addition of a small dose of T$_3$ (0.0125 mg) combined with a decrease in thyroxine of 0.05 mg was shown to improve memory, mood, and other symptoms in one small study.

In patients with an intact hypothalamic–pituitary axis, the adequacy of thyroid replacement can be followed with serial assessments of TSH. However, changes in TSH levels lag behind serum levels of thyroid hormone. Evaluation of TSH levels should be performed no earlier than 4 weeks after an adjustment in thyroid doses. Full effects of thyroid replacement on TSH may not be present until after 8 weeks of therapy.

For patients who have pituitary insufficiency, measurements of free T$_4$ and T$_3$ can be performed to ensure patients remain euthyroid. The goal in these patients is to maintain free thyroid levels in the middle to upper ranges of normal to ensure adequate replacement.

With age, thyroid binding decreases with drops in serum albumin and doses may need to be reduced by up to 20%. Therefore, although less than annual monitoring could be justified in younger adult patients whose weight is stable, annual monitoring in older patients is necessary to avoid overreplacement.

Bunevicius R et al: Effects of thyroxine as compared with thyroxine plus triiodothyronine in patients with hypothyroidism. New Engl J Med 1999;340:424.

Grebe SKG et al: Treatment of hypothyroidism with one weekly thyroxine. J Clin Endocrinol Metab 1997;82:870.

Singer PA et al: Treatment guidelines for patients with hyperthyroidism and hypothyroidism. JAMA 1995;273:808.

HYPERTHYROIDISM

Symptoms & Signs

Hyperthyroidism usually presents with progressing nervousness, tremor, palpitations, weight loss, dyspnea on exertion, and difficulty concentrating. Physical findings include a rapid pulse and elevated blood pressure with the systolic pressure increasing to a greater extent than the diastolic pressure, creating a wide pulse–pressure hypertension. Additionally, cardiac dysrythmias such as atrial fibrillation may be evident on examination or electrocardiogram (ECG). A resting tremor may be noted on physical examination.

Thyroid storm represents an acute hypermetabolic state associated with the sudden release of large amounts of thyroid hormone. This occurs most often in Graves' disease, but can occur in acute thyroiditis conditions. Individuals with thyroid storm present with confusion, fever, restlessness, and sometimes with psychotic-like symptoms. Physical examination shows tachycardia, elevated blood pressure, and sometimes fever. Cardiac dysrhythmias may be present or develop. They will have other signs of high output heart failure (dyspnea on exertion, peripheral vasoconstriction) and may exhibit signs of cardiac or cerebral ischemia. Thyroid storm is a medical crisis requiring prompt attention and reversal of the metabolic demands from the acute hyperthyroidism.

Pathogenesis

Graves' disease is the most common cause of hyperthyroidism. Like most of the autoimmune conditions noted in thyroiditis, Graves' disease is more common in women. Graves' disease is an autoimmune disorder caused by immunoglobulin G (IgG) antibodies that bind to TSH receptors initiating the production and release of thyroid hormone. In addition to the usual hyperthyroid symptoms, about 50% of patients with Graves' disease also exhibit exopthalmosis.

The second most common cause of hyperthyroidism is an autonomous nodule that is secreting thyroxine. Although thyroid tissue usually produces thyroid hormone under the influence of TSH, these nodules do not rely on TSH stimulation. The nodules continue to excrete large amounts of thyroxine despite low, or nonexistent, circulating TSH.

Another cause of hyperthryoidism is the acute release of thyroid hormone in early phases of thyroiditis. In these cases, symptoms are generally transient and resolve in a matter of weeks. Once it has been determined that symptoms of hyperthyroidism are due to thyroiditis, symptomatic treatment with a β-blocker can be used temporarily with little need for long-term therapy.

Laboratory & Imaging Evaluation

Hyperthyroidism can be confirmed by an elevated free thyroxine level usually with a corresponding low TSH. Once hyperthyroidism is identified, further testing for autoimmune antibodies and radionucleotide scanning of the thyroid can determine whether the problem is related to Graves' disease, an autonomous nodule, or thyroiditis.

Radionucleotide imaging provides both a direct image of the thyroid and an indication of thyroid functioning. Imaging is performed using either an isotope of technetium (^{99m}Tc) or iodine (^{123}I). These radionucleotides are taken up by the active thyroid and, in the case of ^{123}I, incorporated into thyroid hormone. ^{99m}Tc is preferred over radiolabeled iodine for scanning for a couple of reasons. First, the radiation dose from ^{99m}Tc is much lower than that delivered by ^{123}I. Second, uptake of radioactive iodine is altered by the use of thyroid-suppressing medications. In cases in which patients have had their hyperthyroidism controlled by thyroid-suppressing drugs, the medications must be withdrawn before an adequate scan can be completed. Use of ^{99m}Tc is not affected by thyroid-suppressing medications, avoiding any risk to patients from the temporary discontinuation of their medications.

Imaging of the thyroid after the administration of one of these agents allows visualization of active and inactive areas of the thyroid as well as an indication of the level of activity in that area of the thyroid gland. In patients with Graves' disease, there will be diffuse hyperactivity with large amounts of uptake. In contrast, nodules demonstrate very limited areas of uptake with surrounding hypoactivity. In thyroiditis, there is patchy uptake with overall diminution of activity reflecting the release of existing hormone rather than overproduction of new thyroxine.

The single diagnostic test that differentiates Graves' disease from other causes of hyperthyroidism is the detection of thyroid-receptor antibodies, which are specific for Graves' disease.

Treatment

Radioactive iodine is the treatment of choice for Graves' disease in adult patients who are not pregnant. Radioactive iodine should not be used in children or breast-feeding mothers. There is also concern that the administration of radioactive iodine in patients with active ophthalmopathy may accelerate progression of eye disease. For this reason, some experts initially treat Graves' disease with oral suppressive therapy until the ophthalmological disease has stabilized.

Antithyroid drugs are well tolerated and successful at blocking the production and release of thyroid hormone in patients with Graves' disease. These drugs work by blocking the organification of iodine. Propylthiouracil (PTU) also prevents peripheral conversion of T_4 to the more active T_3. PTU must be given in divided doses (two or three times a day), whereas methimazole and carbimazole can be administered once a day. The most serious side effect of these drugs is agranulocytosis, which occurs in 3 per 10,000 patients per year. All of these drugs are relatively safe in pregnancy, but associations of carbimazole with aplasia cutis and the decreased release of PTU in breast milk make PTU the favored treatment in pregnant or potentially pregnant women. Antithyroid drugs are especially useful in adolescents where Graves' disease may go into spontaneous remission after 6–18 month of therapy.

Surgery is reserved for patients in whom medication and radioactive iodine ablation are not acceptable treatment strategies or in whom a large goiter is present that compresses nearby structures or is disfiguring. Surgical results for Graves' disease after 1 year show that approximately 80% of patients will be euthyroid, 20% may be hypothyroid, and 1% remain hyperthyroid. Recurrence of hyperthyroidism occurs at a rate of 1–3% per year. Complications of surgery include damage to the superior laryngeal nerve (1–2% of cases) and possible hypocalcemia from inadvertent removal of parathyroid tissue.

For patients with thyroid storm, aggressive initial therapy is essential to prevent complications. Treatment should include the administration of high doses of PTU (100 mg every 6 h) to quickly block thyroid release and reduce peripheral conversion of T_4 to T_3. In addition, high doses of β-blockers (propranalol 1–5 mg intravenously or 20–80 mg orally every 4 h) can be used to control tachycardia and other peripheral symptoms of thyrotoxicosis. Hydrocortisone (200–300 mg/day) also is used to prevent possible adrenal crisis.

THYROID NODULES & THYROID CANCER

Symptoms & Signs

Most thyroid nodules are asymptomatic and are found on routine health examinations. In rare cases, the nodule may be very large and may compress nearby structures. Most benign nodules grow slowly. Small nodules (under 4 cm in size) are rarely malignant. Most thyroid nodules are not associated with hyper- or hypothyroidism. However, autonomously functioning adenomas can cause hyperthyroidism. In this condition, the thyroid-producing adenoma does not reduce thyroid hormone production in response to low levels of TSH and may continue to secrete thyroid hormones despite excessively high levels.

Pathogenesis

The most common type of nodule is a simple colloid cyst (about 40%). Other types of nodules include adenomas, carcinomas (see below), metastatic disease from breast, kidney, or prostate tumors, lymphomas, or a benign neoplasm such as a neurofibroma, hamartoma, or teratoma.

Thyroid cancer is less common in women than in men and is more common in patients with familial colonic polyposis and hamartomas (Cowden's syndrome). Previous breast, renal, or central nervous system cancer also increases the risk for a primary thyroid cancer.

Two types of primary thyroid cancer exist: medullary cancer (10% of all cancers) and adenocarcinomas. Adenocarinoma is the most common type of thyroid cancer and can be subcategorized into four different groups: papillary (60% of all cancers), follicular (25%), medullar, Hurthle cell, and anaplastic carcinomas (<5%).

Although papillary carcinoma is the most common adenocarcinoma, it also is the least aggressive form of thyroid cancer. Follicular cancers with some papillary components also behave like papillary carcinomas. These tumors tend to remain in the thyroid gland and, if they do spread, metastasize only to local lymph nodes. Follicular cancer, on the other hand, metastasizes to lung and bone. These two kinds of cancer combined have a 97% cure rate when treated with surgery, radioactive iodine, and thyroid suppression. In contrast, anaplastic thyroid tumors have a very bad prognosis. These are very aggressive tumors that rapidly invade adjacent tissue. Surgery, chemotherapy, and iodine radiation are usually ineffective at preventing metastases. Patients rarely survive more than 6 months after diagnosis.

Medullary carcinoma is more aggressive and is often part of the multiple endocrine neoplasia (MEN) syndrome. Surgical resection may initially control symptoms, but is not curative. Other chemotherapeutic agents can help slow the spread of disease.

A final category of thyroid cancer is non-Hodgkin's lymphoma (NHL) of the thyroid. There is a relationship between chronic lymphocytic (Hashimoto's) thyroiditis and NHL, so as the prevalence of chronic lymphocytic thyroid disease increases, NHL should increase as well. This type of tumor should be suspected when patients with chronic lymphocytic thyroiditis develop superimposed thyroid nodules. Surgery is the primary therapeutic option with supplemental radiation and chemotherapy.

On examination, most benign nodules are soft and cystic and may be tender. Nodules over 4 cm should also be suspected of being malignant. Cervical lymph nodes should not be enlarged. Nodules suggestive of thyroid cancer are often hard and fixed and may involve adjacent cervical tissue. Paralysis of the vocal cords and/or cervical lymphadenopathy are other concerning signs.

Laboratory & Imaging Evaluation

Radionucleotide imaging is usually the first step in evaluating the thyroid nodule or suspected thyroid mass. Adenomas will take up the radiotracer, producing a so-called "hot nodule" because it will be more active than surrounding thyroid tissue. When a nodule demonstrates thyroid hormone-producing activity on scan, the next step is to determine whether the nodule is under the influence of TSH. To accomplish this, exogenous L-thyroxine can be administered and the scan repeated several weeks later to determine if the nodule is suppressed. Nodules that suppress their secreting function in response to exogenous thyroid administration are under the control of TSH whereas those that do not are autonomous and likely to result in hyperthyroid symptoms.

Colloid cysts and tumors do not take up the radiotracer and are "cold" in contrast to the surrounding active thyroid. Consequently, the finding of thyroid activity on a thyroid scan is a good indication that it is benign.

If a cold nodule has been identified, further evaluation is necessary to distinguish a colloidal cyst from a potential tumor. The initial test for distinguishing a colloidal cyst from a solid or semisolid tumor is thyroid ultrasound. Ultrasound can differentiate a cystic structure (colloidal cyst) from solid or solid-cystic structures that are more typical of cancer. Definitive diagnosis can be made with fine needle aspiration.

When the thyroid mass is not well-defined, further imaging can be accomplished with magnetic resonance imaging (MRI). MRI is superior to computed tomography (CT) scanning in evaluating neck masses.

Treatment

As noted above for functional nodules, an attempt at suppression with exogenous thyroid is indicated to determine if the nodule is under the control of TSH. Functioning adenomas that respond to TSH will be suppressed after administration of exogenous thyroid. These types of nodules can be controlled with small doses of thyroid hormones. Autonomous nodules are not suppressed and may cause symptoms of hyperthyroid. These nodules may need to be treated with antithyroid medications or radioactive iodine. For large nodules, surgical excision may be considered.

Cystic adenomas require no therapy unless they become large and unsightly. In these cases, subtotal thyroidectomy can be performed to remove the area that contains the cyst.

The management of thyroid cancers should be accomplished in collaboration with surgical and medical oncologists familiar with the management of these tumors.

■ ADRENAL DISORDERS

ADRENAL INSUFFICIENCY

Symptoms & Signs

Adrenal insufficiency presents with a wide range of symptoms and signs, including weakness, malaise, anorexia, hyperpigmentation (especially of the gingival mucosa, scars, and skin creases), vitiligo, postural hypotension, abdominal pain, nausea and vomiting, diarrhea, constipation, myalgia, and arthralgia. The most specific sign of primary adrenal insufficiency is hyperpigmentation of the skin and mucosal surfaces. Another specific symptom of adrenal insufficiency is a craving for salt. Autoimmune adrenal disease can be accompanied by other autoimmune endocrine deficiencies, such as thyroid disease, diabetes mellitus, pernicious anemia, hypoparathyroidism, and ovarian failure (Table 35–4).

Pathogenesis

Although adrenal insufficiency was once most closely associated with tuberculosis, the most common cause of primary adrenal insufficiency is now autoimmune adrenalitis (Addison's disease). In addition, the acquired immune difficiency syndrome (AIDS) and the antiphospholipid syndrome are other causes to consider for adrenal insufficiency.

Secondary adrenal insufficiency may result from pituitary or hypothalamic disease as discussed earlier. Iatrogenic tertiary adrenal insufficiency caused by suppression of hypothalamic–pituitary–adrenal function secondary to glucocorticoid administration is a more common secondary cause of adrenal insufficiency.

In acute adrenal failure, adrenal crisis occurs. Adrenal crisis is characterized by hypotension, bradycardia, fever, hypoglycemia, and a progressive deterioration in mental status. Abdominal pain, vomiting, and

Table 35–4. Causes of adrenal insufficiency.

Primary
Autoimmune adrenalitis
Tuberculosis
Adrenomyeloneuropathy
Systemic fungal infections
AIDS
Metastatic carcinoma
Isolated glucocorticoid deficiency
Adrenal hemorrhage, necrosis, or thrombosis
Secondary
Pituitary or metastatic tumor
Craniopharyngioma
Pituitary surgery or radiation
Lymphocytic hypophysitis
Sarcoidosis
Histiocytosis
Empty-sella syndrome
Hypothalamic tumors
Long-term glucocorticoid therapy
Postpartum pituitary necrosis (Sheehan's syndrome)
Necrosis or bleeding into pituitary macroadenoma
Head trauma, lesions of the pituitary stalk
Pituitary or adrenal surgery for Cushing's syndrome

After Oelkers W: Adrenal insufficiency. New Engl J Med 1996;335: 1206.

diarrhea also may be present. In the patient with spontaneous adrenal insufficiency, acute adrenal hemorrhage and adrenal-vein thrombosis should be considered.

Laboratory & Imaging Evaluation

Laboratory abnormalities occur in nearly all patients. These abnormalities include hyponatremia, hyperkalemia, acidosis, slightly elevated plasma creatinine concentrations, hypoglycemia, hypercalcemia, mild normocytic anemia, lymphocytosis, and mild eosinophilia.

The diagnosis of adrenal insufficiency relies on a finding of inadequate cortisol production. Plasma cortisol concentration fluctuates throughout the day in a diurnal pattern that is normally high in the early morning and low in the late afternoon. Coritsol levels also increase with stress. A low plasma cortisol level of <3 µg/dL (83 nmol/L) either in the morning or at a time of stress provides presumptive evidence of adrenal insufficiency. Conversely, a level of 550 nmol/L (20 g/dL) or greater rules out adrenal insufficiency. An intermediate plasma cortisol level between 3 and 19 µg/dL (83–525 nmol/L) is not diagnostic.

For most patients in whom adrenal insufficiency is considered, a short ACTH stimulation test should be performed. In this test, a low-dose ACTH (1 g or

0.5 g/1.73 m² surface area) is given and the patient's blood is tested 30 and 60 min later to confirm a corresponding increase in plasma cortisol. A rise in plasma cortisol concentration after 30 or 60 min to a peak of 55 nmol/L (20 g/dL) or more is considered normal. No increase in serum cortisol or a blunted response after ACTH administration confirms adrenal insufficiency. If the test is slightly abnormal, an insulin or a metyrapone test using 30 mg/kg of metyrapone with a snack at midnight should be performed.

For the evaluation of suspected secondary adrenal insufficiency, three other tests are recommended. An insulin stress test causes hypoglycemia that normally results in the release of ACTH. In this test, a blood sugar level less than 40 mg/dL is induced by the intravenous injection of regular insulin in doses of 0.1–0.15 μg/kg, stimulating the entire hypothalamic–pituitary–adrenal axis; plasma cortisol concentrations should increase to at least 20 μg/dL. A second test, the short metyrapone test, measures the plasma levels of 11-deoxycortisol (a cortisol precursor) and cortisol at 8 AM after the oral administration of metyrapone (an adrenal 11-hydroxylase inhibitor) at midnight. Normally, the plasma level of 11-deoxycortisol increases. A final test is a corticotropin-releasing hormone (CRH) challenge test. CRH stimulates the production of ACTH so that normally plasma cortisol level rises and usually peaks 30–45 min after the injection of CRH. However, CRH stimulates cortisol secretion less strongly that does insulin-induced hypoglycemia or metyrapone, making it a less sensitive test for secondary adrenal insufficiency.

In patients with adrenal insufficiency, radiological procedures may be indicated. In patients having headaches and visual disturbances, an MRI should be performed to investigate for a possible pituitary or hypothalamic tumor. In patients with suspected primary adrenal insufficiency, a CT scan of the adrenal glands should be performed to rule out hemorrhage, adrenal vein thrombosis, or metastatic disease as the cause for the adrenal dysfunction.

Treatment

For patients with symptomatic adrenal insufficiency, hydrocortisone or cortisone should be given in divided doses early in the morning and afternoon to simulate the dirunal release of cortisol by the adrenal gland (Table 35–5). The smallest dose that relieves the patient's symptoms should be used so that weight gain and risk of osteoporosis are minimized. During febrile illnesses, acute injury, or other periods of physiological stress, the dose of hydrocortisone should be doubled or tripled temporarily. Patients with primary adrenal insufficiency should also receive fludrocortisone as a substitute for aldosterone.

Table 35–5. Initial doses of medications used in treating adrenal insufficiency.

Replacement	
Hydrocortisone	Adults: 25 mg (divided into doses of 15 and 10 mg)
	Children: 25 mg/m²/day in three divided doses
Cortisone	Adults: 37.5 mg (divided into doses of 25 and 12.5 mg)
	Children: 32 mg/m²/day divided three times daily
Fludrocortisone (substitute for aldosterone)	Adults: 50–200 μg (single daily dose)
	Children: 50–150 μg (single daily dose)
Emergency therapy	
Hydrocortisone	Adults: 100 mg bolus dose followed by infusion of 100–200 mg/24 h
	Children: 25–50 mg/m²/24 h

Adapted from Oelkers W: Adrenal insufficiency. New Engl J Med 1996;335:1206.

Patients with acute adrenal insufficiency need immediate treatment with high-dose intravenous hydrocortisone. During this initial phase of treatment, other supportive care may need to be implemented (ie, isotonic saline for hypovolemia and hyponatremia).

Davenport J et al: Addison's disease. Am Fam Phys 1991;43;1338.

Oelkers W: Adrenal insufficiency. New Engl J Med 1996;335;1206.

CUSHING'S SYNDROME

Symptoms & Signs

Cushing's syndrome refers to overproduction of cortisol due to any cause, ie, adrenal hyperplasia, exogenous steroid use, etc. Cushing's disease is a more specific term that refers to excessive cortisol resulting from excessive ACTH produced by pituitary corticotroph tumors. The most common signs of Cushing's syndrome are the relative sudden onset of central weight gain, often accompanied by thickening of the facial fat, which rounds the facial contour ("moon facies"), and a florid complexion due to telangiectasia. Other concomitant signs that can accompany Cushing's syndrome include an enlarged fat pad, or "buffalo hump," hypertension, glucose intolerance, oligomenorrhea or amenorrhea in premenopausal women, decreased libido in men, and spontaneous ecchymoses (Table 35–6).

Overall, Cushing's syndrome is rare with a prevalence estimated at about 10 per 1 million persons. Cushing's disease is four- to six-fold more prevalent in

Table 35–6. Clinical symptoms and signs of Cushing's syndrome.

General:
  Central obesity
  Proximal muscle weakness
  Hypertension
  Headaches
  Psychiatric disorders

Skin
  Wide (>1 cm), purple striae
  Spontaneous ecchymoses
  Facial plethora
  Hyperpigmentation
  Acne
  Hirsutism
  Fungal skin infections

Endocrine and metabolic derangements
  Hypokalemic alkalosis
  Osteopenia
  Delayed bone age in children
  Menstrual disorders, decreased libido, impotence
  Glucose intolerence, diabetes mellitus
  Kidney stones
  Polyuria

Elevated white blood cell count

After Meier CA, Biller BM: Clinical and biochemical evaluation of Cushing's syndrome. Endocrinol Metab Clin North Am. 1997;26: 741.

women, whereas ectopic ACTH secretion is more common in men, largely due to the higher incidence in men of bronchogenic lung cancers that produce ACTH.

Pathogenesis

ACTH-producing tumors account for 80% of cases with Cushing's disease accounting for 70–80% of these cases. Adrenal tumors, such as adenomas, carcinomas, and micronodular and macronodular hyperplasia, autonomously producing glucocorticoids are found in 20% of patients with Cushing's syndrome.

Laboratory & Imaging Evaluation

The evaluation of suspected excessive glucocorticoid production includes screening and confirmatory tests for the diagnosis and the localization of the source of hormone excess.

Tests that can be used to confirm excessive glucocorticoid production include a 24-h urinary free cortisol test, an overnight dexamethasone suppression test, and a midnight cortisol level determination. The 1-mg overnight dexamethasone suppression test (DST) has

been considered the screening test of choice, but problems associated with its low specificity have led to the urinary free cortisol (UFC) excretion rate as the preferred test for many patients.

The determination of the 24-h UFC is based on the measurement of the cumulative excretion of unbound plasma cortisol. It is the most sensitive (95–100%) and specific (98%) screening test for Cushing's syndrome if the collection is adequate as documented by creatinine excretion. Most studies report a sensitivity of greater than 98%, particularly when multiple 24-h urine collections are performed. UFC values of greater than 250–300 µg/24 h (700–840 nmol/24 h) determined on several occasions are considered virtually diagnostic. The rate of UFC excretion can be determined by radioimmunoassay, competitive protein binding after solvent extraction, or high-performance liquid chromatography (HPLC).

Affective psychiatric disorders (ie, major depression) and alcoholism can be associated with the biochemical features of Cushing's syndrome and, therefore, may decrease the reliability of test results.

Another laboratory finding that suggests Cushing's syndrome is a flattening of the circadian secretion pattern or a high afternoon plasma cortisol level. However, the lack of validated reference ranges available for individual interpretation makes these tests unsuitable for confirming the diagnosis.

Following confirmation of Cushing's syndrome, further imaging studies that are appropriate include a pituitary MRI to look for adenomas followed by an adrenal CT for adrenal tumors. If both of these studies are negative, chest x-ray or CT scanning should be performed to look for ectopic sources of ACTH production.

Treatment

For patients with a pituitary adenoma (Cushing's disease), the treatment of choice is transsphenoidal microadenomectomy assuming that a circumscribed microadenoma can be identified and resected. If an adenoma cannot be clearly identified, patients should undergo a subtotal (85–90%) resection of the anterior pituitary. If patients wish to preserve pituitary function so that they can have children, they should be treated with pituitary irradiation. If radiation does not decrease exogenous ACTH production, bilateral total adrenalectomy is a final treatment option. For adult patients not cured by transsphenoidal surgery, pituitary irradiation is the most appropriate choice for the next treatment.

Patients who have a nonpituitary tumor that secretes ACTH are cured by resection of the tumor. Unfortunately, most nonpituitary tumors that secrete ACTH are not amenable to resection. In these cases, cortisol excess can be controlled with adrenal enzyme inhibitors, alone or in combination, with the proper dose determined by measuring plasma and urinary cortisol.

For patients with adrenal hyperplasia, bilateral total adrenalectomy is required. Patients with an adrenal adenoma or carcinoma can be managed with unilateral adrenalectomy. Patients with hyperplasia or adenomas almost invariably have recurrences that are not amenable to either radiation or chemotherapy.

Kvols LK, Buck M: Chemotherapy of endocrine malignancies: a review. Semin Oncol 1987;14:343.

Meier CA, Biller BM: Clinical and biochemical evaluation of Cushing's syndrome. Endocrinol Metab Clin North Am 1997;26:741.

Orth DN: Cushing's syndrome. New Engl J Med 1995;332;791.

Tsigos C, Chrousos GP: Differential diagnosis and management of Cushing's syndrome. Annu Rev Med 1996;47:443.

STEROID DEPENDENCE

Pathogenesis

Systemic corticosteroid therapy is indicated for many disease states. After several weeks of therapy with corticosteroids, the hypothalamic–pituitary–adrenal axis may become depressed. In this situation, the corticosteroid dose must be reduced gradually to limit the adverse effects of corticosteroid therapy withdrawal (Table 35–7).

Several factors should be considered when determining whether a "tapering" regimen should be implemented: the length and amount of steroid and whether a single or divided doses were given. Currently, the general consensus is that if high doses are given for more than 7–10 days, symptomatic adrenal suppression may occur.

Treatment

Initially, the dose of corticosteroid should be gradually reduced until the patient can safely tolerate a dosage equivalent of 20 mg of hydrocortisone/day. During this taper, the patient may experience some mild withdrawal symptoms, including fatigue, anorexia, nausea, and orthostatic lightheadedness. If the patient experiences acute stress during this period (ie, minor surgery, infection), the steroid dose should be increased to 100–500 mg of hydrocortisone in divided doses, depending upon the situation. Once the stress has resolved, the corticosteroid dosage should again be tapered to a dosage equivalent of 20 mg of hydrocortisone per day. This dosage should be continued for at least 4 weeks.

Continuing decreases in steroids can be performed as shown in Table 35–7.

HYPERALDOSTERONISM

Symptoms & Signs

Patients with hyperaldosteronism present with hypertension and hypokalemia. Other complaints include headaches, muscular weakness or flaccid paralysis caused by hypokalemia, or polyuria. Inappropriate hypersecretion of aldosterone is an uncommon cause of hypertension, accounting for fewer than 1% of cases. Any patient presenting with hypertension and unprovoked hypokalemia should be considered for the evaluation of

Table 35–7. Suggested protocol for glucocorticoid withdrawal.

Step	Interval	Observation	Result	Glucocorticoid and Dose
I	Variable	Underlying disease	Worsening underlying disease; symptoms and signs of steroid withdrawal	Gradual decrements in dose to equivalent of hydrocortisone, 20 mg/day
II	4 weeks	8 AM plasma cortisol	Plasma cortisol When < 10 μg/dL	Taper hydrocortisone by 2.5 mg/day once per week to 10 mg every morning
			When > 10 μg/dL	Stop hydrocortisone; supplement for stress
III	4 weeks to indefinite	8 AM cosyntropin challenge (250 μg/dL intramuscularly)	Plasma cortisol increment < 6 μg/dL or max. < 20 μg/dL (or both)	Supplement for stress
IV	4 weeks to indefinite	8 AM cosyntropin challenge (250 μg/dL intramuscularly)	Plasma cortisol increment > 6 μg/dL and max. >20 μg/dL	Stop supplementation for stress

From Byyny RL: Withdrawal from glucocorticoid therapy. New Engl J Med 1976;295:30.

hyperaldosteronism. Hypertension may be severe, although malignant hypertension is rare. The peak incidence occurs between 30 and 50 years of age, and most patients are women.

Pathogenesis

Primary hyperaldosteronism accounts for 70–80% of all cases of hyperaldosteronism and is usually caused by a solitary unilateral adrenal adenoma. Other causes of hyperaldosteronism include bilateral adrenal hyperplasia, so-called idiopathic hyperaldosteronism, and glucocorticoid-remediable hyperaldosteronism. Adrenal carcinoma and unilateral adrenal hyperplasia are rare causes.

Laboratory & Imaging Evaluation

Initially, laboratory evaluation is used to document hyperaldosteronemia and suppressed renin activity. Further diagnostic tests, including imaging procedures, are used to determine whether the etiology is amenable to surgical intervention or requires medical management.

Screening aldosterone measurements can be made on plasma or 24-h urine collection. Plasma aldosterone is usually measured after 4 h of upright posture. Plasma renin activity should be measured in the same sample. A ratio of plasma aldosterone concentration to plasma renin activity greater than 20 to 25 is very suspicious for hyperaldosteronism.

In the hypertensive patient with hypokalemia and/or kaliuresis or with an elevated plasma aldosterone–renin ratio, the diagnosis of hyperaldosteronism is confirmed by demonstrating failure of normal suppression of plasma aldosterone. Urine aldosterone excretion of more than 30 nmol (14 µg)/day after oral sodium loading over 3 days establishes the diagnosis.

The intravenous saline suppression test is also widely used to confirm hyperaldosteronism. In this test, isotonic saline is infused intravenously at a rate of 300–500 mL/h for 4 h, after which plasma aldosterone and renin activity are measured. Aldosterone levels normally fall to less than 0.28 nmol/L (10 ng/dL) and renin activity is suppressed. Failure to suppress normally identifies patients with aldosterone-producing adenomas, as most patients with secondary forms of hyperaldosteronism suppress normally. False-negative results are most often seen in patients with bilateral hyperplasia.

Once the diagnosis is established, it is necessary to distinguish between aldosterone-producing adrenal adenoma and bilateral adrenal hyperplasia. A widely used test is based on the less complete suppression of renin activity in hyperaldosteronism caused by bilateral hyperplasia. Plasma renin activity rises slightly and aldosterone concentration increases significantly after the stimulation of 2–4 h of upright posturing in these patients. In contrast, renin remains suppressed and aldosterone does not rise in patients with adenomas, in whom plasma aldosterone level may fall.

Imaging procedures can assist in differentiating causes of hyperaldosteronism and lateralizing adenomas. The diagnostic accuracy of high-resolution CT scans is only about 70% for aldosterone-producing adenomas, largely because of the occurrence of nonfunctioning adenomas. MRI is no better than CT in differentiating aldosterone-secreting tumors from other adrenal tumors. Scintigraphic imaging with ^{131}I-labeled cholesterol derivatives during dexamethasone suppression provides an image based on functional properties of the adrenal. Asymmetric uptake after 48 h indicates an adenoma, whereas symmetric uptake after 72 h indicates bilateral hyperplasia. Diagnostic accuracy is 72%. However, if the adrenal CT is normal, iodocholesterol scanning is unlikely to be helpful.

Treatment

For adrenal adenoma, total unilateral adrenalectomy is the treatment of choice and provides a cure in most cases. Although some patients with primary bilateral hyperplasia may benefit from subtotal adrenalectomy, these patients cannot be accurately identified preoperatively. Following surgery, the electrolyte imbalances usually correct rapidly, whereas blood pressure control may take several weeks to month.

Medical therapy is indicated for most patients with bilateral adrenal hyperplasia or for those patients with adrenal adenomas who are unable to undergo adrenalectomy. Spironolactone controls the hyperkalemia, although it is not a very potent antihypertensive agent. Amiloride and calcium channel blockers are often used to control blood pressure.

Bravo EL: Primary aldosteronism: issues in diagnosis and management. Endocrinol Metab Clin North Am 1994;23:271.

■ PARATHYROID DISORDERS

HYPERPARATHYROIDISM

Symptoms & Signs

Hyperparathyroidism refers to excessive production of parathyroid hormone (PTH). Primary parahyperparathyroidism refers to the overproduction of PTH in an inappropriate fashion resulting usually in hypercalcemia. Primary hyperparathyroidism is more common in postmenopausal women. Most patients have nonspecific complaints that may include aches and pains, constipation, muscle fatigue, generalized weakness, psychiatric disturbances, and polydipsia and polyuria. The hypercalcemia can cause nausea and vomiting, thirst, and anorexia. A history of peptic ulcer disease or hypertension is not uncommon, and there may be accompanying constipation, anemia, and weight loss. Precipitation of calcium in the corneas may produce a band keratopathy and patients may also experience recurrent pancreatitis. Finally, skeletal problems can result in pathological fractures.

Secondary hyperparathyroidism, on the other hand, refers to appropriate additional production of PTH because of hypocalcemia related to other metabolic conditions such as renal failure, calcium absorption problems, or vitamin D deficiency.

Pathogenesis

The most common cause of primary hyperparathyroidism is a benign solitary parathyroid adenoma. Adenomas account for approximately 80% of all cases. Another 15% of patients have diffuse hyperplasia of the parathyroids, a condition that tends to be familial. Carcinoma of the parathyroid occurs in less than 1% of cases.

Laboratory & Imaging Evaluation

Hypercalcemia (serum calcium >10.5 mg/dL when corrected for serum albumin levels) is the most important clue to the diagnosis. In the situation of an elevated calcium with no apparent cause, serum PTH should be determined using a two-site immunometric assay. An elevated PTH level in the presence of hypercalcemia confirms the diagnosis of primary hyperparathyroidism.

Other findings may include a low serum phosphate (<2.5 mg/dL) with excessive phosphaturia. Urine calcium excretion may be high or normal. Alkaline phosphatase levels are elevated only in the presence of bone disease, and elevated plasma chloride and uric acid levels may be seen.

With chronic hyperparathyroidism, there may be diffuse bone demineralization, loss of the dental lamina dura, and subperiosteal resorption of bone (particularly in the radial aspects of the fingers) apparent on x-rays. Cysts may be noted throughout the skeleton, and "salt and pepper" appearance of the skull may be seen. Pathological fractures can occur, and renal calculi and soft tissue calcification may be visualized.

Imaging studies are usually reserved for patients with resistant or recurrent disease. In these cases, ultrasonography, CT scanning, MRI, and thallium-201–

technetium-99m scanning may be useful at locating ectopic parathyroid tissue.

Treatment

Treatment of severe hypercalcemia and parathyroidectomy are the mainstays for therapy. When hypercalcemia is severe, treatment includes aggressive hydration and correction of any underlying hyponatremia and hypokalemia should be initiated along with administration of a loop diuretic to accelerate calcium clearance. Other medications that can be effective in reducing hypercalcemia include etidronate, plicamycin, and calcitonin. Any medications or other products that increase calcuim levels, such as estrogens, thiazides, vitamins A and D, and milk, should be avoided

In addition to management of acute hypercalcemia, surgical removal of parathyroid tissue should be undertaken. Surgical resection provides the most rapid and effective method of reducing serum calcium in these patients. Hyperplasia of all glands requires removal of three glands along with subtotal resection of the fourth. Surgical success is directly related to the experience and expertise of the operating surgeon.

For mild cases and poor surgical candidates, conservative therapy with adequate hydration and long-term pharmacological therapy is recommended. Individuals should avoid drugs and products that elevate calcium and have their serum calcium monitored closely.

HYPOPARATHYROIDISM
Symptoms & Signs

Hypoparathyroidism results from an underproduction of PTH. The lack of PTH results in hypocalcemia, which produces most of the symptoms associated with hypoparathyroidism. Symptoms associated with hypocalcemia include tetany, carpopedal spasms, paresthesias of the lips and hands, and a positive Chvostek's sign or Trousseau's sign. Patients may also exhibit less specific symptoms such as anxiety, depression, or fatigue. Additionally, hyperventilation, respiratory alkalosis with or without respiratory compromise, laryngospasm, hypotension, and seizures may occur with severe hypocalcemia.

Pathogenesis

The most common cause of hypoparathyroidism is the removal of the parathyroid glands during a thyroidectomy or following surgery for primary hyperparathyroidism. Less commonly, hypoparathyroidism is idiopathic, familial, or the result of a congenital absence of the parathyroids (DiGeorge's syndrome). Patients with idiopathic hypoparathyroidism often have antibodies against parathyroid and other tissues, and an autoimmune component may play a role. Other unusual causes of hypoparathyroidism include previous neck irradiation, magnesium deficiency, metastatic cancer, and infiltrative diseases.

Laboratory & Imaging Evaluation

On laboratory evaluation, patients with hypoparathyroidism have a low serum calcium and elevated serum phosphate with a normal alkaline phosphatase. Urinary levels of calcium and phosphate are decreased. The key finding is a low to absent PTH.

Treatment

Acute hypocalcemia with tetany requires aggressive therapy with multiple drugs. Therapy should be started with calcium gluconate administered in a 10% solution intravenously given slowly until tetany resolves. Oral calcium along with vitamin D should be given after the acute crisis is resolved. Hypomagnesemia also needs to be corrected with intravenous magnesium sulfate administered at a dose of 1–2 g every 6 h. Chronic replacement of magnesium can be accomplished using 600 mg magnesium oxide tablets once or twice daily.

For the maintenance of normal calcium, vitamin D supplementation along with oral calcium should be given. Calcium in the form of calcium carbonate (40% elemental calcium) is the drug of choice administered in a dose of 1–2 g of calcium a day. Serial calcium levels should be obtained regularly (every 3–6 months), and "spot" urine calcium levels should be maintained below 30 mg/dL.

Sherman RG, Lasseter DH: Pharmacologic management of patients with diseases of the endocrine system. Dent Clin North Am 1996;40:727.

■ ANTERIOR PITUITARY DISORDERS

PANHYPOPITUITARISM

Symptoms & Signs

Panhypopituitarism is a rare condition. In most cases (95% of cases), pituitary deficiency is seen later in life as a consequence of pituitary gland destruction from an enlarging macroadenoma or pituitary damage from subsequent treatment of the adenoma with surgery or radiation. Microadenomas, on the other hand, rarely cause significant pituitary injury, but can result in overproduction of selected anterior pituitary hormones, es-

pecially prolactin. In addition to congenital hypopituitarism and hypopituitarism secondary to adenoma, individuals may also develop pituitary insufficiency from ischemia seen in such instances as shock and birth asphyxia. Rarer causes of pituitary deficiency are infiltrative diseases such as hemochromotosis, histiocytosis, and granulomatous diseases.

Pathogenesis

As noted above, acquired hypopituitary problems usually arise secondary to pituitary resection. However, congenital dysfunction or absence of the pituitary also occurs. Congenital hypopituitarism should be suspected when neonates have unrelenting jaundice and/or unexplained hypoglycemia. Hypoglycemia develops because of poor glycogen stores, increased utilization of glucose due to the lack of antagonistic hormones (ie, corticosteroids and growth hormone), and decreased gluconeogenesis when hypoglycemia does occur. Often, frequent bottle feedings in the nursery setting may mask the hypoglycemia. With the normal metabolic response to hypoglycemia blunted, as feeding frequency decreases or in early nursing before maternal milk supply is adequate, neonates can develop prolonged and severe hypoglycemia. Because gonadotropins are necessary for appropriate development of male genitalia, another finding in males with congenital absence of the pituitary is micropenis.

Adults with acquired hypopituitarism are more likely than children to present with more classic signs of multiple hormone deficiency (Table 35–8). Of the hormones produced or regulated by the pituitary, adrenal insufficiency is the deficiency most likely to be overlooked since mineralocorticoid production is not altered with pituitary dysfunction. The key to the diagnosis of pituitary insufficiency is that patients present with many different symptoms that suggest multiple hormone deficiencies. In this situation, the absence of one anterior pituitary hormone should prompt evaluation of other hormones to determine if multiple defects are present.

Laboratory & Imaging Evaluation

Evaluation of the patients with suspected pituitary abnormalities is fairly straightforward. In adults, measurement of anterior pituitary hormones will reveal low or nondetectable levels of ACTH, TSH, follicle-stimulating hormone (FSH), luteinizing hormone (LH), and prolactin. Most children with pituitary failure will be identified by low T_4 levels on neonatal screens. However, the diagnosis often is made because of prolonged jaundice or recurrent hypoglycemia before neonatal screening tests are completed. Testing for cortisol and TSH can be performed in the neonatal period and will

Table 35–8. Symptoms of pituitary insufficiency.

Hormone Deficiency	Symptoms
ACTH (corticotropin)	Acute deficiency: fatigue, weakness, nausea, vomiting, hypotension
	Chronic deficiency: fatigue, pallor, weight loss, hypoglycemia
	Children: growth retardation
	Laboratory findings: hyponatremia, hypoglycemia
Thyroid-stimulating hormone (TSH)	Adults: weight gain, fatigue, depression/mental status changes, dry skin, hair loss
	Children: growth retardation, delayed intellectual development (mental retardation if untreated)
	Laboratory findings: hyponatremia
Gonadotropin deficiency (FSH/LH)	Children: micropenis, delayed puberty
	Women: amenorrhea, infertility/anovulation, loss of libido, osteoporosis, premature atherosclerosis
	Men: loss of libido, impaired sexual functioning, decreased muscle mass and hair growth
Growth hormone	Children: growth retardation, hypoglycemia
	Adults: decreased muscle mass and strength, central obesity, fatigue, premature atherosclerosis
Prolactin	None
Melanocyte-stimulating hormone	None

After Lamberts SWJ, De Herder WW, van der Lely AJ: Pituitary insufficiency. Lancet 1998;352:127.

demonstrate low to undetectable levels. Further testing is not indicated at that time since the replacement of hormones other than corticosteroids and thyroid is not necessary until later in life.

In some situations, provocative testing is used to differentiate pituitary insufficiency from primary endocrine organ failure such as Addison's disease. To differentiate primary adrenal insufficiency (Addison's disease) from secondary adrenal insufficiency (pituitary insufficiency), an ACTH stimulation test can be performed. In this test, serum cortisol is measured before and 30–60 min after intravenous infusion of 250 μg of synthetic ACTH. With primary adrenal insufficiency, no increase in cortisol is found; in secondary adrenal insufficiency, a rise in cortisol to over 550 nmol/L occurs after ACTH administration.

Growth hormone levels will also be low, but are often low in healthy individuals. To confirm that the anterior pituitary does not make growth hormone appropriately, provocative testing may be necessary. In most situations, provocative testing is not necessary. Growth hormone is usually deficient when multiple (two or more) pituitary hormones are abnormal. Further evidence of growth hormone deficiency is the finding of low levels of circulating insulin-like growth factor I (IGF-I). If other pituitary hormones are low and IGF-I is low, then further testing for growth hormone deficiency is not worthwhile.

If provocative testing for growth hormone deficiency is necessary, the usual approach is insulin-hypoglycemia stimulation. For this test, insulin is administered intravenously and both glucose and growth hormone are measured. Individuals with normal growth hormone production respond to hypoglycemia with a rise in

growth hormone of 3–5 μg/L. If growth hormone does not rise with hypoglycemia, then a diagnosis of growth hormone deficiency is established.

Once pituitary insufficiency is diagnosed, unless the cause for this condition is evident, such as surgical excision or radiation, evaluation of the pituitary is warranted. Imaging of the anterior pituitary is important to evaluate for macroadenomas. The failure to remove these adenomas can result in visual disturbances as the enlarging adenoma compresses the optic chiasm.

Treatment

Medication therapy for pituitary insufficiency is summarized in Table 35–9.

Treatment of pituitary insufficiency focuses on replacing the hormones normally controlled by the anterior pituitary. The most crucial hormones that must be replaced are cortisol and thyroxine. Replacement of growth hormone is not critical and replacement is not necessary until the child experiences delays in growth.

In most individuals, cortisol is given three times a day with half the dose provided in the morning and the remaining half split in the afternoon and evening. This produces a more physiological response by producing a morning peak and lower, more steady levels throughout the remainder of the day. In young children, three times a day dosing may be impractical; a better schedule is twice a day dosing with the daily required dose split into equal doses given in the morning and the late afternoon. Under times of physiological stress, such as severe injury, surgery, or febrile illnesses, steroid doses must be adjusted. In these cases, the dose should be doubled or

Table 35–9. Hormone therapy in pituitary insufficiency.

Deficiency	Replacement Recommendations
ACTH (corticotropin)	**Adults** Cortisone acetate (25 mg AM/12.5 mg PM) *or* hydrocortisone (20 mg AM/10 mg PM) *or* prednisone (4–7.5 mg/day) *or* dextromethosone (0.25–0.5 mg/day) **Children** Cortisone acetate *or* hydrocortisone 0.5–0.75 mg/kg/day given in two or three divided doses **Crises** Hydrocortisone 100–150 mg/day in adults and 30–60 mg/m^2/day in children
Thyroid-stimulating hormone (TSH)	**Adults** Thyroxine (100–150 μg/day; start at 25–50 μg/day in patients with risk of ischemic heart disease and advance slowly over 6–8 weeks) adjusted by free T_3 or free T_4 **Children** Thyroxine 8–10 μg/kg/day adjusted by free T_3 or free T_4 assessed every 3 months
Gonadotropins	**Premenopausal women** *No fertility desired:* Cyclic estrogen/progesterone as in oral contraceptives *Fertility desired:* Cyclic human menopausal gonadotropin (hMG) with human chorionic gonadotropin (hCG) used to induce ovulation **Postmenopausal women** Estrogen (eg, conjugated estrogen 0.625 mg/day) with methoxyprogesterone 5 mg/day for women with an intact uterus **Men** Testosterone by injection (250 mg every 3 weeks) or implantable testosterone pellets (600–800 mg subcutaneously) every 4–5 months
Growth hormone	**Adults** Weekly maintenance dose of 0.04–0.08 mg/kg subcutaneously (start with lower weekly dose of 0.02 mg/kg and advance weekly) **Children** Daily administration of 0.1 IU/kg or 0.2–0.3 mg/kg/dose adjusted every 3 months for changes in weight
Prolactin	No replacement recommended
Melanocyte-stimulating hormone	No replacement recommended

tripled. Also, when individuals are vomiting or cannot take their cortisol orally for any other reason, families should have injectable steroids on hand for administration. Injectable hydrocortisone at a dose of 50–150 mg for children and 100–150 mg for adults should be given under these circumstances. Because vomiting can be a sign of hypocortisolism, any episode of repeated vomiting should be treated with a dose of parenteral steroids.

Thyroid may be given once a day with the adequacy of replacement assessed by following free thyroid levels. Following a TSH in this group is not effective as patients do not produce TSH. In older patients or those with risk factors for ischemic heart disease or dysrhythmias, replacement should start with a low dose (eg, 25 μg/day) and increase slowly over a couple of month to target levels. Free T_3 and/or T_4 can be used to assess adequate replacement in both adults and children.

For children, growth hormone will be necessary for the attainment of normal height. Without growth hormone, most children will make only minimal interval growth and quickly fall below the 10th percentile for their age. Growth hormone is administered in a single day by subcutaneous injection that is adjusted for weight. Because even recombinant growth hormone is extremely expensive, physicians often have to work closely with families and their insurance companies to ensure that children receive their medications appropriately. Growth hormone should be considered when growth curves fall below the 10th percentile for age. The dose of growth hormone is adjusted by weight and does not have to be changed during puberty. Replacement doses are stopped when children reach acceptable adult height. At that time, maintenance doses may be continued weekly. Although not all adults receive maintenance growth hormone, there is evidence that a small dose given weekly will reduce fatigue, improve body image, and prevent muscle wasting.

For gonadotropin deficiency replacement of estrogen and testosterone is usually necessary for continued sexual development and menstrual function. Replacement of gonadotropins is necessary only if fertility is desired. Because gonadotropins are expensive, testosterone or estrogen is administered instead at age 12–14 to initiate puberty. In girls and premenopausal women, estrogen therapy with a combination birth control pill that includes 20–35 µg of estrogen will usually stimulate puberty. In males, testosterone proprionate given intramuscularly at a dose of 200 mg every 2 weeks provides sufficient replacement. Alternatively, transdermal testosterone can be administered via a scrotal or nonscrotal patch system. These deliver 4–6 mg of testosterone each day and must be changed daily.

If fertility is desired in panhypopituitary women, gonadotropins can be administered as human menopausal gonadotropin (hMG) with human chorionic gonadotropin (hCG) used in a pulsatile fashion to stimulate ovulation. Pregnancy can usually be achieved in about 50% of women. If pituitary deficiency is secondary to hypothalamic dysfunction rather than pituitary abnormalities, gonadotropin-releasing hormone (GnRH) administered in pulsatile subcutaneous doses is also effective. For men who wish to become fertile, the dosing and frequency of hormone administration vary considerably. Prolactin and melanocyte-stimulating hormone are not replaced in individuals with pituitary insufficiency.

As with patients with adrenal insufficiency, patients with pituitary insufficiency should wear medical identification bracelets that alert emergency workers of their condition and that alert health care providers that the person is steroid dependent.

Choo-Kang, LR, Sun CJ, Counts DR: Cholestasis and hypoglycemia: manifestations of anterior hypopituitarism. J Clin Endocrinol Metab 1996;81:2786.

Cuneo RC: Current strategies for hormone replacement therapy for the hypopituitary patient. Med J Aust 1995;163:539.

Lamberts SWJ, De Herder WW, van der Lely AJ: Pituitary insufficiency. Lancet 1998;352:127.

Powrie J, Weissberger A, Sonksen P: Growth hormone replacement therapy for growth hormone-deficient adults. Drugs 1995; 49:656.

Yazigi RA, Quintero CH, Salameh WA: Prolactin disorders. Fertil Steril 1997;67:215.

PITUITARY ADENOMAS

The two most common adenomas that occur in the pituitary are prolactin-secreting and growth hormone-secreting tumors.

Symptoms & Signs

Prolactin adenomas are the most common type of tumor and are classified either as microadenomas (<1 cm) or macroadenomas (>1 cm). In general, macroadenomas produce more prolactin than smaller tumors although this is not universally true as up to 15% of macroadenomas may produce only very small amounts of prolactin. Symptoms that occur with prolactin adenomas include amenorrhea and galactorrhea in women and decreased libido and erectile dysfunction in men. With rapidly enlarging macroadenomas, visual field defects or headaches may be presenting symptoms. Clinical symptoms of prolactin deficiency in the presence of an elevated prolactin level without evidence of hypothyroidism or drugs that induce hyperprolactinemia should prompt further evaluation for an adenoma.

Growth hormone-producing adenomas account for about 15% of all clinically diagnosed pituitary adenomas. Excessive growth hormone in children causes giantism. In adults whose growth plates have closed, overproduction of growth hormones results in acromegaly. Symptoms and physical features of acromegaly include fatigue, large hands and feet, forehead bossing, parotid gland enlargement, decreased libido and erectile dysfunction, paresthesias and nerve entrapment syndromes, and arthralgias. Biochemical abnormalities include glucose intolerance. A later complication of untreated acromegaly is congestive heart failure.

Laboratory & Imaging Evaluation

In prolactin-secreting tumors, measurement of prolactin levels usually reveals elevated prolactin. Other causes of elevations in prolactin should also be explored, including a large number of medications such as antipsychotic agents, narcotics, estrogens/androgens, and cimetidine.

Growth hormone levels are more difficult to assess. Because growth hormone is released in a pulsatile fashion and responds to stress and hypoglycemia, growth hormone itself may not be reliable. Instead, measurement of serum IGF-I may be more sensitive and specific for the detection of excessive growth hormone production. Because release of IGF-I is dependent on growth hormone, levels of IGF-I correlate with growth hormone availability. High levels of IGF-I indicate excessive growth hormone.

Once excessive production of the hormone is established, MRI with attention to the sella turcica is the test of choice for evaluating the pituitary for an adenoma. CT is less sensitive for these small tumors. Plain films of the skull or the sella turcica are not useful.

Treatment

If the tumor is large and the symptoms unbearable, surgery is the treatment for pituitary adenomas. Evidence of local invasion, compression of nearby structures, and eccentric location that could compromise carotid sinuses are indications for surgical removal. In some patients, the symptoms may be minimal and the tumor small and located in a position less amenable to surgical excision. In these situations, medical treatment can be attempted to reduce symptoms.

For prolactin-secreting tumors, suppression of prolactin release with dopamine agonists such as bromocriptine can reduce galactorrhea. Bromocriptine therapy can be started with 2.5 mg at bedtime to minimize side effects with an additional 2.5 mg added in the morning with the dose gradually increased until reaching acceptable clinical responses. In addition to a pill form, a vaginal suppository of bromocriptine is also available. Side effects of bromocriptine include nausea, flushing, headaches, hypotension, nasal congestion, and hallucinations. Within 6 month of the start of dopaminergic therapy, approximately 80% of women will also resume normal ovulation. Those who do not ovulate with bromocriptine may require induction of ovulation with clomiphene. If women become pregnant and wish to breast-feed postpartum, bromocriptine should be stopped. The increase in prolactin levels during breast-feeding (usually 10-fold higher than in non-breast-feeding women) is much higher than usually seen from microadenomas. Once breast-feeding has been stopped, bromocriptine can be resumed to prevent galactorrhea.

Dopaminergic agents are also useful for the suppression of growth hormone. In studies using a wide range of dosages of bromocriptine, about 70% of patients with acromegaly showed improvement. Octreotide, a synthetic version of somatostatin, has also been shown to be effective in between 60% and 70% of patients with acromegaly with fewer side effects than bromocriptine. Octreotide reduces the release of growth hormone, glucogon, and insulin. It is effective at reducing the headaches and other symptoms associated with acromegaly. The drug is given by subcutaneous injection of 100 μg three times a day. Like growth hormone, octreotide is expensive; 300 μg daily costs about $7,500 a year. Side effects include hypoglycemia, nausea, diarrhea, and fat malabsorption. Long-term use is associated with gallstone formation. Patients who do not respond optimally to either bromocriptine or octreotide can be treated with combination therapy of both drugs.

Ezzat S: Acromegaly. Endocrinol Metab Clin North Am 1997;26:703.

Maugans TA, Coates ML: Diagnosis and treament of acromegaly. Am Fam Physician 1995;52:207.

■ POSTERIOR PITUITARY DISORDERS

DIABETES INSIPIDUS

Symptoms & Signs

Diabetes insipidus is a fairly uncommon disorder, affecting approximately 3 out of 100,000 people. This disorder, due to a temporary or chronic deficiency or ineffectiveness of vasopressin (antidiuretic hormone or ADH), is characterized by excretion of excessive quantities of dilute urine and excessive thirst due to a compromise in the ability to conserve free water. Diabetes insipidus is easily distinguished from other causes of polyuria by the absence of a solute load (particularly glucose) and abnormally low urine concentration.

Patients with diabetes insipidus present with marked polyuria and associated persistent thirst and polydipsia. These symptoms are usually well tolerated. Nocturia is usually the presenting complaint, often causing enuresis in children.

Pathogenesis

Two types of diabetes insipidus are recognized: neurogenic (central) and nephrogenic (peripheral) (Table 35–10). Numerous underlying conditions can result in each form of diabetes insipidus (Table 35–11). Neurogenic diabetes insipidus is more common and can be either idiopathic or secondary to an intracranial event. In one case series of adults, 25% of cases were idiopathic, 20% were related to benign brain tumors, 17% were related to blunt head trauma, 9% were related to neurosurgery, 6% were related to ischemic or toxic brain injury, and 8% were related to metastatic cancer. In

Table 35–10. Classification of diabetes insipidus.

Cause	Name
Decreased arginine vasopressin (AVP) secretion	Neurogenic
	Cranial
	Central
	Hypothalamic
	Vasopressin responsive
Decreased AVP effect	Nephrogenic
	Vasopressin resistant
Excessive water intake	Primary polydipsia
Increased AVP metabolism	Gestational

Adapted from Robertson GL: Diabetes insipidus. Endocrin Metab Clin North Am 1995;24:549.

Table 35–11. Causes of diabetes insipidus.

Neurogenic Causes	Nephrogenic Causes
Idiopathic	Familial
Acquired	Acquired
Neoplastic	Drug induced
Craniopharyngioma, lymphoma, meningioma, metastatic carcinoma, other brain tumor	Lithium, demeclocycline, methoxyflurane
	Metabolic
Head trauma	Hypokalemia, hypercalciuria, usually with hypercalcemia
Neurosurgery	
Ischemia	Renal disease
Shock, cardiac arrest, Sheehan's syndrome (postpartum pituitary necrosis), aneurysms, sickle cell crisis	Polycystic kidneys, obstructive uropathy, chronic pyelonephritis, sickle cell nephropathy, sarcoidosis, chronic renal failure, multiple myeloma, Sjögren's disease, analgesic nephropathy
Granulomatous	
Sarcoid, histiocytosis	
Infectious	
Tuberculosis, encephalitis, meningitis	
Autoimmune	
Familial	

Adapted from Adam P: Evaluation and management of diabetes insipidus. Am Fam Physician 1997;55:2146.

children, central diabetes insipidus is idiopathic in only 8% of cases; most cases in children are caused by tumors, neurosurgery and trauma, or a sequela of meningitis. Idiopathic diabetes insipidus is invariably permanent, affecting males more often.

Laboratory & Imaging Evaluation

Other than a low urinary specific gravity, diabetes insipidus in not associated with any abnormality on physical examination or routine laboratory testing. Severe disturbances in hydration, usually found in patients who are comatose, lack a normal thirst mechanism, or are too young to regulate their own water intake, occur infrequently.

The water deprivation test has been the standard used to confirm the presence of diabetes insipidus and to differentiate between central and nephrogenic forms. In a controlled state, a mild form of dehydration is induced, with hourly monitoring of urine osmolality, urine specific gravity, serum sodium, and serum osmolality. Adequate dehydration is documented by a weight loss of 1.3–2.25 kg (3–5 lb) or two sequential urine osmolality values that differ by less than 30 mOsm/kg. Serum antidiuretic hormone level is then determined, and the patient is given 5 U of subcutaneous antidiuretic hormone (ADH). Urine and serum osmolality values are determined several times at hourly intervals (Table 35–12).

The key to diagnosing diabetes insipidus and distinguishing between nephrogenic and central diabetes insipidus lies not in the absolute test results but in the association between urine and serum osmolality and antidiuretic hormone level in response to dehydration. Circulating ADH levels can be measured directly by radioimmunoassay and may be more convenient for the patient, especially children. However, the water deprivation test is so accurate that in most cases direct measurement of ADH is unnecessary.

A closely monitored trial of desmopressin (DDAVP) also may be used to diagnose diabetes insipidus. If a standard dose of DDAVP (2–4 µg subcutaneously every 12 h) for 2 days resolves the polydipsia and polyuria without causing water intoxication, the patient has central diabetes insipidus.

If a patient is diagnosed with central diabetes insipidus, the underlying cause must be determined. MRI of the head is indicated in patients who are otherwise asymptomatic, for possible hypothalamic tumor. MRI is thought to be 80–95% sensitive in detecting microadenomas, with CT scan only slightly less sensitive.

Treatment

Patients with central diabetes insipidus are treated with intranasal or oral DDAVP, a synthetic analog of vasopressin without pressor or uterine effects. DDAVP is

Table 35–12. Laboratory tests in the differential diagnosis of diabetes insipidus.

Type	Urine Specific Gravity	Urine Osmolality (mOsm/kg)	Plamsa Osmolality (mOsm/kg)	After ADH[1]
Normal	≥1.015	700–1400	285–295	No change
Central diabetes insipidus (complete)	< 1.010	50–200	310–320	Doubles
Central diabetes insipidus (partial)	1.010–1.015	250–500	295–305	Increases
Nephrogenic diabetes insipidus	<1.010	100–200	310–320	No change

Adapted from Adam P: Evaluation and management of diabetes insipidus. Am Fam Physician 1997;55:2146.
[1] One hour after administration of 5 U aqueous ADH subcutaneously.

the formulation of ADH that is best tolerated, easiest to administer, and most consistent with its antidiuretic effect. The duration of relief ranges from 8 to 20 h and varies between patients but remains constant for individual patients.

The starting dose of 10 μg at night is usually sufficient to relieve nocturia, and a morning dose may be added if symptoms persist during the day. The actual dose delivered can be titrated by using a special nasal catheter. DDAVP is expensive, with a typical bottle of 50 doses costing $100. Patients are encouraged to undertreat themselves to guard against volume overload and hyponatremia.

Patients with partial pituitary diabetes insipidus may respond to the hypoglycemic drug chlorpropamide, which stimulates ADH secretion and potentiates its effects on the kidneys. Clofibrate and carbamazepine may also stimulate ADH secretion and may be used as treatment in patients with partial diabetes insipidus.

In patients with nephrogenic diabetes insipidus, ADH replacement is ineffective. Certain drugs improve polyuria and thus reduce polydipsia. Diuretics, such as thiazides, amiloride, or both, function by depleting total body salt, thus increasing the isotonic absorption of water in the proximal tubule. However, this effect can be countered by a diet heavy in salt. Most patients respond to a daily dosage of 50–100 mg of hydrochlorothiazide.

Adam P: Evaluation and management of diabetes insipidus. Am Fam Physician 1997;55:2146.

Robertson GL: Diabetes insipidus. Endocrinol Metab Clin North Am 1995;24:549.

Singer I, Oster JR, Fishman LM: The management of diabetes insipidus in adults. Arch Intern Med 1997;157:1293.

Common Upper & Lower Extremity Fractures

36

David A. Nikovits, MD, Richard E. Rodenberg, Jr., MD, Thomas D. Armsey, & Robert G. Hosey, MD

■ UPPER EXTREMITY FRACTURES

CLAVICLE FRACTURES

Clinical Findings

A. SYMPTOMS AND SIGNS

A direct blow to the clavicle or a fall on the lateral shoulder may cause a clavicular fracture. Fractures of the clavicle occur in the middle (80%), distal (15%), and medial (5%) thirds. Patients will hold the affected arm adducted and resist motion. Typically, there is swelling and tenderness over the fracture site and a visible and palpable deformity.

B. IMAGING STUDIES

Imaging studies should include an anteroposterior (AP) view. Sometimes an apical lordotic view (AP view 45° cephalad) will help visualize the clavicle without rib interference. A distal third fracture with articular involvement may require cone views or a lateral view. Likewise, at times a medial third fracture is seen with cone and lateral views. A computed tomography (CT) scan helps visualize articular fractures.

Complications

Complications include subclavian vascular injuries and nerve root avulsion or contusion. Middle third fractures may develop malunion, excessive callus formation, and nonunion (no x-ray signs of healing in 4–6 months). Displaced distal third fractures with torn coracoclavicular ligaments may lead to delayed union (no x-ray signs of healing after 3 months). It may require years for a large callus to remodel. Articular surface involvement in either the medial or distal third can lead to degenerative arthritis.

Treatment

Treatment includes ice, analgesics, sling immobilization, and physical therapy. Typically the sling may be discontinued after 6 weeks. Contact sports should be avoided for 2 months. On initial x-rays, there will only be an early callus or none at all. At 2-week follow-up, x-rays should be obtained to evaluate for displacement and angulation. A callus forms between 4 and 6 weeks, along with disappearance of the fracture line. If the fracture is not clinically healed, recheck the x-ray at 6–8 weeks. If the fracture is clinically and radiographically healed at 8–12 weeks, discontinue x-rays. The patient may return to normal activity when the clavicle is painless, the fracture is healed on x-ray, and the shoulder has a full range of motion and near normal strength. This is usually 6 weeks after the injury. The patient may return to contact sports when the x-ray reveals a solid union, after approximately 4–6 months.

Displaced fractures, open fractures, nonunion, and persistent pain 6–8 weeks postfracture are indications for referral.

Eiff MP:Management of clavicle fractures. Am Fam Physician 1997;55(1):121. [PMID:9012272].

WEB SITES

www.emedicine.com/orthoped/byname/clavicle-fractures.htm
www.orthoteers.co.uk/Nrujp-ij33lm/Orthoclaviclefrac.htm

COLLE'S FRACTURES— DISTAL RADIUS FRACTURE

Clinical Findings

A. SYMPTOMS AND SIGNS

A fall-on-outstretched-hand (FOOSH) injury can lead to a Colle's fracture. Patients typically present with pain, swelling, and tenderness at the distal forearm. On examination a "dinner fork" deformity (dorsal displacement of the distal fragment and volar angulation of the distal intact radius with radial shortening) may be identified.

B. IMAGING STUDIES

Imaging studies consist of AP and lateral x-rays (Figure 36–1). Concomitant fracture of the ulnar styloid process may be present. With immobilization, the fracture becomes stable in 6–8 weeks.

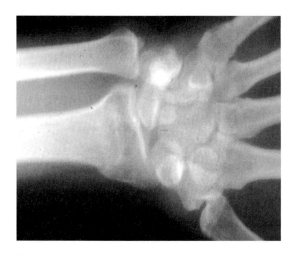

Figure 36–1. Distal radius fracture. (Courtesy of Kentucky Sports Medicine, Dr. Mary Lloyd Ireland.)

Complications

There are early and late complications of Colle's fractures. The early complications include median nerve compression, tendon damage, ulnar nerve contusion or compression, compartment syndrome, and fragment displacement with loss of reduction. Patients may develop a decreased range of motion of the wrist and prolonged swelling. The possible late complications are stiffness of the fingers, shoulder, or radiocarpal joint, shoulder–hand syndrome, cosmetic defects, rupture of the extensor pollicis longus, malunion, nonunion, flexor tendon adhesions, and chronic pain of the radioulnar joint with supination. If there is distal radial ulnar joint (DRUJ) disruption and radial shortening, decreased grip strength, decreased range of motion with supination, and difficulty writing may develop.

Treatment

A nondisplaced distal radial fracture or minimally displaced fracture with little comminution can be managed by the primary care provider. Treatment steps include anesthesia, reduction of the fracture with traction and manipulation, and immobilization with casting. Afterward, postreduction radiographs are taken to ensure proper alignment.

Reduction is necessary to maintain radial length and volar tilt. A short arm cast may be used in an elderly patient and for others with a nondisplaced fracture. All others should be placed in a long arm cast for 3–6 weeks followed by a short arm cast. Physical therapy is helpful for maintaining elbow range of motion. The cast should extend to the proximal palmar crease

volarly and to the metacarpal phalangeal (MCP) prominences dorsally to allow finger and MCP motion and allow opposition. There must be adequate padding around the edges of the cast.

At 2 weeks, AP and lateral x-rays may show little or no callus formation. These should be compared to the original x-rays. Rereduction may be necessary. At the 4- to 6-week follow-up visit, x-rays may show a bridging callus. If there is adequate callus on the x-ray and no tenderness or motion at the fracture site then discontinue the cast. Physical therapy for wrist and elbow range of motion should be started. For support at night, use a bivalve cast or cock-up splint. If there is residual tenderness or motion at the fracture site and inadequate callus, replace this with a short arm cast. At 6–8 weeks a bridging callus should be seen. The fracture line will be less distinct. The x-ray should be checked for malunion, radial shortening, and delayed union as well as for functionality of the wrist. The cast should be discontinued if criteria at the 4- to 6-week follow-up are met. At the 8- to 12-week follow-up, callus should be seen on the x-ray and the fracture line should begin to disappear. The x-ray should be checked for malunion and delayed union. Nonunion occurs with no healing at 4–6 months postinjury.

Indications for referral include fractures with radiocarpal or radioulnar joint involvement, significantly comminuted fractures, and displaced articular fractures. Also, a distal radial fracture with dissociative dorsal intercalary segment instability (DISI), usually caused by scapholunate dissociation, should be referred for percutaneous pinning.

SCAPHOID FRACTURES

Clinical Findings

A. SYMPTOMS AND SIGNS

Scaphoid fractures are caused by a forceful hyperextension of the wrist. This is typically due to a FOOSH with wrist dorsiflexed and radially deviated. Fracture locations are the distal pole, waist, proximal pole, and tubercle. Another important factor is stability of the fracture. A scaphoid fracture is stable unless there is (1) displacement greater than 1 mm, (2) scapholunate angulation greater than 60°, or (3) radiolunate angulation greater than 15°. Associated injuries to look for include perilunate dislocation, lunate dislocation, trapezium fractures, triquetrum fractures, radial styloid fractures, distal radius fractures (Colle's fractures), metacarpals I and II fractures, and capitate fractures. Patients will present with a painful wrist and may report swelling or parasthesias of the affected hand. On examination, there is maximal tenderness in the anatomical snuff box, pain with radial deviation of the wrist, and pain with axial compression of the thumb.

Bone healing occurs at different rates depending on the location of the fracture. A tuberosity fracture usually heals in 4–6 weeks. A scaphoid waist fracture will typically heal in 10–12 weeks. A proximal pole fracture can require 16–20 weeks for healing. Greater than 4–6 months without healing constitutes a nonunion.

B. IMAGING STUDIES

Imaging studies include AP (hand in neutral position), AP (tube tilted 40° distally), lateral (distal arm elevated 15°), and oblique (hand in 10° supination and maximal ulnar deviation) x-ray views. Occasionally, right and left oblique views or a scaphoid view may be necessary. It is appropriate to order a bone scan 3 days after injury if a fracture is clinically suspected, but x-rays are negative. Studies have shown bone scans to be 100% sensitive and 98% specific. Further imaging with a CT scan is appropriate if the bone scan is positive or if a fracture is clinically suspected, but x-rays are negative and the patient needs to return to activity as early as possible.

Complications

There are a number of complications associated with a scaphoid fracture: delayed union (no healing, no trabeculae crossing the fracture line, at 3 months), avascular necrosis (x-rays show sclerosis and cyst development), compartment syndrome (rarely), and compression neuropathy (rarely). Of utmost concern is malunion or nonunion (absence of evidence of healing at 4–6 months). Malunion resulting in a humpback deformity can lead to carpal instability, loss of wrist extension, weakness of grip, carpal collapse, and degenerative changes in the wrist. The most common type of carpal instability is a DISI pattern. On lateral x-rays, this DISI pattern allows palmar flexion of the scaphoid and dorsiflexion of the lunate.

Treatment

Nondisplaced or minimally displaced (<1 mm) scaphoid fractures are placed in a thumb spica cast. A short arm cast is used for tuberosity fractures and long arm casts for all other nondisplaced or minimally displaced scaphoid fractures. When casting, the wrist should be in a neutral flexion/extension, neutral to radial deviation with the thumb included. A long arm cast is used for 6 weeks and is then replaced with a short arm cast for another 6 weeks.

Follow-up should occur at 2 weeks with AP, lateral, and oblique x-ray views. Check for step-offs, angulation, and displacement. At this point no callus and possible fracture site resorption are seen. Later at 4–6 weeks there

is no callus because there is no periosteal membrane. However, trabecular bone may be visible across the fracture line. At 8–12 weeks the fracture line begins to disappear. The normal trabecular bone pattern returns in 12–16 weeks. Rehabilitation takes 3–6 months. Union rates vary; for a nondisplaced fracture the rate is 100%. Angulated fracture union rates are 65% and displaced rates are 45%. The proximal one-third fracture union rate range is 60–70% with immobilization.

Consultation is required for open reduction and internal fixation for displaced, delayed union, and nonunion scaphoid fractures. Referral is also appropriate for a patient initially presenting more than 3 weeks after the injury.

WEB SITES

www.physsportsmed.com/issues/1996/06_96/gutierez.htm

METACARPAL FRACTURES

Clinical Findings

A. SYMPTOMS AND SIGNS

Metacarpal fractures are caused by direct trauma to the hand. These fractures can be stable or unstable. Stable fractures can be impacted or isolated fractures with little or no displacement. Unstable fractures are comminuted, displaced, oblique, or spiral, often multiple fractures. Patients present with tenderness and swelling.

Special fractures include the following:

- Bennett's fracture—two-part intraarticular fracture of the base of the first metacarpal.
- Rolando's fracture—three-part intraarticular fracture of the base of the first metacarpal.
- Reverse Rolando's fracture—three-part intraarticular fracture of the base of the fifth metacarpal.
- Boxer's fracture—fifth metacarpal neck fracture.

B. IMAGING STUDIES

AP and lateral x-rays are needed and comparison views are sometimes helpful. However, it is recommended that initial x-rays of fractures of the fourth and fifth metacarpals be AP and oblique pronated views. Additional lateral x-rays are helpful only after confirmation of a proximal comminuted fracture or signs of a pronounced AP dislocation. A CT scan may be helpful for metacarpal head and base fractures.

Complications

Complications are many and include decreased grip strength, arthritis if the articular surface is involved, prolonged swelling, reflex sympathetic dystrophy, compartment syndrome, decreased MCP prominence with metacarpal shaft dorsal prominence, and decreased range of motion.

Treatment

Treatment will depend on a variety of factors. Casting is appropriate for the following situations: no degree of rotational deformity; an intraarticular fracture, with no more than a 1- to 2-mm step-off; stable neck and shaft fractures; extraarticular metacarpal base fractures; comminuted metacarpal head fractures; and second, third, and fourth intraarticular metacarpal base fractures. Certain angular restrictions must be adhered to.

For shaft fractures:

- First digit—no more than 30° of apex dorsal angulation.
- Second and third digits—no more than 10° of apex dorsal angulation.
- Fourth and fifth digits—no more than 20° of apex dorsal angulation.

For neck fractures:

- Second digit—no more than 10° of apex dorsal angulation.
- Third digit—no more than 20° of apex dorsal angulation.
- Fourth digit—no more than 30° of apex dorsal angulation.
- Fifth digit—no more than 40° of apex dorsal angulation.

If the metacarpal fracture meets the above conditions it may be casted or splinted. The affected digit is buddy taped. The wrist is casted in 30° of extension. The MCP joints are flexed 60–90°. The distal and proximal interphalangeal joints are placed in 5–10° of flexion. The cast should be trimmed to allow visualization of the tip of the injured digit and the adjacent buddy-taped digit. This step facilitates checking capillary refill. Recheck for loss of correction after casting.

At 2 weeks postcasting, an x-ray will not show any callus formation but needs to be checked for loss of correction. A bridging callus should be seen at 4–6 weeks. Again, check for loss of correction. If there is tenderness, motion, or inadequate callus formation, recast and recheck every 2 weeks. If there is no tenderness, no motion at the fracture site, and adequate callus formation is noted consider a protective splint for 1–2 weeks. Consider a night splint for aggressive physical therapy. At the 6- to 8-week follow-up, a bridging callus should

be seen. The fracture line will be less distinct. At 8–12 weeks check the x-rays for malunion and delayed union (no sign of healing on the x-ray 3 months after injury) Discontinue the x-rays if there is abundant callus or the disappearance of the fracture line. Check for nonunion and failure to heal by 4–6 months.

Physical therapy is needed to limit stiffness. Motion is started before complete bony union. However, this puts the fracture at risk of displacement or loss of alignment.

Unstable metacarpal neck or shaft fractures should be referred to an orthopedic surgeon. Also, most intraarticular fractures of the base of the first and fifth metacarpals need referral. The above cases will likely be treated by closed reduction and percutaneous pinning. Open reduction and internal fixation are indicated for intraarticular fractures of the metacarpal base that cannot be maintained by closed reduction and metacarpal head fractures with mild comminution.

RADIAL HEAD FRACTURES

Clinical Findings

A. SYMPTOMS AND SIGNS

Radial head fractures can be caused by a FOOSH while pronated or partially flexed. Another mechanism of injury is a valgus force on the elbow forcing the humeral capitellum into the radial head. Patients will present with elbow pain and swelling. Physical findings are tenderness over the radial head, pain increased with supination, reduced range of motion, and swelling secondary to a hemarthrosis. Swelling in the center of a triangle formed by the lateral epicondyle, olecranon, and radial head may occur. Evaluate the patient for neurovascular compromise, checking capillary refill, sensation, and posterior interosseous nerve function. The medial collateral ligament (MCL) should be evaluated for tenderness and opening with valgus stress.

B. IMAGING STUDIES

Check the wrist with AP and lateral views to rule out distal radial ulnar joint disruption. Imaging studies of the elbow include AP, lateral (Figure 36–2), and radiocapitellar (45° from the lateral toward the radial head) views. Look for the radiocapitellar line and a fat pad sign. Follow-up x-rays at 2 weeks will not show a callous. However, at 4–6 weeks a bridging callous should be noted. Bone healing is visible between 6 and 8 weeks. Begin rehabilitation as soon as the fracture is stable, to maintain functional range of motion. At 8–12 weeks there should be abundant bridging callous and a resolving fracture line. In the rare case of nonunion, the patient will report pain and examination will reveal tenderness.

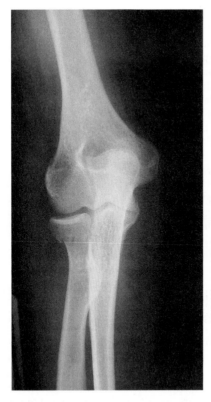 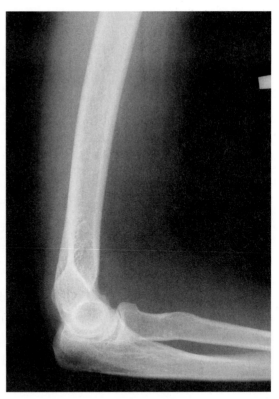

Figure 36–2. AP and lateral view of radial head fracture. Negative fat pad sign.

Complications

Possible complications include reflex sympathetic dystrophy, compartment syndrome of the elbow and forearm, heterotropic ossification, increased carrying angle of the elbow, arthritis with restricted range of motion, deformity, valgus instability, decreased grip strength, posterior interosseous or median nerve injury, and brachial artery injury.

Classification (Mason)

Type I—Nondisplaced

Type II—Marginal fractures with displacement, depression, or angulation.

Type III—Comminuted fractures of the entire head or completely displaced fractures of the radial head.

Type IV—Type I, II, or III with elbow dislocation.

Treatment

The primary care physician can treat Type I (nondisplaced radial head) fractures. Treatment includes aspiration (to decrease the hematoma and capsular disten-

tion—injection of anesthetic may aid in evaluation), early range of motion, and a sling for 5 to 7 days. Bone healing typically occurs in 6–8 weeks. Range of motion rehabilitation should be started as soon as possible, when the fracture is stable.

Elite athletes and younger patients will usually be treated with open reduction with internal fixation (ORIF). On the other hand, elderly patients with a stable elbow may be treated with early radial head excision and range of motion exercises. If there are fracture fragments, excision will be needed. Based on the Mason classification, Type II fractures (displacement 2–3 mm, greater than 25° involvement of the articular surface) require ORIF. Additionally, Type III fractures (nonreparable comminuted) will require radial head excision. Patients with Type IV fractures (posterior dislocation) also need referral.

WEB SITES

www.orthoseek.com/articles/fractman.html
www.physsportsmed.com/issues/1996/06_96/cordas.htm
www.worldortho.com/database/sgt/tr4a.pdf

■ LOWER EXTREMITY FRACTURES

STRESS FRACTURES

General Considerations

Stress fractures were first described in Prussian army recruits by a Prussian surgeon, Breithraupt, in 1855. Over the next 100 years stress fractures were predominantly studied in military recruits. The first athletic stress fracture was described in 1958. Since that time the diagnosis of stress fracture has become well recognized and widely reported.

Management of traumatic fractures of the lower extremity long bones is relatively straightforward if a few simple rules are recognized. Orthopedic referral will be required for any traumatic fracture that is displaced or involves a joint line. If the primary care physician would like to obtain competence in acute traumatic fracture management, requiring casting, then other references must be sought. The goal of this section of the chapter will be to guide the primary care physician through a basic understanding of concepts surrounding bone stress pathogenesis including epidemiology, clinical signs and symptoms, physical examination, radiographic diagnostic aids, and treatment of four difficult-to-treat areas of stress reaction in the lower extremities. The population most at risk for stress reaction is the athlete. This population presents therapeutic challenges secondary to their increased activity, predilection to overuse injury, and the ultimate desire to return to competition with as little down time as possible, often competing before full resolution of the stress injury.

Stress fractures are estimated to make up 10% of all athletic injuries. Ninety-five percent of stress injuries occur in the lower extremities secondary to the extreme repetitive weight-bearing loads placed on these bones. The peak incidence occurs in people 18–25 years of age. However, with recent emphasis on exercise for the elderly, the diagnosis of stress fracture should not be neglected in this population. There is a decreased incidence of stress fracture in men secondary to greater lean body mass and overall bone structure. It has been estimated that women military recruits have a relative risk of 1.2–10 times greater for stress fracture as compared to men with the same training volume. In athletic populations a gender difference is not as evident, possibly because athletic women are more fit and conditioned. Incidence is estimated to be comparable for all races.

Stress fracture is most common after changes in an athlete's training regimen. Injury is especially prevalent in nonconditioned runners who increase their training regimen. Training error, which can include increased quantity or intensity of training, introduction of a new activity, poor equipment, and change in environment (ie, surface), is the most important risk factor for stress injury. Low bone density, dietary deficiency, abnormal body composition, menstrual irregularities, hormonal imbalance, sleep deprivation, and biomechanical abnormalities also place the athlete at risk. Keeping this in mind and recognizing the increasing incidence of female athletic triad (amenorrhea, eating disorder, and osteoporosis), it is easy to understand why women can have an increased risk for stress injury.

Clinical Findings

A. SYMPTOMS AND SIGNS

Stress fractures are related to a maladaptive process between bone injury and bone remodeling. Bone reacts to stress by early osteoclastic activity (old bone resorption) followed by strengthening osteoblastic activity (new bone formation). With continued stress, bone resorption outpaces new bone formation and a self-perpetuating cycle occurs with continued activity allowing weakened bone to be more susceptible to continued microfracture and ultimately progressing to frank fracture. The initiation of stress reaction is unclear. It has been postulated that excessive forces are transmitted to bone when surrounding muscles fatigue. The highly concentrated muscle forces act across localized area of bone, causing mechanical insults above the stress-bearing capacity of bone. These insults occur at the insertion of tendons and lead to insults in the bone that may propagate into a stress fracture.

Athletic stress fracture follows a crescendo process. Symptoms start insidiously with dull, gnawing pain at the end of physical activity. Pain increases over days to the point where the activity cannot be continued. At first pain decreases with rest, then shorter and shorter duration of activity causes pain. More time is then needed for pain to dissipate until it is present with minimal activity and at night. After a few days of rest, pain resolves, only to return once again with resumption of activity. More specific historical and physical examination findings will be discussed in conjunction with specific anatomical regions.

B. IMAGING STUDIES

The diagnosis of stress fracture is primarily clinical and is based on history and physical examination. It is prudent to start with plain radiographs, which have poor sensitivity but high specificity, as the initial study. The presence of stress reaction is confirmed by the presence of periosteal reaction, intramedullary sclerosis, callus, or obvious fracture line. Usually plain films will reveal no obvious abnormality unless symptoms have been present for at least 2–3 weeks. Some stress injuries will never show changes on plain film.

The technetium triple-phase bone scan is the diagnostic gold standard with high sensitivity and poor specificity. Stress reactions can often be visualized within 48–72 h from symptom onset. Triple-phase bone scan can differentiate soft tissue and bone injury. The first phase flow image immediately after intravenous injection of tracer shows perfusion in bone and soft tissue. The second phase (static blood pool phase), taken 1 min after injection, reflects the degree of hyperemia and capillary permeability of bone and soft tissue showing acute inflammation. In the third phase (delayed image), taken 3-4 h after injection of tracer, approximately 50% of the tracer has concentrated in the bone matrix. All three phases can be positive in an acute fracture. In soft tissue injuries, with no bony involvement, the first two phases are often positive, whereas the delayed image shows minimal or no increased uptake. In conditions such as medial tibial stress syndrome (MTSS), in which there is early bony stress reaction, the first two phases are negative and the delayed image is positive. Bone scan does not visualize the fracture and is not used to monitor healing secondary to delayed images showing uptake 12 months after initial studies.

CT scans can identify conditions that mimic stress fracture on bone scan, confirm fracture suspected on bone scan, or help to make treatment decisions as with navicular stress fractures.

MRI is not superior to bone scan. It is highly specific. It offers the advantage of visualizing soft tissue changes in anatomic regions in which the soft tissue structures often cloud the differential diagnosis. Bone stress is identified as marrow edema, whereas frank stress fracture can be visualized as a line at the cortex surrounded by an intense zone of edema in the medullary cavity. Clinically the high sensitivity of bone scan and MRI is necessary only when the diagnosis of stress fracture is in question or the exact location or extent of injury must be known in order to determine treatment.

Brukner P, Cradshaw C, Bennell K: Managing common stress fractures: let risk level guide treatment. Physician Sportsmed 1998;26(8):39.

Knapp TP, Garrett WE: Stress fractures: general concepts. Clin Sports Med 1997;16(2):339. [PMID: 9238314]. (Guidelines for managing common stress fractures.)

Perron AD, Brady WJ, Keats TA: Management of common stress fractures: when to apply conservative therapy, when to take an aggressive approach. Postgrad Med 2002;111(2):95. [PMID: 11868316]. (Guidelines for management and referral of common stress fractures.)

1. Femoral Stress Fractures

General Considerations

Stress fractures involving the femur can occur in a variety of locations, most commonly the femoral shaft and neck. A study by Matheson et al looking at 320 athletes with bone scan-positive stress fractures revealed the femur to be the fourth most frequent site of injury.

Theories for site-specific causes of these fractures are thought to be secondary to insufficiency and fatigue mechanisms. The insufficiency mechanism is the result of bone wear from normal muscular activity on deficient bone producing tension at the biopsy site. During fatigue, repetitive stresses wear in normal bone. The question of which mechanism precedes the other has not been answered.

Differential Diagnosis

The symptom most commonly encountered with stress fractures of the femur is pain at the anterior aspect of the hip. Differentiating the diagnosis can be difficult secondary to the multiple number of structures in the hip that have the potential to produce similar pain syndromes and the deep nonpalpable structures of the anatomical region. The differential diagnosis is broad but must include consideration of disease processes such as apophyseal and epiphyseal injury in the adolescent population, arthritis in the adult population, along with inflammatory arthritides, muscle strains, tendinitis, stress fractures, sports hernia with nerve entrapment, osteitis pubis, and acetabular labral tears across all age groups. Because the diagnosis can be made complex by the multiple array of structures in this region from which pain may emanate, the physician must be astute to the history, as mentioned previously, to narrow the differential down to a list in which stress fracture is prominent. This is important in order to avoid severe complications associated with fractures of the femoral neck.

Femoral Shaft Fractures

Femoral shaft fractures are more common than expected. The incidence of femoral shaft stress fractures in athletes was found to be 3.7%. Onset of pain can be gradual over a period of days to weeks. Average time from symptom onset to diagnosis was found to be 2.2 weeks. The fulcrum test was well suited to act as a guide for ordering radiological tests and thereby decreasing time to diagnosis. It was also found to be a good clinical test to assess healing. For this test, the athlete is seated on the examination table with legs dangling as the examiner's arm is used as a fulcrum under the thigh. The examiner's arm is moved from the distal to proximal thigh as gentle pressure is applied to the dorsum of the knee with the opposite hand. A positive test is elicited by sharp pain or apprehension at the site of the fracture. Plain films usually are not sensitive in detecting stress fractures within the first 2–3 weeks of symptoms. The technetium triple-phase bone scan is the gold standard for diagnosis. However, MRI has been shown to be more specific than bone scan and gives the added benefit of looking at soft tissue structures of the anterior hip. The most common site of injury in athletes was the midmedial or postereomedial cortex of the proximal femur.

Once diagnosis is confirmed, treatment depends on the underlying causes responsible for the injury. If the fracture is consistent with a compression-sided fracture, treatment consists of rest with gradual resumption of activity (Figures 36–3 and 36–4). This usually is adequate for healing of nondisplaced fractures. Treatment protocols are based on empiric data gathered from clinical observation. An example of a treatment protocol may consist of rest for a period of 1–4 weeks of toe-touch weight bearing progressing to full weight bearing. This would be followed by a phase of low-impact activity (ie, biking/swimming). Once patients are able to

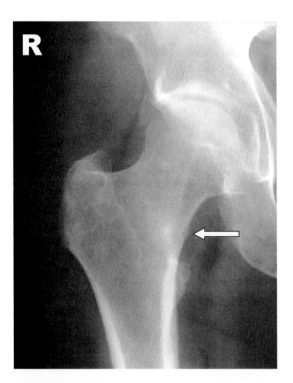

Figure 36–3. Compression-sided stress fracture of the right femoral neck indicated by the white arrow at the site of periosteal reaction.

perform low-impact activity for a prolonged time without pain, they may gradually advance to high impact. Resumption of full activity averages between 8 and 16 weeks. Surgical treatment would be considered should there be displacement of the fracture, delayed union, or nonunion following conservative therapy.

Femoral Neck Fractures

Stress fractures of the femoral neck are uncommon but carry a high complication rate if the diagnosis is missed or the fracture is improperly treated. The primary presenting symptom is pain at the site of the groin, anterior thigh, or knee. Pain is exacerbated by weight-bearing or physical activity. The athlete may have an antalgic gait or painful/limited hip range of motion in internal rotation or external rotation. MRI is the diagnostic modality of choice for evaluating femoral neck stress fractures. Stress fractures of the femoral neck are divided into two categories: compression and tension type. Compression fractures are more common in younger patients. The fracture line, if seen on the x-ray, can propagate across the femoral neck. A nondisplaced, incomplete compression fracture is treated with rest until the patient is pain free with full motion. Non-weight-bearing ambulation with the patient on crutches follows until radiographic healing as shown on plain films is complete. Frequent radiographs may need to be obtained to monitor propagation of the fracture. If the compression fracture becomes complete, or fails to heal with rest, then internal fixation may be necessary (Figure 36–5). Nonsurgical treatment may take several months before full activity is achieved. Tension (distraction)-sided femoral neck fractures are an emergency because of the potential for complications (ie, nonunion or avascular necrosis). The patient is immediately made non-weight-bearing and will acutely need internal fixation. If the fracture is displaced the patient will need ORIF urgently.

Boden BP, Speer KP: Femoral stress fractures. Clin Sports Med 1997;16(2):307. [PMID: 9238312]. (Guidelines for recognition and management of femoral stress fractures.)

Fullerton LR: Femoral neck stress fractures. Sports Med 1990;9(3): 192. [PMID: 2315577]. (Guidelines for recognition and management of femoral stress fractures.)

Johnson AW, Weiss CB, Wheeler DL: Stress fractures of the femoral shaft in athletes—more common than expected. Am J Sports Med 1994;22(2):248. [PMID: 8198195]. (Guidelines for recognition and management of femoral stress fractures with description of clinical diagnostic test.)

Matheson GO et al: Stress fractures in athletes: a study of 320 cases. Am J Sports Med 1987;15(1):46. [PMID: 3812860].

O'Kane JW: Anterior hip pain. Am Fam Physician 1999;60(6): 1687. [PMID: 10537384]. (Guidelines for differentiating and treating causes of anterior hip pain.)

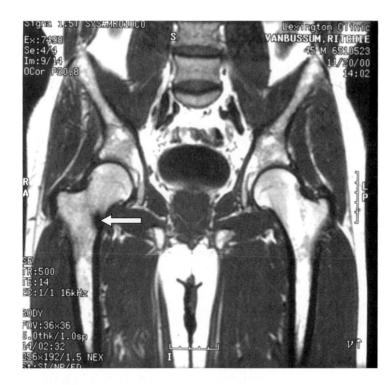

Figure 36–4. Compression-sided stress fracture of the right femoral neck as indicated on MRI by the white arrow.

2. Tibial Stress Fractures

General Considerations

Tibial stress fractures account for 50% of stress fractures diagnosed as demonstrated in a large series by Matheson et al. The tibia is therefore the number one site for stress fractures to occur. Most tibial stress fractures, in athletes, are secondary to running. An average of 3–6 weeks of overtraining has been shown to be associated with increased incidence of tibial stress fractures.

Two sites located within the tibia are most commonly associated with stress fractures. The first most common site affected is between the middle and distal third of the tibia along the posteromedial border. This type of injury is most commonly associated with running. The second site of fracture is along the middle third of the anterior cortex. This injury is most commonly associated with activities involving a great deal of jumping (ie, dancing, basketball, gymnastics).

Clinical Findings

A. SYMPTOMS AND SIGNS

On history the patient will commonly describe pain occurring in the region of the fracture with activity (ie, running/jumping) and resolving with rest. The pain will eventually progress and last longer after the activity until the patient is symptomatic at rest. Physical examination will often reveal localized pain to palpation. Sometimes persistent thickening, secondary to periosteal reaction, can be appreciated by palpation along the tibia.

B. IMAGING STUDIES

Diagnosis by radiographic plain film may be possible if symptoms have been present for at least 4–6 weeks. Triple-phase bone scan is very sensitive and may allow

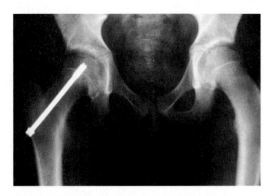

Figure 36–5. Intramedullary screw fixation of a femoral neck stress fracture.

diagnosis within 48–72 h of symptom onset. Tibial stress fractures can be seen clearly on MRI with sensitivity comparable to triple-phase bone scan. Both bone scan and MRI allow differentiation of medial tibial stress syndrome and stress fracture.

Differential Diagnosis

Medial tibial stress syndrome (MTSS) is the most commonly confused diagnosis in the classification of tibial stress injuries with stress fracture. MTSS usually occurs diffusely along the middle and distal third of the posteromedial tibia and is commonly seen in runners. This condition, however, can also be seen with activities involving persistent jumping. The symptom spectrum commonly progresses, as does that of stress fractures, with continued activity. MTSS represents a stress reaction within bone where the usual remodeling process becomes maladaptive. This injury responds well to rest in a shorter time period as compared to stress fracture and is easily differentiated from stress fracture on triple-phase bone scan. If symptoms do not resolve or are consistent with distal numbness or in a region of nerve traversing one of the four involved compartments of the lower leg, the diagnosis of chronic compartment syndrome must be considered.

Treatment

Once the diagnosis of tibial stress fracture has been made, a distinction between a compression versus tension-sided injury must be made. Fractures along the posteromedial border are considered compression stress injuries and respond well to conservative therapy (Figure 36–6). The average recovery time for this injury is approximately 12 weeks when the patient is treated with rest alone. Most guidelines for treatment of this injury involve relative or absolute rest. These stress fractures can be effectively treated in a pneumatic leg brace. Athletes treated in the pneumatic brace (long leg air cast) showed decreased time to pain-free symptoms (14 ± 6 days) and time to competitive participation (21 ± 2 days) versus traditional mode non-weight-bearing treatment (77 ± 7 days). Athletes in the brace may continue exercising but modifications of the training routine must be made to maintain pain-free activities. Patients are progressed based on a functional activity progression as outlined by Swenson et al. Partial weight bearing with crutches is sometimes necessary for the athlete who continues to complain of pain in the air cast, but this is the exception to the rule.

Tibial stress fractures of the mid-anterior cortex, also known as "the dreaded black line," radiographically (Figure 36–7), are very difficult to manage conservatively. This fracture occurs at the tension side of the tibial cortex, most commonly in athletes who jump. Two

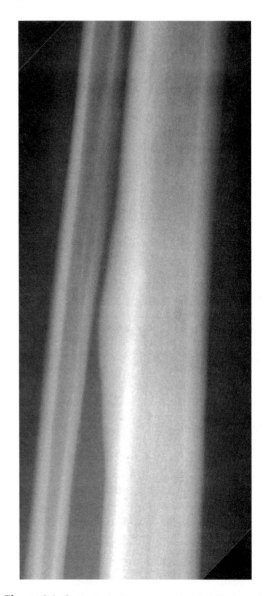

Figure 36–6. Periosteal stress reaction (white arrow) at the posterior medial aspect of the tibia.

significant complications including delayed union and complete fracture plague this fracture site. Rettig et al revealed in a study that average time to symptom-free return to activity from symptom onset was 12.7 months with conservative care. Conservative treatment revolves around rest and/or immobilization. The duration of treatment was modestly helped by addition of pulsed electromagnetic field (PEMF). Patients who do not respond to conservative treatment or are involved in activities (career or competitive athletics) are

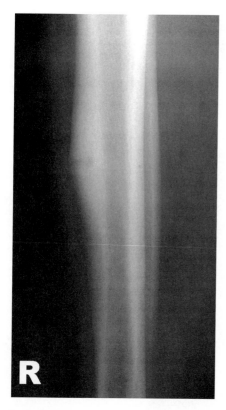

Figure 36–7. Dreaded black line at the anterior medial aspect of the tibia.

individuals in whom surgical treatment with tibial intramedullary nailing would be beneficial (Figure 36–8). These fractures, secondary to the prolonged treatment and risk of complication, should be referred to a sports medicine specialist.

Beck BR: Tibial stress injuries: an aetiological review for the purpose of guiding management. Sports Med 1998;26(4):265. [PMID: 9820925]. (Review for treatment of tibial stress injuries.)

Chang PS, Harris RM: Intramedullary nailing for chronic tibial stress fractures: a review of five cases. Am J Sports Med 1996; 24(5):688. [PMID: 8883694]. (Surgical options for tibial stress fracture.)

Couture CJ, Karlson KA: Tibial stress injuries: decisive diagnosis and treatment of "shin splints." Physician Sportsmed 2002;30(6):29. [Guidelines for differentiating and treating causes of generic term shin splints (tibial stress injuries).]

Matheson GO et al: Stress fractures in athletes: a study of 320 cases. Am J Sports Med 1987;15(1):46. [PMID: 3812860].

Perron AD, Brady WJ, Keats TA: Management of common stress fractures: when to apply conservative therapy, when to take an aggressive approach. Postgrad Med 2002;111(2):95. [PMID: 11868316]. (Guidelines and treatment of common stress fractures.)

Rettig AC et al: The natural history and treatment of delayed union stress fractures of the anterior cortex of the tibia. Am J Sports Med 1988;16(3):250. [PMID: 3381982]. (Description of treatment options for delayed union anterior tibial stress fractures.)

Swenson EJ et al: The effect of a pneumatic leg brace on return to play in athletes with tibial stress fractures. Am J Sports Med 1997;25(3):322. [PMID: 9167811]. (Use of pneumatic leg brace to speed return to play in athletes suffering from posterior medial tibial stress injuries.)

3. Tarsal Navicular Stress Fractures

General Considerations

Tarsal navicular stress fractures are an underdiagnosed source of prolonged, disabling foot pain predominantly seen in active athletes involved in sprinting and jumping. In a study involving 111 competitive track and field athletes, Bennell et al found that navicular stress fractures are the second most common lower extremity stress fracture.

Clinical Findings

A. Symptoms and Signs

These fractures are prone to misdiagnosis secondary to the vague nature of pain. The pain may radiate along the medial arch and not directly over the talonavicular joint. Sometimes pain radiates distally, causing the physician to suspect Morton's neuroma or metatarsalgia. The pain often disappears with a few days of rest, often tricking the athlete into not believing the potential seriousness of the diffuse foot pain. The diagnosis is also clouded because the fractures are rarely seen on plain film.

Imaging Studies

A retrospective multicenter study by Khan et al looking at 86 fractures of the tarsal navicular bone, all with CT confirmation of clinical diagnosis, reported a range in time of diagnosis from symptom onset to be 3–60 months (average 4 months). Symptoms suggesting a clinical diagnosis consisted of (1) insidious onset of vague pain over the dorsum of the medial midfoot or over the medial aspect of the longitudinal arch, (2) ill-defined pain, soreness, or cramping aggravated by activity and relieved by rest, (3) well-localized tenderness to palpation over the navicular bone or medical arch, and (4) little swelling or discoloration. Certain foot abnormalities including short first metatarsal and metatarsus adductor and /or limited dorsiflexion of the ankle may concentrate stress on the tarsal navicular region, predisposing to stress reaction.

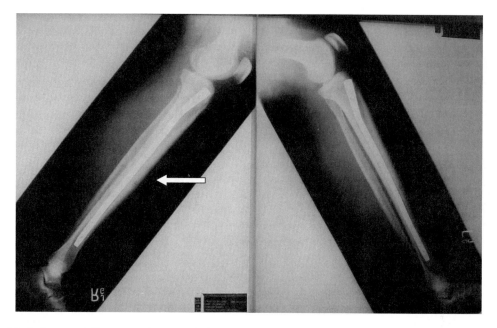

Figure 36–8. Intramedullary screw fixation of bilateral anterior medial tibial stress fractures.

Treatment

The study by Khan et al reaffirmed the best treatment modality as proposed by Torg et al in 1982 was 6–8 weeks of non-weight-bearing cast immobilization. This retrospective study also offered guidelines for treatment, the CT appearance of the fracture after conservative treatment, and parameters used to follow fracture healing. When seriously considering diagnosis of tarsal navicular stress fractures, plain film radiographs should be obtained in an AP, lateral, and oblique standing position (Figure 36–9). If the x-ray is normal a bone scan should be obtained. If the bone scan is positive and the x-ray is negative, a CT scan to confirm stress fracture as opposed to stress reaction should be obtained. The CT slices must be no wider than 1.5 mm apart and include the dorsal proximal cortical surface. Most fractures are located in the sagittal plane and in the central third of bone along the proximal articular surface corresponding to angiographic studies indicating this to be a relatively avascular region (Figure 36–10).

Data indicate that 6–8 weeks of non-weight-bearing cast immobilization compares favorably with surgical treatment for failed weight-bearing treatment. Surgery is recommended for a displaced, complete fracture with a small transverse fragment (ossicle), or failure of conservative management. Conservative management, however, may be warranted initially for these fractures. Complete fracture with a large dorsal transverse fracture

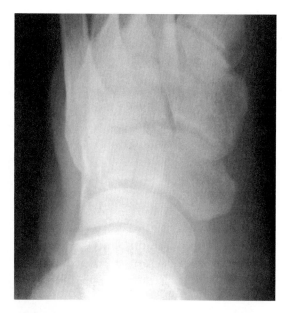

Figure 36–9. Radiograph revealing stress fracture of the tarsal navicular (Courtesy of Kentucky Sports Medicine, Dr. Mary Lloyd Ireland.)

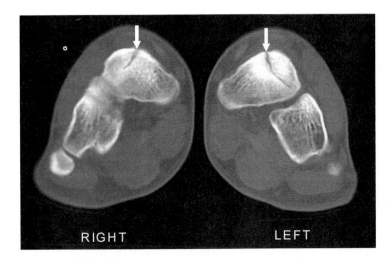

Figure 36–10. CT scan of bilateral tarsal navicular stress fractures (white arrows). (Courtesy of Kentucky Sports Medicine, Dr. Mary Lloyd Ireland.)

has been found to progress to union with conservative treatment and not require excision of the fragment. Surgical treatment often consists of either bone graft or screw fixation (Figure 36–11) followed by non-weight-bearing cast immobilization for 6 weeks.

After 6 weeks of non-weight-bearing cast immobilization the fracture is followed clinically by palpation of the fracture site along the dorsal proximal region of the navicular bone. Persistent tenderness over this "N"

spot requires an additional 2 weeks of non-weight-bearing immobilization before reassessment. If the fracture site is not tender after casting, the patient may begin weight bearing. The patient may feel some diffuse foot pain at first that is different from the original pain. This pain can usually be attributed to stiffness of crural, subatalar, and midtarsal joints. Plain films do not provide a reliable indication of fracture healing secondary to low sensitivity. Bone scan will often remain positive long

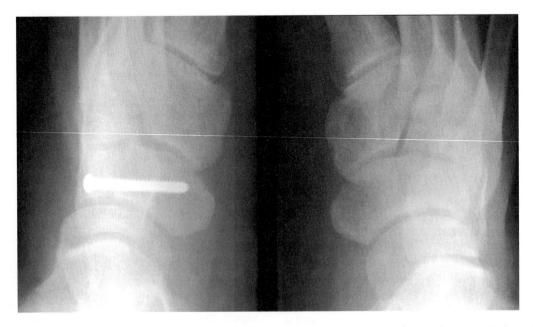

Figure 36–11. X-Ray of screw fixation of a tarsal navicular stress fracture. (Courtesy of Kentucky Sports Medicine, Dr. Mary Lloyd Ireland.)

after clinical union. A CT scan up to 3–6 months from therapy, although asymptomatic, can show blurring of the fracture line and cortical bridging. The CT scan may not show complete obliteration on 3-month repeat films. For this reason the recommendation is not to repeat the CT scan but instead to rely on clinical examination (palpation of the "N" spot).

Of note is the topic of "bone strain." During this phenomenon the bone scan may be positive but the patient is asymptomatic. This can be seen when the bone scan is ordered to assess MTSS and activity is picked up in the navicular bone. The CT scan remains normal. Persistent training results in progression to stress fracture. Treatment of bone strain does not require cast immobilization. This condition can be managed successfully with 6 weeks of strict limitation of activity with weight bearing.

Bennell KL et al: The incidence and distribution of stress fractures in competitive track and field athletes: a twelve-month prospective study. Am J Sports Med 1996;24(2):211. [PMID: 8947404].

Khan KM et al: Outcome of conservative and surgical management of navicular stress fracture in athletes: eighty-six cases proven with computerized tomography. Am J Sports Med 1992;20 (6):657. [PMID: 1456359]. (Treatment guidelines for navicular stress fractures.)

Torg JS, Pavlov H, Torg E: Overuse injuries in sport: the foot. Clin Sports Med 1987;6(2):306. [PMID: 2891450]. (Guidelines for recognition and treatment of tarsal navicular stress injuries.)

4. Metatarsal Stress Fractures

General Considerations

Metatarsal stress fractures in athletes are very common. Depending on the study referenced they are either third or fourth in incidence. These fractures are also known as "March fractures" because of the large numbers of military recruits who obtained these fractures after sudden increases in their level of activity. The second metatarsal is the most common location followed by the third and fourth metatarsals. The second metatarsal is subjected to three to four times body weight during loading and push-off phases of gait.

Clinical Findings

A. Symptoms and Signs

Clinical suspicion for this injury is raised when the athlete complains of forefoot or mid-foot pain of insidious onset. On examination these injuries present as areas of point tenderness overlying the metatarsal shaft.

Imaging Studies

Radiographs are usually sufficient to document stress fracture, which is visualized as a frank fracture or periosteal reaction at the affected site. As with most stress fractures the patient may be symptomatic 2–4 weeks prior to visualizing the fracture on x-ray. If the diagnosis is in question, bone scan and MRI have significantly higher sensitivity and specificity for detecting these injuries at an earlier time frame.

Treatment

Treatment is easily managed by the primary care physician. The injury is treated symptomatically, allowing the athlete to participate in activities that are not painful. Immobilization in the form of a steel shank insole or stiff, wooden-soled type shoe may be necessary for a limited time, until no longer painful. At times the patient may benefit from a short leg walking cast or removable walking boot for severe pain. Four weeks of rest is usually sufficient for healing. During these 4 weeks, the athlete may continue modified conditioning with non-weight-bearing exercises (ie, swimming and pool running), followed by cycling and stair climbing.

Although most of these fractures heal well with conservative management, fractures of the proximal fifth metatarsal have a high incidence of delayed union and nonunion. A thorough understanding of the classification and anatomy of fractures in this location is required for proper identification to determine conservative versus surgical treatment.

Fractures of the Proximal Fifth Metatarsal

Fractures of the proximal fifth metatarsal include tuberosity avulsion fractures, acute Jones' fractures, and diaphyseal stress fractures. Diaphyseal stress fractures in this area can further be classified as early, delayed union, and nonunion fractures.

The fifth metatarsal consists of a base tuberosity, shaft (diaphysis), neck, and head. The tuberosity protrudes plantarward from the base. The metaphysis tapers to the diaphysis. There are three articulations including the cuboid fourth metatarsal, cuboid fifth metatarsal, and the fourth and fifth intermetatarsal articulation in this region. The proximal fifth metatarsal serves as the insertion of the lateral band of the plantar fascia, peroneus brevis tendon, and peroneus tertius tendon (Figure 36–12).

A. Tuberosity Fractures

Tuberosity fractures are typically known as dancer fractures because they are usually associated with an ankle inversion plantar flexion injury. It was commonly

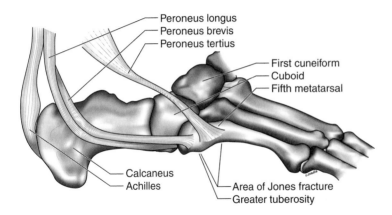

Figure 36–12. Anatomy of the proximal fifth metatarsal. (Courtesy of Ellsworth C. Seeley, M.D.)

thought that these injuries were associated with tearing of the peroneus brevis tendon insertion. However, this injury is more likely secondary to the plantar aponeurosis pulling from the base of the fifth metatarsal. Nondisplaced fracture carries an excellent prognosis, almost always healing in 4–6 weeks with conservative therapy. The athlete's treatment consists of limited weight bearing to pain with modified activity such as that used with second, third, and fourth metatarsal injuries. If needed the athlete can be immobilized in a walking cast, wooden (or steel shank) soled shoe, or walking boot. The immobilization can usually be removed by 3 weeks (average 3–6 weeks) in favor of modified footwear if pain has diminished. The patient then gradually may return to vigorous activity with most athletes returning to full sports activity in 6–8 weeks. Bony union usually takes place by 8 weeks. Orthopedic referral is needed for displaced fractures or comminuted fractures involving >30% of the cubometatarsal articular surface or step-off greater than 2 mm. Sometimes small displaced fractures at this site may require surgical removal if bony union does not occur secondary to chronic irritation. As a side note, be aware that certain conditions, such as apophysis of the tuberosity and accessory ossicles (os peroneum and os vesatranium), may radiographically mimic an avulsion fracture. Usually, these entities have smooth radiolucent lines on x-ray as compared to that of a fracture.

B. JONES' FRACTURES

Jones' fractures, first described by Sir Robert Jones in 1902, consist of a transverse fracture at the junction of the diaphysis and metaphysis corresponding to the area between the insertion of the peroneus brevis and tertius tendons without extending past the fourth and fifth intermetatarsal articulation (Figure 36–13).

The Jones' fracture is believed to occur when the ankle is in plantar flexion and a large adduction force is applied to the forefoot. It is important to realize this is a mid-foot injury with no prodromal symptoms. Therefore, the injury is classified as acute.

Torg et al showed that this fracture, in nonathletes, could heal in 6–8 weeks with strict non-weight-bearing immobilization. However, secondary to low vascularization and high stresses at the site of the Jones' fracture, the injury is associated with a poor outcome; it is

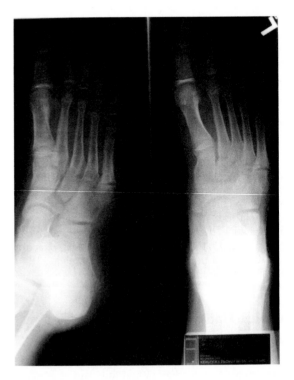

Figure 36–13. Jones' fracture.

plagued by delayed union and nonunion if treated conservatively in athletic patients. Many athletes are unwilling to tolerate non-weight-bearing ambulation for this extended period of time. Failure to heal by 12 weeks in this population is not uncommon. Those who undergo conservative treatment are placed on a non-weight-bearing immobilization protocol, in a plaster cast, for 6–8 weeks. If there is lack of clinical healing by 6–8 weeks, therapy is individualized. If clinical healing is present by 6–8 weeks, immobilization is continued in a fracture brace with range of motion and gradual weight bearing. If there are no signs of clinical healing, treatment must be individualized either with continued cast immobilization or surgical intervention. Surgical intervention for Jones' fracture consists of either intramedullary screw fixation (first choice; Figure 36–14) or bone grafting.

C. DIAPHYSEAL FRACTURES

Stress fractures distal to the site of Jones' fractures and acute on chronic fractures occurring in the same position as Jones' fractures are commonly seen in athletes who run. Pain is usually over the lateral aspect of the foot, over the fifth metatarsal base. Usually no significant trauma has been associated with these fractures. Prodromal symptoms occurring weeks to months in advance of an acute injury can often be elicited in the history.

Torg et al classified these stress fractures into three types based on radiographic appearance. By adhering to this classification, much of the guesswork for determining treatment can be avoided. Type I can show minimal periosteal reaction, indicating early stress reaction with no intramedullary sclerosis. Type II shows features of delayed union represented by a fracture line involving both cortices with associated periosteal bone union, a widened fracture line with adjacent radiolucency related to bone reabsorption, and, most importantly, evidence of intramedullary sclerosis. Type III represents nonunion fractures revealing a widened fracture line, new periosteal bone and radiolucency, and complete obliteration of the medullary canal by sclerotic bone. Acute or chronic injuries will show a fracture line at the same site as a Jones' fracture but also evidence of stress injury as described above. Careful history reveals the patient had a prodrome of symptoms consisting of intermittent pain.

Treatment of choice for acute nondisplaced diaphyseal stress fracture is non-weight-bearing immobilization. Ninety three percent of Torg's series healed within 7 weeks. Treatment for Type II stress fractures is individualized. Conservative treatment may take up to 20 weeks and result in nonunion. Complications of prolonged immobilization include recurrence of fracture and significant dysfunction from muscle atrophy and loss of range of motion. For athletes, surgical options are recommended. Symptomatic nonunion fracture or Type III fractures require surgical treatment. Casting and prolonged immobilization of acute or chronic fractures frequently fail, giving rise to delayed or nonunion fractures. Surgery is often needed and is the recommended procedure of choice.

The difference between screw fixation and bone grafting is recovery time. It takes up to 12 weeks to return to prefracture activity with grafting versus 6–8 weeks with screw fixation. Grafting carries a higher failure rate. Screw fixation is now recommended first and bone grafting if fixation fails.

Lawrence SJ, Botte MJ: Jones' fractures and related fractures of the proximal fifth metatarsal. Foot Fellow's Rev 1993;14(6):358. [PMID: 8406253]. (Guidelines for recognition and management of fractures of the fifth metatarsal.)

Nunley JA: Fractures of the base of the fifth metatarsal: the Jones fracture. Orthoped Clin North Am 2001;32(1):171. [PMID: 11465126]. (Guidelines for recognition and management of fractures of the fifth metatarsal.)

Strayer SM, Reece SG, Petrizzi MJ: Fractures of the proximal fifth metatarsal. Am Fam Physician 1999;59(9):2516. [PMID: 2891450]. (Guidelines for recognition and management of fractures of the fifth metatarsal.)

Torg JS, Pavlov H, Torg E: Overuse injuries in sport: the foot. Clin Sports Med 1987;6(2):298. [PMID: 2891450]. (Guidelines for recognition and management of fractures of the fifth metatarsal.)

Yu WD, Shapiro MS: Fractures of the fifth metatarsal. Physician Sportsmed 1998;26(2):47.

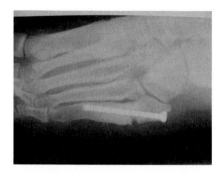

Figure 36–14. Intramedullary screw fixation for Jones' fracture. (Courtesy of Kentucky Sports Medicine, Dr. Mary Lloyd Ireland.)

SECTION IV

Geriatrics

Healthy Aging

37

Cynthia M. Williams, DO

Introduction

The population of the United States is aging. In 1900 4% of the population was 65 years or older. It is now over 13% of the population with a projection to be over 20% by 2030 (Figure 37–1). These aging demographics also reveal that the "oldest old," those persons age 85 years and older, are the most rapidly growing group within the population. This aging population is heterogeneous. Most research tends to group this population by ages with 65–74 years old being considered "young-old," 75–84 years old considered "old," and those 85 years and older "old-old." Those with the poorest health are considered "frail" or "at-risk" elders. These divisions, however, are arbitrary and do not take into account functional abilities, comorbidities, or the presence of other infirmities.

In the rapidly changing fields of health care financing and delivery, services that promote or improve functional abilities, prevent or delay disease progression, and improve the overall health status of this aging population are needed. Little information and evidence are available about what constitutes the best practices in health promotion, prevention, and counseling for older adults. This chapter will discuss the concepts of successful and healthy aging as well as make recommendations for preventive services, counseling, physical activity, and nutrition.

Federal Interagency Forum on Aging-Related Statistics: *Older Americans 2000: Key Indicator of Well-Being. Federal Interagency Forum on Aging-Related Statistics.* U.S. Government Printing Office, 2000.

Successful Aging

In a highly heterogeneous population, some individuals are ravaged early by a multitude of chronic conditions and disabilities, whereas others appear to have excellent health with a high level of functioning. Aging has been characterized as either usual (those individuals who exhibit typical nonpathological age-associated changes) or successful (those individuals who exhibit little or no loss in function relative to the average of their younger counterparts). Successful aging includes three factors: low probability of disease and disability, high cognitive and physical functioning, and active engagement with life. All three are important, but active engagement (interpersonal relations and productive activity) appears to represent the concept of successful aging most fully. Older adults who are actively engaged in life by being involved in such endeavors as volunteer activities have been found to enjoy a better quality of life.

There are many factors at work that determine how one individual will age compared to another. Genetic factors, although important in early life, become less dominant the longer one lives past the age of 75 years. Environmental and behavioral factors such as diet, exercise, education, nutrition, alcohol consumption, social supports, and coping styles are the key determinants in the development of disease and disability and therefore play a central role in successful, healthy aging. Successful aging has been associated with higher rated life satisfaction and with those older individuals who report their health as good to excellent.

Although successful and healthy aging is a goal for all individuals, there is a potential "risk" of having a population age successfully. The risks of potentially increasing life expectancy could pose a significant challenge to the health care system. It has been estimated that for every year of extra life expectancy added, an individual may spend on average 80% of that time in a disabled state. Another risk of successful aging involves the increased burden to society to care for an older more vulnerable population of survivors, with much of

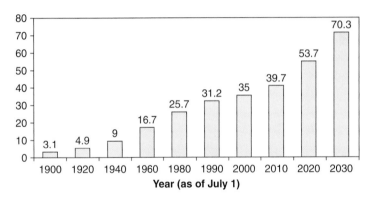

Figure 37–1. Number of persons 65 and older, 1900–2030 (numbers in millions). (From *Projections of the Total Resident Population by 5 Year Age Groups, Race, and Hispanic Origin with Special Age Categories: Middle Series, 1999 to 2000.* U.S. Census. Internet Release Date: January 13, 2000 with *Population Projections of the United States by Age, Sex, Race and Hispanic Origin: 1995–2050.* Current Population Reports, P25-1130. Data for 2000 are from the 2000 Census.)

that burden falling to aging family members to provide the primary support for aging parents and grandparents.

Cassel CK: Successful aging: how increased life expectancy and medical advances are changing geriatric care. Geriatrics 2001; 56:35.

Vaillant GE, Mukamal K: Successful aging. Am J Psychiatry 2001; 158:839.

Epidemiology of Aging

The majority of older adults are healthy and independent, and contribute to the society in which they live. The epidemiology of aging evaluates not only the demographic changes associated with aging but also evaluates those diseases causing excess morbidity and mortality and as well as those conditions that cause disability and decline in independent function. Many epidemiological studies on aging focus on prevention in an attempt to establish a scientific basis for minimizing the illness associated with aging and its related burden. Health status in the elderly is a function of the chronic diseases associated with aging as well as the "geriatric syndromes" most commonly associated with this population (Table 37–1). One measure of functional well-being is the number of restricted activity days an individual has because of illness or injury. On average for noninstitutionalized individuals over age 65, 6 restricted activity days were associated with falls, 4 days each for heart disease and arthritis, and 2 days each for cerebrovascular disease, hypertension, and visual impairments. It is obvious that the overall health status or well-being of older adults is highly complex, resulting from many interacting processes including risk factor exposure (tobacco, alcohol, drugs, diet, sedentary lifestyle), underlying biological age-related changes, progressive development of impairments, the consequences of these impairments, the risk that changes in health and function confer, and the interactions of underlying health status with acute clinical conditions. Many of the conditions previously thought of as "normal aging" are now known to be modifiable or even preventable if disease prevention and health promotion strategies are taken seriously not only by health care providers but by the patients for whom they care.

Fried LP: Epidemiology of aging. Epidemiol Rev 2000;22:95.

Prevention & Health Promotion

Prevention in geriatrics attempts to focus on those elements of life-style, environment, and health care management that will delay the onset of clinical expression of chronic diseases until the upper limit of the human life span is reached. This concept of a "compression" of morbidity and disability until the last years of life is a primary goal of any medical practice caring for older individuals. The primary strategy for prevention lies in the alteration of life-style and environmental factors that contribute to the development of chronic disease.

Table 37–1. Most common conditions associated with aging.

Arthritis
Hypertension
Heart disease
Hearing loss
Influenza
Injuries
Orthopedic impairments
Cataracts
Chronic sinusitis
Depression
Cancer
Diabetes mellitus
Visual impairments
Urinary incontinence
Varicose veins

In attempting to delay or prevent the onset of chronic, disabling disease, a strategy to promote health must become part of the provider–patient contract.

Health promotion does not necessarily equate with disease prevention. Health promotion is a broad term with the objectives of improving or enhancing the individual's current health status; if health is promoted early enough in life, disease may be prevented. The purpose of health promotion, especially as applied to the elderly, is the prevention of avoidable decline, frailty, and dependence.

Frailty as a concept is beyond the scope of this chapter, but it is important to understand that the purpose of health promotion is the delay or prevention of frailty. Frailty has been described as a multifaceted condition that is most likely associated with the pathophysiological affects of an altered metabolic balance, manifested by cytokine overexpression and hormonal decline. It can be thought of as the midway point between independence and near death in which the older adult becomes more vulnerable and is at highest risk for adverse health outcomes. The trajectory of frailty is one in which an older adult goes from independence to coping and needing assistance to "the dwindles" and functional decline. This leads to "frailty" with its attendant failure to thrive, disability, failure to cope, dependence, taking to bed, cachexia, and eventual death. Frailty has been associated with numerous conditions, many of which may be preventable if recognized early (Table 37–2).

Traditionally, preventive strategies have been thought of in terms of primary prevention or avoidance of disease occurrence, secondary prevention or detection of disease in its earliest asymptomatic state, and tertiary prevention or forestalling the further consequences of clinically manifest disease. Prevention for older adults, however, needs to be addressed within the framework of disability prevention or, put another way, function preservation.

For health promotion to be effective with older adults it needs to be individualized in terms of age of the patient, functional status, patient preference, and culture. Culture is especially important as it may be a barrier preventing an older adult from even contemplating a change in behavior to following through with preventive tests such as Pap smears, mammograms, and fecal occult blood testing. Culture is also important in understanding the older adult's health belief system. Without this understanding, a health care provider may not be able to negotiate a treatment strategy (including prevention practices) that is acceptable to the patient and the provider. Another important factor to consider is the socioeconomic status of the older adult, as persons with lower socioeconomic status tend to use preventive services less often and minority women tend to have higher rates of disability, indicating a vulnerable population, especially in terms of functional independence.

Secondary prevention including cancer screening is considerably uncertain for older adults. There is a paucity of evidence due to the lack of randomized clinical trials in patients older than 75 years old with most prevention/health promotion recommendations being extrapolated from younger subjects and reported as average effectiveness. When considering a screening test for older adults the risk of dying from the disease process, the benefits of the screening, the harms resulting from the screening, and the patient's values and preferences need to be weighed (Table 37–3). A patient who gets peace of mind from a screening test may warrant one but a patient who may become upset or agitated by the test or refuse further treatment should not be screened.

The United States Preventive Services Task Force (USPSTF) has set the standard for providing recommendations for clinical practice on preventive interventions including screening tests, counseling interventions, immunizations, and chemoprophylactic regimens. These standards were established by a review of the scientific evidence of the clinical effectiveness of each preventive service. In considering screening strategies,

Table 37–2. Conditions associated with frailty.

Advanced age, usually 85 years and older
Functional decline
Falls and associated injuries (hip fracture)
Polypharmacy
Chronic disease
Dementia and depression
Social dependency
Institutionalization or hospitalization
Nutritional impairment

Adapted from Hammerman D: Toward an understanding of frailty. Ann Intern Med 1999;130:945.

Table 37–3. Potential downside of screening tests.

There is no single operational definition for cancer
Aggressive cancers can be missed
Test results may be ambiguous requiring additional testing
Pseudodisease may be detected
Unnecessary treatments may be started
Following screening protocols may distract the physician
   from issues important to the patient

From Welch GH: Informed choice in cancer screening. JAMA 2001;285:2776.

major causes of death (Table 37–4) and remaining life expectancy of the older adult should be considered. A healthy 65-year-old individual has a life expectancy of another 15 to 20 years but an 85 year old has a life expectancy of 5 to 7 years, with most averaging 3 to 5 years. It has therefore been recommended that for healthy older adults screening can be stopped at 85 years, especially for those individuals who have had repeated negative screening in the past, who are frail or demented, or who have a limited quantity and quality of life remaining.

Many of the leading causes of death in this population are amenable to both primary and secondary preventive strategies, especially if targeted early in life. The major targets of prevention should therefore be focused at the major causes of death including coronary heart disease, cancer, and stroke, with the goals of reducing premature mortality caused by acute and chronic illness, maintaining function, enhancing quality of life, and extending active life expectancy. A priority in screening should be given to those preventive services that are easy to delivery with beneficial outcomes. Tables 37–5 and 37–6 outline the recommended preventive services and screening for individuals age 65 years and older. Details of preventive services can be found in the references noted within the tables with frequent updates found online at http://www.ahrq.gov and at http://members.aol.com/TGoldberg/prevrecs .htm.

The two health promotion activities that correlate the strongest with healthy and successful aging are physical activity and nutrition. However, they receive little attention by most health care providers even though they are of vital importance in averting frailty and in maintaining overall quality of life throughout the life span.

Brown M et al: Physical and performance measures for the identification of mild to moderate frailty. J Gerontol Med Sci 2000; 55A:M350.

Ostchega Y et al: The prevalence of functional limitations and disability in older persons in the US: data from the National Health and Nutrition Examination Survey III. J Am Geriatr Soc 2000;48:1132.

Thomas DR: The critical link between health-related quality of life and age-related changes in physical activity and nutrition. J Gerontol Med Sci 2001;56A:M599.

Physical Activity in Older Adults

You are never too old to start a physical activity program. Exercise received an **A** grading from the USPSTF recommending that older adults should be counseled on the benefits of aerobic and resistance exercise. Exercise either in the forms of aerobic training, resistance training, or life-style modification has many benefits in older adults, even the oldest-old.

Sixty percent of the American public is sedentary even though the human genome has been programmed for activity. Only 11% of the adult population in the United States reports engaging in regular, vigorous physical activity for 20 min or longer more than twice per week. The long-term effects of a sedentary life-style are numerous including functional limitations from chronic disease, obesity, diabetes mellitus, and cardiovascular disease. It has been estimated that 35% of deaths from coronary heart disease, 32% from colon cancer, and 35% from diabetes could be prevented if all Americans exercised.

Exercise seems too hard and dangerous and so many older adults will not even begin to contemplate a program of physical activity. From the risks of sudden death from cardiac causes and silent ischemia in master athletes to the possibility of overuse injuries and environmental hazards, exercise can appear hazardous to older adults. Older adults, however, are fairly resilient with respect to cardiovascular endurance and strength even after a period of detraining.

Factors associated with older adults participating in regular aerobic exercise include age, positive health perception, higher levels of education and income, and less than two chronic health conditions. Other predictors of physical performance in the elderly include prior exercise behavior and a supportive social network. Factors associated with physical inactivity, in addition to fear of undue harm caused by the activity itself, include caregiving responsibilities, lack of energy to exercise, absence of enjoyable scenery, and infrequent observations of others exercising in the neighborhood.

Exercise as a form of primary prevention has many benefits even for sedentary older adults. Exercise improves functional limitations, decreases progression to disability, reduces blood pressure and cardiovascular disease, reduces abdominal fat and glucose-stimulated insulin response, reduces falls in selected populations, minimizes or reverses physical frailty, improves overall sense of well-being and self-esteem, prevents hip fractures, improves longevity, reduces cardiovascular risk, improves bone density, decreases congestive heart fail-

Table 37–4. Preventable major causes of death associated with aging.

Cause of Death	Percentage of All Deaths
Cardiovascular disease	47
Cancer	20
Stroke	11
Lung disease	6
Accidents/falls	2
Diabetes mellitus	2

Adapted from Rubenstein LZ: Update on preventive medicine for older adults. Generations, Winter 1996–1997;20:47.

Table 37–5. Health promotion and preventive screening for older adults.[1]

Screening of Asymptomatic Older Adults[2,3]	Recommendation	Grade[4]	Notes
Blood pressure[a–c]	Every exam, at least every 1–2 years	A	Goal for primary prevention 140/80; treat systolic BP >160 mm Hg
Lipid disorders[d]	Screen men aged 35 and older and women aged 45 and older for total cholesterol and HDL-C; screen every 5 years until age 65	A	Those with CVD and DM need individualized management http://www.nhlbi.nih.gov.
Physician breast exam[5]	Annually beginning at age 40	A	
Mammogram[5,a,b,e,f]	Annually beginning at age 40 (ACS) or every 1–2 years ages 50–69 (USPSTF) or continue every 1–3 years ages 70–85 (AGS, USPSTF)	A C > 69 years old	Older women who undergo regular mammography are diagnosed with early stage disease and are less likely to die from breast cancer[g] http://www.americangeriatrics.org
Pap smear/pelvic exam[5,a,b,h,i]	Every 1–3 years after two or three negative exams; annual exams can be decreased or discontinued after ages 65–70	A C > 65 years old	No need to do a Pap smear in a women who had a complete hysterectomy (including cervix) http://www.americangeriatrics.org
Fecal occult blood testing[5,a,b,e,j,k]	Annually ≥ 50 years old	B	ACS recommends a total colon examination (air-contrast barium enema or colonoscopy) every 10 years; or fecal occult blood testing annually and sigmoidoscopy every 5 years http://www.cancer.org and http://www.gastro.org
Sigmoidoscopy	Every 5 years ≥50 years old	B	See above
Problem drinking[a,l]	Periodically	B	Counsel on drinking and driving; encourage men to limit drinking to 2 drinks per day and women to 1 drink per day (1 glass wine = 4 oz, 12 oz beer, or 1½ oz 80-proof spirits)
Hearing impairment[a,b]	Periodically	C	Inquire; use office audioscope
Vision/glaucoma screening[a,b,m]	Periodically by eye specialist age 65 years and older	C	
Glucose[6,n]	Periodic in high-risk groups	C	Every three years starting age 45 (American Diabetic Association); http://www.diabetes.org
Thyroid function test (TSH)[a,o]	TSH every 5 years for women over age 50 years	C	American College of Physicians; http://www.acp.org
Electrocardiogram[p]	Periodically 40–50 years	C	AHA; http://www.heart.org
Cognitive impairment[q,r,s]	As needed, be alert for decline	C	Follow-up based on caregivers concerns or informal descriptions of decline; assessment may be based on individual complaint of memory loss
Exam of mouth, nodes, testes, skin, heart, lung[e,p]	Annually	C	http://www.cancer.org http://www.heart.org

(continued)

Table 37–5. Health promotion and preventive screening for older adults.[1] (*Continued*)

Screening of Asymptomatic Older Adults[2,3]	Recommendation	Grade[4]	Notes
Bone mineral density (osteoporosis)[5,j,t]	If needed for treatment decision	C	Counsel perimenopausal women concerning calcium intake and hormone replacement http://www.nof.org
Prostate exam/PSA[5,a,e,u]	Annually age 50 and older if greater than 10 year life expectancy; not recommended by USPSTF	C–D	http://www.auanet.org; http://www.cancer.org USPSTF recommends counseling patients about potential benefits and harm of early detection and treatment
Chest x-ray[a,b]	Not recommended	D	

[1]ACS, American Cancer Society; AGS, American Geriatric Society; AHA, American Heart Association; bp, blood pressure; CVD, cardiovascular disease; DM, diabetes mellitus; HDL-C, high-density lipoprotein cholesterol; PSA, prostate-specific antigen; TSH, thyroid-stimulating hormone; USPSTF, United States Preventive Services Task Force.

[2]References:

[a]U.S. Preventive Services Task Force: *Guide to Clinical Preventive Services,* ed 2. Williams & Wilkins, 1996/2001. Updates available online at http://www.ahrq.gov.

[b]Institute for Clinical Systems Improvement: ICSI Health Care Guideline. Institute for Clinical Systems Improvement, 2001. http://www.ICSI.org.

[c]Smith SC et al: AHA/ACC guidelines for preventing heart attack and death in patients with atherosclerotic cardiovascular disease: 2001 update. Circulation 2001;104:1577.

[d]Agency for Healthcare Research and Quality: Screening for lipid disorders: recommendations and rationale. Article originally in Am J Prevent Med 2001;20(3S):73. http://www.ahrq.gov/clinic/aspmsuppl/lipidrr.htm.

[e]Smith RA et al: American Cancer Society guidelines for the early detection of cancer. CA 2000;50:34.

[f]American Geriatric Society Clinical Practice Committee: Breast cancer screening in older women. J Am Geriatr Soc 2000;48:842.

[g]McCarthey EP et al: Mammography use, breast cancer state at diagnosis, and survival among older women. J Am Geriatr Soc 2000;48:1226.

[h]Goldberg TH, Chavin SI: Preventive medicine and screening in older adults. J Am Geriatr Soc 1997;45:344.

[i]American Geriatric Society Clinical Practice Committee: Screening for cervical carcinoma in elderly women. J Am Geriatr Soc 2001;49:655.

[j]Goldberg TH: Update: preventive medicine and screening in older adults. J Am Geriatr Soc 1999;47:122.

[k]Ransohoff DF, Sandler RS: Screening for colorectal cancer. New Engl J Med 2002;346:40.

[l]Fingerhood M: Substance abuse in older people. J Am Geriatr Soc 2000;48:985.

[m]Smeeth L, Iliffe S: Community screening for visual impairment in the elderly (Cochrane Review). In: *The Cochrane Library,* Issue 3: Update Software, 2001.

[n]The Expert Committee on the Diagnosis and Classification of Diabetes Mellitus: Report of the Expert Committee on the Diagnosis and Classification of Diabetes Mellitus. Diabetes Care 2002;25(Suppl 1):S5.

[o]American College of Physicians: Screening for thyroid disease: clinical guideline, part 2. Ann Intern Med 1998;129:141. http://www.acponline.org.

[p]Grundy SM et al: Assessment of cardiovascular risk by use of multiple-risk-factor assessment equations: a statement for healthcare professionals from the American Heart Association and the American College of Cardiology. Circulation 1999;100:1481.

[q]Petersen RC et al: Practice parameter: early detection of dementia: mild cognitive impairment (an evidence-based review). Neurology 2001;56:1133.

[r]Knopman DS et al: Practice parameter: diagnosis of dementia (an evidence-based review). Neurology 2001;56:1143.

[s]Doody RS et al: Practice parameter: management of dementia (an evidence-based review). Neurology 2001;56:1154.

[t]National Osteoporosis Foundation: *Physicians Guide to the Prevention and Treatment of Osteoporosis.* html//www.nof.org/professional/clinical/clinical.htm.

[u]American Urological Society: Prostate-specific antigen (PSA) best practice policy. Oncology 2000;14:267.

[3]Screening recommendations for asymptomatic older adults; clinical judgment should be used always, especially with regard to patients >85 years old, who are frail, or who have a limited quality and quantity of life.

[4]A–B, do; C, equivocal; D, don't.

[5]Covered by Medicare.

[6]Medicare covers diabetes self-management.

Table 37–6. Chemoprophylaxis and counseling for older adults.[1]

Chemoprophylaxis/ Counseling[2]	Recommendation	Rating[3]	Notes[4]
Exercise[a-f]	Encourage aerobic and resistance exercise as tolerated	A	Encourage a minimum of 30 min of moderate-intensity exercise (brisk walking) daily; this may be done in intermittent or short bouts (~10 min) of activity throughout the day to total 39 min
Nutrition and weight management[a,b,f-n]	Limit intake of fat and cholesterol and maintain caloric balance; encourage a well-balanced diversified diet low in saturated fat and high in fiber	A–B	Health care providers should enlist the help of registered dietitians or qualified nutritionists; BMI = weight in kilograms divided by height in meters squared
Tobacco cessation counseling[a,b,f,g]	Complete history of tobacco use and assessment of dependence	A	The most effective clinician message is a brief, unambiguous, and informative statement on the need to stop using tobacco
Falls prevention[i]	Discuss measures to reduce the risk of falling including exercise to improve balance; environmental hazard reduction and monitoring medications	B–C	High-risk elders for falls include >75 years old or persons aged 70–74 using benzodiazepines, antihypertensives, or more than four medications; impaired cognition, strength, balance, and gait
Aspirin[g,j]	Discuss use with adults who are at increased risk of CHD including men > 40 years; postmenopausal women; and those with hypertension, diabetes, and current smokers	A	75 mg/day Discuss benefits—prevention of MI Discuss risks—GI and intracranial bleeding Most trials included men 40–75 years old Current benefits and harms may not be reliable for women and older men Older adults may derive greatest benefit because of their risk for CHD and stroke, but bleeding risks may also be greater
Tetanus–diphtheria vaccine[a,b]	Primary series then booster every 10 years	A	
Influenza vaccine[5,a,g]	Annually 65 years and older or if chronically ill	B	
23-Valent pneumococcal vaccine[5,a,b]	At least once at age 65 years	B	

(continued)

Table 37–6. Chemoprophylaxis and counseling for older adults.[1] (*Continued*)

Chemoprophylaxis/Counseling[2]	Recommendation	Rating[3]	Notes[4]
Calcium[a,k]	800 to 1500 mg/day	B	National Osteoporosis Foundation
Estrogen/estrogen receptor-modifying agent (SERM)/or bisphosphonate[k,l]	Postmenopausal women	B	Osteoporosis prevention and treatment National Osteoporosis Foundation

[1]BMI, body mass index; CHD, coronary heart disease; GI, gastrointestinal; MI, myocardial infarction.

[2]References:

[a]U.S. Preventive Services Task Force: *Guide to Clinical Preventive Services,* ed 2. Williams & Wilkins, 1996/2001. Updates available online at http://www.ahrq.gov.

[b]Institute for Clinical Systems Improvement: *ICSI Health Care Guideline.* Institute for Clinical Systems Improvement, 2001. http://www.ICSI.org.

[c]Pate RR et al: Physical activity and public health: a recommendation from the Centers for Disease Control and Prevention and the American College of Sports Medicine. JAMA 1995;273:402.

[d]Fletcher CF et al: Statement on exercise: benefits and recommendations for physical activity programs for all Americans: a statement for health professionals by the Committee on Exercise and Cardiac Rehabilitation of the Council on Clinical Cardiology. American Heart Association. Circulation 1996;94:857.

[e]Mazzeo RS et al: American College of Sports Medicine Position Stand: exercise and physical activity for older adults. Med Sci Sports Exerc 1998;30:992.

[f]Institute of Medicine Health and Behavior: *The Interplay of Biological, Behavioral, and Societal Influences.* National Academy Press, 2001.

[g]Smith SC et al: AHA/ACC guidelines for preventing heart attack and death in patients with atherosclerotic cardiovascular disease: 2001 update. Circulation 2001;104:1577.

[h]Institute of Medicine: *The Role of Nutrition in Maintaining Health in the Nation's Elderly.* National Academy Press, 2000.

[i]Feder G et al: Guidelines for the prevention of falls in people over 65. Br Med J 2000;321:1007.

[j]Agency for Healthcare Research and Quality: *Aspirin for the Primary Prevention of Cardiovascular Events. Recommendations and Rationale,* January 2002. http://www.ahrq.gov/clinic/3rduspstf/asprin/asprr.htm.

[k]National Osteoporosis Foundation: *Physicians Guide to the Prevention and Treatment of Osteoporosis.* html//www.nof.org/professional/clinical/clinical.htm.

[l]Goldberg TH: Update: preventive medicine and screening in older adults. J Am Geriatr Soc 1999;47:122.

[3]A–B, do; C, equivocal.

[4]Web sites of interest: http://www.ctfphc.org (Canadian Task Force on Preventive Health Care), http://www.ahrq.gov (Agency for Health Care Research and Quality), and http://www.ICSI.org (Institute for Clinical Systems Improvement).

[5]Covered by Medicare; Medicare also covers hepatitis B vaccine.

ure, protects against cardiac electrical instability and sudden death, improves blood lipids, modifies obesity, and improves osteoarthritis.

Physical activity, exercise, and physical fitness have distinct definitions that in and of themselves may be barriers to how health care providers counsel their older adults concerning the merits of engaging in some form of physical activity (Table 37–7). Life-style physical activities that are more unstructured as compared to a formal exercise plan are being shown to increase levels of physical activity in sedentary populations.

Patients who are counseled on risk-reducing behaviors such as diet and exercise tend to be more compliant than those who are never counseled. However, in a recent Centers for Disease Control and Prevention (CDC) analysis of seven states and Puerto Rico only 40% of patients received risk-reduction counseling. Health care providers may not feel comfortable giving information about physical activity to older adults because of the misperception of potential harm and the misperception that to reap the benefits of exercise vigorous, endurance training must be undertaken. It has now been shown that promoting changes in life-style physical activity can improve function and quality of life.

Gardner MM, Robertson C, Campbell AJ: Exercise in preventing falls and fall related injuries in older people; a review of randomized controlled trials. Br J Sports Med 2000;34:7.

Gregg EW et al: Physical activity and osteoporotic fracture risk in older women. The Study of Osteoporotic Fractures Research Group. Ann Intern Med 1998;129:81.

Hambrecht R et al: Regular physical exercise corrects endothelial dysfunction and improves exercise capacity in patients with chronic heart failure. Circulation 1998;98:2709.

Miller ME et al: Physical activity, functional limitations, and disability in older adults. J Am Geriatr Soc 2000;48:1264.

Penninx B et al: Physical exercise and the prevention of disability in activities of daily living in older persons with osteoarthritis. Arch Intern Med 2001;161:2309.

Pescatello LS: Exercising for health: the merits of lifestyle physical activity. West J Med 2001;174:114.

Pescatello LS, VanHeest JL: Physical activity mediates a healthier body weight in the presence of obesity. Br J Sports Med 2000;34:86.

Shephard RJ: *Aging, Physical Activity and Health.* Human Kinetics, 1997.

Shephard RJ, Balady GJ: Exercise as cardiovascular therapy. Circulation 1999;99:963.

Promoting Life-style Physical Activity in Older Adults

For an older adult to make the expected change in physical activity the importance of the change should be made clear. The overall benefits of exercise and the potential risks of engaging in exercise need to be explained, with emphasis on the benefits that the individual will gain. A detailed exercise history should be obtained to include the patient's lifelong pattern of activities and interests; activity level in the past 2–3 months to determine a current baseline; concerns and perceived barriers regarding exercise including issues regarding lack of time, unsafe environment, cardiovascular risks, and limitations of existing chronic diseases; level of interest and motivation for exercise; and social preferences regarding exercise. The discussion should be documented with a recommendation by the American Heart Association for an informed consent for exercise training to be placed in the patient's record. A physical examination should be performed with emphasis on cardiopulmonary systems and any other limiting conditions the patient may have including visual or musculoskeletal impairments. The American

Table 37–7. Definitions of exercise, physical activity, physical fitness, and life-style physical activity.

Term	Definition
Physical activity	Any bodily movement produced by skeletal muscles that results in energy expenditure. Physical activity is a behavior. People who are physically active tend to have a higher level of physical fitness.
Exercise	Physical activity that is planned, structured, repetitive, and purposeful with the objective to improve or maintain physical fitness. Exercise is a subset of physical activity.
Physical fitness	The ability to perform prolonged work that is measured by maximal oxygen intake ($\dot{V}o_2$) and includes cardiovascular fitness, muscle strength, body composition, and flexibility. Physical fitness is a characteristic that people strive to achieve.
Life-style physical activity	The daily accumulation of at least 30 min of moderate intensity self-selected activities including all leisure, occupational, and household activities. These activities may be planned or unplanned and are part of everyday life.

Adapted from Pescatellow LS: Exercising for health: the merits of lifestyle physical activity. West J Med 2001;74:114 and Shephard RJ, Balady GJ: Exercise as cardiovascular therapy. Circulation 1999;99:963.

College of Sports Medicine recommends stress testing for any older adult who intends to begin a vigorous exercise program such as strenuous cycling or running (Table 37–8). Conditions that are absolute and relative contraindications to exercise stress testing or embarking on an exercise program should be evaluated (Table 37–9). Finally an exercise prescription should be written on a prescription pad to strengthen the endorsement for increased physical activity. The prescription should include frequency, intensity, type, and time of exercise.

It is important to "start low and go slow," especially if the older adult has been relatively sedentary. It is more important to get the older adult to do any physical activity than to prescribe something that is unattainable. The health of older adults may be better served if they perform a little more exercise or activity than the previous week, attempting to incorporate the activity into their normal daily lives such as walking to a store or gardening. The goal should be for the person to feel "pleasantly" tired a few hours after the activity with the aim to increase the activity slowly until a desired level of fitness is obtained.

Christman C, Andersen RA: Exercise and older patients: guidelines for the clinician. J Am Geriatr Soc 2000;48:318.

Fletcher GF et al: AHA Scientific Statement: Exercise standards for testing and training; a statement for healthcare professionals from the American Heart Association. Circulation 2001;104:1694.

The Exercise Prescription

The exercise prescription should include both aerobic and resistance exercise. Aerobic exercise in the form of walking from a more moderate to a vigorous pace is very attainable for most if not all community-dwelling elders, especially if barriers of environment and safety are taken into account. Aerobic exercise should be performed on most days of the week with the goal of achieving 30 min of moderate to vigorous intensity exercise daily. This can also be achieved by splitting the 30-min goal into two or three sessions.

Resistance training is necessary to counter the muscle atrophy of aging. Current research indicates that for healthy persons of all ages, even those with chronic diseases, a single set of 15 repetitions performed a minimum of 2 days per week can develop and maintain muscle mass, endurance, and strength. Each workout session should consist of 8–10 different exercises that train the major muscle groups. To minimize the possibility of orthopedic risk the exercise should start at a lower intensity level such as 10 repetitions, start with low weight, and progress slowly over 2–4 weeks. These exercises do not need special equipment and can be done at home with light-weight dumbbells and ankle weights, heavy household objects such as plastic milk jugs filled with water or gravel, food cans of various weights, or inner tubes and elastic bands.

Table 37–8. Graded exercise test (GXT) recommendations according to coronary heart disease (CHD) risk factors[1] and exercise stratification.

Risk	Moderate Intensity Exercise	Vigorous Intensity Exercise
	Walking at 3–4 mph Cycling for pleasure <10 mph Moderate effort swimming Racket sports Pulling or carrying golf clubs	Walking briskly uphill or with a load Cycling fast or racing >10 mph Swimming, fast tread or crawl Singles tennis or racquetball
Low Men <45 years old and women <55 years old with ≤1 CHD risk factor and asymptomatic	GXT not necessary	GXT not necessary
Moderate Men ≥54 and women ≥55 years old or those with ≥2 CHD risk factors	GXT not necessary	GXT recommended
High Individuals with symptoms of disease or known metabolic, cardiovascular, or pulmonary disease	GXT recommended	GXT recommended

Adapted from American College of Sports Medicine: *ACSM's Guidelines for Exercise Testing and Prescription*, ed 6. Lippincott Williams & Wilkins, 2000.
[1]CHD risk factors: family history, cigarette smoking, hypertension, dyslipidemia, impaired fasting glucose tolerance, obesity, sedentary life-style.

Table 37–9. Absolute and relative contraindications to exercise stress testing or starting an exercise program.

Absolute Contraindications	Relative Contraindications
Acute myocardial infarction within 2days	Left main coronary stenosis
Critical or severe aortic stenosis	Moderate stenotic valvular heart disease
Active endocarditis	Tachyarrhythmias or bradyarrhythmias
Decompensated heart failure	Atrial fibrillation with uncontrolled ventricular rate
High-risk unstable angina	Hypertrophic cardiomyopathy
Active myocarditis or pericarditis	Electrolyte abnormalities
Acute pulmonary embolism or infarction	Mental impairment leading to an inability to cooperate
Serious cardiac arrhythmias causing hemodynamic compromise	High-degree atrioventricular block
Acute noncardiac condition that may affect exercise performance or may exacerbate the condition (infection, renal failure, thyrotoxicosis)	
Physical disability that precludes safe and adequate test performance	
Inability to obtain consent	

Adapted from Fletcher GF et al: Exercise standards for testing and training: a statement for healthcare professions from the American Heart Association. Circulation 2001;104:1649.

Promotion of an active life-style is important at all ages and the benefits to older adults are numerous. Health care providers need to realize that for exercise to be beneficial it need not be strenuous or prolonged. Just encouraging patients to get up out of their chairs and start moving will improve not only the quality but the quantity of disabled free years.

Feigenbaum MS, Pollock ML: Prescription of resistance training for health and disease. Med Sci Sports Exerc 1999;31:38.

Snell PG, Mitchell JH: Physical inactivity: an easily modified risk factor? Circulation 1999;100:2.

Nutrition

Nutrition has been named a priority for Healthy People 2010. As individuals age, chronic diseases, functional impairments, polypharmacy, and age-related physiological and socioeconomic changes may all act in concert to make an older adult nutritionally at risk. Good general nutrition beginning early in life and maintained throughout the life span is important for overall health and is one approach to successful aging. Nutrition has been associated with a reduction in disability and death from heart disease and with its social and nurturing aspects that may lead to increased physical activity, physical functioning, independence and overall quality of life. Health care providers, however, rarely take the time to consider the diet and nutritional status of their patients.

A. Problems in Older Adults

Many disorders that affect older adults are related to nutritional status. Poor nutritional status may be the result of too little dietary intake leading to malnutrition, too much dietary content for actual expenditure leading to obesity, and inappropriate dietary intake exacerbating such conditions as diabetes, hypertension, and renal insufficiency. With aging weight tends to increase until the seventh decade when it stabilizes or declines. Obesity tends to be a problem for the "young-old," whereas undernutrition is commonly encountered in the "old-old." Although animal studies have indicated increased longevity with lower body weight and caloric restriction without malnutrition, studies on the relative risk of obesity to mortality in older adults are inconsistent, ranging from a protective effect for hip fractures to increased functional disability.

A multitude of interrelated factors can place an older adult at nutritional risk (Table 37–10). Oral health contributes greatly to poor nutrition and can be a causative factor in malnourished older patients. Among edentulous individuals, not wearing dentures or wearing defective dentures is associated with malnutrition. For individuals with natural dentition, those with fewer occluding pairs of teeth and the presence of mobile teeth are also associated with poor nutritional status.

Many older adults, especially minority and rural populations, are at nutritional risk from inadequate intake of key nutrients including vitamin B_6, vitamin C, vitamin E, calcium, phosphorus, and zinc. There is low consumption of fiber, fruits and vegetables, breads, and other grain products within more economically deprived populations. Other dietary nutritional needs not being met by older adults regardless of their ability to acquire safe and nutritious foods include niacin, riboflavin, vitamin B_{12}, magnesium, and iron. Many of these nutritional factors are important for bone health,

Table 37–10. Nutrients, requirements with signs of excess and deficiency.

Nutrient	Requirement	Signs of Deficiency	Signs of Excess
Vitamin A	Requirements **decrease** with advancing age 3333 IU for men 2667 IU for women	Loss of bright, moist appearance of eyes; dry conjunctiva; gingivitis	Toxic effects include headache, lassitude, anorexia, reduced white blood cell count, impaired hepatic function, and bone pain with hypercalcemia; hip fracture
Vitamin B_1 (thiamine)	1.1–1.2 mg/day	Common in alcoholic elderly and institutionalized elderly; disordered cognition (delirium), neuropathies, and cardiomegaly	Liver damage and exacerbation of peptic ulcer disease especially with those using megadoses
Vitamin B_2 (riboflavin)	1.1–1.3 mg/day	Cheilosis, angular stomatitis, gingivitis; changes to tongue papillae	
Vitamin B_6 (pyroxidine)	1.5–1.7 mg/day	Glossitis, peripheral neuropathy, and dementia especially related to alcohol abuse	Liver damage and nervous system dysfunction especially with those using megadoses
Vitamin B_{12}	2.4 µg/day	Pallor, optic neuritis, hyporeflexia, ataxia, anorexia; loss of proprioception, vibratory sense, and memory loss; megaloblastic anemia	
Vitamin C		Gingival hypertrophy, bleeding gums, petechiae, and ecchymoses	Megadose use can cause diarrhea, oxalate kidney and bladder stones; impaired absorption of vitamin B_{12}; interfere with serum and urine glucose testing; false-negative hemoccult testing
Vitamin D	10–15 µg/day (400–600 IU/day)	Osteomalacia; severe bone pain and osteoporosis; muscular hypotonia; pulmonary macrophage dysfunction	Nausea, headache, anorexia, weakness, and fatigue; interferes with vitamin K absorption
Vitamin K	Widely distributed in food and provided by synthesis of intestinal bacteria; supplements advised for fat malabsorption syndromes and long-term antibiotic therapy	Hemorrhages in skin or gastrointestinal tract; unexplained prolongation of prothrombin time	Unknown
Folic acid	400 µg/day	Pallor, stomatitis, glossitis, memory impairment, depression	
Vitamin E	400 IU/day	Deficiency is rare; abundant in diet	Interfere with vitamin K metabolism; thrombophlebitis; gastrointestinal (GI) distress; possible reduction in wound healing
Niacin	14–16 mg/day	Fissured tongue; dry; thickened; scaling; hyperpigmented skin; diarrhea; dementia	Histamine flush; liver toxicity
Calcium	1200–1500 mg/day	Osteoporosis	

(continued)

Table 37–10. Nutrients, requirements with signs of excess and deficiency. (*Continued*)

Nutrient	Requirement	Signs of Deficiency	Signs of Excess
Iron		Rare secondary to increased iron stores; usually secondary to pathological blood loss	Constipation; excess iron usually given when anemia of chronic disease is misdiagnosed as iron deficiency anemia; some association between neoplasia and coronary artery disease
Zinc		Impaired wound healing; diarrhea; decreased vision, olfaction, insulin, and immune function; anorexia; impotence	GI disturbance; sideroblastic anemia from impaired copper absorption; adverse effect on cellular immunity; interfere with other vitamin absorption

Adapted from Johnson L: Vitamins and aging. In: Morley JE et al (editors). *The Science of Geriatrics,* Vol. 2. Springer Publishing, 2000, p 379 and Dywer JT, Gallo JJ, Reichel W: Assessing nutritional status in elderly patients. Am Fam Physician 1993;47:613.

especially regarding the intake of potassium, magnesium, and fruits and vegetables with a higher bone mineral density in both men and women. Over 5% of households with older adults struggle to meet basic food needs. Physical signs of nutritional deficiencies and excess are important to recognize in older individuals (Table 37–11).

Optimal weight for enhanced longevity in an aging population is controversial as is the relationship between body mass index (BMI: weight in kilograms divided by height in meters^2) and mortality. For 60- to 69-year-old men and women, the lowest mortality is associated with a BMI of 26.6 kg/m^2 and 27.3 kg/m^2, respectively. Studies have shown that decreases in free fat mass and total body fat occur in older people even in the absence of disease and that weight loss rather than weight gain has a greater affect on mortality and functional status. Seidell et al reported that extremes of weight or BMI <24 kg/m^2 or >30 kg/m^2 may increase mortality, especially in men. In nonsmoking older adults a BMI <24 kg/m^2 was associated with higher mortality, whereas a higher BMI showed no relationship to mortality even in individuals with cardiovascular disease and other potential risk factors. Stevens et al reported that increased BMI was associated with increased mortality between the ages of 30 and 74, and that the relative risk of increased body weight was higher in younger subjects. It also appears that a BMI >27 kg/m^2 and the associated increased risk of mortality may not be related to body habitus per se but to a sedentary life-style and physical inactivity. Finally, a BMI <22 kg/m^2 was found to be related to dependency in activities of daily living and lower overall survival.

B. REQUIREMENTS FOR OLDER ADULTS

Physiological changes associated with aging can have an impact on the older adult's nutritional requirement. Some of these changes include the following:

1. Changes in taste and smell that may affect palatability of food and decrease intake; a progressive loss of taste buds predominantly in the anterior tongue for sweet and salt; decreased saliva production.

2. Decrease in basal metabolic rate most likely from a decrease in lean body mass and a sedentary life-style leading to decreased caloric consumption.

3. Decreased gastrointestinal motility with slower gastric emptying leading to a sensation of early satiety.

4. Decreased ability to concentrate urine leading to decreased thirst and dehydration.

Energy requirements are decreased in the elderly. The recommended daily allowance (RDA) is 2300 kcal for a 77-kg male and 1900 kcal for a 65-kg female. It has been suggested there is a need for a 10% reduction based on basal energy expenditure between ages 51 and 75 with an additional 10–15% reduction after age 75. Therefore, men between the ages of 51 and 75 would require 2070 kcal and women would require 1710 kcal. After age 75 men would require approximately 1800 kcal and women approximately 1500 kcal. Protein intake to meet the needs of a community-dwelling older population is 0.8–1 g/kg/day or about 12–14% of total calories. The recommended amount of dietary carbohydrate is between 50 and 100 g/day (55–60% of total calories) with an increase in proportion of com-

Table 37–11. Risk factors associated with poor nutritional status and weight loss in older adults.

Psychosocial	Environmental	Behavioral	Pathological	Physiological
Dementia	Nursing home	Physical inactivity	Cancer	Decreased lean body mass with associated lower basal energy expenditure
Depression	Inability to cook or purchase food	Functional impairments	Chronic cardiac, renal, or pulmonary failure	Constipation
Bereavement	Unappealing food preparation	Personal dietary restrictions	Diabetes mellitus	Decreased taste and smell
Isolation		Idiosyncratic food preferences	Drug–nutrient interactions	Decreased thirst
Poverty		Religious restrictions	Alcoholism	Dental changes
Caregiver fatigue		Prescribed dietary modifications	Malabsorption	Lactose intolerance
Neglect			Swallowing disorders	Anorexia of aging associated with loss of appetite, predisposing stress and weight loss
Abuse			Chronic infections	
Suicidality			Thyroid disease	
			Medications Prescribed/over the counter Polypharmacy Nutritional supplements	

Adapted from Fiatrarone M: Nutrition in geriatric patients. Hosp Pract 1990;Sept 30:38 and Lipschitz DA: Approaches to the nutritional support of the older patients. Clin Geriatr Med 1995;11:715.

plex carbohydrates to simple sugars. A prudent diet should have 30% or less calories as fat with less than 10% saturated fats (fats that are solid at room temperature such as butter, lard, salt pork, meat fat, coconut or palm oil, hydrogenated margarine or shortening), 10–15% monounsaturated fats, and not more than 10% polyunsaturated fats (fats that are liquid at room temperature). Dietary cholesterol should be limited to 300 mg or less per day. Little is known about fiber requirements of adult diets but it is recommended that intake be 25 g/day.

Dehydration is a particular problem of the elderly and often goes unrecognized. Dehydration may be responsible of 7% of hospitalizations. It may be due to excessive losses or inadequate intake of fluids. Those who are chronically ill, demented, and have poor bladder control often do not drink enough fluids. Fever, diarrhea, malabsorption, vomiting, and hemorrhage can lead to excessive loss of fluid as may therapy with diuretics and laxatives. The recommendation is to drink 30 ml/kg/day or on average six to eight cups of water per day.

C. OBESITY

The significance of mild to moderate obesity in the elderly is unclear. Individual consideration is required. Height/weight charts for ideal body weight based on life insurance tables are probably relevant only to the age of 54. Recommending weight loss especially to an older individual must be done with caution as weight loss in general carries poor prognosis. For patients under the age of 70 who are 20% above ideal body weight, prudent weight loss should be recommended. For patients over the age of 70, if a medical condition is likely to be significantly improved by prudent dieting then it should be recommended. Such conditions would include severe hypertension, back pain from obesity, degenerative joint disease, gait and balance problems, and diabetes mellitus. Dietary management of hypercholesterolemia is controversial, especially if the individual is already close to or at ideal body weight. Severe restriction of fat may lead to weight loss, causing more harm than good. A dietician should be utilized in formulating a weight loss program for older patients with a goal of 0.5 to 1 pound of weight loss per week.

D. Undernutrition

Undernutrition and weight loss can be significant in older persons and are associated with increased mortality. Undernutrition can result either from lack of calories or poor protein intake. When calories are insufficient but protein is normal, older adults insidiously and unintentionally lose weight. Treatment is aimed at increasing calories by ensuring palatable meals that are high in both carbohydrates and fat. Frequent small meals, using caloric dense nutritional supplements as snacks, or meal replacements can be of benefit as well as a rehabilitative program of physical therapy and exercise. Failure to gain weight is associated with a poor prognosis.

The other cause of undernutrition is protein energy undernutrition (PEU). A BMI <17 kg/m^2 is considered definitive for chronic PEU and a BMI between 17 kg/m^2 and 20 kg/m^2 is considered to be consistent with but not diagnostic of PEU. It is more common in hospitalized and institutionalized older adults and is a response to stress associated with an increased need for calories and protein. A hallmark of protein–energy malnutrition is an albumin level of <3.0 g/dL. Weight loss may not be present and by anthropometric measures these individuals may be obese. It is important to monitor the nutritional status of acutely hospitalized older adults. Dehydration should be corrected; adequate voluntary food intake should be ensured with a nutrient goal of 35 kcal/kg body weight with 20% of those calories from protein. Staff and/or family should be available to assist in feeding those who are functionally impaired. In some cases enteral, peripheral, or percutaneous gastrostomy tube placement may be necessary to ensure adequate nutritional support.

The old adage "we are what we eat" is applicable to our aging population. Recently in a small study of older adults it was shown that energy intake from protein, carbohydrate, or fat enhanced memory independently of elevations in blood glucose. These findings along with the known affects of macronutrient deficiencies on cognition should give the primary care clinician another reason and opportunity to promote nutritional health in older adults.

American Dietetic Association: Position of the American Dietetic Associaiton: nutrition, aging and the continuum of care. J Am Diet Assoc 2000;100:580.

Calle EE et al: Body-mass index and mortality in a prospective cohort of U.S. adults. New Engl J Med 1999;341:1097.

Kaplan RJ et al: Dietary protein, carbohydrate, and fat enhance memory performance in the healthy elderly. Am J Clin Nutr 2001;74:687.

Seidell JC et al: Overweight, underweight and mortality. Arch Intern Med 1996;156:958.

Stevens J et al: The effect of age on the association between body-mass index and mortality. New Engl J Med 1998;338:1.

U.S. Department of Health and Human Services: *Healthy People 2010: Understanding and Improving Health.* U.S. Department of Health and Human Services, 2000.

Common Geriatric Problems

38

Daphne P. Bicket, MD, MLS

The syndromes of failure to thrive, pressure ulcers, and falls, common in the elderly, share several criteria that make them particularly challenging. Their etiologies are multifactorial; they require an interdisciplinary approach to maximize care; and they often herald disability, institutionalization, and death. Maintaining open communication with patients and/or caregivers is vital. It not only empowers them to play a role in their care, but also focuses their expectations realistically. Clinicians should continually reassess their objectives, remembering that in elders concern is as much for independence and quality of life as it is for cure.

FAILURE TO THRIVE

General Considerations

Failure to thrive (FTT), a syndrome of community-dwelling elders, is also known as the dwindles, wasting, or end-stage frailty. Typically the patient is brought in because of weight loss, apathy, and overall functional and social decline. The National Institute on Aging defines it "as a syndrome of weight loss, decreased appetite and poor nutrition, and inactivity, often accompanied by dehydration, depressive symptoms, impaired immune function, and low cholesterol."

Pathogenesis

Despite this formal definition, geriatricians are still investigating and refining the concept of this syndrome and its causes. The condition of sarcopenia, the loss of muscle with age, has been implicated as one of several contributors to the syndrome and bears mention not only because of its potential contribution, but also because weight training and nutritional supplementation have been found to be effective. Of note, loss of lean body mass also diminishes the acute phase response to physiological stress and decreases immune competence. Not all individuals experience sarcopenia, however, so its application in FTT is not universal. Weight loss has been further studied in other contexts.

Weight loss was followed for 4 years in a cohort of 247 community-dwelling male veterans 65 years of age. A 4% annual weight loss was the cutoff for defining clinically important involuntary weight loss and was seen in 13% of the subjects. This group also experienced higher mortality: 28% in weight losers versus 11% in nonlosers. Interestingly, anthropometric decrements occurred in centrally distributed fat, not muscle. In another study an annual weight loss of ≥3% in a cohort of nuns was associated with a 2.7–3.9 times greater likelihood of becoming dependent in activities of daily living. Finally, Framingham data show that a body mass index of <21.40 is a significant predictor of subsequent nursing home placement for elderly women. Thus, it remains unclear as to what kind of weight loss is correlated with decline and mortality, and whether it heralds or follows another process that itself initiates FTT.

Clinical Findings

A. SYMPTOMS AND SIGNS

Weight loss is only one aspect of FTT. Commonly recurring features are impaired physical functioning, malnutrition, depression, and cognitive impairment. A useful working definition requires that three criteria be met: biopsychosocial failure, weight loss or undernutrition, and no immediate explanation for the condition, eg, no underlying terminal disease. This framework provides a practical structure for the evaluation and treatment of the syndrome.

B. UNDERLYING PRINCIPLES

In approaching the patient, several caveats bear review. First, baseline functional data are the foundation of eldercare and should be obtained annually on all elders. Geriatric assessment is covered in Chapter 40. Second, although function declines predictably over time, it does so at a **variable rate** based on known age-associated metabolic parameters such as forced expiratory volume at 1 s (FEV_1), basal metabolic rate (BMR), and glomerular filtration rate (GFR). Third, as in infants, FTT can occur from organic and nonorganic causes, thus necessitating an approach that includes medical, psychological, functional, and social domains. Finally, conceptualizing FTT as a model initiated by a "trigger" event that impacts all four domains sets a framework for the evaluation and management of the process.

C. History and Physical Examination

The history and physical examination are the cornerstones of evaluation. The history provided by the patient and caregiver is a key in establishing the onset of the condition and uncovering potential triggers. Common acute medical problems include infections, constipation, peptic ulcer disease, and exacerbation of chronic diseases. Common chronic diseases include congestive heart failure, ischemic heart disease, chronic obstructive pulmonary disease, cancer, uncontrolled endocrine disease, tuberculosis, dementia, and depression.

Drugs must be reviewed to identify any new additions from other physicians, over-the-counter drugs, unforeseen drug interactions, changes in renal–hepatic function, or drug–food interactions. Levels are nonspecific in this setting; normal therapeutic levels can also have adverse effects (see Table 38–1 for drugs that con-

Table 38–1. Drugs that contribute to anorexia or FTT.

Alendronate
Antibiotics
Antiarrhythmics
Antihistamines
α-Antagonists
Benzodiazepines
β-Blockers
Calcium antagonists
Digoxin
Diuretics
Glucocorticoids
Iron supplements
Metformin
Metronidazole
Neuroleptics
Nonsteroidal antinflammatory drugs
Narcotics
Selective serotonin reuptake inhibitors
Tricyclic antidepressants
Xanthines
More than six prescription drugs

See Zhan C et al: Potentially inappropriate medication use in the community-dwelling elderly: findings from the 1996 medical expenditure panel survey JAMA 2001;286:2823; Huffman GB: Evaluating and treating unintentional weight loss in the elders. Am Fam Physician 2002;65:640; and Verdery RB: Clinical evaluation of failure to thrive in older people. Clin Geriatr Med 1997;13:769.

tribute to anorexia, weight loss, and FTT). A recent survey revealed that between 2.6% and 13.3% of Medicare recipients had drugs prescribed that are generally thought to be harmful to elders. More women than men are at risk as well as patients reporting poor health status and those using more than 14 prescriptions in a year. Physicians should consider alcohol ingestion and its potential influence on medications being prescribed and should review how and when the patient is taking medication.

A psychosocial history is particularly important. Do patient and/or caregiver note increased memory loss or depression? Has there been a recent change in the social structure such as a death of a person or pet or the moving away of a key friend or family member? Are there signs of caregiver burnout? Is there a recent environmental change either in the home, neighborhood, church, or community? Are there new financial concerns for the patient? Does the patient have access to adequate, appropriate foods and the means to prepare and eat them? Elders are often too proud to reveal their needs; if the history does not supply sufficient information, a housecall can provide further data.

A comprehensive physical examination is important. Special emphasis should be placed on those items noted in Table 38–2. Table 38–3 lists ancillary test recommendations.

Table 38–2. Physical examination details and considerations.[1]

Vital signs: BMI <21 or percentage of weight loss since last visit, BP and HR in two positions, pulse for 60 s; abnormal if >88/min, respiratory rate and effort
Ears: hearing defects or tinnitus lead to social isolation
Eyes: cataracts/vision disturbance lead to depression and isolation
Oral health: tooth or gum disease impairs eating
Swallowing: aspiration and cough can negatively impact eating; have patient swallow liquid in your presence if any question of aspiration
JVD: most sensitive marker for CHF exacerbation
Breast mass: will often be unnoticed by the patient
Abdomen: masses, constipation, urinary bladder distention
Skin: sacrum and feet, axillae, panniculus, and groin for breakdown/candida/impetigo
Feet: any condition causing gait or balance disturbance
Motor: gait: bradykinesia, consider Parkinson's disease; shoulder/hip weakness, consider polymyalgia rheumatica
Mental status: test for variance from baseline and screen for depression

[1]BMI, body mass index; BP, blood pressure; HR, heart rate; JVD, jugular venous distention; CHF, congestive heart failure.

Table 38–3. Standard tests to evaluate FTT.[1]

Test	Condition
CBC	Anemia, vitamin or iron deficiency, infection, or hematopoietic or lympho-proliferative disorder
Serum electrolytes, calcium, BUN, creatinine	Hypo- or hypernatremia or kalemia, acid–base disorder, osmolality, renal failure, dehydration
Glucose	Diabetes
Serum bilirubin and transaminase levels	Liver failure, hepatitis
Thyroid-stimulating hormone level	Hypo- or hyperthyroidism
Fecal occult blood	Cancer
Urinalysis	Infection
ESR	Active inflammation
PPD	Tuberculosis

See Huffman GB: Evaluating and treating unintentional weight loss in the elders. Am Fam Physician 2002;65:640; and Verdery RB: Clinical evaluation of failure to thrive in older people. Clin Geriatr Med 1997;13:769.

[1]CBC, complete blood count; BUN, blood urea nitrogen; ESR, erythrocyte sedimentation rate; PPD, purified protein derivative.

Treatment

A. Assessment and Plan

When the diagnosis of FTT is confirmed, the life expectancy of the patient should be assessed. Physicians need to determine which symptoms and conditions are reversible and address these methodically. Risk–benefit assessment should be included in all interventions and physicians should collaborate with the patient and family on decision making. As medical interventions become more limited, palliative measures can be initiated. The physician can maintain a therapeutic relationship with the patient and the family beyond the time medical therapies are effective.

B. Team Approach

Physicians must make sure prescribing is in line with current standards of care. Eliminating, substituting, or changing the administration time of drugs may reveal if side effects are contributing to the problem. Physicians should consult a PharmD and utilize specialists by phone or referral to optimize chronic disease management. If depression is an issue, patients should be aggressively treated and referred to psychiatry if no improvement is seen at 4–6 weeks. Selective serotonin

reuptake inhibitors remain the drugs of choice in treating subsyndromal and major depression in the elderly.

A social worker (SW) either from the hospital, home health agency, or Area Agency on Aging [www.aoa.dhhs.gov or (800) 677-1116] should be involved. The SW can assist by identifying and coordinating services for the patient and the caregiver. Caregiver issues in fact may be the crux of the patient's FTT. Caregiver education and respite services have been shown to delay institutionalization for patients with Alzheimer's dementia. Although this has not been proved for other disabling diseases, at the very least, quality of life for the caregiver may be improved. Concerns about neglect or abuse should be discussed openly and frankly with the family and caregiver and reported if appropriate. Elder abuse or neglect is reportable to the local Area Agency on Aging.

A nutritionist should be consulted to assess and counsel the patient. Malnutrition in the nonterminal state is correctable. Other health professionals of potential value include a dentist, audiologist, speech therapist, pain specialist, psychologist, occupational therapist, and physical therapist. Church members and pastors may provide valuable support.

Lonergan ET (editor): *Extending Life, Enhancing Life: A National Research Agenda on Aging.* National Academy Press, 1991.

Markson EW: Functional, social, and psychological disability as causes of loss of weight and independence in older community-living people. Clin Geriatr Med 1997;13(4):639.

Sarkisian CA, Lachs MS: Failure to thrive in older adults. Ann Intern Med 1996;124:1072.

Tully CL, Snowdon DA: Weight change and physical function in older women: findings from the nun study. J Am Geriatr Soc 1995;53:1394.

Wallace JI et al: Involuntary weight loss in older outpatients; incidence and clinical significance. J Am Geriatr Soc 1995;43:329.

Zhan C et al: Potentially inappropriate medication use in the community-dwelling elderly: findings from the 1996 medical expenditure panel survey. JAMA 2001;286:2823.

PRESSURE ULCERS

General Considerations

Pressure ulcers, formerly known as pressure sores or decubitus ulcers, are challenging for many reasons. First, they are harbingers of death: development of an ulcer is associated with a 4-fold increase in in-hospital mortality and nonhealing ulcers carry a 6-fold increase in mortality. Second, even with assiduous prevention they occur at an incidence of 2.7–29.5% in hospitals and 13% in long term-care settings the first year, increasing in subsequent years. Third, they are difficult to heal: stage 1–2 ulcers typically take 4–8 weeks and stage 3–4 ulcers take many months. Healing is dependent on nonphysician interventions and thus success is related to a multitude of caregivers and factors. Finally, there is scant evidence from randomized controlled trials on which interventions work. A wide range of pressure-relieving devices and topicals contribute to the over $8 billion/ year industry in the United States. Pressure ulcers account for 17,000 lawsuits annually with awards up to $50 million in judgments. It is deemed such a significant problem that prevention of pressure ulcers in institutionalized elders is one of the goals of *Healthy People 2010*.

To date we continue to rely on the Agency for Heathcare Research and Quality guidelines, now over a decade old. Although built on consensus opinion rather than evidence, they remain the current standard of care. The recently published *Quality Indicators for Assessing Care of Vulnerable Elders (ACOVE)* is a practical addition to the guidelines, reflects the best available evidence, and provides specific indicators to monitor quality.

Pathogenesis

Extrinsic and intrinsic factors cause pressure ulcers. The presence and duration of pressure are the most significant extrinsic factors and must be present for breakdown. Experimentally, 2 h of pressure at 32 mm Hg (capillary pressure) will cause tissue ischemia. Clinically, though, it takes more than that to create a pressure ulcer. Contributors are friction, shearing forces, moisture, maceration, and prolonged immobilization. Intrinsic causes are the susceptibility of aged skin (less thickness and elasticity), loss of sensation, circulatory compromise, and, possibly, malnutrition (Table 38–4).

Prevention

Of elders who develop pressure ulcers 56–92% do so within the first 2 weeks of a hospital stay. *ACOVE* recommends that individuals admitted to the hospital who cannot reposition themselves be assessed for ulcer risk and, if at risk, be placed on a prevention protocol within 12 h of admission. Commonly used screening tools for ulcer risk are the Braden and Norton scales. The Braden scale contains six subscales: sensory perception, skin moisture, activity level, mobility, nutritional status, and friction and shear. A perfect score is 23, with a score of 16 or lower predicting pressure sore development. Braden has good interrater reliability and has been used in acute and long-term settings. The Norton scale includes mental condition; impaired cognitive status is a significant contributor to ulcer development.

Hospitalized elders identified at risk should be placed on a foam or gel overlay mattress, otherwise known as a Group 1 support surface, turned every 2 h

Table 38–4. Risk factors for pressure ulcers.

Advanced age
Arteriosclerotic disease
Cognitive impairment
Dehydration
Delirium
Moisture: perspiration, urine, feces
Immobilization
Incontinence
Neuropathy
Sensory impairment
Surgery/postoperative period

See Lonergan ET (editor): *Extending Life, Enhancing Life: A National Research Agenda on Aging.* National Academcy Press, 1991; Fiatarone MA et al: High intensity strength training in nonagenarians: effects on skeletal muscle. JAMA 1990;236:3029; Fiatarone MA et al: Exercise training and nutritional supplementation for physical frailty in very elderly people. New Engl J Med 1994;330:1769; and Wallace JI et al: Involuntary weight loss in older outpatients; incidence and clinical significance. J Am Geriatr Soc 1995;43:329.

if immobile, and provided with appropriate protective gear to prevent bony surfaces from pressure. A clock on the wall with 2-h intervals identified with the appropriate position change will help caregivers. The dietitian should assess the patient for protein–calorie malnutrition and institute corrective therapy. Although no studies have shown that adequate nutrition prevents pressure ulcers, there is indirect evidence that prevention of malnutrition will reduce the risk of ulcer formation.

At the time of admission, the physician should document the condition of the elbows, sacrum, ischia, greater trochanters, heels, and malleoli, and in patients with kyphosis, thoracic vertebrae. Extra vigilance is needed in cognitively or sensory impaired elders who have support stockings, casts, or other orthopedic devices. This baseline documentation is important for medical and legal reasons. In addition, patients and families should be informed about risk for ulcer development and their part in preventing it (Table 38–5).

Clinical Findings

If a patient is admitted with an ulcer or if one occurs during hospitalization, the physician must document its stage, size, depth, and location (see Figure 38–1 for assessment and classification). A stage 1 ulcer should be evaluated by palpating the ulcer to ensure the absence of fluctulance, crepitance, or soft tissue breakdown beneath the surface. A stage 2 or above ulcer should be probed with a sterile Q-tip moistened with normal saline to identify undermining or sinus tracts. Stage

Table 38–5. Guidelines for pressure ulcer prevention.

1. During admission assess patient for risk of pressure ulcer development
2. Institute repositioning and pressure reduction within 12 h in patients at risk
3. Inspect high-risk patients daily and document condition of all bony prominences, sacrum, and heels
4. Inspect skin at contact sites of casts and other orthopedic devices
5. Keep skin clean using mild soap and water
6. Minimize skin exposure to moisture
7. Use topical agent with moisture barrier for incontinent patients
8. Minimize friction and shear through correct repositioning and turning and use lift-sheet and/or bed trapeze
9. Post a written turning schedule near patient
10. Place at-risk patients on approved pressure-relieving devices
11. Provide heel pressure relief for bed-bound patients using inflatable heel elevators
12. Avoid doughnut cushions
13. Maintain head of the bed flat when possible; this minimizes pressure on the sacrum and greater trochanter
14. Reposition chair-bound patients every hour and weight shift every 15 min; use pressure-relieving seat cushion
15. Maintain and promote mobility
16. Institute medical nutrition plan for hypoalbuminemic, anemic, underweight, and obese patients
17. Educate patient and family about pressure ulcer prevention

See Coletta EM: Pressure ulcers: practical considerations in prevention and treatment. In: *Reichel's Care of the Elderly, Clinical Aspects of Aging,* ed 5. Gallo J et al (editors). Lippincott, Williams & Wilkins, 1999; Bennett RG: *Pressure Ulcers.* Geriatric Review Syllabus, American Geriatric Society, 1999; Berlowitz D: Prevention and treatment of pressure ulcers. UpToDate, www.uptodate.com, January 9, 2002; Agency for Healthcare Research and Quality (AHRQ): *Pressure Ulcer Treatment, Quick Reference Guide for Clinicians.* AHRQ, 1994 [can be downloaded from the AHRQ web site (www.ahrq.gov) or obtained from AHRQ Publications Clearinghouse, P.O. Box 8547, Silver Spring, MD 20907 or by telephone: 800-358-9295]; Bates-Jensen B: Quality indicators for prevention and management of pressure ulcers in vulnerable elders: (ACOVE). Ann Intern Med 2001;135 [8 (part 2), Suppl]:744; and Houston S et al: Adverse effect of large-dose zinc supplementation in an institutionalized older population with pressure ulcers. J Am Geriatr Soc 2001;49(8):1120.

1–2 ulcers are often referred to as partial thickness and stage 3–4 ulcers as full thickness. Almost 50% of partial-thickness ulcers will heal by 30 days and 75% by 60 days. Only 59% of stage 3 and 33% of stage 4 ulcers heal by 6 months. Stage 3–4 ulcers are often better drawn or photographed in addition to being measured. Measurements should be length × width × depth. Staging cannot be done if eschar is present; it must first be removed. The one exception is the heel. All stage 2–4 ulcers will be colonized with skin flora; therefore, cultures are of limited value; use of antibiotics will be covered under treatment.

Treatment

A. THE WOUND

A stage 1 ulcer is nonblanchable erythema of intact skin. It should be kept clean and dry. A protective ointment is appropriate (product descriptions are given in Table 38–6). It does not need a dressing unless exposed to friction; then a thin transparent film will suffice. The site should be pressure free via any number of creative repositioning strategies and/or protective gear. Doughnut cushions can worsen the ulcer and are no longer used; bunny boots are also out of favor and have been replaced by inflatable heel elevators. A foam or gel overlay provides appropriate support for beds or chairs.

Stage 2 ulcers involve loss of the epidermis or dermis but do not break the fascia. If the wound is superficial, clean, and without drainage (essentially a break in the skin), a transparent film is appropriate. For more extensive wounds with scant to minimal exudate, a hydrocolloid or hydrogel wafer is appropriate and can be left on for up to 7 days. Cleansing should be done with normal saline only. Old favorites such as hydrogen peroxide, betadine, liquid detergent, acetic acid, and hypochlorite solutions are potentially toxic to both fibroblasts and white blood cells. The wound bed should be kept moist and the surrounding skin dry. The immobile patient should be on a Group 1 surface and all pressure should be off the wound.

Stage 3 and 4 ulcers require a staged approach. First, they should be debrided of devitalized tissue. The only exception to debriding is stable heel ulcers, which should left alone and protected from pressure. Debridement may be done (1) using sharp instruments such as a scalpel or scissors; (2) using enzymes such as collagenase, papain, fibrinolysin, or deoxyribonuclease; (3) mechanically by irrigation or wet-to-dry dressings; or (4) by autolytic debridement using a hydrocolloid or other occlusive product. Extensive debridement should be performed by a general surgeon in the operating room. When sharp debridement involves bleeding, a dry dressing should be applied for the first 8–24 h.

Patient Name_____ Date:_____ Time:_____

Ulcer 1:

Site_____

Stage[a]_____

Size (cm)

   Length_____

   Width_____

   Depth_____

	No	Yes
Sinus Tract	☐	☐
Tunneling	☐	☐
Undermining	☐	☐
Necrotic Tissue	☐	☐
Slough	☐	☐
Eschar	☐	☐
Exudate	☐	☐
Serous	☐	☐
Serosanguineous	☐	☐
Purulent	☐	☐
Granulation	☐	☐
Epithelialization	☐	☐
Pain	☐	☐

Surrounding Skin:

Erythema	☐	☐
Maceration	☐	☐
Induration	☐	☐

Ulcer 2:

Site_____

Stage[a]_____

Size (cm)

   Length_____

   Width_____

   Depth_____

	No	Yes
Sinus Tract	☐	☐
Tunneling	☐	☐
Undermining	☐	☐
Necrotic Tissue	☐	☐
Slough	☐	☐
Eschar	☐	☐
Exudate	☐	☐
Serous	☐	☐
Serosanguineous	☐	☐
Purulent	☐	☐
Granulation	☐	☐
Epithelialization	☐	☐
Pain	☐	☐

Erythema	☐	☐
Maceration	☐	☐
Induration	☐	☐

Description of Ulcer(s):

_____

_____

Indicate Ulcer Sites:

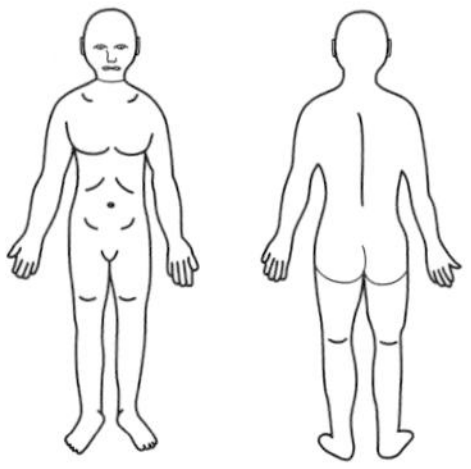

Anterior   Posterior

(Attach a color photo of the pressure ulcer[s] [Optional])

[a]Classification of pressure ulcers:

Stage I: Nonblanchable erythema of intact skin, the heralding lesion of skin ulceration. In individuals with darker skin, discoloration of the skin, warmth, edema, induration, or hardness may also be indicators.

Stage II: Partial thickness skin loss, involving epidermis, dermis or both.

Stage III: Full thickness skin loss involving damage to or necrosis of subcutaneous tissue that may extend down to, but not through, underlying fascia. The ulcer presents clinically as a deep crater with or without undermining adjacent tissue.

Stage IV: Full thickness skin loss with extensive destruction, tissue necrosis, or damage to muscle, bone, or supporting structures (e.g., tendon or joint capsule).

Figure 38–1. Pressure ulcer assessment and classification. [From the Agency for Healthcare Research and Quality (AHRQ): *Pressure Ulcer Treatment, Quick Reference Guide for Clinicians.* AHRQ, 1994.

Table 38–6. Product list and use.

Product	Use	Example
Incontinence cleanser	Cleanse peri area (incontinence)	Periwash, Aloe Vest Cleansing Foam, Proshield Foam & Spray
Moisture barrier	Protect against incontinence (prevention/mild)	Proshield, Hollister Moisture Barrier Ointment, Carrington Moisture Barrier
Extra protection barrier	Moderate/severe excoriation (incontinence)	Citric-Acid, Triple Care, Baza, Balmex, Desitin, zinc oxide
Emollient lotion	Moisturize/protect dry skin	Lubriderm, Eucerin
Wound cleanser	Cleanse wounds	Normal saline, Technicare, Dermal wound cleanser
Transparent dressing	Protect from friction, promote moisture	Bioclusive, Op-site, Tegaderm
Hydrogel	Moist wound healing	Intrasite, Carrington gel, Curasol
Hydrogel sheet	Moist wound healing for superficial wounds	Nu-Gel, Vigilon
Hydrogel-impregnated gauze	Moist wound healing in deeper wound	Solostie, Carrasyn
Hydrocolloid dressing	Promote moist wound healing and autolytic	Duoderm, Restore
NaCl-impregnated dressing	Absorbent dressing; aids in debridement	Mesalt
Island dressing	Absorbent semipermeable, self-adhesive, secondary	Alldress, Primapore
Foam dressing	Absorbent nonadherent dressing	Hydrosorb, Allevyn
Absorbent dressing	Absorbent for high exudate	Kalstat, Sorbsan, Aquacel

From UPMC McKeesport Policy and Procedure Manual, 2001.

Otherwise, all wounds should be kept moist. Appropriate dressings for minimal exudate were noted above. They are both autolytic and moisture retentive. When the wound has moderate to heavy exudate, calcium alginates and foam dressings should be used and changed daily for 3–5 days as they become saturated. Cleansing should be done at every dressing change with normal saline using a water pic at number 1 setting or a 35-mL syringe with a 19-gauge catheter; both of these provide adequate pressure between 4 and 15 pounds per square inch. Whirlpool treatments are helpful if the site is extensive, has copious exudate, or has necrotic tissue. They should be discontinued once the ulcer is clean.

B. THE PATIENT

When setting treatment goals the patient's ability to comply with the plan must be considered. Improvement in cognitive or affective status through medications such as acetylcholinesterase inhibitors or selective seratonin reuptake inhibitors may enhance healing. Mobility should be reassessed and physical and/or occupational therapy enlisted to maximize gait, balance, transfers, and weight shifting or to recommend and provide orthotics. Incontinence complicates treatment of pressure ulcers and should be treated aggressively. A Foley catheter may become necessary in patients whose incontinence is not medically managed or for those who do not have access to around the clock personal care. Short-acting narcotics should be offered prior to dressing changes or procedures as an adjunct to around-the-clock pain management. Patient and caregiver education should be provided in the inpatient setting and continued by Home Health in the outpatient setting. If healing does not occur at the anticipated rate, a house-call can determine whether additional assistance is needed. First- and second-hand smoke should be eliminated.

C. NUTRITION

Nutrition should be reassessed and a medical nutrition plan instituted. Although vitamin C and zinc have been used for years in wound healing, no studies have demonstrated their efficacy. The recommended daily allowance for zinc has been reduced (50 mg/day) and new research reveals a more modest margin between zinc deficiency and toxicity. A recent study showed that oral zinc supplementation (100/mg/day as zinc sulfate) in a group of institutionalized older patients was associated with significant and clinically adverse events: nausea, vomiting, and a higher incidence of infection, without obvious benefits. Slim-Fast, Carnation Instant Breakfast, and a multivitamin with minerals are inexpensive sources of added nutrients that may help in healing. Protein intake of 1.0–1.2 g/kg/day is recommended for all patients with pressure ulcers. Unless restricted by heart or renal failure, fluids should be encouraged.

D. Support Surfaces

Support surfaces are categorized into three groups; because of the complexity of their use and reimbursement, a wound care nurse should guide the physician through the process. Briefly, Group 1 surfaces are used for prevention in at-risk patients and treatment. The surfaces are a purchase item, with Medicare paying 80% and coinsurance normally paying the remaining 20%. Group 2 surfaces are appropriate for multiple stage 2 ulcers, a prior comprehensive treatment program for 1 month, worsening of stage 3–4 ulcers, skin graft or previous use of a group 2 surface in the inpatient, or a long-term care setting. Group 2 surfaces are rental. Group 3 mattresses are for an elite group of patients who meet complex criteria. If this type of mattress is proposed, a wound care team should be involved. Most equipment suppliers do not provide this level of bed due to problems with reimbursement; they are rented directly through the manufacturer or home care agency (example: HillRom, KinAir, FluidAire, etc). All surfaces require a physician's order.

E. Infection and Other Complications

Sixty thousand patients die a year from pressure ulcer–related complications. If the patient is clinically infected, ie, fever without other known cause, mental status change, leukocytosis, or advancing cellulitis, systemic antibiotics should be instituted. At this stage wound culture is not appropriate because it will be colonized with multiple organisms. Gram-positive organisms should be covered based on local susceptibilities. If improvement does not occur with systemic coverage methicillin-resistant *Staphylococcus aureus* and culture by needle aspiration or punch biospy should be considered. Although the literature recommends bone biopsy if osteomyelitis is suspected, this is rarely done practically. If there is suspicion of osteomyelitis an infectious disease specialist should be involved; various approaches for diagnosing osteomyelitis are beyond the scope of this chapter but are reviewed by Coletta. Finally, deep wounds may harbor tetanus; for a patient with no proof of recent booster or tetanus series, immunization should be instituted.

F. Other Therapies

Platelet-derived growth factors were introduced in the 1990s. One study has shown improved healing of pressure ulcers but the subjects were spinal cord injury patients aged 28–70 years. No study to date has shown improved healing in the elderly patient with the multiple risk factors noted earlier. Furthermore, these growth factors are very expensive. A 15-day application of becaplermin (Regranex gel) costs $437.74. Neither hyperbaric oxygen, infrared, ultraviolet, low energy, and laser irradiation, nor ultrasonography has been shown to enhance healing. Electrical stimulation therapy was thought to enhance healing but a recent systematic review concluded that there was insufficient reliable evidence to recommend it. Despite this review, many wound specialists believe this modality promotes more healing.

Agency for Healthcare Research and Quality (AHRQ): *Pressure Ulcer Treatment, Quick Reference Guide for Clinicians.* AHRQ, 1994. [This can be downloaded from the AHRQ web site (www.ahrq.gov) or obtained from AHRQ Publications Clearinghouse, P.O. Box 8547, Silver Spring, MD 20907 or by telephone: 800-358-9295.]

Bates-Jensen B: Quality indicators for prevention and management of pressure ulcers in vulnerable elders: (ACOVE). Ann Intern Med 2001;135[8 (part 2), Suppl]:744.

Bello YM: Recent advances in wound healing. JAMA 2000;283 (6):716.

Coletta EM: Pressure ulcers: practical considerations in prevention and treatment. In: *Reichel's Care of the Elderly, Clinical Aspects of Aging,* ed 5. Gallo J et al (editors). Lippincott, Williams & Wilkins, 1999.

Cullum N. Nelson EA, Flemming K: Systematic review of wound care management: (5) beds; (6) compression; (7) laser therapy, therapeutic ultrasound, electrotherapy and electromagnetic therapy. Health Technol Assess 2001;5:1.

U.S. Department of Health and Human Services: *Healthy People 2010.* DHHS, 2000.

FALLS

General Considerations

Postural instability and falls are a major and modifiable syndrome of the elderly. They exact an enormous toll in terms of quality of life and cost. One-third of community-dwelling elders will fall in a year; 5–15% of those falls will result in serious injury, 75% of which are fractures. The estimated lifetime cost for fall-related injuries in those over 65 years is $12.6 billion. Other sequelae include fear of falling, anxiety, social isolation, and physical deconditioning. Primary prevention starts with education. Patients registering for a visit should be given The American Geriatric Society *Fall Prevention* pamphlet (available free from the Society at 350 Fifth Avenue, Suite 801, New York, NY 10118).

Framework for Evaluation

Whether addressing falls during an acute visit for which it is the chief complaint or for those at risk identified by geriatric assessment, a multidimensional approach is warranted. A practical working construct incorporates (1) postural stability, (2) medical comorbidities, (3) overall function, and (4) environment.

Postural stability is maintained in three phases: input, processing, and output. Input includes vision, vestibular apparatus, and proprioception. Processing requires an intact nervous system: both central processing and competent efferent command. Output requires a motor system characterized by strength, flexibility, absence of pain, and cardiovascular endurance. Impairment of any **one** increases the risk for falls and the risk is cumulative. Conversely, interventions to modify any of these impairments will decrease the risk for falls.

Chronic diseases, and the **medications** used to treat them, constitute the second key area of assessment. Conditions and drugs that affect the components of postural stability are suspect and there are usually more than one.

Finally, the concept of **functional thresholds** places the data into a framework that identifies the point at which a particular patient exceeds his or her compensatory abilities. A detailed history and focused physical/performance examination will provide key information on function. For those frail elders who most commonly fall at home, a home assessment will complete the evaluation.

Clinical Findings

A. SYMPTOMS AND SIGNS

The history should elicit details of the fall as precisely as possible. "When did the fall or near-fall occur (post-prandial, what time of day), where were you (outside, inside), what were you doing (stairs, turning, reaching, stooping, micturition), did you have pain at the time, were there other symptoms, and finally what medications had you just taken?" Medication changes from other physicians, eye drops, over-the- counter medications, and alcohol intake should be noted.

Pinpointing the patient's subjective complaints of instability or of the fall is also helpful. Lightheadedness or a near faint is consistent with cerebral ischemia and would suggest orthostasis, arrhythmias, and other cardiovascular conditions. Muscular weakness, the sense that their legs cannot hold them up, would be more consistent with de-

Table 38–7. Conditions and drugs that increase risk for falls.

Syncope
Seizures
Orthostasis
Dysrhythmia
Vertibrobasilar insufficiency
Cervical degeneration
Carotid sinus syndrome[1]
Vertigo
Parkinson's disease
Movement disorder
Cerebrovascular accident
Intracranial mass or hydrocephalus
Peripheral neuropathy
Myopathy
Deconditioning from any cause
Pain
History of previous falls
Vision impairment
Depression
Cognitive impairment
Polypharmacy (more than four medications)
Psychotropics
Benzodiazepines, short and long acting
Narcotics
Antiarrhythmics
Digoxin
Diuretics
Selective seretonin reuptake inhibitors[2]
Tricyclic antidepressants
Antihypertensives
Anticholinergics

From the American Geriatrics Society, British Geriatrics Society, and American Academy of Orthopaedic Surgeons Panel on Falls Prevention: Guideline for the prevention of falls in older persons. J Am Geriatr Soc 2001;49:664.
[1]Davies AJ, Steen N, Kenny RA: Carotid sinus hypersensitivity is common in older patients presenting to an accident and emergency department with unexplained falls. Age Ageing 2001; 30:289 and Kenny RA et al: Carotid sinus syndrome: a modifiable risk factor for nonaccidental falls in older adults (SAFEPACE). J Am Coll Cardiol 2001;38:1491.
[2] Thapa PB, Gideon P, Cost TW: Antidepressants and the risk of falls among nursing home residents. New Engl J Med 1998;339: 875 and Liu B, Anderson G, Mittmann N: Use of selective serotonin-reuptake inhibitors or tricyclic antidepressants and risk of hip fractures in elderly people. Lancet 1998;351:1303.

conditioning, or neuromuscular disease. Dysequilibrium or the sensation of no coordination between the legs and the walking surface is suggestive of vestibulospinal tract, proprioception, somatosensory, and cerebellar lesions. Finally, the sensation of movement within the patient or of the room spinning is true vertigo.

Table 38–7 lists the chronic conditions and medications that can contribute to postural instability and falls.

B. Physical Examination

The physical examination should be problem focused as noted in Table 38–8.

Treatment

A. Performance Assessment

It is helpful to categorize the patient as frail, intermediate, or robust for performance assessment. In general, vigorous elders will fall outside the home, while doing complicated activities such as stairs or challenging themselves with tasks that displace the center of mass. Frail elders generally fall at home doing activities of daily living. Most studies show equal injury rates in both, although the frail fall more often. Gait speed is currently the best predictor of mobility problems and correlates with future disability in activities of daily living.

Table 38–8. Focused physical examination.

Vital signs: orthostatic blood pressure and heart rate, sitting and standing. Pulse for 1 min.

Height: loss of height and kyphosis indicate osteoporosis. Intervention may reduce fracture risk.

Body mass index: if below 21, patient is at risk of malnutrition and/or depression. Decreased padding leads to increased injury risk.

Vision: visual acuity, field testing, pupillary size, depth perception. Visual field loss and depth perception have a much greater impact on mobility and vision function than acuity. Dark adaptation time increases with age and is contingent on pupil size; lens opacification and duration and brightness of light aggravate the problem further.[1] An annual ophthalmological examination is recommended for all elders; alert the ophthalmologist to your concerns.

Vestibular function: have patient march in place with eyes closed. Abnormal response is moving more than a few degrees or moving more than a foot in any direction.[2]

Cardiovascular: assess for dysrhythmia, valvular disease, congestive heart failure.

Neuromuscular

Proximal muscle weakness suggests polymyalgia rheumatica, polymyositis, adrenal, thyroid, or parathyroid disease.

Distal muscle weakness is more suggestive of peripheral neuropathy.

Peripheral neuropathy: up to 20% of elders will have peripheral neuropathy: common causes are diabetes, alcohol, chronic lung disease, monoclonal gammopathy, neoplasm, medication (dilantin, lithium, isoniazid, vincristine), renal disease, thyroid disease, and vitamin B_{12} deficiency. Neuropathy occurs before weakness or ataxia. Further testing includes vibratory sense: patients should be able to feel a 128-Hz tuning fork at the malleolus for 10 s. Absence of position sense and heel jerk helps confirm the diagnosis.[3]

Generalized muscle weakness: consider toxic myopathy from alcohol, glucocorticoids, HMG coenzyme A reductase inhibitors, and colchicine. Atrophy suggests deconditioning; overall weakness suggests electrolyte imbalance.

Muscle tone and postural reflexes should be assessed to rule out Parkinson's disease or movement disorders.

Range of motion: joint, neck, spine, hip, knee, and ankle should be assessed; restriction impairs reflex time and precision. Cervical spondylosis is a significant cause of falls.

Feet: in addition to peripheral neuropathy, check for deformities such as bunions, calluses, ulcers, hammertoes, and nail pathology. Achilles reflex suggests peripheral neuropathy but is absent in up to 70% of normal aged individuals.[4] Note footwear; thick, soft-soled shoes increase fall risk.

Cognitive ability can be screened by three-item recall, Mini-mental status examination, or clock draw.

See King MB, Tinetti ME: A multifactorial approach to reducing injurious falls. Clin Geriatr Med 1996;12:745; Berg K, Norman KE: Functional assessment of balance and gait. Clin Geriatr Med 1996; 12:705; and Alexander N: Differential diagnosis of gait disorders in older adults. Clin Geriatr Med 1996;12:689.

[1] Maino JH: Visual deficits and mobility: evaluation and management. Clin Geriatr Med 1996;12:803.

[2] Studenski S, Rigler SK: Clinical overview of instability in the elderly. Clin Geriatr Med 1996;12:679.

[3] Richardson JK, Ashton-Miller JA: Peripheral neuropathy, an often overlooked cause of falls in the elderly. Postgrad Med 1996; 99:161.

[4] Klein RB, Knoefel JE: Neurologic problems in the elderly. In: *Reichel's Care of the Elderly, Clinical Aspects of Aging,* ed 5. Gallo J et al (editors). Lippincott, Williams & Wilkins, 1999.

For robust elders, patients should tandem walk and stand on one leg with the other leg flexed for 30 s. If they have no problems, risk reduction counseling is all they need. If they have difficulty, the focus should be on peripheral neuropathy as a potential and remediable culprit. Its onset is insidious, it affects an estimated 20% of elders, and it significantly increases the risk of falling. Intermediate patients should be asked to climb stairs, step over objects, rise from a chair with their arms folded, and stand on one leg for 10 s. The 10-s stand is a more sensitive screen than the Romberg. Difficulty with these tasks may represent deconditioning, a neuromuscular disorder, and/or peripheral neuropathy.

For frail elders the "Up and Go" and functional reach should be performed. The timed "Up and Go" is a simple, well-validated office tool for assessing gait and balance disturbance in frail elders. Patients should sit in a straight-back chair, rise and walk 10 m, turn, walk back, and sit in the chair. They may use whatever assistive device they normally use and should be allowed one trial before being timed. Under 10 s represents no risk and can be expected from nonfrail elders. A score of 10–19 s represents minimal risk, 20–29 s moderate risk, and >30 s a definite risk for falling. Referral to physical therapy is warranted if the score is ≥20 s. The functional reach is described in Chapter 40.

B. Environmental Assessment

A home assessment is warranted for frail elders and for anyone who has fallen at home. Although the evidence is mixed on the effectiveness of modifying the home environment after a fall, prudence dictates that anyone discharged from the hospital after a fall should have a home evaluation as part of a multidimensional targeted intervention. This may be done by the physician or occupational therapist and should include the environment itself as well as a replay of the circumstances of the fall (Table 38–9).

For frail patients a review of their activities in the home can be informative. The patient should be asked to simulate daily activities from getting out of bed to navigating the bathroom, kitchen, and basement stairs, and entering and leaving the house including locking the door. The more frail the individual, the greater the benefit of reducing environmental demands through both redesigning and providing assistive devices. Any modification that reduces risk *and* allows for maintenance of the patient's activities of daily living is of benefit.

C. Targeted Interventions

Risk reduction includes advice on appropriate footwear (hard soled, flat, closed-toed shoes), adequate lighting for all activities, and caution with any activity that re-

Table 38–9. Environmental checklist.

Approach outside: uneven sidewalk or walkway, exterior lighting, steps, ease of opening screen/storm/front door, proximity of steps to front door, ease of unlocking door.
Interior lighting: especially on stairs and thresholds, loose electrical cords, accessibility of light switches.
Carpets: scatter rugs, frayed or worn or high-pile carpets.
Floors: slippery, polished, unkempt (water, oil, clutter).
Bathroom: toilet height and ease of use, grab bars or bilateral grab bars if needed, bathing site including ease of entry, lighting, surface features, visibility of shower threshold. For overall safety ask about water temperature at this time; should be no more than 120°F.
Kitchen: location of most commonly used items, reaching and stooping, unstable stools, chair, or pedestal or glass table. Smoke alarm.
Stairs: lighting, handrail, condition of steps, ease of use, non-skid surface.
Furnishings: sharp edges, location in trafficked areas, height of bed and chairs.
Assistive devices: good repair, appropriate height for patient, stored out of the way when not in use.

See Connell BR: Role of the environment in falls prevention. Clin Geriatr Med 1996;12:859 and Scanameo AM, Fillit H: House calls: a practical guide to seeing the patient at home. Geriatrics 1995;50(3):33.

quires balance. For example, seniors should not climb stairs without a hand on the railing and stairs should be well lit and in good repair. Climbing ladders should be discouraged. Vigorous seniors should be cautioned about activities (skiing, skating, etc) that increase their risk for falls, hence putting them at greater risk for fractures. Patients identified as having balance difficulty or who have had multiple falls benefit from balance training (there is less evidence for benefits of resistance and aerobic training). Successful programs are a minimum of 10 weeks and should be sustained for lasting benefit. Tai Chi may reduce the risk of a fall but further studies are needed. When possible, medications should be reduced and psychotropics eliminated. Assistive devices may prevent falls when used correctly within a targeted intervention. Environmental modification is of known benefit as part of an overall targeted intervention in the subgroup of older patients that is at known risk for falls. It has not been proved to reduce risk in and of itself, although implementing it certainly makes good sense (see Table 38–10 for the American Geriatric Society's recommendations and level of evidence).

American Geriatrics Society, British Geriatrics Society, and American Academy of Orthopaedic Surgeons Panel on Falls Prevention: Guideline for the prevention of falls in older persons. J Am Geriatr Soc 2001;49:664.

Table 38–10. Strength of evidence for interventions.

Recommendation	Strength of Recommendation[1]
Gait training and appropriate use of assistive devices	B
Review and modification of medications, especially psychotropics	B
Exercise programs with balance training	B
Treatment of postural hypotension	B
Modification of environmental hazards	C
Treatment of cardiovascular disorders, including cardiac arrhythmias	D (note: recommendation prior to SAFEPACE study)[2]

See American Geriatrics Society, British Geriatrics Society, and American Academy of Orthopaedic Surgeons Panel on Falls Prevention: Guideline for the prevention of falls in older persons. J Am Geriatr Soc 2001;49:664.
[1]**Categories of evidence:** Class I: Evidence from at least one randomized controlled trial or a meta-analysis of randomized controlled trials. Class II: Evidence from at least one controlled study without randomization or evidence from at least one other type of quasiexperimental study. Class III: Evidence from nonexperimental studies, such as comparative studies, correlation studies, and case-control studies. Class IV: Evidence from expert committee reports or opinions and/or clinical experience of respected authorities. **Strength of recommendation:** A: Directly based on Class I evidence. B: Directly based on Class II evidence or extrapolated recommendation from Class I evidence. C: Directly based on Class III evidence or extrapolated recommendation from Class I or II evidence. D: Directly based on Class IV evidence or extrapolated recommendation from Class I, II, or III evidence.
[2]Kenny RA et al: Carotid sinus syndrome: a modifiable risk factor for nonaccidental falls in older adults (SAFEPACE). J Am Coll Cardiol 2001;38:1491.

Berg K, Norman KE: Functional assessment of balance and gait. Clin Geriatr Med 1996;12:705.

Connell BR: Role of the environment in falls prevention. Clin Geriatr Med 1996;12:859.

King MB, Tinetti, ME: A multifactorial approach to reducing injurious falls. Clin Geriatr Med 1996;12:745.

Klein RB, Knoefel JE: Neurologic problems in the elderly. In: *Reichel's Care of the Elderly, Clinical Aspects of Aging,* ed 5. Gallo J et al (editors). Lippincott, Williams & Wilkins, 1999.

Thapa PB, Gideon P, Cost TW: Antidepressants and the risk of falls among nursing home residents. New Engl J Med 1998; 339:875.

Urinary Incontinence

39

Robert J. Carr, MD

General Considerations

Urinary incontinence has been defined as the involuntary loss of urine so severe as to have social and/or hygienic consequences. It is a very common problem in family medicine with a prevalence in community dwelling elderly as high as 35%, and significantly higher rates among institutionalized patients. Despite this high prevalence, studies have shown that about half of all incontinent persons have never discussed the problem with a physician. This is likely because of embarrassment, a belief that incontinence is normal with aging, or an assumption that nothing can be done to help. Incontinence is associated with significant medical morbidity including infection, sepsis, pressure ulcers, and falls. It is also associated with significant psychological stress and social isolation. Incontinence causes significant caregiver burden, and is frequently cited as a reason for deciding to abandon home care efforts in favor of nursing home placement. The economic burden of incontinence is also substantial with an estimated direct cost in the United States of $16.3 billion per year.

Because of its high prevalence, significant morbidity, and high psychosocial impact, it is important for family physicians to accurately identify, assess, and treat incontinent patients. The large majority of patients with incontinence can be diagnosed and managed effectively by family physicians in the primary care setting.

A. Physiology of Normal Urination

A basic understanding of the normal physiology of urination is important to understand the potential causes of incontinence, and the various strategies for effective treatment.

The lower urinary tract consists primarily of the bladder (detrusor muscle) and the urethra. The urethra contains two sphincters, the internal urethral sphincter (IUS), composed predominantly of smooth muscle, and the external urethral sphincter (EUS), which is primarily voluntary muscle. The detrusor muscle of the bladder is innervated predominantly by cholinergic neurons from the parasympathetic nervous system, the stimulation of which leads to bladder contraction. The sympathetic nervous system innervates both the bladder and the IUS. Sympathetic innervation in the bladder is primarily β-adrenergic and leads to bladder relaxation, whereas α-adrenergic receptors predominate in the IUS, leading to sphincter contraction. Thus, in general, sympathetic stimulation of the urinary tract promotes bladder filling (relaxation of the detrusor with contraction of the sphincter), whereas parasympathetic stimulation leads to bladder emptying (detrusor contraction and sphincter relaxation).

The EUS, on the other hand, is striated muscle and primarily under voluntary (somatic) control. This allows for some ability to voluntarily postpone urination by tightening the sphincter and inhibiting the flow of urine. Additional voluntary control is provided by the central nervous system through the pontine micturition center. This allows for central inhibition of the autonomic processes described above, and for further voluntary postponement of the need to urinate until the circumstances are more socially appropriate or until necessary facilities are available.

The physiological factors influencing normal urination are summarized in Table 39–1, and will be important to keep in mind when discussing urinary disorders and treatment.

B. Age-Related Changes

Contrary to common perception, urinary incontinence is not inevitable with aging. Most elderly patients remain continent throughout their lifetimes, and a complaint of incontinence at any age should receive a thorough evaluation and not be dismissed as "normal for age." Nonetheless, many common age-related changes do predispose elderly patients to incontinence, and increase the likelihood of its development with advancing age.

The frequency of involuntary bladder contractions (detrusor hyperactivity) increases in both men and women with aging. In addition, total bladder capacity decreases, causing the voiding urge to occur at lower volumes. Bladder contractility decreases, leading to in-

Table 39–1. Physiological factors influencing normal urination.

Bladder filling	Sympathetic nervous system	β-Adrenergic	Detrusor relaxation
		α-Adrenergic	IUS[1] contraction
Bladder emptying	Parasympathetic nervous system	Cholinergic	Detrusor contraction
Voluntary control	Somatic nervous system	Striated muscle	EUS[1] contraction
	Central nervous system	Pontine micturition center	Central inhibition of urinary reflex

[1]IUS, internal urethral sphincter; EUS, external urethral sphincter.

creased postvoid residuals and increased sensation of urgency or fullness. Elderly patients excrete a larger percentage of their fluid volume later in the day than younger persons. This, in addition to the other changes listed, often leads to an increase in the incidence of nocturia with aging with more frequent nighttime awakenings.

In women, menopausal estrogen decline leads to urogenital atrophy and a decrease in the sensitivity of α-receptors in the IUS. In men, prostatic hypertrophy can lead to increased urethral resistance, and varying degrees of urethral obstruction.

It is important to remember that these age-related changes are found in many healthy, continent persons as well as those who develop incontinence. It is not completely understood why the predisposition to urinary problems is stronger in some patients than in others, which emphasizes the multifactorial basis of incontinence.

C. CULTURAL ISSUES

The cultural impact of incontinence on quality of life is only beginning to be appreciated and studied. Patients often associate incontinence with impending incompetence and declining independence. This leads to low self-esteem and a perceived need to hide their incontinence so as not to compromise their competence in the eyes of others. These feelings of low self-esteem may be more pronounced among certain ethnic groups in which "cleanliness" is associated with religious or cultural purity. In a recent pilot study, it was shown that incontinence led to religious restriction for both Jewish and Muslim women that was related to the cleanliness needed for prayer. A study among Pakistani women demonstrated similar findings, and led to an increase in secretiveness and isolation in an effort to hide their incontinence. Further study on cultural differences and perceptions is needed, and a multicultural urinary incontinence-specific quality of life measure has recently been standardized and translated into 11 languages. This will enhance the ability of researchers to study diverse international and ethnic populations, and to de-

velop a better understanding of the cultural influences impacting patients with incontinence.

Chaliha C, Stanton SL: The ethnic, cultural, and social aspects of incontinence—a pilot study. Int Urogynecol J Pelvic Floor Dysfunct 1999;10(3):166.

Herzog AR, Fultz NH: Prevalence and incidence of urinary incontinence in community dwelling populations. J Am Geriatr Soc 1990;38:273.

Herzog AR et al: Methods used to manage urinary incontinence by older adults in the community. J Am Geriatr Soc 1989;37:339.

National Institutes of Health Consensus Development Statement: Urinary incontinence in adults. NIH 1988;7(5).

Patrick DL et al: Cultural adaptation of a quality-of-life measure for urinary incontinence. Eur Urol 1999;36(5):427.

Wyman JF, Harkins SW, Fantl JA: Psychosocial impact of urinary incontinence in the community-dwelling population. J Am Geriatr Soc 1990;38(3):282.

Clinical Findings

A. SYMPTOMS AND SIGNS

1. Incontinence outside the urinary tract—Incontinence is often classified based on whether it is related to specific urogenital pathology or to factors outside the urinary tract. Terms such as *transient versus established, acute versus persistent,* and *primary versus secondary* have been used to highlight this distinction. A mnemonic, DIAPPERS, developed by Resnick (Table 39–2), is helpful in remembering the many causes of incontinence that occur outside the urinary tract. These "extraurinary" causes are very common in the elderly, and it is important to identify and/or rule them out before proceeding to a more invasive search for primary urogenital etiologies.

Delirium, depression, and disorders of excessive urinary output generally require medical and/or behavioral management of the primary cause rather than strategies relating to the bladder. Once the primary causes are corrected, the incontinence often resolves. Urinary tract infections, although easily treated if discovered, are a relatively infrequent cause of urinary incontinence in

Table 39–2. Causes of urinary incontinence without specific urogenital pathology.[1]

D	Delirium/confusional state
I	Infection (symptomatic)
A	Atrophic urethritis/vaginitis
P	Pharmaceuticals
P	Psychiatric causes (especially depression)
E	Excessive urinary output (hyperglycemia, hypercalcemia, CHF)
R	Restricted mobility
S	Stool impaction

[1]Also known as transient, acute, or secondary incontinence.

the absence of other classic symptoms (dysuria, urgency, frequency, etc). Asymptomatic bacteruria, which is common even in well elderly, does not cause incontinence.

Pharmaceuticals are a particularly important and very common cause of incontinence. When we remember the many neural receptors that are involved in urination (Table 39–1), it is easy to understand why so many medications used to treat other common problems can readily affect continence. Medications frequently associated with incontinence are listed in Table 39–3. It is important to note that many of these medications are available over the counter and in combination (Table 39–4). In addition, commonly used substances such as caffeine and alcohol can contribute to incontinence by virtue of their diuretic effects or the effects they have on mental status. Because of this, some

medications and substances associated with a patient's incontinence may not be considered important or readily volunteered during a medication history unless the physician specifically asks about them.

Restricted mobility or the inability to physically get to the bathroom in time to avoid incontinence is also referred to as "functional" incontinence. The incontinence may be temporary or chronic depending on the nature of the physical or cognitive disability involved. Physical therapy and/or strength and flexibility training may be helpful, as well as simple measures such as a bedside commode or urinal.

Stool impaction is very common in the elderly, and may cause incontinence both through its local mass effect and by stimulation of opioid receptors in the bowel. It has been reported to be a causative factor in up to 10% of patients referred to incontinence clinics for evaluation. Continence can often be restored by a simple disimpaction.

2. Urological causes of incontinence—Once secondary or transient causes have been investigated and ruled out, further evaluation should focus on specific urological pathology that may be causing incontinence.

The urinary tract has two basic functions: the emptying of urine during voiding and the storage of urine between voiding. A defect in either of these basic functions can cause incontinence, and it is useful to initially classify incontinence by whether it is primarily a defect of storage or of emptying. An *inability to store* urine occurs when the bladder contracts too often (or at inappropriate times), or when the sphincter(s) cannot contract sufficiently to allow the bladder to store urine and

Table 39–3. Pharmaceuticals contributing to incontinence.

Pharmaceutical	Mechanism	Effect
α-Adrenergic agonists	IUS[1] contraction	Urinary retention
α-Adrenergic blockers	IUS relaxation	Urinary leakage

Anticholinergic agents
  Antidepressants
  Antihistamines
  Antipsychotics
  Sedatives
	Inhibit bladder contraction, sedation, immobility	Urinary retention and/or functional incontinence

β-Adrenergic agonists	Inhibits bladder contraction	Urinary retention
β-Adrenergic blockers	Inhibits bladder relaxation	Urinary leakage, urgency
Calcium channel blockers	Relaxes bladder	Urinary retention
Diuretics	Increases urinary frequency, urgency	Polyuria
Narcotic analgesics	Relaxes bladder, fecal impaction, sedation	Urinary retention and/or functional incontinence

[1]IUS, internal urethral sphincter.

Table 39–4. Nonprescription agents contributing to incontinence.

Agent	Mechanism	Effect	Common Examples
Alcohol	Diuretic effect, sedation, immobility	Polyuria and/or functional incontinence	Beer, wine, liquor, some liquid cold medicines
α-Agonists	IUS[1] contraction	Urinary retention	Decongestants, diet pills
Antihistamines	Inhibit bladder contraction, sedation	Urinary retention and/or functional incontinence	Allergy tablets, sleeping pills, anti-nausea medications
α-agonist/antihistamine combinations	IUS contraction *and* inhibition of bladder contraction	Marked urinary retention	Multisymptom cold tablets
Caffeine	Diuretic effect	Polyuria	Coffee, soft drinks, analgesics

[1]IUS, internal urethral sphincter.

keep it from leaking. Thus the bladder rarely, if ever, fills to capacity and the patient's symptoms are generally characterized by frequent incontinent episodes of relatively small volume. An *inability to empty* urine occurs when the bladder is unable to contract appropriately, or when the outlet or sphincter(s) is partially obstructed (either physically or physiologically). Thus the bladder continues to fill beyond its normal capacity and eventually overflows, causing the patient to experience abdominal distention and continual or frequent leakage.

Determining whether the primary problem is the inability to store or the inability to empty can often be done easily during the history and physical examination based on the patient's pattern of incontinence (intermittent or continuous) and whether abdominal (bladder) distention is present. Determination of postvoid residual, which will be discussed in the "Physical Examination" section below, will also be helpful in making this distinction. This initial classification will be impor-

tant in narrowing down the specific etiology of the incontinence, and in ultimately deciding on the appropriate management strategy.

3. Symptomatic classification—Once it is determined whether the primary problem is with storage or with emptying, incontinence can be further classified according to the type of symptoms that it causes in the patient. The most common categories will be discussed below. The first two types, urge incontinence and stress incontinence, result from an inability to store urine. The third type, overflow incontinence, results from an inability to empty urine. A patient may have a single type of incontinence, or a combination of more than one type (mixed incontinence). Table 39–5 summarizes the major categories of incontinence, the underlying urodynamic findings, and the most common etiologies for each.

Urge incontinence is the most common type of incontinence in the elderly. Patients complain of a strong,

Table 39–5. Types and classification of urinary incontinence.

Underlying Defect	Symptomatic Classification	Most Common Urodynamics	Possible Etiologies
Inability to store urine	Urge (U)	Detrusor hyperactivity	Uninhibited contractions; local irritation (cystitis, stone, tumor); central nervous system causes
	Stress (S)	Sphincter incompetence	Urethral hypermobility; sphincter damage (trauma, radiation, surgery)
Inability to empty urine	Overflow (O)	Outlet obstruction	Physical (benign prostatic hyperplasia, tumor, stricture); neurological lesions, medications
		Detrusor hypoactivity	Neurogenic bladder (diabetes, alcoholism, disc disease)
	Functional (F)	Normal	Immobility problems; cognitive deficits
	Mixed	U + S, U + F	

and often immediate, urge to void followed by an involuntary loss of urine. It is often not possible to reach the bathroom in time to avoid incontinence once the urge occurs, and patients often lose urine while rushing toward a bathroom or trying to locate one. Urge incontinence is most frequently caused by involuntary contractions of the bladder, often referred to as *detrusor instability* (DI). These involuntary contractions increase in frequency with age, as does the ability to voluntarily inhibit them. Although the symptoms of urgency are a hallmark feature of this type of incontinence, DI can sometimes result in incontinence without these symptoms. Although most patients with DI are neurologically normal, uninhibited contractions can also occur as the result of neurological disorders such as stroke, dementia, or spinal cord injury. In these cases it is often referred to as *detrusor hyperreflexia*. DI and urgency can also be caused by local irritation of the bladder as with infection, bladder stones, or tumors.

Stress incontinence is much more common among women than men, and is defined as a loss of urine associated with increases in intraabdominal pressure (Valsalva maneuver). Patients complain of leakage of urine (usually small amounts) during coughing, laughing, sneezing, or exercising. In women, it is most often caused by urethral hypermobility resulting from weakness of the pelvic floor musculature, but can also be caused by intrinsic weakness of the urethral sphincter(s) most commonly following trauma, radiation, or surgery. Stress incontinence is rare in men, unless they have suffered damage to the sphincter through surgery or trauma. In making the diagnosis of stress incontinence, it is important to ascertain that the leakage occurs exactly *coincident with* the stress maneuver. If the leakage occurs several seconds after the maneuver, it is more likely caused by an uninhibited bladder contraction that has been triggered by the stress maneuver, and is urodynamically more similar to urge incontinence. This is sometimes known as *stress-induced detrusor instability*.

Overflow incontinence is a loss of urine associated with overdistention of the bladder. Patients complain of frequent or constant leakage or dribbling, or they may lose large amounts of urine without warning. It may result either from a defect in the bladder's ability to contract (*detrusor hypoactivity*) or from obstruction of the bladder outlet or urethra. Detrusor hypoactivity is most commonly the result of a *neurogenic bladder* secondary to diabetes, chronic alcoholism, or disc disease. It can also be caused by medications, primarily muscle relaxants and β-adrenergic blockers. Outlet obstruction can be physical (prostatic enlargement, tumor, stricture), neurological (spinal cord lesions, pelvic surgery), or pharmacological (α-adrenergic agonists). Because neurogenic bladder is relatively rare in the geriatric population, it is important to rule out possible causes of obstruction whenever the diagnosis of overflow incontinence is made.

Functional incontinence is a term used to describe physical or cognitive impairments that interfere with continence even in patients with normal urinary tracts. This has been described above in the "Restricted Mobility" section of the DIAPPERS mnemonic.

Mixed incontinence describes various combinations of the above four types, and when present can make the diagnosis and management of incontinence more difficult. The term is most frequently used to describe patients who present with a combination of stress and urge incontinence, although other combinations are also possible. Functional incontinence, for example, can coexist with stress, urge, or overflow incontinence further complicating the treatment of these patients. Side effects of medications being used to treat other comorbidities can also cause a mixed picture when combined with underlying incontinence of any type. Mixed stress and urge incontinence is particularly common among elderly women. When present, it is helpful to focus on the symptom that is most bothersome to the patient, and to direct your initial therapeutic interventions in that direction.

Cultural differences exist in the relative rates and types of incontinence among various ethnic groups. African-American women have lower rates of genuine stress incontinence than Hispanic, white, or Asian women but have higher rates of detrusor instability than all three groups. This is felt to be caused by functional and morphological differences in the urethral sphincteric and pelvic support systems among the different ethnic groups.

B. HISTORY AND PHYSICAL FINDINGS

The history and physical examination of a patient presenting with incontinence should have the following goals:

1. To evaluate for and rule out causes of incontinence outside the urinary tract (DIAPPERS).

2. To determine whether the primary defect is an inability to store urine or an inability to empty urine.

3. To determine the type of incontinence based on the patient's symptoms and likely etiologies.

4. To determine the pattern of incontinence episodes and its effect on the patient's functional ability and quality of life.

1. History—A thorough medical history should include special focus on the neurological and genitourinary history of the patient as well as any other medical problems that may be contributing factors (Table

39–2). Information on any previous evaluation(s) for incontinence, as well as their degree of success or failure, can be helpful in guiding the current evaluation and in determining patient expectations. A careful medication history is very important, focusing on the categories of medications listed in Table 39–3, and remembering to include nonprescription substances (Table 39–4). Finally, the pattern of incontinence is important in helping to classify its type and in planning appropriate therapy. This includes episode frequency, timing, precipitating factors, and volume of urine lost as well as a determination of the symptoms that are most bothersome to the patient and their impact on his or her life. A voiding diary or bladder record can be a very useful tool in obtaining this information. The patient or caretaker is given a set of forms and is asked to keep a written record of each incontinent episode for several days. A sample form is shown in Table 39–6.

Table 39–6. Sample voiding record.

Bladder Record

Name:
_____

Date:
_____

Instructions: Place a check in the appropriate column next to the time you urinated in the toilet or when an incontinence episode occurred. Note the reason for the incontinence and describe your liquid intake (for example, coffee, water) and estimate the amount (for example, one cup).

Time interval	Urinated in toilet	Had a small incontinent episode	Had a large incontinent episode	Reason for incontinence episode	Type/amount of liquid intake
6–8 a.m.					
8–10 a.m.					
10–noon					
Noon–2 p.m.					
2–4 p.m.					
4–6 p.m.					
6–8 p.m.					
8–10 p.m.					
10–midnight					
Overnight					

Number of pads used today: _____
Number of episodes: _____
Comments:

Incontinent episodes are recorded in terms of time, estimated volume (small or large), and precipitating factors. Fluid intake, as well as any episodes of urination in the toilet, is also recorded. When completed accurately, the bladder record can often elucidate the most likely type of incontinence and provide a clue to possible precipitating factors. Continuous leakage, for example, may be more consistent with overflow incontinence, whereas multiple, large-volume episodes may be more consistent with urge. Smaller-volume episodes associated with coughing or exercise may be more consistent with stress incontinence, whereas incontinence occurring only at specific times each day may suggest an association with a medication or other non-urinary tract cause. Although other information from the physical and laboratory evaluations will obviously be needed, the physician can often make significant progress toward determining the type of incontinence and possible precipitating factors from the history and voiding record alone.

2. Physical examination—In addition to a thorough search for nonurological causes of incontinence, the physical examination should focus on the abdominal, genital, and rectal areas. Evidence of bladder distention on abdominal examination should raise suspicion for overflow incontinence. Genital examination should include a pelvic examination in women to assess for evidence of atrophy or mass, as well as any signs of uterine prolapse, cystocele, or rectocele. A rectal examination is helpful in ruling out stool impaction or mass, as well as in evaluating sphincter tone and perineal sensation for evidence of a neurological deficit. A prostate examination is usually included, but several studies have demonstrated a poor correlation between prostate size and urinary obstruction. A neurological examination focusing on the lumbosacral area will be helpful in ruling out a spinal cord lesion or other neurological deficits.

Two additional tests, specific to the diagnosis of incontinence, should be added to the general physical. The first is provocative stress testing. This attempts to reproduce the symptoms of incontinence under the direct visualization of the physician, and is useful in differentiating stress from urge incontinence. The patient should have a full bladder, and preferably be in a standing position (although a lithotomy position is also acceptable for patients unable to stand). The patient should be told to relax, and then to cough vigorously while the physician observes for urine loss. If leakage occurs simultaneously with the cough, a diagnosis of stress incontinence is likely. A delay between the cough and the leakage is more likely caused by a reflex bladder contraction and is more consistent with urge incontinence.

The next test is the measurement of postvoid residual (PVR), and should be performed for incontinent patients suspected of urinary retention and potential obstruction. PVR measurement is traditionally done by urinary catheterization; however, portable ultrasound scanners are now available for this purpose that also provide very accurate readings. These ultrasound devices minimize the risks of instrumentation and infection that are inherent in catheterization, especially in male patients. Prior to measurement, the patient should be asked to empty the bladder as completely as possible. Measurement of residual urine in the bladder should be made within a few minutes after emptying using either in-and-out catheterization or ultrasound. A PVR of less than 50 mL is normal, whereas a PVR of greater than 200 mL indicates inadequate bladder emptying and is consistent with overflow incontinence. PVRs from 50 to 199 mL can sometimes be normal but may also exist with overflow incontinence, and results should be interpreted in light of the clinical picture. Patients with elevated PVRs should generally be referred for further evaluation and to rule out obstruction prior to treatment of the incontinence symptoms.

Other diagnostic maneuvers or "bedside urodynamics" have often been recommended to help in the diagnosis of incontinence. The best known of these are the Q-tip test to diagnose pelvic laxity and the Bonney (Marshall) test to determine whether surgical intervention will be helpful. Although these tests may be useful in some settings, recent studies have cast doubt on their predictive value, and in the family practice setting they are unlikely to add clinically useful information to that obtained from the history and physical examination as described above. Likewise, bedside urodynamics to assess bladder contractions and function will not likely add useful information to help in sorting out the small percentage of patients whose diagnosis remains unclear after a thorough history and physical examination.

C. Laboratory Evaluation

Like the history and physical examination, the laboratory evaluation should be focused on ruling out the nonurological causes of incontinence. A urinalysis is very helpful in screening for infection as well as in evaluating for hematuria, proteinuria, or glucosuria. It must be remembered, however, that asymptomatic bacteriuria is very common in the elderly, and is not a cause of incontinence. Antibiotic treatment of asymptomatic bacteriuria has not been shown to reduce morbidity or to improve incontinence either in the institutionalized elderly or in ambulatory women. Thus antibiotic treatment in the face of incontinence and bacteriuria should be reserved for patients whose incontinence is of recent onset, has recently worsened, or is accompanied by other signs of infection. Hematuria, in the absence of infection, should be referred for further evaluation to rule out carcinoma.

Additional laboratory studies that are recommended and may be helpful include measurement of renal function [blood urea nitrogen (BUN) and creatinine] and evaluation for metabolic causes of polyuria (hypercalcemia, hyperglycemia).

Radiological studies are not routinely recommended in the initial evaluation of most patients with incontinence; however, a renal ultrasound will be useful in patients with obstruction to evaluate for hydronephrosis.

Abrutyn E et al: Does asymptomatic bacteriuria predict mortality and does antimicrobial treatment reduce mortality in elderly ambulatory women? Ann Intern Med 1994;121(11)901.

Brandeis GH, Resnick NM: Urinary incontinence. In: *Practice of Geriatrics,* ed 3. W.B. Saunders, 1998.

Escobar del Barco L et al: Value of the Q-tip test in patients with urinary incontinence. Obstet Mex 1996;64:117.

Fantl JA et al: Urinary incontinence in adults: acute and chronic management. Clinical Practice Guideline No. 2, 1996 Update. U.S. Department of Health and Human Services. Public Health Service, Agency for Health Care Policy and Research. AHCPR Publication No. 96-0682, 1996.

Ouslander JG, Johnson TM: Incontinence. In: *Principles of Geriatric Medicine and Gerontology,* ed 4. Hazzard WR et al (editors). McGraw-Hill, 1999.

Ouslander JG et al: Use of a portable ultrasound device to measure post-void residual volume among incontinent nursing home residents. J Am Geriatr Soc 1994;42(11):1189.

Resnick NM: Urinary incontinence. Lancet 1995;346:94.

Treatment

If nonurological or functional causes are found as major contributors to the patient's incontinence, treatment should be targeted at the underlying illnesses and improving any functional disability. In addition to medical management of the underlying disorder(s), physical therapy and/or the use of assistive devices may be helpful in improving the patient's level of function and his or her ability to reach the bathroom prior to having an incontinent episode. For the ambulatory patient, a home visit is often useful in assessing for environmental hazards that may be contributing to functional incontinence.

Simple life-style modifications may be helpful in mild cases of urinary incontinence. Fluid restriction and avoidance of caffeine and alcohol, especially in the evening, can be recommended as an initial step. Weight loss can be recommended if the patient is obese, and the use of a bedside commode or urinal can also be helpful. For patients with more severe incontinence, however, including most patients with urological causes, further treatment measures will usually be necessary.

Treatment for urinary incontinence is divided into three categories: behavioral/nonpharmacological, pharmacological, and surgical. Alternative and complementary therapies that have been described in the literature will also be discussed.

A. BEHAVIORAL/NONPHARMACOLOGICAL THERAPIES

Behavioral therapies should be the first line of treatment in most patients with urge or stress incontinence, as they have the advantages of being effective in a large percentage of patients with few, if any, side effects. Behavioral therapies range from those designed to treat the underlying problem and restore continence (eg, bladder training, pelvic muscle exercises) to those designed simply to promote dryness through increased attention from a caregiver (eg, timed voiding, prompted voiding). The former category requires a motivated patient who is cognitively intact, whereas the latter category can be used even in patients with significant cognitive impairment.

Bladder training is a technique designed to help patients control their voiding reflex by teaching them to void at scheduled times. The patient is asked to keep a voiding record for approximately 1 week to determine the pattern of incontinence and the interval between incontinent episodes. A voiding schedule is then developed with a scheduled voiding interval significantly shorter than the patient's usual incontinence interval. (For example, if the usual time between incontinent episodes is 1–2 h, the patient should be scheduled to void every 30–60 min.) The patient is asked to empty the bladder as completely as possible at each scheduled void whether or not an urge is felt. Patients who get the urge to void at unscheduled times should try to stop the urge through relaxation or distraction techniques until the urge passes, and then void at the next scheduled time. If the urge between scheduled voids becomes too uncomfortable, the patient should go ahead and void, but should still void again as completely as possible at the next scheduled time. As the number of incontinent episodes decreases, the scheduled voiding intervals should be gradually extended each week, until a comfortable voiding interval is reached.

Fantl et al, in a well-publicized albeit relatively small trial of bladder retraining, demonstrated significant improvement in both the number of incontinent episodes and the amount of fluid lost in incontinent elderly women. Although the benefit was greatest in women with urge incontinence, women with stress incontinence also demonstrated improvement. In a later study, their group also demonstrated a significant improvement in quality of life following institution of bladder training. Studies in a family practice setting, in a home nursing program, and in a health maintenance organization also demonstrated significant benefit from a program of bladder training. The latter, a randomized controlled trial published in 2002, included patients with stress, urge, and mixed incontinence. Overall, patients had a 40% decrease in their incontinent episodes with 31% being 100% improved, 41% at least 75% improved, and 52% at least 50% improved.

Pelvic muscle exercises, also known as Kegel exercises, are designed to strengthen the periurethral and perivaginal muscles. They are most useful in the treatment of stress incontinence, but may also be effective in urge and mixed incontinence. Patients are initially taught to recognize the muscles to contract by being asked to squeeze the muscles in the genital area as if they were trying to stop the flow of urine from the urethra. While doing this, they should be sure that only the muscles in the front of the pelvis are being contracted, with minimal or no contraction of the abdominal, pelvic, or thigh muscles. Once the correct muscles are identified, patients should be taught to hold the contraction for at least 10 s followed by 10 s of relaxation. The exercises should be repeated between 30 and 80 times per day. Patients are then taught to contract their pelvic muscles before and during situations in which urinary leakage may occur to prevent their incontinent episodes from occurring.

A recent systematic review of 43 published clinical trials concluded that pelvic muscle exercises are effective for both stress and mixed incontinence, but that their effectiveness for urge incontinence remains unclear. Biofeedback has been used effectively to improve patients' recognition and contraction of pelvic floor muscles, but required equipment and expertise can make this impractical in a primary care setting. Weighted vaginal cones and electrical stimulation have also been used to enhance pelvic muscle exercises. These modalities are provided by many physical therapy or geriatric departments and can be considered as additional options for women who are unsuccessful with pelvic muscle exercises or who have obtained only partial improvement. The Cochrane group concluded that weighted vaginal cones, electrostimulation, and pelvic muscle exercises are probably similar in effectiveness. There was not enough evidence to conclude that the effectiveness of cones plus pelvic muscle exercises is different than either one alone.

Timed voiding is a passive toileting assistance program that is caregiver dependent, and can be used for patients who are either unable or unmotivated to participate in more active therapies. Its goal is to prevent incontinent episodes rather than to restore bladder function. The caregiver provides scheduled toileting for the patient on a fixed schedule (usually every 2–4 h) including at night. There is no attempt to motivate the patient to delay voiding or resist the urge to void as there is in bladder training. The technique can be used both for patients who can toilet independently as well as those who require assistance. It has been used with

success in both male and female patients and has achieved improvements of up to 85%. Timed voiding has also been used effectively in postprostatectomy patients as well as in patients with neurogenic bladder. A variation of timed voiding, known as *habit training,* uses a voiding schedule that is modified according to the patient's usual voiding pattern rather than an arbitrarily fixed interval. The goal of habit training is to preempt incontinent episodes by scheduling the patient's toileting interval to be shorter than the usual voiding interval. Both timed voiding and habit training are most commonly used in the nursing home setting, but may also be used in the home setting if a motivated caregiver is available.

Prompted voiding is a technique that can be used for patients with or without cognitive impairment, and has also been studied most frequently in the nursing home setting. Its goal is to teach patients to initiate their own toileting through requests for help and positive reinforcement from caregivers. Approximately every 2 h, caregivers prompt the patients by asking whether they are wet or dry and suggesting that they attempt to void. Patients are then assisted to the toilet if necessary, and praised for trying to use the toilet and for staying dry. A recent systemic analysis of controlled trials of prompted voiding concluded that the evidence was suggestive, although inconclusive that prompted voiding provided at least short-term benefit to incontinent patients. The addition of oxybutynin to a prompted voiding program may provide additional benefit for some patients. A recent nursing home trial demonstrated that prompted voiding is most effective for reducing daytime incontinence, and that routine nighttime toileting was not effective in reducing incontinent episodes during the night.

B. PHARMACOLOGICAL THERAPY

Medications may be used alone or in conjunction with behavioral therapy when degree of improvement has been insufficient. There are very few studies comparing drug therapy with behavioral therapy, but both have been found more effective than placebo. It is important to have an accurate diagnosis of the type of incontinence to choose appropriate pharmacological therapy for each patient.

For *urge incontinence,* anticholinergic medications are the drugs of choice with oxybutynin and tolterodine being the most widely used. Both are now available in once-a-day formulations (oxybutynin = Ditropan XL 5–10 mg daily; tolterodine = Detrol LA 2–4 mg daily). Oxybutynin is also available in a generic formulation that is significantly less expensive, but requires dosing (2.5–5 mg) two to four times a day. No direct trial has yet been published comparing the long-acting forms of the two drugs. A recent study of long-acting oxybutynin versus short-acting tolterodine found oxybutynin was modestly more effective with a similar side effect profile and cost. A recent meta-analysis of four comparative trials (looking mainly at the short-acting formulations) concluded that oxybutynin is superior in efficacy, but that tolterodine is better tolerated with fewer dropouts because of medication side effects. Major side effects of both drugs (although less with tolterodine) include dry mouth, urinary retention, and delirium. The tricyclic antidepressant imipramine has also been widely used to treat urge incontinence, but its use has now largely been supplanted by these newer agents with more favorable side effect profiles and better documented efficacy.

For *stress incontinence,* medical treatment is most effective for patients with mild to moderate incontinence and without a major anatomic abnormality. The α-agonist pseudoephedrine is the drug of choice for patients without contraindications at a dosage range of 15–60 mg three times a day. Side effects include nausea, dry mouth, insomnia, and restlessness. Studies using phenylpropanolamine (now removed from the market) demonstrated improvement in 19–60% of women and cure in 9–14%. One study indicated that a significant number of patients referred for surgical intervention could avoid surgery with α-agonist therapy.

Traditionally, estrogen therapy has been used in conjunction with α-agonists to increase α-adrenergic responsiveness and improve urethral mucosa and smooth muscle tone. The recent HERS trial, however, demonstrated estrogen therapy to be less effective than placebo for symptoms of urinary incontinence with only 20.9% of the treatment group reporting improvement and 38.8% reporting worsening of their incontinence (compared to 26% improvement and 27% worsening in the placebo group). Data from the Women's Health Initiative study indicating that patients on an estrogen/progestin combination demonstrated increased risk for heart disease, stroke, breast cancer, and pulmonary embolism also cast significant doubt on the advisability of chronic estrogen use for this indication. Although the risks and benefits of topical estrogen are still not completely known, it would be prudent to use caution when considering its use until more conclusive data are available.

Overflow incontinence associated with outlet obstruction is generally not treated with medications, as the primary therapy is removal of the obstruction. In males, outlet obstruction is most commonly caused by prostatic enlargement secondary to infection (prostatitis), benign hyperplasia (BPH), or prostate cancer. Prostatitis can be treated with a 2- to 4-week course of a fluoroquinolone or trimethoprim-sulfamethoxazole. Once prostate cancer has been ruled out, BPH may be treated with α-blockers, finasteride, surgery, or transurethral microwave ther-

motherapy. α-Blockers have been shown to be ineffective in "prostatism-like" symptoms in elderly women.

Medical treatment of overflow incontinence caused by bladder contractility problems is usually not highly efficacious. The cholinergic agonist bethanechol may be useful subcutaneously for temporary contractility problems following an overdistention injury, but is generally ineffective when given orally or when used long term.

C. Surgical Therapy

Surgical therapy may be indicated for patients with incontinence resulting from anatomic abnormalities (eg, cystocele, prolapse), with outlet obstruction resulting in urinary retention, or for patients in whom more conservative methods of treatment have not provided sufficient relief.

Beyond the correction of anatomic abnormalities or obstruction, surgical therapy is most effective for stress incontinence or for mixed incontinence where stress incontinence is a primary component. Numerous surgical options are available for the management of stress incontinence including injection of periurethral bulking agents, transvaginal suspensions, retropubic suspensions, slings, and sphincter prostheses. Choice of procedure is based on the relative contributions of urethral hypermobility versus intrinsic sphincter deficiency, urodynamic findings, the need for other concomitant surgery, the patient's medical condition and life-style, and the experience of the surgeon.

Surgical management of refractory urge incontinence is generally more difficult. Options include sacral root neuromodulation procedures and augmentation enterocystoplasty, both of which offer substantial success rates in properly selected patients.

D. Primary Care Treatment versus Referral

Once the information from the history, physical examination, voiding record, provocative stress testing, PVR measurement, and laboratory data is available, a presumptive diagnosis can be made in the large majority of patients. If the patient has uncomplicated urge or stress incontinence, or a mixture of urge and stress, primary treatment can be initiated by the family physician. If the patient has overflow incontinence, manifested by an elevated PVR, referral is indicated to rule out obstruction prior to attempting medical or behavioral management. In the minority of patients in whom the type or cause of incontinence still remains unclear, referral for urodynamic testing is indicated if a specific diagnosis will be helpful in guiding therapy. Urodynamic testing in the routine evaluation of incontinence is not indicated, as studies have not shown an improvement in clinical outcome between patients diagnosed by urodynamics and patients treated based on history and physical examination.

Other indications for referral include incontinence associated with recurrent symptomatic urinary tract infections, hematuria without infection, history of prior pelvic surgery or irradiation, marked pelvic prolapse, suspicion of prostate cancer, lack of correlation between symptoms and physical findings, and failure to respond to therapeutic interventions as would be expected from the presumptive diagnosis.

E. Pads, Garments, Catherization, and Pessaries

The use of absorbent pads and undergarments is extremely common among the elderly. Although they are not recommended as primary therapy before other measures have been tried, they may be useful in patients whose incontinence is infrequent and predictable, who cannot tolerate the side effects of medications, or who are not good candidates for surgical therapy. The main purposes of these pads and garments is to contain urine loss and prevent skin breakdown. However, there are very few studies comparing the numerous absorbent products available and their degree of success or failure in meeting these objectives. A recent Cochrane review concluded that disposable products may be more effective than nondisposable products in decreasing the incidence of skin problems and that superabsorbent products may perform better than fluff pulp products. More comparative studies are needed in this area to assist patients and caregivers in making better informed decisions.

Although urethral catheterization should be avoided as a general rule, it is sometimes indicated in cases of overflow incontinence or in patients for whom no other measures have been effective. External collection devices (eg, Texas catheters) are preferable to indwelling catheters, but acceptable external devices are not widely available for women and adverse reactions such as skin abrasion, necrosis, and urinary tract infection are not uncommon. When internal catheterization is needed, intermittent or suprapubic catheterization has been shown to be preferable to indwelling catheterization in reducing the incidence of bacteriuria and its consequent complications. Indwelling urethral catheterization should be limited to very few circumstances including comfort measures for the terminally ill, prevention of contamination of pressure ulcers, and for patients with inoperable outflow obstruction.

Pessaries are intravaginal devices used to maintain or restore the position of the pelvic organs in patients with genitourethral prolapse. Although there are few comparative data on their use in incontinence, they can sometimes be useful in patients with intractable stress incontinence who are poor candidates for, or who do not desire, surgery.

F. Alternative and Complementary Therapies

The use of biofeedback, electrical stimulation, and pelvic muscle exercises in the treatment of incontinence has been discussed in the section on "Behavioral/Nonpharmacological Therapies." Magnetic stimulation and botulism toxin have also been described as potential therapies for urge incontinence, although large controlled trials on their risks and benefits for this indication are lacking. Buzhongyiqitang, an old Chinese prescription, provided relief from stress incontinence in 78% of patients in one small study (23 patients), but this remedy is not readily available in the United States. Hypnotherapy has been reported to be effective in a small group of patients with urge incontinence who failed to respond to other therapies. Acupuncture has also been used with some success in various types of urinary incontinence. Serenoa repens, the extract of the saw palmetto tree, provides mild to moderate improvement in urinary symptoms and flow measures in patients with BPH, but long-term safety and effectiveness are still unknown. Additional controlled trials of these complementary methods are needed so that clinicians can make informed decisions about incorporating them into a comprehensive treatment plan.

Appel RA et al: Prospective randomized controlled trial of extended-release oxybutynin chloride and tolterodine tartrate in the treatment of overactive bladder: results of the OBJECT study. Mayo Clinic Proc 2001;76:358.

Benson JT: New therapeutic options for urge incontinence. Curr Womens Health Rep 2001;1(1):61.

Blaivas JG, Groutz A: Urinary incontinence: pathophysiology, evaluation, and management overview. In: *Campbell's Urology,* ed 8. Walsh PC (editor). W.B. Saunders, 2002.

Eustice S et al: Prompted voiding for the management of urinary incontinence in adults (Cochrane Review). In: *The Cochrane Library,* Issue 3. Update Software, 2002.

Fantl JA et al: Efficacy of bladder training in older women with urinary incontinence. JAMA 1991;265:609.

Glazener CMA, Lapitan MC: Urodynamic investigations for management of urinary incontinence in adults (Cochrane Review). In: *The Cochrane Library,* Issue 3. Update Software, 2002.

Godec, CJ: Timed voiding: a useful tool in the treatment of urinary incontinence. Urology 1994;23(1):97.

Grady D et al: Postmenopausal hormones and incontinence: The Heart and Estrogen/Progesterone Replacement Study. Obstet Gynecol 2001;97(1):116.

Harvey MA et al: Tolterodine versus oxybutynin in the treatment of urge urinary incontinence: a meta-analysis. Am J Obstet Gynecol 2001;185:56.

Hay-Smith EJC et al: Pelvic floor muscle training for urinary incontinence in women (Cochrane Review). In: *The Cochrane Library,* Issue 3. Update Software, 2002.

Madersbacher H et al: Conservative management in the neuropathic patient. In: *Incontinence: First International Consulta-*

tion on Incontinence. Recommendations of the International Scientific Committee: the Evaluation and Treatment of Urinary Incontinence. Abrams P, Khoury S, Wein A (editors). Health Publication Ltd., 1999.

Shirran E, Brazzelli M: Absorbent products for containing urinary and/or faecal incontinence. In: *Cochrane Database of Systemic Reviews,* Issue 3. Update Software, 2002.

Subak LL et al: The effect of behavioral therapy on urinary incontinence: a randomized controlled trial. Obstet Gynecol 2002; 100(1):72.

Writing Group for the Women's Health Initiative Investigators: Risks and benefits of estrogen plus progestin in healthy postmenopausal women. Principal results from the Women's Health Initiative randomized controlled trial. JAMA 2002; 288(3):321.

Assessing the Vulnerable Elderly

40

Cynthia M. Williams, DO

Introduction

Geriatric assessment has been called the heart and soul of geriatric care and a gateway to care for frail or vulnerable older adults. A major focus of geriatric assessment is on function and functional decline. Health care providers by clinical judgment alone can diagnose severe functional impairment, but have difficulty in identifying moderate impairments, which are more likely to affect a community-dwelling older population. The multitude and complexity of problems a vulnerable older adult may have require more than just management of their diseases. It requires a team approach to care either in a multidisciplinary (many different disciplines are involved) and/or interdisciplinary (different disciplines work together in a coordinated fashion for patient centered-goals) manner (Table 40–1) and a focus that is concerned as much with caring as it is with curing.

The education of physicians and even social service professionals in the United States has inadequately prepared them to care for vulnerable elders, especially in using the collective knowledge of the team approach. The health care system within the United States is so complex that no one individual has the requisite knowledge to navigate through it. To provide quality care for the elderly the family physician needs to become knowledgeable in many areas of health care that go outside the "comfort zone" of a medical model. Quality care of the elderly also requires elderly patients and their caregivers to become involved with recommendations and decisions and it requires effective coordination of care and close follow-up either in the home or office or by telephone.

One of the goals of geriatric assessment is to identify those individuals who will benefit from a comprehensive care plan. It is important to identify elders who may be frail or vulnerable in outpatient clinical practice. The vulnerable elderly has been defined as adults over the age of 65 years who are at risk for functional decline and death. Family physicians assessing this population should strive to identify those conditions and

clinical situations most affecting this group (Table 40–2). In general, geriatric assessment attempts to obtain a "big picture" in order to provide quality care for the elderly (Table 40–3). Geriatric assessment is often necessary to accurately define an older person's problems, develop interventions, and serve as a baseline from which to measure outcomes of treatment.

The five original goals of multidimensional or comprehensive geriatric assessment were to improve diagnostic accuracy, guide selection of interventions to restore or preserve health, recommend an optimal environment (nursing home placement), predict outcomes, and monitor clinical change. However, outcomes for geriatric assessment, especially comprehensive geriatric assessment (CGA), are mixed. In a meta-analysis of CGA it was found that survival and function were improved if strong long-term follow-up and management were utilized. CGA also has other associated limitations including availability of the assessment and the length of the assessment, which tend to be slow, inefficient, and disruptive, especially to frail elderlys. Finally, the outcomes of CGA have been questioned in terms of the expectations of patients, caregivers, physicians, and case managers (Table 40–4).

For the family physician in community practice, several issues concerning care of older adults need addressing. First and foremost, caring for older adults is different from caring for younger individuals. The primary goal of care is maintenance of function and independence in an attempt to delay disability until the last years of a person's natural life.

The Assessing Care of Vulnerable Elders (ACOVE) Project has developed quality assessment tools to guide care for vulnerable elders. Phase 1 of this project yielded 22 quality indicators that should be applied to ensure quality care to community-dwelling older adults 65 years and older. These indicators were developed using systematic literature reviews, expert opinion, and the guidance of expert groups and stakeholders. The indicators and background information to the ACOVE project can be found online at http://www.acponline.org/sci-policy/acove.

Table 40–1. The role of team members in assessing vulnerable older adults in a clinical setting.

Health Care Provider	Required Training	Responsibility
Physician	FP/IM/geriatrics trained	History, physical, functional, cognitive, and affective assessment; laboratory testing; good geriatric prescribing practices; monitor therapy, communicate with physicians and other consultants, conference team leader
Nurse	RN/NP/nurse specialist	Nursing assessment including functional assessment; home visits, coordinate care plan; patient education
Social worker	LCSW	Mental status evaluation; liaison with family and community agencies; elder's family advocate; coordinate care plan
Geropsychiatrist	Physician	Psychiatric consultation, psychopharmacological management
Clinical psychologist/ neuropsychologist	PhD	Psychotherapy; caregiver support; neuropsychological testing
Pharmacist	Pharm D	Patient education, monitor compliance and changes
Physical therapist	MPT, licensed (some certificate in aging/gerontology preferred)	Assessment of rehabilitation potential; mobility and balance training; canes, walkers, wheel chairs; HCFA documentation regulations
Occupational therapist	Registered, licensed, certificate in aging preferred	Teach or reteach everyday skills to function in home and the community; knowledge of ADL, IADL scales; MMSE and GDS; adaptive devices; environmental evaluation; documentation regulations

From Elon R et al: General issues and comprehensive approach to assessment of elders. In: *Comprehensive Geriatric Assessment.* Osterweil D, Brummel-Smith K, Beck JC (editors). McGraw-Hill, 2000.

Table 40–2. Common chronic syndromes among vulnerable elderly.

Continuity and coordination of care
Dementia
Depression
Diabetes mellitus
End-of-life care
Falls and mobility disorders
Hearing impairment
Heart failure
Hospital care
Hypertension
Ischemic heart disease
Malnutrition
Medication management
Osteoarthritis
Osteoporosis
Pain management
Pneumonia and influenza
Pressure ulcers
Screening and prevention
Stroke and atrial fibrillation
Urinary incontinence
Vision impairment

From Wegner NS. et al, (eds.): Quality indicators for assessing care of vulnerable elders. Ann Intern Med 2001;135 [suppl (8; pt. 2)]: 641. Online at http://www.acponline.org/sci-policy/acove/.

Solomon D: Introduction: In: *Comprehensive Geriatric Assessment.* Osterweil D, Brummel-Smith K, Beck JC (editors). McGraw-Hill, 2000.

Wegner NS et al: Quality indicators for assessing care of vulnerable elders. Ann Intern Med 2001;135[suppl 8 (pt 2)]:641.

Who Needs Assessment?

The question always asked is "which older person needs a geriatric assessment and what is the best approach to implement this screening?" Because geriatric assessment is an attempt to gain a complete picture of the health status of an older individual, the primary care provider

Table 40–3. Goals of geriatric assessment.

To define the functional capabilities and disabilities of older patients
To appropriately manage acute and chronic diseases of frail elders
To promote prevention and health
To establish preferences for care in various situations (advance care planning)
To understand financial resources available for care
To understand social networks and family support systems for care
To evaluate an older patient's mental and emotional strengths and weakness

Table 40–4. Goals of geriatric assessment as expressed by patients, caregivers, physicians, and case managers.

Patients	Family Caregiver	Physicians	Case Managers
General health and well-being	Education/referrals	Education/referrals	Education/referrals
Functioning/independence	Social/family relations/activities	Functioning/independence	Medication issues
Social/family relations/activities	Functioning/independence	Social/family relations/activities	Social/family relations/activities
Medical issues	Supervision	Supervision	Medical issues
Education/referrals	General health and well-being	Medical issues	Supervision
Caregiver burden	Medication issues	Medication issues	Functioning/independence
Supervision	Medical issues	Emotional issues	Emotional issues
Emotional issues	Cognitive issues	Behavioral issues	Cognitive and behavioral issues
Health behaviors	Emotional issues	Health behaviors	Health behaviors
Medications	Health behaviors	Driving	Driving

From Bradley EH et al: Goals in geriatric assessment: are we measuring the right outcomes. Gerontologist 2000;40:191.

must become involved not only in diagnosing and treating medical problems but also in all the factors that affect the health of older patients. A geriatric assessment is a **diagnostic tool,** not a therapeutic intervention for the cure of chronic disease and the reversal of disability. Table 40–5 details the components of a geriatric assessment.

What is fortunate for most primary care providers is that the majority of older adults do not need an extensive assessment, but more of a screen to uncover problems. If screening uncovers a problem or problems, a more extensive evaluation can be instituted and a plan of treatment and/or management can be implemented. A common screening tool (Table 40–6) that can be used by nonphysician office staff to screen ambulatory older patients is available. This instrument attempts to uncover those common areas in which an older patient may be having difficulties. It addresses vision, hearing, leg mobility, incontinence, nutrition, memory, depression, and physical disability. It can be administered in 8–12 min, has been found to have good validity and reliability, and can be easily implemented in an ambulatory practice. If the older patient is found to have difficulties in one of the functional areas defined by the screen, then further evaluation by the physician can be instituted.

For a family physician, the ability to identify vulnerable elders is important. Health care organizations taking on the financial risk of older adults want to identify those high-risk elders in order to avert a health crisis and to provide the special care and management needed

Table 40–5. Components of geriatric assessment.

Functional assessment
  Basic activities of daily living (BADLs)—fundamental to independent living: bathing, dressing, toileting, transfers, feeding
  Instrumental activities of daily living (IADLs)—complex daily activities: transportation, shopping, meal preparation, housework, finances
  Advanced activities of daily living (AADLs)—"functional signature"
  Gait-mobility and balance
  Upper extremity evaluation
Cognitive and affective assessment
  Dementia
  Depression
  Suicide
  Alcohol misuse
Sensory impairments
Nutrition
Incontinence
Social assessment (caregivers, environment, finances)
Driving
Sexuality
Advance care planning

From Gallo JJ et al: *Handbook of Geriatric Assessment,* ed 3. Aspen Publishers, 2000.

Table 40–6. A geriatric screening for impaired ambulatory elderly.

1. Medications
   Did the patient bring in all bottles or a list of medications?
   List all medications
   Remember to ask about over-the-counter medications
   Remember to ask about supplements and herbs
2. Nutrition
   Weigh patient and record
   Have you lost more than 10 lb in the last 6 months?
   Positive screen: 10 lb weight loss or < 100 lb
   Intervention: Further evaluation with the Mini-Nutritional Assessment
3. Hearing
   Use handheld audioscope at 40 dB and screen both ears at 1000 and 2000 Hz
   Positive screen: Patient unable to hear 1000 or 2000 Hz frequency in *both* ears *or* unable to hear the 1000 and 2000 Hz frequency in *one* ear
   Intervention: Evaluate for cerumen impaction; refer to audiology
4. Vision
   Ask: "Do you have any problems driving, watching TV, reading, or doing any of your activities because of your eyesight?" If yes
   Do Snellen eye chart
   Positive screen: 20/40 or greater
   Intervention: Refer to optometry or ophthalmology
5. Mental Status
   Ask to remember three objects—"ball, car, and flag" (have them repeat objects after you)
   Positive screen: Unable to remember all three items after 1 min
   Intervention: Administer more formal mental status testing such as the 7-Minute Neurocognitive Screening Battery or MMSE; assess for causes of cognitive impairment including delirium, depression, and medications
6. Depression
   Ask: "Are you depressed?" or "Do you often feel sad or depressed?"
   Positive screen: Yes
   Intervention: Perform a more thorough depression screen (Geriatric Depression Scale); evaluate medications; consider pharmacological treatment and/or refer to psychiatry
7. Urinary Incontinence
   Ask: "In the last year have you ever lost urine or gotten wet?" if *yes*
   Ask:" Have your lost urine in at least 6 separate days?"
   Positive screen: Yes to both
   Intervention: Initiate workup for incontinence; consider urology referral
8. Physical Disability
   Ask: Are you able to do strenuous activities like fast walking or biking? Heavy work around the house like washing windows, floors, and walls? Go shopping for groceries or clothes? Get to places out of walking distance? Bathe, either sponge bath, tub bath or shower? Dress, like putting on a shirt, buttoning and zipping, and putting on your shoes?
   Positive screen: Unable to do any of the above independently or able to do only with assistance from another
   Intervention: Corroborate responses if accuracy uncertain with caregivers; determine reason for inability to perform task; institute appropriate medical, social, and environmental interventions. Patient may benefit from physical and/or occupational therapy and a home visit
9. Mobility
   Ask: "Do you fall or feel unbalanced when walking or standing?"
   Positive Screen: Yes
   Intervention: "Up and Go" test: Get up from the chair, walk 20 feet, turn, walk back to the chair, and sit down (walk at normal, comfortable pace)
   Positive screen: Unable to complete the task in 15 s
   Intervention: Refer to physical therapy for gait evaluation and assistance with use of appropriate adaptive devices; home safety evaluation. Patient may need to be instructed in strengthening of both upper and lower extremities

(*continued*)

Table 40–6. A geriatric screening for impaired ambulatory elderly. (*Continued*)

10. Home Environment
    Ask: Do you have trouble with stairs either inside or outside of your house? Do you feel safe at home?
    Positive Screen: Yes
    Intervention: Supply the older patient or caregiver with a home safety self-assessment check list; consider making a home visit or use a visiting nurse or other community resource to evaluate the home; make appropriate referrals to help remediate safety issues
11. Social Support
    Ask: Who would be able to help you in case of an illness or emergency?
    Record identified person(s) in medical record with contact information
    Intervention: Become familiar with available resources for the elderly within your community or know who can provide you with that assistance

Adapted from Lachs MS et al: A simple procedure for general screening for functional disability in elderly patients. Ann Intern Med 1990;112:699 and Moore AA, Siu AL: Screening for common problems in ambulatory elderly: a clinical confirmation of a screening instrument. Am J Med 1996;100:438.

to optimize health. Three screening methods to identify high-risk elders are available for organizations and groups to use to survey their older populations: periodic survey screening by telephone or mail, clinician recognition, and analysis of administrative data. None of these methods alone is sufficient to identify all high-risk seniors in a population.

Two population screening instruments to assist in identifying at-risk or vulnerable elders are the P_{ra} (probability of repeated admissions to a hospital in the future) and the vulnerable elders survey. In several longitudinal studies the P_{ra} screening has been shown to identify those high-risk elders who use twice as many health services as low-risk seniors. The vulnerable elders survey identified 32% of a nationally represented sample as vulnerable. This group was found to have 4.2 times the risk of death and functional decline over 2 years. Attempting to identify those high-risk elders may allow for better targeting of services not only to vulnerable elders but to the caregivers.

Boult C, Pacala JT: Care of older people at risk. In: *New Ways to Care for Older People: Building Systems Based on Evidence.* Calkins E et al (editors). Springer Publishing, 1999.
Saliba D et al: The vulnerable elders survey: a tool for identifying vulnerable older people in the community. J Am Geriatr Soc 2001;49:1691.

The Importance of Function

The ability to function independently in the community is an important public health and quality of life issue for all older adults. A recent trend toward declining disability has been noted among older persons, especially those with a higher level of education. The overall health status of older Americans is also improving with regard to physical functioning, social activities, and regular exercise. Older adults who walk a mile at least once per week have a greater probability of improvement and show less of a decline in functional limitations and disability than their sedentary counterparts. However, these trends are not indicative of the total population. Non-Hispanic black and Mexican-American men and women generally report more functional limitations and disability and represent a vulnerable subpopulation within the United States.

Several predictors of functional decline and mortality have been reported. Health status belief and decreased abilities in activities of daily living (ADL) appear to be important predictors of mortality. Older individuals (both men and women) with high depressive symptomology have increased risk of ADL disability, as it appears depressive symptoms undermine efforts to maintain physical functioning. Social networks may have a negative impact on ADLs by provoking dependency and a sense of "learned" helplessness, especially in older men.

Kivela SL, Pahkala K: Depressive disorder as a predictor of physical disability in old-age. J Am Geriatr Soc 2001;49:290.
Ostchega Y et al: The prevalence of functional limitations and disability in older person in the US: data from the National Health and Nutrition Examination Survey III. J Am Geriatr Soc 2000;48:1132.

Functional Assessment

Assessment of function is at the core of caring for older adults. The capacity to perform functional tasks necessary for daily living can be used as a surrogate measure of independence or a predictor of decline and institutionalization. A specific evaluation of functional status is necessary in older individuals, as functional impairment cannot be predicted by an individual's medical diagnoses. Functional status needs to be assessed directly and independently of medical and laboratory abnormalities or cognitive impairment, as specific functional loss is not disease specific and cognitive impairment does not necessarily imply inability to function independently in a familiar environment. Functional assessment can help focus on an older individual's capabilities and by noting changes in these can search for possible illness such as cognitive impairment, depression, substance abuse, adverse drug events, or sensory impairment, and then intervene with the appropriate support and resources.

Functional assessment can be seen as a hierarchy. The basic activities of daily living (BADL) are those self-care activities that are at the most basic level of functioning, such as bathing, dressing, toileting, transfers, continence, and feeding (Table 40–7). An older adult may be fully independent, need assistance, or be fully dependent in any or all of these activities. Individuals may move in and out of needing assistance or dependence, especially at the time of and after the onset of an acute illness or disease process.

Assessment of BADL items allows the primary care provider to focus on functional abilities, thus matching services to needs. The hierarchy for loss of BADL abilities is associated with increasing age and appears to be dependent on lower extremity strength, such that bathing, mobility, and toileting are lost before dressing and feeding, which rely on upper extremity strength. Of all of the BADL measures, dependence with regard to going to the toilet has been shown to be an indicator

Table 40–7. Basic and instrumental activities of daily living.

ADL (self-care)
Bathing
Dressing
Toileting
Transfers
Continence
Feeding
IADL (independent community living and interactions)[1]
Housework—Can you do your own housework?
Traveling—Can you get places outside of walking distance?
Shopping—Can you go shopping for food and clothing?
Money—Can you handle your own money?
Meal preparation—Can you prepare your own meals?

Adapted from Katz S et al: Studies of illness in the aged: the index of ADL: a standardized measure of biological and psychosocial function. JAMA 1963;185:914 and Fillenbaum G: Screening the elderly: a brief instrumental activities of daily living measure. J Am Geriatr Soc 1985;33:683.
[1]In order of most difficult to least difficult—knowing a person can perform one item indicates they can perform item below it.

of overall performance and the need for overall higher levels of assistance.

The next higher level of functioning is known as the instrumental activities of daily living (IADL). These activities are required for independent living within the community and include a set of more complex and demanding tasks (Table 40–7). Older individuals living in the community who cannot perform IADLs may have difficulty functioning at home. The more IADLs that are impaired in a community-dwelling elder, the greater the likelihood of developing dementia within 1 year.

The advanced activities of daily living (AADL) are those tasks that may be considered the "functional signature" of a well community-dwelling older individual. These tasks include voluntary social, occupational, or recreational activities. An older person who does not successfully participate in such activities may not be dysfunctional, but an assessment that uncovers significant involuntary loss of such function may be an important risk factor for further functional losses. Globally knowing how an elderly person spends his or her days can give the physician a reference point for potential functional decline at subsequent visits.

Gallo JJ et al: *Handbook of Geriatric Assessment,* ed 3. Aspen Publishers, 2000.

Sherman FT: Functional assessment: easy to use screening tools to speed initial office work-up. Geriatrics 2001;56:36.

Gait-Mobility & Balance

Direct observation of physical performance by the physician in the office setting can provide an assessment of function and may disclose deficits that go unreported by the patient. Performance measures for gait, balance, transfers, and joint function are particularly valuable tools to the physician who is attempting to correlate self-report with direct observation of abilities. Physical performance measures are tests in which the individual is asked to perform a specific task in an objective uniform manner using predetermined criteria. Many performance measures that have been developed for research are not applicable to a primary care practice and have no practical meaning if an older individual is able to function within his or her environment. However, because the ability of an older individual to live independently in the community requires the capacity to maneuver through the environment safely and effectively, observations for impairment in mobility may detect an individual at risk for injury, falls, nursing home placement, or mortality.

Knowledge of performance with respect to gait and balance is an important part of the functional as well as physical assessment of an older adult and may allow the primary care physician to identify an elderly individual at risk for falling. Falls are more likely to occur in frail individuals who are over 80 years old and have gait and balance abnormalities, cognitive impairment, depression, poor upper and lower body strength, and poor vision. Nondisabled older persons with poor lower extremity function have been estimated to constitute 10% of the 70- to 90-year-old population and are at risk for increased disability. The ACOVE quality indicator on falls states that all vulnerable elderly should have documentation at least annually about the occurrence of recent falls and that basic gait-mobility and balance evaluations should be done and documented. Assessment of gait and balance can be easily done in an ambulatory setting. A recent review of interventions to prevent falls found muscle strengthening, balance retraining, and health and environmental risk factor screening were valuable to the vulnerable older adult.

Ostchega Y et al: Reliability and prevalence of physical performance examination assessing mobility and balance in older persons in the US: data from the Third National Health and Nutrition Examination Survey. J Am Geriatr Soc 2000;48:1136.

A. THE "GET-UP AND GO" TEST

The "Get-up and Go" (GUG) test was devised to evaluate balance disturbances in frail elderly older adults in an attempt to identify individuals at risk for falls. The test can be scored or timed; however, what is important is that it is incorporated into the physical evaluation of an elderly patient. To do this test the older patient is seated in a straight back high-seated chair. Sitting balance and transfers from sitting to standing are noted. The older patient is instructed to rise from the chair (without using armrests if possible), stand still momentarily, walk forward approximately 10 feet, turn, walk back to the chair, turn around, and sit back down. The primary care provider should be observing for any evidence that the older adult may potentially fall (Table 40–8). It has been noted that self-selected gait speed is the single greatest predictor of self-perceived function and overall physical performance in a wide range of abilities.

B. BALANCE

Standing balance can be evaluated by observing the response to position stress, loss of visual input, and displacement. The patient first stands with eyes open and feet comfortably apart, then with eyes closed. Stability is observed and the patient should be asked if he or she feels steady. A light nudge to the sternum assesses the response to displacement. These maneuvers may identify causative factors such as osteoarthritis, peripheral neuropathy, foot problems, atherosclerosis, weakness, stroke, pain, or contractures.

Table 40–8. Observations during the "Get-up and Go" test.

Unsafe or incomplete transfers
Poor sitting balance
Difficulty or unsafe sitting down
Difficulty rising
Instability on first standing
Short, discontinuous steps
Slowness and hesitancy
Staggering on turns
Excessive truncal sway
Grabbing for support
Stumbling
Unsafe maneuvers

Adapted from Fleming KC et al: Practical functional assessment of elderly persons: a primary-care approach. Mayo Clin Proc 1995;70:890.

The Functional Reach Test can also be used to assess balance. The older patient is asked to stand with one shoulder close to a wall, to extend the fist along the wall directly frontward, and then to lean forward, fist extended in front as far as possible without taking a step or losing balance. The patient should be able to move the fist forward a distance of 6 inches. A lesser distance indicates a significant risk for falls and is a strong predictor of frailty.

Upper-Extremity Evaluation

The upper extremities of older patients need evaluation, especially with reference to hand and shoulder function. Age-related changes in the shoulder may result in limited range of motion with decreased strength, mobility, and chronic pain. A simple evaluation of shoulder function is to have older patients put both hands behind their head and then put both hands together behind their back. Hand grasp can be evaluated by asking patients to squeeze two of the examiner's fingers with each hand. Any pain or limitation in shoulder and/or hand function should prompt further evaluation and referral.

Assessment of Cognitive Impairment & Depressed Mood

Cognitive impairment is uncommon in community-dwelling elders 65–74 years old, but rises substantially in those 85 years old and older. It is estimated to affect 10% of community-dwelling elders and up to 50% of institutionalized older adults. Primary care providers are likely to encounter cognitive impairment and depressive disorders in day-to-day practice. The importance of screening will allow for detection, management, and treatment of newly diagnosed disease. In the case of memory complaints the provider can offer reassurance if cognitive impairment is not found, look for potential reversible causes of dementia, provide prognostic information to the patient and family, and use newer medications if warranted for the impairment diagnosed. The ACOVE quality indicators recommend a multidimensional assessment of cognitive and functional abilities if a vulnerable elder is admitted to the hospital or is new to a physician's practice.

A. Cognitive Impairment

Common screening tools for detection of cognitive impairment include the Mini-Mental State Examination (MMSE), 3-item recall (subset of the MMSE), clock drawing test, time and change test, and 7-minute screen. A recent evidence-based review of early detection of patients with mild cognitive impairment recommended that those individuals be routinely followed with an instrument such as the MMSE as long as language other than English, cultural differences, and educational level including reading level are taken into account.

If elderly patients have difficulty with 3-item recall, have difficulty managing finances or balancing a checkbook, get lost driving, frequently forget names of relatives, frequently repeat stories or statements, or have poor judgment, then the primary care physician should be highly suspicious of early Alzheimer's disease and undertake a more formal assessment and evaluation. Other indicators of dementia from functional assessment include difficulties with telephone use and managing medications.

Solomon PR et al: A 7-minute neurocognitive screening battery highly sensitive to Alzheimer's disease. Arch Neurol 1998;55: 349.

Tierney MC et al: Prediction of probable Alzheimer's disease in patients with symptoms suggestive of memory impairment: value of the mini-mental state examination. Arch Fam Med 2000;9:527.

B. Depression

Depression is the most common psychiatric condition in primary care and is underreported and undertreated in older adults. As noted earlier, depression as well as cognitive impairment can impair functioning, increase risk for cardiac mortality, and lead to increased health service use and costs. The prevalence of depressive symptoms ranges from 16% to 35% using self-reported questionnaires with the oldest-old often neglected in the investigation of geriatric depression. ACOVE quality indicators recommend asking about depression and starting treatment if a vulnerable elder presents with new onset of sad mood, feeling down, insomnia or difficulties with sleep, anhedonia, complaints of memory loss, and unexplained weight loss or fatigue and low energy.

Screening for depression is done by simply asking the elderly patient: "Do you often feel sad or depressed?" This question has a positive predictive value of 85% and a negative predictive value of 90%. If an elderly patient answers in the affirmative to this question or has any of the other ACOVE indicators, then a more thorough evaluation for depression should be undertaken. The Geriatric Depression Scale (GDS) has three versions ranging from 30 items to 5 items for the detection of depression. These scales are reliable and valid and allow for independent patient completion.

Hoyl MT et al: Development and testing of a five-item version of the Geriatric Depression Scale. J Am Geriatr Soc 1999;47: 873.

Alcohol Misuse

Alcohol consumption and alcoholism are commonplace among the elderly with 10.5% of men and 3.9% of women in one primary care practice reporting problem alcohol use. Detection of alcoholism in the elderly is difficult for numerous reasons, including the idea that elderly patients do not see alcoholism as a disease, but rather as a sign of weakness. Physicians create their own barriers to the diagnosis including uncertainty of the diagnosis, pessimism concerning treatment, and possible subconscious hostility toward the alcoholic older patient. ACOVE quality indicators for preventive care include screening all vulnerable elders at least once to detect problem or hazardous drinking by taking a history of alcohol use and using a standard screening questionnaires such as the 4-item CAGE or the 10-item AUDIT.

American Medical Association: Alcoholism in the Elderly: Diagnosis, Treatment, and Prevention: Guidelines for Primary Care Physicians. The American Medical Association, 1995.

Driving

Evaluating the driving competence of an older patient is a challenge for physicians. The automobile is the ultimate symbol of freedom and the most important source of transportation for older adults. The ability to drive or be driven is closely linked to independence and self-esteem, allowing the older adult to maintain important links within the community. Those who are unable to drive or stop driving risk social isolation, depression, and functional decline. Driving is an instrumental activity of daily living composed of complex tasks that require not only physical but mental integrity. As the population ages, it is estimated that by 2020, 15% of all drivers will be over 65. A recent analysis of traffic-related fatalities among older drivers and passengers found that adults over the age of 65 will account for 27% of all automobile fatalities in 2015, an increase of 373% since 1975.

In an attempt to reduce risk, many older drivers alter their driving habits by driving shorter distances, driving only during daylight, and avoiding rush hour, major highways, and inclement weather. However, not all older drivers avert risk. One study found that older adults with diagnosed Alzheimer's dementia and those needing help with dressing and bathing still persisted in driving. Adults who voluntarily stop driving are usually older (over 85 years), female, nonwhite, and had driven less than 50 miles per week. Heart disease and hearing impairment are more often associated with reports of adverse driving events. Driving accidents with older adults rarely involve high speeds or alcohol. Their accidents are usually related to issues involving visual–spatial difficulties and cognitive and motor skills.

Assessment of the older driver is made all the more difficult because chronic illness, functional status, or even cognitive impairment cannot consistently predict adverse driving events. An assessment of the older driver should include a review of the driving record; medications; alcohol use; and functional measures including vision, hearing, attention (spell WORLD backward), visual–spatial skills (clock drawing), muscle strength, and joint flexibility. Older drivers should be advised on the importance of safety restraints, obeying speed limits, avoidance of drinking and driving and the use of cellular telephones while driving, use of a helmet if riding a motorcycle or bicycle, and taking a driving refresher course. It is important for primary care physicians to know the laws of their state with regard to driving and reportable medical conditions.

Carr DB: The older adult driver. Am Fam Physician 2000;61:141.

Foley KT, Mitchell SJ: The elderly driver: what physicians need to know. Cleveland Cl J Med 1997;64:423.

Sensory Impairments

Vision and hearing impairments are prevalent in the elderly. Normal vision is associated with decreased visual acuity, visual field defects, and retinal diseases. The aging lens causes light to scatter at night, leading to increased glare and reduced nighttime safety. Cataracts, glaucoma, and macular degeneration increase with age and can lead to progressive visual loss. Impairment of vision has been related to increased risk of nursing home placement ("legally blind"), falls, and even mortality. Of individuals 65 years and older, 18% have a vi-

sual impairment of 20/70 or greater and 20% of adults over 85 years of age have difficulty seeing with glasses. Screening for visual impairment can be done by having older adults read a Snellen eye chart. Failure to read all letters at the 20/40 line should alert the physician to refer this patient for a thorough ophthalmological evaluation. ACOVE quality indicators recommend that all vulnerable elderly be offered an eye evaluation every 2 years.

Hearing impairment is the most common sensory impairment of the elderly, affecting 24% to almost 70% of older adults. Hearing impairment affects cognitive, emotional, social, and physical functioning and has been implicated along with visual impairment as a risk for increased mortality. Hearing impairment is poorly recognized and undercorrected. The ACOVE quality indicators recommend that all vulnerable elderly have their hearing screened as part of the initial evaluation.

Screening by using the whisper or watch test is highly inadequate. The recommendation is to screen for hearing impairment using a handheld audioscope that delivers pure tones at 40 dB at four frequencies—500, 1000, 2000, and 4000 Hz. A patient who is unable to hear either 1000-Hz or 2000-Hz tones in both ears or 1000-Hz and 2000-Hz tones in one ear fails the screen. Referral to an audiologist should be offered for further evaluation for aural rehabilitation as amplification devices lead to improved function and quality of life. A recently developed brief self-report of hearing impairment has been found to be 80% sensitive and specific in predicting hearing loss. This tool could easily be incorporated into a screening evaluation of all older adults.

Jerger J et al: Hearing impairment in older adults: new concepts. J Am Geriatr Soc 1995;43:928.

Keller BK et al: The effect of visual and hearing impairments on functional status. J Am Geriatr Soc 1999;47:1319.

Nutrition

Maintaining optimal nutrition is important for healthy aging but requires particular attention in vulnerable older adults. The two most common nutritional problems in the elderly are obesity (a problem of the young-old) and energy undernutrition (a problem of the old-old). Many factors place older adults at nutritional risk including inability to acquire and prepare nutritious meals, drug–food interactions, and aging physiology (see Chapter 37). The ACOVE quality indicators recommend screening for malnutrition by weighing all community-dwelling vulnerable elders at each physician visit and documenting the weight. If the vulnerable elder has involuntary weight loss equal to or greater than 10% of body weight in 1 year or less, the weight loss should be documented and an evaluation initiated. New patients to a physician's office can be asked: "Without trying have you lost 10 pounds in the past 6 months?"

A brief assessment can also include the calculation of the patient's body mass index (BMI: weight in kilograms/height in meters^2). A BMI <17 kg/m^2 is associated with protein–energy undernutrition. Also, a serum albumin of 3.5 mg/dL or less can be a simple indicator of possible malnutrition. Finally, the "Checklist to Determine Your Nutritional Health" from the Nutrition Screening Initiative can be given to the older adult in the waiting room as a self-assessment of nutritional risk and can provide additional insight for the older adult, caregivers, and physician concerning potential nutritional problems. However, this checklist is neither sensitive nor specific in accurately identifying nutritional risk. Other factors that may alert the provider to possible malnutrition include eating problems, polypharmacy, eating a special diet, and functional limitations.

Jensen GL et al: Screening for hospitalization and nutritional risks among community-dwelling older persons. Am J Clin Nutr 2001;74:201.

Incontinence

Urinary incontinence is common in the elderly. It is underreported by women and underrecognized by physicians. Common reasons women do not report incontinence are embarrassment and a misconception that it is a common part of aging best controlled with pads. Minor incontinence may have few medical concerns but many social ramifications for the older woman or man. Severe incontinence can lead to skin breakdown, ulcers, increased caregiver burden, and if the person is frail or demented may lead to institutionalization.

The ACOVE quality indicators recommend that all vulnerable elders should have the presence or absence of urinary incontinence documented at the initial visit. Screen by asking: "In the last year, have you ever lost urine or gotten wet?" If the older adult answers yes, then a targeted history and physical examination are indicated (see Chapter 39).

Social Assessment

An important aspect of caring for older persons, especially vulnerable older persons, is to have an understanding of their social environment. Social assessment includes the sources and kinds of help available to the older adult and assessment of the primary caregiver, often called the "hidden patient." The social assessment is important in the development of an effective care plan and all parts of the social assessment should be covered, usually over several patient visits. The elements of the social assessment are listed in Table 40–9.

Social Support

It is important to understand the social networks of an older person. The social networks consist of informal supports such as family and close longtime friends, formal supports such as social welfare and other social service and health care delivery agencies, and semiformal supports such as church groups, neighborhood organizations, and clubs. Relationships with family and friends are intricate and can have consequences for the vulnerable elder. The availability of assistance from family or friends frequently determines whether a functionally dependent elder remains at home or is institutionalized. Knowing who would be available to help the elder if he or she becomes ill is important to document even for healthy elders. Other important information to obtain from older persons is outlined in Table 40–10. For a more formal assessment of social support the Norbeck Social Support Questionnaire or the Lubben Social Network Scale should be considered.

Caregiver Burden

For individuals caring for a frail, often cognitively impaired elder, the demands can be overwhelming. Caregiver burden has been defined as the strain or load borne by the person who cares for an elderly, chronically ill, or disabled family member or other person. Caregivers are at higher risk for mortality if there is increased mental or emotional strain. Caregiver burden is linked to the caregiver's ability to cope and handle stress. The physician should be alert for signs of possible caregiver burnout including multiple somatic complaints, increased stress and anxiety, circular thinking, social isolation, depression, and weight loss. More for-

Table 40–9. Elements of social assessment.

Social support
Caregiver burden
Elder mistreatment
Economic
Environment
Sexual health
Spiritual
Suicide
Advanced care planning (values history, living will, durable power of attorney)

From Gallo JJ et al: *Handbook of Geriatric Assessment*, ed 3. Aspen Publishers, 2000.

Table 40–10. Social support screening.

How many relatives do you see or hear from in the course of a month?

Tell me about the relative with whom you have the most contact.

How many relatives do you feel close to—such as to discuss private matters?

How many friends do you see or hear from in the course of a month?

Tell me about the friend with whom you have the most contact.

When you have an important decision to make, do you have someone you can talk to about it?

Do you rely on anybody to assist you with shopping, cooking, doing repairs, cleaning house, etc?

Do you help others with shopping, cooking, transportation, child-care, etc?

Do you live alone?

With whom do you live?

From Gallo JJ et al: *Handbook of Geriatric Assessment,* ed 3. Aspen Publishers, 2000.

mal assessment tools include the Caregiver Strain Index and the Zarit Burden Interview, for which a short version and screening version are available.

Bedard M et al: The Zarit Burden interview: a short version and screening version. Gerontologist 2001;41:652.

Kasuya RT, Polgar-Bailey P, Takeuchi R: Caregiver burden and burnout: a guide for primary care physicians. Postgrad Med 2000;108:119.

Schulz R, Beach SR: Caregiving as a risk factor for mortality: The Caregiver Health Effects Study. JAMA 1999;282:2215.

Economic Assessment

Economic factors have important consequences with respect to an older person's health, nutrition, and living environment. Understanding the impact of financial status of the elderly may provide insight into how the individual copes, such as buying food versus medications. The primary care provider should have a working knowledge of Medicare and state and local assistance programs and know where the older person could go to obtain needed assistance in applying for appropriate financial benefits. The physician can inquire by asking if older individuals have enough financial resources to meet their needs. The physician needs to know if the proposed treatment will be an economic burden on the individual.

Environmental Assessment

The physical environment of the older person, including home environment, neighborhood, and transporta-

tion system, is critical to maintaining independence. Environmental hazards within the home are high and can be a potential constraint not only on the day-to-day functioning of frail elders but also on those older persons without any specific physical deficits. Common environmental hazards within the home include loose throw rugs, curled carpet edges, obstructed pathways, lack of grab bars in tub and shower, and low and loose toilet seats. These hazards could lead to an increased risk of falls and fractures. The physician should inquire about the safety of the neighborhood and ask if older persons have transportation or transportation services available in close geographic proximity to where they live. This is especially important for elders dependent in IADLs and still living within the community.

Older persons often have problems not easily detected during an office visit. A home visit either by the physician or a community agency provider such as a visiting nurse can reveal problems in the living situation, such as wandering, household and bathing hazards, social isolation and loneliness, family stress, nutrition problems, financial concerns, and even alcohol abuse. An environmental checklist that the older person or family member can use for a self-assessment can be found at the National Safety Council's web site (www.nsc.org).

Unwin BK, Jerant AF: The home visit. Am Fam Physician 1999; 60:1481.

Sexual Health Assessment

Sexuality late in life is a normal and important part of aging. Primary care providers need to be aware of their own comfort level in taking a sexual health history from older adults. Older adults prefer that the provider initiate the discussion surrounding sexual functioning. Using open-ended questions allows the individual to give as much or as little information as is comfortable. The physician needs to have an understanding of what the older adult's normal sexual patterns and interests have been and what if any changes have occurred that affect sexual functioning and intimacy such as health problems, medications, physical disabilities, or cognitive impairments.

The physician should inquire into the nature of the older person's sexual quality of life by asking about how affection is displayed and how physical intimacy is expressed. Because not all older persons are in committed heterosexual relationships, it is vitally important that the physician express openness to answers conveyed. It is important for the physician to gain an understanding of what the older adult perceives about changes that may have occurred with regard to sexual function with aging. Issues concerning the quality of erections and orgasm for men or concerns about erectile dysfunction should be discussed. Women may have concerns about their sexual cycle and issues surrounding lubrication and orgasm.

If a problem is uncovered it should be documented and a more thorough assessment and evaluation should be undertaken. Finally, issues surrounding safer sex practices should be discussed with those older adults who are sexually active and not in a committed monogamous relationship.

Zeiss Am, Zeiss RA, Davies H: Assessment of sexual function and dysfunction in older adults. In: *Handbook of Assessment in Clinical Gerontology.* Lichtenberg PA (editor). John Wiley, 1999: 270.

Spirituality

Assessing an older person's spirituality is important to understanding the overall well-being of that individual. It is important to ascertain what religion or spirituality means to older adults and what role it plays in their lives. The spiritual assessment should include the older person's concept of God or deity, religious practices, beliefs about spirit and hell, and value and meaning in life. Older adults can suffer from spiritual distress that may be expressed as depression, crying, fear of abandonment, or hopelessness, anxiety, and despair. This distress may occur after a loss of a significant other, after a family or personal disaster, or when there is a

Table 40–11. Five steps to successful advanced care planning.

Steps	Process
1. Introduce the topic	During a wellness visit or some other time when the individual is in a good state of health Explain the purpose and nature of the discussion Inquire into how familiar the individual is with advanced care planning and define terms as necessary Be aware of the comfort level of the patient—give information and be supportive Suggest that family members, friends, or even members of the community explore how to manage potential burdens Discuss the identification of a proxy decision maker Encourage the patient to bring the proxy decision maker to the next visit
2. Engage in structured discussions	Convey commitment to patients to follow their wishes and protect patients from unwanted treatment or undertreatment Involve the potential proxy decision maker in discussions and planning Allow the patient to specify the role he or she would like the proxy to assume if the patient is incapacitated—follow patient's explicit wishes or allow the proxy to decide according to the patient's best interests Elicit the patient's values and goals Use a validated advisory document available at http//www.medicaldirective.org
3. Document patient preferences	Review advanced directives with patient and proxy for inconsistencies and misunderstandings Enter the advanced directives into the medical record Recommend statutory documents be completed by the patient that comply with state statutes Distribute directives to hospital, patient, proxy decision maker, family members, and all health care providers Include advanced directives in the care plan
4. Review and update the directive regularly	
5. Apply directives to actual circumstances	Most advanced directives go into affect when the patient can no longer direct his or her own medical care Assess the patient's decision-making capacity Never assume advanced directive content without reading it thoroughly Advanced directives should be interpreted in view of the clinical facts of the case Physician and proxy decision maker will need to work together to resolve ambiguous or uncertain situations If disagreements between physician and proxy cannot be resolved—seek the assistance of an ethics consultant or committee

Adapted from Emanuel LL, von Guten CF, Ferris FD: Advance care planning. Arch Fam Med 2000;9:1181.

disruption in usual religious activities. Religion and spirituality are a source of comfort for patients. Inquiring into the spirituality of patients requires empathy on the part of the physician, strong interpersonal skills, and a closely established physician–patient relationship.

Advanced Care Planning

Advanced care planning is a process of planning for the medical future in which the patient's preferences will guide the nature and intensity of future medical care, particularly if the patient is unable to make his or her own decisions. As part of the assessment of the older person it is important for the physician to learn about the patient's goals and preferences for care. This is especially important for the frail elderly as it will ultimately influence management decisions. The ACOVE quality indicators recommend that the outpatient record of all vulnerable elders should include either an advanced directive indicating the patient's surrogate decision maker, documentation of a discussion about who would be a surrogate decision maker or a search for a surrogate, or an indication that no surrogate has been identified. The process of advanced care planning helps patients identify their personal values and goals about health and medical treatment. They should indicate the care they would and would not want to receive in various situations. Advanced care planning is designed to ensure that the patient's wishes are known, even if the patient is unable to participate in those decisions.

Fewer than 25% of seriously ill patients have discussed preferences for cardiopulmonary resuscitation with their physician and over 50% of those patients were not interested in doing so. Involving patients in the process of planning can build trust between patient, physician, and proxy. It can also allow patients to reflect upon and understand their own values, goals, and preferences, relieve anxiety and fear, and avoid potential future confusion and conflicts. Table 40–11 outlines five steps for successful advanced care planning. By following these guidelines common problems can be avoided such as failure to plan, vague or misunderstood patient wishes, failure to involve the proxy in planning and decision making, and failure to follow the written directive as set out by the patient. Advance care planning should be a standard practice and part of all routine geriatric assessments.

Emanuel LL, von Guten CF, Ferris FD: Advance care planning. Arch Fam Med 2000;9:1181.

Depression in Older Patients

41

Charles F. Reynolds III, MD[1,2]

General Considerations

Depression is common in elderly primary care patients, with clinically significant symptoms affecting about 15–20% of patients aged 60 years and above at any time. Depression in later life usually coexists with other chronic medical illnesses (especially diabetes, arthritis, hypothyroidism, coronary artery disease, congestive heart failure, chronic obstructive lung disease, and neurodegenerative disorders such as Alzheimer's or Parkinson's), amplifying the disability and burden of care giving occasioned by these illnesses. Depression diminishes quality of life, leads to nonadherence with self-care (diet, exercise, taking medication as prescribed), increases other medical services use, is a risk factor for suicide (especially in older white males), and is frequently associated with cognitive impairment. Because of time constraints and inadequate reimbursement for provision of mental health services, depression in later life often does not compete well for time in primary care practices and may go unrecognized and untreated. However, depression in the elderly *is* treatable, and most elderly actually prefer to be treated in the general medical sector, rather than be referred out to specialty care. Moreover, many if not most primary care physicians feel that treating depression in their elderly patients is properly a part of their clinical expertise and responsibility.

Of particular clinical relevance to general medical and family medicine practice, depression in later life is very much a "family affair," in the sense that family members are critically important in getting patients to

treatment and keeping them in treatment long enough to do some good. At the same time, the burden of care giving to an elderly family member with depression is considerable, with the result that family members need information about the illness and how best to care for themselves. Hence, we advocate a patient-focused and family-centered approach to care. As we elaborate below, depression in late life is usually a chronic illness, often following a relapsing course. We tell our patients that *getting well is not enough—it is staying well that counts.* To achieve this objective, it is usually medically appropriate to institute maintenance treatment, beyond the acute treatment of the episode, to prolong recovery and prevent recurrence. Notwithstanding the advances in the science of treatment of depression in late life, reimbursement policies are discriminatory (reflecting a look of mental health parity) and represent a major obstacle to the implementation of good care. As well, further research is very much needed on ways of improving cultural competence of providers, practice structures, and incentives to optimize depression care in older Americans.

Diagnosis

The initial assessment procedures should include a focused psychiatric history and examination, including a brief clinical cognitive examination. In addition, a medical history, physical examination, and focused neurological examination are preferred as part of the assessment. The most important symptoms in diagnosing depression in an older patient include sad, downcast mood, frequent tearfulness, loss of pleasure, and recurrent thoughts of death or suicide. Other important tip-offs include diminished interest in pleasurable activities and hobbies, feelings of hopelessness and emptiness, feelings of guilt, avoiding social interactions or engagements outside the home, psychomotor agitation or retardation, difficulty making decisions, and difficulty initiating new projects.

Additional important domains to assess include level of functioning and disability, loss and grief, and the pa-

[1]With The Pittsburgh Late Life Depression Treatment Research Collaborative Network: Charlotte Brown, PhD, Mario Cruz, MD, Ellen G. Detlefsen, DLS, David Hall, MD, Kathy Homrok, MD, Amy Kilbourne, PhD, Brenda Lee, Eric Lenze, MD, Mark D. Miller, MD, Benoit H. Mulsant, MD, Jeffrey Palmer, Edward P. Post, MD, PhD, Charles F. Reynolds III, MD, Grant Shevchik, MD, Francis X. Solano, MD, Gregory Spence-Jones, PhD, and Jeannette South-Paul, MD.
[2]Supported in part by NIMH Grants P30 MH52247, R01 MH59318, and K23 MH01879. Dr. Kilbourne is supported by a VA Health Service Career Development Award.

tient's environment and psychosocial situation. We have found that several instruments are useful for screening for depressive symptoms in primary care practice, including the Center for Epidemiologic Studies depression scale (CES-D), the Patient History Questionnaire (PHQ)-9, and, for diagnostic purposes, the mood disorders module of the PRIME-MD. Similarly, the Folstein Mini-mental state examination is a useful "bedside" screen for cognitive impairment. Scores of 23 or lower on the Folstein raise the possibility of cognitive impairment that needs further assessment. Table 41–1 lists the key symptoms of depression.

Assessing *risk factors for suicide* is an essential part of the diagnostic process. The most important risk factors for suicide in older patients include severity of depression, presence of psychotic depression, alcoholism and other substance abuse, recent loss or bereavement, abuse of sedative hypnotics, and development of disability. Abuse of painkillers is also important. Elderly white males have the highest rates of suicide, almost always related to depression. In 70% of these cases, handguns are used to commit suicide, underscoring the importance of asking about access to lethal means and working with family members to *remove handguns from the home environment.* Up to three-quarters of suicide victims will have seen a primary care physician in the month before death, signaling an opportunity for lifesaving interventions. Always watch for the red flag of hopelessness when assessing suicidality.

Pathogenesis

There are multiple pathways to depression in old age. In the clinical samples reported in many of our National Institutes of Health (NIH)-sponsored investigations, about half of the subjects report onset of depression earlier in life, with recurrences in old age. The role of genetic liability to depression seems to figure more prominently in earlier onset illness. About half of our subjects experience clinical depression for the first time after the age of 60, if not even later. Late-onset depression has a complex and often multifactorial etiology. In some cases, there are clear psychosocial correlates, such

Table 41–1. Tip-offs to clinical depression in the elderly.

Persistent low mood, sadness
Lack of pleasure in usual activities
Suicidal ideation and death wishes
Increased worrying
Increasing dependency
Numerous inexplicable somatic complaints
Increased utilization of health services

---

as spousal bereavement, major role transitions (such as retirement or relocation into a nursing home), or major life events such as medical illnesses (myocardial infarction, stroke, macular degeneration) that occasion loss of independence. In other late-onset cases, depression may herald the onset of a dementing disorder or be the product of cerebrovascular disease, including but not limited to stroke. Some cases of depression in old age may represent subclinical cerebrovascular disease, with white matter hyperintensities on magnetic resonance imaging (MRI) scan and prominent apathy and executive dysfunction clinically. Some depression in old age is iatrogenic, the result of inappropriate sedative hypnotic use, and some is an unwanted side effect of medications such as steroids.

Prevention

Over the past decade we have learned that antidepressant treatments can have a very favorable impact on the long-term course of depressive illness, preventing recurrences of disease (ie, tertiary prevention). This topic is discussed below in the section on "Treatment." There is increasing interest in early preventive interventions (secondary prevention) with patients who are at high risk for developing depression in the wake of medical events such as stroke, myocardial infarction, macular degeneration, interferon therapy, and arthritis. Some of these interventions could take the form of using selective serotonin reuptake inhibitors (SSRI) pharmacotherapy in patients with elevated symptoms of depression either before or after a medical insult, as well as the use of problem-solving therapies to help patients cope more effectively with growing limitations. Efforts to research primary prevention strategies could be usefully focused on other high-risk groups of elderly, such as the recently bereaved (20–30% of spousally bereaved elderly develop clinically significant depression), those who provide care to family members with mild cognitive impairment (MCI) or Alzheimer's dementia, those with chronic insomnia (itself a risk factor for the subsequent development of depression), and those advancing into the final years of life with increasing frailty. In these circumstances, it seems likely that prevention packages may include multicomponent interventions such as psychoeducation about the particular psychosocial challenge being confronted, stress-coping techniques and affective self-management, and education in health sleep practices. As the bard of Avon noted hundreds of years ago, sleep "knits up the raveled sleeve of care." Protecting sleep quality through better sleep practices may be an important component of helping the elderly successfully meet the challenges of growing old, such as coping with bereavement, care giving, or loss of independence.

Clinical Findings

Because depression in older patients often occurs in the context of medical and neurological illnesses, somatic symptoms such as changes in sleep and appetite, although important, have limited diagnostic utility. More emphasis is appropriately placed on sad, downcast mood, recurrent thoughts of death or suicide, and diminished interest in pleasurable activities. Typically, these symptoms have been present for weeks, if not months, and are associated with anguish and diminished functioning. An elderly person presenting with numerous seemingly unrelated somatic complaints is likely to have an underlying depression or anxiety disorder. Those somatic symptoms often improve and distressed help-seeking decreases with effective treatment of the underlying depression and/or anxiety.

Although the majority of older depressed patients are treated in primary care settings, some cases are especially difficult to manage in general medical clinics. Specialized psychiatric care is strongly indicated if clinical findings support a diagnosis of psychotic depression, bipolar disorder, depression accompanied by active suicidal ideation/planning and easy access to lethal means such as handguns, depression with comorbid substance abuse, depression with comorbid dementia, or other needs for more specialized assessment.

Differential Diagnosis

The most important comorbid conditions to assess include current alcohol and substance-use disorders, medications that can cause mood disturbances (eg, prednisone), and other central nervous system (CNS) illnesses, especially Alzheimer's dementia.

Depending on the clinical presentation, physicians should also assess the patient for a variety of general medical problems (eg, cerebrovascular disease and metabolic problems such as hypothyroidism) that could be contributing to mood symptoms. Accidental misuse of medications and physical, verbal, or emotional abuse by care givers or relatives should also be evaluated. Chronic pain, myocardial infarction, orthostatic hypotension, hypertension, diabetes, congestive heart failure, coronary artery disease, neoplasms, hypothyroidism, and chronic obstructive pulmonary disease (COPD) also are among the most important comorbid conditions to assess.

Depression in later life usually coexists with cognitive impairments. In our clinical research experience, close to 60% of elderly patients treated to remission of depression qualify for a diagnosis of MCI (amnestic or other subtypes). The U.S. Preventive Services Task Force has determined that the evidence is insufficient to recommend for or against routine screening for dementia in older adults. However, the task force has said that primary care physicians should be vigilant for signs of dementia whenever cognitive deterioration is suspected based upon the physician's direct observation; a patient's own report; or concerns raised by family members, friends, or caretakers. The full recommendation and rationale are found at http://www.ahrq.gov/clinic/3rduspstf/dementia/dementrr.htm. The key practice point is that depression and dementia frequently coexist. Treating depression in the cognitively impaired elder usually benefits mood, cognition, and behavior.

Complications

If unrecognized and untreated, depression in old age generally does not resolve on its own and may in fact worsen over time with respect to symptom burden and impact on functional status and quality of life. Depression also impacts cognition in many ways, for example, by reducing the speed of information processing, interfering with attentional and memory capacities, and, quite prominently, undermining executive control functions. Because depression amplifies the disability associated with coexisting medical illness, depressed elderly can get caught up in a "vicious circle" of noncompliance with medical treatment, a downward spiral of disability and depression, and early mortality (including, but not limited to, suicide). We also view depression in old age as a "contagious" illness, one that burdens (and burns out) family members and care givers, and erodes social networks. Depression produces isolation no less than being the consequence of isolation. Finally, depression is now recognized as a risk factor for both coronary artery disease and for Alzheimer's dementia. Given that late-life depression is a risk factor or prodrome to dementia, it is important to avoid or to minimize the use of medications that impair cognition, especially anticholinergic drugs.

Treatment

A. Working with Minority Elders Suspected of Having Psychiatric or Cognitive Disorders

Providers must keep in mind that patients and providers have unique backgrounds that tailor how they understand the meaning of illness in their lives and what symptoms constitute disease. Providers and patients must develop a relationship of openness and trust to feel comfortable in exploring the unique meaning of illness in their lives for accurate diagnosis and treatment plans that are understandable from the patient's perception. Ethnic diversity in America is growing at a fast pace. In 2010, almost 50% of the population in America will be non-White, with Hispanic Americans being the largest minority group. With this shift in population demographics, health care providers must acquire cross-cultural competency skills to ensure optimal care for all individuals they will see. Cross-cultural competency entails *knowledge* of the attitudes, values, beliefs, and behaviors of certain ethnic groups; *sensitivity and awareness* of one's own cultural identity, ethnic biases that are created as a result of one's own cultural background that foster the tendency to stereotype individuals from another ethic group, and the appreciation for diverse health values, beliefs, and behaviors; and the *communication skills* that are essential to eliciting patients' explanatory models (what patients believe is causing their illness) and agendas (what patients' seek from treatment), the role of family members in their lives and how those family members will react to the patient being treated for a mental illness, and how patients perceive taking medicine for depression and sharing some of their darkest secrets with someone outside of their usual group of confidants.

Providers must also have the sensitivity to recognize, particularly with elderly individuals, how real world experiences of racism and prejudice have sensitized them to be suspicious of diagnoses that do not require radiological or laboratory examinations to prescribe treatment. The communication skills of the provider to address the above mentioned issues and the capacity to convey humility, empathy, respect, and compassion will be the deciding factors in the accurate diagnosis and treatment of depression in ethnically diverse populations.

Health communications research has shown that recognition of depression is improved if providers pursue questions related to depression early in appointments rather than later. So, when evaluating patients for depression, ask questions pertaining to the symptoms of depression, eg, sleep disturbance, appetite disturbance, recent losses, and lack of interest in daily activities, near the beginning of the visit if clinical suspicion is high so that there will be time to explore the cultural and racism issues discussed earlier.

Also, patients prefer appointments in which the provider balances the query between assessing symptoms, gathering history, health education, and discussing the social/interpersonal influences in their lives and the effect these influences have upon their psychological well-being. This balance between symptom assessment and exploration of psychosocial beliefs will help develop an effective treatment plan to which the patient is capable of adhering.

The last issue is related to an important element of treatment effectiveness. That is, activation of the patient as a participant in his or her own treatment. Patient activation ensures that patients understand that depression is a medical and treatable illness, how depression has negatively influenced their lives, and that treatment effectiveness is contingent on adhering to the agreed-upon treatment recommendations and returning for future appointments. There is less adherence to treatment recommendations for depression in nonwhite American patients. Health communications research studies have shown that providers dominate discussions in sessions and have shorter visits with nonwhite American patients, which limit patients' ability to actively participate in their care. It leaves patients with the impression that the provider has little interest in them. This can result in patients having minimal interest in adhering to treatment recommendations. To ensure patients are motivated to participate in their care, they must have enough time to speak, ask questions, and discuss different treatment alternatives (Table 41–2).

Depressive disorders are underdiagnosed in African-Americans, Latinos, and Asian-Americans. Misdiagnosis can be the result of misinterpretation of illness presentation or miscommunication between doctors and patients. Some Latinos and Asians will express distress in sometimes vivid and highly emotional narratives, particularly those individuals for whom English is not their first language. If the provider does not speak the patient's native language, a trained health care interpreter should be used to ensure that accurate information is obtained.

The psychiatric diagnostic evaluation emphasizes the interpretation of the patient's appearance, behavior, language, and thought content, all of which are considered highly sensitive to cross-cultural misinterpretation. When diagnosing mental illness in individuals of ethnic groups different from one's own, guard against "category fallacy," the application of categories or terms to describe a patient's presentation in Western European terms without ensuring that the category or term is valid in the patient's local culture. Category fallacy also applies to African-Americans.

Table 41–2. Useful strategies for working with minority elderly with suspected mental illness.

Confidentiality is even more important than usual because of the persisting stigma of mental illness (dementia falls into this category as well).

Although families will accept as normal higher levels of mental and emotional dysfunction than might be seen in the rest of the population, families may be totally unable to cope and require rescue once the threshold is reached.

Be prepared for and support sharing the management of mental disorders with the clergy. Seek information regarding faith belief models and feedback as to how such beliefs are influencing care.

Carefully elicit data regarding mental status. Minority elderly who feel questions infantilize them often become angry with how they perceive they are being treated.

To guard against category fallacy, the *Diagnostic and Statistical Manual of Mental Disorders,* 4th edition, recommends that the diagnostic evaluation include a cross-cultural formulation. This would include an assessment of (1) the cultural identity of the individual (eg, does the patient have a Western view of life or is it different?); (2) cultural explanations of the individual's illness; (3) cultural factors related to psychosocial environment and level of functioning; (4) cultural elements of the relationship between the individual and the clinician; and (5) overall cultural assessment for diagnosis and care.

B. MEDICATIONS AND PSYCHOTHERAPY

In elderly patients with severe unipolar nonpsychotic major depression, expert consensus is to combine antidepressant medication with psychotherapy as the treatment of choice, with medication alone as another first-line strategy. Electroconvulsive treatment (ECT) is an alternative strategy for severe depression, especially if the patient is actively suicidal, psychotic, or treatment resistant. Psychotherapy should not be used alone for severe depression. A combination of medication and psychotherapy is also recommended as first-line treatment for milder cases of depression, but either treatment modality could be used alone, depending partly on patient preference. SSRIs are the medications of choice for treating depression in old age. Venlafaxine XR is another first-line option, which may also be useful in SSRI failures. Second-line alternatives include bupropion and mirtazepine, as well as nortriptyline or desipramine for more severe depression.

With respect to the choice of specific medication within classes, expert opinion favors citalopram, escitalopram, sertraline, or paroxetine among the SSRIs and nortriptyline or desipramine among the tricyclic antidepressants (TCAs). Antidepressants best avoided in the elderly, because of side effects and other safety concerns, include amitriptyline, imipramine, and doxepine. Adequate dosing of antidepressants is tabulated in Table 41–3.

C. FREQUENTLY ASKED QUESTIONS

A frequently asked question concerns the *general strategy for managing depression in the context of a medical condition* known to contribute to depression, eg, hypothyroidism. The strategy preferred is to use antidepressant medication plus medication for the comorbid medical condition from the outset. The strategy of first treating the comorbid medical condition (ie, prescribing antidepressant medication if depressive symptoms persist) usually produces only partial remission of depression.

If the major depressive episode coexists with alcohol or benzodiazepine abuse, the preferred strategy is to treat the substance abuse first and then prescribe an antidepressant if depressive symptoms persist. There is less consensus on this point, however, than with respect to other medical comorbid conditions. Although drug–drug interactions are generally not problematic, if coumadin is coprescribed with SSRIs, its dosage may need to be adjusted downward.

A second frequently asked question is *how long to wait before making a change* in the treatment regimen (ie, switching to a different agent) for an older patient who is having an inadequate response to initial treatment. If the physician has already raised the dose to the maximum level the patient is able to tolerate, expert opinion calls for waiting 3–5 weeks if there is a partial response to a low dose and 4–7 weeks if there is a partial response to a high dose. Guidelines published by the Agency for Healthcare Policy and Research recommend continuing for 6 weeks if there is little or no response or 12 weeks if there is partial response. Further consultation with a local mental health specialist on second-line treatment for poorly or partially responding patients is advisable.

With respect to the choice of *psychosocial interventions,* the preferred psychotherapy techniques include cognitive-behavioral therapy, supportive psychotherapy, problem-solving psychotherapy, and interpersonal psychotherapy. Additional psychosocial interventions optimally include a range of psychoeducation, family counseling, visiting nurse services to help with medica-

Table 41–3. Adequate dose of antidepressants in elderly patients.

Antidepressant	Average Starting Dose (mg/day)	Average Dose after 6 Weeks (mg/day)	Usual Highest Dose (mg/day)
Bupropion SR	100	150–300	300–400
Citalopram	10–20	20–30	30–40
Desipramine	10–40	50–100	100–150
Escitalopram	10	20	20
Fluoxetine	10	20	20–40
Mirtazepine	7.5–15	15–30	30–45
Nortriptyline	10–30	40–100	75–125
Paroxetine	10–20	20–30	30–40
Phenelzine	15	30–45	30–75
Sertraline	25–50	50–100	100–200
Venlafaxine XR	25–75	75–200	150–300

tion, bereavement groups, and use of senior citizen centers.

With respect to *evaluating treatment outcomes,* the most important indicators are presence and severity of suicidal ideation, severity of depressive symptoms, and level of disability (functional deficits). Although rating scales are useful for assessing response, such as the Hamilton Depression Rating Scale, another more practical suggestion is that the primary care physician write down two to four target symptoms (eg, "depressed 90% of the time, poor sleep almost nightly, and feelings of hopelessness"), as well as functional status (eg, unable to do housework), and document changes in these target symptoms as treatment progresses.

If an older patient is in remission after a single lifetime episode of major depression, the preference is to continue with antidepressant medication for 1 year; if the patient has had two episodes, continue medication at least 2 years if not longer; and if the patient has had three or more episodes, there is broad agreement to continue antidepressant medication at least 3 years and probably indefinitely. The preferred strategy in any scenario is to continue using the dose of antidepressant medication that was effective during acute treatment. Lowering the dose may put the patient at risk for partial or complete relapse.

D. Management of the Elderly in Primary Care Settings

Recent multisite clinical trials with elderly depressed patients conducted in primary care settings demonstrated the efficacy and usefulness of placing depression care managers in primary care practices to improve the recognition and treatment of depression in the elderly. For example, in the PROSPECT study collaborative care between depression care managers (master's level psychiatric nurses, social workers, or psychologists) and primary care physicians enabled the Agency for Health Care Policy and Research (AHCPR, now AHRQ) guideline-based care to be implemented successfully, with significantly higher rates of treatment response than seen in usual care. This model of collaborative care for depression in later life views depression as a condition that, like diabetes or hypertension, is a chronic disease in which patients and their families need information and education about the illness and its treatment to boost compliance with appropriate medical care. As well, by providing on-target and on-time input to the primary care physician, the depression care manager facilitates achievement of better short- and longer-term outcomes. The challenge now will be to effect changes in reimbursement policy to allow this type of service to be covered.

Prognosis

The good news is that depression in later life responds to treatment. Most patients can be treated to remission, especially if medication and psychotherapy are combined. Depression in later life is a chronic, relapsing illness; however, treatment works not only to get patients well, but also to keep them well. Treatment prevents relapse and recurrence, prolongs recovery, and facilitates functional recovery as well as symptomatic relief. Good depression treatment also ameliorates suicidal ideation in the majority of patients; however, in about 20% of patients, suicidal ideation persists and may require additional specialized treatment beyond routine depression care.

An area of active ongoing research addresses the relationship between depression in old age and dementia. Evidence suggests that depression in old age is a risk factor for the subsequent onset of dementia and may, in some cases, be an early harbinger of dementia. Treatment of depression in old age generally improves cognitive functioning but often does not normalize it completely. Additional research is needed to determine if the coprescription of antidepressant medication and cognitive enhancers such as cholinesterase inhibitors would help to further improve and stabilize cognition in late life depression.

Alexopoulos GS et al: Pharmacotherapy of depressive disorders in older patients. The Expert Guideline Series. *Postgraduate Medicine.* McGraw-Hill, 2001. (This includes guidelines for primary care physicians and mental health specialists and guides for patients and families.)

American Psychiatric Association: *Diagnostic and Statistical Manual of Mental Disorders,* ed 4, *Text Revision.* American Psychiatric Association, 2000.

Carney PA et al: How physician communication influences recognition of depression in primary care. J Fam Pract 1999;48 (12):958.

Charney DS et al: Depression and bipolar support alliance consensus statement on the unmet needs in diagnosis and treatment of mood disorders in late life. Arch Gen Psychiatry (in press).

Cooper-Patrick L et al: Patient-physician race concordance and communication in primary care. J Gen Intern Med 2000;15: 106.

Institute of Medicine: *Unequal Treatment: Confronting Racial and Ethnic Disparities in Healthcare.* Smedley BD, Stith AY, Nelson AR (editors). The National Academies Press, 2003.

Miller MD, Reynolds CF: *Living Longer Depression Free.* Johns Hopkins University Press, 2002. (This book was written for consumers and family members.)

Snowden LR: Bias in mental health assessment and intervention: theory and evidence. Am J Public Health 2003;93(2):239.

Szanto K et al: Occurrence and course of suicidality during short-term treatment of late-life depression. Arch Gen Psychiatry 2003;60:610.

Thomas L et al: Response speed and rate of remission in primary and specialty care of elderly patients with depression. Am J Geriatr Psychiatry 2002;10:583.

Unutzer J et al: IMPACT Investigators. Improving Mood-Promoting Access to Collaborative Treatment. Collaborative care management of late-life depression in the primary care setting: a randomized controlled trial. JAMA 2002;288(22): 2836.

WEB SITES

Alzheimer's Association
www.alz.org

American Association for Geriatric Psychiatry
www.aagpgpa.org
Depression and Bipolar Support Alliance
www.dbsa.org
Intervention Research Center for Late Life Mood Disorders, University of Pittsburgh
www.latelifedepression.org
National Alliance for the Mentally Ill
www.nami.org
National Institute of Mental Health
www.nimh.nih.gov

Elder Abuse

42

Deborah J. Bostock, MD, Cynthia M. Williams, MD, & Cheryl Woodson, MD

As hidden as the other forms of family violence may be, domestic elder abuse is even more concealed within our society. Elder abuse was first described in the literature in 1975, when the first reports of "granny battering" appeared. Vastly underreported, only one in four domestic elder abuse incidents (excluding the incidents of self-neglect) come to the attention of authorities.

Physicians are not equipped to address this important social and medical problem. In 1995, a random survey of emergency physicians showed that of emergency departments only 27% had elder abuse protocols available as compared to 75% that were prepared for child abuse. In a study of four counties in Michigan, physicians reported an average of only 2% of all incidents of suspected elder mistreatment. Primary care physicians in counties with low physician-to-population ratios are more active in reporting mistreatment of older people.

Family physicians are particularly positioned to assist in identifying and managing elder abuse. Except for the primary caregivers, they may be the only ones to see an abused elderly patient. Older victims who suffer from neglect, self-neglect, or physical abuse are likely to seek care from their primary care physician or gain entry into the medical care system through an emergency department.

Definition & Types of Abuse

Elder abuse is an all-inclusive term to describe all types of mistreatment and abuse behaviors toward older adults. The mistreatment can be either acts of commission (abuse) or acts of omission (neglect). Labeling a behavior as abusive, neglectful, or exploitative can depend on the frequency, duration, intensity, severity, consequences, and cultural context. Currently, state laws define elder abuse and the definitions vary considerably from one jurisdiction to another.

There are three basic categories of elder abuse: (1) domestic elder abuse, (2) institutional elder abuse, and (3) self-neglect or self-abuse. The National Center on Elder Abuse (NCEA) describes seven different types of elder abuse: physical abuse, sexual abuse, emotional abuse, financial exploitation, neglect, abandonment, and self-neglect (Table 42–1). These different types of abuse are based on an analysis of existing state and federal definitions of elder abuse, neglect, and exploitation conducted by the NCEA in 1995.

Prevalence & Incidence

More than 5% of the nation's elderly may be victims of moderate to severe abuse but because of underreporting, poor detection, and differing definitions the true estimate of elder abuse may be far greater. According to a survey of states by the Subcommittee on Health and Long-Term Care, only one of every eight cases of elder abuse is reported.

From 1986 to 1996, there was a steady increase in the reporting of domestic elder abuse nationwide from 117,000 reports in 1986 to 293,000 reports in 1996. This represents an increase of 150% over a 10-year reporting period. In the most widely quoted prevalence study, the incidence of elder abuse in a random sample in the metropolitan Boston area was estimated at 32 cases per 1000 adults older than age 65 living in the community. An NCEA study in 1996 estimated that approximately one million elders were victims of various types of domestic elder abuse, excluding abuse due to self-neglect. The National Elder Abuse Incidence Study reported that in 1996 approximately 450,000 elderly persons in domestic settings were abused or neglected and when self-neglect was added, the number increased to approximately 550,000, of which 21% were reported to adult protective services (APS) and the remainder went unreported. This study also found that elderly females were abused at higher rates than elderly males; adults 80 years and older were abused and neglected at two to three times their proportion of the elderly population; the perpetrator of the abuse was known in almost 90% of the cases with two-thirds of the perpetrators being spouses or adult children; and victims of self-neglect were depressed, confused, or extremely frail. In the past two decades several community surveys have

Table 42–1. Elder abuse: definitions.

Physical abuse	Use of physical force that may result in bodily injury, physical pain, or impairment
Sexual abuse	Nonconsensual sexual contact of any kind with an elderly person
Emotional abuse	Infliction of anguish, pain, or distress through verbal or nonverbal acts
Financial/material exploitation	Illegal or improper use of an elder's funds, property, or assets
Neglect	Refusal, or failure, to fulfill any part of a person's obligations or duties to an elderly person
Abandonment	Desertion of an elderly person by an individual who has physical custody of the elder or by a person who has assumed responsibility for providing care to the elder
Self-neglect	Behaviors of an elderly person that threaten the elder's health or safety

Data from Tatara T: *Understanding Elder Abuse in Minority Populations.* Brunner/Mazel, 1999.

been conducted that show 4–6% of older adults report experiencing incidences of domestic elder abuse, neglect, and financial exploitation. These surveys are summarized in Table 42–2.

In reported cases of domestic elder abuse, 66.4% of the victims were white, 18.7% were African-American, and 10% were Hispanic. The proportions of Native Americans and Asian Americans/Pacific Islanders were each less than 1%. Neglect— the failure of a designated caregiver to meet the needs of a dependent elderly person—is the most common form of elder maltreatment in domestic settings. The most frequent abusers of the elderly in domestic settings are spouses or adult children, with almost 33% of the substantiated cases of elder abuse in 1991 involving adult children as the perpetrator.

Risk Factors

A number of theories about the origins of elder mistreatment exist: overburdened caregivers, dependent elders, mentally disturbed caregivers, a history of childhood abuse and neglect, and the marginalization of elders in society. Other risk factors usually cited for elder mistreatment are listed in Table 42–3.

From the Indicators of Abuse Screen, a profile of the abuser has been developed that can identify abuse cases 78–85% of the time. The salient features of the profile are detailed in Table 42–4.

Table 42–2. Elder abuse in domestic settings.

Study[1]	Area	Overall Prevalence Rate (%)	Types of Abuse Reported	Perpetrator
Pillemer and Finkelhor (1988)	Metropolitan area surrounding Boston, MA	3.2	Physical abuse 2%, verbal aggression 1.1%, neglect 0.4%, financial exploitation, NA[2]	Spouse 58%, adult child 24%
Podnieks (1992)	Canada	4.0	Financial exploitation 2.5%	
Ogg and Bennett (1992)	Great Britain		Verbal aggression 5.6%, physical abuse 2.0%, financial abuse 2.0%	Family member or relative
Kurrle et al (1992)	Australia			
Comijs et al (1998)	Amsterdam, the Netherlands	5.6 (1-year prevalence)	Verbal aggression 3.2%, physical aggression 1.2%, financial mistreatment 1.4%, neglect 0.2%	Relative 60%, friend, housekeeper, or professional caregiver 40%

[1]Studies: Pillemer K, Finkelhor D: The prevalence of elder abuse: a random sample survey. Gerontologist 1988;28:51. Kurrle SE, Sadler PM, Cameron ID: Patterns of elder abuse. Med J Aust 1992;157:673. Comijs HC et al: Elder abuse in the community: prevalence and consequences. J Am Geriatr Soc 1998;46:885.

[2]NA, not studied.

Table 42–3. Risk factors for elder abuse.

Overall poor health (neglect)
Living with someone (physical and verbal abuse)
Lack of access to resources (neglect and financial abuse)
Social isolation or living alone (financial abuse and neglect)
Impaired activities of daily living performance (physical abuse and neglect)

A typology of abusers has also been suggested to better delineate who may perpetrate abuse. Five types of offenders have been postulated:

1. Overwhelmed offenders are well intentioned and enter caregiving expecting to provide adequate care; however, when the amount of care expected exceeds their comfort level, they lash out verbally or physically. The maltreatment is usually episodic rather than chronic. This type of offender is often seen in long-term care settings.

2. Impaired offenders are well intentioned, but have problems that render them unqualified to provide adequate care. The caregiver may be of advanced age and frail, have physical or mental illness, or have developmental disabilities. This type of maltreatment is usually chronic and the caregiver is unable to recognize the inadequacy of the care. Neglect is frequently observed in these cases.

3. Narcissistic offenders are motivated by anticipated personal gain and not the desire to help others. These individuals tend to be socially sophisticated and gain a position of trust over the vulnerable elder. Maltreatment is usually in the form of neglect and financial exploitation and is chronic in nature. These offenders will also use psychological abuse and physical maltreatment to obtain their objective. This type of offender may work in a long-term care facility and become involved in stealing from the residents.

4. Domineering or bullying offenders are motivated by power and control and are prone to outbursts of rage, believing their actions are justified by rationalizing that the victim "deserved it." These offenders know where and when they can get away with abuse. This abuse is chronic, multifaceted, and ongoing with frequent outbursts of temper. Abuse takes the form of physical, psychological, and even forced sexual coercion. Their victims are fearful and the abuser may lash out when confronted or attempt to manipulate those who confront them.

5. Sadistic offenders derive feelings of power and importance by humiliating, terrifying, and harming others. They have sociopathic personalities and inflict severe, chronic, and multifaceted abuse. Signs of this type of abuse include bite, burn, and restraint marks and other signs of physical and sexual assault. Their victims are fearful and experience terror. If confronted the abuser may attempt to charm and manipulate or intimidate and threaten the accuser in an attempt to control professionals who are trying to stop the abuse.

Clinical Evaluation

A number of medical and social factors make the detection of elder abuse more difficult than other forms of family violence. One major issue for the physician is denial that the reason for the presentation into the health care system could be attributable to abuse. Given the higher prevalence of chronic diseases in older adults, signs and symptoms of mistreatment may be misattributed to chronic disease, leading to "false negatives," such as fractures that are ascribed to osteoporosis instead of physical assault. Alternatively, sequelae of many chronic diseases may be misattributed to elder mistreatment, creating "false positives," such as weight loss in a patient because of cancer ascribed instead to intentional withholding of food (Table 42–5).

Table 42–4. Profiles of elder abusers.

Personal Abusive Caregiver Characteristics	Interpersonal Caregiver Characteristics	Abused Elder Characteristics
Abuses alcohol or other substance	Has poor relationships generally or with the elder	Was abused in the past
		Lacks social support
Is depressed or has a personality disorder	Has current marital or family conflict	
Has other mental health problems	Lacks empathy and understanding for the elder	
	Is financially dependent on the elder	
Has behavioral problems		
Caregiving inexperience or is reluctant to give care		

From Reis M, Nahmiash D: Validation of the Indicators of Abuse screen. Gerontologist 1998;38:471.

Table 42–5. Physician barriers to reporting elder abuse.

Lack of consistent definitions
Unfamiliarity with mandatory reporting laws
Lack of required training to recognize abuse
Time constraints
Concerns with offending patients
Unaware of available resources
Subtle presentation
Reluctance/fear of confronting the abuser
Abused elder requests abuse not be reported
Cultural issues
Isolation of victims
Fear of jeopardizing relationship with hospital or nursing
  facility

From Swagerty DL, Takahashi PY, Evans JM: Elder mistreatment. Am Fam Physician 1999;59:2804. Kleinschmidt KC: Elder abuse: a review. Ann Emerg Med 1997;30:463. Rosenblatt DE, Cho K, Durance PW: Reporting mistreatment of older adults: the role of physicians. J Am Geriatr Soc 1996;44:65.

Screening

The American Medical Association recommends that all older patients be asked about family violence even when evidence of such does not appear to exist. A careful history is crucial to determining if suspected abuse or neglect exists. The elderly dependent patient may fear retaliation from the abuser and may be reluctant to come forward with information. The physician should interview the patient and caregiver separately and alone. General questions about feeling safe at home and who prepares meals and handles finances can open the door to more specific questions about disagreements with the caregiver and how these disagreements are handled, such as the caregiver yelling, hitting, slapping, kicking, or punching, making the elder wait for meals and medications, or confining the elder to a room. It is also important to inquire about the possibility of sexual abuse (unwanted touching), financial abuse (stolen money, signing legal documents without understanding the consequences), and finally threats of institutionalization. Table 42–6 lists important questions to ask when screening for suspected abuse.

The caregiver interview should avoid confrontation and blame. The physician needs to appear sympathetic and understanding of the abuser's perceived burden in caregiving. The physician should be alert to a caregiver who has poor knowledge of a patient's medical problems, has excessive concerns about costs, who dominates the medical interview, or who is verbally aggressive either to the patient or physician during the interview. A caregiver with substance abuse or mental health problems and one who is financially dependent

Table 42–6. Questions to elicit information about elder abuse.

Physical abuse
Are you afraid of anyone at home?
Have you been struck, slapped, or kicked?
Have you been tied down or locked in a room?

Psychological abuse
Do you ever feel alone?
Have you been threatened with punishment, deprivation, or institutionalization?
Have you received "the silent treatment"?
Have you been force-fed?
Do you receive routine news or information?
What happens when you and your caregiver disagree?

Sexual abuse
Has anyone touched you without permission?

Neglect
Do you lack aids such as eyeglasses, hearing aids, or false teeth?
Have you been left alone for long periods?
Is your home safe?
Has anyone failed to help you care for yourself when you needed assistance?

Financial abuse
Is money stolen from you or used inappropriately?
Have you been forced to sign a power of attorney, a will, or another document against your wishes?
Have you been forced to make purchases against your wishes?
Does your caregiver depend on you for shelter or financial support?

From Kleinschmidt K: Elder abuse: a review. Ann Emerg Med 1997; 30(4):464.

on the elder should also alert the physician to a greater potential for abuse.

Clinical Detection

A thorough physical examination is the initial invitation to recognizing and documenting elder abuse. Particular attention to the functional and cognitive status of the elder is important to understanding the degree of dependency that the elder may have on the caregiver. The primary care physician may be confronted with subtle forms of ongoing abuse or mistreatment in which neglect and psychological abuse predominate. Behavioral observations of withdrawal, a caregiver who treats the elder like a child, or a caregiver who insists on giving the history should heighten the clinician's suspicions. Table 42–7 lists the basic features of the physical

Table 42–7. Physical examination and possible signs of abuse or mistreatment.

Focus of Examination	Possible Signs of Abuse/Mistreatment	Type of Abuse
General	Hygiene, cleanliness of clothing, weight loss, dehydration	Neglect
Skin and mucous membranes	Skin turgor and signs of dehydration Multiple skin lesions in various stages of healing Bruises, welts, bite marks, burns Pressure ulcers	Neglect Physical Neglect
Head and neck	Traumatic alopecia, scalp hematomas Lacerations or abrasions Poor oral hygiene	Physical Neglect
Trunk and extremities	Bruises and welts; wrist or ankle lesions suggesting restraint use; immersion burns	Physical
Musculoskeletal	Occult fractures, pain; observe gait	Physical
Genitorectal/urinary	Vaginal, rectal bleeding, itching, pain or bruising; sexually transmitted disease; torn, stained, or bloody underwear Poor hygiene; inguinal rash, urine burns, fecal impaction	Sexual Neglect
Neurological and psychiatric status	Thorough cognitive evaluation; look for depression and anxiety; cognitive impairment suggesting delirium or dementia that can affect decision-making capacity Behaviors such as rocking, sucking, antisocial or borderline, or conduct disorders	All forms Psychological
Imaging/laboratory	As indicated from clinical examination; albumin, creatinine, blood urea nitrogen, possible toxicology screen	
Social and financial	Inquire about other members of social network and who can assist and about financial resources and who handles finances	

From Kleinschmidt KC: Elder abuse: a review. Ann Emerg Med 1997;30:463. Lachs MS, Pillemer K: Abuse and neglect of elderly persons. New Engl J Med 1997;332:437.

examination for assessing suspected elder mistreatment or abuse.

Detailed documentation of the physical examination is important as it may be used as evidence in a criminal trial. Documentation must be complete and legible with accurate descriptions and annotations on sketches or, when possible, with the use of photo documentation.

Intervention & Reporting

Once elder abuse is suspected all health care providers and administrators are legally obligated to report the abuse to the appropriate authorities. The laws differ from state to state and the specific reporting requirements of each state should be determined. By emphasizing the diagnosis and treatment of the health consequences of the mistreatment or the abuse, the elderly patient and caregiver may feel less threatened. Reporting should be done in a caring and compassionate manner in order to protect the autonomy and self-worth of the elder while ensuring their continued safety.

The victim and the caregiver should be told that a referral will be made to Adult Protective Services (APS). The law enforcement implications of APS should be downplayed and the social support and services offered by APS should be offered as part of the medical management of the victim. Victims may deny the possibility of abuse or fail to recognize its threat to their personal safety. In the event of financial abuse the victim and/or the offender may not acknowledge the abuse. If the victim or caregiver refuses the APS referral, the clinician should explain that they are bound to adhere to state laws and regulations in making the referral and that the regulations were developed to help those older persons who were not receiving the care they needed for whatever reason.

The safety of the patient is the most important consideration in any case of suspected abuse. If the abuse is felt to be escalating, as may occur with physical abuse, law enforcement as well as APS should be contacted. Hospitalization of the elder may be the only temporary solution to removing the victim from the abuser.

For those elders who are competent and not cognitively impaired, their wishes to either accept interventions for suspected abuse or refusal of those interventions must be respected. If an abused elder refuses to leave an abusive environment the primary care physician can help by providing support and whatever interventions the older person will accept. Helping the older victim to develop a safety plan such as when to call 911 or installing a Lifeline emergency alert system may be part of the management plan. Close follow-up should be offered.

For those older victims who no longer retain decision-making capacity the courts may need to appoint a guardian or conservator to make decisions about living arrangements, finances, and care. This is typically coordinated through APS. The physician's role in these cases is to provide documentation not only of the physical findings of abuse but also of impaired decision-making capacity.

Hirsch C, Stratton S, Loewy R: The primary care of elder mistreatment. West J Med 1999;170:353.

Kleinschmidt K: Elder abuse: a review. Ann Emerg Med 1997;30 (4):464.

Lachs M, Pillemer K: Abuse and neglect of elderly persons. New Engl J Med 1997;332:437.

Lachs M et al: The mortality of elder mistreatment. JAMA 1998; 280:428.

Ramsey-Klawsnik H: Elder-abuse offenders: a typology. Generations 2000;24:17.

Reis M: The IOA Screen: an abuse-alert measure that dispels myths. Generations 2000;24:13.

Reis M, Nahmiash D: Validation of the Indicators of Abuse screen. Gerontologist 1998;38:471.

Rosenblatt D, Cho K, Durance P: Reporting mistreatment of older adults: the role of physicians. J Am Geriatr Soc 1996;44(1): 65.

Tatara T, Kuzmeskus LM: *Types of Elder Abuse in Domestic Settings.* National Center on Elder Abuse, 1997.

Tatara T, Kuzmeskus LM: *Reporting of Elder Abuse in Domestic Settings.* National Center on Elder Abuse, 1997.

Wolf R: The nature and scope of elder abuse. Generations 2000; 24:6.

Pharmacotherapy

Melissa A. Somma, Pharm.D., CDE, & Nicole T. Ansani, Pharm.D.[1]

Medication therapy is an integral part of almost all medical disciplines and patient care. Family physicians, front-line providers of patient care, are positioned to make a large impact on the medication regimen of the patient. With an increasingly aging population, an estimated 4 billion prescriptions will be filled in the year 2004. A meta-analysis noted that adverse drug events have an incidence of 15.1% for hospitalized patients, with 76.2% thought to be preventable. Recent studies noted that 50% of adverse drug events are preventable in the nursing home population and 27.6% are preventable in the ambulatory setting. This provides an even stronger reason for the physician to have a heightened understanding of pharmacotherapy.

Taking a Medication History

The most important element to begin with is the *patient.* Bedell et al discovered a 76% discrepancy in adherence between the medications the patients were actually taking and those prescribed by their physician. No one method of improving adherence has been found to be consistently effective. Improving patient medication adherence should improve patient outcomes. The National Council on Patient Information and Education (NCPIE) refered to nonadherence as "America's other drug problem."

Nonadherence to medications involves patients who take the wrong dose or forget to take a dose, take the medication at the wrong time, stop the drug therapy too soon, or simply do not have the prescription filled. Reasons patients choose not to take their medications as prescribed include cost, misunderstanding, inconvenience, "I'm taking too many," or "it won't help me," among others. By knowing why patients are nonadherent, the physician can provide them with patient-specific reasons as to what regimen may be optimal or can

appropriately alter the regimen to suit their life-style needs.

A. Step 1: Open-Ended Questions

To obtain an accurate medication history, the physician should start by asking open-ended questions, for example, "What medications are you taking?" This approach avoids the common mistake of assuming the patient is taking all medications as prescribed. Patients often feel they need to please their physician. Although using open-ended questions to obtain a medication history may take more time, it may ultimately prevent over- or underprescribing and, through better communication, improve the doctor–patient relationship.

B. Step 2: Over-the-Counter Medications, Herbal Products, and Vitamins

It is essential to inquire in a nonjudgmental manner if patients are taking any over-the-counter (OTC) medications, herbal products, or vitamin supplements. From a U.S. survey by Eisenberg et al, an estimated 12.1% of the population take herbal products on a yearly basis, but only 38.5% of patients report use of any alternative therapy to their physician. Reasons for using herbal products include feeling a "sense of control" for taking action against a condition, dissatisfaction with traditional medicine, or the patient's belief that conventional medicine has failed them. Partnering with the patients in discussing any use of herbal products may allow the physician to discover untreated indications or patient health concerns and potentially avoid unwanted adverse effects or drug–drug interactions. The long-term effects or the occurrence of adverse drug reactions or drug–drug interactions with herbal products are not well documented. Although herbal products may help the patient, provide positive effects, and be worthwhile in their treatment, health care professionals have the responsibility to diligently examine their use, safety, and efficacy in the overall context of the patient's medication regimen. A variety of herbal resources are summarized later in this chapter.

[1]The authors would like to graciously thank Gary Matzke, Pharm.D., and Terry McKaveney for their thoughtful suggestions and review of this chapter.

C. STEP 3: SOCIAL HISTORY

Information about the patient's history of smoking and alcohol and illicit drug use factors into the overall selection of specific medications. A history of long-term alcohol use, and subsequently potential liver function abnormalities, nonadherence, and nutritional deficiencies, must be considered in selecting medications. Smoking induces the cytochrome P-450 3A4 system, speeding up the metabolism of agents such as theophylline. Illicit drug use, such as alcohol consumption, leads to potential changes in liver and kidney function, nonadherence, and concerns about the potential for addiction.

D. FOLLOW-UP: ASSESSING THE NEED FOR COMPLIANCE AIDS

A thorough medication history may uncover the need for compliance aids. Considering that the average patient adherence to taking prescribed medications is 40%, even patients who seemingly understand may need some assistance in remembering how and when to take their medications. One of the most useful tools in explaining the proper timing of medication administration is a medication chart, which lists the name of the medication, its strength, a dose schedule (including morning, noon, evening, and bedtime), and the reason for the use of the medication.

There are other compliance aids available including medication calendars and medication boxes. At the very least, providing patients with a list of medications, their indications, and the appropriate time and sequence of administration serves to aid patients in adhering to their medication regimen. Written patient education information in the form of handouts and brochures and proper instructions printed on the written prescription will all aid patients in understanding their medication regimen.

Bedell SE et al: Discrepancies in the use of medications: their extent and predictors in an outpatient practice. Arch Intern Med 2000;160(14):2129.

Eisenberg DM et al: Trends in alternative medicine use in the United States, 1990–1997: results of a follow-up national survey. JAMA 1998;280(18):1569.

Field TS et al: Risk factors for adverse drug events among nursing home residents. Arch Intern Med 2001;161:1629.

Lewis RK et al: Patient counseling—a focus on maintenance therapy. Am J Health-Syst Pharm 1997;54(18):2084.

McDonald HP, Garg AX, Baynes RB: Interventions to enhance patient adherence to medication prescriptions: scientific review. JAMA 2002;288:2868.

National Council on Patient Information and Education (NCPIE): *The Other Drug Problem: Statistics on Medicine Use and Compliance.* Bethesda, MD, 1997. Available at www.talkaboutrx.org/compliance.html. Accessed March 9, 2003.

Nichols-English G, Poirier S: Optimizing adherence to pharmaceutical care plans: nonadherence can be viewed as a behavioral

disorder—a condition that is best treated by identifying individual risk factors and designing targeted interventions. J Am Pharm Assoc 2000;40(4):475.

Medication Regimen

A. POLYPHARMACY

With an aging population, the availability of more medications, and patients consuming more medications, the concept of polypharmacy has become a major factor in patient care. Defined as the concurrent use of multiple medications or the prescribing of more medications than are clinically indicated, polypharmacy can be minimized by a thorough medication regimen review. Table 43–1 lists five main, simple steps to a medication review.

Seemingly simple, a thorough regimen review aids in ensuring that the appropriate medications are prescribed. Consider a diabetic patient with elevated blood glucose not controlled by diet, hypertension, and hyperlipidemia. According to the 2003 American Diabetes Association Guidelines, an aspirin, antidiabetic agent, antihypertensive agent, and antihyperlipidemic agent should be prescribed. This amounts to four or five medications, not including medications for any other conditions the patient may have. As in this example, polypharmacy may be unavoidable, but with a good medication regimen review, adverse drug reactions, drug–drug interactions, and duplication of therapy may be avoided. This is also an opportunity to work with a pharmacist to best outline a patient's medication regimen.

B. EVALUATION AND CHANGE

Having reviewed the patient's medication regimen, the physician can begin to consider altering the regimen or adding a new therapy based on a new diagnosis. The considerations that impact the selection of an optimal drug therapy regimen are multifaceted. It is important to consider general treatment guidelines, the utility of nonpharmacological treatment options (diet, exercise, weight loss), patient-specific issues such as overall medication use, social history, and medication compliance (discussed above), managed care formulary considerations, and finally actual drug cost.

Table 43–1. Reviewing a medication regimen.

1. Match the medication with the diagnosis
2. Review the regimen for duplication of therapy
3. Elicit from patients if they are taking the medicine
4. Review laboratory work and patient history for efficacy/toxicity of the regimen
5. Strive to remove any unnecessary agents from the regimen

One discipline that has greatly added to our knowledge of medicine utilization is evidence-based medicine (EBM), defined as "the conscientious, explicit, and judicious use of the current best evidence in making decisions about the care of individual patients." EBM entails obtaining the best external evidence to support clinical decisions, and is, therefore, not restricted solely to randomized trials and meta-analysis. Further, EBM does not rest solely on the skills and aptitude of literature evaluation and application of data, but must also incorporate clinical experience. Shaughnessy el al state that "good clinical practice should be performed like good jazz, with the physician blending the structure of evidence based medicine with the appropriate improvisation of clinical experience."

The goal of EBM is to appropriately allocate effective and efficient care to all patients. By staying current with the literature, evaluating appropriate resources, and relying on practice guidelines and drug formularies practitioners can obtain the basic knowledge and skills needed to provide a high level of quality care to their patients based on proven, explicit, and sound evidence-based medicine decisions.

"The strength of a profession lies in its expert generation of information and better management of it than other social groups" (E.J. Huth, MD). How does a generalist manage to keep up with the wealth of medical information available? It is estimated that over six million references are published in over 4000 journals in the National Library of Medicine's database, MEDLINE. Further, it is estimated that this number increases by approximately 400,000 new MEDLINE entries yearly. Busy practitioners need to develop a system of staying current with the literature, without creating information overload. Slawson and Shaughnessy propose that the practitioner should approach this "information jungle" with a basic equation:

$$\text{Usefulness} = (\text{Relevance} \times \text{Validity})/\text{Work}$$

Simple mathematics illustrate that to maximize the usefulness of information, it is necessary to provide the highest level of relevance and validity with the minimum amount of work. Relevance is directly proportional to the relationship/similarities of the information with the patient population most commonly encountered, or its applicability to the physician's practice. It also includes a measure of the impact of change the information creates in the way medicine is practiced. Validity relates to the intrinsic methodology, study design, and conclusions. Thus, by maximizing the principles of the usefulness equation, it is possible to locate the best source of information.

American Diabetes Association: Clinical Practice Recommendations 2003. Standards of Medical Care for Patients with Diabetes Mellitus. Diabetes Care 2003;26(Suppl 1):28.

Sackett DL: Evidence-based medicine. Spine 1998;23;1085.

Shaughnessy AF, Slawson DC, Becker L: Clinical jazz: harmonizing clinical experience and evidence-based medicine. J Fam Pract 1998:47;425.

Shaughnessy AF, Slawson DC, Bennett JH: Becoming an information master: a guidebook to the medical information jungle. J Fam Pract 1994;39;489.

Slawson DC, Shaughnessy AF: Teaching information mastery: creating information consumers of medical information. J Am Board Fam Pract 1999;12:444.

Slawson DC, Shaughnessy AF: Becoming an information master. Using "medical poetry" to remove the inequities in health care delivery. J Fam Pract 2001;50;51.

Steward RB, Cooper JW: Polypharmacy in the aged: practical solutions. Drugs Aging 1994;4:449.

WEB SITES

Agency for HealthCare Research and Quality
http://www.ahrq.gov
Bandolier
http://www.jr2.ox.ac.uk/Bandolier/index.html
Centre for EBM
http://www.cebm.net
The Cochrane Library
http://www.updateusa.com/clibhome/clib.htm
Journal of Family Practice POEMS
http://www.jfponline.com or http://www.medicalinforetriever.com
Netting the Evidence
http://www.shef.ac.uk/~scharr/ir/netting

Exploring the Evidence: Use of Guidelines & Formularies

The need for systematic reviews, summary documents, and formulary systems to stay abreast of the current best evidence is apparent. Keeping up with the flood of primary literature publications is difficult due to lack of organization of the thousands of articles published.

Based on the increase in information and variability in sources, guidelines and formulary systems have been developed to improve health care outcomes, reduce unnecessary practice variations, and potentially contain costs. A guideline is defined by the Institute of Medicine as a "systematically developed statement to assist physicians in patient decisions about appropriate health care for specific clinical circumstances." Drug formularies may be defined as "a continuously revised list of medications that are readily available for use within an institution and reflect the current clinical judgment of the medical staff." These systems provide an organized, evidence-based approach to care. Guidelines and formulary systems have demonstrated beneficial effects in improving the process of care, improving patient outcomes, and promoting cost containment and/or cost-effective care. In fact, the United States Presidents' Advisory Commission on Consumer Protection and Quality in the Health Care Industry has included in their recommendation that the "continued development and dissemination of evidence-based information can help guide practitioners' actions."

Four types of evidence-based guidelines exist and the strength of evidence varies depending on the type of guideline. Evidence-based clinical practice guidelines incorporate recent literature regarding the effectiveness of therapy and clinical experience. Expert consensus guidelines may be the simplest type of guideline; however, a limitation to this approach is inherent author bias and limited evidence-based sources. Outcomes-based guidelines incorporate measures of effectiveness to validate a positive impact on patient care. Lastly, preference-based guidelines combine evidence-based and outcomes-based guidelines with patient preferences. These comprise the least common type of guideline, but provide information on patients' values in guiding decisions.

Regardless of the type of guideline format used, it is imperative to test the validity and applicability of the guidelines and, subsequently, the validity of information by which the guideline was developed. To assess these characteristics of guidelines, it is necessary to consider a number of factors as listed in Table 43–2.

The strength of a guideline or guideline recommendation is directly proportional to the strength of the evidence used to formulate the recommendations. Although the strength of evidence is important in developing guidelines, there are times when a definite answer does not exist and/or the data support is limited. In such cases, reliance on expert consensus guidelines may be necessary.

The Cochrane Collaboration is an example of a system used to provide sound clinical practice guidelines. Cochrane was one of the founders of a system that determines levels of evidence and provides systematic and objective reviews. Currently, the Cochrane Collaboration provides systematic reviews, maintains a registry of trials, and is a leading provider of evidence-based guidelines. Cochrane reviews may be located in the Cochrane Library, Cochrane Collaboration, or Cochrane Reviews' Handbook at http://www.update-software.com/cochrane/cochrane-frame.html or http://www.cochrane.org.

In addition to the Cochrane Collaboration, many medical/professional societies, Health Maintenance Organizations (HMOs), and the Agency for Health Care Policy and Research provide practice guidelines and Internet links to the guidelines.

Table 43–2. Evaluating the usefulness of clinical guidelines.

1. *Does the guideline clearly define the subject area and clearly state the question to be answered?* This is essential to ensure the applicability of the guideline to practice and to assess the validity of the conclusions.
2. *What criteria were used to determine inclusion of articles/information?* This helps to provide an assessment of methodological standards that determines whether these standards are similar to the guideline criteria.
3. *How was the search conducted and what criteria were used to assess inclusion of the information?* This ensures completeness of subject material.
4. *Was the level of information to be included assessed?* It is critical to ensure the quality of information reviewed in order to provide a quality recommendation/end point. An assessment of the level of information should include the validity of the study methodology, assessment of the reproducibility of the studies, and the homogeneity of the study results.
5. *What are the results/recommendations?* Are the results statistically and clinically significant, are the results precise, are the recommendations feasible, and will they change practice? Can this recommendation be applied to your specific practice?
6. *When was the guideline updated?* As new evidence is rapidly becoming available, how is this incorporated to ensure the best and most current practice?

From Snaders GD, Nease RF, Owens DK: Published web-based guidelines using interactive decision models. J Eval Clin Pract 2001;7:175; Oxman AD, Cook DJ, Buyatt GH: Users' guide to the medical literature. VI. How to use an overview. JAMA 1994; 272:1367; Siwek J et al: How to write an evidence-based clinical review article. Am Fam Physician 2002;65:251; and Liberati A et al: Which guidelines can we trust? West J Med 2001;174:262.

As the demand for published, evidence-based guidelines is growing, so too is the need for outcomes-focused formulary systems that consider effectiveness, safety, and cost implications to practice. Drug formulary systems are fundamental tools of hospitals, health systems, and managed care organizations to designate preferred products and provide rational, cost-effective prescribing decisions. A formulary system is a fundamental process used to manage the quality and cost of pharmaceuticals. Traditional formulary decisions are based on comparative efficacy, safety, drug interactions, dosing, pharmacology, pharmacokinetics, and cost.

Pharmacy and Therapeutics (P&T) Committees guide the formulary decision process. The P&T Committees are composed of physicians, pharmacists, nurses, and administrators, representing all major disciplines of practice. The goal of the committee is to provide high-quality, safe, cost-effective prescribing. By reviewing new medications, drug classes, literature, and safety data, the P&T Committee frames the structure of a formulary system. Essential elements of a formulary system are outlined in Table 43–3.

Physicians may consider developing a personal formulary as well. A personal formulary includes methodological selection and routine use of one or two drugs for a clinical condition or from a drug class. Methods of selection reflect information from both primary and tertiary information sources as well as clinical experience. Selection of agents should be based on similar criteria, as noted in the P&T Committee review, be evidence-based, and consider safety parameters such as adverse drug reactions and the potential for drug interactions. Rational use of medication requires meeting the patient's clinical needs through appropriate medication selection as well as providing care in the most cost-effective manner. Evidence-based guidelines and formulary systems can promote patient care when applied appropriately, analyzed properly, and evaluated recognizing the needs of the individual patient.

Crane VS et al: Presenting drug cost information to a board of directors: a case example. Formulary 2001;36:857.

LeGrand A, Hogerzeil HV, Haaijer-Ruskam FM: Intervention research in rational use of drugs: a review. Health Pol Planning 1999;14:89.

Malone PM et al (editors): *Drug Information Second Edition: A Guide for Pharmacists.* McGraw-Hill, 2001.

Scalzitti DA: Evidence-based guidelines: application to clinical practice. Phys Ther 2001;81:1622.

Stoelwinder JU: EBM in healthcare: management and policy. Med J Aust 2001;174:644.

Table 43–3. Essential elements of a formulary system.

---

1. Decisions are based on sound scientific and economic evidence.
2. Methods such as drug use review, monitoring of outcomes, and continuous quality improvement are employed.
3. An active, multi-disciplinary P&T Committee is instrumental in developing and maintaining drug use decisions and oversight.
4. Policies regarding conflict of interest and disclosure are available.
5. Educational programming and communication occurs.
6. Processes to obtain non-formulary designated medications are available.

From LeGrand A, Hogerzeil HV, Haaijer-Ruskam FM: Intervention research in rational use of drugs: a review. Health Pol Planning 1999;14:89.

WEB SITES

Agency for HealthCare Research and Quality
http://www.ahrq.gov/clinic
Clinical Evidence, BMJ Publishing Group
http://www.clinicalevidence.org
Health Web
http://www.uic.edu/depts/lib/health/hw/ebhc
Institute for Clinical Systems Improvement
http://www.ICSI.org
Medical Matrix
http://medmatrix.org
National Guideline Clearinghouse
http://www.guidelines.gov/index.asp
Primary Care Clinical Practice Guidelines
http://medicine.ucsf.edu/resources/guidelines

Balancing the Evidence with the Patient: Managing Medication Cost

Medication costs are soaring. In 2001, the average price of a single prescription was $49.84. In the United States a total of $175.2 billion was spent on drug therapy during that same year. With our aging population and the ever changing face of managed care, the issue of drug cost was put on the major campaign issue list during the 2000 U.S. presidential election. Although the elderly (patients ≥65 years of age) comprise only 13% of the U.S. population, they account for 34% of all prescriptions filled, or 42% of prescription costs. Family physicians, like pharmacists, face the issue of medication cost daily. To tackle this patient care problem, there are a few steps physicians can take.

First, it is important to determine whether a patient has insurance. Based on 2002 estimates of the U.S. population ≥65 years of age, it was determined that 63.1% had private insurance and 7.6% had Medicaid, both of which may carry prescription coverage, while 26.7% had Medicare only, with no prescription coverage. If the patient does have prescription insurance coverage, physicians should be aware of the prescribing or formulary suggestions. If medically appropriate, an attempt should be made to prescribe within the formulary to aid in decreasing the patient's copayment. Patients with insurance may often complain that their copayments are too high, but because they already have insurance, there are few other funding options. Here is where a careful review of the medication regimen with the intention of decreasing numbers of medications, if medically appropriate, is vital.

For the estimated 43 million patients who do not have insurance, there are a few options physicians can pursue to aid them in obtaining medications at a reduced cost.

1. Determine if the patient qualifies for any government, state, or military operated program. Having a basic understanding of the income requirements can assist the physician in guiding the patient in the right direction.

2. Have contact information available for state Medicaid programs.

3. Consider applying for medication assistance programs sponsored by the pharmaceutical manufacturers. In 2002, the pharmaceutical manufacturers supplied free or low-cost medications to over 5.5 million people in the United States. A number of Internet sites are available to aid in obtaining information on how to use these programs including www.needymeds.com, www.rxhope.com, and www.themedicineprogram.com.

Medication samples were not mentioned because of two inherent challenges: (1) these are often the newest and most expensive medications available and (2) physicians are not guaranteed a consistent supply of these medications. Physicians should always attempt to choose the most effective agent for their patients at the most reasonable cost.

Beers MH: Explicit criteria for determining potentially inappropriate medication use in the elderly: an update. Arch Intern Med 1997;157:1531.

WEB SITES

National Center for Health Statistics (NCHS): Health, United States, 2002.
www.cdc.gov/nchs/fastats/elderly.htm.
Pharmaceutical and Research Manufacturers of America (PhRMA)
www.helpingpatients.org

Ensuring Medication Safety

In 1998, the meta-analysis published by Lazarou et al entitled "Incidence of Adverse Drug Reactions in Hospitalized Patients" obtained national attention via the media. It was the first pointed and extensive publication noting the number of adverse drug reactions (ADR) occurring in the United States population. ADRs as defined by the World Health Organization (WHO) include "any noxious, unintended, and undesired effect of a drug, which occurs at doses used in humans for prophylaxis, diagnosis, or therapy." This study and others have largely resulted in an appropriate heightened awareness of medication safety.

The Lazarou meta-analysis reviewed 39 prospective studies of ADRs. It concluded that the majority, 76.2% of ADRs, were Type A or "dose dependent" and therefore were potentially preventable. With the direct costs of ADRs estimated to be between $1.56 and $4 billion and the estimation that ADRs are the fourth to sixth leading cause of death, there is a significant need for a greater understanding of the mechanisms of these reactions. Most recently, Gurwitz et al published a cohort study of outpatient elderly Medicare patients measuring the number of adverse drug events, their severity, and potential preventability. They found 27.6% of the adverse drug events were preventable, 42% of which were life-threatening or fatal. Although health care professionals need to better understand the detection and prevention of ADRs, there is also a need for health system-wide changes to help protect patients.

ADRs are reported to be the cause of 5% of hospital admissions. A number of studies have noted that many ADRs are dose dependent and preventable. Patients at the highest risk of experiencing ADRs include those on multiple medications (five or more) and who have various medical conditions, those hospitalized or in nursing home facilities, diabetic patients, cancer patients, and those with renal or hepatic impairment. Additionally, the classes of drugs most commonly associated with ADRs include nonopioid and opioid analgesics, antibiotics, cardiovascular agents, anticoagulants, and diuretics. Careful monitoring of these patients, ensuring proper indication of individual medications, and patient counseling can help reduce potential ADRs.

There are some basic inquiries, as listed in Table 43-4, that can aid physicians in determining if an ADR is truly linked to a particular drug. It is vitally important to report the ADR no matter how minor or major. One of the primary reasons for not understanding the significance of ADRs is lack of data. During premarketing trials, if 1500 patients or more are exposed to a drug, the most common ADRs will be detected. But it

Table 43–4. Identifying ADRs.

1. Are there any previous reports of an ADR occurring with this agent?
2. Consider the timing of the ADR. Does it match the drug's pharmacokinetic profile for onset of effect?
3. Was there a recent dosage increase or decease?
4. Was a new medication recently added or removed from the regimen?
5. If serum drug levels were available, were they in the toxic range?
6. Has the patient had a similar reaction to medications in the past, especially those of the same class?
7. Are there other drugs or disease conditions that could also cause the symptoms of the event?
8. When the drug was discontinued, did the symptoms resolve?

From Stephens M, Talbot J: *The Detection of New Adverse Drug Reactions,* ed 2. Stockton Press, 1998.

takes over 30,000 patients to be exposed to the drug in the postmarketing period to detect an ADR in one patient with a power of 0.95 to discover an incidence of 1 in 10,000. This is why postmarketing reporting of ADRs is so vital. There are two simple ways physicians can anonymously report ADRs: (1) www.fda.gov/MEDWATCH or call 800-FDA-1088 and (2) if in a hospital or nursing home setting, by contacting the pharmacy.

Gurwitz JH et al: Incidence and preventability of adverse drug events among older persons in the ambulatory setting. JAMA 2003;289:1107.

Kohn L, Corrigan J, Donaldson M (editors): *To Err Is Human: Building a Safer Health System.* Institute of Medicine, 2000.

Lazarou J, Pomeranz D, Corey P: Incidence of adverse drug reactions in hospitalized patients. JAMA 1998;279(15):1200.

Pirmohamed M et al: Fortnightly review: adverse drug reactions. Br Med J 1998;316(7140):1295.

Stricker BHC: *Drug-Induced Hepatic Injury,* ed 2, Vol 5. Elsevier Science, 1992.

WHO: Technical Report Series No. 425, 1996.

WEB SITE

Federal Food and Drug Administration (FDA) Safety Information and Adverse Drug Reporting Program
http://www.fda.gov/MEDWATCH/

Matching the Patient & the Drug: Pharmacokinetic & Pharmacodynamic Principles

Although a subset of ADRs is unpredictable, those that are preventable include drug–drug interactions. A grasp of basic pharmacokinetic and pharmacodynamic principles is needed to prevent such interactions. Pharmacokinetics characterizes the rate and extent of absorption, distribution, metabolism, and elimination of a drug. Pharmacodynamics is the study of the relationship between the drug concentration at the site of action and the response of the patient. Where these concepts come together for the physician is at the point of deciding the best drug and/or dose for a particular patient.

There are five categories of patient characteristics for which the pharmacokinetics of a particular agent must be considered:

- **Age:** Most drugs have been studied on the adult patient. Special considerations therefore need to be made for the pediatric patient who may need a higher dose per kilogram than the adult or a geriatric patient who may need a lower dose per kilogram than the younger adult patient due to decreased drug metabolism and elimination.

- **Gender:** Although data are limited, male and female patients can metabolize and eliminate drugs differently, so the optimal drug dosages may differ.

- **Weight:** For patients who are obese or cachectic, there are often drug clearance (rate at which a drug is removed from the body) or volume of distribution (estimated volume a drug occupies in a patient) changes necessitating adjustments in drug dosage.

- **Disease conditions:** Three disease conditions must be approached with special caution:

  —*Congestive heart failure (CHF)*: as CHF ensues, bodily organ blood flow declines, thus drug clearance declines, leading to the need for lower drug dosages of many agents.

  —*Renal disease*: as organ function declines, renal elimination of drugs can decrease, leading to decreased drug dosages of renally cleared agents.

  —*Hepatic disease*: as organ function declines, hepatic metabolism and elimination of drugs can decrease, leading to decreased drug dosages of hepatically metabolized and cleared agents.

- **Genetics:** Pharmacogenomics is the study of the relationship between genetics in drug metabolism and adverse drug reactions. Much of our understanding is credited to The Human Genome Project. In a systematic review by Phillips et al of 27 drugs known to frequently cause ADRs, 59% were known to be influenced by individual patient genetic characteristics.

Collins F, McKusick V: Implications of the Human Genome Project for Medical Science. JAMA 2001;285:540.

Hanlon JT et al: Geriatrics. In: *Pharmacotherapy,* ed 5. DiPiro JT et al (editors). McGraw-Hill, 2002.

Phillips KA et al: Potential role of pharmacogenomics in reducing adverse drug reactions: a systematic review. JAMA 2001;286:2270.

Sitar DS: Clinical pharmacokinetics and pharmacodynamics: In: *Clinical Pharmacology: Basic Principles in Therapeutics,* ed 4. Carruthers SG et al (editors). McGraw-Hill, 2000.

Drug–Drug Interactions: Utilizing Pharmacokinetic & Pharmacodynamic Principles

Once the patient-specific characteristics above have been established, the physician can begin to examine the drug-specific characteristics. The pharmacokinetic characteristics of a drug can aid in choosing the best drug for the patient and potentially can aid the physician in predicting and understanding adverse drug reactions and drug–drug interactions. Not all drug interactions have adverse consequences; thus, adverse drug reactions are not synonymous with drug–drug interactions.

As might be expected, the more medications a patient takes, the higher the likelihood a drug–drug interaction may occur. The pharmacokinetic and pharmacodynamic principles that help to predict drug responses also help to predict drug–drug interactions. The physician needs to consider first the time course and second the properties of the two drug entities: the precipitant drug (the drug causing a change in the action of another drug) and the object drug (the drug whose action is affected by the precipitant drug).

The time course of the drug interaction involves a number of factors. First, note the time of onset of the interaction, the predicted time to maximum effect of each drug, and the time required for dissipation of the interaction. To determine the time course to dissipation of the interaction, take notice of the half-lives of the drugs involved. If the time to achievement of the steady-state concentration of the precipitant drug is long, the time to onset of the interaction will in turn be delayed. If the half-life of the object drug is long, the time to achievement of a new steady-state concentration of this drug will also take longer. Thus, to predict the time course of a drug interaction, it is important to take note of the individual characteristics of the drug. Table 43–5 summarizes potential pharmacokinetic and pharmacodynamic interactions.

Drug–drug interactions that occur due to alterations in drug metabolism deserve an extended discussion. The main enzymatic system responsible for drug metabolism is the cytochrome P-450 (CYP) system. The CYP system is the enzyme system most widely responsible for the oxidative metabolism of many drugs. Metabolism through the CYP system occurs mainly in the liver, but CYP isozymes are also found in the intestines and other organs. The nomenclature to designate specific isozymes is described by "CYP" with an Arabic number, letter, and another Arabic number following (ie, CYP 3A4).

Identifying different CYP isozymes is an area of ongoing research. There are six isozymes in particular about which there is a reasonable amount of understanding. These isozymes include CYP 1A2, 2C9, 2C19, 2D6, 3A4, and 2E1. Understanding this system allows physicians to predict drug–drug interactions among many patients. To do this, it is necessary to identify which drugs are metabolized by the CYP 450 system and how they interact with the enzyme system. There are three ways a drug can interact with the enzymes:

- Substrate: the drug is metabolized by an enzyme that is specific for an individual CYP receptor.

- Inducer: the drug "revs up" the enzyme system, allowing a greater metabolic capacity.

- Inhibitor: the drug(s) competes with another drug(s) for a specific enzyme-binding site, rendering the enzyme inactive.

A review of the patient's medication list can reveal drugs that may compete or use the same enzyme system. A change in drug selection may prevent a drug interaction. Table 43–6 matches medications with their interaction with the CYP 450 enzyme system. This table can be used as a reference when determining potential drug–drug interactions.

Knowing and predicting drug–drug interactions can be a daunting task. Identifying patients most at risk for drug–drug interactions and adverse drug reactions, carefully monitoring drugs with narrow therapeutic windows (such as warfarin, phenytoin, and theophylline), using lower dose therapies when appropriate, and employing systems to identify and prevent drug–drug interactions at the point of patient care all have the potential to reduce adverse drug reactions from drug–drug interactions.

Gex-Fabry M, Balant-Gorgia AE, Balant LP: Therapeutic drug monitoring databases for postmarketing surveillance of drug-drug interactions. Drug Safety 2001;24(13):947.

Hansten PD, Horn JR: Pharmacokinetic drug interaction mechanisms and clinical characteristics: In: *Hansten and Horn's Drug Interactions Analysis and Management.* Applied Therapeutics, 1997.

Wright JM: Drug interactions. In: *Clinical Pharmacology: Basic Principles in Therapeutics,* ed 4. McGraw-Hill, 2001.

Keeping up with the Literature

Subscribing to survey services is one way to stay current with the pertinent literature, while decreasing the amount of work and time required. Such services provide a quick summary of recent articles that may be delivered electronically to your e-mail system. This mechanism represents an efficient means of reviewing a plethora of medical journals and articles. A limitation of these services may be the tendency to overemphasize positive conclusions or draw conclusions that are not fully supported by the data. The conclusions and recommendations presented by such services should be evaluated before incorporating the information to practice. The relevance and validity of the data must be verified. The true value of these survey systems lies in the ability to focus time and energy to specific areas of interest.

Three basic categories of survey services exist: (1) abstracting services, (2) review services, and (3) true newsletters. Abstracting services for family medicine

Table 43–5. Classification and examples of mechanisms of drug–drug interactions.

Type of Interaction	Basic Description	Time Course	Example
Absorption	Precipitant drug binds to the object drug Object drug concentration decreases	Hours Rate of concentration of object drug declines dependent on object drug half-life	Antacids taken with digoxin, quinolones, and tetracyclines; antacids absorb drugs in the gastrointestinal tract leading to decreased concentration of those drug entities
Distribution	Precipitant drug *displaces* the object drug from a particular binding site Object drug concentration increases	A day to a week Usually a self-limited interaction; after initial interaction, an equilibrium is reached between object drug concentration in the plasma and at the binding site	Sulfamethoxozole/trimethoprim (SMP/TMX) taken with warfarin; SMP/TMX is more highly protein bound than warfarin and will displace warfarin from its binding sites leading to an increase in unbound warfarin
Metabolism	Induction Precipitant drug induces (speeds up) the metabolism of the object drug Object drug concentration decreases	Usually within 2 days, but less than 1 week	Some of the most common precipitant agents responsible for induction of hepatic microsomal drug-metabolizing enzymes include carbamazepine, phenytoin, rifampin, troglitazone; they will induce the hepatic metabolism of agents that require the same hepatic microsomal drug-metabolizing enzymes for metabolism
	Inhibition Precipitant drug inhibits the metabolism of the object drug Object drug concentration increases	Hours	Many exist; some of the most common precipitant agents responsible for inhibition of hepatic microsomal drug-metabolizing enzymes include erythromycin, fluconazole, ketoconazole, nefazadone, and ritonavir; they will inhibit the hepatic metabolism of agents that require the same hepatic microsomal drug-metabolizing enzymes for metabolism
	Competition Precipitant and object drugs compete for metabolic enzymes Both drug concentrations may be altered	Variable	When two drugs use the same hepatic microsomal drug-metabolizing enzymes, competition may occur leading to alterations of either or both serum drug concentrations
Elimination	Precipitant drug competes with the object drug for excretion Both drug concentrations may be altered	Hours	There are three primary methods of renal excretion: glomerular filtration, active tubular secretion, and passive tubular reabsorption; interactions can occur during all three processes; one example is the combination of hydrochlorizide and lithium carbonate; hydrochlorizide causes an increase in sodium reabsorption leading to an increase in lithium reabsorption and thus an increase in the concentration of lithium

(continued)

Table 43–5. Classification and examples of mechanisms of drug–drug interactions. (*Continued*)

Type of Interaction	Basic Description	Time Course	Example
Pharmacodynamic	Additive Precipitant drug together with the object drug produce a heightened therapeutic or toxic response.	Hours to weeks	There are many; consider two drugs with an adverse effect in common (two sedating agents); together they produce a more pronounced adverse effect (sedation)
	Antagonistic Precipitant drug antagonizes (cancels out) the effect of the object drug		Nonsteroidal antiinflammatory drugs when given with an antihypertensive agent can cause a rise in the patient's blood pressure over the course of a few weeks, thus antagonizing the desired effect of the blood pressure agent

From Gex-Fabry M, Balant-Gorgia AE, Balant LP: Therapeutic drug monitoring databases for postmarketing surveillance of drug-drug interactions. Drug Safety 2001;24(13):947; and Hansten PD, Horn JR: Pharmacokinetic drug interaction mechanisms and clinical characteristics. In: *Hansten and Horn's Drug Interactions Analysis and Management.* Applied Therapeutics, 1997.

practitioners include, but are not limited to, the *ACP Journal Club, The Journal of Family Practice,* and *Journal Watch. ACP Journal Club* http://www.acpjc.org is published by the American College of Physicians–American Society of Internal Medicine. The goal of this service is to provide brief, high-level summaries of current original articles and systematic reviews in a structured abstract format in a timely manner. *The ACP Journal Club* reviews over 100 journals and uses prestated criteria to select and evaluate data. Pertinent information summaries are provided to subscribers on a bimonthly bases. *The Journal of Family Practice* http://www.jfponline.com provides family practice physicians with timely, reliable information supplemented by expert commentary. The goal of this service is to provide evidence-based information on clinically applicable topics in a timely fashion. *Journal Watch Online* http://www.jwatch.org is supported by the publishers of the *New England Journal of Medicine.* The goal of this service, similar to the others, is to provide current summaries of the most important research in a timely fashion. An editorial board, composed of physicians from many specialty areas, reviews, analyzes, and summarizes 55–60 critically important articles. The summaries are published on a bimonthly basis. In addition, this service features Clinical Practice Guidelines Watch and editorials of the year's top medical stories.

Review services provide a concise summary of the specific topic areas, rather than a survey of the literature. One example of a review service is *The Medical*

Letter http://www.medletter.com. *The Medical Letter* is published by an independent nonprofit organization. It provides critical appraisals of new medications or new uses for medications in a clinical context, comparing and contrasting the new medications with similar established agents. This publication is printed bimonthly and provides a concise summary of clinical issues. The goal of this publication is to provide "unbiased, reliable, and timely information on new drugs to busy health care professionals." Another example of a review service is *Primary Care Reports* http://www.ahcpub.com/ahc_root_html/products/newsletters/pcr.html. This service is printed bimonthly and is intended to provide review articles on critical issues in primary care; treatment recommendations are provided with each review.

True newsletters provide concise reviews of current literature with topics from news media and other sources. Examples of true newsletters include, but are not limited to, *The Drug and Therapeutics Bulletin* and *Therapeutics Letter. The Drug and Therapeutics Bulletin* http://www.which.net/health/dtb/main.html is a concise monthly bulletin, targeted for physicians and pharmacists, providing evaluations of medications. These articles summarize randomized, controlled clinical trials and consensus statements. The goal of this service is to provide informed and unbiased assessments of medications and their overall place in therapy. *The Therapeutics Letter* http://www.ti.ubc.ca/pages/letter. html is a bimonthly newsletter that targets problematic therapeutic issues. This newsletter provides evidence-based reviews

Table 43–6. Drugs metabolized by CYP 450 isozymes.

Isozyme	Substrates	Inducers	Inhibitors

2D6	Antidepressants
	  Amitriptyline
	  Clomipramine
	  Fluoxetine
	  Imipramine
	  Mirtazapine
	  Nortriptyline
	  Paroxetine
	  Trazadone
	  Venlafaxine
	Antipsychotics
	  Clozapine
	  Fluphenazine
	  Haloperidol
	  Olanzapine
	  Perphenazine
	  Quetiapine
	  Risperidone
	  Thioridazine
	β-Blockers
	  Bisoprolol
	  Carvedilol
	  Metoprolol
	  Pindolol
	  Propranolol
	  Timolol
	Pain medications
	  Codeine
	  Fentanyl
	  Hydrocodone
	  Morphine
	  Oxycodone
	  Propoxyphene
	  Tramadol
		Antiseizure agents
		  Carbamazepine
		  Phenobarbital
		  Phenytoin
		  Primidone
		  Rifampin
		Others
		  Ethanol
		  Ritonavir
		  St. John's wort
			Antidepressants
			  Proxetine > fluoxetine > sertraline > fluvoxamine
			  Nefazodone
			  Venlafaxine
			Antipsychotics
			  Haloperidol
			  Perphenazine
			  Thioridazine
			Other
			  Cimetidine

3A4	Antidepressants
	  Amitriptyline
	  Sertraline
	  Venlafaxine
	Benzodiazepines
	  Aloprazolan
	  Triazolam
	  Midazolam
	Calcium blockers
	Carbamazepine
	Cisapride
	Dexamethasone
	Erythromycin
	Ethinyl estradiol
	Glyburide
	Ketoconazole
	Protease inhibitors
		Antiseizure agents
		  Carbamazepine
		  Phenobarbital
		  Phenytoin
		Others
		  Dexamethasone
		  Rifampin
			Antibiotics
			  Clarithromycin
			  Erythromycin
			Antidepressants
			  Nefazodone > fluvoxamine > fluoxetine > sertraline
			  Paroxetine
			  Venlafaxine
			Antifungals
			  Ketoconazole > itraconazole > fluconazole
			Others
			  Cimetidine
			  Diltiazem
			  Protease inhibitors

(continued)

Table 43–6. Drugs metabolized by CYP 450 isozymes. (*Continued*)

Isozyme	Substrates	Inducers	Inhibitors
	Ritonavir Saquinavir Indinavir Nelfinavir Testosterone Theophylline Verapamil		
1A2	Amitriptyline Clomipramine Clozapine Imipramine Propranolol Warfarin Theophylline Tacrine	Antiseizure agents Phenobarbital Phenytoin Omeprazole Rifampin Smoking	Fluvoxamine Grapefruit juice Quinolone antibiotics Ciprofloxacin Enoxacin > norfloxacin > ofloxacin > lomefloxacin
2E1	Acetaminophen Ethanol	Ethanol Isoniazid	Disulfiram
2C9	Nonsteroidal anti- inflammatory agents Phenytoin Warfarin Torsemide	Rifampin	Antifungals Fluconazole Ketoconazole Itraconazole Others Metronidazole Ritonavir
2C19	Clomipramine Diazepam Imipramine Omeprazole Propranolol	Not known	Antidepressants Fluoxetine Sertraline Others Omeprazole Ritonavir

From Hansten PD, Horn JR: Pharmacokinetic drug interaction mechanisms and clinical characteristics. In: *Hansten and Horn's Drug Interactions Analysis and Management.* Applied Therapeutics, 1997; Cupp MJ, Tracy TS: Cytochrome P450: new nomenclature and clinical implications. Am Fam Physician 1998;57(1):107; Michalets EL: Update: clinically significant cytochrome P-450 drug interactions. Pharmacotherapy 1998;18:84; and Flockhart DA, Tanus-Santos JE: Implications of cytochrome P-450 interactions with prescribing medication for hypertension. Arch Intern Med 2002;162:405.

written and edited by a team of specialists and working groups of the International Society of Drug Bulletins.

Although all of these services provide concise, factual, evidence-based information, it is recommended that these services be used as a scanning system to determine which primary literature articles are critical to read in-depth. It is also important to note that information alone is not equivalent to working knowledge. Knowledge is gained by interpretation and synthesis of information. Ultimately, the goal of information processing is to gain wisdom, which implies an appropriate application of knowledge to a clinical situation. Survey services provide the information, but it is the clinician's responsibility to analyze, interpret, and apply this information to make optimal patient care decisions. The goal of information sourcing is to maximize the usefulness score: increase validity and relevance while minimizing the workload.

Slawson DC, Shaughnessy AF, Bennett JH: Becoming a medical information master: feeling good about not knowing everything. J Fam Pract 1994;38:505.

WEB SITES

ACP Journal Club
http://www.acpjc.org
Drug and Therapeutics Bulletin
http://www.which.net/health/dtb/main.html
Journal of Family Practice
http://www.jfponline.com
Journal Watch Online
http://www.jwatch.org
Medical Letter
http://www.medletter.com
Primary Care Reports
http://www.ahcpub.com
Therapeutics Initiative Evidence Based Drug Therapy
www.ti.ubc.ca

Drug Information/ Pharmacotherapy Textbooks

Application of the usefulness score detailed previously supports textbooks as an information source that provides relevant information in a succinct and efficient summary (low workload). Textbooks are one of the most common sources of information used by medical professionals. Because drug inquiries are one of the most frequent categories of clinical questions, it is important to review drug information texts.

Despite the ease and convenience of use, texts have inherent limitations to their information, including the following:

1. Currency of information: in the vastly growing information era, textbooks quickly become out of date, primarily due to lag time associated with publishing.
2. Insufficient detail: due to the lack of space and limited literature search, important points may be undervalued.
3. Bias: the author and/or manufacturer may have conflicts of interest or inherent bias with regard to subject material.
4. Lack of expertise of the author regarding the particular content.
5. Errors in transcription and/or incorrect interpretation by the author and/or during the publication process.

When evaluating the validity of a textbook, consider the following:

1. Is this the most recent and timely edition?
2. Are statements and facts appropriately referenced?

3. Is the information source likely to contain relevant information (ie, are you searching for a drug interaction in an adverse drug reaction textbook)?
4. Is the language clear, concise, and appropriate?

There are a number of drug information textbooks and resources available to address general or specific pharmaceutical categories (eg, adverse drug reactions, drug interactions, therapeutic use, and dosing). The most common drug information resource used by family medicine practitioners is the *Physicians' Desk Reference (PDR)*. A survey conducted by the Medical Economics Company reports 82–90% of physicians consider the *PDR* their most useful resource. It is estimated that the average U.S. physician uses the *PDR* eight times per week.

The *PDR* is a compilation of drug information from manufacturer product information. It contains information regarding prescription drug indications, dosing, pharmacology and pharmacokinetics, contraindications and precautions, drug interactions, adverse drug reactions, availability, and manufacturer information.

Other commonly used drug information resources include, but are not limited to, *American Hospital Formulary Services (AHFS), MICROMEDEX, Drug Facts and Comparisons (Facts & Comparisons)*, and *The Drug Information Handbook*.

AHFS contains prescribing drug formulary monographs. The categories of information contained in these monograph are similar to the *PDR*. However, *AHFS* contains detailed therapeutic information, including off-label indications and dosing for those indications. *AHFS* also contains detailed drug information and adverse drug reaction summaries, often providing cautionary guidance and recommendations. The *AHFS* is published yearly, with quarterly updates.

MICROMEDEX is a computerized drug information resource that contains facts from the *DRUGDEX* Information System. This is a well-referenced, easily searchable, expansive drug information reference, housing information on prescription, nonprescription, and herbal products. The categories of information contained in *DRUGDEX* are similar to *AHFS* and *PDR*, and also include detailed information on off-label indications, dosing, and management of adverse drug reactions and potential drug interactions.

Facts & Comparisons contains information on prescription and nonprescription medications. Medications are listed by category with summary sections that provide tables and comparative drug class data. Information in specific monographs includes dosing, administration, contraindications and precautions, and inert ingredients. This reference is updated monthly.

The *Drug Information Handbook* is a pocket-sized reference that includes referenced drug monographs.

The monographs are listed alphabetically and include indications, dosing (including dosing in special populations), adverse drug reactions, drug interactions, and monitoring parameters. This reference also contains comparative charts and dosing equivalence tables. This is updated annually.

Table 43–7 summarizes commonly used textbooks and their limitations. This table also assigns the textbooks a "usefulness score," which is based on the opinions of the Drug Information Center at the University of Pittsburgh School of Pharmacy.

Textbooks focusing on herbal and dietary supplements have also become increasingly important as the use of these agents is widespread. The Natural Medicines Comprehensive Database and the Natural Pharmacists are two electronic references of consistently high quality that provide valid natural production information.

Other general drug information resources include, but are not limited to, the following:

1. *Clinical Pharmacology,* which is available free on the internet at http://cp.gsm.com.

2. *Handbook of Clinical Drug Data,* which is a pocket-sized reference that includes brief drug class monographs and off-label indications.

3. *Martindale: The Complete Drug Reference,* which summarizes U.S. and foreign drug products.

4. *USPDI,* which is published as a three-volume set: Volume 1, *Drug Information for HealthCare Professionals;* Volume 2, *Advice for the Patient;* Volume 3, *Approved Drug Products and Legal Requirements.*

Anderson PO, Knober JE, Troutman WG (editors): *Handbook of Clinical Drug Data.* Appleton & Lange, 1999.

Burnham TH et al (editors): *Drug Facts and Comparisons.* Facts and Comparisons, 2002.

Cohen JS, Insel PA: The physicians' desk reference: problems and possible improvement. Arch Intern Med 1996;156:1375.

Cohen JS: Dose discrepancies between the physicians' desk reference and the medical literature, and their possible role in the high incidence of dose-related adverse drug events. Arch Intern Med 2001;16:957.

Ferguson AK, Smith MM (editors): *USP DI.* The United States Pharmacopeial Convention, Inc. 1998.

Table 43–7. Summary of commonly used drug information textbooks.

Textbook	Comments	Limitations	Usefulness Score[1]
Physicians' Desk Reference[2]	Contains a list of FDA-approved indications	Manufacturer bias **Limited clinical trial data** Limited dosing modifications data Potential for outdated ADRs and other information	2
American Hospital Formulary Services[3]	Contains detailed clinical data and off-label drug use information	Lacks consistent, comprehensive drug class summaries/comparisons	3
Micromedex/Drugdex[4]	Easily searchable computerized reference	**Expensive**	3
Facts & Comparisons[5]	Contains prescriptions and nonprescription medication information	Limited clinical data	2
Drug Information Handbook[6]	Pocket-sized reference; easy to use (alphabetized)	Limited clinical data Updated annually	2

[1]Rating scale = 0–3 (not useful to very useful); based on estimation of relevance and validity of information. This rating scale reflects the opinion of the Drug Information Center at the University of Pittsburgh School of Pharmacy.
[2]Murray L et al (editors): *Physicians' Desk Reference.* Medical Economics Company, 2002; Cohen JS, Insel PA: The Physicians' Desk Reference: problems and possible improvement. Arch Intern Med 1996;156:1375; Cohen JS: Dose discrepancies between the Physicians' Desk Reference and the medical literature, and their possible role in the high incidence of dose-related adverse drug events. Arch Intern Med 2001;16:957.
[3]McEvoy GK et al (editors): *American Hospital Formulary Service.* America Society of Health-System Pharmacists, Inc, 2002.
[4]Hutchison TA, Shahan DR (editors): *DRUGDEX® System.* MICROMEDEX (edition expires June 2003).
[5]Burnham TH et al (editors): *Drug Facts and Comparisons.* Facts and Comparisons, 2002.
[6]Lacy CF et al (editors): *Drug Information Handbook.* Lexi-Comp Inc. 2000.

Hutchison TA, Shahan DR (editors): *DRUGDEX® System.* MICROMEDEX (edition expires June 2003).

Information Mastery Working Group: The near future of medicine: "Just-in- time" information at the point-of-care. University of Virginia School of Medicine, 2002.

Lacy CF et al (editors): *Drug Information Handbook.* Lexi-Comp Inc, 2000.

McEvoy GK et al (editors): *American Hospital Formulary Service.* America Society of Health-System Pharmacists, Inc., 2002.

Melmon KL et al: *Clinical Pharmacology.* McGraw-Hill, 1999.

Murray L et al (editors): *Physicians Desk References.* Medical Economics Company, 2002.

Reynolds JEF et al: *Martindale the Extra Pharmacopoeia.* London Pharmaceutical Company, 1999.

Rothschild JM et al: Clinician use of a palmtop drug reference guide. J Am Med Inform Assoc 2002;9:223.

WEB SITE

Therapeutic Research Faculty. Natural Medicines Comprehensive Database

www.naturaldatabase.com

Utilization of Drug Information at Hand: Personal Digital Assistants

Most commonly, the types of questions asked by medical residents relate to treatment or diagnosis of a patient; textbooks and colleagues are utilized as their primary information source. A study published in 2000 evaluated the medical residents' approach to answering 280 clinical questions. This study revealed that only 29% of the questions were pursued and eventually answered; lack of time was the most frequent reason (60%) given. Of the questions answered, the average time spent per response was approximately 15 min (confidence interval 11–18 min).

Lack of time for pursuing clinical questions reinforces the need for "just-in-time" information, defined as highly filtered information with rapid access and ease of use. Some "delivery" systems have been shown to provide information in under 1 min. One method of providing "just-in-time" information at the point of care is through hand-held technology, or a personal digital assistant (PDA). It is estimated that PDAs are used by 30% of U.S. physicians. It is predicted that this use will increase to over 50% by the year 2005. PDAs can provide a convenient resource that may act as an extension of the personal computer. PDA devices allow the health care professional to store, retrieve, and analyze large amounts of medical information at their fingertips. PDAs also permit sharing of information sources. Due to their portability, PDAs can also provide an efficient means of documentation of clinical data, such as medication lists, medical conditions, and allergies.

Although these systems provide rapid ease of information gathering, studies have shown limitations to obtaining "just-in- time" medical information. One of the primary limitations is the lack of standard information technology, prohibiting the ability to cross-reference or link various sources. Several types of operating systems exist, including, but not limited to, the Palm Operating System (PalmOS) and the Pocket Personal Computers (Pocket PCs). The PalmOS has largely captured the market with approximately 85% market share estimated in 2002. However, it is predicted that by 2004, this market share will drop to approximately 45%, shifting to Pocket PC systems. One of the largest differences between these operating systems as applied to the health care professional is the limited medical and pharmacy-related applications available for the Pocket PCs. An estimated 700 medical and pharmacy applications are currently available for the PalmOS systems, whereas approximately 200 are available for the Pocket PC. The Pocket PCs, however, allow the user to toggle between many open applications, whereas the PalmOS systems require that each application be run individually. Lastly, more medication "free ware" and "share ware" are available for the PalmOS systems.

One of the most important features of the hand-held technology to the medical professional is the medical and pharmacy-related software, and the flexibility, accessibility, and usability of these systems. Drug information retrieval systems are a type of commonly used hand-held programs. Several drug information sources are available, and currently there is no official rating system to determine the best fit for a physician's needs. When evaluating drug information sources, the following must be considered: user friendliness, comprehensiveness, accuracy, time interval of updates, free-hand writing capabilities, memory requirements, and cost.

A study was conducted to examine the breadth, clinical dependability, and ease of use of various hand-held drug information software programs. Nine systems were evaluated: LexiComp Platinum, Tarascon's Pharmacopoeia, Mosby Drugs, ePocrates, Davis's Drug Guide for Physicians, *PDR* 2001, Physicians' Drug Handbook, A to Z Drug Facts, and Mobile Micromedex. The expansiveness of the information source (breadth) was calculated by the percentage of questions (from a prepared list of 56 questions) that could be addressed. LexiComp Platinum provided answers to 75% of the questions posed and was the most comprehensive system, whereas Mobile Micromedex could answer the least number of questions. Factual completeness (clinical dependability) was evaluated as the percentage of questions providing a complete response. The LexiComp Platinum system was again the leader in this category, and Mobile Micromedex again failed to produce clinically dependable responses compared to the other systems. Lastly, ease of use, or the time needed to locate an answer, showed that Davis's Drug Guide provided information in the shortest amount of time (12.1 s). All systems, however, provided information in less than 30 s on average.

This study illustrates the differences in breadth, completeness, and ease of use. Other considerations in evaluating systems include current information or timeliness of updating the sources and queries and allowing ease of search by providing several search strings (drug name, drug class, indication, etc). Although Enders et al provided comparative information on nine systems,

several hundred are available. Table 43–8 summarizes commonly used drug information systems.

In addition to drug information systems, medical calculators and patient information documentation systems may be purchased to use with the hand-held systems. With the wealth of different systems available, it is important to consider the key elements of breadth, dependability, and ease of use. One method to determine the system that is best for you is to obtain a test application or trial period before purchasing. There are many web sites available from which to purchase, get demo models, or obtain information on PDA devices and applications.

Table 43–8. Commonly used drug information systems for PDAs.

System	Content	Comments
A to Z Drugs, by Drug Facts and Comparisons	Provides general dosing, adverse drug event data, and indications via drug monographs	This system includes prescription and over-the-counter drugs and is updated quarterly
AHFS Drug information	Provides over 1000 comprehensive drug monographs, including clinically relevant information	This system is costly and may require memory expansion
DrDrugs	This system includes drug monographs for over 1000 agents and provides information on herbal products	Based on *Davis's Drug Guide for Physicians;* limitations to this system are poor documentation of drug–drug interactions and monitoring parameters
ePocrates	This system contains information on over 2500 drugs and is updated daily; multiple drug–drug interaction screening is one of the capabilities as well as DocAlert e-mails on drug recalls, clinical issues, etc	Commonly used program that is currently provided free of charge; although this system is expansive, it often lacks comprehension and extensive information
ePocrates RxPro	This program has all of the functionality of ePocrates plus calculators and clinical guidelines	Upgraded version of ePocrates, provided for a cost
InfoRetriever	This system provides clinical decisions rules, diagnostic testing information, calculators, and Cochrane systematic review abstracts	Provides evidence-based medicine summaries, with software versions targeted specifically to primary care and family medicine
LexiComp Drugs Platinum	Provides information on U.S. and Canadian drugs; this system is comprehensive and includes special patient population parameters (such as geriatric and pediatric information), clinical monitoring, drug costs, and pregnancy information	Frequently updated; limitation: presentation of information on the screen does not provide a condensed view; rated as one of the most comprehensive and clinically dependable systems
PDR Drugs	This system utilizes manufacturer-prescribing information	Based on the *Physicians' Desk Reference;* possesses inherent bias of the available package information
Physicians' Drug Handbook	Provides information on over 5000 drugs and treatment options for common disease states	Drug–drug interactions and monitoring data are limited

From Keplar KE, Urbanski CJ: Personal digital assistant applications for the healthcare provider. Ann Pharmacother 2003;37:287; and Hatton R, Reents S: Hand-held drug information applications for hospital pharmacists. J Am Pharm Assoc 2000:40;841.

PDA use is increasing among health care professionals. The multitude of applications and information sources delivered at the point of care provides useful and efficient information resources. In the information era, it is critical to provide evidence-based medicine decisions. Hand-held technology allows this to be delivered "just in time."

Enders SJ, Enders JM, Holstad SG: Drug-information software for palm operating system personal digital assistants: breadth, clinical dependability, and ease of use. Pharmacotherapy 2002;22:1036.

Felkey BG, Fox BI: Palm OS or Pocket PC? Hosp Pharm 2002; 37:545.

Green ML, Ciampi MA, Ellis PJ: Residents' medical information needs in clinic: are they being met? Am J Med 2000;109:218.

WEB SITES

Hand-Held Software

http://www.doctorsgadgets.com
http://www.handango.com
http://www.handheldmedical.com
http://www.handmedical.com
http://www.healthypalmpilot.com
http://www.medicalpiloteer.com
http://www.mobilecomputing.com
http://www.palmgear.com
http://www.pdamd.com
InfoPOEMs The Clinical Awareness System
http://www.infopoems.com

Movement Disorders

44

Goutham Rao, MD

General Considerations

A movement disorder can be defined as any condition that disrupts normal voluntary movements of the body (eg, a disturbance in gait) or that consists of one or more abnormal movements (eg, tremor).

Movement disorders can be classified as *hypokinesias,* characterized by overall slowness of movement (bradykinesia), lack of movement (akinesia), or difficulty in initiating movement, and *hyperkinesias,* characterized by extra or exaggerated movements (eg, tremor). Common hypokinesias and hyperkinesias are listed in Table 44–1.

Though less frequently encountered by family physicians than chronic diseases such as hypertension, diabetes, and asthma, movement disorders are nevertheless fairly common, especially among the elderly. Parkinson's disease, for example, has an estimated prevalence of 150–200/100,000 members of the general population. It affects 1% of those over 65 and 2% of those over 85 years of age.

Movement disorders present special challenges to family physicians for several reasons. Symptoms and signs are often very subtle. A variety of complex presentations are common among patients suffering from the same movement disorder. The normal process of aging is associated with changes in movement that can be mistaken for a more serious disorder. Finally, laboratory and radiological testing is often of limited value in the diagnosis of movement disorders.

Management is equally challenging. Although drug therapy and specialized therapies are often administered by specialists, family physicians must help patients cope with the broad impact of their illness. Movement disorders have a substantial impact on other medical conditions as well as on the psychological well being of patients and the families that care for them.

The complex nature of movement disorders makes it impossible for family physicians to become familiar with all aspects of these diseases. Most patients with progressive or debilitating movement disorders should be managed in partnership with a neurologist. Family physicians should limit their role to a few important tasks to which their expertise is well suited.

1. Family physicians should become familiar with the common presenting signs and symptoms of the most common movement disorders (eg, Parkinson's disease) and seek the help of a specialist in ordering further tests and establishing a diagnosis.

2. Family physicians should be familiar with how to make use of clinical practice guidelines and other systematically developed resources for the management of common movement disorders. Some patients should be managed in partnership with a specialist.

3. Family physicians should have some knowledge about how to gauge the severity of disease and be aware of side effects of therapies.

4. As mentioned, many movement disorders have a broad and profound impact. Family physicians should become adept at counseling patients and their families about prognosis and the availability of support groups and community resources.

5. The management of certain conditions including Parkinson's disease is rapidly changing. Family physicians should have some awareness of emerging and alternative therapies for this and other movement disorders and knowledge of where to find the latest information about emerging therapies.

O'Brien CF: Movement disorders for the primary care physician. Fam Pract Issues Neurol 1999;10(2). http://www.thecni.org/reviews/10-2-p04-obrien.htm. Accessed July 18, 2002.

Table 44-1. Movement disorders.

Hypokinetic Disorders	Hyperkinetic Disorders
Parkinson's disease	Tremor (eg, essential tremor, dys-
Secondary parkinsonism	tonic tremor, drug-induced
Progressive supranuclear	tremor, physiological tremor)
palsy (PSP)	Tic disorders [eg, Tourette's syn-
Multisystem atrophy	drome (TS)]
(MSA)	Chorea (eg, Huntington's disease)
	Myoclonus
	Dystonia
	Ataxia

■ HYPOKINESIAS

PARKINSON'S DISEASE

ESSENTIALS OF DIAGNOSIS

- Tremor.
- Rigidity.
- Bradykinesia.
- Postural instability.
- Positive glabella tap reflex.

General Considerations

Parkinson's disease is the most common neurodegenerative disease, affecting millions around the world. Symptoms and signs appear as neurons and dopamine are lost from the substantia nigra and intracytoplasmic inclusions (Lewy bodies) proliferate. Although it was first described nearly 200 years ago, diagnosis still remains a challenge. In one study, among 43 patients diagnosed with Parkinson's disease by experienced neurologists, the disease was confirmed at autopsy in only 31 (76%). Imaging studies show some promise in increasing the accuracy of diagnosis.

Clinical Findings

Symptoms and signs of Parkinson's disease typically first appear among men and women in their fifties and sixties. A number of "classic" features of the disease have been described and remain the basis upon which diagnosis is made. These include tremor, rigidity, bradykinesia, and postural instability. A diagnosis of

Parkinson's disease is usually made when two or more of these features are present.

Although the disease as a whole is classified as a hypokinesia, tremor, a hyperkinetic feature, affects roughly 75% of patients with Parkinson's disease. It is usually a resting tremor with a frequency of 4–6 Hz that disappears or becomes less prominent during purposeful movements. Tremor usually first appears in the upper extremities but may also affect the legs, chin, and lips. The tremor of Parkinson's disease can be made worse by physical or emotional stress. It usually disappears during sleep.

Rigidity refers to resistance to passive movements. Patients with Parkinson's disease often display "cogwheel rigidity" in which there is intermittent resistance during passive motion of a limb—like the cogs of a wheel.

Bradykinesia refers to overall slowing of active movement or slowness in initiating movement. Patients complain of difficulty with tasks such as rising from a chair and turning in bed. Gait is affected and patients take slow, small, shuffling steps. Bradykinesia can also affect the face, which takes on a blank look ("masked" facies). Speech can become softer or slurred. Fine motor tasks are affected. Patients report difficulty buttoning buttons and opening jars. Handwriting becomes smaller or illegible.

Postural instability usually appears late in the course of disease and refers to the loss of postural reflexes and the consequent inability of patients to maintain a particular posture. It is the most disabling feature of Parkinson's disease. Patients lose their balance and have a tendency to fall. They may accelerate forward or backward involuntarily (festination).

Although not a "classic" feature, the glabella tap reflex should be evaluated in all patients with suspected Parkinson's disease. It is tested by percussing over the forehead, which causes reflex blinking of both eyes. The blinking normally stops after 5–10 repeated taps. Many patients with Parkinson's disease continue to blink—a "positive" response known as Myerson's sign.

Although many patients with Parkinson's disease will present with more than one or all of these classic features and the glabella tap test in different combinations and to different degrees or ways, it is important to keep in mind that making the diagnosis is difficult and often takes several assessments over time to confirm. A number of "secondary" manifestations such as depression, sleep disturbances, and dementia complicate the diagnosis. Table 44–2 summarizes clinical features that are useful, when present, in confirming the diagnosis of Parkinson's disease. A helpful diagnostic approach consists of a thorough inquiry into symptoms of bradykinesia with a focus on everyday tasks and observation of speech and facies, asking about and observing a resting

Table 44–2. Features useful in the diagnosis of Parkinson's disease.

Tremor	Resting tremor of 4–6 Hz. Made worse by emotional or physical stress. Attenuated by sleep and purposeful movements.
Bradykinesia	Slowness of movements or difficulty initiating movements manifested as difficulty rising from a chair, turning in bed, opening jars, and buttoning as well as "masked" facies, "shuffling" gait, slurred speech, and micrographia.
Rigidity	Manifested as resistance to passive motion. Often presents as "cogwheel" rigidity in limbs whereby resistance is intermittent.
Postural instability	Inability to maintain posture as postural reflexes are lost. Manifested as loss of balance, tendency to fall, and festination.
Glabella tap test	Light tapping of the forehead elicits a blinking response in patients with Parkinson's disease that does not extinguish with repeated tapping.

tremor, examining the patient for rigidity, performing a glabella tap test, and observing the patient's gait and posture. A sample of writing may be helpful in confirming the presence of micrographia. An experienced neurologist should be consulted to help confirm the diagnosis.

Treatment

Clinical practice guidelines for the management of Parkinson's disease are scarce, but the recently published treatment guidelines by Olanow et al provide a rational approach to the use of medications and other therapies. The recommendations in this section are based on these guidelines.

A. PHARMACOTHERAPY

Pharmacological therapy has been shown to reduce morbidity and mortality and is the mainstay of treatment for Parkinson's disease. The goals of pharmacotherapy are two-fold: neuroprotection, the protection of neurons and slowing or stopping of disease progression, and symptomatic therapy.

The selective monoamine oxidase B (MAO-B) inhibitor selegiline has been studied extensively as a neuroprotective agent. It has been shown to delay functional impairment and the progression of signs and symptoms. Selegiline is also effective in relieving symptoms of Parkinson's disease. It is unclear, therefore, whether this disease-modifying effect is due to neuroprotection or the effect of selegiline on symptoms, which may mask disease progression. The use of selegiline, therefore, is controversial. Further evidence is needed to confirm its benefit. In the interim, if it is to be used at all, selegiline should be administered early in the course of disease. Rasagiline is another MAO-B inhibitor whose effect on Parkinson's disease is now being studied.

Unlike neuroprotective therapy, which is administered as soon as the diagnosis is made, symptomatic therapy should be started only when the patient begins to experience "functional impairment." There are no strict rules as to what constitutes functional impairment but clinicians should consider the following questions before starting such therapy:

1. Do the patient's symptoms affect the dominant or nondominant hand? Symptoms affecting the dominant hand make the need for symptomatic therapy more likely.

2. Is the patient employable and how do the patient's symptoms affect the patient's ability to work?

3. What specific features of Parkinson's disease are present (eg, bradykinesia is more disabling than tremor)?

4. How does the patient feel about symptomatic therapy? Minor symptoms may be troubling enough to warrant symptomatic therapy for some patients. Other patients may choose to cope with more disabling symptoms without medication therapy.

Three important classes of medications are currently used in symptomatic therapy. *Dopamine agonists* are dopamine-like compounds that are able to stimulate dopamine receptors. These include bromocriptine, pergolide, and pramipexole (Table 44–3). They were once used only for adjunctive therapy, but their favorable side effect profile has made them useful for initial symptomatic therapy.

Levodopa remains the most effective drug for relieving symptoms. It is usually combined with the decarboxylase inhibitor *carbidopa,* which blocks the conversion of levodopa to dopamine outside the blood–brain barrier, and consequently reduces the incidence of nausea and vomiting. Unfortunately, long-term administration of levodopa is associated with serious adverse effects including dyskinesia and psychosis.

Even when combined with carbidopa, a large amount of levodopa is converted by the enzyme catechol-*O*-methyltransferase (COMT) to the inert metabolite 3-methyldopa (3-OMD). Only 10% of levodopa

Table 44–3. Drugs for symptomatic therapy of Parkinson's disease.

Class	Use	Drug	Usual Dosage Range (mg/day)
Dopamine agonists	Initial therapy or as adjunct to levodopa	Bromocriptine	7.5–40
		Pergolide	0.75–6
		Pramipexole	0.75–3
		Ropinirole	9–24
		Cabergoline	0.5–5
		Lisuride	0.5–5
Levodopa	Initial therapy ± COMT inhibitor; can be used in combination with dopamine agonists; administered in preparations that include carbidopa	Different strengths of car-bidopa–levodopa (Sinemet) are available: 10 mg car-bidopa/100 mg levodopa (10/100), 25/100, and 25/250	300–400 (levodopa)
COMT inhibitors[1]	As adjuncts to levodopa therapy only	Tolcapone	300–600
		Encapone	200 mg given with each dose of levodopa

[1]COMT, catechol-*O*-methyltransferase.

reaches the brain intact. To overcome this limitation, levodopa can be administered together with a COMT inhibitor. Two COMT inhibitors are currently available.

Other classes of medications such as anticholinergics and amantadine today have limited usefulness in the symptomatic treatment of Parkinson's disease. Family physicians may still encounter patients taking these medications.

B. Disease Monitoring

Caring for patients with Parkinson's disease involves long-term assessment of disease severity and monitoring for side effects of therapy, usually levodopa. Levodopa-induced side effects include motor fluctuations and dyskinesias. Motor fluctuations are alterations in the severity of impairment of movement that occur due to a fluctuating response to levodopa. Patients respond well to medication during "on periods" and poorly during "off periods." Fluctuations become more rapid as the disease progresses. Dyskinesias induced by levodopa can include choreiform movements, dystonia, and myoclonus.

The "Unified Parkinson's Disease Rating Scale," although very detailed, is a useful tool for the assessment of disease severity and side effects of therapy with which family physicians should have some familiarity. The scale includes checklists for the assessment of the broad impact of Parkinson's disease and can therefore help remind family physicians of exactly what should be assessed. Completion of the scale is also a practical way for

family physicians to communicate with specialists about the severity of their patient's illness. The scale is divided into several sections designed to assess mentation, mood, behavior, activities of daily living, motor function, and complications of therapy. The complete scale is available from http://www.wemove.org/par_rs.html.

C. Counseling

The overall impact of Parkinson's disease on the quality of life of patients and families is profound. Family physicians should be aware of the psychological needs of patients. Depression and disturbance of sleep are particularly common. It is also extremely important to be aware of the needs of caregivers. Stress, insomnia, depression, and financial hardship are common problems among caregivers about which family physicians should inquire. There is evidence that a good understanding of caregiver needs facilitates better care of patients.

Since the functional impairment in Parkinson's disease is progressive, discussion of advance directives is appropriate with all patients. Education and support are important ways patients with Parkinson's disease can cope with their illness. The information they receive from health professionals can be supplemented by one or more excellent books or Internet web sites. A number of one-on-one peer and support groups address the needs of patients. Information on local groups can be obtained from the American Parkinson Disease Association.

D. Emerging Therapies

Three surgical therapies have been used successfully to treat patients with very severe Parkinson's disease and represent an option for patients who fail medical therapy. All are often associated with dramatic improvement of parkinsonian symptoms, especially tremor. *Ablation* involves using radiofrequency waves, heat, or chemicals to make destructive lesions in very specific targets in the brain including the ventral intermediate nucleus of the thalamus (Vim nucleus) and the globus pallidus pars interna (GPi). Deep brain stimulation (DBS) of the Vim nucleus, Gpi, or subthalamic nucleus (STN) involves inserting an electrode in the target region that is connected to a pulse generator placed subcutaneously over the chest wall. High-frequency stimulation of the brain targets by the electrode is associated with functional benefits comparable to those of ablative surgery. DBS, however, has the advantage of not involving destruction of brain tissue. Ablative surgery has been widely available for some time. DBS has been used in Europe for over 15 years. It has recently been approved for the treatment of Parkinson's disease by the U.S. Food and Drug Administration. Its use is expected to become more frequent in coming years.

Transplantation of fetal dopaminergic neurons into the sustantia nigra of patients with severe Parkinson's disease has shown promising results in improving functional impairment. At present, however, this remains an experimental procedure.

Argue J: *Parkinson's Disease and the Art of Moving.* New Harbinger Publications, 2000.

Colcher A, Simuni T: Clinical manifestations of Parkinson's disease. Med Clin North Am 1999;83(2):327.

Olanow CW, Watts RL, Koller WC: An algorithm (decision tree) for the management of Parkinson's disease (2001): treatment guidelines. Neurology 2001;56(Suppl 5):S1.

Weiner WJ, Shulman LM, Lang AE: *Parkinson's Disease: A Complete Guide for Patients and Families.* Johns Hopkins University Press, 2001.

WEB SITES

American Parkinson Disease Association, Inc.

1-800-223-2732

info@apdaparkinson.org

Lexi-Comp Inc.

http://www.diseases-explained.com/Parkinsons/index.html

National Institute of Neurological Disorders and Stroke

http:// www.ninds.nih.gov/health_and_medical/disorders/ parkinsons_disease.htm

WeMove

http://www.wemove.org

SECONDARY PARKINSONISM, PROGRESSIVE SUPRANUCLEAR PALSY, & MULTISYSTEM ATROPHY

It is important to distinguish between "parkinsonism" and Parkinson's disease. Parkinsonism refers to any clinical syndrome in which two or more common clinical features (eg, tremor and rigidity) are present. Parkinson's disease is the "primary" or idiopathic form of parkinsonism. Secondary or acquired parkinsonism has a variety of causes including drugs such as neuroleptics, hydropcephalus, and head trauma. Although a detailed discussion of secondary parkinsonism is beyond the scope of this chapter, family physicians should keep secondary causes in mind when assessing patients with possible Parkinson's disease.

Multiple system atrophy (MSA) (which encompasses the diagnoses Shy–Drager syndrome, olivopontocerebellar atrophy, and striatonigral degeneration) and progressive supranuclear palsy (PSP) are sometimes referred to as "parkinsonism plus" syndromes and share some common features. Family physicians should have some familiarity with these diagnoses, but both are relatively uncommon. Like Parkinson's disease, MSA often presents with asymmetric rigidity and akinesia. Only a minority of patients, however, have tremor. Of patients with MSA 50% present with autonomic dysfunction and cerebellar symptoms and 25% demonstrate a transient response to levodopa. Rigidity, postural instability, and a positive response to levodopa are common among patients with PSP; tremor is uncommon.

Alder CH: Differential diagnosis of Parkinson's disease. Med Clin North Am 1999;83(2):349.

■ HYPERKINESIAS

TREMOR

Tremor can be defined as any rhythmical, involuntary oscillatory movement of a body part. Tremors can be classified by type or by the disease syndrome in which they appear. There are two main types of tremors: rest tremors, which occur in a body part that is not voluntarily activated and is fully supported against gravity, and action tremors, which are produced by any voluntary contraction of muscle. Action tremors can be further subdivided intro postural and kinetic tremors. There are several types of kinetic tremors. This typological classification is shown in Table 44–4. Three common tremor syndromes are the tremor of Parkinson's disease, physiological tremor (tremor not associated with a neurological pathology), and essential tremor (Table 44–5).

Table 44–4. Typological classification of tremors.

Rest tremors	Tremors occurring in a body part that is not voluntarily activated and is supported completely against gravity.
Action tremors Postural tremors	Tremors that occur while voluntarily maintaining a position against gravity.
Kinetic tremors[1] Simple kinetic tremors	Tremors occurring during voluntary movements that are not target directed.
Intention tremors	Tremors whose amplitudes increase during visually guided movements (eg, finger-to-nose test).
Task-specific kinetic tremors	Tremors that appear or are exacerbated by specific tasks (eg, writing).
Isometric tremors	Tremors that occur during voluntary muscle contraction against a rigid stationary object (eg, squeezing examiner's hand).

[1]Tremors occurring during any voluntary movement.

ESSENTIAL TREMOR

ESSENTIALS OF DIAGNOSIS

- *Tremor of moderate amplitude present in at least one arm.*
- *Interference in activities of daily living.*
- *Medications, thyroid disease, alcohol, and other neurological diseases ruled out as cause of tremors.*

Table 44–5. Three common tremor syndromes.

Tremor of Parkinson's disease	Slow-frequency (4–6 per second) tremor at rest. Tremor inhibited during movement and sleep. Aggravated by emotional and physical stress. "Pill rolling quality."
Classic essential tremor	Bilateral, usually symmetric postural or kinetic tremor. Family history of tremor is common. Attenuated by alcohol.
Physiological tremor	Present to differing degrees in all normal subjects. Enhanced form is easily visible, mainly postural, and has a high frequency (8–12 per second). No evidence of underlying neurological disease. Cause is usually reversible (eg, caffeine).

General Considerations

Essential tremor is the most common of all movement disorders, affecting 1.3–5% of people over 60 years of age.

Clinical Findings

Essential tremor is a clinical diagnosis and there have been several attempts to develop accurate diagnostic criteria. Some general features are given in Table 44–5. In addition, patients are said to have "definite" essential tremor if they manifest the following: (1) postural tremor of moderate amplitude present in at least one arm; (2) tremor of moderate amplitude present in at least one arm during at least four tasks such as pouring water, drinking water, or using a spoon; (3) interference by tremor in at least one activity of daily living; and (4) no evidence that medications, thyroid disease, alcohol, or other neurological diseases are the cause of tremor. Patients are said to have "probable" essential tremor when (1) tremor of moderate amplitude is present in at least one arm during at least four tasks or head tremor is present, and (2) there is no evidence that medications, thyroid disease, alcohol, or other neurological diseases are the cause of tremor.

A thorough history is crucial in making the diagnosis of essential tremor. It should begin with an inquiry about the age at onset (essential tremor usually appears after the age of 50) and if and how the tremor interferes with common tasks and activities of daily living. Many patients have a family history of tremor, although this is not a criterion for diagnosis. Essential tremor often improves with drinking alcohol. As enhanced physiological tremor can be confused with essential tremor, it is important to ask about consumption of caffeine, smoking of cigarettes, and use of other stimulants and in-quire about use of medications (eg, inhaled β_2-agonists, levothyroxine, lithium) that are known to cause or en-hance physiological tremor.

Careful observation of the patient with suspected es-sential tremor is necessary. Essential tremor usually has a frequency of 4–12 per second and affects the hands in 95%, the head in 34%, and the lower extremities in 20% of patients. Tremor in the lower extremities, how-ever, is usually asymptomatic. The patient should be observed while performing common tasks such as drinking from a glass.

Patients under the age of 40 years in whom essential tremor is suspected should also be evaluated for Wil-son's disease, a disorder of copper metabolism with a number of manifestations including action tremor.

Treatment

Systematically developed clinical practice guidelines are unavailable. What follows are general recommendations from the medical literature.

A. PHARMACOTHERAPY

Pharmacotherapy constitutes the main approach to treatment. It is not needed in mild cases of essential tremor that do not interfere with functional well-being. First-line therapies include the β-blocker propanolol and the anticonvulsant primidone. These are roughly equally efficacious in reducing tremor symptoms. Of patients 45–75% report that propanolol is effective. A mean reduction of 75% in tremor amplitude has been found among patients taking primidone. The precise mechanism of action of either medicine in reducing the severity of tremor is unclear. Propanolol is more effec-tive than selective β_1-blockers such as atenolol and metoprolol.

Gabapentin is another anticonvulsant and can be used as a second-line agent. Compared with propanolol and primidone, experience with gabapentin is limited. There is evidence that it is well tolerated and as effec-tive as propanolol as a single agent. Starting and usual effective doses of these three medications are listed in Table 44–6. Benzodiazepines, calcium channel block-ers, and theophylline have also been used to treat essen-tial tremor with questionable results. Their use should not be routine.

B. DISEASE MONITORING

The patient's report of symptoms and ability to per-form daily tasks, rather than the severity of tremor de-tected on physical examination, should serve as guides to adjustment of therapy. As many patients are treated with propanolol and primidone, it is important to monitor patients for side effects of these medications.

Table 44–6. Therapy for essential tremor.

Medication	Usual Starting Dose (mg/day)	Usual Therapeutic Dose (mg/day)
Propranolol	30	160–320
Primidone	62.5	62.5–1000
Gabapentin	300	1200–3600

Propanolol is associated with fatigue, headaches, brady-cardia, impotence, and depression. An acute reaction to primidone consisting of nausea, vomiting, or ataxia oc-curs in many patients. Of patients 20% are forced to discontinue the medication as a result. Long-term treat-ment with primidone, however, is well tolerated.

C. COUNSELING

The impact of essential tremor on quality of life is often underestimated. In a study by Deuschl et al all patients with hereditary essential tremor reported some degree of physical disability, 85% felt that essential tremor handicapped them socially, and 25% were forced to change jobs or retire as a result of tremor. Disability also increased with time. Family physicians need to be aware of the potential impact of essential tremor and advise patients to inform them of possible social and occupational problems. Patients should be offered ag-gressive adjustment of treatment when the impact is se-vere.

D. EMERGING THERAPIES

As with therapy for Parkinson's disease, both deep brain stimulation and ablation of the ventral intermedi-ate nucleus of the thalamus (Vim nucleus) are effective for patients with tremor that is refractory to medical therapy. The use of intramuscular injections of botu-linum toxin A into the hand has been studied but the results have not yet been shown promising enough to recommend this therapy.

Deuschl G et al: Consensus statement of the Movement Disorder Society on tremor. Mov Disord 1998;13(Suppl 3):2.

Elble RJ: Diagnostic criteria for essential tremor and differential di-agnosis. Neurology 2000;54(Suppl 4):S2.

Louis ED: Essential tremor. New Engl J Med 2001;345(12):887.

TIC DISORDERS

A tic can be defined as a brief, intermittent, repetitive, nonrhythmic, unpredictable, purposeless movement (motor tic) or sound (vocal tic). Unlike other move-ment disorders, tics are preceded by a conscious urge and can be voluntarily suppressed to some degree. Suppressing the urge to carry out a tic, however, leads to stress. Stress is relieved once the tic is executed. Tics occur transiently in 20% of children under the age of 10 years. A number of inherited conditions including Wilson's disease, tuberous sclerosis, and neuroacanthocytosis are associated with tics. Secondary causes include infections (eg, encephalitis), drugs (eg, amphetamines), and toxins (eg, carbon monoxide). The focus of this discussion is on the serious, chronic tic disorder known as Tourette's syndrome.

TOURETTE'S SYNDROME

ESSENTIALS OF DIAGNOSIS

- *Multiple motor tics and one or more vocal tics must be present.*
- *Tics occur several times a day for at least 1 year.*
- *Disease onset is before the age of 21 years.*
- *Other causative medical considerations have been ruled out.*

General Considerations

Tourette's syndrome is the most common tic disorder, affecting roughly 5–10 of every 10,000 children. Four times as many boys as girls are affected. The average age of onset is 5.6 years, with 96% of cases having begun before the age of 11 years. Fortunately, 50% of patients have no tics by age 18. A precise cause is yet to be identified, although heredity is thought to play a major role.

Clinical Findings

The Tourette Syndrome Classification Study Group has developed precise diagnostic criteria for this disorder. A definite diagnosis can be made if a patient has the following:

1. Multiple motor tics and one or more vocal tics must be present at some time during the illness, although not necessarily concurrently.
2. Tics must occur several times a day on most days for a period of at least 1 year.
3. Tic characteristics, including the body part(s) involved, frequency, complexity, and severity, must change over time.

4. The onset of disease must occur before the age of 21 years.
5. Tics must not be explainable by other medical conditions.
6. Tics must be observed by a reliable witness or recorded on video.

There are a number of different types of tics. "Simple" vocal tics consist of meaningless sounds such as grunts, squeaks, barks, or sucking sounds. "Complex" vocal tics include the uttering or shouting of obscenities (known as coprolalia), repetition of someone else's words (echolalia), or repetition of one's own words (palilalia). Tics get worse during periods of stress, excitement, boredom, or fatigue. They may even persist during sleep.

Although Tourette's syndrome is defined solely on the presence of tics, the majority of affected children suffer from other conditions as well. Half have coexistent attention-deficit hyperactivity disorder (ADHD) and 30–50% have accompanying obsessive-compulsive symptoms. Migraine headaches have been reported in more than 25% of patients. ADHD and obsessive-compulsive symptoms often cause more functional impairment than tics.

Treatment

A. EDUCATION

Systematically developed clinical practice guidelines are unavailable. Treatment begins with the creation of a supportive environment for the patient. This involves educating the patient, family, teachers, classmates, and others about the patient's illness. Tourette's syndrome can have a devastating impact on the ability of children to function in school and participate in social activities. An environment that is unsupportive or even hostile to a child with Tourette's syndrome can only make the functional impairment worse.

Behavioral approaches have been tried for the treatment of tics with some success but the most effective and long-lasting treatments today are pharmacological.

B. PHARMACOTHERAPY

Pharmacotherapy should be started only if symptoms cause some degree of functional impairment. The dopamine receptor blockers haloperidol and pimozide are widely used for the treatment of tics and are very effective. The α-receptor agonists clonidine and guanfacine are effective in treating mild tics. Both are known to improve symptoms of accompanying ADHD.

Drugs commonly used to treat tics with accompanying doses are shown in Table 44–7.

Because ADHD and obsessive-compulsive symptoms coexist with Tourette's syndrome in so many patients, treatment of these accompanying conditions is

Table 44–7. Drugs commonly used to treat tics.

Drug	Initial Dose (mg/day)
Dopamine receptor blockers	
Pimozide	2.0
Haloperidol	0.5
Fluphenazine	1.0
Risperidone	0.5
α-Receptor agonists	
Clonidine	0.1
Guanfacine	1.0

absolutely necessary. Methylphenidate hydrochloride (Ritalin), a psychostimulant, is commonly used to treat ADHD. Selective serotonin reuptake inhibitors (SSRIs) are effective in controlling obsessive-compulsive symptoms. A more detailed discussion of conditions accompanying Tourette's syndrome is beyond the scope of this chapter.

C. DISEASE MONITORING

The severity and nature of tics among patients with Tourette's syndrome change with time. It is important, therefore, for family physicians to carefully and frequently monitor symptoms and adjust therapy accordingly. Tics may be more severe in some environments. Children, for example, may exhibit more tics at home than in school or vice versa. Teachers and others in addition to parents may provide family physicians with valuable information about disease severity.

Patients on medication need to be carefully monitored for side effects. Haloperidol, pimozide, and other dopamine receptor blockers are associated with lethargy, tardive dyskinesia, parkinsonism, and akathisia (restlessness). Clonidine and guanfacine are, by comparison, associated with few serious adverse effects.

D. COUNSELING

As mentioned, education is an important priority for family physicians. Therapy is used to diminish the severity and frequency of tics. Patients and their families should be aware that treatment is unlikely to eliminate tics completely. Families with a child with even very severe symptoms, however, should be advised that it is likely that symptoms will improve or disappear with time. Tics that persist beyond the teen years have a poorer prognosis and realistic expectations for treatment of teens or adults should be conveyed to the patient and his or her family.

E. EMERGING THERAPIES

Botulinum toxin injections have been successfully used to control tics that are unresponsive to conventional treatment. Encouraging results have also been found with the muscle relaxant baclofen, the benzodiazepine clonazepam, the dopamine agonists pergolide and talipexole, and nicotine patches and gum. High-frequency deep brain stimulation of the thalamus was used successfully to control tics in a 42-year-old man. More evidence is needed before any of these therapies can be widely recommended. At present they should be considered only when conventional therapy fails.

Kossoff EH, Singer HS: Tourette syndrome: clinical characteristics and current management strategies. Paediatr Drugs 2001; 3(5):355.

Robertson MM, Stern JS: Tic disorders: new developments in Tourette syndrome and related disorders. Curr Opin Neurol 1998;11:373.

Tourette Syndrome Classification Study Group: Definitions and classification of tic disorders. Arch Neurol 1993;50:1013.

WEB SITE

The Tourette Syndrome Association
http://www.tsa-usa.org

CHOREA

Chorea can be defined as an unpredictable, irregular, nonrhythmic, brief, jerky flowing or writhing movement. Although involuntary, chorea can be consciously incorporated into voluntary movements. These semipurposeful movements are known as parakinesias. Chorea has numerous causes including drugs (eg, some anticonvulsants and antipsychotics), Wilson's disease, stroke, encephalitis, hyperglycemia, and as part of an immunological reaction after streptococcal infection (Sydenham's chorea). The focus of this discussion is on the most common cause of chorea among adults, the inherited form that occurs in Huntington's disease.

HUNTINGTON'S DISEASE

ESSENTIALS OF DIAGNOSIS

- *Movement abnormalities (chorea and abnormal voluntary movements).*
- *Gait disturbances, abnormal eye movements, dysarthria, dysphagia, rigidity.*
- *Cognitive and mood disturbances; dementia.*

- *Genetic mutation of the IT15 gene on chromosome 4b.*

General Considerations

Huntington's disease is inherited in an autosomal dominant pattern. Although it affects only 4–10 of every 100,000 persons, its impact can be devastating. Men and women are affected in equal numbers. The disease is characterized by movement abnormalities as well as cognitive and emotional disturbances.

Clinical Findings

The onset of Huntington's disease may be at any age, though symptoms first appear in patients aged 35–50 years. There are two types of movement abnormalities: chorea and abnormal voluntary movements. The latter include uncoordinated fine motor movements, gait disturbances, abnormal eye movements, dysarthria (impaired speech), dysphagia, dysdiadochokinesis (clumsiness in performing repeat alternating movements), and rigidity. The disease usually begins insidiously. Patients may complain of clumsiness, difficulty writing, or frequently dropping things. Difficulties with voluntary movements get worse with time. The severity of chorea may stabilize after several years and even diminish in the latter stages of the disease. Death usually occurs 15–20 years after disease onset secondary to falls, suicide, aspiration, or starvation.

Cognitive problems include difficulties with memory, visuospatial abilities, and judgment. Patients with advanced Huntington's disease develop a global dementia similar to that of patients with Alzheimer's disease. The most common psychiatric problem is depression, which affects about 40% of patients. Roughly 12.7% of patients commit suicide. Depression among patients is thought to be due to the effect of the disease itself, rather than a reaction to the impact of the disease on quality of life. Other psychiatric disturbances among patients include bipolar disorder (affects about 25% of patients) and obsessive-compulsive disorder.

The signs and symptoms of Huntington's disease overlap with many other conditions including Alzheimer's disease and other movement disorders, making clinical diagnosis difficult. Huntington's disease is caused by a genetic mutation of the IT15 gene located on chromosome 4b. Fortunately, a simple, accurate direct triplet repeat gene test (tests for the abnormal repeat DNA sequences that characterize Huntington's disease) that uses a polymerase chain reaction (PCR) is now widely available. Appropriate use of the test is discussed under "Counseling."

Treatment

No treatment is available to slow the progression of disease. Treatment should target the signs and symptoms and be adjusted according to disease severity. Clinical practice guidelines that specifically address Huntington's disease are not available. Chorea can interfere with daily activities such as eating, drinking, and walking. Its impact on patients' desire to socialize can also be profound.

A. Pharmacotherapy

Chorea does respond to haloperidol and fluphenazine (in doses of 0.5–1.0 mg/day) but such treatment often makes voluntary movements worse. The dopamine-depleting drugs reserpine and tetrabenazine are also effective in treating chorea. Reserpine can cause depression or exacerbate preexisting depression. Clonazepam is also helpful in controlling chorea. Wrist weights decrease the amplitude of chorea and can improve the ability of patients to function. This nonpharmacological therapy should be tried before medications.

The cognitive and mood disturbances in patients with Huntington's disease can be more devastating than the abnormalities of movement. There are no effective treatments for the dementia associated with the disease. Keeping the patient well-oriented and using sedating medications cautiously can minimize the impact of dementia in patients with Huntington's disease, like that due to any other cause. Depression should be aggressively treated with conventional antidepressants (eg, SSRIs).

B. Disease Monitoring

Huntington's's disease leads to progressive functional impairment. Treatment for chorea should be adjusted according to the patient's perception of disability. Some patients with obvious chorea, for example, may not be terribly troubled by it and may not need pharmacotherapy. Given the high prevalence of depression among Huntington's disease patients and the high incidence of suicide, monitoring patients for depressive symptoms and suicidality should be the utmost priority for family physicians.

C. Counseling

The primary counseling responsibility of family physicians is to understand the role of genetic testing and offer testing to affected and asymptomatic individuals in a responsible manner. The Huntington Disease Society of America has developed detailed guidelines for genetic testing: http://www.hdfoundation.org/testread/hdsatest.htm.

Genetic testing can be used to help confirm the clinical diagnosis, especially when a family history of disease is uncertain. In many cases, patients with a family history of Huntington's disease request testing to determine if they will develop the disease. Prenatal testing to determine if a fetus carries the defective gene is available. It is even possible for an asymptomatic mother to determine if her baby carries the defective gene without having to know her own status.

Testing should be carried out in "high-risk" patients (those with a family history of disease) when the patient is well informed and under no significant life stressors (eg, loss of job, marital difficulties). Patients should be aware of the risks and benefits of testing. They should know that although genetic testing has improved dramatically in recent years, ambiguous results do occur. It is also impossible to determine when exactly symptoms will begin to appear and how severe they will be. Results should always be delivered in person. Those caring for those undergoing the testing process should be acutely aware of symptoms of depression.

Testing should be carried out together with a detailed neurological examination to detect subtle signs of the disease.

D. Emerging Therapies

The outlook for effective emerging therapies is grim. Coenzyme Q and remacemide hydrochloride were recently studied as potential disease-modifying agents. Neither was shown to significantly slow the progression of Huntington's disease. Gene therapy may hold the promise of an effective approach to treatment in the distant future.

Huntington Study Group: A randomized, placebo-controlled trial of coenzyme Q_{10} and remacemide in Huntington's disease. Neurology 2001;57:397.

Ross CA et al: Huntington disease and the related disorder, dentatorubral-pallidoluysian atrophy (DRPLA). Medicine 1997;76 (5):305.

WEB SITES

Huntington Disease Society of America
http://www.hdfoundation.org
WeMove
http://www.wemove.org/hd_epi.html

OTHER MOVEMENT DISORDERS

Other movement disorders family physicians may encounter include myoclonus, dystonia, and ataxia.

1. Myoclonus

Myoclonus is defined as brief, sudden, "shock-like" movements caused by involuntary muscle contractions or lapse of muscle contraction (negative myoclonus or *asterixis*). Negative myoclonus becomes evident when an affected limb is maintained in a sustained posture.

There are several ways to classify myoclonus. It can be classified according to how much of the body is involved. Generalized myoclonus, for example, refers to synchronous "jerks" in many body parts. Focal myoclonus affects a single body part. Myoclonus can be classified according to when it occurs (eg, rest versus voluntary movement) or by its temporal profile (eg, continuous jerks, intermittent single jerks, intermittent multiple jerks). From the standpoint of family physicians, an etiological classification scheme is most useful.

Physiological myoclonus refers to benign movements that occur in many people and that are not associated with functional disability. The most common example is "sleep jerks"—sudden "jerking" during sleep or while falling asleep. *Essential* myoclonus, of which there are hereditary forms, is similar to physiological myoclonus except that jerking is more frequent, can occur at any time, and does interfere with social or physical function. *Epileptic* myoclonus refers to jerks that occur during epileptic seizures. The most common form of myoclonus is *symptomatic* or *secondary*. This refers to the broad variety of causes including drugs (eg, lithium), toxins, metabolic conditions (eg, asterixis in patients with advanced liver disease), infections (eg, human immunodeficiency virus), neurodegenerative syndromes (eg, dementia), brain lesions, and paraneoplastic syndromes.

The workup of clinically significant myoclonus includes a careful search for secondary causes. If found, treatment should be directed at the underlying disorder. Essential myoclonus can be treated symptomatically with clonazepam (2–6 mg/day).

Caviness JN: Primary care guide to myoclonus and chorea. Postgrad Med 2000;108(5):163.

2. Dystonia

Dystonia is defined as a syndrome that includes sustained muscle contractions that often cause twisting, repetitive movements, and abnormal postures. Dystonic movements, unlike myoclonus or chorea, usually follow a particular direction or pattern. Although dystonic movements are involuntary, they can be diminished by specific maneuvers known as "sensory tricks" or "geste antagonists." In spasmodic torticollis, a form of dystonia that affects the muscles of the neck, for example, placing a hand on the chin, side of the face, or occiput often reduces the severity of dystonia.

Dystonia is rare and there are numerous causes. Evaluation should be performed in partnership with a neurologist. There are two main forms of *primary* dystonia. Early-onset primary dystonia becomes apparent before the age of 21 years and is generally focal in distribution. It causes, for example, difficulties with writing, torticollis, or blepharospasm. It is inherited in an autosomal dominant pattern with a penetrance of 30–40%. Late-onset primary dystonia, which is also often hereditary, occurs in older adults and involves multiple body parts. *Secondary* dystonia includes a very large number of causes. It may occur as part of other inherited conditions such as gangliosidoses, Wilson's disease, metachromatic leukodystrophy, and Lesch–Nyhan syndrome. Dystonia sometimes occurs among patients with Parkinson's disease, PSP, and MSA. Most secondary dystonia can be attributed to exogenous factors including dopamine receptor blockers (tardive dystonia, the most common secondary cause), stroke, tumor, trauma, cerebral anoxia, and encephalitis.

Treatment for dystonia should address the underlying cause. Early-onset primary dystonia can be treated successfully with high doses of anticholinergics such as trihexiphenidyl often in combination with baclofen. As with the assessment of dystonia, its treatment should be conducted in partnership with a neurologist.

3. Ataxia

Ataxia refers to a wide-based, unsteady gait usually associated with cerebellar problems and/or proprioceptive sensory deficits. There are inherited forms of ataxia including Freidreich's ataxia and spinocerebellar ataxia. The most common forms family physicians are likely to encounter, however, are secondary. These include ataxia secondary to stroke, trauma, alcoholic degeneration, hydrocephalus, vitamin B_{12} deficiency, cervical stenosis, toxin exposures, and multiple sclerosis. In these cases an ataxic gait is usually only one of a number of presenting signs and symptoms. Evaluation and treatment, therefore, should not be carried out with ataxia alone as its focus, but with the greater context of disease in mind. An alcoholic with an ataxic gait, for example, may also suffer from cognitive impairment, liver disease, and other problems. His or her ataxia may be secondary to vitamin B_{12} deficiency, alcoholic degeneration, or stroke.

Hearing & Vision Impairment in the Elderly

45

Pamela M. Williams, MD, & Alan Williams, MD

Family physicians are keenly aware of the joy that comes from interacting with the world around them. Many elderly patients are deprived of parts of this world because of hearing and vision impairment. Although the degree of disability is variable, it is clear that many geriatric patients are suffering. Hearing and vision impairment can adversely affect the quality and quantity of a patient's life and should be actively evaluated when discovered.

Sensory impairment affects up to two-thirds of the geriatric population. The prevalence of vision and hearing impairment increases with age. Exact percentages will vary with definitions. In one study of outpatients in a general practice, 37% of patients over age 60 years had *undiagnosed* hearing loss. In patients over 90 years of age, 39% are visually impaired and 17% are functionally blind. In the Salisbury Eye Evaluation Study over 50% of visually impaired patients aged 65–84 years were found to have either surgically treatable or potentially preventable conditions. African-Americans were more likely to have blinding diseases, particularly those amenable to intervention, and were less likely to have seen an eye care provider.

The primary focus of this chapter is diagnosis, evaluation, and management of the most common causes of chronic hearing and vision impairment in the elderly, as listed in Table 45–1. Discussions of screening and prevention will also be covered, along with the impact of these conditions on patient function and the doctor–patient encounter. Acute hearing loss and vision loss are generally medical urgencies or emergencies and are not covered in this chapter. Patients presenting with these complaints require immediate evaluation, which is beyond the scope of this discussion.

Functional Impact of Sensory Impairments

The same objective level of sensory impairment will result in different levels of disability depending on the needs and expectations of a patient. Hearing loss in a mature cardiologist can end his or her career while presbyopia in an older accountant requires only the use of glasses. Although objective levels are easily measured, the functional impairment is mostly up to patients and

their families to determine. There are times, however, when the family physician may shed light on functional impairment that was previously unrecognized or under-recognized by the patient.

Research on geriatric hearing and vision loss demonstrates the impact of these disabilities. Vision and hearing impairments have been shown to be linked with the wish to die in elderly patients. Hearing impairment is associated with depression as well as decreased quality of life, mental health, and physical, social, and cognitive functioning. The degree of dysfunction correlates with the degree of hearing impairment.

Mild vision impairment increases the risk of death more than twofold. Vision impairment is associated with an increased risk of falling and hip fracture, impaired visual processing and glaucoma with an increased incidence of older driver crashes, and sensory impairment with an increased risk of occupational injuries.

Hearing and vision impairment may adversely affect the doctor–patient relationship. Hearing impairment can lead to misunderstandings and nonadherence to therapy. Shouting can undermine patient confidentiality. Vision impairment can make it difficult for patients to consistently take the correct medication. Because all elderly patients are at risk for sensory impairment, identification, evaluation, and treatment of these conditions may improve their quality and quantity of life.

Screening Assessment

The goals of screening for disease and impairments include early detection, early treatment, and improved outcomes. Given the functional impact of undetected and untreated hearing and vision impairments, many arguments have been made for population-based screening. Although research has yet to demonstrate that community-based screening of asymptomatic older people results in improvements in vision or hearing, consensus opinions do provide guidance for the family physician to apply in daily practice. Disease-specific screening recommendations, when applicable, will be presented later in the chapter.

Vision impairment is typically defined as a visual acuity of less than 20/60, with correction, whereas a vi-

Table 45–1. Common causes of geriatric hearing and vision impairment.

Common Causes of Geriatric Hearing Impairment	Common Causes of Geriatric Vision Impairment
Presbycusis	Presbyopia
Noise-induced hearing loss	Age-related macular degeneration
Cerumen impaction	
Otosclerosis	Glaucoma
Central auditory processing disorder	Senile cataract
	Diabetic retinopathy

Table 45–2. Hearing Handicap Inventory in the Elderly—Screening Questionnaire.[1]

Question	Yes (4)	No (0)	Sometimes (2)
1. Does a hearing problem cause you to feel embarrassed when you meet new people?			
2. Does a hearing problem cause you to feel frustrated when talking to members of your family?			
3. Do you have difficulty hearing when someone speaks in a whisper?			
4. Do you feel handicapped by a hearing problem?			
5. Does a hearing problem cause you difficulty when visiting friends, relatives, or neighbors?			
6. Does a hearing problem cause you to attend religious services less often than you would like?			
7. Does a hearing problem cause you to have arguments with family members?			
8. Does a hearing problem cause you difficulty when listening to TV or radio?			
9. Do you feel that any difficulty with your hearing limits or hampers your personal or social life?			
10. Does a hearing problem cause you difficulty when in a restaurant with relatives or friends?			

[1]Interpretation of total scores: 0–8, no self-perceived handicap; 10–24, mild to moderate handicap; 24–40, severe handicap.
Adapted from Ventry I, Weinstein B: Identification of elderly people with hearing problems. ASHA 1983;25:37.

sual acuity of less than 20/200 with correction is defined as legal blindness in the United States. Patients with a visual field of 20° or less are also categorized as legally blind. Many individuals who are legally blind still retain some limited visual ability. Screening tests available for the detection of various conditions include the *Snellen eye chart* for visual acuity, *ophthalmoscopy* for cataracts, *funduscopy* for age-related macular degeneration and diabetic retinopathy, and *tonometry* for testing for increased intraocular pressure. The American Academy of Family Physicians recommends Snellen acuity testing in asymptomatic elderly patients. The U.S. Preventative Task Force (USPTF) also recommends Snellen acuity testing for the elderly (B recommendation), but notes that insufficient evidence is available to recommend a specific frequency of screening, specific screening questions for the clinician to use, or the routine use of screening ophthalmoscopy. The USPTF does note that people at higher risk for glaucoma may benefit from early detection and treatment and that referral of these individuals to an ophthalmologist is warranted in such cases. The American Academy of Ophthalmology recommends comprehensive eye examinations, including screening for visual acuity and glaucoma, every 1–2 years in patients older than 65 years of age who do not have conditions requiring intervention at an earlier age.

Screening for hearing impairment has been critically evaluated. No randomized, controlled trial has yet proven its effectiveness. Although audiometry is considered the gold standard for assessing hearing loss, multiple screening tests exist including finger rub, whispered voice test, tuning fork, audioscope for limited pure tone audiometry, and self-assessment screening measures such as the Hearing Handicap Inventory for the Elderly—Screening Version (HHIE-S) (Table 45–2). The recommendations of major authorities are limited. The American Academy of Family Physicians recommends that clinicians question elderly adults about hearing impairment and counsel them about the avail-

ability of treatment when appropriate. The American Speech-Language-Hearing Association suggests that the clinician may choose to use a hearing handicap questionnaire, pure-tone audiometry, or both. The rationale behind recommending both lies in the fact that compliance with hearing rehabilitation is often greater when individuals perceive their hearing loss to be a handicap. The U.S. Preventative Services Task Force gives a B recommendation to periodic questioning of elderly patients about perceived hearing impairment, informing them about hearing aid devices, and making referrals for abnormalities when appropriate. Routine audiometry receives only a C recommendation.

Hearing Impairment

A. CAUSES

The majority of patients with hearing impairment will present with complaints unrelated to their sensory deficit. In the course of an office visit, it may become obvious that a patient is in need of hearing screening. However, in a quiet examination room with face-to-face conversation, patients can overcome significant hearing loss and avoid detection from even a keen clinician. Table 45–3 provides one definition of hearing impairment and aids in understanding why patients with even moderate hearing loss may not seek medical care or may escape detection. Family members are often more concerned about the hearing loss than the patient. The inability to have phone conversations, fights over television volume, and complaints of other people mumbling may be family jokes, but they are also clues that a patient may benefit from formal hearing evaluation.

The initial office screening for general hearing loss can be reliably performed with a questionnaire such as the HHIE-S. The whisper test, although simple, is crude and fraught with inconsistency as a screening test. Limited, office-based, pure tone audiometry, although somewhat cumbersome, is more accurate in identifying patients who would benefit from formal audiometry. These tests have been shown to be valid and reliable for evaluating older adults with concomitant depression and dementia.

Below are the most common causes of geriatric hearing impairment. A brief background discussion for each problem, its clinical presentation, and initial evaluation will be provided. The subsequent section will address treatment, prevention, and rehabilitation.

1. Presbycusis—Presbycusis is age-related sensorineural hearing loss typically associated with both selective high-frequency loss and difficulty with speech discrimination. The term simply means "old man's hearing" and can be alternatively termed presbyacusis, prebyacusia, or presbyacousia. Although it has been described for more than a century, the exact pathophysiological cause remains uncertain.

Presbycusis is the most common form of hearing loss in the elderly. Because it often goes unrecognized, exact prevalence data are lacking. This disorder is more likely to occur with advancing age and in patients with a positive family history. It is a mulitfactorial disorder related to a combination of structural and neural degeneration and genetic predisposition. Purported insults related to presbycusis include diet, cholesterol levels, blood pressure, exercise, smoking, and cumulative noise exposure. Studies to date have not established a definitive link between these possible contributing factors and presbycusis.

Presbycusis is separated into four main subtypes, which are based on specific audiometric patterns and are likely associated with specific anatomic areas of hearing dysfunction. *Sensory presbycusis* is associated with atrophy of the organ of Corti as well as subsequent neural degeneration. Speech discrimination tends to be less affected in sensory presbycusis. Neural atrophy of cochlear neurons is termed *neural presbycusis,* which is actually a specific form of central auditory processing disorder. *Strial presbycusis* is due to cochlear atrophy in the stria vascularis. These patients have flatter pure tone response, but retain speech discrimination. Finally, *cochlear conductive prebycusis* exhibits a descending straight line on audiometric testing. In this subtype, the loss of speech discrimination parallels the degree of hearing loss. Complicating this organizational system is the fact that up to 25% of patients with presbycusis do not have characteristic findings and must be termed indeterminate. For the family physician, these distinctions may be beyond the needs of a routine clinic visit. However, they serve to illustrate the varying etiologies contributing to diminished hearing.

Presbycusis remains a diagnosis of exclusion. Patients with this disorder may present with a chief com-

Table 45–3. Levels of hearing loss and their functional impact.

Degree of Loss	Level of Loss (dB)	Difficulty Understanding	Need for Hearing Aid
Normal	<25	None	None
Mild	26–40	Normal speech	Specific situations
Moderate	41–55	Loud speech	Frequent
Severe	56–80	Anything but amplified speech	For all communications
Profound	>81	Even amplified speech	Hearing aid, plus lip reading, sign language, etc

plaint of hearing loss and difficulty understanding speech. However, prebyscusis is often diagnosed after complaints are raised by close patient contacts, or hearing loss is noted on routine screening in a patient without hearing-related complaints. The physical examination of the ears of patients with presbycusis is normal. Generally, a medical history that does not reveal suspicion for another cause combined with an audiogram showing bilaterally symmetric high-frequency hearing loss is sufficient to make the diagnosis. The expectation of slow progression of this hearing loss should be communicated to the patient. This pattern of hearing loss over time further serves to confirm the diagnosis. Complete deafness, however, is not an expected end result of presbycusis.

2. Noise-induced hearing loss—Since the industrial age, our world has become an increasingly louder place. Hearing loss due to exposure to noise is related to the level of noise and the duration of exposure. It is essentially a wear-and-tear phenomenon that can occur with either industrial or recreational noise exposure. The force of sound is what moves the stereocilia of the hair cells, initiating the nerve impulse that transmits the incoming sound to the brain. Excessive shear force from loud sounds or long exposure results in cell damage, cell death, and subsequent hearing loss. Noise-induced hearing loss is the second most common sensorineural hearing loss after presbycusis. Up to one-third of patients with hearing loss will have some component of their deficit that is noise induced. This is particularly significant given the preventable nature of this condition.

Much public health emphasis has been placed on protecting workers from this threat. Patients whose exposure predates these initiatives, those who were noncompliant or exposed away from the workplace, or those in whom protective measures failed will still present with noise-induced hearing loss. Although the damage from noise typically occurs in the younger years, the problems of hearing loss may not become apparent until presbycusis drops the hearing threshold to a symptomatic level.

Patients will typically present with tinnitus, difficulty with speech discrimination, and problems hearing with background noise. Further testing with a formal audiogram is generally indicated. Audiometric evaluation of noise-induced hearing loss reveals a bilateral notch of sensorineural hearing loss between 3000 and 6000 Hz. The physical examination of a patient with noise-induced hearing loss is otherwise normal.

3. Cerumen impaction—The impaction of wax in the external auditory canal is a common, frequently overlooked problem in the elderly that may produce a transient, mild conductive hearing loss. Twenty-five to 35% of institutionalized or hospitalized elderly are affected by impacted cerumen. Removal of cerumen has been demonstrated to significantly improve hearing ability.

The incidence of cerumen impactions increases in the elderly population due to age-related changes occurring in the external auditory canal. Tragi hairs—coarse, large hairs in the ear canal—are a secondary sex characteristic that become increasingly prominent in the third and fourth decade, particularly in men. Cerumen glands are modified apocrine sweat glands that open both directly onto the skin and into hair follicles. Within the hair follicles, sebum, apocrine secretions, and desquamated epithelial cells compound to form wet or dry cerumen depending on a person's phenotype. In the elderly patient, cerumen gland atrophy results in drier wax that is more likely to become trapped by the large tragi hairs in the external ear canal, leading to an increased frequency of impactions of wax in the older individual. These changes are further exacerbated by hearing aid use.

Patients presenting with a cerumen impaction may complain of sudden or gradual hearing loss affecting one or both ears. Examination of the external canal of the patient will reveal complete or near complete occlusion of the ear canal with cerumen.

4. Otosclerosis—Otosclerosis, also known as otospongiosis, is an autosomal dominant disorder of the bones in the inner ear. It results in progressive conductive hearing loss with onset most commonly in the late 20s through the early 40s. Speech discrimination is typically preserved. This disorder is mentioned here because geriatric patients with hearing loss may have this condition complicating their presentation.

Otosclerosis is twice as common in women as in men and occurs more often in white than in African-American patients. Approximately 10% of the general population have evidence of histological otosclerosis. Only about 10% of these, or 1% of the population, will have actual hearing loss from this condition. Immobilization of the stapes by new bone growth is the primary pathophysiological process. Advanced disease can involve the cochlea and present with additional sensorineural hearing loss.

The slow progression of this disease can result in profound deficits that are unrecognized by the patient. The disease can occur unilaterally or in both ears. It is often associated with tinnitus, although the severity of ringing does not correlate with the level of hearing loss. Patients will be found to have conductive hearing loss with or without a sensorineural component depending on the degree of cochlear involvement. The Rinne test will demonstrate the conductive hearing loss with findings of bone conduction greater than air conduction.

5. Central auditory processing disorder—Central auditory processing disorder (CAPD) is the general term for conditions involving hearing impairment that results from central nervous system (CNS) dysfunction. CAPD can be the end result of any insult to the nervous system. Because CAPD may coexist with other forms of hearing impairment, it is difficult to determine its exact prevalence.

The disorder is characterized by a loss of speech discrimination that is more profound than the associated loss in hearing sensitivity. It is most easily recognized by audiometric testing that includes speech audiometry and pure-tone testing. Because CAPD represents the end result of CNS damage, it will often present in concert with other conditions such as stroke and dementia. These additional clinical concerns may be more life threatening than the associated hearing impairment, so evaluation of CAPD may be delayed.

The patient with CAPD will have difficulty understanding spoken language, but may be able to hear sounds well. These patients may avoid notice if the history is taken mainly from a caretaker with only smiles and nods of assent from the patient. The office physical examination of these patients will be normal, or possibly reveal additional neurological signs. The patient may have difficulty following verbal instructions but understands written ones.

B. Treatment and Prevention

1. Presbycusis—After diagnosing presbycusis, a determination of the level of disability should be made in discussion with the patient and his or her close contacts. Treatment consists of hearing rehabilitation that often involves fitting for binaural hearing aids. Cochlear implantation is reserved for patients with profound hearing loss unresponsive to hearing aids. Classes in lip reading may be useful. Additional tools, which may help these patients, include sound-enhancing devices for concerts, church, or other public gatherings, and telephone amplifiers for patients who do not want or do not need hearing aids. Finally, television closed captioning has become increasingly available. Because the needs of each individual patient will vary significantly, a combined approach involving the patient, hearing loss specialist, the family physician, and close contacts of the patient is likely to produce the best overall treatment plan.

In addition to revealing the number of untreated patients with hearing loss, recent literature has shed light on the number of patients who own hearing aids but do not use them. This represents both a drain on the health care system, as well as another opportunity to assist patients with their problems. Asking patients about the functionality of their assistive devices during clinical visits can be very enlightening. Studies show that patients who perceive their hearing loss as a disability, as measured by hearing assessment questionnaires, are more likely to be compliant with therapy.

Until the exact pathophysiology of presbycusis is understood, attempts at prevention will be limited. Although a number of studies have evaluated the role of vitamins, antioxidants, and diet in preventing presbycusis, there have been no conclusive findings.

2. Noise-induced hearing loss—Treatment of noise-induced hearing loss ideally involves prevention via hearing protection. Massive campaigns for workplace hearing protection are in place in the military and other large employers whose workers are exposed to noise. Education about the risks of exposure to loud noise should begin when patients are still young. Hearing loss can occur from any exposure to loud noise including hobbies and concerts. There is nothing that can be done to reverse the cell death from noise-induced hearing loss. Some patients exposed to brief episodes of loud noise exhibit only hair cell injury and may recover hearing over time. These patients are more susceptible to noise-induced hearing loss on reexposure, however. If prevention fails, then treatment involves hearing rehabilitation as outlined in the management of presbycusis.

3. Cerumen impaction—The management of impactions may be approached in a variety of different manners. When the wax is soft, gentle irrigation of the canal with warm water may be sufficient to remove the offending material. In the case of firmer wax, ceruminolytic agents may be applied, followed by irrigation. Any cerumen remaining after these maneuvers may be removed using a curette in combination with an otoscope. Care should be taking to avoid trauma to the skin, which may lead to bleeding, hematoma, or infection.

Cerumen impactions may be prevented by the regular use of agents that soften wax. Readily available household agents such as water, mineral oil, cooking oils, hydrogen peroxide, and glycerin may be utilized. Commercially available ceruminolytic compounds, such as carbamide peroxide, triethanolamine polypeptide, and docusate sodium liquid, can also be used but have not been shown to be significantly more efficacious.

4. Otosclerosis—Because this disorder is progressive, patients with otosclerosis should have interval audiometric testing. Geriatric patients with previously unrecognized otosclerosis may become symptomatic from presbycusis earlier due to their existing condition. Stapedotomy or stapedectomy with prosthetic replacement of the stapes improves hearing by 15 dB in up to 90% of patients. Surgical intervention is recommended for patients with a 20-dB gap between air and bone conduction and for patients with bilateral involvement. Hearing rehabilitation, including hearing aids, may be of benefit in patients who are not surgical candidates, especially those with mild disease. There are no known preventive measures for this condition.

5. Central auditory processing disorder—Once the diagnosis of CAPD has been made, there is little direct treatment available. If the CNS dysfunction is caused by a reversible entity, such as infection or acute stroke, then treatment for the underlying cause should be rapidly initiated. For most cases, however, the best the family physician can do is identify and treat other causes of sensory impairment that may be exacerbating the CAPD. Typically, it is a patient's CAPD that limits the effectiveness of auditory rehabilitation.

No studies have investigated the prevention of CAPD. It may be postulated that the protection to the nervous system gained by aspirin therapy and hypertension control could decrease the incidence of CAPD, although as yet there are no data to support or refute this.

Vision Impairment

A. CAUSES

Vision loss in the elderly is a significant health care problem. Multiple impairments involving varying structures within the eye may cause disability due to a loss of central vision, a loss of peripheral vision, or a decrease in visual acuity. The degree of disability in a patient will depend upon the relative contribution of each impairment.

The initial office screening of the patient with suspected vision impairment will typically begin with the Snellen wall chart for distant visual acuity and a hand-held card, such as the Snellen near acuity card, for near visual acuity. Further evaluation using ophthalmoscopy, funduscopy, or tonometry will depend upon the patient's symptoms, underlying medical problems, and clinical risk factors. Screening questionnaires may also be useful.

Four disorders account for the majority of conditions leading to vision loss in the elderly: macular degeneration, glaucoma, cataracts, and diabetic retinopathy. These conditions, along with a discussion of presbyopia, are presented here.

1. Presbyopia—By the fourth decade of life, most individuals find it increasingly difficult to focus on near objects while their distant vision remains completely normal. This loss of lens power or accommodation for near vision is termed *presbyopia* and its incidence increases with age. The cause of this disorder is the ongoing increase in the diameter of the lens within the eye as the result of continued growth of the lens fibers. This thickened lens accommodates less responsively to the contraction of muscles in the ciliary body, limiting its ability to focus on near objects.

Patients presenting with this disorder will frequently complain of eye strain or of blurring of their vision when they try to quickly change from looking at a nearby object to one that is far away, or say that their "arms are too short" to hold objects at their new focal point. On examination, the only abnormality noted is a decrease in near vision. The ability to see distant objects remains unchanged.

2. Macular degeneration—Age-related macular degeneration (AMD) is the leading cause of severe vision loss in older Americans. It is characterized by atrophy of cells in the central macular region of the retinal pigment epithelium resulting in the loss of central vision. Peripheral vision generally remains intact. This condition is always progressive, but is never completely blinding.

The pathophysiology of AMD has yet to be delineated. The location of the disease within the eye is debated with some investigating the neural retina (the actual rods and cones) and others the retinal pigment epithelium (the cell layer that provides nutrition to the rods and cones). Risk factors for this disorder have been extensively studied, with age, sex, family history, ethnicity, eye color, exposure to sunlight, history of cardiovascular disease, cigarette smoking, and low dietary intake of antioxidant nutrients all being implicated. Of these, only increasing age and tobacco abuse have consistently been associated with age-related macular degeneration.

AMD is typically classified as early or late, with the late disease being further divided into atrophic (dry) or exudative (wet) forms. In early disease, the most common abnormality seen is the presence of drusen, yellowish colored deposits deep in the retina. Changes in the retinal pigmentation may also occur. In late disease of the atrophic type, the macula is found to have areas of depigmentation. In the exudative form, fluid accumulates beneath the retina, as a result of subretinal neovascularization, which leaks fluid, lipids, or blood. Vision loss is usually sudden. Although this process occurs in only 10% of patients with AMD, it is responsible for the vast majority of severe vision loss related to the disease.

The incidence of AMD has been extensively evaluated in a variety of population-based epidemiological studies. In the Framingham Eye Study, drusen were noted in 25% of all participants over 52 years of age. The Third National Health and Nutrition Examination Survey, a population-based survey of a representative sample of the U.S. population aged 40 years and older, evaluated the presence of AMD by grading fundus photographs in over 4000 individuals. The prevalence of AMD in this civilian, noninstitutionalized population was 9.2%. The prevalence was highest in non-Hispanic whites (9.3%) compared with non-Hispanic blacks (7.4%) and Mexican-Americans (7.1%). Early AMD was found to be more prevalent in persons 60 years of age and older than in persons 40–59 years of age. Late disease was found only in persons aged 60 years and older.

Patients presenting with vision loss due to AMD may report an onset of blurred vision that is either gradual or acute. Patients often note wavy or distorted central vision, known as metamorphopsia. Further, intermittent shimmering lights may be noted. Central blind spots, termed scotoma, may occur. Clinical signs of the disorder include decreased visual acuity and Amsler grid distortion (Figure 45–1). The diagnosis of AMD is a clinical diagnosis based upon the presence of visual disturbances in association with characteristic findings on dilated examination of the macula. An ophthalmologist may employ fluorescein angiography to confirm the diagnosis and to help determine whether a patient has an atrophic or exudative form of the disease.

3. Glaucoma—Glaucoma is the term given to a group of optic neuropathies that can occur in all ages. Although glaucoma is most often associated with elevated intraocular pressure, it is the optic neuropathy that defines the disease. Traditionally, glaucoma is first divided into open- or closed-angle types. The aqueous humor of the eye flows from the posterior chamber through the pupil to the anterior chamber. The majority of outflow occurs in a filtration process through the trabecular meshwork in the corner angle of the anterior chamber. If this angle is blocked, or abnormally narrowed, the resulting disorder is termed closed-angle glaucoma. Patients without physical findings of angle closure, but with characteristic optic neuropathy, have open-angle glaucoma.

Normal intraocular pressure (IOP) is generally accepted to be between 10 and 21 mm Hg. The majority of patients with an IOP >21 mm Hg will not develop glaucoma and 30–50% of patients with glaucoma will have an IOP of less than 21 mm Hg. Despite these facts, it has been clearly shown that as IOP increases, so does the risk of developing glaucoma.

Glaucoma is the second leading cause of blindness in the United States. Octagenarians are 60 times more likely to develop open-angle glaucoma in a given year when compared to patients in their 40s. African-Americans and Mexican-Americans are more likely to develop open-angle glaucoma than whites, and glaucoma is the number one cause of blindness in these groups. Asian patients are also at increased risk for glaucoma, especially for closed-angle glaucoma. In addition to elevated IOP, other risk factors for glaucoma include family history and advancing age. Although some studies have shown that hypertension and diabetes are risk factors for glaucoma, the data are not yet conclusive.

Acute angle-closure glaucoma typically presents with unilateral intense pain and blurred vision. It is three to four times more common in women than in men, occurs more often in patients 55–70 years of age, and can be precipitated by pupil dilation. The patient may report seeing halos around light sources and complain of photophobia, headache, nausea, and vomiting. Physical examination shows a mid-dilated pupil, conjunctival injection, and lid edema. The patient will generally have a markedly elevated IOP, usually between 60 and 80 mm Hg. Acute angle-closure glaucoma is a medical emergency that requires immediate ophthalmological referral and treatment.

Open-angle glaucoma is a much more insidious disease. There is a long asymptomatic phase when screening may detect the disorder. Left undetected, patients may notice a gradual loss of peripheral vision. At this stage, significant nerve damage has occurred. Although the characteristics of this disease make it amenable to screening, a best method of detection has not yet been identified.

The evaluation of a patient with suspected glaucoma is a stepwise process involving the measurement of IOP, visual field testing, and examination of the optic discs. Direct examination of the optic disc is more time consuming than the measurement of IOP. However, this examination has the ability to screen for other diseases while also identifying patients who have glaucoma with a normal IOP. Direct ophthalmoscopy, fundi photography, and computer-aided screening are all

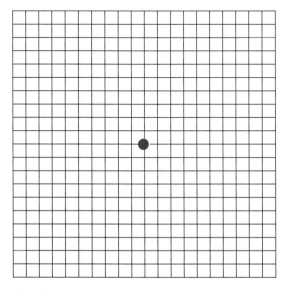

Figure 45–1. Amsler grid for evaluating progression of age-related macular degeneration.

used to directly examine the optic disc. Diagnostic findings include symmetrically enlarged cup-to-disc ratio, cup-to-disc ratio asymmetry between the two eyes, or a highly asymmetric cup in one eye.

There are a variety of tools available to the family physician for measuring IOP, the most readily available being the physician's hand. Palpation of the globe through a lightly closed lid can reveal asymmetric hardness or bilaterally firm eyeballs. Although this is a very gross measure of IOP, this manual assessment is always at hand. More accurate screening tools include tono-pen, Goldman's applanation tonometry, and pneumotonometry (puff test). As screening tools, these are all limited by the fact that IOP is not the sine qua non for glaucoma. Tonometry screening for glaucoma has a sensitivity of 50% and specificity of 90%.

The routine measurement of intraocular pressure by primary care providers to screen for glaucoma is not recommended. The American Academy of Ophthalmology recommends screening for glaucoma by an ophthalmologist every 3–5 years in African-Americans aged 20 to 39 years, and in all individuals every 2–4 years between ages 40 and 64, and every 1–2 years after age 65. The American Academy of Family Physicians does not make any specific recommendations regarding screening for this disorder. Finally, the USPTF does not offer any specific screening guidelines, citing insufficient evidence to recommend for or against routine screening by primary care clinicians for elevated IOP or early glaucoma. The USPTF notes only that effective screening for glaucoma is best performed by eye specialists.

4. Cataracts—Any opacification of the lens is termed a cataract. Although the primary cause of cataracts can be variable, 90% of them are age-related, or senile, cataracts. Cataract disease is the most common cause of blindness worldwide. In the Framingham Eye Study, the incidence of cataracts increased from 2.2% of 55–59 year olds to 46% of patients between 80 and 84 years of age, making cataracts the most common eye abnormality in the elderly.

Age-related cataracts occur as the result of several interactive processes. The addition of layers of lens fibers continues throughout life, leading to a dehydrated opaque lens nucleus. Further, outer layers may hydrate and become more opaque with resultant vision impairment. They are described as nuclear, cortical, posterior subcapsular, and dense white based on both their location in the lens as well as the characteristics of the opacification itself. Risk factors for cataracts include advancing age, ultraviolet B light exposure, smoking, diabetes, and chronic steroid use. Because cataracts tend to develop slowly, the patient may not be fully aware of the degree of vision impairment, and because cataracts

are so common in the elderly, it is not unusual to find them coexisting with other forms of vision impairment. Determining which condition is causing the majority of the vision impairment can be difficult.

Symptoms of cataract include blurring of vision, "ghosting" of images, difficulty seeing in oncoming lights (glare), and monocular diplopia. The patient may also complain of a decrease in color perception and even note "second sight," which is an improvement in near vision with a nuclear cataract. Examination of the eye reveals the opacification of the lens. The cataracts may be easier to see with dilation of the eye and a direct ophthalmoscope held 6 inches from the patients on +5 diopters setting.

5. Diabetic retinopathy—Diabetic retinopathy is the leading cause of blindness in working-aged adults in the United States. However, it is important to consider diabetic retinopathy as a disease of the aging eye since prevalence increases with duration of diabetes. The risk of blindness due to this disorder is greatest after 30 years of illness. Thus, diabetic retinopathy is a serious disease for the elderly.

The earliest clinically apparent manifestations of diabetic retinopathy are classified as nonproliferative or background retinopathy. Abnormalities in the retinal circulation result in microaneurysms, dot and blot hemorrhages, hard and soft exudates (cotton-wool spots), venous dilation and beading, and intraretinal microvascular abnormalities. Although these changes do not impair vision, a maculopathy may result when microaneurysms leak intravascular fluid into the retinal tissue with the fluid accumulating within the fovea. The resultant macular edema may impair central vision. The more severe form of diabetic retinopathy is the proliferative form, which is manifested by neovascularization of the optic disc, retina, or iris as a result of widespread retinal ischemia, fibrous proliferation, preretinal and vitreous hemorrhages, and retinal detachment. Left untreated, this form is relentlessly progressive, leading to significant vision impairment and blindness.

Most patients presenting with diabetic retinopathy will be free of symptoms; even those with the severe proliferative form may have 20/20 visual acuity. In others vision may decrease slowly or suddenly, unilaterally or bilaterally. Scotomata are reported, as are floaters. Ophthalmoscopic examination reveals microaneurysms, dot and blot intraretinal hemorrhages, hard exudates, cotton-wool spots, neovascularization, boat-shaped preretinal hemorrhages, and/or venous beading.

Because patients with retinopathy are often asymptomatic and because photocoagulation treatment is more effective in reducing visual loss when applied at asymptomatic stages, specific guidelines for screening have been developed for the diabetic population. Early detection and treatment offer the best opportunity to reduce loss of vision associated with diabetic retinopathy. Current guidelines recommend that diabetic patients have an initial dilated and comprehensive eye examination by an ophthalmologist shortly after the diagnosis of diabetes is made in patients with type II diabetes. Any patient with visual symptoms or abnormalities should be referred for evaluation. Subsequent examinations should be repeated annually by an ophthalmologist who is experienced in diagnosing the presence of diabetic retinopathy and is knowledgeable about its management. More frequent examinations are needed if the retinopathy is progressive. Patients with any level of macular edema, severe nonproliferative retinopathy, or any proliferative retinopathy require prompt care by an ophthalmolgist experienced in their management and treatment.

B. TREATMENT

1. Presbyopia—In patients with normal distant vision, treatment for this disorder is as simple as purchasing reading glasses over the counter. For patients requiring correction of their distance vision, rehabilitative options include spectacle correction with bifocal or trifocal lenses, monovision contact lenses in which one eye is corrected for distance vision and the other eye for near vision, or contact lens correction of distance vision and simple reading glasses for near vision. As this process is progressive, stronger reading glasses may become necessary over time. The stronger the power of the lens, the narrower the working range for the wearer. As a result, most people are happiest maintaining a weaker prescription until they experience eye fatigue or an inability to hold reading material far enough from the eyes to focus.

Because the effects of presbyopia continue to progress as an individual ages, this condition is not amenable to treatment with radial keratotomy or laser-assisted *in situ* keratomileusis (LASIK) surgery. Other surgical procedures to treat this disorder are currently in Phase I trials.

2. Macular degeneration—Care of the patient with known or suspected AMD will be performed by an ophthalmologist. Patients presenting with suspected or known AMD associated with *acute* visual changes should be referred to an ophthalmologist within 24 h.

Daily Amsler grid (Figure 45–1) testing is an effective tool for detecting progression of AMD. The Amsler grid tests the central 10° of visual field of each eye. When the patient fixates one eye on the black central dot of the white checkerboard from a distance of 12 inches (35 cm), the grid is projected on the central retina (macula). The patient maps wavy lines (metamorphopsia), blind spots (scotomata), and other irregularities in the checkerboard. The procedure is repeated for each eye. The patient performs this test daily and is instructed to contact the physician if metamorphopsia or scotomata are detected and persist for 1–2 days.

Treatments with proven effectiveness include laser photocoagulation and photodynamic therapy. In the Macular Photocoagulation Study Group, a large multicenter prospective randomized clinical trial, laser photocoagulation has been shown to be effective in the treatment of eyes with exudative disease and well-defined subretinal neovascularization. Unfortunately, these findings are present in only about 15% of patients with exudative disease. Treatment may reduce the risk of further vision loss but does not typically restore vision. Laser treatment is an outpatient procedure requiring only topical anesthesia. Photodynamic therapy is a newer treatment that takes advantage of the fact that neovascular vessels appear to preferentially retain dye. Injected dye is subsequently excited by a laser, resulting in the formation of free radicals that close down leaky vessels. Two clinical trials (performed by the same investigators and sponsored by the manufacturer of the dye, verteporfin) revealed that individuals with choroidal neovascularization who underwent this treatment had a lower rate of vision loss than those treated with placebo.

Although treatment is currently grounded in the field of ophthalmology, prevention of AMD remains in the office of the family physician. Because smoking has been so strongly implicated as a risk factor for the disease and continued tobacco use is associated with a poorer response to laser photocoagulation, smoking cessation should be highly recommended. Hypertension has also been linked to a worse response to laser therapy; thus, good blood pressure control is desired as well. The use of antioxidants for the prevention or treatment of AMD is controversial. Observational studies have supported the value of eating foods that are high in antioxidants; however, until recently clinical trials had not yet provided definitive evidence as to the effectiveness of antioxidant vitamin and mineral supplementation in halting the progression of AMD. The Age-Related Disease Study Research Group, a randomized, double-blind, placebo-controlled trial, demonstrated that patients with moderate or advanced AMD had a lower risk of progression to advanced AMD and visual acuity loss if they took both zinc and antioxidants (vitamin C, vitamin E, and β-carotene). These results may begin to clarify the use of these supplements in the management of AMD.

Vision rehabilitation is the cornerstone to helping patients maximize their remaining vision and maintain their level of function for as long as possible. Low-vision professionals along with social workers can be of great assistance in recommending optical aids and devices and accessing local, state, and federal resources for the visually impaired. Direct illuminating devices, magnifiers, high-power reading glasses, telescopes, closed-circuit television, large-print publications, and bold-lined paper are a few of the many devices that can be employed.

3. Glaucoma—The treatment of glaucoma consists of pharmacological and surgical interventions aimed at decreasing the IOP. Although elevated IOP is not required for the diagnosis of glaucoma, it has been shown that reduction of IOP in patients with glaucoma slows the progression of disease. The exact target IOP will vary with each individual case. Even patients with normal pressures can benefit from reduction in IOP. Although uncommon, there are cases of glaucoma that continue to progress despite reduction of IOP to single-digit levels. An ophthalmologist will manage patients with glaucoma.

Patients with glaucoma who are also under the care of a family physician will fall into three general groups. The first group of patients with suspected acute-angle closure need immediate referral to an ophthalmologist. Treatment may be initiated by the family physician, but this action will depend on the specific clinical situation and should be determined in consultation with an eye specialist. The second group consists of patients with significant risk factors or physical findings raising concern for glaucoma. These patients will also need referral to an ophthalmologist for further evaluation and confirmation of diagnosis. These patients will generally not need immediate pharmacological treatment or referral. A discussion of the clinical concerns, referral to an ophthalmologist, and education about the likely diagnoses are all that is required. Finally, the family physician plays an active role in the ongoing care of a patient who has already been diagnosed with glaucoma and who has begun treatment. Topical glaucoma agents have varying degrees of systemic absorption. These medications are fully capable of producing systemic side effects and drug–drug interactions. Thus, it is important to specify all ocular glaucoma medications on a patient's medication list. Asthma, diabetes, chronic obstructive pulmonary disease, coronary disease, thyroid disease, and myasthenia gravis are just a few of the many concomitant disorders that can be affected by topically applied glaucoma medications.

The initial treatment plan for glaucoma typically involves ocular medications. All pharmacological treatments for glaucoma attempt to improve the balance of the creation of aqueous humor to its outflow and, thus, reduce IOP. They may be used alone or in combination. The general classes of medications, their pharmacological effect on the eye, and their potential side effects are listed in Table 45–4.

When medical management is unsuccessful, surgical intervention is considered. Surgical treatments have the same goals as medical management: to improve outflow or decrease production of aqueous humor. Laser trabeculoplasty and laser or conventional trabeculectomy are the most commonly performed procedures.

4. Cataracts—The treatment of cataracts is predominantly surgical. Although small cataracts may be treated by an updated eyeglass prescription or by dilating the eye, most patients with significant symptoms from a cataract will benefit from surgical removal and replacement of the lens. Cataract removal is the most common ocular surgery and is one of the most frequently performed surgical procedures in the United States. The prognosis is excellent with up to 95% of patients obtaining improved vision after surgery. Techniques vary, but phacoemulsification is the most often used technique. The lens is pulverized with a laser and removed through a small incision. A foldable replacement lens is inserted to complete the procedure. Research on techniques to decrease secondary tissue damage and improve the implanted lens (eg, bifocal lens) is ongoing.

Indications for cataract surgery include improving the patient's vision and quality of life, as well as prevention of a secondary glaucoma or uveitis. Ophthalmologists will also recommend removal of cataracts to allow better visualization of the retina and optic nerve in patients at risk for other ocular diseases or in patients who need to undergo retinal surgery or laser treatment. Deciding when to have cataract surgery is a problem that many patients may face. They may turn to their family physician to assist in making this decision. There is no clear point at which a patient must have surgery. Factors that should be considered include life expectancy, current level of disability, status of other medical illnesses, family and social situations, and patient expectations.

The role of the family physician will be to aid patients in understanding the surgery and to assist with preoperative management. Cataract surgery is often accomplished under local anesthesia with minimally invasive techniques. In this case, there is no need to discontinue anticoagulation for the procedure. Communication with the operating surgeon is encouraged to clarify the techniques that will be used. The utility of preoperative evaluation for cataract surgery has been reviewed. Schein et al published a report showing that the routine use of laboratory testing and electrocardiogram screening has not improved surgical outcome. Individuals should receive a routine physical examination and history prior to undergoing surgery, but additional testing is recommended only if findings are abnormal.

Prevention of cataracts is aimed at the modifiable risk factors. Physicians should use steroids at as low a dose as is therapeutic and discontinue them whenever possible. Patients should be advised to avoid ultraviolet (UV) light exposure by using sunglasses with UV pro-

Table 45–4. Agents for treating glaucoma.

Medication Class	Mechanism of Action	Precautions[1]
Carbonic anhydrase inhibitors (oral, topical), eg, acetazolamide, brinzolamide, dorzolamide	Decrease aqueous humor production by inhibiting carbonic anhydrase	Use with caution in renal failure; potentiates salicylate toxicity; may decrease excretion of medications, eg, procainamide, tricyclic antidepressants, and quinidine
Nonselective β_1- and β_2-adrenergic antagonists, eg, levobunolol, timolol, carteolol, metipranolol	Decrease aqueous humor production by blocking β-adreneric receptors	May cause bradycardia, heart block, hypotension, asthma or COPD exacerbation, CHF; interaction with systemic β-blockers, digoxin, calcium channel blockers, and quinidine
Selective β_1-adrenergic antagonists, eg, betaxolol	Decrease aqueous humor production by blocking β-adrenergic receptors	Same as nonselective β-blocker and may also impact diabetes, hyperthyroidism, and myasthenia gravis
Cholinergic agents, cholinesterase inhibitors, eg, physostigmine, carbachol, pilocarpine	Miotic agents that increase aqueous humor outflow	Potential drug interactions with tricyclic antidepressants, amantadine, antihistamines, other cholinergic agents
α_2-Adrenergic agonists, eg, brimonidine	Decrease aqueous humor production by stimulating α_2-receptors	May cause hypotension, fatigue, dry mouth or nose
Epinerprine preparations	Increase aqueous humor outflow	May cause arrhythmias and hypertension
Prostaglandin analog, eg, unoprostone, latanoprost, bimatoprost, travoprost	Increase aqueous humor outflow	May cause changes in eye color

[1]COPD, chronic obstructive pulmonary disease; CHF, congestive heart failure.

tection when outdoors. The possibility of antioxidants providing a protective effect regarding cataracts has been investigated, but results are not conclusive. Aspirin therapy also does not seem to impact cataract development.

5. Diabetic retinopathy—The treatment for diabetic retinopathy has been well established by several multicenter, prospective, randomized controlled studies that demonstrated that intervention with laser photocoagulation surgery or vitrectomy can preserve vision in certain patients. These studies include the Early Treatment of Diabetic Retinopathy Study (ETDRS), which demonstrated the efficacy of focal or grid photocoagulation surgery for diabetic macular edema; the Diabetic Retinopathy Study (DRS), which demonstrated the efficacy of panretinal photocoagulation surgery for proliferative diabetic retinopathy; and the Diabetic Retinopathy Vitrectomy Study (DRVS), which demonstrated a benefit for early vitrectomy in selected patients with dense vitreous hemorrhage or severe neovascular proliferation.

Although the above therapeutic modalities require the expertise of an experienced ophthalmologist or retinal specialist, the primary care physician plays a central role in the early detection and prevention of this disorder. Prevention involves careful attention to glycemic and blood pressure control. The Diabetes Control and Complication Trial (DCCT), a randomized, multicenter, controlled clinical trial, demonstrated that meticulous glycemic control decreased the development and progression of retinopathy in patients with type I diabetes. Subsequent trials have demonstrated similar benefits in patients with type II diabetes. Additional studies have also demonstrated that tight control of blood pressure significantly reduced a patient's risk of requiring retinal photocoagulation and deterioration of baseline retinopathy. The applicability of glycemic control in the elderly patient with diabetes has been examined in a longitudinal cohort study of patients over 60 years of age in Japan with type II diabetes. Poor glycemic control, as measured by $HgbA_{1c}$, was found to be the only significant risk factor for the progression of retinopathy.

Caring for the Patient with Hearing/ Vision Impairment

Patients who have hearing and/or vision impairments have a limited ability to receive, process, and respond to information. Optimal care by family physicians working with these patients will include steps to minimize barriers. The standard clinical setting is frequently filled with cacophonous sounds, finely printed forms, and dimly lit rooms that challenge both providers and patients, most especially the hearing and vision impaired.

When working with the hearing impaired, evaluating the patient in a quiet, well-lit examination room may significantly improve communication. Minimizing extraneous background noise helps to improve speech comprehension. Bright lights reduce shadows on the face of the speaker and allow the impaired individual maximal opportunity to read lips and assess nonverbal cues. A physician should educate the hearing impaired to identify the sources of extraneous noise, to position their better ear away from that source and toward the speaker, and to turn toward the speaker's face so that the mouth may be viewed for lip reading. Teaching the impaired individual to request that a speaker look directly at them and enunciate clearly will help train the patient to advocate for himself or herself.

The physician should ensure that he or she has the patient's attention before beginning to speak. The speaker should address the better ear at a distance of 2–3 feet utilizing slow, clear speech in low tones as presbycusis diminishes hearing mainly in the higher range and should avoid shouting. Shouting distorts language sounds, is uncomfortable to the listener, and may inadvertently convey an impression of anger. If a patient fails to understand a word or sentence, paraphrase, rather than repeat, the information. Pausing at the end of phrases or ideas and alerting patients to a change in subject may help them to follow the conversation more readily. Reinforcement of speech through other channels such as gestures, simple diagrams, and written materials may also improve comprehension. Asking the patient to repeat the main points addressed in a conversation aids in assessing the patient's understanding of what was said. Judicious use of assisted listening devices should also be considered, especially in a practice with a predominantly geriatric population.

The care of the patient with vision impairment will also be improved by providing well-lit reception, waiting, and examination rooms. Consideration should be given to printing selected standard clinical forms in large print to make them easier to read. Similarly, offers to assist in completion of necessary forms can be helpful. When using printed materials for reinforcement, make sure the type is large enough and the typeface is easy to read. As the font size on preprinted instructions and medication labels is frequently quite small, reproducing these in large font may assist the impaired patient in complying with directions. A physician should determine early in an encounter if the patient has brought and is wearing his or her glasses. If the patient has significant trouble reading, consider alternatives to written media such as tape-recording instructions or providing large pictures or diagrams.

American Academy of Family Physicians: *Summary of Policy Recommendations for Periodic Health Examination.* American Academy of Family Physicians, 2001.

American Diabetes Association: Position statement: diabetic retinopathy. Diabetes Care 2001;24(Suppl 1):S73.

Cacciatore F et al: Quality of life determinants and hearing function in an elderly population: Osservatorio Geriatrico Campano Study Group. Gerontology 1999;45:323.

Coleman AL, Wilson MR: Glaucoma diagnosis and management. Ophthalmol Clin North Am 2000;13:349.

Diabetic Retinopathy Study Research Group: Photocoagulation treatment of proliferative diabetic retinopathy. Clinical application of Diabetic Retinopathy Study (DRS) findings, DRS report number 8. Ophthalmology 1981;88:583.

Fong DS: Age-related macular degeneration: update for primary care. Am Fam Physician 2000;61:3035.

Keller BK et al: The effect of visual and hearing impairments on functional status. J Am Geriatr Soc 1999;47:1319.

Leibowitz H et al: The Framingham Eye Study Monograph; an ophthalmological and epidemiological study of cataract, glaucoma, diabetic retinopathy, macular degeneration, and visual acuity in a general population of 2631 adults, 1973–1975. Surv Ophthalmol 1980;24(Suppl):335.

McCarty CA, Nanjan MB, Taylor HR: Vision impairment predicts 5-year mortality. Br J Ophthalmol 2001;85:322.

Munoz B et al: Causes of blindness and visual impairment in a population of older Americans: The Salisbury Eye Evaluation Study. Arch Ophthalmol 2000;118:819.

Realini T, Fechtner RD: Target intraocular pressure in glaucoma management. Ophthalmol Clin North Am 2000;13:407.

Schein OD et al: The value of routine preoperative medical testing before cataract surgery. New Engl J Med 2000;342:168.

Smith W et al: Risk factors for age-related macular degeneration: pooled findings from three continents. Ophthalmology 2000; 108:697.

Strawbridge WJ et al: Negative consequences of hearing impairment in old age: a longitudinal analysis. Gerontologist 2000; 40:320.

Treatment of Age-Related Macular Degeneration with Photodynamic Therapy (TAP) Study Group: Photodynamic therapy of subfoveal choroidal neovascularization in age-related macular degeneration with verteporfin: one-year results of 2 randomized clinical trials—TAP report. Arch Ophthalmol 1999; 117:1329.

U.S. Preventative Task Force: *Guide to Clinical Preventive Services,* ed 2. International Medical Publishing, 1996.

WEB SITES

Lighthouse International (Health information on vision disorders, treatment, and rehabilitation services.)

http://www.lighthouse.org/index.html

National Institute on Aging (Patient education handout on the aging eye and hearing loss.)

http://www.niapublications.org/engagepages/eyes.asp

http://www.niapublications.org/engagepages/hearing.asp

National Institute on Deafness and Other Communication Disorders (Patient education materials on a wide variety of hearing impairment-related topics including presbycusis and hearing aids.)

http://www.nidcd.nih.gov/index.asp

Oral Health

Wanda Gonsalves, MD

Although the nation's oral heath is believed to be the best it has ever been, oral diseases remain common in the United States. In May 2000, the first report on oral health from the U.S. Surgeon General, *Oral Health in America: A Report of the Surgeon General,* called attention to a largely overlooked epidemic of oral diseases that is disproportionately shared by Americans: this epidemic strikes in particular the poor, young, and elderly. The report stated that although there are safe and effective measures for preventing oral diseases, these measures are underused. It also revealed that more than 108 million Americans do not have dental insurance: for every child without medical insurance, 2.6 children do not have dental insurance; for every adult without medical insurance, three do not have dental insurance. The report called for improved education about oral health, for a renewed understanding of the relationship between oral health and overall health, and for an interdisciplinary approach to oral health that would involve primary care providers.

This chapter will describe the three most prevalent oral health conditions (dental caries, periodontal disease, and oral cancer); will discuss their risk factors, prevention, and treatment; and will provide suggestions for referral to a dental health provider.

Dental Anatomy & Tooth Eruption Pattern

In utero, the 20 primary teeth evolve from the expansion and development of ectodermal and mesodermal tissue at approximately 6 weeks of gestation. The ectoderm forms the dental enamel and the mesoderm forms the pulp and dentin. As the tooth bud evolves, each unit develops a dental lamina that is responsible for the development of the future permanent tooth. The adult dentition is composed of 32 permanent teeth. Figure 46–1 shows the anatomy of the tooth and supporting structures. Table 46–1 provides the eruption pattern of the teeth.

DENTAL CARIES

General Considerations

Dental caries (tooth decay) is the single most common chronic childhood disease, five times more common than asthma and seven times more common than hayfever among children 5–7 years of age. More than 50% of children aged 5–9 years have at least one cavity or filling, and this percentage increases to 78% by the time children reach the age of 17. In addition, one-third of persons of all ages have untreated decay, two-thirds of adults aged 35–44 years have lost at least one permanent tooth to dental caries, and many older adults suffer from root caries.

Pathogenesis

Dental caries is a multifactorial, infectious, communicable disease caused by the demineralization of tooth enamel in the presence of a sugar substrate and of acid-forming cariogenic bacteria that are found in the soft gelatinous biofilm (plaque; Figure 46–2). Thus, the development of caries requires a susceptible host, an appropriate substrate (sucrose), and the cariogenic bacteria found in plaque. More than 150 bacterial strains have been found in dental pulp, and approximately 500 bacterial strains have been identified in dental plaque, specifically *Streptococcus mutans* [also known as mutans streptococci (MS)], which is considered to be the primary strain causing decay. Additionally, when plaque is not regularly removed, it may calcify to form calculus (tartar) and cause destructive gum disease.

Finally, the development of caries is a dynamic process that involves an imbalance between demineralization and remineralization of enamel. When such an imbalance is caused by environmental factors such as low pH or inadequate formation of saliva, dissolution of enamel occurs and caries results.

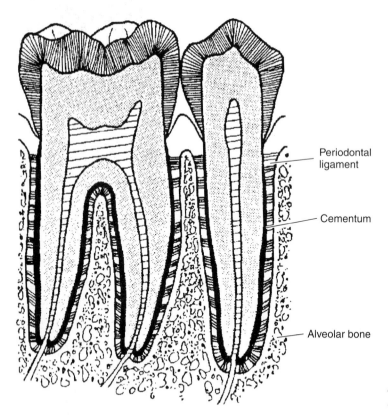

Periodontal ligament

Cementum

Alveolar bone

Figure 46–1. Anatomy of the tooth and supporting structures

Clinical Findings

A. Symptoms and Signs

When enamel is repeatedly exposed to the acid formed by the fermentation of sugars in plaque, demineralized areas develop on the tooth surfaces, between teeth, and on pits and fissures. These areas are painless and appear clinically as opaque or brown spots (Figures 46–3, 46–4, and 46–5). If infection is allowed to progress, a cavity forms that can spread to and through the dentin (the component of the tooth located below the enamel) and to the pulp (composed of nerves and blood vessels; an infection of the pulp is called pulpitis), causing pain, necrosis, and, perhaps, an abscess.

B. Diagnosis

Carious lesions progress at various rates and occur at many different locations on the tooth, including the sites of previous restorations. These factors make it difficult for any one diagnostic modality to detect all forms of caries. Demineralized lesions (white or brown spots) generally occur at the margins of the gingiva and can be detected visually; they may not be seen on radiographs. Advanced carious lesions such as those spread through dentin can be detected clinically or, if they occur between the teeth, by radiographs. Root caries, commonly seen in older adults, occur in areas from which the gingiva has receded.

Dental professionals use a dental explorer to detect early caries in the grooves and fissures of posterior teeth. To diagnose secondary caries (caries formed at the site of restorations), dental professionals use digitally acquired and postprocessed images. Future modalities may include fiberoptic transillumination and light and laser fluorescence.

Risk Assessment

A. Infancy through Childhood

Caries can develop at any time after tooth eruption. Early teeth are principally susceptible to caries caused by the transmission of MS from the mouth of the caregiver to the mouth of the infant or toddler. This type of caries is called early childhood caries (ECC) or baby bottle tooth decay (BBTD). According to the American Academy of Pediatric Dentistry, ECC "is defined as 'the presence of one or more decayed (noncavitated or

Table 46–1. Eruption pattern of teeth.

Teeth	Eruption Date
Primary dentition	
Mandibular central incisor	6 months
Maxillary central incisor	7 months
Mandibular lateral incisor	7 months
Maxillary lateral incisor	9 months
Mandibular first molar	12 months
Maxillary first molar	14 months
Mandibular canine	16 months
Maxillary canine	18 months
Mandibular second molar	20 months
Maxillary second molar	24 months
Permanent dentition	
Mandibular central incisors	6 years
Maxillary first molars	6 years
Mandibular first molars	6 years
Maxillary central incisors	7 years
Mandibular lateral incisors	7 years
Maxillary lateral incisors	8 years
Mandibular canines	9 years
Maxillary first premolars	10 years
Mandibular first premolars	11 years
Maxillary second premolars	11 years
Mandibular second premolars	11 years
Maxillary canines	11 years
Mandibular second molars	12 years
Maxillary second molars	12 years
Mandibular third molars	17–21 years
Maxillary third molars	17–21 years

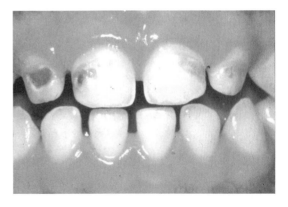

Figure 46–3. Brown spots indicating demineralized areas in enamel

cavitated lesions), missing (due to caries), or filled tooth surfaces' in any primary tooth in a child 71 months of age or younger." In children younger than 3 years, any sign of smooth-surface caries is called severe early childhood caries (S-ECC). Children with a history of ECC or S-ECC are at a much higher risk of subsequent caries in primary and permanent teeth. Dietary practices that increase the risk of dental caries include frequent consumption of liquids containing sugars (juice, milk, formula, soda), consumption of sticky foods, frequent bottle feeding at night, breast-feeding on demand, and repetitive use of a "sippy cup" containing drinks with sugar. Other factors that predispose the child to caries

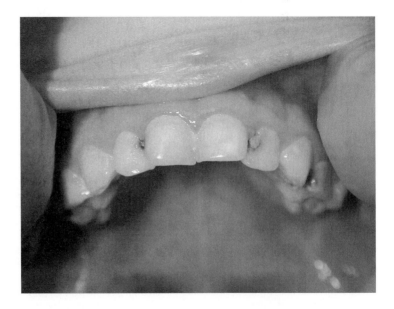

Figure 46–2. Dental caries due to plaque

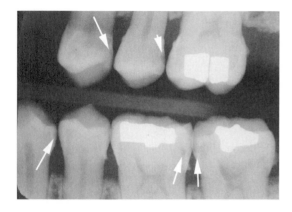

Figure 46–4. Opaque areas indicating demineralized areas in enamel

are maternal and sibling caries, poor dental hygiene, inadequate fluoride in water, and lack of dental visits. Categories of caries risk factors are shown in Table 46–2. Using Table 46–2, the primary care provider can categorize the child's risk status for caries as low, moderate, or high.

The decay rate among preschool populations is nearly 40%, reaching epidemic proportions among certain minority populations. ECC contributes to other health problems, including chronic pain and poor nutritional practices that could result in poor health and weight gain. It also contributes to poor appearance, which may lead to lack of self-esteem among older children and a great reduction in their ability to succeed in life (Table 46–2).

B. ADULT

The risk factors for adult caries are similar to those for childhood caries. However, conditions that compromise good oral hygiene, such as physical and medical disabilities, the presence of existing restorations or oral

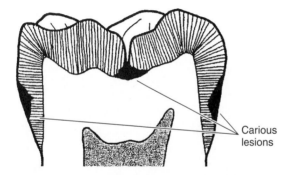

Figure 46–5. Dental caries

appliances, and medical conditions such as Sjögren's syndrome, are associated with an increased risk of caries. The risk of caries is also increased by the use of pharmacological agents that produce dry mouth and of therapeutic radiation to the head and neck that results in a decrease of salivary flow. Gingival recession increases the risk of root caries in the elderly. The risk of caries in this population is also increased by low socioeconomic status and its association with reduced access to medical and dental care.

Prevention & Treatment

One method of preventing dental caries is fluoridation. Fluoride is the ionic form of the element fluorine. Fluoride slows or reverses the progression of existing tooth decay by (1) being incorporated into the enamel before tooth eruption, (2) inhibiting demineralization, (3) enhancing remineralization, and (4) inhibiting bacterial activity in plaque. Water fluoridation is widely accepted as a safe and effective practice for the primary prevention of dental caries. Unfortunately, one-third of the U.S. population has no access to community water fluoridation. Systemic fluoride supplements (tablets, drops, lozenges) are recommended for children older than 6 months who are at high risk of the development of caries, for infants with ECC, and for adults whose water is not fluoridated. Topical fluoride supplements such as gels and varnishes are highly concentrated fluoride products that are professionally applied by a dental health provider or a parent (for gels). Varnishes are applied once or twice a year by disposable brushes, cotton-tipped applicators, or cotton pellets (Table 46–3).

Before prescribing supplemental fluoride, the primary care provider must determine the fluoride concentration in the child's primary source of drinking water. If fluoridated water is not available in the community, natural sources of fluoride are well water exposed to fluorite minerals and certain fruits and vegetables grown in soil irrigated with fluoridated water. Although fluoride supplementation is not recommended for persons who live in communities whose water is optimally fluoridated (0.7–1.2 ppm or >0.6 mg/L), the bottled water used by many families contains only low levels of fluoride. Parents and caregivers should be educated about the benefits of fluoride and the possible side effects of too much fluoride, a condition called fluorosis. Fluorosis results when too much fluoride is obtained from any source when the tooth is forming (Figure 46–6). The benefits and side effects of fluoride use should be weighed against the risk of tooth decay among children at high risk of caries.

A second method of preventing dental caries is proper oral hygiene. Before the teeth erupt, a parent may use a washcloth or cotton gauze to clean a baby's

Table 46–2. Categories of caries risk factors.

Category	Factors
I. Routinely assessed by history and clinical examination	Demographic data: age, race/ethnicity, socioeconomic status, family history, education status Medical history: general health, specific diseases, medications Dental history: presence of caries/restorations, initiation/frequency of dental visits Iatrogenic factors: presence of appliances (orthodontic/prosthetic) Behavioral factors: oral hygiene practices, dietary habits (sugar consumption, frequency), bottle use, breast-feeding practices Dental tissue factors: tooth morphology (deep pits and fissures), enamel defects, gingivitis as indicator of poor oral hygiene Current caries activity: severity of lesions, nature of caries (acute, chronic, arrested), speed of lesion formation Fluoride exposure: level of fluoride in primary drinking water source, use of professionally and self-applied products
II. Special tests	Microbiological testing: salivary mutans streptococci and lactobacilli testing Salivary flow rate: stimulated and unstimulated whole saliva Salivary buffering capacity Plaque index Diet history: 24-h recall, 3-day, 5-day, and 7-day diet diaries
III. Not currently used in clinical practice	Advanced sialometry Salivary composition Pooled and site-specific plaque and plaque fluid analyses Tooth characteristics: acid solubility, fluoride and trace element content Oral clearance/retention profiles

Adapted from Moss ME, Zero DT: An overview of caries risk assessment, and its potential utility. J Dent Educ 1995;59:932, with permission.

mouth and to transition the child to tooth brushing. Parents should supervise brushing and should discourage children younger than 3 years old from using fluoridated dentifrices because of the risk that toothpaste may be swallowed during brushing. A pea-sized amount of toothpaste is recommended for brushing.

Another intervention that has been shown to be beneficial in preventing caries is the use of antimicrobials such as chlorhexidine gels applied by custom-fitted trays, by toothbrush (older children), or by a dental professional. Chlorhexidine reduces the concentration of MS in the saliva. There is no evidence that chlorhexidine supports the primary prevention of secondary caries, the primary prevention of either occlusal or interproximal caries among adults, or root caries. Caution is advised for adults using chlorhexidine because it binds tannins and can cause dental staining among patients who drink coffee, tea, or red wine.

Dental sealants, first introduced in the 1960s, are plastic films that coat the chewing surfaces of primary

Table 46–3. Supplemental fluoride dosage schedule.

Age	Concentration of Fluoride in Water		
	<0.3 ppm F	0.3–0.6 ppm F	>0.6 ppm F
Birth to 6 months	0	0	0
6 months to 3 years	0.25 mg	0	0
3 to 6 years	0.50 mg	0.25 mg	0
6 to at least 16 years	1.00 mg	0.50 mg	0

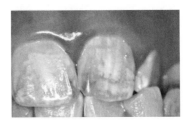

Figure 46–6. Fluorosis

or permanent teeth. Sealants prevent decay from developing in the pits and fissures of teeth. Dental professionals often use sealants in combination with topical fluorides. *Healthy People 2010* states that as many as 50% of all U.S. children should be treated with dental sealants. The cost of sealants is covered by state Medicaid programs (Figure 46–7).

The American Academy of Pediatric Dentistry encourages the following measures for preventing caries among infants and toddlers (Table 46–4):

1. Infants should not be put to sleep with a bottle. *Ad libitum* nocturnal breast-feeding should be avoided after the first primary tooth begins to erupt.

2. Parents should be encouraged to have infants drink from a cup as they approach their first birthday. Infants should be weaned from the bottle at 12–14 months of age.

3. Consumption of juices from a bottle should be avoided. When juices are offered, they should be in a cup.

4. Oral hygiene measures should be implemented by the time the first primary tooth erupts.

5. A visit to an oral health provider is recommended within 6 months of eruption of the first tooth and no later than the age of 12 months. The purpose of this visit is to educate parents and provide anticipatory guidance for prevention of dental disease.

6. An attempt should be made to assess and decrease the mother's or primary caregiver's MS levels so as to decrease the transmission of cariogenic bacteria and lessen the child's risk of ECC.

Older children and adults should avoid frequent consumption of drinks and snack foods containing sugars. Chewing sugar-free gum or cheese after meals has a saliva buffer effect that may counter plaque acids.

Council on Clinical Affairs, American Academy of Pediatric Dentistry: Clinical guidelines on baby bottle tooth decay/early childhood caries/breastfeeding/early childhood caries: unique

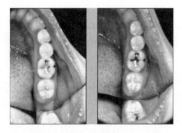

Figure 46–7. Dental sealants

Table 46–4. Guide for routine pediatric dental care within "well child visits."

0 to 6 months
Provide information about teething
Assess risk factors for caries
Counsel about proper cleaning of erupting teeth: twice a day use a washcloth, pea size of toothpaste
Assess need for fluoride supplementation
Explain importance of *no bottle in bed*
Give pacifier and thumb sucking information: ok until age 5

7 to 11 months
Reinforce previous information, especially *no* bottle in bed
Nutrition counseling—limit/dilute juice, sweets
Encourage introduction of cup

12 to 24 months
Thorough examination of teeth for early childhood caries
Refer if caries or early signs of decay noted
First dental visit by age 2; if high risk as soon as identified or age 1
Reinforce nutrition advice, fluoride supplements, and twice a day brushing *by parent* (introduce soft bristle toothbrush)
Encourage use of cup only after 12 months

25 months to 6 years
Reinforce fluoride supplementation—dose change at ages 3 and 6
Reinforce dental visits every 6–12 months
Reinforce nutrition and twice a day brushing advice (children should be supervised until age 5)

7 years and older
Introduce flossing
Stress mouth guards, helmets, and seatbelts for safety
Alcohol and tobacco counseling as indicated
Reinforce previous brushing, nutrition, and dental visit advice

challenges and treatment options. J Am Acad Pediatr Dent (Special Issue: Reference Manual) 2001–02;23(7):29.

Diagnosis and Management of Dental Caries Throughout Life: NIH Consensus Statement Online 2001 March 26–28; 18(1):1. Located at http://consensus.nih.gov/cons/115/115_statement.htm. Last accessed on March 7, 2003.

Domoto PK, Oberg D: Healthy babies-healthy smiles. Infant and toddler dental examinations. WSDA News Special Section. February 1998;1.

Holt R, Roberts G, Scully C: ABC of oral health. Dental damage, sequelae, and prevention. Br Med J 2000;320:1717.

National Center for Chronic Disease Prevention and Health Promotion, Centers for Disease Control and Prevention: *Oral Health Resources. Oral Health 2000: Facts and Figures.* Located at http://www.cdc.gov/OralHealth/factsheets/sgr2000-fs1.htm. Last accessed on March 7, 2003.

Office of Disease Prevention and Health Promotion, U.S. Department of Health and Human Services: *Healthy People 2010.*

Located at http://www.healthypeople.gov/document/html/objectives/21-08.htm. Last accessed on March 11, 2003.

U.S. Department of Health and Human Services: *Oral Health in America: A Report of the Surgeon General—Executive Summary.* U.S. Department of Health and Human Services, National Institute of Dental and Craniofacial Research, National Institutes of Health, 2000. Located at http://www.nidr.nih.gov/sgr/execsumm.htm. Last accessed on March 7, 2003.

PERIODONTAL DISEASE

General Considerations

Periodontal diseases are the most common oral diseases in adults. Although periodontal diseases are not common among young children, they affect 60% of adolescents. Like dental caries, periodontal diseases are caused by bacteria in dental plaque that create an inflammatory response in gingival tissues (gingivitis) or in the soft tissue and bone supporting the teeth (periodontitis). Risk factors that contribute to the development of periodontal disease include poor oral hygiene, environmental factors such as crowded teeth and mouth breathing, steroid hormones, smoking, comorbid conditions such as weakened immune status or diabetes, and low income.

Severe gum disease is defined as a 6-mm loss of attachment of the tooth to the adjacent gum tissue. Severe gum disease affects approximately 14% of adults aged 45–54 years and 23% of those aged 65–74 years. Approximately 30% of adults 65 years of age or older no longer have any natural teeth. The severity of periodontal disease does not increase with age. Rather, the disease is believed to occur in random bursts after periods of quiescence.

Pathogenesis

A. GINGIVITIS

Gingivitis is caused by a reversible inflammatory process that occurs as the result of prolonged exposure of the gingival tissues to plaque. No special tests are needed to diagnose gingivitis; rather, the disease is diagnosed by clinical assessment. Simple or marginal gingivitis may be painless and is treated by good oral hygiene practices such as tooth brushing and flossing. This type of gingivitis occurs in 50% of the population aged 4 years or older. The inflammation worsens as mineralized plaque forms calculus (tartar) at and below the gum surface (sulcus). The plaque that covers calculus causes destruction of bone (an irreversible condition) and loose teeth, which result in tooth mobility and tooth loss. Gingivitis may persist for months or years without progressing to periodontitis; this fact suggests that host susceptibility plays an important role in the development of periodontitis. Steroid hormones encourage the growth of certain bacteria in plaque during puberty and pregnancy and in women taking birth control pills.

Gingivitis (Figure 46–8) can be either acute or chronic. A severe form, acute necrotizing ulcerative gingivitis (ANUG), also known as Vincent's disease or trenchmouth, is associated with anaerobic fusiform bacteria and spirochetes. ANUG (Figure 46–9) is painful, ulcerative, and edematous and produces halitosis and bleeding gingival tissue. Predisposing factors include conditions that contribute to a weakened immune status, such as human immunodeficiency virus (HIV) infection, smoking, malnutrition, viral infections, and, possibly, stress. Chronic gingivitis affects more than 90% of the population and results in gingival enlarge-

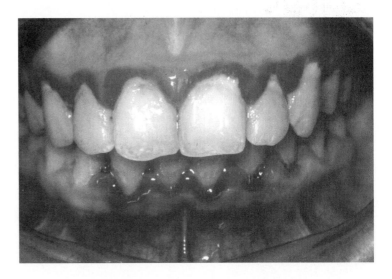

Figure 46–8. Gingivitis

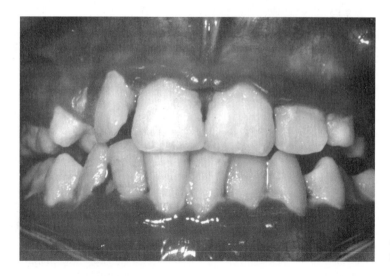

Figure 46–9. Acute necrotizing ulcerative gingivitis (ANUG)

ment or hyperplasia that resolves when adequate plaque control is instituted. Generalized gingival enlargement or swelling may be caused by drugs (calcium channel blockers, phenytoin, and cyclosporin) (Figure 46–10), pregnancy, or systemic diseases such as leukemia, sarcoidosis, and Chrohn's disease.

B. PERIODONTITIS

Periodontitis is caused by chronic inflammation of gingival soft tissue and supporting structures by plaque microorganisms, specifically Gram-negative bacteria that affect gingival soft tissues and supporting structures, with resultant loss of periodontal attachment and bony destruction. Periodontitis is common in adults, affect-

ing more than 50% of the population. Adult-onset periodontitis begins in adolescence and is reversible if treated in its early stages, when minimal pockets (gaps) have formed between the tooth and the periodontal attachment. Severe periodontitis is characterized by a 6-mm loss of tooth attachment as detected by the dental health professional by means of dental probes.

If periodontitis is found in children or young adults or if it progresses rapidly, the primary care provider should be alert to the possibility of a systemic cause. A less common, rapidly progressing form of adult periodontitis begins in patients in the third or fourth decade of life and is associated with severe gingivitis and rapid bone loss. Several systemic diseases, including

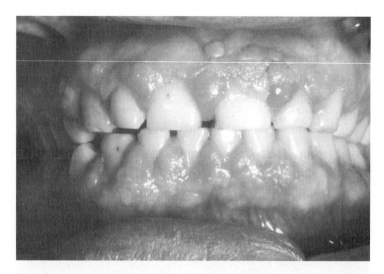

Figure 46–10. Gingival enlargement due to drugs

diabetes, HIV infection, Down's syndrome, and Papillon-Lefevre's syndrome, have been associated with this rare form of periodontitis. Localized juvenile periodontitis (LJP) and localized prepubertal periodontitis (LPP) are forms of early-onset periodontitis seen in teenagers (LJP) and young children (LPP) without evidence of systemic disease. LJP is more common among African-American children. It affects the first molars and incisors, with rapid destruction of bone. It may be inherited as an autosomal dominant trait. Both LJP and LPP are believed to be the result of a bacterial infection (specifically implicated is *Actinobacillus actinomycetemcomitans*) and, possibly, host immunological deficits. Systemic diseases associated with periodontal problems in children may include diabetes, Down's syndrome, hypophosphatasia, neutropenia, leukemia, leukocyte adhesion deficiency, and histiocytosis.

Clinical Findings

A. SYMPTOMS AND SIGNS

Clinical signs of gingivitis and periodontitis include interdental papillae edema, erythema, and bleeding on contact during tooth brushing or dental probing (Figure 46–11). The amount of gingival inflammation and bleeding and the probing depth of gingival pockets determine the severity of periodontal disease. Tartar, gum recession, and loose teeth are characteristics of severe periodontal disease. For children younger than 4 years of age, loss of primary teeth may be the first clinical sign of periodontal disease and the systemic manifestation of hypophosphatasia. Dental probing by the dental health professional will detect sulcus depth.

B. IMAGING STUDIES

Bone loss can be detected by radiographs and bone density scans.

Periodontal Health & Systemic Disease

Emerging evidence, particularly from the dental literature, suggests that periodontal disease may be a risk factor for systemic conditions such as cardiovascular disease and diabetes and for the adverse pregnancy outcomes of preterm labor and low birth weight. However, many of these published reports came from observational studies or experimental animal studies; many of these studies were not rigorously designed, nor were their findings carefully interpreted. Therefore, it is too early for specific recommendations or interventions because no strong evidence exists to support a causal relationship between periodontal disease and these systemic conditions.

Overall, current evidence supports a bidirectional relationship between diabetes and periodontal disease. Periodontal disease is a risk factor for poor glycemic control among diabetics, and diabetes is associated with increased severity of periodontal disease. Studies showing the relationship between periodontal disease and cardiovascular disease have proposed that patients with chronic bacterial infection or periodontitis may have (1) a bacteria-induced platelet-aggregation defect that contributes to acute thrombolic events, (2) injury to vascular tissue by bacterial toxins, or (3) vascular injury resulting from a host inflammatory response that predisposes the patient to a systemic disorder such as atherosclerosis. Additionally, the link between periodontal

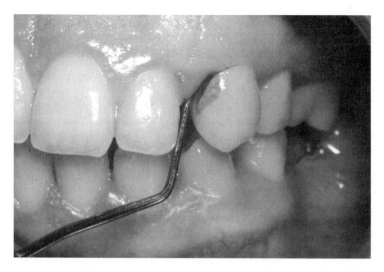

Figure 46–11. Gingival inflammation and bleeding

disease and preterm labor has several proposed biological mechanisms, one of which is the infection that is mediated by prostaglandins and cytokines among patients with severe periodontitis. This infection causes decreased fetal growth and premature labor.

Prevention & Treatment

Good oral hygiene is essential for the prevention and control of periodontal diseases. Gingivitis, the mildest form of periodontal disease, is reversible with regular tooth brushing and flossing. An added benefit is provided by over-the-counter and prescription antimicrobial mouth rinses, such as a 0.1–0.2% chlorhexidine gluconate aqueous mouthwash used twice a day. Caution is advised when chlorhexidine is used because it causes superficial staining of the teeth of patients who drink tea, coffee, or red wine. The treatment of periodontitis includes professional care to remove tartar and may require periodontal surgery.

Because tobacco use is an important risk factor for the development and progression of periodontal disease, patients should be counseled about tobacco cessation. Systemic diseases such as diabetes that may contribute to periodontal disease should be well controlled.

National Center for Chronic Disease Prevention and Health Promotion, Centers for Disease Control and Prevention: *Oral Health Resources: Oral Health 2000: Facts and Figures.* Located at http://www.cdc.gov/OralHealth/factsheets/sgr2000-fsl.htm. Last accessed on March 7, 2003.

Teng YT et al: Periodontal health and systemic disorders. J Can Dent Assoc 2002;68(3):188.

U.S. Department of Health and Human Services: *Oral Health in America: A Report of the Surgeon General—Executive Summary.* U.S. Department of Health and Human Services, National Institute of Dental and Craniofacial Research, National Institutes of Health, 2000. Located at http://www.nidr.nih.gov/sgr/execsumm.htm. Last accessed on March 7, 2003.

Zeeman GG, Veth EO, Dennison DK: Focus on primary care: periodontal disease: implications for women's health. Obstet Gynecol Surv 2001;56:43.

ORAL & OROPHARYNGEAL CANCERS

General Considerations

In the United States, cancers of the oral cavity and oropharynx compose approximately 3% of all cancers among men (the sixth most common cancer among men) and 2% of all cancers among women. The prevalence of these cancers increases with the age of the patients. The American Cancer Society estimates that approximately 28,000 new cases of cancer of the oral cavity and pharynx will be diagnosed in 2002 (18,900 among men and 10,000 among women) and that 7400 people will die of these diseases. Since the 1970s, the incidence of these cancers and the death rates associated with them have been slowly decreasing, except among African-American men, for whom the incidence and 5-year mortality estimates are nearly twice as high as for white men.

The overall survival rate for patients with oral and oropharyngeal cancers is only about 51% and has not changed substantially over the past 20 years. However, the 5-year survival estimate for patients with lip carcinoma is more than 90%; this high survival rate is due in part to early detection. Most oral and oropharyngeal cancers are squamous cell carcinomas that arise from the lining of the oral mucosa. These cancers occur most commonly (in order of frequency) on the tongue, the lips, and the floor of the mouth. Sixty percent of oral cancers are advanced by the time they are detected, and about 15% of patients will have another cancer in a nearby area such as the larynx, esophagus, or lungs. Early diagnosis, which has been shown to increase survival rates, depends on the discerning clinician who recognizes risk factors and suspicious symptoms and can identify a lesion at an early stage.

Table 46–5 shows the risk factors associated with oral and oropharyngeal cancers. Tobacco use and heavy alcohol consumption are the two principal risk factors responsible for 75% of oral cancers. The incidence of oral cancer is higher among persons who smoke or drink heavily than among those who do not.

Prevention

All forms of tobacco, including cigarette, pipe, chewing, and smokeless, have been shown to be carcinogenic in the susceptible host. Alcohol has been identified as another important risk factor for oral cancer, both independently and synergistically when heavy consumers of alcohol also smoke. Therefore, primary prevention in the form of reducing or eliminating the use of tobacco and alcohol has been strongly recommended. The U.S.

Table 46–5. Risk factors associated with oral and oropharyngeal cancer.

Tobacco use (smoking or using smokeless tobacco or snuff)
Excessive consumption of alcohol
Viral infections (HSV, HIV, EBV)[1]
Chronic actinic exposure
Betel quid use
Lichen planus
Plummer–Vinson or Paterson–Kelly syndrome
Immunosuppression
Dietary factors (low intake of fruits and vegetables)

[1]HSV, herpes simplex virus; HIV, human immunodeficiency virus; EBV, Epstein–Barr virus.

Preventive Services Task Force (USPSTF) has not endorsed annual screening (secondary prevention) for asymptomatic patients, stating, "there is insufficient evidence to recommend for or against routine screening" and "clinicians may wish to include an examination for cancerous and precancerous lesions of the oral cavity in the periodic health examination of persons who chew or smoke tobacco (or did so previously), older persons who drink regularly, and anyone with suspicious symptoms or lesions detected through self-examination." However, the American Cancer Society and the National Cancer Institute's Dental and Craniofacial Research Group support efforts that promote early detection of oral cancers. The American Cancer Society recommends annual oral cancer examinations for persons aged 40 years or older.

Because primary care providers are more likely than dentists to see patients at high risk of oral and oropharyngeal cancers, providers need to be able to counsel patients about their behaviors and to be knowledgeable about performing oral cancer examinations. The primary screening test for oral cancer is the oral cancer examination, which includes inspection and palpation of extraoral and intraoral tissues (Table 46–6).

Clinical Findings

A. SYMPTOMS AND SIGNS

Early oral cancer and the more common precancerous lesions (leukoplakia) are subtle and asymptomatic. They begin as a white or red patch, progress to a superficial ulceration of the mucosal surface, and later become an endophytic or exophytic growth. Some lesions are solitary lumps. Larger, advanced cancers may be painful and may erode underlying tissue.

According to the definition of the World Health Organization (WHO), leukoplakia is "a white patch or plaque that cannot be characterized clinically or pathologically as any other disease." The lesions may be white, red, or a combination of red and white (called speckled leukoplakia or erythroleukoplakia). Multiple studies have shown that these lesions undergo malignant transformation. Biopsies have shown that erythroplakia and speckled leukoplakia are more likely than other types of leukoplakia to undergo malignant transformation with more severe epithelial dysplasia. Figures 46–12 and 46–13 show leukoplakia.

Other white lesions sometimes confused with leukoplakia include frictional keratoses, hyperkeratotic lesions that develop as the result of chronic cheek chewing or when exposed edentulous sites receive more irritation during mastication (Figure 46–14). Nicotine stomatitis and tobacco pouch keratoses have a known cause and should not be confused with leukoplakia. Nicotine stomatitis, a very rare disorder, is character-

Table 46–6. Components of an oral cancer examination.[1]

Extraoral examination
 Inspect head and neck
 Bimanually palpate lymph nodes and salivary glands
Lips
 Inspect and palpate outer surfaces of lip and vermilion border
 Inspect and palpate inner labial mucosa
Buccal mucosa
 Inspect and palpate inner cheek lining
Gingiva/alveolar ridge
 Inspect maxillary/mandibular gingiva and alveolar ridges on both the buccal and lingual aspects
Tongue
 Have patient protrude tongue and inspect the dorsal surface
 Have patient lift tongue and inspect the ventral surface
 Grasping tongue with a piece of gauze and pulling it out to each side, inspect the lateral borders of the tongue from its tip back to the lingual tonsil region
 Palpate tongue
Floor of mouth
 Inspect and palpate floor of mouth
Hard palate
 Inspect hard palate
Soft palate and oropharynx
 Gently depressing the patient's tongue with a mouth mirror or tongue blade, inspect the soft palate and oropharynx

[1]A good oral examination requires an adequate light source, protective gloves, 2 × 2 gauze squares, and a mouth mirror or tongue blade.

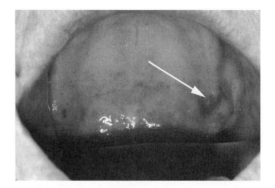

Figure 46–12. Leukoplakia

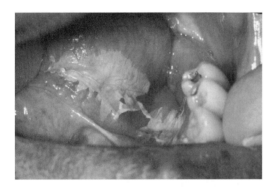

Figure 46–13. Leukoplakia

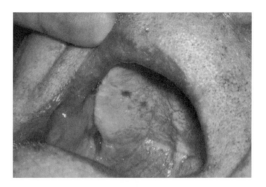

Figure 46–15. Nicotine stomatitis

ized by thickened hyperkeratotic epithelial changes on the hard palate that result from prolonged cigar smoking or cigarette smoking. These changes are due to the intense heat generated by smoking. Similar findings may result from drinking hot beverages (Figure 46–15). Nicotine stomatitis is not considered premalignant and is reversible when tobacco use is discontinued. Tobacco pouch keratosis is associated with the use of smokeless tobacco and chewing tobacco. Lesions appear wrinkled with a grayish-white appearance and are usually located in the buccal or labial vestibule where the tobacco is held. Dysplasia is uncommon; however, if the lesion remains after the use of tobacco has been discontinued for 2–6 weeks, a biopsy should be performed.

Oropharyngeal carcinomas can be found in the intraoral cavity, the oral cavity proper, and the oropharyngeal sites. The most common intraoral site is the tongue: lesions frequently develop on its posterior lateral border. Lesions also occur on the floor of the

mouth and, less commonly, on the gingiva, buccal mucosa, labial mucosa, or hard palate.

A common cancer of the oral cavity proper is lower lip vermilion carcinoma. These lesions arise from a precancerous lesion called actinic cheilosis, which is similar to an actinic keratosis of the skin. Dry, scaly changes appear first and later progress to form a healing ulcer, which is sometimes mistaken for a cold sore or fever blister. Figure 46–16 shows actinic cheilosis.

Oropharyngeal carcinomas commonly arise on the lateral soft palate and the base of the tongue. Presenting symptoms may include dysphagia, painful swallowing (odynophagia), and referred pain to the ear (otalgia). These tumors are often advanced at the time of diagnosis. More rare neoplasms, such as adenoid cystic and mucoepidermoid carcinomas, arise from accessory salivary glands. Clinically, these lesions are painless masses or nodules that appear in persons between the ages of 20 and 50 years.

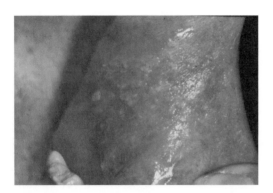

Figure 46–14. Frictional keratoses

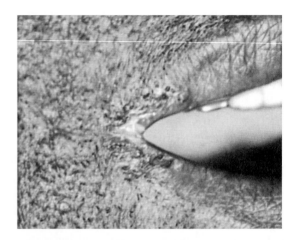

Figure 46–16. Actinic cheilosis

Oral cancer metastasizes regionally to the contralateral or bilateral cervical and submental lymph nodes. Distant metastases are commonly found in the lungs, but oral cancer may metastasize to any other organ.

B. Diagnosis

All patients whose behaviors put them at risk of oral cancer should undergo a thorough oral examination that involves visual and tactile examination of the mouth, full protrusion of the tongue with the aid of a gauze wipe, and palpation of the tongue, the floor of the mouth, and the lymph nodes in the neck. Because oral cancer and precancerous lesions are asymptomatic, primary care providers need to carefully examine patients who are at risk of oral or oropharyngeal carcinomas. Using a scalpel or small biopsy forceps, the primary care physician should perform a biopsy of any nonhealing white or red lesion that persists for more than 2 weeks. Alternatively, the patient may be referred to a dentist, an oral surgeon, or a head and neck specialist, who can perform the biopsy. Patients with large lesions or advanced disease should undergo a complete head and neck examination, because 15% of these patients will have a second primary cancer at the time of diagnosis. Neck nodules with no identifiable primary tumor may be evaluated by fine-needle aspiration.

C. Imaging Studies

Imaging studies such as computed tomography (CT) with contrast and magnetic resonance imaging (MRI) of the head and neck are used to determine the extent of disease and involvement of the cervical lymph nodes for the purposes of staging.

Treatment

Treatments for oral and lip cancers include chemotherapy, surgery, radiation, or some combination of these therapies, depending on the extent of the disease. These treatments can cause severe stomatitis (inflammation of the mouth), xerostomia (dry mouth), disfigurement, altered speech and mastication, loss of appetite, and increased susceptibility to oral infection. The management of these complications requires a multidisciplinary team approach by the clinician, oral surgeon, oncologist, and speech therapist. Early diagnosis allows better treatment, cosmetic appearance, and functional outcome and increases the probability of survival. Patients should be encouraged to visit their dental health provider before beginning cancer therapy so that existing health problems can be treated and some complications can be prevented.

American Cancer Society: *What Are The Key Statistics About Oral Cavity and Oropharyngeal Cancer?* Located at http://www.cancer.org/docroot/CRI/content/CRI_2_4_1X_What_are_the_key_statistics_for_oral_cavity_and_oropharyngeal_cancer_60.asp?sitearea=&level=. Last accessed March 7, 2003.

Mashberg A, Samit A: Early diagnosis of asymptomatic oral and oropharyngeal squamous cancers. CA Cancer J Clin 1995;45:328.

Neville BW, Day TA: Oral cancer and precancerous lesions. CA Cancer J Clin 2002;52:195.

Silverman S Jr: Demographics and occurrence of oral and pharyngeal cancers. The outcomes, the trends, the challenge. J Am Dent Assoc 2001;132;7S.

U.S. Preventive Services Task Force: *Guide to Clinical Preventative Services,* ed 2. Williams & Wilkins, 1996.

Weinberg MA, Estefan DJ: Assessing oral malignancies. Am Fam Physician 2002;65:1379.

WEB SITES

Academy of General Dentistry
www.agd.org
American Association of Public Health Dentistry
www.aaphd.org
American Dental Association
www.ada.org
Children's Dental Health Project
www.childent.org
Health Resources and Services Administration (HRSA) Oral Health Initiative
www.hrsa.gov/oralhealth
National Maternal and Child Oral Health Resource Center
www.mchoralhealth.org
U.S. Surgeon General's Report on Children's Oral Health
www.nidcr.nih.gov/sgr/sgr.htm

SECTION V
Psychosocial Disorders

Depression

Karl O. Moe, PhD, & Charles Privitera, MD[1]

Depression is one of the most common problems presenting in the primary care clinic and one of the most disabling. The *Diagnostic and Statistical Manual of Mental Disorders,* 4th edition (*DSM-IV*), identifies several variations of mood disorders all of which are likely to be referred to as "depression" in routine conversation with a patient and all of which deserve attention by the family physician. The key elements are either depressed mood or loss of interest and pleasure in most or all normally enjoyable activities. The Agency for Health Care Policy and Research (AHCPR) treatment guidelines suggested that the point prevalence of major depression disorders (MDD) in the primary care setting is between 4.8% and 8.6%. The point prevalence for the other depression spectrum disorders deserving attention and treatment is 10%. Although similar estimates have been provided, numbers ranging as high as a prevalence of 22.6% have been suggested. In fact, depression may be the most common problem (15% of patients) encountered by primary care providers. Whether that is true or not, over 50% of depression-related health care in the United States occurs in the offices of family physicians, general internists, and other general medical providers, whereas only approximately 20% of depression-related health care occurs in specialty mental health care settings. Indeed, 80% of the prescriptions for antidepressants are written by nonpsychiatrists. Patients with MDD often present to their doctors with vague physical symptoms rather than emotional complaints. The result can be that MDD is never even suspected. Primary care physicians miss the diagnosis in over 50% of their patients suffering from MDD, and when they recognize it, the quality of care for depression is often less than optimal. MDD assumes particular importance among the working age population because it affects both young and old equally (and affects women two times as often as men), in contrast to many other chronic diseases that affect older people more than younger people.

Depression is becoming recognized as not only quite prevalent but also very costly. Depressed primary care patients use 50–75% more health care services than other patients, with less than 25% of the excess costs due to mental health treatment. The problem of cost is further exacerbated by the apparent fact that when more than one problem is presented at an appointment or when a serious problem other than depression is presented, depression is dramatically less likely to be diagnosed.

Depression is costly beyond the medical resources involved. It is as common as hypertension in the primary care setting and is as disabling as unstable angina, advanced arthritis, and diabetes mellitus. The risk of mortality is also significant. In fact, the risk of suicide may be as much as 100 times greater for a person who is depressed than for the general population. This risk alone makes it worth attending to depression in any setting.

What Is Depression?

Depression is a "whole body" illness. It has physical symptoms, emotional symptoms, behavioral symptoms, and cognitive symptoms. The diversity of symptoms makes a biopsychosocial model of depression especially appropriate and helpful. In talking with patients, it can be useful to identify three broad categories of problems: cognitive, behavioral, and physical. It is important to note that these are not competing theories of depres-

---

[1] The opinions and recommendations expressed in this chapter are solely those of the authors and are not necessarily endorsed by the Department of Defense, the Uniformed Services University of the Health Sciences, or the United States Air Force.

sion. They are interacting aspects of the same disorder and it is helpful to use all these aspects for conceptualizing, explaining, and intervening.

The *cognitive* component is well described in the work of Aaron Beck and his colleagues. Beck's early work, which describes a "negative triad" of beliefs, continues to be relevant. First, depressed people show a predilection to view themselves as worthless, inadequate, unlovable, and generally deficient. Second, there is a strong tendency to think in very negative ways about the world in general and everyone in it. Third, depressed people tend to have negative, dark, and hopeless beliefs about the future. These negative, depressogenic beliefs can be addressed effectively through cognitive therapy.

Friends, family, and patients themselves will be aware of the *behavioral* indications of depression. There are changes in activity level. More often there is a decline in activity. However, a depressed patient occasionally presents an agitated, restless picture. Either way, there will be an identifiable decrease in pleasurable events. There are often corresponding increases in unhealthy behavior, such as substance abuse, smoking, and caffeine use, as well as changes in eating patterns. Additionally, decreases in healthy behavior, such as exercise, relaxation, and social events, are likely. Finally, reduced social involvement and frank withdrawal are often part of the presenting picture.

The *physical* aspects of depression are likely to be the presenting complaint that brings the patient into the primary care clinic. Depressed patients commonly experience, and may complain about, insomnia and poor sleep, fatigue and low energy, and a variety of pains.

Diagnosis

There are no medical tests that will definitively identify depression. The diagnosis must be made on the basis of interview and history. However, in the primary care setting, a physical examination and laboratory tests should be considered. These can be helpful in identifying other medical conditions that may be affecting mood.

It is important to recognize that diagnosis of an MDD requires more than a change in mood. *DSM-IV* provides a set of neurovegetative signs and symptoms that when combined in sufficient number and duration warrants a formal diagnosis of an MDD. The mnemonic SIGECAPS (with an M added to the beginning) is a common device for recalling the diagnostic criteria for depression and aiding in its diagnosis. Table 47–1 provides a sample of useful interview questions that address the following diagnostic criteria:

- **M**ood. The patient describes a depressed mood for most of the day nearly every day for at least 2 weeks.

In children or adolescents, as well as in depressed adults, the mood may be simply irritable. This is one of two symptoms that are a key to making the diagnosis of MDD.

- **S**leep changes. Early morning awakening has been a classic sign of depression. This means waking 2–3 h earlier than is needed or wanted and not being able to return to sleep. However, initial insomnia and sleep maintenance insomnia may also be indications of depression. This will be particularly true in the case of depression that presents with anxiety. Sleep changes must be present nearly every night over the same 2 weeks as the depressed mood (or decreased interest). Additionally, hypersomnia may be a sign of depression, particularly in the case of a seasonal affective disorder.

- **I**nterest. Loss of interest is the second of the two symptoms that are key for diagnosing an MDD. Decreased interest in sex is a specific but certainly not the only example. Either loss of interest in usually enjoyable activities or the mood symptom described above must be present to justify a diagnosis of MDD.

- **G**uilt or feelings of worthlessness. The symptoms related to self-image of an MDD are unreasonably low self-esteem and/or profound and unreasonable levels of guilt most of the time during the preceding 2 weeks. It is important to ask about both feelings of worthlessness and feelings of guilt.

- **E**nergy. The energy criterion is being too fatigued or too lacking in energy to get done what needs to be done.

- **C**oncentration. The inability to think well or concentrate adequately or indecisiveness nearly every day for at least the past 2 weeks is a disabling and disruptive symptom of MDD. Concentration can be assessed formally by using the Digit Span test (repeating six digits forward and four backward is normal) or informally by asking whether the patient can follow conversations and reading.

- **A**ppetite. There is significant weight loss or gain (eg, a change of 5% or more in body weight in a month) or lack of appetite or hyperphagia. Hyperphagia, especially with a craving for carbohydrates, is common for a seasonal affective disorder.

- **P**sychomotor speeding or slowing may be observed by others and is probably very observable in the context of the clinical interview.

- **S**uicidal thoughts, plans, and/or intent or thoughts about death and dying are the most worrisome signs and symptoms of MDD.

For a diagnosis of MDD, the patient must have at least five of the signs and symptoms summarized in the MSIGECAPS mnemonic and must also experience

Table 47–1. Interview questions for diagnosing major depression disorder (MDD).

Question	Criterion	Diagnostic Indications
How have you been sleeping lately?	Sleep changes	Initial insomnia of 20+ min most nights for 2 weeks Sleep maintenance insomnia—wakes for more than 20 min a night most nights for 2 weeks Terminal insomnia—wakes
How's your appetite? So you enjoy your food? Are you gaining weight? Losing weight? Staying the same?	Appetite and weight	Gained or lost 10% of body weight in a month without trying to do so Should be able to think of some food that sounds good
How's your energy? Are you able to get done the things you have to do?	Energy	Unable to get essential work done would meet criteria for MDD
What are you doing for fun? Hobbies? Pastimes? Things you do for fun?	Interest and libido	Being unable to even identify interesting activities would meet criteria for MDD. It is not necessarily to be engaged in fun
How's your sex drive been?		A change in interest in sex—not activity—would meet criteria for MDD
How's your concentration seem? Can you repeat back a phone number if I give it to you?	Concentration	Should be able repeat six digits forward and four digits backward Informally, inability to read or follow a conversation could meet criteria for MDD
How are you feeling about yourself? Do you feel especially guilty about anything?	Self-worth and feelings of profound guilt	Feelings of inadequacy or worthlessness could meet criteria for MDD Profound, unreasonable gult would meet criteria for MDD
Is anyone telling you that you seem to be slowing down or speeding up?	Psychomotor speeding or slowing	Reports of patient or others could meet criteria for MDD Observaton of lethargy and flat affect or of agitation and restlessness could meet criteria for MDD
I have found that when people tell me some of the things you have described, they are sometimes having thoughts about death, dying, or maybe hurting themselves or someone else. Is that true for you?	Death, dying, suicidal thoughts	Even passive but serious thoughts of death could meet criteria for MDD Suicidal thoughts need to be explored more fully for intent and plans

"clinically significant distress or impairment in social, occupational, or other important areas of function" (*DSM-IV*). This impairment must have been applied to most or all aspects of life and potential sources of enjoyment for at least 2 weeks.

Although a review of these specific diagnostic criteria for MDD is fairly easy and straightforward, it is unlikely that they will be reviewed effectively during every appointment. There are a number of potential barriers to diagnosing depression. These include time needed to diagnose, somatization by patients, and coexistence of other medical disorders. When patients present with more than one problem, providers tend to ignore or miss the diagnosis of depression. Use of depression screening questionnaires can help compensate for this possibility. Paper and pencil screens can be used as part

of the check-in procedure for each appointment. Common screening instruments for depression are listed in Table 47–2. Some screen for a number of mental health and behavioral disorders. These last points can be covered by another provider (eg, a psychologist), nurse, or technician. They can also be assessed by using a paper and pencil questionnaire.

The Department of Defense has initiated a comprehensive approach that could be adopted in other managed care organizations. Each year every beneficiary completes the Health Enrollment Assessment Review (HEAR), which is a questionnaire that requests information regarding a wide variety of physical health areas, preventive practices, mental health, and substance abuse. These results are filed in the patient's health record and can be scanned quickly during an appointment. If there

Table 47–2. Screeners for depression.

1. PRIME MD: Primary care evaluations of mental disorders—depression questions (two items)[1]
2. CES-D: Center for Epidemiological Studies—Depression scale (five items) (modified for geriatrics)[2]
3. Zung Depression Rating Scale[3]
4. BDI: Beck Depression Inventory (21 items)[4]
5. MOS: Medical Outcomes Study—depression questions (four items)[5]
6. Ham-D: Hamilton Depression Rating Scale (21 items)[6]

[1]Spitzer RL et al: Health-related quality of life in primary care patients with mental disorders: results from the PRIME-MD 1000 study. JAMA 1995;274:1511. Spitzer RL et al: Utility of a new procedure for diagnosing mental disorders in primary care: the PRIME-MD 1000 study. JAMA 1994;272:1749.
[2]Lewinsohn PM et al: Center for Epidemiological Studies Depression Scale (CES-D) as a screening instrument for depression among community-residing older adults. Psychol Aging 1997; 12(2):277.
[3]Zung wwk: A Self-Rating Depression Scale. Arch Gen Psychiatry 1965;12:63.
[4]Beck AT et al: An inventory for measuring depression. Arch Gen Psychiatry 1961;4:53.
[5]Rost K, Burnam MA, Smith GR: Development of screeners for depressive disorders and substance disorder history. MedCare 1993;31(3):189.
[6]Hedlung JL, Vieweg BW: The Hamilton rating scale for depression. J Operation Psychiatry 1979;10(2):149.

are indications of depression, the provider can investigate further or schedule a follow-up appointment. Additionally, many medical treatment facilities have a nurse or senior technician review the HEARs as they are completed. This allows patients whose results suggest a health concern to be contacted.

If an organizational approach to screening is not available, providers should have a few screening questions that they use routinely if anything suggests the possibility of depression. Two of the most common are listed in Table 47–3. For an oral screening, Preskorn suggests a series of three questions that help ensure a thorough review of all neurovegetative signs of depression:

Table 47–3. Screening questions from PRIME-MD.[1]

1. During the past month, have you often been bothered by feeling down, depressed, or hopeless?
2. During the past month, have you often been bothered by little interest or pleasure in doing things?

[1]Yes to either question suggests further assessment.

1. "You have been having problems with [use the patient's words] (eg, "depression," "insomnia," "stress at work")." Here the interviewer is looking for signs and symptoms of depression, ie, MSIGECAPS.
2. "I understand that you have been feeling [using the patient's words] (eg, "depressed," "sad," "hopeless," "overwhelmed"). Has this affected you physically?" This shifts the attention to physical signs and symptoms and can help complete the review of MSIGECAPS.
3. "Since you have been [using the patient's words] (eg, "depressed," "bothered by headaches"), have you also been having problems with:
   a. Mood (being depressed, irritable, anxious)
   b. Sleep (too little or too much)
   c. Appetite (too little or too much)
   d. Energy (subjective)
   e. Activity (objective)
   f. Interest
   g. Motivation
   h. Concentration/attention
   i. Sex drive?"

Assessment for & Treatment of Suicidality

In 1999, suicide was the eleventh leading cause of death in the United States ahead of homicide, human immunodeficiency virus-related illnesses, liver disease, and hypertension. The lifetime risk of suicide for those who experience an MDD has been reported to be 15%, or 100 times the risk of the general population. Even though more recent research has suggested that the lifetime risk may be lower than 15%, the risk of suicide is still substantial and needs to be assessed in an individual who is depressed. If there are signs of depression, it is important for all health care providers to assess for suicidality.

Simon suggests that the following beliefs, behaviors, and events are serious risk factors for suicide and intentional self-injury:

- The presence of active depression or psychosis and/or the presence of substance abuse.
- A past history of suicidal acts.
- Formulation of a plan.
- A stated intent to carry out the plan.
- The feeling that the world would be better off if the patient were dead.
- Availability of the means for suicide (firearms, pills, etc).
- Disruption of an important personal relationship.
- Failure at an important personal endeavor.

The presence of these factors often constitutes a psychiatric emergency and must always be taken seriously. The Department of Defense and the Veterans Health Administration (DoD/VA) guidelines suggest three areas of inquiry when there are concerns about suicidality: (1) eliciting suicidal ideation or intent, (2) gathering data on risk factors for completed suicide, and (3) weighing items one and two to assess safety. The DoD/VA guidelines go on to suggest a sequence of questions to elicit necessary information (Table 47–4).

For physicians practicing in the primary care setting, it is most appropriate to refer a potentially suicidal patient to a mental health colleague. However, knowing what the treatment of suicidality involves (Box 47–1) allows primary care providers to furnish their patients with information and makes it easier to follow along as the treatment progresses.

Clinical Findings

A. SYMPTOMS AND SIGNS

Depression does not produce diagnostic physical findings. However, there are a variety of diseases and medications that can result in depressive symptoms. These possibilities should be assessed.

First it makes sense to address and rule out psychosis and substance abuse.

A number of medical conditions associated with depression should be considered and evaluated as appropriate (Table 47–5). Simultaneous treatment is often required for both the medical problem and mental health symptoms. Additionally, there is often a strong association between the level of disability from the

---

Box 47–1. Treatment for Suicidality.

When patients threaten suicide and the possibility of suicide is imminent due to the presence of an organized plan, availability of lethal means, extreme hopelessness, and/or psychosis (especially hallucinations commanding the patient to act violently or self-destructively), immediate and decisive action is required. Hospitalization, including involuntary commitment, if needed, should be accomplished. The patient should never be left alone for even a moment.

If the risk of intentional self-injury is judged to include several suicidal risk factors but no imminent plans or intent, management can focus more on the longer term and on an overall therapeutic plan. This might include removing lethal means, especially access to any and all guns; treatment for any mental health or substance abuse conditions; with permission, involvement of family members or other individuals who can provide support; and staying in close touch with the patient. However, the longer term goals for patients who have suicidal thoughts, plans, or intent are to help them address their problems and improve their coping skills. In line with this, a "No Suicide Contract" is often initiated by the provider and signed by the patient. A good contract goes far beyond simply agreeing not to commit suicide or self-injury. As part of the contract, the patient will normally agree to engage in a number of self-care, problem-solving, and coping behaviors before contacting the mental health provider or going to an emergency department.

The general goal in treating a suicidal patient is to help the patient learn to address the problems in ways that are effective. Returning the patient to the primary care provider for long-term follow-up should be part of this goal. For this reason, even if a mental health provider is treating the patient's suicidality and depression, frequent follow-up by the primary care provider is important.

Table 47–4. Sequence of questions to elicit information about suicidal potential.[1]

Are you discouraged about your medical condition (or social situation, etc)?

Are there times when you think about your situation and feel like crying?

During those times, what sorts of thoughts go through your head?

Have you ever felt that if the situation did not change, it would not be worth living?

Have you reached a point that you've devised a specific plan to end your life?

Do you have the necessary items for completion of that plan readily available?

[1]Management of Major Depressive Disorder Working Group: *VHA/DOD Clinical Practice Guideline for the Management of Major Depressive Disorder in Adults*, Version 2. West Virginia Medical Institute, Inc., 2000.

---

medical condition and the depressive symptom requiring treatment. A useful mnemonic adapted from The Management of Major Depressive Disorder Working Group can help recall the possible pathobiological processes that may contribute to depressive symptoms: $[TIC]^2P^2M^2D^3$.

- Trauma
- Tumor
- Infection
- Immune and autoimmune
- Cardiac/vascular
- Congenital/hereditary
- Pain
- Physiological—seizure

Table 47–5. Medical conditions that produce depressive symptoms.

Cardiovascular	Chronic pain	Degenerative diseases
Coronary artery disease	Fibromyalgia	Presbyopia
Congestive heart failure	Reflex sympathetic dystrophy	Presbycusis
Anemia	Low back pain	Alzheimer's disease
Stroke	Chronic pelvic pain	Parkinson's disease
Vascular dementia	Bone- or disease-related pain	Huntington's disease
		Other neurodegenerative diseases
Immune system disease	**Metabolic/endocrine conditions**	**Neoplasm**
HIV (both primary and infection related)	Malnutrition, vitamin deficiencies	Pancreatic cancer
Multiple sclerosis	Hypo/hyperthyroidism	Central nervous system cancer
Systemic lupus erythematosis	Addison's disease	Any cancer
Sarcoidosis	Diabetes mellitus	
	Hepatic disease (cirrhosis)	**Infectious diseases**
	Electrolyte disturbances	Systemic inflammatory response
	Acid-base disturbances	syndrome
	Chronic obstructive pulmonary disease	Meningitis
	or asthma	Lyme disease
	Hypoxia	

- Metabolic
- Malignancy
- Degenerative
- Drug toxicity
- Demyelinating.

It is also important to consider the possibility that one or more prescription medications or over-the-counter (OTC) drugs may be causing or contributing to depressive symptoms (Table 47–6). This should include alternative medicines such as herbs, vitamins, or nutritional supplements.

B. LABORATORY FINDINGS

No laboratory studies will lead to a diagnosis of depression but appropriate laboratory studies can rule out

Table 47–6. Drugs that commonly cause depression.[1]

Cardiovascular drugs	Hormones	Psychotropics
Angiotensin-converting enzyme	Anabolic steroids (+)	Benzodiazepines
inhibitors	ACTH (corticotropin) and glucocorticoids (++)	Neuroleptics
α-Methyldopa (+/–)	Gonadotropin-releasing agonists	
Clonidine	Oral contraceptives	
Digitalis		
Guanethidine		
Propanolol (+/–)		
Reserpine (++)		
Thiazide diuretics		
Anticancer agents[2]	**Antiinflammatory/antiinfective agents**	**Others**
Cycloserine	Baclofen	Amphetamine withdrawal
	Disulfiram	Antihyperlipidemics
	Ethambutol	Cimetidine, ranitidine
	Interferons	Cocaine withdrawal (++)
	Metoclopramide	Levodopa
	Nonsteroidal antiinflammatory agents	L-Dopa (+/–)
	Sulfonamides	Methyldopa
		Topiramate

[1]Adapted from *Depression in Primary Care, Clincal Practice Guideline #5,* AHCPR, 1993 and modified with information from Management of Major Depressive Disorder Working Group, 2000.
[2]Until proven otherwise, consider all anticancer agents as causing or increasing depression.

medical disorders that may cause symptoms of depression. These include complete blood count (CBC), chemistry profile, thyroid studies, and toxicology screen. For patients over the age of 40, an electrocardiogram may be useful.

Treatment

There are two equally effective treatments for depression—psychotherapy and medications. There are a number of choices of empirically supported psychotherapy and a number of choices of effective medication. There are also a number of treatment guidelines available to help choose the precise treatment plan to use with a given patient.

A. PSYCHOTHERAPY

For the most part, psychotherapy is likely to require more time than is available in the schedule of primary care providers in the current practice environment. However, with appropriate training, psychotherapy conducted by the family physician may be an appropriate choice for a specific case. In fact, interpersonal therapy, which focuses on one or two interpersonally relevant problems such as interpersonal deficits, role transition, or dispute resolution, can be adapted to 20-min blocks and extended over 12–16 weeks for use in the primary care setting. However, in most other cases, referral to a psychologist or social worker may be the best choice. In making a referral, it is helpful to know enough about psychotherapy and the referral source to describe the process and the therapist to the patient.

A number of empirically supported forms of psychotherapy are effective for treating depression. Cognitive therapy focuses on the relationships between patients' beliefs, thoughts, and values and how they feel. There are effective approaches for developing ways of thinking that provide for feeling better. Behavior therapy focuses on increasing behaviors that are associated with a sense of accomplishment or reward while reducing behaviors that are associated with adverse consequences. Interpersonal therapy focuses on the relationship aspects of patients' lives, especially role disputes, social isolation, prolonged grief, and/or role transitions. Brief dynamic therapy and marital psychotherapy may also be helpful in treating depression in appropriately selected cases.

Psychotherapy has been shown to be as effective as medication interventions. It is important to note that these approaches do not include all psychotherapeutic traditions. Perhaps most notably, long-term psychodynamic approaches and brief, supportive therapy have not been empirically demonstrated to be effective.

B. MEDICATION

Antidepressant medications, first discovered over 40 years ago, are now divided into seven or eight major categories. In either case, it is interesting to note that all antidepressant medications are equally effective in clinical trials at treating depression. The clinically important differences among the various classes of antidepressant medications primarily have to do with their decidedly different side effect profiles, on which, in fact, treatment decisions are in large part based. Other factors that affect selection of an antidepressant medication include safety in overdose, history of prior response by the patient or family members, other medical conditions, type of depression, and cost per dose. Stahl provides a good review of the monoamine theory of depression and a helpful summary of the differences among the various categories of antidepressant medications. The recent treatment guidelines produced by a joint working group for the DoD/VA, which is readily available online, also provide a comprehensive summary of information about the various antidepressant agents and their use. The treatment guidelines developed by the American Psychiatric Association are stated in Table 47–7.

There are benefits and drawbacks to both the psychotherapy and medication approach to treating depression. For psychotherapy the most prominent benefits include the possibility of benefits that last beyond the duration of treatment, a reduced or obviated need for antidepressant medications with their attendant side effects, and the opportunity to make meaningful self-improvements and life changes. The principal drawbacks include the need to consistently keep appointments for several months and the possibility that a therapist with training in empirically validated treatments may not be locally available. For a medication approach the clearest benefit is the possibility of a rapid response to initial treatment. In addition, some patients prefer this approach. The drawbacks include the need to take medications as prescribed; the potential for side effects, which can affect adherence or even produce medical complications; and the likely need to take medication for an extended period of time.

Treatment for depression shares some of the problems common to treatment for other chronic diseases. A number of specific suggestions for prescribing effectively are given in Table 47–8. They address many of the problems encountered in using a medication approach to treat any chronic disease.

C. COLLABORATIVE CARE

The quality of treatment for depression in the primary care setting is negatively affected by inadequate patient education, poor patient adherence to treatment regimens, poor follow-up by the patient, and lack of a close

Table 47–7. American Psychiatric Association medication guidelines for treating depression.[1]

Commonly Used Antidepressant Medications (Generic Name)	Starting Dose [2]	Usual Dose (mg/day)
Tricyclics and tetracyclics		
Amitriptyline	25–50	100–300
Clomipramine	25	100–250
Doxepin	25–50	100–300
Imipramine	25–50	100–300
Trimipramine	25–50	100–300
Secondary amine tricyclics		
Desipramine[3]	25–50	100–300
Nortriptyline[3]	25	50–200
Protriptyline	10	15–60
Tetracyclics		
Amoxapine	50	100–400
Maprotiline	50	100–225
Selective serotonin reuptake inhibitors[3]		
Citalopram	20	20–60[4]
Fluoxetine	20	20–60[4]
Fluvoxamine	50	50–300[4]
Paroxetine	20	20–60[4]
Sertraline	50	50–200[4]
Dopamine-norepinephrine reuptake inhibitors		
Bupropion[3]	150	300
Bupropion, sustained release	150	300
Serotonin-norepinephrine reuptake inhibitors		
Venlafaxine[3]	37.5	75–225
Venlafaxine, extended release	37.5	75–225
Serotonin modulators		
Nefazodone	50	150–300
Trazodone	50	75–300
Norepinephrine-serotonin modulator		
Mirtazapine	15	15–45
Monoamine oxidase inhibitors (MAOIs)		
Irreversible, nonselective		
Phenelzine	15	15–90
Tranylcypromine	10	30–60
Reversible MAOI-A		
Moclobemide	150	300–600
Selective noradrenaline reuptake inhibitor		
Reboxetine	—[5]	—[5]

[1]American Psychiatric Association: Practice guidelines for major depressive disorder in adults. Am Psychiatry 1993;150(4)(Suppl):1. Also available at http://www.psych.org/clin_res/Depression2e.book-7.cfm#table1.
[2]Lower starting doses are recommended for elderly patients and for patients with panic disorder, significant anxiety or hepatic disease, and general comorbidity.
[3]These medications are likely to be optimal medications in terms of the patient's acceptance of side effects, safety, and quantity and quality of clinical trial data.
[4]Dose varies with diagnosis; see text for specific guidelines.
[5]Food and Drug Administration approval is anticipated. When available, consult manufacturer's package insert or the *Physician's Desk Reference* for recommended starting and usual doses.

Table 47–8. Seven habits of highly effective psychopharmacologists.[1]

1. "Begin with the end in mind." That is, have complete remission as the target. This is an achievable goal with depression and anxiety. Establish measurable outcomes. Identify, for example, "Three things you would be doing if you were not depressed." After recovery, relapse may be signaled by discontinuance of these activities.
2. "Synergize." That is, if drugs that are active in just one monoamine pathway (eg, a selective serotonin reuptake inhibitor) are not completely effective, add a drug that is primarily active in a different pathway.
3. "Sharpen the saw." That is, attend high-quality continuing education and learn to identify the information that can be applied to improving diagnosis and prescription practice.
4. "Put first things first." That is, pay attention to the difference between nonadherence due to troublesome side effects, which often occur before therapeutic results are present, as well as unhelpful beliefs versus nonadherence due to resistance. Communicate this difference to nonadherent patients.
5. "Think win-win." That is, develop a negotiation-oriented and collaborative relationship with patients. This helps when adverse side effects seem to be sabotaging treatment. It is then possible to consider another medication or to look for a drug that cancels adverse side effects.
6. "Become proactive." That is, psychiatric conditions are well known to be underdiagnosed in the primary care setting and, when diagnosed, are inadequately treated. Proactively go after mental health diagnoses and take the time required to deliver effective care—usually 9–12 months.
7. "Understand and be understood." Listen carefully to the patient's presenting complaints. This will lead to better communication and a better relationship. Both of these characteristics lead to better adherence and treatment outcomes. Communication is enhanced by having clear written instructions on medications. It can be further enhanced through collaborative care models in which a behavioral health provider collaborates on an overall treatment plan in the primary care setting.

[1]From Stahl SM: Basic psychopharmacology of antidepressants, Part 1: antidepressants have seven distinct mechanisms of action. J Clin Psychiatry 1998;59(Suppl 4):5.

consulting and referral relationship between primary care providers and mental health providers. Pearson et al suggest that collaborative models of care offer significant promise for addressing these barriers to treatment in late-life depression. There is no reason to suspect that collaborative approaches would not address the same barriers for younger patients as well.

One version of the collaborative care program developed by Katon and colleagues is a multifaceted intervention including the following components:

1. An educational book and videotape concerning effective management of depression.
2. Two to four consultation visits with a liaison psychiatrist practicing in the primary care clinic.
3. Algorithm-based adjustment of antidepressant pharmacotherapy.
4. As-needed referral to psychosocial treatment or community resources.
5. Ongoing monitoring of adherence to the medication regimen.

During this period of collaborative care, most patients alternated follow-up visits with the liaison psychiatrist and primary care physician. After 3–4 months, responsibility for ongoing care of depression was transferred back to the primary care physician (with specialty mental health services available as in usual care). Liaison psychiatrists continued to monitor treatment adherence and provide as-needed consultation to the primary care physicians throughout the follow-up period. The result was 16.7 fewer days of depression over the first 6 months of treatment. The cost, approximately $22 dollars per day free of depression, compares very favorably with interventions for other debilitating disorders and diseases.

A recent review of the AHCPR guidelines lends further support to the notion of collaborative care. Schulberg et al note that although both antidepressant medication and time-limited psychotherapies for depression are efficacious in the primary care setting, improvements in delivery are needed. Specifically, they suggest better organized treatment programs, regular follow-up, and monitoring of adherence. They also recommend a prominent role for behavioral health providers in the primary care setting to help facilitate these suggestions. Clarifying the picture a bit, it was found that primary care physicians are able to follow the AHCPR guidelines despite their complexity. However, keeping patients in treatment is difficult. Suggested solutions include greater flexibility in the treatment regimens and increased follow-up support.

Robinson and colleagues developed one of the most extensive and successful approaches to providing care for depression in the primary care setting. The integrated care programs they developed have been demonstrated to be effective and are acceptable to both patients and primary care providers. Behavioral health specialists, primarily psychologists and clinical social workers, are available in the primary care setting to see patients who are referred by their primary care provider—typically within the last day or two. They are also immediately available for "curb side consults" on patients who are still in the examination room. Variations of this model have been shown to be effective in obtaining superior treatment outcomes. Recently, the United States Air Force has adapted this model for their Behavioral Health Optimization Project, which places mental health providers in the primary care setting to help attend to behavioral and emotional issues.

D. PATIENT EDUCATION

Many patient education brochures are available from pharmaceutical companies and a number have been produced in conjunction with treatment guidelines. In evaluating the usefulness of specific patient education material Robinson's research group found that educational materials, including printed brochures and videotapes, have the potential to significantly improve the outcome of treatment for depression in the primary care setting. A version of the printed materials is included in the manual for treating depression in primary care settings by Robinson et al.

One of the important educational issues addressed by the DoD/VA guidelines has to do with helping the patient choose the initial course of treatment. One of the first choices has to do with whether to start with medications or with psychotherapy. The pros and cons of both approaches, as detailed above, can be distilled into a handout and discussed with patients.

E. COMPLEMENTARY AND ALTERNATIVE THERAPIES

There are two well-known "alternative" therapies for the treatment of depression: St John's wort (*Hypericum perforatum*) and the use of light therapy for seasonal affective disorder. Exercise as a form of therapy may, at the least, prove useful as an adjunctive treatment.

St. John's wort, which has a 2000-year history of being used medically, probably acts as a weak selective serotonin reuptake inhibitor with fewer side effects. Reviews of current knowledge of the pharmacology, sites of action, and therapeutic effectiveness for St. John's wort tend to be positive, but conclude that the available data are not definitive. In general, St John's wort is recommended as a treatment for mild to moderate depression. However, its therapeutic effect is unclear, in part due to the variable quality of the reported research. It is clear that use of St. John's wort is not completely accepted as an effective treatment for depression and there are certainly medical and ethical questions that still need to be addressed.

Light therapy has become reasonably well known as the diagnosis of seasonal affective disorder (SAD) has become better known. Actually, the *DSM-IV* identifies SAD as a variant of MDD rather than a diagnosis all by itself. SAD is identified primarily by a seasonal variation in mood with depression normally occurring nearly every winter but not linked to psychosocial stressors that occur in the winter, such as school or seasonal unemployment. Prominent characteristics include hy-

persomnia, hyperphagia with a craving for carbohydrates, and a lethargic lack of energy.

A proposed model for understanding SAD draws on research demonstrating seasonal variation in a number of biochemical processes. Specifically, postmortem studies of nonpsychiatric patients showed that hypothalamic serotonin levels are sharply lower during the fall and winter months. There are, of course, a variety of possible explanations for why this might occur but, in any case, lower levels of serotonin are entirely in line with the monoamine theory of depression. Later work has confirmed this model.

Light therapy has typically consisted of sitting very close (90–180 cm) to a fluorescent light source of bright (approximately 2500 lux) white, full-spectrum light for up to 3 h before dawn and up to 3 h after sunset. For mild to moderate depression results have primarily been positive, although many patients have required additional treatment in the form of antidepressants or presumably psychotherapy. Additionally, many patients find it difficult to just sit for many hours a day.

F. CULTURAL ISSUES

Age as well as cultural and ethnic factors all affect the prevalence, diagnosis, and treatment of depression.

1. Age—There is considerable room to improve treatment of depression in older adults seen in the primary care setting. About 25% of elderly patients seen in the primary care setting have serious symptoms of depression, but only 12–25% of those patients who should be treated for depression are actually treated. Further, of patients treated with antidepressants, less than 30% receive adequate doses. As people get older they take more medications and the possibility of drug–drug contraindications increases. This makes nondrug interventions for treatment of depression more attractive. Research demonstrates that a range of psychotherapies is as effective as antidepressant medication for older depressed patients. In fact, older adults are generally positive with regard to psychotherapy and may prefer this form of treatment to pharmacotherapy. Offering cognitive or behavioral therapy as a first-line intervention for mild to moderately depressed older adults could be the most cost-effective approach in most settings.

Age is a risk factor for suicide. The elderly and especially elderly white males are at increased risk for suicide. Assessing for suicidality is particularly relevant for primary care providers because far more patients visit their primary care provider than visit a mental health provider.

2. Culture and race—Patients treated in agency-run clinics, especially minority group patients, rely much more on their primary care providers for evaluation and treatment of depression. A recurring concern is that nonwestern cultures tend to somatize their depression and distress, resulting in lower rates of recognition of depression than actually exist. Although it has been argued that somatization is a ubiquitous rather than a "nonwestern" characteristic, it is a barrier to diagnosis and does seem to be more common among nonwestern European and non-Euro-American cultures. This makes it important to remain sensitive to the notion that somatic symptoms can be part of a language of distress.

Although African-Americans seemed to have poorer functional outcomes when treated for depression, both African-American as well as white patients can be effectively treated with both standardized psychotherapy and pharmacotherapy. Interestingly, African-Americans may prefer counseling and psychosocial interventions to medication.

G. INDICATIONS FOR REFERRAL AND/OR ADMISSION

There are a number of situations that are best referred to specialty mental health care. Referral is appropriate if the patient shows indications of psychosis (serious delusions, hallucinations, incoherence, confusion, catatonia, extreme negativism, mutism, or inappropriate/bizarre affect), past mania or hypomania, or comorbid psychiatric conditions. It may also be appropriate if there are concerns about mental health that persist even though the primary care provider cannot identify symptoms of depression. After 12 weeks of treatment for depression without remission, it may be appropriate to refer for specialty care.

Some cases are simply a complex mix of personality, marital, family, and interpersonal problems. These cases may be appropriate to refer at any point.

Hospital admission for depression alone is rarely needed. Admission may be clearly indicated if the patient represents a risk to self or others. Specific questions regarding suicidality are suggested in Table 47–4.

Agency for Health Care Policy and Research: *AHCPR Clinical Practice Guideline, Number 5*. U.S. Department of Health and Human Services, Public Health Service. AHCPR publication No. 93-0550, March 1993.

American Psychiatric Association: *Diagnostic and Statistical Manual of Mental Disorders,* ed 4. American Psychiatric Association, 1994.

Beck AT et al: *Cognitive Therapy of Depression.* Guilford Press, 1987.

Blair-West GW et al: Lifetimes suicide risk in major depression: sex and age determinants. J Affect Disord 1999;55:171.

Field HL et al:. St. John's wort. Int J Psychiatry Med 2000;30(3): 203.

Freudenstein U et al: Treatments for late life depression in primary care—a systematic review. Fam Pract 2001;18(3):321.

Jacobson N, Hollon S: Cognitive-behavior therapy versus pharmacotherapy: now that the jury's returned its verdict, it's time to present the rest of the evidence. J Consult Clin Psychol 1996; 64:74.

Kirmayer LJ: Cultural variations in the clinical presentation of depression and anxiety: implications for diagnosis and treatment. J Clin Psychiatry 2001;62:22.

Management of Major Depressive Disorder Working Group: *VHA/DOD Clinical Practice Guideline for the Management of Major Depressive Disorder in Adults,* Version 2. West Virginia Medical Institute, Inc., 2000. http://www.oqp.med.va.gov/cpg/MDD/MDD_cpg/content/mddintro_fr.htm.

Mischoulon D et al: Management of major depression in the primary care setting. Psychother Psychosom 2001;70(2):103.

Office for Prevention and Health Services Assessment: *Primary Behavioral Health Care Services Practice Manual,* Version 2. USAF Medical Operations Agency, 2002.

Pearson JL, Conwell U, Lyness JM: Late-life suicide and depression in the primary care setting. New Direct Mental Health Serv 1997;76:13.

Persons JB, Thase ME, Crits-Chrisoph P: The role of psychotherapy in the treatment of depression. Arch Gen Psychiatry 1996;53(4):283.

Preskorn SH: *Outpatient Management of Depression: A Guide for the Practitioner.* Professional Communications, Inc. 1999.

Reynolds CF et al: Treatment of 70(+)-year-olds with recurrent major depression. Excellent short-term but brittle long-term response. Am J Geriatr Psychiatry 1999;7(1):64.

Robinson P, Wischman C, Del Vento A: *Treating Depression in Primary Care: A Manual for Primary Care and Mental Health Providers.* Context Press, 1996.

Robinson P et al: The education of depressed primary care patients: what do patients think of interactive booklets and a video. J Fam Pract 1997;44(6):562.

Rost AJ et al: The role of competing demands in the treatment provided primary care patients with major depression. Arch Fam Med 2000;9(2):150.

Rush AJ, Hollon SD: Depression. In: *Integrating Pharmacotherapy and Psychotherapy.* Beitman BD, Klerman GL (editors). American Psychiatric Press, 1991.

Schulberg HC et al: Treating major depression in primary care practice: an update of the Agency for Health Care Policy and Research Practice Guidelines. Arch Gen Psychiatry 1998;55 (12):1121.

Schuyler D: Depression comes in many disguises to the providers of primary care: recognition and management. J S C Med Assoc 2000;96(6):267.

Simon RI: Clinical risk assessment of suicidal patients: assessing the unpredictable. In: *Clinical Psychiatry and the Law.* The American Psychiatric Press, 1992.

Stahl SM: Basic psychopharmacology of antidepressants, part 1: antidepressants have seven distinct mechanisms of action. J Clin Psychiatry 1998;59(Suppl 4):5.

U.S. Preventive Services Task Force: *Screening for Suicide Risk. Guide to Clinical Preventive Services,* ed 2. U.S. Preventive Services, 1996.

Anxiety Disorders

48

Philip J. Michels, PhD, Jamee Lucas, MD, & Scott McKay, MD

General Considerations

Anxiety is a diffuse, unpleasant, and often vague subjective feeling of apprehension accompanied by objective symptoms of autonomic nervous system arousal. The experience of anxiety is associated with a sense of danger or a lack of control over events. The psychological component varies from individual to individual and is strongly influenced by personality and coping mechanisms.

Anxiety is pathological when it occurs in situations that do not call for fear or when the degree of anxiety is excessive for the situation. Anxiety may occur as a result of life events, as a symptom of a primary anxiety disorder, as a secondary response to another psychiatric disorder or medical illness, or as a side effect of a medication.

We live in a rapidly changing culture with nonending technological advancements and a proliferation of ever refined information. Mass media, adult-oriented media, and the video game industry saturate their programming with violence and/or sexuality to an expanding degree unparalleled in history, encouraging violence and shallow relationships and increasing fear of becoming victimized.

In today's workplace significant trends toward downsizing, restructuring, merging, and specialization are emerging. Despite the anticipated availability of work, insecurity evolves from transient work relationships and from a decline or elimination of ongoing benefits such as health insurance and retirement provisions. Insecurity is not likely to diminish.

The majority of individuals with mental disorders receive psychiatric care from primary care settings, whereas less than 20% receive care in specialized mental health settings. Among mental disorders, anxiety disorders have the highest overall prevalence rate, yet only 23% of anxious patients receive treatment. Patients with anxiety disorders are at increased risk for other medical comorbidities, longer hospital stays, more procedures, higher overall health care costs, failure in school, low-paying jobs, and financial dependence in the form of welfare or other government subsidies.

Mendlowicz MV, Stein MB: Quality of life in individuals with anxiety disorders. Am J Psychiatry 2000;157(5):669.

Pathogenesis

A. Biomedical

Because the symptoms of anxiety are so varied and prevalent, a number of etiologies exist to explain them. A recent meta-analysis revealed a significant genetic component, especially for panic disorder, generalized anxiety, and phobias. Temperament, which has genetic roots, is a broad vulnerability factor for anxiety disorders.

The inhibitory transmitter γ-aminobutyric acid (GABA) occupies about 40% of all synapses and is clearly implicated in the anxiety disorders, as is the endocrine system. Exposure to a stressor activates the release of an endogenous opioid, β-endorphin (BE), which is co-released with adrenocorticotrophic hormone (ACTH).

A number of physical illnesses mimic symptoms of anxiety. The clinician must rule out psychiatric disorders and ascertain if symptoms of anxiety are secondary to a medical illness or to a side effect of a medication. If anxiety did not predate a medical illness, subsequent anxiety may represent an adjustment disorder with anxious mood. The most likely organic cause of anxiety is alcohol and drug use (withdrawal or intoxication). Caffeine toxicity and increased sensitivity to caffeine also commonly mimic symptoms of anxiety.

B. Psychological

Family dysfunction and parental psychopathology are involved in the development and maintenance of anxiety. Families of anxious children are more involved, controlling, and rejecting, and less intimate than are families who do not manifest anxiety. Parents of anxious children promote cautious and avoidant child behavior.

Behavioral and cognitive explanations define anxiety as a learned response. Anxiety develops in response to neutral or positive stimuli that become associated with a noxious or aversive event. Fearful associations develop from the situational context and the physical sensations present at the time.

The patient may generalize (ie, classify objects and events based on a common characteristic) and thereby establish new cues to trigger anxiety. Previously neutral situations become feared and avoided. By avoiding anxiety-arousing stimuli, anxiety is diminished.

As panic and avoidance become more chronic, the behaviors involved become more habitual and awareness of one's thoughts in relation to these anxiety states diminishes. Information-processing prejudices such as selectively attending to threatening stimuli become involuntary and unconscious. A person's appraisal of an event, rather than intrinsic characteristics of that event, defines stress, evokes anxiety, and influences the ability to cope. Failure to cope elicits fear and vulnerability.

Hettema J, Neale MC, Kendler KS: A review and meta-analysis of the genetic epidemiology of anxiety disorders. Am J Psychiatry 2001;158:1568.

Kagan J, Snidman N: Early childhood predictors of adult anxiety disorders. Biol Psychiatry 1999;46:1536.

Prevention

Training in stress inoculation, relaxation training, and cognitive–behavioral therapy can be implemented through an integrated curriculum in public education during the early and middle years. School settings provide furtive environments for group modeling and an opportunity to reach large numbers of people. The work of Dr. Martin Seligman (Gillham et al) demonstrates the sizable advantages of such school-based programs.

Clinical Findings

A. Symptoms and Signs

Examination of the patient will usually yield few clues to assist with establishing the diagnosis of an anxiety disorder. Diagnosis is complicated by the amount of symptoms and their overlap with other disease states. Table 48–1 lists various symptoms of anxiety.

Despite the variety and diffuse nature of many of these symptoms, anxiety disorders need not be diagnoses of exclusion. The symptoms of each anxiety disorder are sufficiently specific to arrive at the diagnosis by observation. Recognition of anxiety subtypes leads to differential treatment options with proven efficacy.

B. Laboratory Findings

There are no "gold standard" laboratory studies to diagnose anxiety disorders. It is reasonable to perform a limited empiric evaluation to identify the etiology of the symptoms as well as evaluate for comorbid medical problems that may complicate the treatment. This eval-

Table 48–1. Somatic symptoms of anxiety.

System	Symptoms
Musculoskeletal	Muscle tightness, spasms, back pain, headache, weakness, tremors, fatigue, restlessness, exaggerated startle response, jitters
Cardiovascular	Palpitations, rapid heartbeat, hot and cold spells, flushing, pallor
Gastrointestinal	Dry mouth, diarrhea, upset stomach, lump in throat, nausea, vomiting
Bladder	Frequent urination
Central nervous	Dizziness, paresthesias, light-headed
Respiratory	Hyperventilation, shortness of breath, constriction in chest
Miscellaneous	Sweating, clammy hands

From Sharma R, Andriukaitis S, Davis JM: Anxiety states. In: *Psychiatry: Diagnosis and Treatment.* Flaherty JA, Davis JM, Janicak PG (editors). Appleton & Lange, 1993.

uation may include a complete blood count, electrolyte, glucose, creatinine, calcium, liver panel, and thyroid function test. Further testing should be tailored on an individual case basis depending on the clinical circumstances.

C. Imaging Studies

Although functional magnetic resonance imaging may eventually let us identify the specific neural events underlying symptom reports, there are no imaging studies that diagnose anxiety disorder. Imaging studies are done to preclude any type of organic disease that may mimic anxiety or panic and/or laboratory abnormalities to include but are not limited to thyroid scan and cardiac diagnostics.

D. Special Tests

Psychological tests resort to self-report of symptoms and are major assessment tools for anxiety. This is unfortunate given that most other medical diagnoses (eg, diabetes) rely on both symptom self-report and systematic biomedical measurements (eg, the glucose tolerance test).

The State-Trait Anxiety Inventory measures the frequency and intensity of transient anxiety processes and anxiety proneness as a character trait. Other validated measures are the Anxiety Sensitivity Inventory, Agoraphobic Cognitions and Body Sensations Questionnaires, and the Panic Belief Questionnaire.

Comorbidity can comprehensively be assessed by the Minnesota Multiphasic Personality Inventory-II (MMPI-2), a test composed of 567 true–false test items that can be completed in about 2 h. The Profile of Mood States (POMS) primarily measures mood states in psychiatric outpatients. Its advantage over the MMPI-2 is a completion time of about 10 min.

Chambless DL et al: The assessment of fear in agoraphobics: The Body Sensations Questionnaire and the agoraphobic cognitions questionnaire. J Consult Clin Psychol 1984;52:1090.

Gillham JR et al: Prevention of depressive symptoms in schoolchildren: two-year follow-up. Psychol Sci 1995;6:343.

Greenberg RL: Panic disorder and agoraphobia. In: *Cognitive Therapy in Clinical Practice: An Illustrative Casebook.* Scott J, Williams JM, Beck AT (editors). Routledge and Kegan Paul, 1989.

Hathaway SR, McKinley C: *Minnesota Multiphasic Personality Inventory-2.* National Computer Systems, University of Minnesota, 1989.

McNair DM, Lorr M, Droppleman LF: *Profile of Mood States, Revised.* Educational and Industrial Testing Service, 1992.

Peterson RA, Reiss S: *Manual for the Anxiety Sensitivity Index,* ed 2. International Diagnostic Services, 1992.

Spielberger CD: *State-Trait Anxiety Inventory.* Consulting Psychologists Press, 1983.

Differential Diagnosis

Because anxiety is a ubiquitous symptom of numerous medical conditions, family physicians must be alert to the possibility of alternative causes. A thorough investigation helps alleviate patients' concerns that their symptoms are due to other pathological processes.

The first step in planning a diagnostic evaluation is to perform a thorough history and physical examination. Table 48–2 presents the differential diagnosis of other symptom-related medical conditions.

Symptoms of cardiovascular abnormalities such as chest discomfort, shortness of breath, and palpitations are also cardinal symptoms of anxiety. Many anxious patients function poorly because they believe that they have heart disease.

The electrocardiogram can be a useful tool to differentiate anxiety from a significant cardiac abnormality. Further evaluation should be considered based on the patient's symptoms and risk profile. When further cardiac evaluation yields normal results, the anxious patient is more effectively reassured.

A careful auscultatory examination of the heart may reveal evidence of mitral valve prolapse, the most common valvular abnormality in adults. Long-term studies have shown that complications from mitral valve prolapse are rare.

The primary care physician must be alert to acute medical conditions that can present with hyperventilation or dyspnea such as with pulmonary symptoms. The differentiation between these entities can be as

Table 48–2. Differential diagnosis of related medical conditions.

Cardiovascular
    Acute coronary syndrome, congestive heart failure, mitral valve prolapse, dysrhythmia, syncope
Drugs
    β-Agonists, caffeine, digoxin toxicity, levodopa, nicotinic acid, pseudoephedrine, selective serotonin reuptake inhibitors, steroids, stimulants (methylphenidate, dextroamphetamine), theophylline preparations, thyroid preparations
Endocrine disorders
    Hyper/hypothyroidism, hyperadrenalism
Neoplastic
    Carcinoid syndrome, pheochromocytoma, insulinoma
Neurological disorders
    Parkinsonism, encephalopathy, restless leg syndrome, seizure, vertigo
Pulmonary
    Asthma (acute), chronic obstructive pulmonary disease, hyperventilation, pneumonia, pneumothorax, pulmonary edema, pulmonary embolus
Psychiatric
    Affective disorders, drug abuse and dependence/withdrawal syndromes
Other conditions
    Anaphylaxis, anemia, electrolyte abnormalities, porphyria, menopause

simple as checking a pulse oxygen saturation but will often require more advanced diagnostic studies.

Musculoskeletal pain syndromes, psychological problems, and esophageal disorders, including esophageal motility disorders and gastroesophageal reflux disease, are the most common noncardiac explanations of chest pain. A majority of patients with chronic unexplained chest pain have concomitant psychiatric diagnoses, especially anxiety.

Hyperthyroidism and hypoglycemia may be mistaken for anxiety. Hypoparathyroidism, hyperkalemia, hyperthermia, hyponatremia, hypothyroidism, menopause, porphyria, and carcinoid tumors are less common causes of organic anxiety syndromes.

Anxiety exacerbates gastrointestinal conditions such as colitis, ulcers, and irritable bowel syndrome. Treating anxiety often resolves gastrointestinal symptoms. Anxiety, hyperventilation, and dyspnea may accompany recurrent pulmonary emboli with few reliable physical signs.

Depression is the most common psychiatric disorder associated with anxiety. Symptoms that discriminate clinical depression from anxiety include depressed mood and loss of interest and pleasure.

Patients with anxiety disorders commonly drink to excess. Alcohol and drug problems involving dependence rather than abuse are most strongly associated with problems involving anxiety. Anxiety disorder and alcohol disorder can each initiate the other, especially in cases of alcohol dependence. Although many alcoholic patients present with anxiety, these symptoms decrease rapidly when the patient stops drinking. Only a small percentage (perhaps 10%) have persistent symptoms of anxiety.

Kushner MG, Abrams K, Borchardt C: The relationship between anxiety disorders and alcohol use disorders: a review of major perspectives and findings. Clin Psychol Rev 2000;20:149.

Smoller JW, Otto MW: Panic, dyspnea, and asthma. Curr Opin Pulmon Med 1998;4(1):40.

Anxiety Disorders: *DSM-IV* Classification

A description and relevant information about each anxiety disorder found in the *Diagnostic and Statistical Manual of Mental Disorders,* 4th edition (*DSM-IV*), as well as recommended treatments with efficacy outcome literature for each anxiety disorder will be presented.

A. PANIC DISORDER (PD) (300.01)

Recommended treatment includes breath retraining, cognitive restructuring, interoceptive exposure, and relaxation training. If anxiety is short term, benzodiazepines should be used; if anxiety is chronic, paroxetine, fluvoxamine, citalopram, fluoxetine, sertraline, nefazodone, or imipramine should be used.

A **panic attack** involves a discrete period of intense fear or discomfort that has a sudden onset, rapidly builds to a peak, usually in 10 min or less, and is often accompanied by a sense of imminent danger or impending doom and an urge to escape. About 33–50% of panic-stricken people from community samples have **agoraphobia,** a fear of being in places or situations from which escape might be difficult or embarrassing or in which help may not be available. Individuals suffering from panic disorder without agoraphobia have higher success rates than those with agoraphobia.

Although current treatments allow control of panic disorder, full recovery is questionable. Psychological treatments involve lower relapse rates, higher levels of acceptability, and lower attrition rates and are better tolerated than many pharmacological treatments. Exposure and deep breathing work especially well for patients with panic attacks and agoraphobia.

The percentage of patients who become free of panic attacks from medication is generally 50–80% in acute pharmacological trials, and this percentage rises with longer treatment. Selective serotonin reuptake inhibitors (SSRIs) reduced panic attack frequency to zero in 36–86% of patients and were well tolerated over long-term administration. Additionally, because of the high rate of depression comorbidity associated with panic attacks, SSRIs are the pharmacological treatment of choice.

High doses of benzodiazepines, although effective, are less recommended. Benzodiazepines are best used for acute management. In most studies relapse after discontinuation of medications has been relatively high, ranging from one-third to three-fourths of patients, suggesting the need to be on the medications for at least 6 months.

B. SIMPLE PHOBIAS (300.29)

Recommended treatment includes exposure therapy, deep breathing, relaxation training, and cognitive restructuring, as well as short-term use of benzodiazepines.

A **phobia** refers to significant, provoked, and irrational anxiety that a person experiences when near a specific object or situation that is feared. Patients with simple phobias do not usually seek treatment. They avoid the particular object or situation that evokes anxiety.

For those who seek intervention, exposure therapy is the sine qua non treatment. Initial use of benzodiazepines and/or the presence of significant others aids compliance and should be faded out with continued exposure to the feared object or event. Cognitive restructuring enhances maintenance effects.

C. SOCIAL PHOBIA (300.23)

Recommended treatment includes exposure therapy, cognitive restructuring, relaxation training, social skills training, and group therapy; medications that may be helpful include paroxetine, fluvoxamine, sertraline, venlafaxine, clonazepam, buspirone, and β-blockers.

A **social phobia** involves clinically significant anxiety that occurs when an individual is exposed to certain types of social or performance situations. The lifetime prevalence of social phobia is estimated to be as high as 13%. Social phobia affects most areas of life, particularly education, career, and romantic relationships.

When fearing negative evaluation, patients narrow their attention to social threat cues. Cognitive therapy corrects these distortions whereas exposure therapy reduces anticipatory fear. In cognitive–behavioral group settings, 81% of patients had significant improvement that was maintained 5.5 years later.

For social anxiety disorder paroxetine is approved by the Food and Drug Administration (FDA), and fluvoxamine and sertraline have also been shown to be effective. Although β-blockers reduce hand tremor and symptoms of tachycardia without causing cognitive impairment, we know of no placebo-controlled randomized study that has supported this long-held clinical practice. In nongeneralized social anxiety in which performance phobia is involved, β-blockers are considered helpful.

D. Obsessive-Compulsive Disorder (OCD) (300.3)

Recommended treatment includes referral as well as exposure therapy, response prevention, and cognitive restructuring; SSRIs and clomipramine may be used.

Obsessive-compulsive disorder involves intrusive thoughts that cause marked anxiety or distress. Compulsions (compelling acts) neutralize anxiety. The disorder typically stages as Obsession → Anxiety → Compulsion → Relief. The average patient with OCD waits 7 years after symptoms first appear before seeking clinical attention. Onset is usually gradual and the course is typically chronic. Up to 80% of patients with OCD evidence depression, anxiety, substance abuse, and/or work disability.

Behavior therapy and SSRIs are primarily recommended. Homework assignments expose patients to stimuli associated with their obsessions. During **response prevention,** patients refrain from rituals (fixed behaviors that reduce anxiety) for progressively longer intervals until discomfort diminishes.

Significant differences in efficacy among the SSRIs have not been found. Dosages for these medications are usually much higher than for antidepressant dosages (eg, fluoxetine up to 80 mg/day). Tricyclic antidepressants other than clomipramine do not appear to be effective in treating OCD.

E. Posttraumatic Stress Disorder (PTSD)(309.81)

Recommended treatment includes referral as well as individual or group psychotherapy, relaxation training, or cognitive restructuring; eye movement desensitization and reprocessing can be considered. Medications include fluoxetine or bupropion; benzodiazepines may be used based on symptom severity and history of substance abuse.

Posttraumatic stress disorder involves the patient reexperiencing an extremely traumatic event accompanied by symptoms of increased arousal and avoidance of stimuli associated with the trauma. Rape, war-related stress, assault, and accidents commonly precipitate PTSD. The traumatizing effect is linked to the fact that these events are unexpected, uncontrollable, and/or inescapable. Optimally, new experiences are assimilated and expressed.

Like OCD, PTSD is especially hard to treat. Early intervention reduces tendencies for substance abuse, secondary gain, litigation, and malingering. Referral is mandatory.

Some form of exposure/desensitization is essential. Patients put frightening memories into words while receiving new and incompatible information. Systematic exposure to the traumatic memory in a safe environment allows a reevaluation of and habituation to threat cues.

Although there is no established pharmacotherapy for PTSD, about 70% of patients seem to benefit from pharmacotherapy with moderate to marked effects.

SSRIs, especially fluoxetine, appear to have the greatest efficacy of any single class of medications. Clonazepam and buspirone may be helpful in suppressing hyperarousal symptoms. The anticonvulsant carbamazepine has been shown to decrease flashbacks, hyperarousal, and impulsivity. Carbamazepine, lithium, and β-blockers may be helpful in patients with poor impulse control.

Acute **S**tress **D**isorder entails the same PTSD-type symptoms that occur immediately in the aftermath of a traumatic event but resolve within 4 weeks.

F. Generalized Anxiety Disorder (GAD) (300.02)

Recommended treatment includes worry exposure, thought control techniques (mismatch, cognitive restructuring), relaxation training, and cognitive restructuring; venlafaxine, paroxetine, buspirone, or benzodiazepines can be used.

Generalized anxiety disorder involves at least 6 months of persistent and excessive anxiety and worry with an inability to stop worrying. These chronic worriers commonly display insomnia, feel irritable, tense, and tired, and have difficulty concentrating. The degree of comorbidity between GAD and other psychiatric disorders is high. Patients with GAD show higher general medical utilization than patients with depression.

No treatment has been convincingly effective for GAD. Although cognitive–behavioral therapy appears to produce superior results, effects remain variable. Cognitive psychotherapy addresses probability overestimation (ie, overestimating the likelihood of negative events) and catastrophic thinking.

Nonvalidated coping strategies such as physical action, thought replacement, analysis, counterpropaganda, and talking to a friend have been utilized by people. No one strategy was more efficient and none was rated "very efficient." What works well for one person may not work well for another. Thought intensity influenced choice of strategy and efficacy. Talking to a friend may be more efficient when thoughts are intense, whereas thought replacement may work well when intensity is low.

SSRIs are well-demonstrated medications of choice for most anxiety disorders; however, although the SSRIs, notably citalopram, paroxetine, and venlafaxine, have shown promise in the treatment of GAD, their role in this treatment is still under investigation. Response to benzodiazepines is variable. When conspicuous worry, apprehension, irritability, and depression exist, buspirone has been especially effective and has been shown to be comparable to benzodiazepines in multiple studies of GAD.

G. Substance-Induced Anxiety Disorder (292.0)

In substance-induced anxiety disorder, anxiety is due to a direct physiological consequence of a drug of abuse, medication, or exposure to a toxin.

H. Adjustment Disorder with Anxious Mood (309.24)

In adjustment disorder with anxious mood, clinically significant symptoms of anxiety occur in response to an identifiable stressor within 3 months after the onset of the stressor and resolve within 6 months after the termination of the stressor. However, symptoms may persist for a prolonged period if they occur in response to a chronic stressor (eg, a disabling chronic medical condition) or to a stressor that has enduring consequences (eg, financial effects of a divorce). Referral for psychotherapy is recommended.

I. Anxiety Disorder Due to a General Medical Condition (293.89)

Anxiety disorder due to a general medical condition involves prominent symptoms of anxiety judged to be a direct physiological consequence of a general medical condition. It is estimated that up to 20% of medical patients experience anxiety during the course of their medical illness. Anxiety comorbidity with other medical conditions is important because comorbid disorders may moderate treatment outcome, help clarify issues related to diagnostic validity, and indicate the generalizability of certain treatment strategies.

When organic etiology is ruled out of a **somatizing** presentation, the patients involved usually are less educated, have psychiatric disorders, and belong to a culture that deemphasizes emotional displays while focusing on bodily concerns. Many of these patients lack social support and have suffered trauma.

Ballenger JC: Current treatments of the anxiety disorders in adults. Biol Psychiatry 1999;46:1579.

Culpepper L: Generalized anxiety disorder in primary care: emerging issues in management and treatment. J Clin Psychiatry 2002;63:35.

den Boer JA: Pharmacotherapy of panic disorder: differential efficacy from a clinical viewpoint. J Clin Psychiatry 1998;59:30.

Kendall PC, Grady EU, Verduin TL: Comorbidity in childhood anxiety disorders and treatment coutcome. J Am Acad Child Adolesc Psychiatry 2001;40:787.

Raj BA, Sheehan DV: Social anxiety disorder. Med Clin North Am 2001;85(3):712.

Shalev RY: Acute stress reactions in adults. Biol Psychiatry 2002; 51:532.

Wells A: A cognitive model of generalized anxiety disorder. Behav Mod 1999;23(4):526.

Treatment

To embrace psychosocial treatments, the attitudes of the family physician sometimes need to be examined. Physicians often miss psychiatric problems because of a biomedical orientation. Complications include excessive diagnostic tests, increased costs, frustrated patients, and cynical physicians. Seeing the patient more frequently while maintaining the time constraints of a 15-min office visit will improve patient functioning without punishing the busy family physician.

Continuity of care and a sound doctor–patient relationship offer treatment advantages to family physicians in relation to mental health consultants. Positive patient expectations and trust formidably impact prognosis.

Familiarity with a few cognitive–behavioral techniques and several psychotrophic medications allows family physicians to use their influence on patients to enhance outcome. Some of the following cognitive–behavioral techniques can easily be implemented by a busy family physician as supplemental treatment to psychopharmacology. Other interventions can be offered through referral to mental health specialists. If after several 15-min office visits the patient remains unimproved or noncompliant, referral can be made.

A. Medications

Medications provide symptomatic relief rather than cure. Although use of medications is effective and widespread, when medications are discontinued, symptoms usually recur. Prescribing medication should be based on the patient's degree of emotional distress, the level of functional disability, and the side effects of the medication. Table 48–3 provides a summary of the dosage range, indications, and financial costs associated with the preferred drugs used to treat anxiety disorders.

1. Selective serotonin reuptake inhibitors (SSRIs)— SSRIs are now considered the first line of medication treatment. They are easily tolerated, have minimal toxicity in overdose, and are not associated with the withdrawal effects of benzodiazepines.

Recommendations on dosing have been to start low and titrate slowly upward with doses usually in the range of those prescribed for depression. An exception would be the treating of OCD which often requires higher than usual dosing. When a patient exhibits both

Table 48–3. Psychopharmacology management of anxiety disorders.[1]

Classification	Drug	Dose	Indication	Cost
SSRIs	Sertraline (Zoloft)	50–200 mg/day	FDA approved; panic disorder with or without agoraphobia	$60.00
	Paroxetine (Paxil)	20–50 mg/day	FDA approved; generalized anxiety disorder, social phobia, PTSD	$70.00
	Venlafaxine (Effexor XR)	75–225 mg/day	FDA approved; generalized anxiety disorder	$60.00
	Citalopram (Celexa)	20–50 mg/day	OCD, panic	$60.00
	Fluoxetine (Prozac)	20–50 mg/day	OCD, bulimia	$80.00
Aminoketone	Bupropion (Wellbutrin)	75–200 mg twice a day	PTSD, anxiety	$100.00
Benzodiazepine	Alprazolam (Xanax)	0.5–4 mg/day	Situational anxiety, panic	$30.00
	Chlordiazepoxide (Librium)	5–300 mg/day	Situational anxiety	$40.00
	Clonazepam (Klonopin)	1–6 mg/day	Situational anxiety, panic	$30.00
	Diazepam (Valium)	2–20 mg/day	Situational anxiety	$26.00
	Lorazepam (Ativan)	0.5–10 mg/day	Situational anxiety, panic	$25.00
Azaspirodecanedione	Buspirone (BuSpar)	20–30 mg/day two or three times a day	Situational anxiety	$120.00
Neuroleptic	Gabapentin (Neurontin)	300–600 mg three times a day	OCD, augment SSRI in panic, social phobia	$100.00

[1]SSRI, selective serotonin reuptake inhibitors; FDA, Food and Drug Administration; PTSD, posttraumatic stress disorder; OCD, obsessive-compulsive disorder.

depression and anxiety, SSRIs are strongly recommended.

2. Benzodiazepines—Benzodiazepines remain rapid and effective medications to treat panic disorder and have proven efficacy in the treatment of anticipatory anxiety, phobic avoidance, and anxiety resulting from transient situational stress reactions. Despite these advantages, benzodiazepines impair the ability to acquire new information (anterograde amnesia) with accelerated rates of forgetting most apparent within the first 24 h. Drug-induced decrements in processing speed, impaired attention/vigilance, and more accidental injury are associated with benzodiazepine use.

Tolerance to the antianxiety effects is uncommon. The abrupt discontinuation of benzodiazepines, espe-cially those with short half-lives, is associated with withdrawal syndromes of relatively rapid onset. A rebound syndrome similar to but more transiently intense than the original disorder may begin over a few days.

3. Buspirone (BuSpar)—Buspirone does not bind to the benzodiazepine/GABA receptor complex and is not cross-tolerant with benzodiazepines, other sedative-hypnotic agents, or alcohol. Onset of action is delayed by 3–4 weeks. Although there is uncertainty about its clinical effectiveness, buspirone is recommended by many physicians for patients with chronic anxiety problems. If a patient had previously been on a benzodiazepine, patient expectations about the drug should be discussed. Gradually tapering off the benzodiazepine while beginning buspirone enhances compliance.

4. Tricyclic antidepressants—Tricyclic antidepressants may be considered after failed trials of SSRIs, when anxiety attacks are chronic and unremitting, and when the patient has an aversion to benzodiazepines. These drugs are commonly prescribed as sedatives (eg, Elavil) in conjunction with other types of medications when insomnia is chronic. Because of an unattractive variety and severity of side effects, large numbers of patients discontinue treatment.

5. β-Blockers—β-Blockers are safe and effective when prescribed to control peripheral nervous system dysfunction in the treatment of "stage fright." They reduce rapid heart rate, flushing, and sweating. The medication is usually taken about 30 min before the event. Dizziness, drowsiness, and light-headedness are the most common side effects. β-Blockers may be prescribed in combination with other antianxiety medication.

6. Atypical anticonvulsants—Atypical anticonvulsants are also used in refractory anxiety treatment when SSRIs alone have failed to control symptoms. Gabapentin (Neurontin) has been shown to augment SSRI activity in the treatment of panic disorder and obsessive-compulsive disorder and to reduce anxiety associated with chronic pain syndrome.

7. Monoamine oxidase (MAO) inhibitors (MAOIs)—MAOIs produce fewer anticholingeric and sedative effects compared with tricyclic antidepressants; about 8% of patients taking MAOIs experience hypertensive crises. Dietary restrictions are prohibitive. For these reasons MAOIs have lost favor and are last line choices, used only when other pharmacotherapies have been unsuccessful.

B. Psychological

1. Behavior therapy—Behavioral therapy focuses on overt behavior. The "how to" improve is emphasized rather than "why" the problem exists. The role of the family physician is to explain a behavioral procedure and prescribe homework. Time management need not suffer. Fifteen-minute office visits should be sequenced about 1–2 weeks apart.

During **exposure therapy** the patient is repeatedly brought into contact with what is feared until discomfort subsides. The longer the exposure interval and the more intensive the exposure experience (massed trials), the better. Often a significant other is initially present. As exposure continues, the other is gradually removed. Likewise, a benzodiazepine initially may be used to enhance compliance and then gradually eliminated. Exposure treatment alters contingencies.

For example, with escape prohibited, an agoraphobic patient is placed in a shopping mall for 3–4 h each day for several weeks. The patient may initially take a benzodiazepine and/or be accompanied by a significant other until the end of the first week. Within weeks the patient experiences a dramatic reduction in symptoms of agoraphobia and panic.

Although few people are formally educated in stress management, a large repertoire of **coping skills** is available. Table 48–4 offers a partial list of such strategies that can be given as a patient handout.

Numerous types of **relaxation training** are useful in the treatment of all anxiety disorders and also have been shown to assist anger management. Learning to relax is inexpensive and easily accessible. Reduction in the body's consumption of oxygen, blood lactate level (associated with muscle tension), metabolism, and heart and respiration rates occurs during practice. Countless medical conditions from bronchial asthma to high blood pressure have shown significant improvement after regular practice in relaxation training.

Home practice for 20 min or more twice each day in a quiet place produces significant effects. Commercialized relaxation tapes are available for eidetic imagery and progressive muscle relaxation.

Panic attacks can be mediated by **breathing retraining,** which involves slow, deep (diaphragmic) breathing. Slowly inhaling, holding the breath, and slowly exhaling is repeated for 10 or more sequences. During slow, deep breathing the patient is told to substitute realistic thoughts ("I'm having a panic attack and I'm not in any danger") for panic-inducing thoughts ("I'm having a heart attack and I'll die soon"). This provides a sense of self-mastery and restores an oxygen–carbon dioxide balance to the body. Alternatively, breathing into a paper bag, although more conspicuous and embarrassing, rapidly restores the oxygen–carbon dioxide balance.

During an office visit it helps to induce a panic attack by asking the patient to breathe rapidly. The family physician then models the deep breathing exercise

Table 48–4. Effective coping strategies.

Talk or write about stressful problems
Do enjoyable activities
Get enough rest and relaxation
Exercise regularly
Eat properly (beware of caffeine, chocolate, and alcohol)
Plan your time and set priorities
Accept responsibility for your role in a problem
Make expectations realistic
Get involved with others
Build in self-rewards
Utilize a sense of humor
Learn assertiveness
Attend support groups

and thinks rationally out loud while asking the patient to copy his or her example. Despite its simplicity, the combination of deep breathing, cognitive restructuring, and **interoceptive exposure** is impressively effective.

To use the **worry exposure technique** the patient is asked to do the following:

1. Identify (perhaps write down) and distinguish worry thoughts from pleasant thoughts.
2. Establish a 30-min worry period at the same place and time each day.
3. Use the 30-min period to worry about concerns and to engage in problem solving.
4. Postpone worries outside the 30-min worry period with reminders that they can be considered during the next worry period (the patient may choose to write down new worries to avoid worrying about forgetting them).
5. During intrusions replace worries with attention to present moment experiences and/or pleasant memories.

This strategy challenges dysfunctional beliefs about the uncontrollability of thoughts and the dangerous consequences of failing to worry. Delusional jealousy also can be mediated by this approach.

In **mismatch strategy** the physician asks the patient to write a detailed account of the content of the worry (eg, exposure to a particular situation normally avoided) and then asks the patient to worry about what could happen in that situation. Finally, the patient is instructed to enter the situation and observe what really happens to assess the validity of the worry thoughts.

Lastly, the family physician can ask the patient to practice alternative endings for worry sequences. Rather than rehearsing catastrophic outcomes, the patient contemplates positive scenarios in response to worry triggers.

2. Cognitive therapy—Cognitive therapy is behavioral therapy of the mind. Based on the theory that thoughts, images, and assumptions usually account for the onset and persistence of anxiety, cognitive therapy assumes that the way patients perceive and appraise events and interpret arousal-related bodily sensations as dangerous (anxiety sensitivity) provokes symptoms of anxiety. Cognitive changes are the best predictors of treatment outcome for the anxiety disorders.

Achieving thought control is of central importance to mental health. Patients with obsessive-compulsive disorder and generalized anxiety disorder are especially prone to poor thought control. These patients devalue their ability to adequately deal with threats. Homework involving "self-talk" must be believed by the patient to be useful.

Because alternative interpretations and explanations (cognitive restructuring) are always available for upsetting events, patients can assume more control of and accept more responsibility for their adaptation. Acceptance of these assumptions empowers the patient. Documented durable improvement results from **cognitive restructuring** (substituting rational assumptions and perspectives and transforming the meaning of events and physiological arousal cues).

Although it is not possible to control all outside events, it is possible to control one's reaction to any event. As soon as patients are aware of being upset, they should pause and reflect on

1. the event;
2. thoughts about the event;
3. associated feelings; and
4. another way to perceive the event (another meaning) that is also true and makes sense.

When time permits, patients may enter this information in a small notebook for review with the family physician at a subsequent office visit.

C. ALTERNATIVE MEDICINE

Use of alternative therapies is more common among people with psychiatric problems and especially people with self-defined anxiety than among the rest of the population. Most alternative therapies are used without supervision. Because there are so few data on the relative effectiveness of these therapies, most people tend to try a therapist who has been recommended and, by trial and error, find a preferred therapy.

Eisenberg et al reported survey data suggesting that 42% of American people across a wide range of sociodemographic characteristics are paying (out of their own pockets) for alternative medicine. Most patients do not inform their doctor that they use these alternative practices. The most popular forms of alternative medicine in this survey were meditation/yoga, chiropractics, and massage therapy.

Massage therapies can be classified as energy methods, manipulative therapies, and combinations of each. Swedish massage is the most common form of massage and is usually given with oil. Movements called effleurage (smooth stroking) and petrissage (kneading-type movements) are done up and down the back and across many tissues of the body. The Trager method, similar to many other types of massage therapy, involves gentle holding and rocking of different body parts. **Reflexology,** an energy method, could be called a massage therapy because it involves kneading, stroking, rubbing, and other massage procedures. These procedures are centered on particular points of the feet, hands, or ears. Although few controlled studies exist utilizing massage therapy, most people report anxiety-reduction benefits. There are no empiric data on the efficacy of reflexology.

At least seven randomized controlled trials have evaluated the effects of the herb **Kava (*Piper methysticum*)** for the symptomatic treatment of mild anxiety. Although results have been positive, the studies have been criticized because of methodological flaws. Benefits remain uncertain.

Acupuncture has been demonstrated to reduce anxiety across a variety of populations and presenting problems. However, additional double-blind, placebo-controlled studies are needed.

Research indicates the benefits of yoga to quality of life and improved health. Yoga, which involves body postures and *asanas* (body maneuvers), appears to exercise various tissues, organs, and organ systems and provide an avenue to address character armors, attitudes, and tensions. Specific application to stress management is widespread with generally significant positive results. As is the case with acupuncture, however, better controlled research is needed.

D. REFERRAL

Referral may not be necessary when symptoms reoccur or when tapering a medication is difficult. Referral is appropriate when the family physician is uncomfortable with an indicated therapy, when patients are potentially suicidal or are actively abusing drugs, when noncompliance is suspected, or when psychopathology is severe.

If therapy is indicated, the specialized training of a clinical or a counseling psychologist is recommended. When psychopharmacology is warranted, the expertise of a psychiatrist is unmatched. Sound treatment is based on specific and accurate diagnosis and relies on empirically validated procedures that take into account the personality of the patient.

Table 48–5 provides eight referral treatments and their indications for the effective nonpharmacological management of anxiety disorders.

E. SPECIAL POPULATIONS

1. Human immunodeficiency virus-positive (HIV⁺) patients—Anxiety is an almost universal consequence of receiving a diagnosis of HIV⁺. Shock, disbelief, somatic complaints, and suicidal ideation typify reactions. Fears concerning death and multiple illnesses, the high cost of care and denial of insurance, the negative social stigma, the possible loss of job, and adherence to infection control strategies, as well as the need to adapt to pronounced life-style changes, contribute to reactions of anxiety. Referral for psychotherapy, stress management, and/or relaxation training is often recommended.

Family reactions also need attention. Working through shock, anger, guilt, and grief and mediating a family's use of denial are best accommodated through continuity of care with a family physician.

2. Children/youth—Transient fears are common in children of all ages and represent part of the normal developmental process. Normal fears need to be distinguished from the anxiety disorders of adulthood, which are prevalent among children and adolescents. In fact, anxiety disorders are also the most prevalent psychological problems of childhood. For example, panic disorder is very common among the young. Children with anxiety disorders also manifest a high rate of comorbidity, especially with other, secondary anxiety disorders.

Table 48–5. Referral interventions and indications for use.

Type of Intervention	Description	Indications
Psychotherapy		
Individual	Insight, empowerment, support	Privacy, complicated patient
Group	Interactive, common interest	Social skills, support, vicarious learning
Family	Rx environment and patient	Enabling, dysfunctional family
Eye movement desensitization and reprocessing (EMDR)	Follow oscillation movement of object (pencil) thinking of trauma Mixed results	Posttraumatic stress disorder
Hypnosis	Relaxation induction; suggestions	Suggestible patient
Biofeedback	EMG, EKG, EEG monitor physiological parameters to alter activity; cost is a limiting factor	Headaches, tension, blood flow, etc
Stress innoculation/anxiety management	Multifaceted, comprehensive cognitive–behavioral Rx	All anxiety disorders
Assertiveness training	Learn skills to be firm, not nasty	Dependent, unassertive, aggressive patients
Transcranial magnetic stimulation (TMS)	Noninvasive, painless method of brain stimulation via electrical current using changing magnetic fields	Applications are in their infancy

Anxiety is often manifested among children by avoidance behavior, distorted thinking, or subjective distress. The *DSM-IV* anxiety designations of childhood and adolescence include **separation anxiety disorder** (excessive anxiety concerning separation from home or from those to whom the child is attached) and **overanxious disorder** (at least 6 months of persistent and excessive anxiety and worry). Separation anxiety disorder is treated by exposure to the feared event (eg, the child attends school despite the discomfort). Psychotherapy is the treatment of choice for overanxious disorder.

Cognitive–behavioral treatment for children with anxiety disorders is the first-line treatment recommended. Similar approaches to those described for adults are utilized with emphasis on exposure paradigms. Response rates for children have ranged from 70% to 80%.

Family problems include overcontrolling, conflictual, and overly protective parents. In such cases, family involvement in therapy improves outcome.

Caution remains in effect regarding the prominent prescribing of medication for the treatment of childhood anxiety disorders. The International Narcotics Control Board of the United Nations has expressed concern about the inappropriate use of medication to treat social problems in developed countries and the widespread use of drugs to treat behavioral symptoms instead of treating the underlying causes. Further complicating pharmacology considerations is that few data are available on the impact of age on absorption, metabolism, therapeutic levels, or possible drug interactions. It is expected that to achieve the same serum levels in children compared with adults the relative dose would be higher.

Despite this caution, FDA indications for adults with anxiety disorders are often used in children and adolescents. Approximately 50–70% of children with these disorders respond to SSRIs. Benzodiazepine and tricyclic antidepressant treatment trials in childhood anxiety disorders generally have not shown efficacy. Minimal open data are available to guide pediatric use of β-blockers for anxiety.

3. The elderly—Although the most common form of psychiatric condition in the elderly, anxiety disorders are still underdiagnosed. Polypharmacy is often present. Altered pharmacokinetics and pharmacodynamics in the geriatric population lead to greater sensitivity to and prolonged half-life of the medication due to decreased clearance of the drugs.

Because of these drug complications, psychotherapy is attractive. There is a growing literature examining the effectiveness of psychotherapy. Cognitive–behavioral therapy is the best studied.

F. PATIENTS WITH RELATED CONDITIONS

1. Personality disorders—Personality disorders are life-long characterological problems that significantly complicate treatment and outcome. Poor compliance, medication abuse, interpersonal agitation, and poor insight characterize patients with personality disorders. These patients suffer more from anxiety than patients without personality disorders. Prescribing benzodiazepines is counterindicated.

2. Hyperventilation—During hyperventilation excessive rate and depth of breathing produce a marked drop in carbon dioxide and blood alkalinity. These changes can be subtle. A person may slightly overbreathe for a long time. Even a yawn may trigger symptoms, accounting for the sudden nature of panic attacks during sleep. Breathing retraining is recommended.

3. Insomnia—Patients with anxiety disorders commonly have sleep problems that worsen anxiety. Sympathomimetic amines may cause sleep-onset insomnia, whereas alcohol abuse produces sleep-termination insomnia.

Benzodiazepines are frequently prescribed as hypnotic-sedatives. For sleep-onset insomnia, triazolam and zolpidem are rapidly acting short half-life compounds. For sleep maintenance, longer acting drugs such as flurazepam and quazepam are more effective. Tolerance for the sedative effects, alteration of sleep topography, suppression of rapid eye movement (REM; dream sleep), impaired cognitive function, the occurrence of falls, and REM rebound following discontinuation, counterindicate use of benzodiazepines to treat chronic insomnia.

Sleep hygiene suggestions provide an effective *initial* treatment option. Patients are asked to review and alter life-style patterns that interfere with sleep. Table 48–6 outlines these suggestions for patient use. Compliance with recommendations and shift work are limiting factors.

Brown TA, Barlow DH: Long-term outcome in cognitive-behavioral treatment of panic disorder: clinical predictors and alternative strategies for assessment. J Consult Clin Psychol 1995; 63(5):754.

Eich H et al: Acupuncture in patients with minor depression or generalized anxiety disorders: results of a randomized study. Fortscrit Neurol Psychaitrie 2000;68:137.

Eisenberg DM et al: Unconventional medicine in the United States: prevalence, costs, and patterns of use. New Engl J Med 1993;82:246.

Kessler RC et al: The use of complementary and alternative therapies to treat anxiety and depression in the United States. Am J Psychiatry 2001;158:289.

Labellarte MJ et al: The treatment of anxiety disorders in children and adolescents. Biol Psychiatry 1999;46:1567.

Lichstein KL et al: Relaxation and sleep compression for late-life insomnia: a placebo-controlled trial. J Consult Clin Psychol 2001;69(2):227.

Table 48–6. Sleep hygiene recommendations.

Keep a sleep diary for a few weeks and monitor sleep-related activities
Establish a regular sleep–wake cycle (go to bed at about the same time and get up at about the same time)
Get regular exercise
Reduce noise
Avoid all naps
Eat dinner at a reasonable hour to allow time to digest your food
Avoid excessive amounts of caffeine (chocolates, soft drinks, coffee, tea), especially before bedtime
Avoid excessive fluid intake before bed
Avoid in-bed activities such as reading, eating, or watching TV
Avoid clock watching while trying to sleep
If not asleep within 10–15 min after going to bed, get up:
    If you still want to lie down, do so in another room
    When sleepy, go back to bed
    If not asleep in 10–15 min, repeat these steps

Sheikh JI, Cassidy EL: Treatment of anxiety disorders in the elderly: issues and strategies. J Anxiety Disord 2000;14(2):173.

Stewart SH, Kushner MG: Introduction to the special issue on anxiety sensitivity and addictive behaviors. Addict Behav 2001; 26:775.

Wise MG, Griffies WS: A combined treatment approach to anxiety in the medically ill. J Clin Psychiatry 1995;56(Suppl l2):14.

Prognosis

The combination of cognitive–behavioral treatment and SSRI medication provides an excellent prognosis for the majority of anxiety disorders, especially panic disorder, specific phobias, and social phobia. Although these treatments show promise with OCD, GAD, and PTSD, efficacy results are more variable.

Referral for OCD and PTSD is mandatory. Given the expected need to individualize treatment and provide novel treatment options, the busy family physician has neither the time nor expertise to engage in these comprehensive interventions. Nonetheless, attempting the discussed treatment recommendations during multiple 15-min continuity office visits will often render referral unnecessary.

Just 25 years ago, most estimates were that 80% of patients with anxiety disorders would not significantly benefit from available treatment. Today the opposite is true.

WEB SITES

Anxiety Disorders of America
http://www.adaa.org/
Anxiety/Panic Internet Resource
http://www.algy.com/anxiety
Internet Mental Health
http://www.mentalhealth.com/
National Institute of Mental Health
http://www.nimh.nih.gov/anxiety/anxietymenu.cfm

Personality Disorders

49

William Elder, PhD

Personality disorders (PDs) are a heterogeneous group of deeply ingrained and enduring behavioral patterns that manifest as inflexible and extreme responses to a broad range of situations. PDs impinge on medical practice in multiple ways, including self-destructive behaviors, interpersonal disturbances, and noncompliance. Appropriate physician responses and effective treatments exist for many PDs. Borderline personality disorder (BPD) is an extremely debilitating and notoriously difficult to treat disorder. BPD may be misattributed to other PDs, and behaviors of patients in crises may also misleadingly suggest BPD. Correct diagnosis of PDs and proper intervention will help to improve patient outcomes.

ESSENTIALS OF DIAGNOSIS

- *An enduring pattern of inner experience and behavior that deviates from cultural expectations, manifesting in cognition (ways of perceiving and interpreting self, others, and events), affectivity (range, intensity, lability, and appropriateness of response), interpersonal functioning, and impulse control.*

- *The pattern is inflexible and pervasive across a broad range of personal and social situations, leads to clinically significant distress or functional impairment, is stable, of long duration, and traceable at least to adolescence or early adulthood, and is not a manifestation or consequence of another mental disorder or due to the direct physiological affects of substances or general medical conditions.*

Ten PDs are currently distinguished clinically. They are often grouped into three clusters: odd or eccentric, anx-

ious or fearful, and dramatic, emotional, or erratic. These are helpful in broadly categorizing PD difficulties but are limited in their usefulness because they do not signify similarities in etiologies and treatment response. Table 49–1 summarizes the 10 PDs.

General Considerations

PDs are relatively common, with a prevalence of 10–18% in the general population. Patients with PDs may seek help from family doctors for physical complaints, rather than psychiatric help. Higher rates for all types of PDs are found in medical settings. Gender ratios differ among PDs with the ratio of females to males in BPD being 3 to 1. Depending upon the sample, prevalence of BPD in the general community is between 0.2 and 1.8%.

PDs have pervasive impact because they are central to who the person is. They are major sources of long-term disability and are associated with greatly increased mortality. Patients with PDs have fewer coping skills, and during stressful situations may have greater difficulties, which are worsened by poor social competency, impulse control, and social support. Patients with BPD are frequently maltreated in the forms of sexual, physical, and emotional abuse, physical neglect, and witnessing violence. PDs are identified in 70–85% of persons identified as criminal, 60–70% of persons with alcohol dependence, and 70–90% of persons who abuse drugs.

Borderline, schizoid, schizotypal, and dependent PDs are associated with high degrees of functional impairments and greater risk for depression and alcohol abuse. Obsessive-compulsive and narcissistic PDs may not result in appreciable degrees of impairment. Dependent PD is associated with a marked increase in health care utilization.

Pathogenesis

A. PD

PDs are syndromes rather than diseases. Avoidant, dependent, and schizoid PDs appear to be heritable. Simi-

Table 49–1. Clinical features and clusters of 10 *DSM-IV* personality disorders.

Cluster	Personality Disorder	Clinical Features
Cluster A: odd, eccentric	Paranoid	Suspicious; overly sensitive; misinterpretations
	Schizotypal	Detached; perceptual and cognitive distortions; eccentric behavior
	Schizoid	Detached; introverted, constricted affect
Cluster B: dramatic, emotional, erratic	Antisocial	Manipulative; selfish, lacks empathy; explosive anger; legal problems since adolescence
	Borderline	Dependent and demanding; unstable interpersonal relationships, self-image, and affects; impulsivity; micropsychotic symptoms
	Histrionic	Dramatic; attention seeking and emotionality; superficial, ie, vague and focused on appearances
	Narcissistic	Self-important; arrogance and grandiosity; need for admiration; lacks empathy; rages
Cluster C: anxious, fearful	Avoidant	Anxiously detached; feels inadequate; hypersensitive to negative evaluation
	Dependent	Clinging, submissive, and self-sacrificing; needs to be taken care of; hypersensitive to negative evaluation
	Obsessive-compulsive	Preoccupied with orderliness, perfectionism, and control

larly, schizotypal disorder is considered to be heritable, as one end of a schizotypal/schizophrenia spectrum. Twin and adoption studies suggest a genetic predisposition for antisocial PD, as well as environmental influences, via poor parenting and role modeling. Histrionic PD may be related to indulged tendencies toward emotional expressiveness.

B. BPD

BPD may result from both constitutional and environmental factors. Genetically, BPD is five times more common among first-degree relatives of those with the disorder but to say to what degree BPD is heritable is difficult given the reciprocity between family and child that occurs during development. BPD symptoms have been attributed to highly pathological and conflicted interactions between mother and child. The conflict brings great ambivalence about relationships and interferes with the child's ability to regulate affect. More about this process appears in the treatment section on managing termination of care, a very difficult situation for patients with BPD. Child sexual abuse has been thought causal in BPD, but a recent meta-analysis did not support this hypothesis. It is certainly the case that traumatic childhood experiences are frequent for patients with BPD. As a group, patients with antisocial and borderline PDs report higher frequencies of perinatal brain injury, head trauma, or encephalitis.

C. Common Comorbid Conditions

Substance abuse disorders frequently cooccur in community and clinical populations, particularly with antisocial, borderline, avoidant, and paranoid PDs. Anorexia nervosa, bulimia nervosa, and binge eating may be seen in patients who are obsessional, borderline, and avoidant, respectively. Self-injurious skin picking can be conceptualized as an impulse control disorder and has been found with significant frequency in patients with obsessive-compulsive PD and BPD. Up to 50% of patients with BPD will have major depressive disorders or bipolar disorders.

Prevention

Except for efforts to address the roots of criminal behaviors that are common in antisocial PD, there is no literature on prevention of PDs. Primary prevention could consist of better treatment of parental mental illnesses that negatively impact parent–child interactions and public health interventions to reduce prenatal brain insults. Both primary and secondary prevention could occur with increased interventions in family functioning and parenting skills.

Clinical Findings

PDs were once referred to as character disorders. Various descriptive labels have appeared in the literature, such as the oral fixated character, the impulsive personality, and the introverted personality type. Each of these represents a theory of personality (psychoanalytic, developmental, and analytical, respectively) that has been applied clinically.

Currently, there are few points of correspondence between personality theory and diagnosis of PDs. A relatively atheoretical, categorical perspective dominates clinical practice in the United States. In the categorical perspective, PDs represent qualitatively distinct clinical syndromes.

A. THE DIAGNOSTIC AND STATISTICAL MANUAL OF MENTAL DISORDERS, 4TH EDITION (DSM-IV)

The *DSM-IV* exemplifies the categorical perspective. Diagnosis using the *DSM-IV* involves delineating the patient's condition multiaxially. "Clinical" mental disorders appear on Axis I. PDs appear on Axis II; thus PDs may be referred to as "Axis II disorders." The Axis II placement does not imply that PDs are conditions that are less severe than disorders on Axis I. Instead, the additional axis provides a place where pervasive, persisting disorders may be differentially recorded. Mental retardation, similarly pervasive and persistent, is also an Axis II disorder.

Diagnosis of PDs according to *DSM-IV* involves identifying the best match(es) between patient difficulties and criterion symptoms listed for each PD. Frequently, more than one PD is coded. A diagnosis of PD—Not Otherwise Specified (PD-NOS) is available when symptoms are mixed. Patients with significant personality difficulties but an insufficient number of symptoms to meet diagnostic criteria may be identified on Axis II as having a "trend" toward a personality disorder (eg, dependent personality trends). In addition to the PDs appearing in Table 49–1, *DSM-IV* includes two PDs "requiring further study." Depressive PD involves persistent gloominess, pessimism, and anhedonia. Passive-aggressive PD encompasses a wide range of negative attitudes along with alternations between hostility and contrition.

B. SYMPTOMS AND SIGNS

1. PD—Clinical lore about appearance and presentations of PDs exists. Anything extreme in appearance that is not ethnically appropriate or currently fashionable may suggest a PD. Examples include flamboyant jewelry, particularly in males, tattoos and piercing in older males and females, steel-toed boots in males, and excessive cosmetics and large hair ribbons in females.

The patient's style of interacting with the physician can be revealing about personality difficulties. For example, the dependent patient will seek much advice and be unable to make an independent decision. The patient with antisocial PD may be "smooth talking" or threatening. Interactions with patients with BPD can

be very difficult. The patient will switch from extreme idealization to devaluation of the physician. The patient may cause "splitting" among staff, with some people siding with the patient and others extremely angry with the patient. Table 49–2 describes problem behaviors associated with various PDs.

Physician countertransference may be a sign of a PD. Reactions such as anger, guilt, desire to punish, desire to reject, desire to please, sexual fantasies, and a sense that the physician is the "one person" capable of helping the patient are all examples of physician countertransference responses to patient PDs. Reflection and self-awareness are helpful in dealing with the strong feelings and interpersonal conflict encountered in medical care.

No laboratory tests exist for PDs. Structured clinical interviews and personality inventories may be helpful in differentiating PDs and tracking treatment response. Interpretation by a psychologist enhances the value of the results. A consult should be considered in cases of diagnostic uncertainty.

2. BPD—Physicians may overattribute or underattribute patient difficulties to BPD; therefore, it is important to be sensitive to BPD phenomena and to ascertain whether patient difficulties and symptoms represent BPD. BPD diagnostic criteria call for a pervasive pattern of instability in interpersonal relationships, self-image, and affect, and marked impulsivity beginning by early adulthood and present in a variety of contexts as indicated by at least five of the following:

1. Frantic efforts to avoid real or imagined abandonment (not including suicidal behaviors).
2. A pattern of unstable and intense interpersonal relationships characterized by alternating extremes of idealization and devaluation.
3. Identity disturbance: a markedly and persistently unstable self-image or sense of self.
4. Impulsivity in at least two areas that are potentially self-damaging (not including suicidal behaviors).
5. Recurrent suicidal behavior, gestures, threats, or self-mutilating behavior.
6. Affective instability due to a marked reactivity of mood (eg, intense episodic dysphoria, irritability, or anxiety usually lasting a few hours and only rarely more than a few days).
7. Chronic feelings of emptiness.
8. Inappropriate intense anger or difficulty controlling anger.
9. Transient, stress-related paranoid ideation or severe dissociative symptoms.

BPDs make up a heterogeneous group with subgroups consisting of patients differing in affective, impulsive, and micropsychotic symptom clusters. These differences can suggest different treatments, discussed later. Patients with BPD have significantly higher rates of suicidal ideation and 70–80% exhibit self-harming behavior at least once. Suicide attempts are often regarded as manipulative gestures, but suicide rates are very high in this population: 3–9.5% of patients with BPD receiving inpatient care eventually kill themselves. Self-harming behaviors in the form of self-mutilation, such as wrist scratching, are symptomatic of BPD. Nausea and vomiting may be a primary care analog of self-mutilation in some patients with BPD, and a common chief complaint. Obtaining a history suggesting BPD may mitigate the need for extensive and invasive gastrointestinal symptom evaluations, and may suggest more effective treatment strategies directed to personality functioning.

Differential Diagnosis

A. PD

Accurate diagnosis is essential for proper response to and treatment of PDs.

- Histrionic PD patients are dramatic and manipulative, but lack the affective instability of BPD. Impulsivity, when seen, is related to attention seeking and sexual acting out.

- Dependent PD patients fear abandonment, but patients with BPD have much affective instability and impulsivity.

- Schizotypal PD patients have the micropsychotic symptoms of BPD, but are odder and lack the affective instability of BPD.

- Paranoid PD patients have volatile anger, but lack the impulsivity, self-destructiveness, and abandonment issues of the BPD patient.

- Narcissistic PD patients have rages and reactive mood, but have a stable, idealized self-image in contrast to the patient with BPD, who has an unstable identity.

- Antisocial PD patients are often less impulsive than intentionally aggressive for materialistic gains. Patients with BPD act out when needy and to gain support.

B. Other Mental Disorders

A PD is not diagnosed if symptoms are explained by an Axis I condition or substance use. Although PDs may share impulsivity, raging, and grandiosity with bipolar disorder, they seldom have the same intensity and rate of speech or irrationality of thought that a manic episode brings. Substance use disorders differ from antisocial PD when illegal behaviors are restricted to substance use and procurement. Dissociative identity disorder, formerly known as multiple personality disorder, may have a more traumatic etiology similar to BPD. Obsessive-compulsive PD is not on the same spectrum as obsessive-compulsive disorder. Although patients with both disorders are quite orderly and inflexible, patients with obsessive-compulsive PD are comfortable with their behavior whereas patients with obsessive-compulsive disorder recognize that their behavior and thoughts are irrational. A diagnosis of PD does not apply when changes in behavior result from changes in brain function. For example, although personality changes are expected in dementia, a diagnosis of PD is not indicated. An Axis I diagnosis "Personality Change Due to a...[General Medical Condition]" is available when a change in personality characteristics is the direct physiological consequence of a general medical condition. Because transient changes in personality are common in children and adolescents, diagnosis of a PD is not appropriate for a patient younger than 18 years of age unless the behavioral pattern has been present for at least 1 year.

C. Cultural Considerations

Culturally related characteristics may erroneously suggest PDs. Promiscuity, suspiciousness, and recklessness have different norms in different cultures. The degree of physical or emotional closeness sought and the intensity of emotional expression also differ. Manner of dress and health beliefs may seem strange to the conventional Western physician. Passivity, especially with one's elders, is not a sign of dependency in most recently immigrated individuals. Constricted affect is a normal response when entering a new environment. Asking someone from the culture if the behavior is extreme can be helpful, as can evaluating for significant interpersonal difficulties.

Treatment

Miller has described how experienced family physicians differentially and efficiently respond to visits that can be categorized as routine, ceremony, or drama. In some cases, good application of family medicine's care principles may be beneficial psychotherapeutically. (Compare the psychotherapy of PDs described below with the patient-centered method of family practice.) Suggestions for helping patients with PDs in a nonpsychiatric medical setting appear in Table 49–2. Table 49–3 offers suggestions for helping patients who present with BPD.

Common wisdom has held that personality cannot be changed. However, increasingly specific psychopharmacological and psychotherapeutic interventions have brought improved outcomes and some cures. The most effective treatments are multidisciplinary, combining medications, individual and group psychotherapies,

Table 49–2. Problem behaviors associated with personality disorders.

	Personality Disorder				
	Paranoid	**Schizotypal**	**Schizoid**	**Antisocial**	**Borderline**
Patient's perspective	People are malevolent. Situation is dangerous.	Understanding of care may be odd or near delusional.	Illness will bring too much attention and invade privacy.	Threatened if unable to feel "on top." Illness presents opportunity for crime.	Fears abandonment. Overreacts to symptoms and situation.
Problem behaviors	Fearful. Misconstrues events and explanations. Irrational. Argumentative.	Odd health beliefs and behaviors. Poor hygiene. Avoids care.	Unresponsive to kindness. Difficult to motivate. Avoids care.	Acts out to gain control. Malingering. Uses staff and doctors. Superficially charming. Drug seeking.	Idealizes, then devalues care. Self-destructive acts. Splits staff.
Helpful physician responses and management strategies	Be emphatic toward patient's fears, even when they seem irrational. Carefully explain care plan. Provide advance information about risks. Protect patient's independence.	Communicate directly. Avoid misinterpreting patient as intentionally noncompliant. Do not reject patient for oddness. Honor patient's beliefs.	Manage personal frustration at feeling unappreciated. Maintain a low-key approach. Appreciate patient's need for privacy.	Do not succumb to patient's anger and manipulation. Avoid punitive reactions to patients. Motivate by addressing patient's self-interest. Set clear limits that interventions must be medically indicated.	Manage feelings of hopelessness about patient. Avoid getting too close emotionally. Schedule frequent periodic check-ups. Tolerate periodic angry outbursts, but set limits. Monitor for self-destructive behavior. Discuss feelings with co-workers.

and a high level of communication among providers. Comorbid substance dependence, violent acting out toward others, or severely self-harming behaviors must be addressed first, via inpatient care.

A. RISK MANAGEMENT

Physicians should acknowledge the threats and challenges associated with PDs. General risk management considerations include

- having good collaboration and communication with a qualified mental health professional;
- attention to documentation of communications and risk assessments;
- attention to transference and countertransference issues described earlier;
- consultation with a colleague regarding high-risk situations;
- careful management of termination of care, even when it is the patient's decision; and
- informed consent from the patient and, if appropriate, family members, regarding the risks inherent in the disorder and uncertainties in the treatment outcome.

B. RECOMMENDING TREATMENT, CONSULTATION, OR REFERRAL

Consultation or referral should be considered when the following exist:

- The patient has several psychiatric diagnoses.
- The patient has significant problems with self-regulation.
- The patient has moderate to severe substance use disorder(s).
- The diagnosis is uncertain or the presentation is puzzling.
- Initial treatment by the family physician is ineffective.
- The physician and/or staff are unable to compensate for and are overwhelmed by the patient's personality problems.

Patient acceptance of treatment can be difficult. The patient may disagree about what is wrong. Symptomatically, patients with PD may externalize blame for their problems. PD behavioral patterns also tend to be egosyntonic. That is, even patients who agree that their behavior is excessive may believe that the excess is rea-

Histrionic	Narcissistic	Avoidant	Dependent	Obsessive-Compulsive
Illness results in feeling unattractive or presents an opportunity to receive attention.	Illness results in feeling inadequate or is an opportunity to receive admiration.	Illness is personal. Fears exposure.	Fears abandonment. Intensifies feelings of helplessness.	Fears losing control of body and emotions. Feels shame.
Overly dramatic, attention-seeking. Excessively familiar relationship. Not objective—overemphasis on feeling states.	Demanding and entitled attitude. Will overly praise or devalue care providers to maintain sense of superiority.	Missed appointments. Delay seeking care. Extremely nonassertive.	Dramatic and urgent demands for medical attention. May contribute to or prolong illness to get attention.	Unable to relinquish control to health care team. Great difficulty and anger at any change. Excessive attention to detail.
Avoid frustration with patient vagueness. Show respectful and professional concern for feelings, with emphasis on objective issues. Avoid excessive familiarity.	Avoid rejecting the patient for being too demanding. Avoid seeking patient's approval. Generously validate patient's concerns, with attentive but factual response to questions. Protect self-esteem of patients by giving them a role in their care.	Provide empathic response to inadequacy. Be patient with timidity. Work toward clear treatment plans—must obtain patient's view. Treat anxiety disorder.	When exhausted by patient needs, avoid hostile rejection of patient. Give reassurance and consistency. Set limits to availability—schedule regular visits. Help patient obtain outside support.	Avoid impatience. Thorough history taking and careful diagnostic workups are reassuring. Give clear and thorough explanations. Avoid control battles; treat patient as a partner; encourage self-monitoring.

Table 49–3. Working with patients with BPD in medical settings.

1. Recognize the characteristics. The patient fears abandonment and increases demands on the physician. May be noncompliant, manipulative, somatacize, or "split" the health care team.
2. Behavior is need driven. Demands may be overt or covert. Identify needs and motivations. Patient has little insight into problems. Externalization is symptomatic.
3. Tolerate patient's behaviors. Speaking "harshly or strictly" will activate abandonment fears and worsen the situation. Use a nonconfrontational and an educational approach.
4. A long-term plan provides stability for the patient. Follow continuity of care principles. This may be curative for the patient.
5. Titrate closeness and visit frequency. Avoid extremes of constant availability.
6. Set limits. Make clear agreements about call and office visits. Point out to patients that you are almost always involved in solving some type of problem and are unable to give full attention to their problems without an appointment. Suggest that patients schedule fairly frequent visits so that a regular time is available to discuss the problems they are experiencing.
7. Foresee problems related to abandonment fears such as when the social situation is disturbed, when the patient is referred, or when there are changes in physician or staff.
8. Use a multidisciplinary approach. Involve a highly skilled clinical psychologist or clinical social worker in the care. Encourage communication and cooperation among the care team.
9. Monitor your and the staff's reactions. Frustration and anger may be expected. Discuss the situation. Help the staff to recognize the etiology of the frustration might originate in the patient's personality not in the crisis of the moment. Coordinate responses to patients.
10. Set personal limits for the number of these challenging patients that you accept into your practice.

sonable, given their perception of the circumstances. Treatment may also be difficult if it is perceived as an attempt to control the patient; referral may be experienced as devaluing or as abandonment. Thus treatment and referral suggestions should be offered with an understanding of how patients with various PDs may perceive them. Table 49–2 describes patient perspectives on care common to different PDs.

C. PSYCHOPHARMACOLOGICAL INTERVENTIONS

In many cases, medications are effective only as a means to manage stress-exacerbated symptoms. For example, under stress, paranoid, schizoid, or schizotypal patients may experience delusions, distress, and hallucinations, which can be helped with antipsychotic medications. When not stressed, the odd behavior and beliefs of these patients remain unresponsive to treatment. Narcissistic, antisocial, and histrionic PD patients are not helped with current medications, including antidepressants, unless a mood disorder coexists.

Some PDs may be successfully treated with medications. Avoidant personality disorder appears to be an alternative conceptualization of social phobia. It can be treated with selective serotonin reuptake inhibitors (SSRIs) and selective serotonin and norepinephrine reuptake inhibitors (SNRIs). Patients with obsessive-compulsive PD may become less irritable and compulsive with SSRIs. Rejection sensitivity seen in patients with dependent PD may be helped by SSRIs.

Soloff has proposed three symptom-specific pharmacotherapy algorithms for PDs. They are based on differential medication effects on cognitive disturbances, behavioral dyscontrol, and affective dysregulation. Soloff's first algorithm is for treatment of PDs where cognitive-perceptual symptoms are most significant (ie, patients with suspiciousness, paranoid ideation, and micropsychotic symptoms). The second algorithm is for treatment of affective dysregulation (ie, patients with a depressed/angry/anxious/labile mood). The third algorithm is for treatment of impulsive-behavioral symptoms (ie, patients with impulsive aggression, binging, or self-injuring behaviors). Practice guidelines for treatment of BPD were published by the American Psychiatric Association (APA) in October 2001. The guidelines are largely in accord with Soloff's recommendations. Recommendations that follow are based on the APA guidelines. It should be noted that current guidelines are based on a small database that lacks sufficient randomized controlled trials. Therefore, each treatment should be approached as an empirical trial, with the patient as a coinvestigator. Side effects, risk–benefit ratios, conjoint medications, and patient preferences should be considered carefully. Pharmacotherapy is an adjuvant to psychotherapy; medications do not cure character and will never be a substitute for the work of a therapist.

SSRIs and SNRIs are effective with affective dysregulation. Tricyclic antidepressants are no more effective than SSRIs and should not be used, given their cardiotoxic effects with overdose and a possibility of paradoxical worsening of symptoms. Monoamine oxidase inhibitors (MAOIs) were proven useful in treating BPD prior to the advent of SSRIs and offer a second treatment option for affective dysregulation, including rejection sensitivity. Mood stabilizers offer an additional level of treatment. Lithium should be used in conjunction with an antidepressant, whereas valproate and carbamazepine may be offered alone. Although patients suffering BPD will complain of anxiety, benzodiazepines are contraindicated, having been shown to cause increased impulsivity. Clonazepam, a benzodiazepine with anticonvulsant and antimanic properties, is associated with increased serotonin levels and may be useful adjunctively for anxiety, anger, and dysphoric mood.

Antipsychotics are the most researched medications for the treatment of BPDs and should be the first-line treatment where cognitive-perceptual symptoms are significant. Low doses should be tried first. There is no evidence that antipsychotics are helpful for BPD cognitive-perceptual symptoms in the long term. Antipsychotics may also be used adjuvantly with antidepressants for affective dysregulation, particularly with anger. Antipsychotics such as risperidone may exacerbate or induce manic symptoms, although they produce symptom improvement in bipolar disorder when used in conjunction with mood-stabilizing medications. When the recent guidelines were written, there was insufficient evidence that third-generation antipsychotics (eg, risperidone or olanzapine) would be effective with cognitive-perceptual symptoms in BPD, but given side effect profiles of conventional versus third-generation antipsychotics, the newer drugs are being used increasingly, empirically. The atypical antipsychotic clozapine is effective in personality disturbances that are cognitive-perceptual and impulsive but, given its risk for agranulocytosis, should be reserved until several trials of other medications have failed.

Risperidone appears superior to conventional antipsychotics in treatment of impulsivity and aggression, especially in BPD. However, SSRIs at low to moderately high doses should be tried first. If needed, low-dose antipsychotics may then be added to SSRIs, or used more aggressively as a last line of treatment. Mood-stabilizing medications are indicated as midlevel treatment for impulsivity. Lithium is effective, perhaps because of its impact on serotonin levels. The anticonvulsant divalproex sodium has been used to treat irritability and impulsivity in patients with BPD who have failed SSRI therapy, apparently independent of the presence of abnormal electroencephalographic findings.

Carbamazepine is also effective as a mood stabilizer. Use of mood stabilizers requires various laboratory tests to monitor metabolic functioning. Various antipsychotic medications carry risks for extrapyramidal symptoms, tardive dyskinesia, weight gain, diabetes, extended Q-T intervals, etc.

D. PSYCHOTHERAPEUTIC INTERVENTIONS

Some PDs are amenable to some forms of psychotherapy. Treatments of less than 1 year duration probably represent crisis interventions or treatments of concurrent Axis I disorders rather than attempts to address core PD psychopathology. Psychotherapy for borderline and narcissistic personalities tends to take significantly longer. Even with extended duration, treatment goals tend to be for functional improvement such as decreased symptom severity and decreased acting out, rather than complete remission of symptoms. Anxiety-related PDs, such as avoidant and dependent PDs, are most amenable to psychotherapy, followed by BPD, followed by schizotypal PD. Cognitive-behavioral psychotherapy, which challenges irrational beliefs, may be effective with avoidant, dependent, obsessive-compulsive, narcissistic, and paranoid personality disorders. Because individuals with antisocial PD are manipulative and seldom take responsibility for their behavior, psychotherapy is difficult and relatively rare, unless court-order interventions are counted as psychotherapy, which is questionable.

Successful treatment of borderline and narcissistic PDs requires high levels of therapist experience. Skills in managing the therapeutic alliance and creating a stable, trusting relationship are crucial. Insight is less of a focus. Psychotherapy for narcissistic PDs may be highly specialized where the patient's hypersensitivity to slights is confronted only after much trust building and attainment of positive transference.

Group therapy and partial hospitalization are effective for schizotypal and borderline PDs. Dialectical behavior therapy is a unique form of psychotherapy that is effective for BPD. During individual and group therapies the patient's beliefs, contradictions, and acting out are empathically accepted. That is, the patient's personhood is responded to positively, and dysfunctional behaviors are responded to matter of factly, neither sympathizing with, nor punishing, the patient. Sessions focus on learning to solve problems, control emotions, manage anxiety, and improve interpersonal relationships. After many months of this consistent and intensive treatment, limits are set on the patient's behavior.

E. COMPLEMENTARY AND ALTERNATIVE MEDICINE (CAM) INTERVENTIONS

CAM interventions have not been identified for PDs. Preference for CAM is not a sign of PD.

F. TRANSFER AND END OF CARE SEPARATION STRATEGIES

Patients with certain PDs may have great difficulty separating from their family physician. Separation is also difficult for patients with chronic illnesses and other psychiatric disorders or who are socially isolated. Responses to termination can be understood in the context of attachment and loss. According to attachment theory, humans form strong bonds that serve basic biological functions by ensuring that the very young are protected. Separation of the young from their object of attachment results in crying, clinging, increased anxiety, and a possibility of depression or anger upon rapprochement. Even for patients without mental disorders, attachment-related behaviors can resurface during times of stress as panic and anxiety, particularly with the helplessness and dependence that accompany illness and hospitalization or loss of the powerful figure that the physician may represent.

Developmentally oriented theorists have suggested that BPD pathology originates in a disturbed attachment process. Abandonment is extremely traumatic for children. Depression and difficulty forming new relationships result. The notion in BPD is that during the critical period of ages 2–3 when the child typically practices separation from the mother, the parent of the borderline progeny is unable to accept the child's distancing from the parent and is inconsistent upon the child's return, alternatively rejecting or indulging the child. This pattern repeats through childhood and is replicated in adulthood, where there is great ambivalence about relationships. BPD relational patterns seem to approximate the practicing phase of childhood where there is highly emotional approaching and distancing from the pseudoparental object. Tenuous relationships may be formed and abandonment fears are strong. This interpersonal pattern applies to the doctor–patient relationship, as well. The patient, fearing abandonment, will alternate between extremes of overvaluing and devaluing the physician. During times away from the doctor, the patient may be preoccupied with thoughts of the physician and may experience physical distress.

The following suggestions may help to avoid serious problems for patients undergoing separation:

- Inform patients in advance of upcoming separations.
- Review with patients their responses to previous losses. This will give some prediction about how the patient will react to the termination as well as help the physician–patient team identify strengths on which to capitalize and weaknesses to address.
- Take the pending separation as an opportunity to review the patient's health care and the role of the doctor–patient relationship in the process of care.

- Have patients express how the relationship has been beneficial, what they may have learned about themselves in that relationship, and how that could be helpful in future relationships.

- Resist a desire to not say goodbye to your patients. This may happen for a number of reasons, including fear of hurting the patients, reluctance to cause "clinging" behaviors, or anger at noncompliant yet demanding patients.

- Understand the patient's reaction to the news. Some patients may be cool or otherwise noncommittal to the physician's leaving. A patient who does not want to speak about an upcoming separation can be offered the opportunity to speak about it at a future visit. The patient should know that any and all emotional responses are acceptable. Issues of trust and feelings of abandonment warrant explicit discussion.

- Initiate the discussion with a brief statement that the physician is leaving. Follow this with a brief silence that allows patients to understand and respond. If the silence persists, ask patients what they are thinking or feeling. Body language may provide clues. They can be asked to elaborate on their feelings or, if not responding, gently confronted with a question like, "I am wondering what this news is like for you."

- When possible, introduce patients to their new care provider. This meeting facilitates information transfer and symbolizes a turning over of the relationship with the patient.

- Ask new patients how they feel about their previous physician.

G. TERMINATION OF CARE

Despite the physician's best efforts, it is sometimes necessary to terminate care against the patient's wishes. The following steps and policies should be considered:

- Have a clear policy about what circumstances will produce care termination such as repeated drug abuse, violent acting out including threatening, repeatedly missed appointments, physician's opinion that care has reached maximal therapeutic benefit, etc.

- Try contracting with your patient to stop these behaviors first.

- Give your patients written, advanced warning that you are terminating care. Thirty days warning is typical. You may need to provide care in the interim unless circumstances argue otherwise. If not, give directions on where they may receive care.

- Ethical practice includes physician freedom to choose whom they will serve. However, termination of a patient with a mental disorder requires consideration of patient competency and emotional status, or else abandonment is possible. Consulting with a colleague is an appropriate means to ensure that consideration is given to patient needs.

- Be aware of any specific policies or actions required in your state.

Prognosis

Perhaps 50% of patients with PDs currently never receive treatment. Several of the PDs, although pervasive in their negative effects, are perhaps not sufficiently impairing or distressing to warrant treatment. Treatment outcomes are improving for the PDs that are extremely debilitating, such as BPD. PDs with anxiety components have good potential for improvement. There remains debate as to whether any treatment other than incarceration can be effective with antisocial PD, and with this, the effect may come from time, as the person becomes less disruptive as age 40 is approached. Patients with BPD appear to improve by age 40 as well. Patients with BPD who are in treatment improve at a rate seven times their natural course.

American Psychiatric Association: *The Diagnostic and Statistical Manual of Mental Disorders,* ed 4. American Psychiatric Press, 1994.

American Psychiatric Association: *Practice Guideline for the Treatment of Patients with Borderline Personality Disorder.* American Psychiatric Press, 2001.

Beck AT et al: Dysfunctional beliefs discriminate personality disorders. Behav Res Ther 2001;39(10):1213.

Feder A, Robbins SW: Personality disorders. In: *Behavioral Medicine in Primary Care.* Feldman MD, Christensen JF (editors). Appleton & Lange, 1997.

Gross R et al: Borderline personality disorder in primary care. Arch Intern Med 2002;162:53.

Miller WL: Routine, ceremony, or drama: an exploratory field study of the primary care clinical encounter. J Fam Pract 1992;34(3):289.

Perry JC, Banon E, Ianni F: Effectiveness of psychotherapy for personality disorders. Am J Psychiatry 1999;156:1312.

Phillips KA, Gunderson JG: Personality disorders. In: *Synopsis of Psychiatry,* Vol. 8. Hales RE, Yudofsky SC (editors). American Psychiatric Press, 1996.

Roller B, Nelson V: Group psychotherapy treatment of borderline personalities. Int J Group Psychother 1999;49(3):369.

Sansone RA, Widerman MW, Sansone LA: Borderline personality symptomatology, experience of multiple types of trauma and health care utilization. J Clin Psychiatry 1998;59(3):108.

Shah A: Literature review: treatment of bipolar disorder and aggression with risperidone. Janssen Pharmaceut, April 2002.

Skodol A et al: Functional impairment in patients with schizotypal, borderline, avoidant, or obsessive-compulsive personality disorder. Am J Psychiatry 2002;159(2):276.

Soloff PH: Psychopharmacology of borderline personality disorder. Psychiat Clin North Am 2000;23(1):169.

World Health Organization: *The ICD-10 Classification of Mental and Behavioral Disorders: Clinical Descriptions and Diagnostic Guidelines.* WHO, 1992.

Somatoform Symptoms & Disorders 50

William Elder, PhD

Somatoform disorders involve unexplained physical symptoms that bring significant distress and functional impairment. They present one of the more common and most difficult problems in primary care. They are seldom "cured" and should be approached as a chronic disease. Recognition, a patient-centered approach, and specific treatments may help alleviate symptoms and distress. Essential features of somatoform disorders include the following:

- Somatoform disorders involve physical symptoms or irrational anxiety about illness or appearance, where biomedical findings are not consistent with a general medical condition. Somatoform disorders have specific courses, symptoms, and complaints (Table 50–1).
- Symptoms develop with or are worsened by psychological stress and are not intentional.
- Symptoms vary along a spectrum of seriousness. Somatic expression of psychological distress is normal. Comorbid or primary mental disorders are common with somatoform symptoms.
- Patients seek much medical care. Paradoxically, treatment and attempts to reassure them can be counterproductive.
- Somatoform complaints may foster feelings of frustration for the physician. Patients are often seen as "difficult patients."

General Considerations

Ten percent of all medical services are provided to patients with no organic disease. Twenty-six percent of primary care patients meet criteria for somatic "preoccupation": 19% of patients have medically unexplainable symptoms and 25–50% of visits involve symptoms that have no serious cause. Where somatoform disorders are present, cost for ambulatory care is 9 to 14 times greater than controls. With appropriate recognition and treatment, costs of care may be reduced by 50%. Individuals with somatoform disorders undergo numerous medical examinations, diagnostic procedures, surgeries, and hospitalizations. They risk increased morbidity from these procedures. Eighty-two percent stop working at some point because of their difficulties.

Pathogenesis

To some degree, somatoform symptoms should be considered normal. Bodily experiences of emotions are common. Examples include anger in the jaw, tension in the shoulders, loss in the chest, disappointment in the gut, shame in the reddening face, fear in the bowels, etc. Children quickly feel ill when they learn that a friend is sick or when family stress is high. Student's syndrome, experienced by medical students in their first pathology class, is an example of nonpathological fear of having a disease.

Regarding somatoform disorders, some individuals are susceptible to overexperiencing sensations, apparently through a difference in gating, which is worsened by anxiety or psychological stress. Other individuals demonstrate obsessive tendencies. Fears of disease may form. A vicious process of symptom amplification has been demonstrated in hypochondriasis where obsession about the body focuses attention on sensations, which when misinterpreted cause anxiety, increasing sensations and further worsening obsessiveness. Perceptual disturbances and bodily concerns apparent in body dysmorphic disorder are similar to obsessive-compulsive disorders, but when extreme may suggest a mild thought disorder. Genetic factors, demonstrated in adoption studies, appear to play a role in developing somatic sensitivities and obsessive tendencies. Traumatic experiences in the form of sexual, physical, and emotional abuse and witnessing violence are predictive of somatoform disorders and demonstrate the role of anxiety in development of somatic symptoms.

Because families differ in how they respond to symptoms and illnesses, individual differences in health beliefs and illness-related behaviors are to be expected. Families also shape the tendency to experience, display, and magnify somatoform symptoms, where somatoform disorders or malingering are modeled or reinforced by adults. Social factors include single parent-

Table 50–1. Somatoform disorders.

	Symptom Presentation	Type of Symptoms	Prevalence and Gender Ratios	Voluntary Control over Symptoms	Symptom Duration	Age of Onset
Somatization disorder	Sees self as sickly; frequent medical care	Multiple systems or functions of several types, including pain and pseudoneurological	0.2–2% in females; less than 0.2% in males	No	Chronic, recurring and/ or stable	Adolescence or early 20s; rare in aged
Undifferentiated somatoform disorder	Sees self as ill; frequent medical care	Single system of symptom	Common	No	More than 6 months	Early 20s
Conversion disorder	Onset after acute stress	Single, pseudoneurological	0.01–0.1%; females much more common	No	Sudden onset; short duration	Adolescence
Pain disorder	Focus solely on pain; pain behaviors	Pain; low back, neck, pelvic; emotional changes	Common	No	Sudden onset; worsens with time	All ages; 30s–40s most common
Hypochondriasis	Fearful of disease; preoccupied with symptoms; not reassured	Multiple; normal bodily sensations; may be vague	4–9% of medical practices; equal	No	Long history, worsens after actual illness	Any Typically early adulthood; concerns without fears not abnormal in elderly
Body dysmorphic disorder	Excessive concern over imagined defect in appearance	Specific complaints of defect	?	No	Usually several years	Adolescence; early 20s
Factitious disorder with physical symptoms	Multiple operations; infections	Nonhealing and unremitting	Rare	Yes	Chronic; multiple admissions; remits with confrontation	Early adulthood
Malingering	Protest; demand for medical help	Vague pain and/or paralysis common	?	Yes	Multiple episodes of same problem	Early adulthood

hood, living alone, unemployment, and marital and job difficulties.

Gender ratios and prevalence of somatoform disorders differ across cultures. In North America, somatization, conversion, and pain disorders are more frequent in females whereas hypochondriasis and body dysmorphic disorder involve males and females equally. Somatoform symptoms are more prevalent among Chinese-American, Asian, and South American patients.

Cultures have different explanatory models for physical functioning and disease processes. Disorders with somatoform characteristics specific to certain cultures include the *dhat* syndrome in India, which is a concern about semen loss, and koro in Southeast Asia, a preoccupation that the penis will disappear into the abdomen, resulting in death. A nondelusional sense of having worms in the head or burning hands is not uncommon in Africa and Southeast Asia. Cultures influence illness behaviors, such as whether a medical clinician or traditional healer is sought first, or how emotions should be expressed. Cultures also sanction religious and healing rituals that promote behaviors that may appear conversion-like. Symptoms should be evaluated for appropriateness to the patient's social context. Behaviors sanctioned by the culture are typically not considered pathological.

Western medicine's dominant conceptualization of the mechanism of somatoform symptoms is that of somatization, a process in which mental phenomena such as emotions manifest as physical symptoms. As a concept, somatization assumes psychopathology. It originated in psychoanalytic theory, where it was considered a primitive, psychological defense against unconscious conflicts, needs, and desires that the individual was too weak to express. The notion of somatization as a defense has some clinical utility and constitutes an improvement over beliefs that some feminine physical complaints reflect a uterus loose in the body, hence the term hysterical, which is derived from the Greek word for uterus. However, the notion of somatization as pathological ignores the normalcy of physical expression of emotions and the social construction of illness behaviors, including the belief that conventional medical treatments such as medication and surgery can solve most problems.

Clinical Findings

A. Symptoms and Signs

Somatoform symptoms can suggest a large number of general medical conditions. However, in addition to ruling out general medical conditions, diagnosis may also be made by inclusion. The following features should increase suspicion of a somatoform presentation:

- Unexplained symptoms that are chronic or constantly change.
- Multiple symptoms. Four symptoms in males and six in females suggest somatic preoccupation. Fainting, menstrual problems, headache, chest pain, dizziness, and palpitations are the symptoms most likely to be somatoform.
- Vague or highly personalized, idiosyncratic complaints.
- Inability of more than three doctors to make a diagnosis.
- Presence of another mental disorder, especially depressive, anxiety, or substance abuse disorders.
- Distrust toward the physician.
- Physician experience of frustration.
- Paradoxical worsening of symptoms with treatment.
- High utilization including repeated visits, frequent telephone calls, multiple medications, and repeated subspecialty referrals.
- Disproportionate disability and role impairment.
- The specific symptom patterns the course and complaints of somatoform disorders.

B. Diagnostic Criteria

Somatoform disorders are mental disorders that involve physical symptoms or irrational anxiety about illness or appearance, where biomedical findings are not consistent with a general medical condition. Diagnosis requires a finding that the symptoms have brought unneeded medical treatment or that there is significant impairment in social, occupational, or other important areas of functioning. Somatoform disorders cannot be caused by another mental condition or by direct effects of substances. If the disorder occurs in the presence of a general medical condition, complaints or impairment must be in excess of what would be expected from the physical findings and history.

1. Somatization disorder—This is a persisting pattern of recurring, multiple somatic complaints beginning before age 30. Patients view themselves as "sickly." Historically, somatization disorder was referred to as *hysteria* or Briquet's syndrome, a fluctuating mental disorder in young women characterized by frequent complaints of physical illness involving multiple organ systems. Current diagnostic criteria are more extensive, requiring a history of pain related to at least four different sites or functions, two gastrointestinal symptoms other than pain, one sexual symptom other than pain, and one pseudoneurological symptom other than pain. Common sites of pain include the head, abdomen, back, joints, extremities, chest, and rectum and common functions include pain during menstruation, during sexual intercourse, or during urination. Common gastrointestinal symptoms include nausea, bloating, diarrhea, or multiple food intolerances. Sexual symptoms include sexual indifference, sexual dysfunction, and menstrual problems. Pseudoneurological symptoms can be motor related, such as impaired coordination or balance, paralysis or localized weakness, difficulty swallowing including "lump in throat," aphonia, urinary retention, or sensory-perceptual, such as minor hallucinations, loss of touch or pain sensation, double vision, blindness, and deafness. Seizures, amnesia, and loss of consciousness are also possible.

2. Undifferentiated somatoform disorder—This is a residual diagnosis for clinically significant, somatoform complaints persisting for more than 6 months. Examples include chronic fatigue, weakness, and anorexia as well as the symptoms described with regard to somatization disorder, when insufficient in number to meet diagnostic criteria for somatization disorder.

3. Conversion disorder (formerly hysterical conversion disorder)—This consists solely of pseudoneurological symptoms such as those described with somatization disorder (ie, deficits affecting the central nervous system, voluntary motor or sensory functions). Psychological factors in the form of stressors or emotional conflicts are expected and precede the symptoms. Depending on the medical naivete of the patient, symptoms are often quite implausible, not conforming to anatomical pathways or physiological mechanisms. Symptoms may symbolically represent emotional conflicts, such as arm immobility, as an expression of anger and impotence. Other clues indicating that the symptoms are pseudoneurological include worsening in the presence of others, noninjuries despite dramatic falls, normal reflexes, muscle tone, and pupillary reactions, and striking inconsistencies on repeated examinations. Symptoms may be experienced with a relative lack of concern (so-called *la belle indifference*) but dramatic or histrionic presentations are more common. Course is an important consideration. Conversion disorder is rare before age 10 or after age 35 years. Symptoms are transient, rarely lasting beyond 2 weeks, and respond to reassurance, suggestion, and psychological support. Secondary gain, seen in malingering, may be apparent but is not primary in conversion disorders.

4. Pain disorder associated with psychological factors—This disorder is the psychiatric equivalent of chronic nonmalignant pain syndrome, except that no minimum duration of symptoms is required. Psychological factors play a significant role in the pain picture including its onset, severity, exacerbation, and maintenance. Physical pathologies are possible and frequent but organic findings are insufficient to explain the severity of the pain. Common sites for pain include the lower back, neck, pelvis, and head. Patients with this disorder may follow a downward spiral of poor functioning, especially if they lack adequate skills to adaptively cope with their losses of physical functioning and situational changes. The experience of pain will severely disrupt patients' lives; thus functional deficits are common including disability, increased use of the health care system, abuse of medications, and relational and vocational disruptions. Depression or anxiety may be secondary or may also be primary or comorbid, predisposing the patient to an increased experience of pain as well as a deficient ability to cope with the illness situation. Patients with severe depression or with terminal conditions are at increased risk for suicide. Insomnia is frequently associated with pain complaints.

5. Hypochondriasis—The individual with hypochondriasis is preoccupied with fears of having a serious disease. The preoccupation may originate in an overfocus on and misinterpretation of normal physiological sensations (eg, orthostatic dizziness), erroneous attributions about the body (eg, "aching veins"), or obsession about minor physical abnormalities. In the case of concerns about physical abnormalities, the individual must believe that the abnormality indicates the presence of a disease; otherwise a diagnosis of body dysmorphic disorder is more appropriate. Patients are easily alarmed when hearing of new diseases, knowing someone who is sick, or from sensations and occurrences in their own body. Fears persist despite medical reassurance. Doctor shopping is common. Hypochondriacal concerns (ie, attention to symptoms and fear of death) are common in panic disorders.

6. Body dysmorphic disorder—This disorder involves excessive preoccupation with a minor or imagined defect of one or more body parts. Concern may not focus exclusively on obesity, which would indicate an eating disorder. Although many people are concerned about their appearance, the concerns and behaviors associated with this disorder are extreme, distressing, time consuming, and debilitating. Self-consciousness is significant with public exposures avoided, hiding of defects, and nondisclosure to the physician common. Medical, dental, and surgical treatments are sought but may only worsen preoccupations. Concerns about appropriateness of sexual characteristics may be better represented in a diagnosis of gender identity disorder. Concerns about appearance are common during major depressive episodes. Patients who insist that an imagined defect is real and hideous will meet the criteria for delusional disorder, somatic type.

7. Malingering, factitious disorder, and factitious disorder by proxy—These are not somatoform disorders; symptoms are voluntary and deceptive. Deception is obtained by feigning or self-inducing symptoms or by falsifying histories or laboratory findings. Common symptoms include fever, self-mutilation, hemorrhage, and seizures. Malingering and factitious disorder differ by whether symptom gain is primary or secondary. In malingering, symptoms are produced to gain rewards or avoid punishments (secondary gain). Factitious disorder involves production of symptoms in order to assume the sick role (primary gain). Unlike malingering, factitious disorder is considered a mental disorder principally because the need to be in the sick role is abnormal. Factitious disorder by proxy occurs when illness is caused by a caregiver, typically to meet a need for drama and to be a rescuer of the patient. Direct evidence, such as inconsistent laboratory or physical findings or observations (eg, injection of bacteria), may be the first sign that symptoms are intentional. Earlier signs of factitious disorder include patients who are migratory or have no visitors, are comfortable with more aggressive treatments including extended hospitalization, are connected in some manner with the health professions, or whose presentation is exaggerated and quite dramatic (Munchausen's syndrome).

C. SCREENING QUESTIONS AND DIAGNOSTIC MEASURES

Valid diagnostic and screening questionnaires exist, but often lack clinical utility in comparison to an interview. Where doubts remain, a referral for evaluation is probably in order. Asking questions about depressed mood and hopelessness/loss of interest has great sensitivity for depressive disorder, if the depression is not occult. Questions should address cognitive symptoms, such as guilt and lowered self-esteem, endorsement of which may suggest depression even in the absence of sad mood. Questions should also evaluate patients suspected of having body dysmorphic disorder (Table 50–2).

Table 50–2. Questions to evaluate body dysmorphic disorder.

1. Do you worry about the appearance of your face or body? If so, what is your concern?
2. How bad do you think your (face or body part) appears?
3. How much time do you spend worrying about your (face or body part)?
4. Have you done anything to hide or rid yourself of the problem?
5. How does this concern with your appearance affect your life?

Partially adapted with permission from Phillips KA: Body dysmorphic disorder: diagnosis and treatment of the imagined ugliness. J Clin Psychiatry 1996;57(suppl 8):61.

Differential Diagnosis

Diagnosis should be considered tentative and provisional until there is considerable external support. General medical conditions characterized by multiple and confusing somatic symptoms (eg, hyperparathyroidism, porphyria, multiple sclerosis, and systemic lupus erythematosus) should be considered. Conversion disorder, in particular, is often misdiagnosed, with medical diagnoses eventually replacing up to 50% of conversion diagnoses. Shaibani and Sabbagh have described a number of clinical tests that may reveal whether conversion symptoms are pseudoneurological. Onset of multiple physical symptoms in early adulthood suggests somatization disorder but in the elderly suggests a general medical condition. Primary or secondary depression should be considered in any patient suspected of having somatoform disorder. Other mental disorders including anxiety disorders and substance-related disorders are frequently seen with somatoform disorders and in some cases may better explain symptoms and thus constitute the better diagnosis. Personality disorders such as histrionic, borderline, and antisocial personality are frequently associated.

Patients with Somatoform Symptoms as "Difficult Patients"

Characterizing medically unexplained symptoms as pathological may lead physicians to misconstrue patients as solely suffering from a psychiatric disorder. In reality, primary care patients are usually quite different from those seen in specialty psychiatric care. The notion and usefulness of discrete disease entities are problematic to begin with. Primary care patients present with undifferentiated symptoms that are best addressed with a comprehensive approach that includes continuity of care and attention to the doctor–patient relationship. Pathologizing makes patients feel illegitimate, in itself a major source of distress, and produces stereotypes of patients as "crocks, whiners, or difficult." If this happens, the relevance of the patient's experience and the potential of partnership between patient and physician are both obviated. A patient-centered method, so important to family practice, becomes impossible. Patients who consider their physicians as patient centered are more satisfied with care, are referred less, and receive fewer diagnostic tests.

Even without attributions of a mental disorder, somatoform symptoms present one of the most difficult challenges in primary care. Patient characteristics considered as difficult include extensive or exaggerated complaints, noncompliance with treatment recommendations, or behaviors that raise suspicion of seeking drugs. Uncertainties associated with the diagnosis, the sense that the focus is not medical therefore the interaction is inappropriate, patient symptom amplification, and the sense that services are being overused inappropriately contribute to the perception that the patient is difficult.

Treatment

Somatoform symptoms exist on a continuum and should rarely indicate that the patient's difficulties are to be attributed solely to a mental disorder. Comprehensive, continuous, patient-centered care will appropriately address most primary care patient presentations. The following general recommendations apply to such an approach.

A. General Recommendations

1. First visits—A therapeutic alliance should be built by a thorough history and physical examination and by a review of the patient's records. Show curiosity and interest in the patient's complaints. Validate the patient's suffering. Psychogenic attributions should be avoided. To appear puzzled initially is a good strategy. Delivery of a diagnosis is a key treatment step with somatoform disorders. Different disorders require different types of information. Suggestions for statements to be made to the patient appear in Table 50–3.

2. Management—Treat the disorder as a chronic illness. Focus on functioning rather than symptom cure. Expect gradual change, with periods of improvement and relapse. Practice secondary prevention, especially of iatrogenic harm. When new symptoms arise, do at least a limited physical examination. Permit invasive diagnostic and therapeutic procedures only on the objective evidence, not on subjective complaints. Avoid the need for unnecessary tests and procedures by having the patient feel "known" by you.

3. Patient-centered care—Feelings of illegitimacy by patients and common physician attitudes toward patients contribute to power differentials and struggles. These can be avoided by practicing the relational behaviors patients prefer from their providers. Doctors should speak with patients as equals, listen well, ask lots of questions, answer lots of questions, explain things understandably, and allow patients to make decisions about their care. Develop a relationship that is collaborative. Work together with the patient to understand and manage patient problems. Monitor the "common ground" shared by you and the patient. Discuss differences.

4. Structure office visits—Schedule regular, brief appointments. Avoid "as-needed" medications and office visits that make your attention contingent on symptoms. Practical time-related strategies include negotiat-

ing and setting the agenda early in the visit, paying attention to emotional agenda, listening actively rather than in a controlling manner, soliciting the patient's attributions for the problems, and communicating empathetically.

5. Address psychosocial issues—Reassure the patient, but not too soon. Intersperse psychosocial questions with biomedical ones. Explore all issues: physiological, anatomic, social, family, and psychological. Inquire about trauma and abuse. As trust builds, encourage the patient to explore psychological issues that may be related to symptoms. Link symptoms to the patient's life and feelings. Do not overuse the term "stress." Eventually and subtly, patients are likely to reveal their personal side and concerns. The BATHE Technique is an excellent way to probe and briefly counsel emotional issues, usually with the goal of assisting the patient in developing a personally relevant solution to solving conflicts.

6. Involve the family—Invite family members to participate in patient's visits. Occasionally conduct a family conference where several questions should be of value. Ask each person's opinion about the illness and treatment. Ask how family life would be different if the patient were without symptoms. Solicit and constantly return to the patient's and family's strengths and areas of competence.

B. Psychopharmacology

Because these patients may be extremely sensitive to side effects, psychopharmacological agents generally should not be used unless the patient has a demonstrated pharmacologically responsive mental disorder such as major depression, generalized anxiety disorder, panic disorder, or obsessive-compulsive disorder. Selective serotonin reuptake inhibitors (SSRIs), other nontricyclic antidepressants, and benzodiazepines are the medications most frequently used for coexisting psychiatric conditions. Treatment should be initiated at subtherapeutic doses and increased very gradually. Patients should be warned about side effects that are listed in Table 50–4, along with recommended initial doses and therapeutic range of doses.

Hypochondriasis and body dysmorphic disorders are similar to obsessive-compulsive disorder and may benefit directly from higher doses of SSRIs, if side effects are tolerated. Transitorily extreme dysmorphic concerns may benefit from temporary treatment with an atypical neuroleptic. Contrary to standard placebo effect-enhancing practice (ie, enthusiastic recommendation of a medication), psychopharmacological agents should be recommended with a degree of pessimism, with the notion that it is unlikely to be very beneficial, but may be worth a try.

Table 50–3. Delivering the diagnosis in somatoform and related disorders.

Disorder	Statements
Somatization disorder	1. I know that you are experiencing much discomfort and feeling very ill. 2. You have a medical disorder called somatization disorder. 3. This disorder runs in families and has a unique pattern of symptoms. It does not cause physical deterioration or shorten life. 4. It is not curable, but manageable. A specific treatment plan is required.
Conversion disorder	1. Avoid terms "conversion disorder" and "psychogenic." 2. After thorough evaluation, the (symptom name, eg, blindness) will resolve very quickly. 3. It is, in fact, starting to improve at this time.
Pain disorder	1. I have reviewed your records and thoroughly evaluated you. 2. All appropriate interventions have been tried. 3. You have a medical condition called somatoform pain disorder. 4. Your disorder is not life-threatening but I know that you are experiencing much discomfort and (specific function, eg, moving) quite poorly. 5. Our goal must be rehabilitation, not necessarily being pain free. 6. A specific treatment plan is required.
Hypochondriasis	1. Reassurance of nonpathology is unlikely to be helpful. A diagnostic label will be helpful. 2. You have a syndrome of neurological amplification of body sensations. 3. The syndrome is not life-threatening but requires careful monitoring. 4. We need to schedule regular appointments. I want you to discuss your concerns at these appointments and I'll examine you thoroughly.
Body dysmorphic disorder	1. I can see that you are very concerned about this sense that your (body part, eg, nose) is ugly. 2. You get very anxious when you think about people seeing it and want to hide it. You even want to stay away from others because you are so anxious. 3. What I suggest we do for now is try these measures to treat your anxiety so that your suffering is less and you function better, not missing out on things that you would otherwise like to do.
Factitious disorder	1. The physician may decide to directly confront a patient. However, if family or other social situation is available to promote the patient's need to save face, a therapeutic double bind is suggested. A thorough physical examination and attempt to build a therapeutic alliance must be performed before delivering the diagnosis. 2. Sometimes people do things to make themselves ill. We call this problem factitious disorder. 3. You have an unusual problem. I believe it will respond to one more attempt to treat it. If, however, the problem does not respond to this attempt, a diagnosis of factitious disorder will be established.
Malingering	1. Informing the patient that their deception has been detected can be dangerous and should be handled carefully. In some cases it may be better to deprive the patient of any benefits of the sick role, which will extinguish the behavior. 2. I guess I am wondering if there might be some reason for you to be sick right now. 3. Have you thought about what might happen if you continue to do this?

Partially adapted with permission from McCahill ME: Somatoform and related disorders: delivery of diagnosis as first step. Am Fam Physician 1995;52(1):193.

C. SPECIALIST MENTAL HEALTH CARE

A mental health clinician may be helpful to diagnose comorbid mental conditions, offer suggestions for psychotropic medications, and engage some patients in psychotherapy. However, patients are unlikely to see the value of consultation, or may experience referral as an accusation that their symptoms are not authentic. Pressuring the patient to accept a consultation is unlikely to be effective and may render the consultant encounter unproductive. Trust must first be established and psychological issues must be made a legitimate subject for discussion. The idea of referral can be reintroduced later. When possible, it can be more effective to see the patient along with the mental health clinician so

Table 50–4. Pharmacotherapy for coexisting psychiatric conditions in patients with somatoform complaints.

Agent	Initial dose	Therapeutic Range	Side Effects	Indications
Selective serotonin reuptake inhibitors				
Citalopram	10 mg/day	20–40 mg/day	Sexual dysfunction, nausea, dyspepsia, sedation, somnolence, agitation, insomnia, headache, dizziness	Depression, panic disorder, obsessive-compulsive disorder, generalized anxiety disorder
Fluoxetine	5–10 mg/day	20–80 mg/day	Sexual dysfunction, nausea, dyspepsia, sedation, somnolence, agitation, insomnia, headache, dizziness	Depression, panic disorder, obsessive-compulsive disorder, generalized anxiety disorder
Paroxetine	10 mg/day	20–50 mg/day	Sexual dysfunction, nausea, dyspepsia, sedation, somnolence, agitation, insomnia, headache, dizziness	Depression, panic disorder, obsessive-compulsive disorder, generalized anxiety disorder
Sertraline	12.5–25 mg/day	50–200 mg/day	Sexual dysfunction, nausea, dyspepsia, sedation, somnolence, agitation, insomnia, headache, dizziness	Depression, panic disorder, obsessive-compulsive disorder, generalized anxiety disorder
Other antidepressants				
Bupropion	75 mg/day	100–150 mg three times a day	Anxiety, insomnia, agitation, nausea, anorexia, seizures (at high doses)	Depression
Nefazodone	50 mg/day	150–300 twice a day	Sedation, nausea, headache, hypotension, dizziness	Depression
Trazodone	25 mg at bedtime	100–200 mg twice a day	Sedation, orthostasis, nausea, priapism (rare), headache	Depression
Venlafaxine	25 mg twice a day	75–150 mg twice a day	Nausea, anxiety, tremor, insomnia, sexual dysfunction, hypertension (high doses only), discontinuation effects, dizziness	Depression, generalized anxiety disorder
Benzodiazepines				
Alprazolam	0.25 mg/day	0.5–2.0 mg four times a day	Sedation, drowsiness, ataxia, falls (in elderly patients), falls (in elderly patients), memory impairment, confusion (especially in elderly patients), discontinuation effects and symptom rebound, fatigue, weakness, psychomotor impairment	Panic disorder, generalized anxiety disorder (short term)
Clonazepam	0.25 mg/day	0.5–2.0 mg twice a day	Sedation, drowsiness, ataxia, memory impairment, confusion (especially in elderly patients), discontinuation effects and symptom rebound, fatigue, weakness, psychomotor impairment	Panic disorder, generalized anxiety disorder (short term)

Reprinted with permission from Barsky AJ: The patient with hypochondriasis. New Engl J Med 2001;345(19):1395.

that a comprehensive approach continues to be emphasized, the patient does not feel abandoned, and doubts that the patient's concerns are not taken seriously are alleviated. Extreme distress or preoccupations worsening to delusional levels may require inpatient hospitalization.

D. Psychotherapy

Standardized group or individual cognitive-behavioral therapies can be an effective treatment for chronic somatoform disorders, reducing somatic symptoms, distress, impairment, and medical care utilization and costs. Cognitive interventions train the patient to identify and restructure dysfunctional beliefs and assumptions about health. Behaviorally, the patient is encouraged to experiment with activities that are counter to usual practices, such as avoidance, doctor shopping, or excess seeking of reassurance. In addition, patients learn relaxation and meditation techniques to manage symptoms of anxiety.

E. Complementary and Alternative Treatments

It is to be expected that patients with somatoform symptoms often try alternative treatments such as herbals, manipulations, and mind–body and non-Western medical approaches. Conventional treatments appear to have failed. Distrust of physicians may be high. Distress is great. Federal regulations require that label claims and instructions on herbals and supplements address symptoms only; therefore, there are no specific herbals for somatoform disorders, per se. Given the plethora of symptoms that can exist in somatoform disorders, it is not surprising that there are numerous alternative medications that patients may try.

Patients with pain disorder or primary/comorbid anxiety may benefit from body and mind–body interventions such as massage, movement therapies, manipulations, relaxation, guided imagery, and hypnosis. The placebo effect of various remedies may be helpful, particularly if the agents are largely inert, as bothersome side effects seen in conventional medicines will be favorably avoided. Alternative therapies often include "nonspecific therapeutic effects" that go beyond the placebo effect and can be beneficial. Nonspecific effects include warmth and listening skills of the practitioner, empowerment that comes from legitimization of the patient's problem, and an egalitarian approach to care. These may be recognized as important constituents of the patient-centered approach. Physicians may wish to recommend alternative treatments and collaborate with alternative practitioners but should also be prepared to protect the patient by cautioning against treatments that are potentially harmful, excessively expensive, or that circumvent conventional treatments that are needed for demonstrated medical conditions.

F. Complications

Unidentified, nonconventional, alternative treatments may potentially have negative pharmacological interactions. Failure to recognize and properly treat somatoform complaints can lead to excessive diagnostic procedures and treatments, which perpetuate patient preoccupations and place the patient at risk for iatrogenic disorders. Sedative and analgesic/narcotic dependencies are common iatrogenic complications.

G. Patient Education Information

The American Academy of Family Physicians has developed a patient education handout for somatoform disorders. Information is similar to and expands on the key statements for somatization disorder appearing in Table 50–3. The web address for the handout is http://www.familydoctor.org/handouts/162.html.

Barksy AJ: A 37-year-old man with multiple somatic complaints. JAMA 1997;278:673.

Barsky AJ: The patient with hypochondriasis. New Engl J Med 2001;345(19):1395.

Blackwell B, DeMorgan NP: The primary care of patients who have bodily concerns. Arch Fam Med 1996;5:457.

Epstein RM, Quill TE, McWhinney IR: Somatization reconsidered: incorporating the patient's experience of illness. Arch Intern Med 1999;159(3):215.

Hahn SR et al: The difficult doctor-patient relationship: somatization, personality and psychopathology. J Clin Epidemiol 1994;47(6):647.

McCahill ME: Somatoform and related disorders: delivery of diagnosis as first step. Am Fam Physician 1995;52(1):193.

Righter EL, Sansone RA: Managing somatic preoccupation. Am Fam Physician 1999;59:3113.

Shaibani A, Sabbagh MN: Pseudoneurologic syndromes: recognition and diagnosis. Am Fam Physician 1998;57(10):2485.

Slaughter JR, Sun AM: In pursuit of perfection: a primary care physician's guide to body dysmorphic disorder. Am Fam Physician 1999;60(6):1738.

Stuart MR, Lieberman JA: *The Fifteen Minute Hour: Practical Therapeutic Inverventions in Primary Care,* ed 3. Elsevier Science, 2002.

Substance Use Disorders

51

Robert Mallin, MD

ESSENTIALS OF DIAGNOSIS

1. Screening positive (answering yes to two or more questions) on the CAGE questionnaire.
2. A pattern of substance misuse during which the patient maintains control over use (abuse) or during which control over use is lost (dependence).
3. The presence of a withdrawal syndrome.
4. A medical history of addiction to drugs or alcohol.
5. Depression, anxiety disorder, sleep disturbances, eating disorders, sexual dysfunction.

The diagnosis of substance use disorders is most typically begun with a screening test that identifies a user at risk. The CAGE questionnaire (Table 51–1) is perhaps the most widely used screening tool for the identification of patients at risk for substance use disorders. When a patient answers yes to two or more questions, the sensitivity of the CAGE is 60–90% and the specificity is 40–60% for substance use disorders. Because a screening test is more predictive when applied to a population more likely to have a disease, clinical clues (Table 51–2) to substance use disorders may be useful indicators in determining who to screen. Once a patient screens positive for a substance use problem it becomes necessary to determine whether the disorder involves abuse or dependence. Substance abuse is a pattern of misuse during which the patient maintains control, whereas in substance dependence, control over use is lost. Physiological dependence, evidenced by a withdrawal syndrome, may exist in either state (see Tables 51–3 and 51–4 for the diagnostic criteria for substance abuse and dependence). The primary means by which the diagnosis of substance abuse or dependence is made is a careful history. However, substance-disordered patients may be deliberately less than truthful in their history, and often the patient's denial prevents the physician from seeing the connection between substance use and its consequences. Biochemical markers may help support the diagnostic criteria gathered in the history, or can be used as a screening mechanism to consider patients for further evaluation (Table 51–5).

Reynaud M et al: Objective diagnosis of alcohol abuse: compared values of carbohydrate-deficient transferrin (CDT), gamma-glutamyl transferase (GGT), and mean corpuscular volume (MCV). Alcohol Clin Exp Res 2000;24(9):1414. [PMID: 11003208].

Staab JP et al: Detection and diagnosis of psychiatric disorders in primary medical care settings. Med Clin North Am 2001;85 (3):579. [PMID: 11349474].

General Considerations

The prevalence of alcohol and drug disorders in primary care outpatients is between 23% and 37%. The cost to society of these disorders is staggering. Each year in the United States substance use disorders are associated with 100,000 deaths and costs of approximately $100 billion. The high prevalence of these disorders in primary care outpatients suggests that family physicians are confronted with these problems daily. These disorders rarely present overtly, however. Patients in denial about the connection between their substance use and the consequences caused by it frequently minimize the amount of their use and often do not seek assistance for their substance use problem.

The epidemiology of alcohol and drug disorders has been well studied, and is most often reported from data of the National Institute of Mental Health Epidemiologic Catchment Area (ECA) Program. Lifetime prevalence rates for alcohol disorders from the ECA survey data were 13.5%. For men the lifetime prevalence was 23.8% and for women 4.7%. The National Comorbidity Survey indicated that lifetime prevalence rates of alcohol abuse without dependence were 12.5% for males and 6.4% for females and with dependence were 20.1% for males and 8.2% for females, The ECA data yield an

Table 51–1. CAGE questions adapted to include drugs.[1]

1. Have you felt you ought to **C**ut down on your drinking or drug use?
2. Have people **A**nnoyed you by criticizing your drinking or drug use?
3. Have you felt **G**uilty about your drinking or drug use?
4. Have you ever had a drink or used drugs first thing in the morning to steady your nerves or to get rid of a hangover or to get the day started? (**E**ye-opener)

Adapted from Schulz JE, Parran T Jr: Principles of identification and intervention. In: *Principles of Addiction Medicine,* ed 2. Graham AW, Shultz TK (editors). American Society of Addiction Medicine, 1998.
[1]Two or more yes answers indicates a need for a more in-depth assessment. Even one positive response should raise a red flag about problem drinking or drug use.

Table 51–2. Clinical clues of alcohol and drug problems.

Social history
    Arrest for driving under the influence of alcohol once (75% association with alcoholism) or twice (95% association)
    Loss of job or sent home from work for alcohol or drug reasons
    Domestic violence
    Child abuse/neglect
    Family instability (divorce, separation)
    Frequent, unplanned absences
    Personal isolation
    Problems at work/school
    Mood swings

Medical history
    History of addiction to any drug
    Withdrawal syndrome
    Depression
    Anxiety disorder
    Recurrent pancreatitis
    Recurrent hepatitis
    Hepatomegaly
    Peripheral neuropathy
    Myocardial infarction < age 30 (cocaine)
    Blood alcohol level >300 or >100 without impairment
    Alcohol on breath or intoxicated at office visit
    Tremor
    Mild hypertension
    Estrogen-mediated signs (telangectasias, spider angiomas, palmer erythema, muscle atrophy)
    Gastrointestinal complaints
    Sleep disturbances
    Eating disorders
    Sexual dysfunction

Table 51–3. *DSM-IV* criteria for substance abuse.

A maladaptive pattern of substance use, leading to clinically significant impairment or distress, as manifested by two (or more) of the following occurring at any time within a 12-month period:

1. Recurrent substance use resulting in failure to fulfill major role obligations at work, school, or home (eg, repeated absences or poor work performance related to substance use; substance-related absences, suspensions, or expulsions from school; neglect of children or household).
2. Recurrent substance use in situations in which it is physically hazardous (eg, driving an automobile or operating a machine when impaired by substance use).
3. Recurrent substance-related legal problems (eg, arrests for substance-related disorderly conduct).
4. Continued substance use despite having persistent social or interpersonal problems caused or exacerbated by the effects of the substance (eg, arguments with spouse about consequences of intoxication, physical fights).

The symptoms have never met the criteria for Substance Dependence for this class of substance.

Modified from American Psychiatric Association: *Diagnostic and Statistical Manual of Mental Disorders,* ed. 4. American Psychiatric Press, 1994.

overall prevalence of drug use disorders of 6.2%. As with alcohol use disorders, the lifetime prevalence rate of drug use disorders is higher in men (7.7%) than in women (4.8%). Characteristics known to influence the epidemiology of substance use disorders include gender, age, race, family history, marital status, employment status, and educational status.

Crum RM et al: The association of depression and problem drinking: analyses from the Baltimore ECA follow-up study. Epidemiologic Catchment Area. Addict Behav 2001;26(5):765. [PMID: 11676386].

Regier DA et al: Prevalence of anxiety disorders and their comorbidity with mood and addictive disorders. Br J Psychiatry Suppl 1998;(34):24. [PMID: 9829013].

Pathogenesis

The difference between abuse and dependence is important. With substance abuse, patients retain control of their use. This control may be affected by poor judgment and social and environmental factors, and mitigated by the consequences of the patients' use. Patients who become dependent (addicted) no longer have full control of their drug use. The brain has been "hijacked" by a substance of abuse that affects the mechanism of control over the use of that substance. This addiction is

Table 51–4. *DSM-IV criteria for
substance dependence.*

A maladaptive pattern of substance use, leading to clinically
significant impairment or distress, as manifested by three (or
more) of the following occurring at any time in the same
12-month period:

1. Tolerance as defined by either of the following:
   a. A need for markedly increased amounts of the sub-
      stance to achieve intoxication or the desired effect.
   b. Markedly diminished effect with continued use of the
      same amount of the substance.
2. Withdrawal, as manifested by either of the following:
   a. The characteristic withdrawal syndrome for the sub-
      stance.
   b. The same (or closely related) substance is taken to re-
      lieve or avoid withdrawal symptoms.
3. The substance is often taken in larger amounts or over a
   longer period than was intended.
4. There is a persistent desire or unsuccessful efforts to cut
   down or control substance use.
5. A great deal of time is spent in activities necessary to obtain the substance, use the substance, or recover from its
   effects.
6. Important social, occupational, or recreational activities are
   given up or reduced because of substance use.
7. The substance use is continued despite knowledge of having a persistant or recurrent physical or psychological
   problem that is likely to have been caused or exacerbated
   by the substance.

Modified from American Psychiatric Association: *Diagnostic and
Statistical Manual of Mental Disorders,* ed. 4. American Psychiatric
Press, 1994.

far more than physical dependence. The need to use the
drug becomes as powerful as the drives of thirst and
hunger. Evidence that the brains of addicted individuals are different from those of nonaddicted persons is
enormous. Many of these abnormalities predate the use
of the substance and are thought to be inherited. In genetically predisposed individuals, substances of abuse
cause changes in the dopaminergic mesolimbic system
that result in a loss of control over substance use. These

changes are mediated by a number of neurotransmitters: dopamine, γ-aminobutyric acid (GABA), glutamate, serotonin, and endorphins. The different classes
of substances of abuse act through one or more of these
neurotransmitters, ultimately affecting the level of
dopamine in the mesolimbic system, otherwise known
as the reward pathway. These changes in the brain are
permanent and are the primary reason for relapse in an
addicted patient trying to maintain abstinence or control of use.

Prevention

Although neurobiology plays a large role in addiction,
the precursors of substance abuse are also environmental in nature and include family, school, community,
and peer factors (Table 51–6). These multiple factors
make effective prevention very difficult. Primary prevention is designed to discourage the use of substances,
thereby making abuse impossible. These programs are
designed primarily for the young. In secondary prevention screening programs are used to identify abuse early
and to redirect the patient's behavior before addiction
becomes overt. In tertiary prevention the focus is on the
treatment of addictive behavior in an effort to prevent
the consequences of compulsive use. Prevention programs can be divided into those that address the four
environmental areas of risk: family, school, peers, and
community. Family physicians can include behaviors
within their practice that support these efforts (Table
51–7).

Botvin GJ, Griffin KW: Life skills training as a primary prevention approach for adolescent drug abuse and other problem
behaviors. Int J Emerg Ment Health 2002;4(1):41. [PMID:
12014292].

Kodjo CM, Klein JD: Prevention and risk of adolescent substance
abuse. The role of adolescents, families, and communities. Pediatr Clin North Am 2002;49(2):257. [PMID: 11993282].

Clinical Findings

The signs and symptoms of substance abuse are varied
and often subtle. This is complicated by the fact that
most patients do not recognize their substance use as

Table 51–5. Biochemical markers of substance use disorders.

Marker	Substance	Sensitivity (%)	Specificity (%)	Predictive Value (%)
Mean corpuscular volume (MCV)	Alcohol	24	96	63
γ-Glutamyltransferase (GGT)	Alcohol	42	76	61
Carbohydrate-deficient transferrin (CDT)	Alcohol	67	97	84

Table 51–6. Environmental risk factors for substance abuse.

Family factors
    Sexual or physical abuse
    Parental or sibling substance abuse
    Parental approval or tacit approval of child's substance use
    Disruptive family conflict
    Poor communication
    Poor discipline
    Poor supervision
    Parental rejection
School factors
    Lack of involvement in school activities
    Poor school climate
    Norms that condone substance use
    Unfair rules
    School failure
Community factors
    Poor community bonding
    Disorganized neighborhoods
    Crime
    Drug use
    Poverty
    Low employment
    Community norms that condone substance use
Peer factors
    Bonding to peer group that engages in substance use or other antisocial behaviors

the cause of their problems and are often quite resistant to accepting evidence that it is. Consequently the family physician must have a high index of suspicion, realizing that the prevalence of substance use disorders in outpatient primary care is as high as 20%. A perspective that recognizes the prevalence of these disorders will enable physicians to interpret signs such as those described in Table 51–2 as potential clues to substance use.

Table 51–7. Family physician's role in substance abuse prevention

1. Support efforts to strengthen parenting skills, family support, and communication.
2. Patient and community education about drug and alcohol use, abuse, and treatment.
3. Screen and assess patients of all ages for substance use disorder in the office and hospital.
4. Support community efforts in substance abuse prevention.
5. Endorse and promote public policy that supports prevention, early detection, and treatment of substance use disorders

Exploring a patient's history of substance use (Table 51–8) when presented with these problems is an effective tool for case finding in substance use disorders. Signs of sedative hypnotic or alcohol withdrawal may be misinterpreted as anxiety disorder. Chronic use of stimulants may present as a psychotic disorder. In fact, in the presence of active substance abuse other psychiatric diagnoses often must await patient detoxification before they can be accurately assessed. Physical dependence, although not always seen with substance abuse, suggests abuse unless the patient is on long-term prescribed addictive medicines. The signs and symptoms of withdrawal from alcohol and other sedative hypnotic drugs are found in Table 51–9. Alcohol withdrawal may be life threatening if not properly treated. Opiate withdrawal (Table 51–10) is not life threatening and neither is withdrawal from cocaine or other stimulants (Table 51–11), although they both may be associated with morbidity and relapse to substance abuse.

In dealing with sedative hypnotic, alcohol, or opiate withdrawal, assessment of the degree of withdrawal is important to determine appropriate use and dose of medication to reduce symptoms and, in the case of sedative hypnotic drugs or alcohol, prevent seizures and mortality. The Clinical Institute Withdrawal Assessment Scale (Table 51–12) allows the signs and symptoms of withdrawal to be quantified in a predictable fashion that allows clinicians to discuss the severity of withdrawal for a given patient and thus choose intervention strategies that are effective and safe.

Differential Diagnosis

Because substance abuse is a behavioral disorder, when considering a differential diagnosis, psychiatric disorders often come to mind. Indeed, there is a high comorbidity between substance use disorders and psychiatric disorders. Approximately 50% of psychiatric patients have a substance use disorder. For patients with addictions, however, the rates of psychiatric disorders are similar to the general population. Problems such as substance-induced mood disorders (frequently noted in alcohol, opiate, and stimulant abuse) and substance-induced psychotic disorders (most frequently associated with stimulant abuse) complicate differentiating the primary psychiatric disorders from those that are primarily substance use disorders. Most clinicians agree that psychiatric disorders cannot be reliably assessed in patients who are currently or recently intoxicated. Thus detoxification and a period of abstinence are necessary before evaluation for other psychiatric disorders may effectively be done.

Other than the dilemma of determining if there is a substance-induced or comorbid psychiatric disorder,

Table 51–8. Elements of the substance use history.

1. Determine the type, frequency, route of administration, and amount of substance use
   a. Alcohol
   b. Tobacco
   c. Other drugs
      i. Cocaine
      ii. Marijuana
      iii. Others
2. Determine consequences of substance use; ask about the following:
   a. Legal problems
      i. Arrests (DUI, public intoxication, disorderly conduct, etc)
      ii. Civil suits for financial problems, bankruptcy, etc
   b. Social problems
      i. Social isolation
   c. Family problems
      i. Marital problems
      ii. Parenting problems
      iii. Domestic violence
      iv. Family members with depression
      v. Divorce
   d. Work or school problems
      i. Frequent absences
      ii. Poor performance
      iii. Frequent job changes
   e. Financial problems
      i. Significant debt
      ii. Selling personal possessions
      iii. Stealing and selling possessions of others
   f. Psychological problems
      i. Agitation
      ii. Irritability
      iii. Anxiety
      iv. Panic attacks
      v. Mood swings
      vi. Hostility
      vii. Violence
      viii. Sleep disturbance
      ix. Sexual dysfunction
      x. Depression
      xi. Blackouts
   g. Medical problems
      i. Gastritis
      ii. Peptic ulcer
      iii. Abdominal pain
      iv. Hypertension
      v. Peripheral neuropathy
      vi. Nasal septum perforation
      vii. Vasospasm
      viii. Dysrhythmias
      ix. Weight loss
      x. HIV
      xi. Skin abscesses
      xii. Trauma

Table 51–9. Signs and symptoms of alcohol withdrawal.

Development of a combination of the following several hours after cessation of a prolonged period of heavy drinking.

1. Autonomic hyperactivity: diaphoresis, tachycardia, elevated blood pressure
2. Tremor
3. Insomnia
4. Nausea or vomiting
5. Transient visual, tactile, or auditory hallucinations or illusions
6. Psychomotor agitation
7. Anxiety
8. Generalized seizure activity

differential diagnosis in substance abuse revolves around the issues of abuse versus dependence. The essential difference is a loss of control over use in dependence that is not present in abuse. This is further complicated by the chronic and waxing and waning nature of substance use disorders. As a result it is necessary to examine the behavior of patients over an extended period of time, looking for evidence of past loss of control of use that may not currently be present. Usually in addiction a pattern of progressively increasing loss of control becomes evident as the consequences of chronic substance abuse unfold.

Complications

The medical complications from substance abuse are legion and profoundly affect the health of our population. The number of deaths attributed to the abuse of substances exceeds 500,000 yearly, with tobacco (see Chapter 52) accounting for 380,000 of these deaths. Cardiovascular disease and cancer lead this list. Alcohol causes approximately 100,000 deaths yearly and is associated with motor vehicle accidents, other accidents,

Table 51–10. Signs and symptoms of opioid withdrawal.

1. Mild elevation of pulse rate, respiratory rate, blood pressure, and temperature.
2. Piloerection (gooseflesh)
3. Dysphoric mood, drug craving
4. Lacrimation and or rhinorrhea
5. Mydriasis, yawning, diaphoresis
6. Anorexia, abdominal cramps, vomiting, diarrhea
7. Insomnia
8. Weakness

Table 51–11. Signs and symptoms of cocaine or stimulant withdrawal.

1. Dysphoric mood
2. Fatigue, malaise
3. Vivid unpleasant dreams
4. Sleep disturbance
5. Increased appetite
6. Psychomotor retardation or agitation

homicides, cirrhosis of the liver, and suicide. Injection drug use is responsible for the fastest growing population of human immunodeficiency virus (HIV) infection (see Table 51–13 for common medical complications from substance abuse). In addition to medical complications, substance abuse causes considerable neuropsychiatric morbidity, both as a primary cause (Table 51–14) as well as by exacerbating existing psychiatric disorders.

Acute substance-induced psychosis is often indistinguishable from a primary psychotic disorder such as schizophrenia in the setting of substance abuse. Neurocognitive states such as dementia may be substance induced and result in permanent brain damage. Depression, commonly diagnosed and treated in the primary care setting, may often be complicated by a substance-induced mood disorder. Often what appears to be treatment-resistant depression is actually the result of persistent substance abuse. Withdrawal syndromes often present as episodes of anxiety, sleep disorders, mood disorders, or seizure disorders.

Mallin R et al: Detection of substance use disorders in patients presenting with depression. Substance Abuse 2002;23(2):115.

Treatment

Many substance use disorders resolve spontaneously or with brief interventions on the part of physicians or other authority figures in the workplace, legal system, family, or society. This occurs because patients with a substance abuse disorder continue to maintain control over their use, and when the consequences of that use outweigh the benefits of the drug, they choose to quit. Patients with substance dependence disorders, on the other hand, have, by definition, impaired control. They rarely get better without assistance.

Substance use disorders can be treated successfully. Brief interventions and outpatient, inpatient, and residential treatment programs reduce morbidity and mortality associated with substance abuse and dependence. Determining the type and intensity of treatment that are best for a given patient may be difficult. The American Society of Addiction Medicine has developed

guidelines for clinicians to help determine the level and intensity of treatment for patients (Table 51–15). Once patients have been adequately assessed treatment can begin. Detoxification, patient education, identification of defenses, overcoming denial, relapse prevention, orientation to 12-step recovery programs, and family services are the goals of substance abuse treatment.

A. INTERVENTION

Once screening and diagnosis are complete, it is time for physicians to share their assessment with the patient. Because of the nature of substance abuse, patients rarely choose to seek help for their alcohol or drug problem until the negative consequences of their addiction far outweigh the positive aspects of treatment. Intervention may be seen as a means of bringing these consequences to the attention of the patient. This can be accomplished by a wide range of approaches, some quite informal and others carefully orchestrated and executed. Physicians or family members can often intervene simply by providing patients with feedback about their behavior, describing the feelings generated by that behavior, avoiding enabling behavior, and offering help.

The traditional intervention for alcohol or drug addiction is a formal process, best accomplished by an addictions specialist trained in this process. This approach is often effective, resulting in positive results in about 80% of cases. Although effective, the traditional, formal model of intervention is often less than ideal for the family physician. Specialist involvement and orchestration of significant relationships of the patient are sometimes difficult to achieve. In addition, if the intervention fails, it may become difficult if not impossible for the physician to continue a relationship with the patient. Another approach to consider is that of the brief intervention. This highly effective approach to intervention is based on motivational interviewing and the stages of change.

1. Stages of change—Underlying the strategy of the brief intervention is the model known as the stages of change. Changing of behavior is described as a process that evolves over time, through a series of changes: precontemplation, contemplation, preparation, action, maintenance, and termination. The individual must progress through each of these stages to get to the next and cannot leap past one to get to another.

In **precontemplation** an individual is not planning to take any action in the foreseeable future. This is the stage most often described as denial. Patients do not perceive their behavior as problematic. In **contemplation** people perceive that they have a problem and believe they should do something about it. Many addicted patients who do not appear to be ready for traditional treatment programs are in this stage. They recognize that they have a substance problem, believe

Table 51–12. Clinical Institute withdrawal assessment scale (CIWA).

Patient_____ Date_____ Time_____ BP___/___

Age_____ Race/Sex_____ Drugs of choice (Primary)_____ Other_____

1. Autonomic hyperactivity:
   Pulse rate/minute
   0 <80
   1 81–100
   2 101–110
   3 111–120
   4 121–130
   5 131–140
   6 141–150
   7 >150
   Sweating (observation)
   0 No sweating
   1 Barely perceptible sweating, palms moist
   2
   3
   4 Beads of sweat obvious on forehead
   5
   6
   7 Drenching sweats

2. Hand tremor: arms extended and fingers spread apart:
   Observation
   0 No tremor
   1 Not visible
   2
   3
   4 Moderate with patient's arms extended
   5
   6
   7 Severe, even with arms not extended

3. Anxiety: Ask, "Do you feel nervous or anxious?"
   Observation
   0 No anxiety, at ease
   1 Mildly anxious
   2
   3
   4 Moderately anxious
   5
   6
   7 Severe, equivalent to panic

   Total Score_____ Max Score = 56

   Rater's initials_____

4. Transient tactile, auditory, or visual disturbances: Ask, "Have you itching, pins, and needle sensations, any burning or numbness, or do you feel bugs crawling on or under your skin?" Are you more aware of sounds around you and are they harsh? Are you hearing things that you kknow are not there? Does the light appear too bright? Does it hurt your eyes? Are you seeing anything that is disturbing to you?
   Observation
   0 Not present
   1 Present but minimal
   2
   3 Moderate
   4 Frequent
   5
   6
   7 Hallucinations almost continuous

5. Agitation:
   Observation
   0 Normal activity
   1 Somewhat more than normal activity
   2
   3
   4 Moderately fidgety and restless
   5
   6
   7 Paces back and forth during most of the interview, or con-stantly thrashes about

6. Nausea or vomiting: Ask, "Do you feel sick to your stomach or have you vomited?" Include recorded vomiting since last observation:
   Observation
   0 Not present
   1 Very mild
   2
   3
   4 Moderate
   5
   6
   7 Severe

7. Headache: Ask, "Does your head feel full?" "Does it feel like there is a band around your head?" Don't rate for lightheadedness. Other-wise rate:
   Severity
   0 Not present
   1 Very mild
   2
   3
   4 Moderate
   5
   6
   7 Severe

Table 51–13. Medical complications of substance abuse.

Drug	Medical Complication
Alcohol	Trauma
	Hypertension
	Cardiomyopathy
	Dysrhythmias
	Ischemic heart disease
	Hemorrhagic stroke
	Esophageal reflux
	Barret's esophagus
	Mallory–Weiss tears
	Esophageal cancer
	Acute gastritis
	Pancreatitis
	Chronic diarrhea malabsorption
	Alcoholic hepatitis
	Cirrhosis
	Hepatic failure
	Hepatic carcinoma
	Nasopharyngeal cancer
	Headache
	Sleep disorders
	Memory impairment
	Dementia
	Peripheral neuropathy
	Fetal alcohol syndrome
	Sexual dysfunction
	Substance-induced mood disorders
	Substance-induced psychotic disorders
	Immune dysfunction
Cocaine (other stimulants)	Chest pain
	Congestive heart failure
	Cardiac dysrhythmias
	Cardiovascular collapse
	Seizures
	Cerebrovascular accidents
	Headache
	Spontaneous pneumothorax
	Noncardiogenic pulmonary edema
	Nasal septal perforations
Injection drug use	Hepatitis C, B
	HIV infection
	Subacute endocarditis
	Soft tissue abscesses

Table 51–14. Neuropsychiatric complications of substance abuse.

Substance-induced mood disorder, depressed/elevated
Substance-induced anxiety disorder
Substance-induced psychotic disorder
Substance-induced personality change
Substance intoxication
Substance withdrawal
Delirium
Wernicke's disease
Korsakoff syndrome (alcohol-induced persisting amnestic disorder)
Transient amnestic states (blackouts)
Substance-induced persisting dementia

abstinence is the generally agreed upon behavior that signifies action. **Maintenance** is the period after action during which the changed behavior persists and the patient works toward preventing relapse. Maintenance often requires a longer sustained effort than patients anticipate, and failure to continue with maintenance behavior is a common cause of relapse. **Termination** describes the stage in which there is no temptation and there is no risk of returning to old habits. In the case of

Table 51–15. American Society of Addiction Medicine placement criteria.

Levels of service

Level 0.5:	Early intervention
Level I:	Outpatient services
Level II:	Intensive outpatient/partial hospitalization services
Level III:	Resident/inpatient services
Level IV:	Medically managed intensive inpatient services

Assessment dimensions
1. Acute intoxication and/or withdrawal potential
2. Biomedical conditions and complications
3. Emotional/behavioral conditions and complications (eg, psychiatric conditions, psychological or emotional/behavioral complications if known or unknown origin, poor impulse control, changes in mental status, transient neuropsychiatric complications)
4. Treatment acceptance/resistance
5. Relapse/continued use potential
6. Recovery/living environment

From Mee-Lee D, Shulman G, Gartner L: *Patient Placement Criteria for the Treatment of Substance-Related Disorders,* ed. 2. American Society of Addiction Medicine, 1996.

that they should stop using the addictive substance, but seem unable to do so. In **preparation** patients have made a decision to change and plan to do so soon, usually within the next month. These patients are ready to enter action-oriented treatment programs. **Action** refers to the stage of change during which patients make specific changes in their behavior. In the case of addiction,

addiction, most patients must work toward a lifetime of maintenance rather than termination. The risk of relapse is such that few truly reach this final stage for the disease of addiction.

2. Brief interventions—Presenting the diagnosis of a substance use disorder by itself may be viewed as a brief intervention. Most physicians who have worked with these patients will not be surprised to learn that as many as 70% of patients are in the precontemplation or contemplation stage when presented with the diagnosis. The resistance associated with these stages tends to force the clinician into one of two modalities—either avoiding the diagnosis or confronting and arguing with the patient. Both of these approaches are futile. One approach in presenting the diagnosis is to use the DEATH glossary (Table 51–16), a list of pitfalls to avoid when presenting the diagnosis of addiction. On a more positive note, the SOAPE glossary (Table 51–17) describes suggestions to use when talking to patients about their addiction.

Table 51–16. DEATH glossary: pitfalls to avoid when presenting the diagnosis.

Drinking or drug use details are not relevant; talking with a drunk is not useful. Patients will often give long and complex explanations for their drug or alcohol use and why they do not have a problem with it. It may be necessary to interrupt these explanations and move on. In addition, patients who are intoxicated cannot process the information given to them and it is appropriate to reschedule them and ask them not to drink prior to that visit.

Etiology: Patients may try to elicit or provide an explanation for their addiction. It is unlikely that this will be useful. Just as when treating other chronic illnesses without clear etiologies, it is important to focus on the evidence for the diagnosis and the plan for treatment, and not be distracted by theoretical discussions of etiology.

Arguments: Arguments can seriously damage the patient–physician relationship and should be avoided at all costs. Respect, sympathy, and support are your best defenses against arguments.

Threats: Threats are a serious cause of damage to the therapeutic relationship; threats, guilt, and shame do not promote recovery.

Hedging: Although arguments are detrimental, there should be no hedging on the diagnosis. If the patient appears unable to accept the diagnosis, an agreement to disagree should be made as well as another appointment to continue the discussion.

Modified from Schulz JE, Parran T Jr: Principles of identification and intervention. In: *Principles of Addiction Medicine,* ed. 2. Graham AW, Shultz TK (editors). American Society of Addiction Medicine, 1998.

Table 51–17. SOAPE glossary for presenting the diagnosis.

Support: Use phrases such as "we need to work together on this," "I am concerned about you and will follow up closely with you," and "As with all medical illnesses the more people you work with, the better you will feel." These words reinforce the physician–patient relationship, strengthen the collaborative model of chronic illness management, and help convince the patient that the physician will not just present the diagnosis and leave.

Optimism: Most patients have controlled their alcohol or drug use at times and may have quit for periods of time. They may expect failure. By giving a strong optimistic message such as "You can get well," "Treatment works," and "You can expect to see improvements in many areas of your life," the physican can motivate the patient.

Absolution: By describing addiction as a disease and telling patients that they are not responsible for having an illness, but that now only they can take responsibility for their recovery, the physician can lessen the burden of guilt and shame that is often a barrier to recovery.

Plan: Having a plan is important to the acceptance of the illness. Using readiness to change categories can help in designing a plan that uses the patient's willingness to move ahead. Indicating that abstinence is desirable, but recognizing that all patients will not be able to commit to that goal immediately can help prevent a sense of failure early in the process. Ask "What do you think you will be able to do at this point?"

Explanatory model: Understanding the patient's beliefs about addiction may be important. Many patients believe this is a moral weakness and that they lack willpower. An explanation that willpower cannot resolve illnesses such as diabetes or alcoholism may go a long way to reassure the patient that recovery is possible.

Modified from Clark WD: Alcoholism: blocks to diagnosis and treatment. Am J Med 1981;71:285.

Even for patients in the precontemplative stage at presentation of the diagnosis, continued use of the brief intervention strategy will ultimately reduce the amount of drug use if not result in abstinence.

Brief interventions should include some of the elements of motivational interviewing. These include offering empathetic, objective feedback of data, meeting patient expectations, working with ambivalence, assessing barriers and strengths, reinterpreting past experience in light of current medical consequences, negotiating a follow-up plan, and providing hope.

B. DETOXIFICATION

Detoxification and treatment of withdrawal and any medical complications must have first priority. Alcohol and other sedative hypnotic drugs share the same neurobiological withdrawal process. Chronic use of this class of drugs results in down-regulation of the GABA receptors throughout the central nervous system. GABA is an inhibitory neurotransmitter that is uniformly depressed during sedative hypnotic use. Abrupt cessation of sedative hypnotic drug use results in an up-regulation of GABA receptors and a relative paucity of GABA for inhibition. The result is stimulation of the autonomic nervous system and the appearance of the signs and symptoms listed in Table 51–9. Withdrawal seizures are a common manifestation of sedative hypnotic withdrawal, occurring in 11–33% of patients withdrawing from alcohol.

Alcohol withdrawal seizures are best treated with benzodiazepines and by addressing the withdrawal process itself. Long-term treatment for alcohol withdrawal seizures is not recommended and phenytoin should not be used to treat seizures associated with alcohol withdrawal. The cornerstones of treatment for alcohol withdrawal syndrome are the benzodiazepines. All drugs that provide cross-tolerance with alcohol are effective in reducing the symptoms and sequelae of alcohol withdrawal, but none has the safety profile and evidence of efficacy of the benzodiazepines (see Table 51–18 for recommendations in the treatment of alcohol withdrawal). Opiate withdrawal may not be life threatening, but the symptoms are significant enough

Table 51–18. Treatment regimens for alcohol withdrawal.

Use the Clinical Institute Withdrawal Assessment (CIWA) for monitoring

    Do the CIWA scale every 4 h until the score is below 8 for 24 h

    For CIWA >10

        Give chlordiazepoxide 50–100 mg or diazepam 10–20 mg or oxazepam 30–60 mg or lorazepam 2–4 mg

    Repeat the CIWA 1 h after the dose to assess the need for further medication

Non-symptom-driven regimens

    For patients likely to experience withdrawal use chlordiazepoxide 50 mg every 6 h for four doses followed by 50 mg every 8 h for three doses, followed by 50 mg every 12 h for two doses, and finally by 50 mg at bedtime for one dose

    Other benzodiazepines may be substituted at equivalent doses

Patients on a predetermined dosing schedule should be monitored frequently both for breakthrough withdrawal symptoms as well as for excessive sedation

---

that without support most patients will not remain in treatment (see Table 51–19 for recommendations in the treatment of opiate withdrawal). The symptoms of cocaine and other stimulant withdrawal are somewhat less predictable and much harder to improve. Despite multiple studies with many different drug classes, no medications have been shown to reliably reduce the symptoms and craving associated with cocaine withdrawal.

C. PATIENT EDUCATION

Patients' knowledge and understanding of the nature of substance use disorders are the key to their recovery. For patients still in control of their use, education about appropriate substance use will help them to choose responsibly if they continue to use. For patients who meet the criteria for substance dependence (addiction), abstinence is the only safe recommendation. Once having made the transition to addiction, patients can never reliably use addictive substances again. The neurobiological changes in the brain are permanent, and loss of control may occur any time the brain is presented with an addictive substance. Unfortunately this loss of control can be unpredictable. Consequently addicted patients may find that they can use for a variable period of time with control, which gives them the false impression that they were never addicted in the first place or perhaps that they have been cured. Invariably if they continue to use addictive substances they will again lose control and begin to experience consequences at or above the level that they did before. Understanding that the problem of addiction is a chronic

Table 51–19. Treatment for opioid withdrawal.

Methadone: A pure opioid agonist restricted by federal legislation to inpatient treatment or specialized outpatient drug treatment programs. Initial dosage is 15–20 mg for 2–3 days, then tapered with a 10–15% reduction in dose daily guided by patient's symptoms and clinical findings.

Clonidine: An α-adrenergic blocker, 0.2 mg every 4 h to relieve symptoms of withdrawal, may be effective. Hypotension is a risk and sometimes limits the dose. It can be continued for 10–14 days and tapered by the third day by 0.2 mg daily.

Buprenorphine: This partial μ receptor agonist can be administered sublingually in doses of 2, 4, or 8 mg every 4 h for the management of opioid withdrawal symptoms.

Naltrexone/clonidine: A rapid form of opioid detoxification involves pretreatment with 0.2–0.3 mg of clonidine followed by 12.5 mg of naltrexone (a pure opioid antagonist). Naltrexone is increased to 25 mg on the second day, 50 mg on Day 3, and 100 mg on Day 4, with clonidine given at 0.1–0.3 mg three times daily.

---

disorder for which there is remission but not cure becomes essential. The question then becomes not whether to remain abstinent but rather how to remain abstinent.

D. IDENTIFICATION OF DEFENSES AND OVERCOMING DENIAL

During this phase of treatment patients typically work in a group therapy setting and are encouraged to look at the defenses that have prevented them from seeking help sooner. Denial can best be defined as the inability to see the causal relationship between drug use and its consequences. Thus patients who believe they drank because they lost their job may be encouraged to consider that they lost their job because they drank.

E. RELAPSE PREVENTION

Once patients are educated about the nature of their disease and have identified destructive defense mechanisms, relapse prevention becomes the primary goal. Identification of triggers for alcohol and drug use, plans to prevent opportunities to relapse, and new ways to deal with problems help patients to maintain their abstinence. In most treatment programs a relapse prevention plan will be developed and individualized for each patient.

F. TWELVE-STEP RECOVERY PROGRAMS

It would be difficult to overstate the contribution 12-step programs make to recovery. Despite millions of dollars in research, and the efforts of a large segment of the scientific community, there has been no treatment, medication, or psychotherapy that has taken the place of the 12 steps (Table 51–20).

Twelve-step recovery has its roots in Alcoholics Anonymous (AA). AA as a fellowship was founded in 1935 by a New York stockbroker and by a physician from Akron who found that they could stay sober by working with each other and helping other alcoholics. The program of AA is the 12 steps that were published and explained in the textbook *Alcoholics Anonymous* in 1939. The steps are best described in the foreword of *The Twelve Steps and Twelve Traditions*: "A.A.'s Twelve Steps are a group of principles, spiritual in their nature, which, if practiced as a way of life, can expel the obsession to drink and enable the sufferer to become happily and usefully whole." The *fellowship* of alcoholics is best described in the preamble: "Alcoholics Anonymous is a fellowship of men and women who share their experience, strength and hope with each other that they may solve their common problem and help others to recover from alcoholism. The only requirement for membership is a desire to stop drinking. There are no dues for AA membership, we are self supporting through our

Table 51–20. The 12 steps of Alcoholics Anonymous.

We:
1. Admitted we were powerless over alcohol—that our lives had become unmanageable;
2. Came to believe that a Power greater than ourselves could restore us to sanity;
3. Made a decision to turn our will and our lives over to the care of God *as we understood Him;*
4. Made a searching and fearless moral inventory of ourselves;
5. Admitted to ourselves, and to another human being the exact nature of our wrongs;
6. Were entirely ready to have God remove all these defects of character;
7. Humbly asked Him to remove our shortcomings;
8. Made a list of all persons we had harmed, and became willing to make amends to them all;
9. Made direct amends to such people wherever possible, except when to do so would injure them or others;
10. Continued to take personal inventory and when we were wrong promptly admitted it;
11. Sought through prayer and meditation to improve our conscious contact with God *as we understand Him,* praying only for knowledge of His will for us and the power to carry that out;
12. Having had a spiritual awakening as the result of these steps, we tried to carry this message to alcoholics, and to practice these principles in all our affairs.

From Alcoholics Anonymous World Service.

own contributions. AA is not allied with any sect, denomination, politics, organization, or institution; does not wish to engage in any controversy; neither endorses nor opposes any causes. Our primary purpose is to stay sober and help other alcoholics to achieve sobriety."

There are over 200 spin-off recovery organizations that have used the 12 steps with some modifications. Important other 12-step programs for patients with substance use disorders include Al-Anon, for friends and family of alcoholics, Narcotics Anonymous (NA), for those with drug problems other than alcohol, and Cocaine Anonymous, for those with cocaine addiction. At the heart of each of these fellowships is the program of recovery outlined in the 12 steps. AA and related 12-step programs are spiritual, not religious in nature. No one is told they must believe in anything including God. Agnostics and atheists are welcome in AA and are not asked to convert to any religious belief. Newcomers in AA are encouraged to go to meetings regularly (daily is wise initially), obtain a sponsor, and begin work on the 12 steps. A sponsor is usually someone of the same sex who is in stable recovery and has worked the steps. The sponsor helps guide the newcomer through the steps and provides a source of information and encouragement. At meetings members share their experience, strength, and hope concerning their recovery. In this fashion, storytelling often becomes the means by which information about strategies for recovery is relayed. AA meetings vary in their composition and structure, given that one of the traditions of AA is that each group is autonomous. Consequently if a patient feels uncomfortable at one meeting another may be more acceptable. There are meetings for women or men only, for young people, for doctors, for lawyers, and for virtually any special interest group in most large cities. There is often a great deal of confusion about what AA does and does not do. AA is not treatment. Despite the close connection many treatment programs have with 12-step recovery fellowships, these fellowships are not affiliated with treatment centers by design. Table 51–21 lists some of the self-described limitations of AA and other 12-step groups.

From multiple sources, it appears clear that AA and other 12-step recovery programs are among the most effective tools we have to combat substance disorders. About 6–10% of the population have been to an AA meeting during their lives. This number doubles for those with alcohol problems. Although 50% of those who come to AA leave, of those who stay for a year 67% stay sober, of those who stay for 2 years 85% stay sober, and of those who stay sober for 5 years, 90% remain sober indefinitely. Outcome studies of 8087 patients treated in 57 different inpatient and outpatient treatment programs showed that those attending AA at 1 year follow-up were 50% more likely to be abstinent than those not attending. Adolescents studied were found to be four times more likely to be abstinent if they attended AA/NA when compared to those who did not. Finally, in an effort to identify which groups in AA did better than others, studies of involvement in AA (defined as service work, having a sponsor, leading meetings, etc) found that those who were involved, as compared to those just attending meetings, did better in maintaining abstinence.

Having a list of AA members willing to escort potential new members to meetings is a powerful tool for physicians to help patients into recovery. Generally in every AA district there is a person identified as the chair of the Cooperation with Professional Community Committee who can help physicians identify people willing to perform this service. Al-Anon and NA have similar contacts. The telephone numbers for most of these 12-step groups can be found in the phone book. These contacts can often supply the physician with relevant literature to help dispel some of the myths patients may hold regarding 12-step recovery. Patients will often use these myths as excuses for why AA will not work for them. Seeing this as resistance and ambivalence about entering a life of recovery is important for the physician. Family physicians are in a unique position to encourage their patients to invest in 12-step recovery. Recovering persons are keenly aware of this fact and physicians are encouraged to attend and are welcomed at open AA and other 12-step meetings to become more familiar with the way they work.

G. Pharmacology

Agents useful in the treatment of withdrawal have already been discussed in the section on detoxification. Here the discussion will be limited to agents used to help prevent relapse into alcohol or other drug use. These drugs attempt to impact drug use by one of several mechanisms:

1. Sensitizing the body's response, resulting in a negative reaction to ingesting the drug and causing an aversion reaction, such as with disulfram and alcohol.

2. Reducing the reinforcing effects of a drug, such as the use of naltrexone in alcoholism.

3. Blocking the effects of a drug by binding to the receptor site, such as naltrexone for opiates.

4. Saturating the receptor sites by agonists, such as the use of methadone in opioid maintainance therapy.

5. Unique approaches such as the creation of an immunization to cocaine.

Drug therapy for addiction holds promise. As our understanding of the neurobiology of addiction im-

Table 51–21. Limitations of 12-step groups.

AA does not solicit members; it will only reach out to people who ask for help.

AA does not keep records of membership (although some AA groups will provide phone lists for group members).

AA does not engage in research.

There is no formal control or follow-up on members by AA.

AA does not make medical or psychiatric diagnoses. Each member needs to decide if he or she is an addict.

AA as a whole does not provide housing, food, clothing, jobs, or money to newcomers (although individual members may do this).

AA is self-supporting through its own members' contributions; it does not accept money from outside sources.

From *A Brief Guide to Alcoholics Anonymous.* Alcoholics Anonymous World Service Inc., 1972.

proves, so does the chance that we can intervene at a molecular level to prevent relapse. At the current level, however, pharmacotherapy to prevent relapse must be relegated to an adjunctive position. No drug alone has provided sufficient power to prevent relapse to addictive behavior. Still in some patients the use of appropriate medication may provide the edge necessary to move closer to recovery.

1. Pharmacological treatment for alcoholism—

a. Disulfram—Disulfram inhibits aldehyde dehydrogenase, the enzyme that catalyzes the oxidation of acetaldehyde to acetic acid. Thus, if a patient taking disulfram ingests alcohol, the acetaldehyde levels rise. The result is referred to as the disulfram–ethanol reaction. This manifests as flushing of the skin, palpitations, decreased blood pressure, nausea, vomiting, shortness of breath, blurred vision, and confusion. The reactions are usually related to the dose of both disulfram and alcohol. This reaction can be severe and with doses of disulfram over 500 mg and 2 ounces of alcohol death has been reported. Common side effects of disulfram include drowsiness, lethargy, peripheral neuropathy, hepatotoxicity, and hypertension.

In the United States, doses of 250–500 mg are most commonly used. Because of individual variability in the disulfram–ethanol reaction, these doses often do not produce a reaction sufficient to deter the patient from drinking. In the United Kingdom, it is common to do an ethanol challenge test to determine the dose needed to result in an aversion effect. Whether disulfram is actually effective in preventing relapse is the subject of some debate. Most studies have failed to show a statistically significant result. On closer examination, it appears that compliance with the medication appears to be the most important factor. In a large Veterans Administration multicenter study, a direct relationship between compliance with drug therapy and abstinence was found. In addition, the involvement of a patient's spouse in observing the patient's consumption of disulfram results in considerable improvement in outcome. It appears that disulfram can be a useful adjunct for patients who have a history of sudden relapse and who have a social situation in which compliance may be adequately monitored.

b. Naltrexone—Naltrexone, an opioid antagonist, has been shown to reduce drinking in animal studies and in human alcoholics. Initial optimism over the potential of this discovery was tempered by several studies indicating that the effects of reducing drinking and preventing relapse diminished over time, and overall failed to reduce relapse to heavy drinking. Still, the effect of naltrexone on the craving for alcohol in alcoholism is promising in that it suggests that the opioid system is

involved, which may open the door for other opioid active drugs to impact on drinking.

c. Serotonergic drugs—Animal studies have consistently shown that selective serotonin reuptake inhibitors (SSRIs) reduce alcohol intake in animal models. The data with respect to humans are less clear or consistent. It appears that the SSRIs do reduce drinking in heavily drinking, nondepressed alcoholics, but probably only about 15–20% from pretreatment levels. When abstinence is the outcome studied, the results are not promising. The SSRIs may eventually find a place in concert with other anticraving medication, however. SSRIs appear to reduce drinking in a more robust fashion in alcoholics with comorbid depression.

d. Acamprosate (calcium acetylhomotaurinate)—Acamprosate is a new drug that has been shown to reduce the craving for alcohol in alcoholics. It appears to affect both GABA and glutamine neurotransmission, both important in alcohol's effect in the brain. Unlike naltrexone, the effects of acamprosate on relapse appear to be greater and longer lasting. Twice as many alcoholics remained abstinent in a 12- month period while taking acamprosate compared to those who took placebo. The addition of disulfram to the regimen appears to increase the effectiveness of acamprosate further. Acamprosate has a very benign side effect profile and appears to be free of any effects on mood, concentration, attention, or psychomotor performance. Acamprosate has been studied extensively in Europe with good results. It is currently undergoing clinical trials in the United States.

In conclusion, it appears that disulfram, naltrexone, possibly other opioid antagonists, SSRIs, and acamprosate may have a place in the prevention of relapse in alcoholism. Acamprosate appears to be the most promising of these medications, and there is some reason to believe that the addition of disulfram to it may increase abstinence further. Clearly, the goal of abstinence for patients addicted to alcohol cannot be met by medication alone at this time. In selected patients medication may improve their chances for stable recovery.

2. Pharmacological treatment for cocaine addiction—Despite great interest in and much activity devoted to finding an effective pharmacological intervention for cocaine and other stimulant addiction, none has withstood the test of rigorous study. Heterocyclic antidepressants, such as desipramine, SSRIs, monoamine oxidase inhibitors, dopamine agonists, such as bromocriptine, neuroleptics, anticonvulsants, and calcium channel blockers have all been tried. Variable results, often positive in animal studies, have resulted in attempts to treat cocaine addicts with these drugs. As each potentially effective drug is studied more rigorously, however, little in the way of positive results is found. These drugs are used to try to ameliorate the craving for cocaine or to mediate the withdrawal symptoms of anhedonia and fatigue. An attempt to use stimulants such as ritalin or amphetamine for cocaine dependence in a manner analogous to the use of methadone maintenance for opiate addiction has produced disappointing results. One of the more interesting approaches to a pharmacological answer to cocaine addiction has been the development of a "vaccine" for cocaine. In this approach, a cocaine-like hapten linked to a foreign protein produces antibodies that attach to cocaine molecules and prevent them from crossing the blood–brain barrier. This approach has had some success in animal models but has yet to be tested on humans. The state of the art in the pharmacological treatment of cocaine addiction makes it difficult to recommend any medication-based treatment with confidence.

3. Pharmacological treatment for opiate addiction—Agonist maintenance with methadone is the primary pharmacological treatment for opioid addiction. The rationale for the use of methadone and its longer acting relative levo-α-acetylmethadol (LAAM) is to saturate the opiate receptors, thus blocking euphoria and preventing the abstinence syndrome. Because methadone and LAAM treatment programs are tightly regulated by the federal government, the average family physician would not be prescribing this drug, but certainly may see patients who are on a maintenance program. Methadone programs are frequently referred to as harm reduction programs because the primary beneficiary of these programs is society. Reductions in crime and in the costs of active intravenous heroin abuse are clearly demonstrated as a result of these programs. The addict also benefits with a dramatic decrease in the risk of death due to addiction and in contraction of HIV disease. There is social stabilization in the addict's life as well, especially when appropriate social services are provided by the maintenance program.

Antagonist maintenance with naltrexone was initially thought to be ideal given its essentially complete blockade of opioid-reinforcing properties. Unfortunately only 10–20% of patients remained in treatment when this approach was used. The most important use of naltrexone at this time appears to be in the management of health care professionals with opioid dependence. Compliance with a naltrexone regimen ensures abstinence and allows health care professionals to work in an environment in which opioids may be accessible. Doses of 350 mg weekly divided into 3 days will provide complete protection from the effects of opioids.

Buprenorphine, a partial opioid agonist with κ antagonist effects, is currently being tested as an alternative to methadone maintenance treatment. Dosing this medication currently is problematic, with 65% of patients remaining abstinent at 16 mg/day compared with 28% abstinence at 4 mg/day. Buprenorphine may also decrease the use of cocaine in opioid-dependent patients. It also has less potential for diversion, making it an attractive alternative to methadone. New regulations allowing maintenance treatment of opioid dependence with buprenorphine in primary care are expected soon.

Anton RF: Pharmacologic approaches to the management of alcoholism. J Clin Psychiatry 2001;62(Suppl 20):11. [PMID: 11584870].

Chang PH, Steinberg MB: Alcohol withdrawal. Med Clin North Am 2001;85(5):1191. [PMID: 11565494].

Kosanke N et al: Feasibility of matching alcohol patients to ASAM levels of care. Am J Addict 2002;11(2):124. [PMID: 12028742].

Krambeer LL: Methadone therapy for opioid dependence. Am Fam Physician 2001;63(12):2404.

Moyer A et al: Brief interventions for alcohol problems: a meta-analytic review of controlled investigations in treatment-seeking and nontreatment-seeking populations. Addiction 2002;97 (3):279. [PMID: 11964101].

Weisner C, Matzger H: A prospective study of the factors influencing entry to alcohol and drug treatment. J Behav Health Serv Res 2002;29(2):126. [PMID: 12032970].

Tobacco Cessation

52

Martin C. Mahoney, MD, PhD, FAAFP, & Andrew Hyland, PhD

General Considerations

The use of brief interventions to facilitate tobacco cessation in clinical settings is reviewed. Evidence-based strategies for using a systematic approach to diagnosing and treating nicotine dependence, including the use of adjunctive pharmacotherapy, are also highlighted.

Nicotine dependence results in an immense burden to patients, their families, and the health care system. Increased efforts to promote smoking cessation are a key element in decreasing the tobacco-related disease burden over the next 20 years. Current treatments for nicotine dependence represent promising opportunities for clinicians to increase cessation and decrease tobacco-attributable morbidity and mortality among their patients.

The primary goals of *Healthy People 2010* are to increase quality and years of healthy life and eliminate health disparities (http://www.health.gov/healthypeople). Because tobacco use varies by income and race and ethnicity, increased smoking cessation will play a key role in realizing these goals. Toward this end, two of the *Healthy People 2010* objectives are to reduce the prevalence of cigarette smoking among adults from 24% to 12% and to increase the number of yearly cessation attempts among smokers from 41% to 75%.

Food and Drug Administration (FDA)-approved pharmacotherapies (nicotine gum, patch, inhaler, spray, lozenges, and bupropion) can double the likelihood of smoking cessation, even when used without psychosocial therapy. However, individuals with lower incomes are less likely to report prior use of such therapies. Increased access to these effective therapies can increase the number of quit attempts. Use of the nicotine patch among individuals with incomes below $10,000 was greater (12%) in states that covered the cost for the patch as part of their public health insurance, compared to states that did not cover the cost (7.7%).

Fiore C et al: *Treating Tobacco Use and Dependence. Clinical Practice Guideline.* U.S. Department of Health and Human Services. Public Health Service, 2000.

Brief Interventions

Smoking cessation treatment often begins with a brief intervention (BI), in which a physician or other health care provider advises smokers to quit and may recommend methods for quitting. For many smokers, the only contact with the health care system may be through their family physician, and office visits often provide the impetus for smokers to attempt to stop smoking.

Meta-analyses report that BIs have significant potential to reduce smoking rates, with even minimal BIs conferring an estimated 30% increased likelihood of cessation. Although previous studies have examined the effect of BIs in a controlled setting, little research has been conducted to examine their effects in nonexperimental settings over an extended period of time. In addition, little is known about the characteristics of who gets a BI, how the effectiveness of BI varies by sociodemographic groups, or about the natural history of receiving BIs over time and how this relates to indicators of smoking cessation that include not only quit attempts and cessation, but other behaviors smokers engage in when trying to stop smoking such as switching to low tar cigarettes, decreasing the number of cigarettes smoked per day, or trying stop smoking pharmacotherapies.

A. Use of Brief Interventions to Promote Smoking Cessation

The updated Agency for Health Research and Quality (AHRQ) smoking treatment guidelines recommend that health care workers screen all patients for tobacco use and provide advice and follow-up behavioral treatments to all tobacco users. Current users are advised to quit and those who are willing to make a quit attempt are given appropriate assistance and a follow-up visit is arranged. Those who are identified as former smokers are given advice to prevent relapse, and primary prevention is engaged for persons who have never used tobacco.

The aim of these guidelines is to increase smoking cessation through improved understanding of the health consequences of smoking, better information about the availability and proper use of treatments, and the provision of encouragement and support.

Controlled studies have found that physician involvement, especially more extensive interventions, increases quit rates. This approach has also been found to be cost effective. Overall, the interventions recommended by AHRQ cost about $2500 per year of life saved, whereas mammography screening costs about $50,000 per year of life saved.

Although studies find that physician interventions are an efficacious and cost-effective way to increase quit rates, patient reports indicate that much of the smoking population does not receive them. The Centers for Disease Control and Prevention (CDC) found that only 70% of smokers had seen a physician in the past year, and only 37% of these reported they were advised to stop smoking, which represents about 25% of all smokers. In another study 91% of participating doctors indicated that providing advice regarding smoking cessation was important, but only 47% of smokers reported that their physicians had advised them to quit. Higher rates have been reported by patients in recent years, but still less than 65% of smokers seeing a doctor were advised to quit.

Some studies offered more encouraging results regarding the extent of physician advice and counseling. Among approximately 280 attempted quitters, the majority reported that they had received counseling on correct patch usage and on possible side effects. In this study, however, BI was part of a more extensive program of community intervention, which might account for its high rate. Based on surveys of 447 managed health care plans covering approximately 60 million Americans, the National Committee for Quality Assurance reported that 64% of physicians advised their patients to quit smoking in 1997.

The rate of BI has increased over time. The CDC found that the rate at which smokers had ever received physician advice increased from 26.4% in 1976 to 56.1% in 1991. More recently, data from the 1996 and 1999 Current Population Survey Tobacco Use Supplements indicate the rate of physician advice increased from 56% in 1996 to 63% in 1999.

Physicians tend to report higher rates of intervention. In one study 95% of physicians reported that they advise all or most of their patients who smoke to quit, but a survey of their patients found that only 29% of those reported receiving advice. Thus, reports from physicians and from patients appear to be at odds. Possible explanations for the discrepancy are that physicians who report giving advice may not provide the advice to all smokers, or physicians provide only perfunctory advice that their patients do not remember and physicians do not follow up.

In population-based settings, it was found that physicians asked about two-thirds of patients if they smoked, but provided counseling to only 21% in 1995. In a study of smokers in California in 1998, 49% reported receiving advice from a doctor to quit smoking in the past year, but of these only 12% reported that their physician suggested a quit date, only 7% received a prescription for nicotine replacement therapy, and only 10% were offered suggestions concerning other assistance. A survey of doctors found that in 1997 only 8% reported that they provided follow-up advice to smokers, and less than 50% were planning on increasing their rate of interventions in the next 6 months. Physicians who advise their patients who smoke to quit once may fail to provide additional advice if the patient has not taken any initiative to quit.

Estimates of prevalence of BI vary. The discrepancies can be attributed in part to methodological differences, the time period examined, whether the survey was based on physician or patient report, how long after the visit the survey was conducted, sample size, and smoker and demographic variations. In particular, attention needs to be directed to demographic differences in the patterns of implementation of BI. Nonetheless, estimates of prevalence indicate that although BIs appear to be cost effective, much of the smoking population does not receive them. Moreover, few data are available on the correlation between the effect of BIs and the type of health care provider who delivers the message (eg, physician, physician assistant, or nurse practitioner).

B. Characteristics of Those Who Receive a Brief Intervention

Limited attention has been directed to examining differences in rates of BI by gender, age, and racial and ethnic group. Reports indicate that in Australia physicians were more likely to offer advice to males, whereas in the United States advice was more likely to be given to females. The CDC found that only 25% of adolescents reported that their physicians had provided advice on smoking. Older patients (50–74 years old) were about five times as likely to receive BIs as younger patients, with those aged 65 and above about 1.5 times as likely to receive advice as those aged 18–24. One study found whites more likely than nonwhites to receive advice, whereas another found whites less likely than blacks and Asians, but more likely than Hispanics and others to receive advice. Recent work indicates that younger, less educated, black or Hispanic males were less likely to receive BIs than other demographic groups.

C. Effectiveness of Brief Interventions

Many studies have examined the effectiveness of BIs. Based on a meta-analysis of seven studies, AHRQ reported that physician advice increased 6-month quit rates by 2.3% (10.2% versus 7.9% for controls). Another meta-analysis of four randomized clinical trials reported that BIs increased 1-year quit rates by 2.7%.

Studies also find that more intensive interventions are more successful. One-year quit rates were found to be higher when physicians offered advice plus follow-up (15.8%) than advice only (12.7%). The most recent AHRQ tobacco treatment guidelines support these findings.

A population-based study of BIs using the 1990 California Tobacco Survey surveyed 9796 current smokers and found that those who had been advised to stop smoking in their most recent physician visit were significantly more likely to attempt to quit (OR = 1.61, 95% CI = 1.31–1.98). There was no significant difference in the number of quit attempts by smokers who had been previously advised to quit but not in their most recent doctor visit and quit attempts by smokers who had never received such advice. Only the intention or attempt to quit was considered and not whether quits were successful. Physician advice to quit was reported to increase the likelihood of making a future quit attempt by 50–100%, with stronger effects among those who received repeated BIs over time.

Although these results generally indicate that even minimal BIs increased quit rates by an estimated 30%, little is known about the effects on specific demographic groups. Few studies have looked at both quitting and quit attempts, and no studies have considered other outcomes such as switching to low-tar cigarettes, decreasing the amount smoked, changes in motivation to stop smoking, or changes in the use of stop smoking pharmacotherapies. In addition, few studies have examined BIs in the general population. Most have been largely based on experimental, controlled interventions with relatively short follow-up durations and few studies have examined the efficacy of repeated interventions over time. Effectiveness may differ in uncontrolled settings, as there is limited guidance on or control of effective implementation. Further, studies conducted in a controlled setting may yield misleading results if the subjects are more motivated or react differently knowing that they are part of a study.

D. Attempts to Encourage Brief Interventions

Interventions designed to increase rates of physician advice and counseling have been shown to be effective. In a study based on the 1993 Community Intervention Trial for Smoking Cessation (COMMIT) survey, it was found that physicians in intervention communities were more likely than those in control communities to advise patients to stop smoking, encourage patients to set a quit date, and recommend use of nicotine replacement therapy. Thus, studies indicate the potential to increase BIs, which has important implications for de-

veloping mechanisms to promote physician BIs as a clinical stop smoking intervention.

Repeated advice with follow-up may be necessary to encourage smokers, particularly heavy smokers, to quit. Smokers generally try to quit repeated times before they are successful. Nevertheless, the incremental effect of advice given a second time may be less than the first time; the percentage of those previously advised to quit who have not yet stopped smoking increases and smokers may become frustrated after trying and failing multiple times. In that case, interventions, especially those that are less extensive, become less effective over time. More extensive interventions may be necessary.

Centers for Disease Control and Prevention: Physician and other health-care professional counseling of smokers to quit—United States, 1991. MMWR 1993;42(44):854.

Centers for Disease Control and Prevention: Use of clinical preventive services by adults aged <65 years enrolled in health-maintenance organizations—United States, 1996. MMWR 1998; 47(29):613.

Cromwell J et al: Cost-effectiveness of the clinical practice recommendations in the AHCPR guideline for smoking cessation. Agency for Health Care Policy and Research. JAMA 1997; 278(21):1759.

Gilpin EA et al: Physician advice to quit smoking: results from the 1990 California Tobacco Survey. J Gen Intern Med 1993; 8(10):549.

Goldstein MG et al: A population-based survey of physician smoking cessation counseling practices. Prev Med 1998;27(5, Pt 1):720.

Hyland A et al: Effect of physician clinical interventions on indicators of cessation. Nicotine Tobacco Res 2003;5(5):781.

Kottke TE et al: Delivery rates for preventive services in 44 midwestern clinics. Mayo Clin Proc 1997;72(6):515.

Ockene JK et al: Tobacco control activities of primary-care physicians in the Community Intervention Trial for Smoking Cessation. COMMIT Research Group. Tobacco Control 1997; 6(Suppl 2):S49.

Thorndike AN et al: National patterns in the treatment of smokers by physicians. JAMA 1998;279(8):604.

Tobacco Use and Dependence Clinical Practice Guideline Panel, Staff, and Consortium Representatives: A clinical practice guideline for treating tobacco use and dependence: A US Public Health Service report. JAMA 2000;283(24):3244.

Diagnosis & Treatment

The Tobacco Use and Dependence Clinical Practices Guideline Panel recommends five specific actions ("the 5 A's") for integration into all clinical practice settings. These systematic approaches to tobacco dependence require less than 3 min to deliver, but the potential yield is enormous. This model is illustrated in Figure 52–1.

- **Ask** about tobacco use at all office visits. Patients with tobacco dependence can be identified by simply

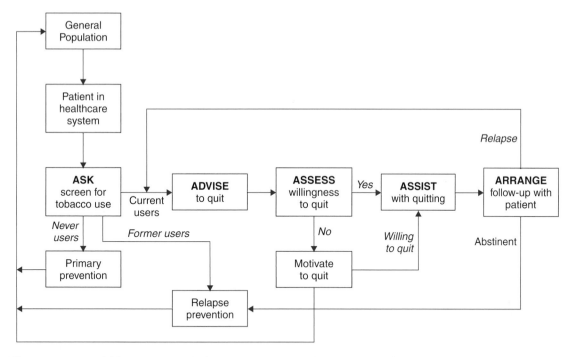

Figure 52–1. Model for treatment of tobacco use and dependence. (Adapted from Fiore C et al: *Treating Tobacco Use and Dependence.* U.S. Department of Health and Human Services. Public Health Service, 2000.)

inquiring about use of tobacco products during the assessment of vital signs. Information on tobacco use should be clearly recorded in the patient's chart. This approach helps to systematize the approach for all patients. Moreover, it is important to make a comprehensive assessment of tobacco use, including use of traditional types of tobacco (eg, cigarettes, cigars, pipe, and smokeless tobacco) as well as use of nontraditional forms that have become increasingly more common among adolescents and young adults (eg, bidis and kreteks).

- **Advise** all tobacco users to quit. Office staff, both physician and nonphysician, should encourage cessation among those identified to be tobacco users. When appropriate, tobacco use can be linked to current health issues.

- **Assess** the willingness of tobacco users to quit by asking if they have thought about quitting. Alternatively, the transtheoretical model can be used to determine readiness to change. This behavioral model assigns patients to one of five stages: precontemplation, contemplation, preparation, action, and maintenance. Brief comments from the physician can be useful in helping patients to move onto the next stage. Patients who are not yet willing to quit use of tobacco should be provided with a brief intervention

to stimulate their interest in quitting and should be reminded of the physician's willingness to support their efforts. Patients who express an interest in quitting smoking should be counseled on use of adjunctive pharmacotheraphy and provided with other information (eg, motivational intervention or referral to behavioral therapy sessions) during that specific office visit. Former users of tobacco products should be encouraged to maintain abstinence and should be offered the opportunity to address problems or threats to continued cessation.

- **Assist** each patient in developing a quit plan. At this point, physicians can provide assistance with setting a quit date, identifying social supports, discussing how to cope with physical and psychological withdrawal symptoms, and identifying patient preferences for adjunctive pharmacotherapies. Patients can be provided with printed materials and referred to community-based cessation classes, internet sites, or toll-free help lines for further information.

- **Arrange** for follow-up soon after the quit date. This can be used as an opportunity to reinforce continued cessation or to recommit to complete abstinence. A brief telephone call from the physician during the first week of cessation may be of great value to patients. An office visit should occur 2–4 weeks after the quit date to discuss successes, challenges, coping strategies, and experiences with pharmacotherapy. Patients should be contacted at about 2 weeks and 4 weeks after their quit dates.

The tobacco dependence guidelines recommend that all smokers receive at least a brief intervention. Although intensive interventions are more effective, they are not likely to be attended by the majority of smokers interested in quitting. Therefore, policies that restrict access to treatment by requiring attendance at intensive smoking cessation clinics are likely to be detrimental to smokers because they discourage quit attempts.

For patients who are currently unwilling to make a quit attempt clinicians should present a brief motivation intervention structured around "the 5 R's":

1. *Relevance*—make tobacco cessation personally relevant (personal medical history, family composition).
2. *Risk*—review the negative effects of quitting (include both immediate and long-term risks).
3. *Rewards*—identify the benefits of quitting (improved sense of taste and smell, personal sense of accomplishment, money saved, health benefits).
4. *Roadblocks*—identify perceived barriers to quitting and ways of overcoming these impediments (symptoms of withdrawal, weight gain, lack of social supports).

5. *Repetition*—repeat this intervention at all office visits.

A. Pharmacotherapy

It can be argued that all tobacco users have a physical dependence on nicotine in addition to a variety of reinforced psychological and social behaviors. The Fagerstrom nicotine dependence scale was developed to aid in quantifying the magnitude of addiction and to aid in selected pharmacotherapy. Alternatives to the Fagerstrom scale include a modified CAGE questionnaire and an abbreviated version of the Fagerstrom scale. The revision to the Fagerstrom Tolerance Scale, the Fagerstrom Test for Nicotine Dependence (FTND), suggests that the time to first daily cigarette represents the single best indicator of nicotine dependence.

An algorithm for identifying and treating nicotine dependence is summarized in Figure 52–2. This emphasizes development of a systematic approach to querying all patients about tobacco use, asking current users about interest in quitting, and motivating never users and former users to remain abstinent.

The United States Public Health Service guideline on management of tobacco dependence recommends sustained release bupropion and all forms of nicotine replacement (eg, resin/gum, inhaler, nasal spray, lozenges, and patch) as first-line agents. A medical chart form to facilitate both patient discussion and documentation relating to use of first-line adjunctive pharmotherapy

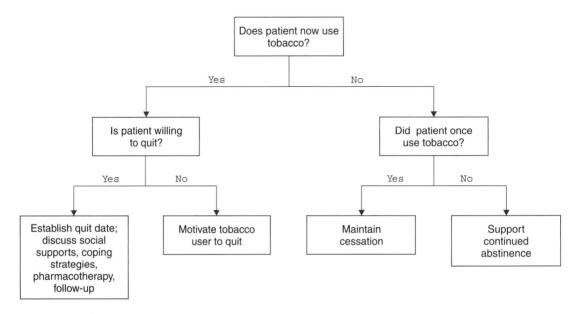

Figure 52–2. Algorithm for treating nicotine dependence. (Adapted from Fiore C et al: *Treating Tobacco Use and Dependence*. U.S. Department of Health and Human Services. Public Health Service, 2000.)

for the treatment of tobacco dependence is given in Table 52–1. The table lists the first-line agents for smoking cessation pharmacotherapy along with recommended starting doses. Patients should be queried about prior use of these agents and their experiences and asked if they are interested in a particular agent. Clinicians are encouraged to apply appropriate clinical judgment when assessing contraindications to the use of a particular agent. Table 52–1 can be used to document the prescription, any discussion of possible side effects, and other instructions given to the patient.

Bupropion (sustained release) is started at a dose of 150 mg daily for 3 days before increasing to 150 mg twice daily on Day 4. Treatment with bupropion is begun 1–2 weeks before the anticipated quit date; its use is contraindicated among patients with a history of seizure disorders, current substance abuse, or other conditions that may lower the seizure threshold. Bupropion can be used in combination with nicotine replacement.

Patients should be counseled to stop smoking completely prior to initiating nicotine replacement therapy (NRT). Nicotine patches, lozenges, and resin are available over the counter, whereas nicotine nasal sprays and the nicotine inhaler systems both require prescriptions. Reduced dose regimens of nicotine replacement might be considered for patients consuming fewer than 10 cigarettes daily or those weighing less than 100 pounds. Using two forms of nicotine replacement (eg, patch and resin) results in higher quit rates and should be recommended if other forms of nicotine replacement are not effective alone.

Clonidine and nortriptyline both represent second-line pharmacotherapy for use among patients in whom first-line line agents have been judged to be inappropriate or ineffective. (Therefore, neither of these products is included in Table 52–1.) Although neither clonidine nor nortriptyline is approved by the Food and Drug Administration as adjunctive therapy for smoking cessation, several studies have demonstrated about a doubling in abstinence rates. Studies of clonidine have reported a variety of doses. It should be noted that the abrupt discontinuation of clonidine can result in rebound hypertension and other symptoms. Only a limited number of studies have examined the use of nortriptyline as a cessation aid and its use is tempered by concerns about potential side effects. Use of either of these agents for smoking cessation requires a clear discussion of risks and benefits with the patient and close monitoring by the treating physician.

Nicotine-containing products are not associated with the occurrence of acute cardiac events. Nonetheless, NRT should be approached cautiously among patients who are within 2 weeks of an acute myocardial infarction, are known to have significant arrhythmias, and who have significant or worsening symptoms of angina.

Pharmacotherapy doubles the effect of any tobacco cessation intervention. Patients who are willing and able to participate in more intensive interventions should be encouraged to use them.

Use of adjunctive pharmacotherapy should be strongly considered for all persons, including hospitalized patients, given the distinct health benefits associated with cessation. Clinical experience with use of these adjunctive agents in pregnant women and adolescents is generally limited. Smokers with concurrent or prior depression may benefit from use of bupropion. Clinical judgment is advised regarding a comprehensive assessment of the risks and benefits associated with use of adjunctive pharmacotherapy in each of these settings.

Use of adjunctive pharmacotherapy may be continued for up to 6 months or longer. Patients should be encouraged to wean themselves off nicotine replacements after about 6–12 weeks of treatment; however, some patients elect to continue nicotine-containing therapy long term.

B. Relapse

Although risk of relapse is greatest immediately following the quit attempt, it can occur months or even years following cessation. Because tobacco use status will be determined for all patients at each visit, physicians should encourage all former tobacco users to remain abstinent and encourage these patients to express specific concerns or difficulties (see Figure 52–2). These topics can be addressed briefly during the scheduled office visit or explored more fully during a subsequent appointment. Approaches can include reassurance, motivational counseling, extended pharmacotherapy, recommendations for exercise, and/or referral to supportive/behavioral therapy.

Centers for Disease Control and Prevention: Youth tobacco surveillance—United States, 1998–1999. MMWR 2000;49(10):1.

Fagerstrom KO: Measuring degree of physical dependence to tobacco smoking with reference to individualization of treatment. Addict Behav 1978;3(3–4):235.

Jorenby DE et al: A controlled trial of sustained-release bupropion, a nicotine patch, or both for smoking cessation. New Engl J Med 1999;340(9):685.

Mallin R: Smoking cessation: integration of behavioral and drug therapies. Am Fam Physician 2002;65:1107.

Okuyemi KS, Ahluwalia JS, Harris KJ: Pharmacotherapy of smoking cessation. Arch Fam Med 2000;9(3):270.

Conclusions

The U.S. Public Health Guideline notes that brief interventions of 3 min or less are effective. Two questions are critical: "Do you smoke?" and "Do you want to

Table 52–1. Chart aid for use of first-line adjunctive pharmacotherapy in smoking cessation.[1]

Stop Smoking Medication	Used in Past	Patient Would Like to Use?	Contraindications	Side Effects	Rx Given (Dose/ Frequency/Number)	Other Instructions Given
Nicotine patch (7, 14, or 21 mg/24 h for 4 weeks, then taper 2 weeks and 2 weeks)	Yes—Rx/OTC No	Yes No	Concurrent smoking	Local skin reaction Insomnia	7/14/21 mg patch every 24 h for 4 weeks then taper every 2 weeks	Counseling (problem solving, skills training) Stop smoking classes Set quit date: ___ F/U appt: ___
Nicotine gum (1–24 cigs/day—2 mg gum or 25+ cigs/day—4 mg gum; max 24 pieces/day for up to 12 weeks)	Yes—Rx/OTC No	Yes No	Concurrent smoking	Mouth soreness Dyspepsia	2 mg gum 4 mg gum Max 24 pieces/day for up to 12 weeks	Counseling (problem solving, skills training) Stop smoking classes Set quit date: ___ F/U appt: ___
Nicotine nasal spray (8–40 doses/day for 3–6 months)	Yes—Rx No	Yes No	Concurrent smoking	Nasal irritation	___ doses/day for 3–6 months	Counseling (problem solving, skills training) Stop smoking classes Set quit date: ___ F/U appt: ___
Nicotine inhaler (6–16 cartridges/day for up to 6 months)	Yes—Rx/OTC No	Yes No	Concurrent smoking	Local irritation of mouth and throat	___ Cartridges/day for ___ months	Counseling (problem solving, skills training) Stop smoking classes Set quit date: ___ F/U appt: ___
Nicotine lozenges (if first cig smoked within 30 min or arising—4 mg lozenge; if first cig after 30 min of arising—2-mg lozenge; max 5 loz/6 h or 20 loz/day for up to 12 weeks)	Yes—Rx/OTC No	Yes No	Concurrent smoking Contains phenylalanine	Mouth soreness Dyspepsia	2-mg lozenge 4-mg lozenge Maximum 20 loz/day for up to 12 weeks	Counseling (problem solving, skills training) Stop smoking classes Set quit date: ___ F/U appt: ___
Zyban/bupropion SR	Yes—Rx No	Yes No	History of seizures History of eating disorder Currently treated for depression Used MAO inhibitor within past 14 days	Local skin reaction Insomnia	150 mg orally every day for 3 days, then 150 mg twice a day	Dosing reviewed Quit on Day 7 Counseling (problem solving, skills training) Stop smoking classes Set quit date: ___ F/U appt: ___
Other	Yes—Rx/OTC No	Yes No				

[1]Rx, prescription; OTC, over the counter; F/U, follow-up; MAO, monoamine oxidase.

quit?" Clinicians can offer interventions during an office visit that can ultimately save a patient's life and reduce comorbidity.

The guideline for treating tobacco use and dependence also notes that "proactive" telephone counseling, in which a clinician counsels the patient over the telephone, is an effective intervention for helping patients stop smoking. Other types of self-help, including quitlines/helplines, can serve to facilitate cessation among callers.

All hospitalized smokers should be approached using the 5 A's—Ask, Advise, Assess, Assist, and Arrange. The guideline also includes a limited discussion of adjunctive pharmacotherapy among specific patient groups including pregnant women, patients with psychiatric conditions and/or chemical dependency, adolescents, and older smokers. However, data regarding use of specific pharmacotherapy among selected patient subgroups are limited.

Several national and regional studies have shown that despite otherwise stated intentions, on average only about 25% of eligible smokers seen in primary care receive tobacco cessation advice. The rates are higher during well visits and for patients with chronic diseases associated with tobacco, but there is much room for improvement.

It is somewhat stunning to note that 9 out of 10 quit attempts end in failure. Thus, only a small proportion of tobacco users achieve permanent abstinence during an initial quit attempt; the majority persist in tobacco use for many years and typically cycle through multiple periods of relapse and remission. Accordingly, a chronic disease model for nicotine dependence has many appealing aspects. This model acknowledges the long-term nature of the disorder with the expectation that patients may have periods of relapse and remission. If nicotine dependence is recognized as a chronic condition, clinicians will better understand the relapsing nature of the ailment and the requirement for ongoing and continuous attention, rather that just acute care. Clinicians should also recognize that despite the potential for relapse, numerous effective treatments are now available.

There is strong evidence to suggest that smoking cessation treatments delivered by clinicians, whether physicians or nonphysicians (eg, a psychologist, nurse, dentist, or counselor), can increase abstinence. Therefore all clinicians should provide smoking cessation interventions.

With the dissemination of the tobacco use and dependence clinical practice guideline all physicians have access to a valuable resource to enhance their skills in successfully delivering office-based tobacco cessation assessment and counseling.

Because of its wide-ranging impact, it is appropriate to view nicotine dependence as a chronic disease requiring assessment, counseling, pharmacotherapy, and follow-up care. Because 70% of all smokers interact with the health care system annually, clinicians can play an important role in reducing tobacco-related morbidity and mortality. Also, nearly 50% of smokers attempt to quit each year. Thus, a systematic approach to tobacco dependence can ensure that all tobacco users are identified and assessed to maximize long-term success.

Recommendations presented in the United States Public Health Service Clinical Practice Guideline on Treating Tobacco Use and Dependence (AHRQ publication No. 00-0032) are also available at http://www.surgeongeneral.gov/tobacco.

Borland R et al: The effectiveness of callback counselling for smoking cessation: a randomized trial. Addiction 2001;96(6):881.

Mahoney MC, Jaen CR: Counseling for tobacco cessation. Am Fam Physician 2001;64(11):1881.

SECTION VI

Doctor–Patient Issues

Communication

Nancy Levine, MD, & Marian Block, MD

Physician–Patient Communication

A. THE THERAPEUTIC ALLIANCE

It is within the context of communication that the therapeutic alliance between physician and patient is formed. When communication with a patient is nonjudgmental, respectful, and genuine, the stage is set for a successful therapeutic alliance. Medical knowledge is vitally necessary, but alone it is not sufficient to accomplish the tasks of caring for a patient. It is the ability of the physician to translate medical knowledge for the patient and to enlist the trust of the patient that will ultimately lead to good health care for the patient.

We know that good communication has a number of beneficial effects on the relationship between the doctor and the patient. It improves patient satisfaction, compliance, and health. It also improves physicians' satisfaction with their work and the accuracy of information they obtain from the patient and it decreases the likelihood that physicians will be sued for malpractice.

B. PATIENT SATISFACTION

The impact of good communication on patient satisfaction is the best studied of these benefits. In *The Medical Interview* Ware et al extensively review the evidence for the validity of using patient satisfaction and other patient rating scales. They conclude, "Patients' ratings of interpersonal aspects of care provide not only useful and valid information for quality assessment but also the best source of data on the interpersonal aspects of care."

Patients generally want more information than their physicians give them. The amount of information given to the patient strongly correlates with patient satisfaction. Doctors spend a small fraction of the time giving information, 1 min out of 20, and believe that they

spend more time than they actually do. Thus the correlation between the amount of information patients receive and their satisfaction with the visit is a strong and consistent observation in the medical literature.

Many other physician behaviors also correlate with satisfaction. These include courtesy, attention, listening, empathy, and sympathy. Patients whose physicians communicate and interpret emotions well and are friendly, concerned, take time to answer questions, and give explanations are more satisfied. Patients rate their physicians positively if they were encouraging, open, and attentive and negatively if they dominated the encounter.

Physicians' personal qualities are rated highly if the encounter centers on the patient rather than on the physician's concerns. Physicians who ask many directive questions and keep tight control over the interaction tend to have patients who feel that their doctors do not listen to them.

C. PHYSICIAN SATISFACTION

Physician satisfaction, although not as well studied as patient satisfaction, is very important for physicians' personal and professional lives. Physicians find reward and meaning in their interpersonal relationships with patients. The quality of those relationships is directly related to physician satisfaction with their work. Good communication with patients will improve the quality of the relationship and thus improve physician satisfaction.

D. ACCURACY OF INFORMATION OBTAINED

In 1988 George Engel said, "the interview is the most powerful, encompassing, sensitive, and versatile instrument available to the physician." In a 1984 study, Beckman and Frankel discovered that physicians frequently interrupted patients before they completely expressed their concerns, and rarely returned to patients' initial concerns. They found that physicians controlled the interview with directive questions and they postulated that these interviewing tactics resulted in a loss of relevant information. They also found that these behaviors resulted in an incomplete clinical picture and disorganized care, thus leading to the collection of inaccurate information. Accurate information is lost when physicians use medical jargon. In one study, 50% of doctor–patient interactions were adversely affected by the physicians' use of medical jargon. Patients frequently believed they understood the jargon, but actually did not.

Other behaviors by the physician interfere with accurate data collection. Excessive control of the interview by the physician limits patients' ability to communicate all of their concerns and their database is flawed. The way a question is asked has an important impact on the information received. Patients who are asked "what concerns you about this problem" give better information than patients who are asked "what worries you about this problem." The use of closed-ended questions (questions that have yes/no answers) limits the ability of patients to describe symptoms in their own words. In summary, physicians can improve the accuracy of their medical interviews if they use open-ended questions, allow patients to fully answer a question before interrupting, and avoid the use of medical jargon.

E. HEALTH OUTCOMES

The relationship between improved health and good communication is more difficult to study than the correlation between patient satisfaction and good communication. Outcomes are influenced by many more variables and are temporally more distant. However, evidence indicates that good communication between doctor and patients correlates with good health outcomes. Patients with peptic ulcer disease who are involved in their own care through shared decision making with their physicians have less functional impairment due to their illness. When there is agreement between doctors and patients about the nature and severity of the patient's health problem, improvement in or resolution of the problem occurs more often. Physicians who are less controlling, give more information, and show more emotion have patients with fewer functional limitations, lower blood pressure, and lower blood sugar. Patients who can express their emotions, both positive and negative, have improved health outcomes; in addition, when the ratio of patient to physician talk is high, patients are healthier. Open-ended questions are superior to directive questions. Patients who are allowed to tell their story in their own words have lower blood pressures. In a study in which anes-

thesiologists were trained to give patients more detailed information about what to expect during their hospitalization, the patients required less pain medicine and left the hospital earlier.

F. MALPRACTICE SUITS

Physicians who communicate well are less likely to be named in a lawsuit. Patients of frequently sued physicians are more likely to say they were rushed, never received explanations, felt ignored, and felt their physicians did not communicate with them. There was no correlation between quality of care and adverse outcomes and malpractice claims in one study. These studies and others suggest that physicians are sued because patients are unhappy with their care and not because of poor quality of care.

G. ADHERENCE

There is ample evidence that good communication leads to better adherence to a physician's advice. Francis et al found a strong association between patient satisfaction and compliance: poor compliance results when parents of young patients have unmet expectations from the visit, when there is a lack of warmth on the part of the physician, and when parents fail to receive an explanation for their child's illness. A number of communication techniques are associated with improved compliance. Patients are more likely to be compliant if they have the opportunity to explain their understanding of their problem and ask questions. When patients are coached to ask more questions they are more likely to keep future appointments. Physicians who recognize nonverbal cues have patients who keep appointments more often.

Communication Skills

All the communication techniques described so far can be easily learned and used in the standard medical interview. A number of excellent textbooks are available for thorough review of these (Coulehan and Block, Smith, and Cole and Bird). The following are especially important.

1. A statement such as "How did you hope I might help you this visit?" will elicit important concerns that patients might not otherwise express.

2. Expressing empathy is an important basic skill. Empathy has three components in the doctor–patient relationship. The first component is knowing how the patient views a problem, the second is understanding that point of view, and the third is acknowledging to the patient that you understand his or her point of view. To be genuinely empathetic the physician needs to accomplish all three of these.

3. Allow patients to completely express their concerns.

4. Ask patients if they have any specific requests.

5. Elicit your patients' explanation of their problem and negotiate a mutual understanding of that problem. A question such as "what do you think is the cause of your problem?" would be helpful.

6. Encourage your patients to express feelings about their illness by asking "How are you feeling about this illness?" It is important for physicians to be aware that they do not need to resolve patients' negative feelings. Simply expressing negative emotions is a relief for patients.

7. Give patients specific information about their health condition.

8. Involve patients in their treatment plan. Patients who are collaborators in their care will feel in control of their illness and this will lead to an improved ability to cope with the illness. Patients who are passive will feel that the illness controls them and may give up on working to improve their health. Physicians can accomplish this by asking questions about how patients feel the proposed treatment plan might work and by giving them choices about the plan.

9. Reassurance is a powerful communication tool. At its best it can allay anxiety and enable patients to cope with difficult health problems. When offered prematurely, however, it can be insincere and worsen anxiety. It is important for the physician to truly understand the patient's concerns and perform a thorough medical evaluation of the problem before offering reassurance.

Special Communication Challenges

There are a number of situations that physicians find especially challenging. Many of these topics are reviewed in detail in other chapters of this book. The focus here is mainly on the communication issues that these special situations pose for clinicians and their patients.

A. The Angry Patient

There are a number of emotional responses that patients have toward their illness that physicians find difficult to deal with, but none poses a greater challenge than the patient who is angry. Anxiety and sadness can be difficult, but it is easier for the physician to be sympathetic or empathetic. The natural reaction to anger is defensiveness, not empathy. It requires considerable communication skills to develop empathy with a patient who is angry.

The clinician must first recognize anger, then acknowledge it, understand it, and respond to it. Recog-

nizing it is easy if patients tell you they are angry, but often they do not. Recognizing anger in a patient often requires that you recognize defensiveness in yourself. If you are feeling defensive, it is likely that your patient is angry. There may be other cues such as patient voice tone or agitation. If you are sensing that the patient is angry, but he or she has not volunteered this, it is important for you to explore the anger. An observation such as "you seem upset" may be helpful in getting the patient to share his or her feelings. Be sure that your language matches what you see in the patient. If the patient seems furious and you say "you seem a little upset," the patient is likely to become more angry. If you say "you seem furious" and the patient is a little piqued, the patient will deny it.

Once the patient has shared with you that he or she is angry, you are now in a position to explore it. There are myriad reasons patients may be angry; most of them have little to do with their physician. Until you understand why the patient is angry, you will be unable to address the anger in any constructive way. Often patients state the reason for their anger in response to your initial reflection "you seem upset." If they do not, you will need to acknowledge the anger and ask specifically about it. "I see that you are upset; are you willing to share with me what it is about?" The answer to this question will determine how you proceed. The patient's anger may be directed at you justifiably and may require an apology. It is more likely to be directed at someone or something else over which you have no control. Your task will now be to empathize with the patient. The patient will now feel understood and you will be able to move the conversation to other areas.

It is important to understand that anger is often displaced, especially when a patient is ill. The sadness and loss of control the patient feels about the illness are directed at those caring for the patient in the form of anger. The anger is really directed at the illness, not the physician. If the patient seems angry with you or another member of the health care team and you genuinely feel that you have done a good job caring for the patient, this may be displaced anger. This anger will also need to be explored and understood. It may not be as easily resolved as other forms of anger. It will be most helpful if the clinician is aware that the anger is displaced, as this will prevent an automatic defensive response on the part of the physician. A defensive response will typically make a patient feel justified in his or her anger. It will be important after exploring the anger to redirect the conversation to the difficulties and frustrations of the patient's illness.

B. Compliance

Compliance is a complex problem for physicians and their patients. Negotiation is one of the key concepts when addressing problems with compliance. The physician and the patient need to agree about the nature of the problem at hand and agree about the evaluation and treatment of it. Without this agreement, there is no reason for the patient to follow the advice of the doctor. We know that patients come to their physicians with certain beliefs about their illness and expectations about its evaluation and treatment. Patients will follow their physician's advice if the advice is consistent with these beliefs. Various communication strategies set the stage for successful negotiation.

Eliciting accurate information about patient compliance is the first step in dealing with noncompliance. If you do not know that your patient is not following your advice, you cannot intervene to help. There are several methods suggested in the medical literature to elicit information about compliance. You can count medication, measure drug levels, look at outcomes, or ask the patient. The most effective method is to ask. With a well-framed question, your patients will give you accurate information about their compliance 80% of the time. Asking a patient "Are you taking your medication?" is unlikely to yield accurate information. The answer to this type of question is an automatic yes. Physicians who ask specific questions about medication names, dosages, and times elicit more accurate information about compliance. Giving your patients permission to be noncompliant with a question such as "Some of my patients have difficulty remembering to take their blood pressure medicine every day; I wonder if you have found this also?" is often fruitful. Patients are relieved to hear that their problem is common and assume from the tone of the question that you are likely to be forgiving.

Once you have established that the patient is not following your advice, your next task will be to determine the reason or reasons. Because these usually have to do with patients' beliefs, goals, and expectations, questions to elucidate these will be important. Patients' beliefs are varied and it is impossible to predict them without asking. A patient might have had a father who took the same medicine you are prescribing and who died of complications of his disease anyway. A patient might believe that she can tell when her blood pressure is high and therefore takes her medicine only on these days. A patient might believe that she has no control over her illness and therefore your treatment will not work. There are a number of useful questions to elicit patients' beliefs, goals, and expectations. "Do you know anyone with your condition?" and if so "How were they treated?" "What happened to them?" "Have you read anything about your condition?" "What have you read?" "What do you think caused what you have?" "How do you think you should be treated?" "What kinds of tests do you think you should have?" "What might prevent you from following my advice?"

These types of questions will quickly demonstrate where you and your patient disagree. The next step will be to come to some common agreement with your patient about how to proceed. The nature of the disagreement will determine how the problem is resolved. It is important to realize that it needs to be resolved in such a way that the physician feels he or she is providing good medical care and the patient feels that he or she is receiving good medical care. To accomplish this, the physician and patient will need to influence each other. There are some common useful strategies for negotiation. The physician can correct misperceptions, refer the patient to a trusted source (friend, family member, article, organization, etc), explore options with the patient, suggest alternatives that are consistent with the patient's beliefs or goals, or compromise.

A word about the use of fear as a motivating tactic is important. It is commonly used by physicians and is usually unsuccessful for a variety of reasons. It greatly increases anxiety, which often encourages the behavior you are trying to stop. For example, the typical response to "If you don't stop smoking you are going to get lung cancer!" is to smoke more in response to the increased anxiety. Fear can make an illness seem more overwhelming and a common response to reduce anxiety is to deny the problem exists; thus compliance is worsened, not improved. Fear tactics are not only ineffective, but are often counterproductive.

Your patients are much more likely to comply if you point out the positive results of following your advice rather than the negative results of not following it. "If you stop smoking you will reduce your chances of lung cancer" is a more powerful motivator than "If you don't stop smoking you might get lung cancer." Focus on your patients' successes, even if they are small, rather than on their failures. Encourage your patients' strengths, attitudes, and actions. Offer hope. When patients are hopeful about their condition they are more likely to be able to make changes in their lives to accomplish the task at hand. When physicians are hopeful they are more effective clinicians.

Patients' behavior is strongly influenced by their social context; thus it is important to explore this. What is their cultural background and do they share the same cultural beliefs about their condition as this group? They might subscribe to a religion that believes that illness is a punishment for bad behavior. They might come from a culture in which herbal remedies are used for their condition. Friends and family are also important. You might have a patient who believes that a weight loss diet will help his heart condition, but he has a wife who does the cooking and who believes that the main way to express her love is to feed her loved ones. A patient may be unable to quit smoking because all of her friends smoke.

In summary, effective communication is the main tool a physician has to assess adherence to advice and to intervene for the good of the patient if the patient is not following that advice. The key principles of good communication concerning compliance include a nonjudgmental exploration of the problem, information giving, encouraging the patient to share beliefs and asking questions, asking about the social context of the problem, and focusing on the positive results of the advice you give to patients.

C. COMMUNICATING WITH PATIENTS WHO HAVE A TERMINAL ILLNESS

Much of caring for patients at the end of life involves communicating with them and their families. Communication revolves around two main areas, giving bad or sad news and discussing goals and wishes for medical care. Certainly all the general rules for communication are important in these circumstances. There are unique and predictable difficulties for patients and physicians when discussing end-of-life care. This discussion will focus on "the bad-news consultation."

The first communication problem a clinician typically encounters is how much to tell the patient about his or her illness. We assume that patients desire full information about their illness and this is usually a correct assumption. However, some patients do not want to know a bad prognosis; thus the physician needs to be skilled at assessing the patient's desire for information. A question such as "If it is bad news, do you want to know?" might be helpful to begin this discussion. If the patient does not want to be given bad news, there are two further areas for discussion. The first is to determine if there is someone else that the patient wants to receive the news and the second is to explore the reasons that the patient does not want to know.

Once you have determined the patient does want to hear the bad news, it is important to set up the interview carefully. When patients are satisfied with this initial interview they are less likely to be depressed later in their illness. Does the patient want anyone else to be present? Is the setting private and free of interruptions? Do you have enough time? Your attitude should be understanding, positive, and reassuring. The main goal of the session should be to give the news. Any further discussion of treatment goals and choices may overwhelm the patient and should be deferred to a future visit.

The next task will be to actually give the news. A "warning" such as "I'm afraid I have some bad news" will help the patient prepare for the information. Then deliver the news in a simple, direct, and straightforward manner. Pause to give the patient time to react and assess the patient's reaction before you proceed. Often the reaction is obvious: the patient may cry or become angry. The patient may, however, be silent, and you may need to ask "How are you feeling about this news?" At this point the patient's reaction will direct the rest of the interview. Regardless of where the discussion goes from this point, the clinician should continuously monitor and respond to the patient's emotions, understanding, and desire for information.

Attention to the end of this interview is important for future care. The physician should inquire about the patient's understanding of his or her illness: "Can you tell me what you understand about your illness?" The physician should communicate continued support: "I'm going to do everything I can to help you through this" and should offer hope, but be realistic: "Let's hope for the best and prepare for the worst." Finally, the patient will need a follow-up visit within a short period of time to discuss options and goals of treatment.

D. PATIENT EDUCATION AND COUNSELING

Effective patient education serves a number of important purposes in the clinical encounter. It satisfies the patient's desire to know about his or her condition, it improves patient satisfaction and compliance, and it relieves the patient's anxiety. It also improves health outcomes and reduces health risks. Physicians must be acutely aware that patients misunderstand and forget much of what they hear from their doctor.

The ultimate goal in patient education is to change behavior in order to improve the health of the patient. To accomplish this goal patients need to understand their illness, recognize behaviors that put them at risk, make decisions about treatment options, and adhere to their physician's advice.

Studies show that patients commonly believe their physician does not give them enough information. Other studies show that patients commonly misunderstand or do not remember the information their physician gives them and that high levels of interpersonal skill on the part of the physician correlate with the amount of information a physician gives to a patient and the amount the patient recalls. There are situations predictably associated with poor recall such as many medical problems discussed at one visit, patient anxiety, more than one medication being prescribed, and new or bad news being given. Techniques a physician can use to improve recall include simplification, repetition, giving specific information, checking the patient's understanding, discussing fewer problems, and limiting new medications. Physicians should also negotiate an agreement with the patient about the nature of and solution to the problem and explore patients' ideas about the problem. More nonverbal immediacy such as closer interpersonal distance, more eye contact, and leaning toward the patient is beneficial. It is also important to assess what a patient wants to know.

These interventions target information giving and recall and are critical. Behavior change, however, is more complicated than simply giving information that the patient can understand and remember. Physicians need to assess patients' understanding of the problem and assess and understand their motivation to change. Questions targeted toward the patient's understanding of the disease such as "What do you know about your condition?" and questions directed at motivation to change such as "What are you willing to do about your condition?" are also useful.

Physicians need to present options and help patients make choices. Patients are more likely to make behavior changes successfully if they have several choices. Too many options, however, may be overwhelming. Statements such as "Your options are. . ." and questions such as "Which option will you choose?" or "How will you go about it?" are helpful. Some additional important areas of communication include continued offers of support from the physician, encouragement of small successes by the physician, and continued reassessment of the problem.

Beckman HB, Frankel RM: The effect of physician behavior on the collection of data. Ann Intern Med 1984;101:692-696.

Buller MK, Buller DB: Physicians' communication style and patient satisfaction. Health Soc Behav 1987;28:375.

Cole S, Bird J: *The Medical Interview: The Three-Function Approach.* Mosby, 2000.

Coulehan J, Block M: *The Medical Interview: Mastering Skills for Clinical Practice.* F.A. Davis, 2001.

Engel GL: In: *The Task of Medicine: Dialogue at Wickenburg.* White KL (editor). Kaiser Family Foundation, 1988.

Francis V, Korsch BM, Morris MJ: Gaps in doctor patient communication. New Engl J Med 1969;28:535.

Gueninger UJ, Goldstein MG, Duffy FD: A conceptual framework for interactive patient education in practice and clinical settings. J Hum Hypertension 1990;4(Suppl 1):21.

Lipkin M, Putnam SM, Lazare A (editors): *The Medical Interview: Clinical Care, Education, and Research.* Springer, 1995.

Smith R: *The Patient's Story: Integrated Patient-Doctor Interviewing.* Little Brown, 1996.

Suchman AL et al: Physician satisfaction with primary care office visits. Med Care 1993;31:1083.

Cultural Competence

Kathleen A. Culhane-Pera, MD, MA, & Sonia Patten, PhD

What Is Cultural Competence?

Family practitioners have recognized the importance of cultural competence for many years. Cultural competence is now gaining acceptance in other areas of medicine and in medical education. Its acceptance is based on the concept that disease, illness, healing, and health involve more than cells, organs, and biochemical systems and that both healers and patients bring their complex social and cultural contexts into the clinical encounter. Several recent governmental and nongovernmental policies, reports, and recommendations require physicians and medical institutions to implement policies, procedures, and educational efforts to improve health care delivery to all.

The U.S. Department of Health and Human Services' (DHHS) 10-year program to improve health, called *Healthy People 2010,* has two goals: (1) to increase the quality and years of healthy life and (2) to eliminate health disparities. To achieve equity in health care and to eliminate health disparities, "*Healthy People 2010* is firmly dedicated to the principle that—regardless of differences in gender, race and ethnicity, income and education, disability, geographic location, and sexual orientation—every person in every community across the Nation deserves equal access to comprehensive, culturally competent, community-based health care systems that are committed to serving the needs of the individual and promoting community health."

In addition, as part of the Initiative to Eliminate Racial and Ethnic Disparities in Health the DHHS approved the *National Standards for Culturally and Linguistically Appropriate Services* (CLAS) in December 2000: "Health care organizations should ensure that patients/consumers receive from all staff members effective, understandable, and respectful care that is provided in a manner compatible with their cultural health beliefs and practices and preferred language." Of the 14 standards, four are requirements for recipients of federal funds, and the others are guidelines or recommendations.

Title VI of the 1964 Civil Rights Act guarantees the right to equal access to federally funded services, regardless of gender, age, race, ethnicity, religion, or national origin. The DHHS interprets this law to include people of limited English proficiency. All health care organizations that receive federal funds must provide linguistically appropriate services (such as interpreters, bilingual workers, and vernacular written materials) to patients with limited English proficiency or face penalties for violation of the Civil Rights Act. In response, some state Medicaid services are providing reimbursement for interpreter services.

In 1998, the American Medical Association adopted recommendations for culturally competent physicians and in 1999 published a compendium of resources: "Culturally competent physicians are able to provide patient-centered care by adjusting their attitudes and behaviors to account for the impact of emotional, cultural, social and psychological issues on the main biomedicine ailment. [R]esources assist physicians in understanding how their own life experiences and emotional makeup and their 'physician culture' affect the care they deliver."

The Institute of Medicine's (IOM) scathing report on the condition of the medical care system, *Crossing the Quality Chasm,* cites six aims for the American medical system: safe, timely, efficient, effective, equitable, and patient-centered care. Equity is defined as "care that does not vary in quality because of personal characteristics, such as gender, ethnicity, geographic location, and socioeconomic status."

In medical education, the Accreditation Council for Graduate Medical Education's (ACGME) *Outcome Project* has defined six general competencies for graduates of residency programs, including professionalism that requires physicians to "demonstrate sensitivity and responsiveness to patients' culture, age, gender, and disabilities."

Given these requirements and recommendations, why is cultural competence so important? What about culture is so important in medicine? And how can physicians provide culturally competent care in clinical settings?

Accreditation Council for Graduate Medical Education: *Outcomes Projects with Six Competencies,* 2001. Retrieved December 29, 2001: http://www.acgme.org/outcome/comp/compFull.asp#5.

American Medical Association (AMA): *Enhancing the Cultural Competence of Physicians. Recommendations from the Council on Medical Education,* Report 5-A-98, 1998. Retrieved December 27, 2001: http://www.ama-assn.org/meetings/public/annual98/reports/cme/cmerpt5.htm.

American Medical Association (AMA): *Cultural Competence Compendium,* 1999. http://www.ama-assn.org/ama/pub/category/4848.html.

Culhane-Pera KA et al: Multicultural curriculum in family practice residencies. Fam Med 2000;32(3):167.

Institute of Medicine: *Crossing the Quality Chasm: A New Health System for the 21st Century,* 2001. Retrieved December 29, 2001: http://www.iom.edu/IOM/IOMHome.nsf.

Why Is Cultural Competence Important?

A. CULTURE INFLUENCES PEOPLE'S VIEWS OF HEALTH, ILLNESS, AND TREATMENT

Health, illness, and treatment are strongly influenced by cultural contexts. It may seem strange to students and practitioners of scientifically based biomedicine that the cultures of providers and patients are major factors in clinical encounters. However, all humans have been socialized from childhood to define and experience the world in ways that are shared with other members of their group. Culture provides concepts, rules, and meanings that are basic to and are expressed in the ways people relate to other people, to the supernatural, and to the environment. Culture provides us with a basis for language, symbols, rituals, art, beliefs, values, and attitudes. It is through culture that we learn to divide the world into categories that render meaning and to interpret the events of the world, rendering the world understandable, orderly, and predictable. Culture is such an intrinsic part of an individual's identity that it can be difficult to contemplate any other way of being human. Keep in mind that culture is a social phenomenon, and that no single individual is a repository for his or her entire culture. Not all members of a cultural group believe, think, or act in the same manner. Individuals vary because of psychological factors and because of the influence of their ethnicity, gender, age, language, formal education, occupation, socioeconomic class, and physical abilities, as well as their religious, political, and sexual orientation.

Interestingly, people become most aware of culture when they are thrust into contact with another cultural group. Experiencing cultural differences can arouse a variety of responses. The temptation is great for people to negatively evaluate, or totally reject, all cultures but their own. Some individuals feel very threatened and may react with fear or anger; some feel puzzled and disoriented; and some are fascinated. Culture shock is a very real phenomenon that can result in psychological discomfort, frustration, depression, and alienation. Individuals who have not learned about cultural differences or have not developed proficiency in communicating across cultures are most likely to experience devastating culture shock.

B. THE DIVERSE AMERICAN POPULATION

The changing demographics of the United States provide compelling reasons for health care providers to consider the impact of cultural factors on health, disease, and health care. The population is diverse; according to the 2000 census, non-Hispanic whites comprise 69.1% of the population, non-Hispanic blacks 12.1%, Hispanics 12.5%, Asians 3.6%, and American Indians 0.7%. The population as a whole will grow more slowly than it has in the past but subgroups within it will have different trajectories, such that the aggregated current ethnic minority populations will eventually outnumber the historic majority of European-Americans. Both differential birth rates and magnitude of immigration are factors that influence the composition of American society. In the 2000 census, foreign-born individuals comprised 13.3% of the total population, with more than half of the residents of some American cities being foreign born. This rate of growth in immigrants, refugees, and undocumented foreign-born residents is a highly politicized issue. For providers, it means that cultural differences are in the foreground in the health care arena.

Historically, racial and ethnic categories were considered fixed biological criteria; they are now widely recognized as social categories that humans create for various purposes (eg, to describe, influence, or control human behavior; to impact policy and law). Presently the terms "race" and "ethnic group" are used in a way that makes them virtually interchangeable.

C. RACIAL AND ETHNIC HEALTH DISPARITIES

The health statistics of minority and lower socioeconomic class populations are markedly worse than those of majority and middle- or upper-class populations. Improvements in infant mortality rates, disease morbidity, and life expectancies for minority Americans of all classes lag behind improvements for majority Americans. This is due to a complex interaction of many factors, including increased exposure to disease and decreased access to health care. People with health insurance and substantial economic resources have better health status than poor people, and a larger percentage of ethnic minority people is poor. Health statistics are best in countries with small differences between rich and poor and with national health insurance policies, such as Costa Rica, Norway, and Japan. The distance between rich and poor in the United States has been increasing, and the disparity in health statistics has been growing. Historical factors of discrimination cannot be ignored as a major contributing factor in this connection.

Even after controlling for the differences in socioeconomic class, however, ethnic minority groups still have worse health status than the majority group. Institutional discrimination and individual discriminatory practices in health care settings have been cited as contributing causes. Comparisons between black and white patients with similar medical conditions have shown that despite the ability to pay, blacks are more frequently admitted to wards than to private rooms, receive less intensive treatment and reduced amounts of pain medication, and have fewer invasive procedures, tests, and operations. Engaging in culturally competent care is an important remedy in redressing discriminatory practices in medical care.

D. PATIENT-CENTERED CARE INCLUDES CULTURALLY COMPETENT CARE

An anthropological perspective that is now rather widely subscribed to within medicine makes a distinction between disease and illness, with physicians focusing on the biological processes of disease and patients focusing on the experience of the illness. It is a challenge for biomedically trained physicians to maintain a focus on the patient as a person while simultaneously using diagnostic technology to explore the disease. A movement toward patient-centered medical care with emphases on improved communication and patient–provider satisfaction has built upon Engel's biopsychosocial model.

Treating a patient in a manner that is neither alienating nor paternalistic involves acknowledgment of and respect for the complexity of cultural, social, and psychological factors that the person brings to health, disease, and treatment endeavors. Working with the power that patients have to improve their health, treat their diseases, and cope with their illnesses requires a patient-centered model of care. Studies show that patients' satisfaction with clinical encounters and health care outcomes is related to their being heard by health care providers, getting their desires met, and having their fears addressed. Working with patients' cultural beliefs, values, and expectations and incorporating their family and social community improve health care outcomes.

The patient-centered care approach requires physicians to elicit and respectfully respond to patients' beliefs, concerns, and experiences with their illnesses—all culturally influenced dimensions. Patient-centered care is therefore compatible with culturally competent care.

Census 2000: Retrieved December 27, 2001: http://www.census.gov.

Engel G: The need for a new medical model: a challenge for biomedicine. Science 1977;196:129.

Graves JL: *The Emperor's New Clothes: Biological Theories of Race at the Millennium.* Rutgers University Press, 2001.

Mayberry RM et al: *Racial and Ethnic Differences in Access to Medical Care: A Synthesis of the Literature.* Morehouse Medical Treatment Effectiveness Center, commissioned by the Henry J. Kaiser Family Foundation, 1999. Retrieved from www.kff.org, search 1526.

Stewart M et al: The impact of patient-centered care on outcomes. J Fam Pract 2000;49:796.

Williams DR: Race, socioeconomic status, and health: the added effects of racism and discrimination. Ann NY Acad Sci 1999; 896:173.

Williams DR, Rucker TD: Understanding and addressing racial disparities in health care. Health Care Financ Rev 2000; 21(4):75.

What about Culture Is Important?

Throughout this section, a case study will be used to illustrate major points.

CASE: MT was a 72-year-old Hmong woman with a severe headache, blurred vision, and gait instability. A computed tomography scan revealed intracerebellar hemorrhage and evidence for an early pontine herniation. Neurologists and neurosurgeons recommended a life-saving craniotomy to evacuate the clot and reduce the pressure. The family refused the operation and taking her left the hospital against medical advice to perform traditional Hmong treatments.

In this situation, and similar situations when patients and physicians have different perspectives about appropriate responses to illness, exploring the cultural issues can be enlightening. In this chapter seven important concepts about the influence of culture on patients and physicians that are pertinent to the provision of medical care in cross-cultural settings are described. After the description of each concept, the information is applied to MT's case.

One word of caution. The following general cultural beliefs and practices need to be considered as information that illustrates the importance of culture and *not* as stereotypical statements about all people from a cultural group. Although cultural groups can generally be described as having certain characteristics, cultural beliefs and practices are variable for individuals within groups.

A. CONCEPTS OF BODILY FUNCTIONS

All cultures have an internally consistent system of beliefs about how the body functions normally, how it is influenced by factors to function abnormally, and how the body can be restored to health. Human beings have created many systems of thought about bodily functions and malfunctions: the Chinese system of balance between yin and yang; the Aryuvedic concept of balance in nature; Western systems of biomedicine, homeopathy, and naturopathy; as well as ethnic groups' traditional systems. Although the systems are vastly different because they are intimately connected with each group's unique perspective on the natural order of the world, the perspectives have striking similarities because each group has been influenced by the diffusion of thoughts, beliefs, and practices around the globe through the centuries.

Each ethnic group's beliefs about the functioning of the natural, social, and supernatural worlds are germane to its ideas about health, illness, and healing. The natural realm includes ideas about the connections between people and the earth's elements of soil, water, air, plants, animals, etc. The social realm is the ideas about individuals and the appropriate interaction between people of different ages, genders, lineages, and ethnic groups. And the supernatural realm includes religious beliefs about birth, death, the afterlife, reincarnation, spirits, and the interaction between the spiritual world and the human world.

To fully understand any ethnic group's perspectives about health and disease, physicians need to place various aspects of culture—from the idea of personhood to the kinship system to the religious meaning of suffering, life, and death—into the context of illness.

Application to the case: Hmong in the United States are refugees from the Vietnam War in Laos. As a Chinese minority, they have concepts that are similar to those of the Chinese. The concepts of health and disease are akin to the Chinese humoral theory of balance between the forces of yin and yang. The kinship system is patrilineal, the residence pattern is patrilocal, and political power lies in the hands of male elders. Hmong religion includes beliefs in multiple souls that may leave the body, thus causing illness, and in ongoing relationships between the living and the spirits of ancestors.

B. CLASSIFICATION OF DISEASES

Each ethnic group has its own system of classifying diseases, which varies from group to group and does not necessarily correspond to the others. This presents problems for translation of words and of ideas between different systems.

Entities that are recognized by certain ethnic groups and not others have been studied as folk illnesses or culture-bound syndromes. These entities are ailments with coherent concepts of etiologies, pathophysiologies, and treatments, but they may also be expressions of mental and/or social distress that have social and symbolic meanings. Examples include Latino *nervios,* Malaysian *amok,* Laotian *latah,* African-American "high blood," and English "colds." Some, such as American premen-

strual syndrome, bulimia, and anorexia nervosa, have moved from folk illness to biomedical diagnosis. Culture-bound syndromes are part of the *Diagnostic and Statistical Manual of Mental Disorders,* fourth edition (*DSM-IV*), but can also be considered as entities in their own right.

Health care providers must be aware that not everyone shares the biomedical system of classifying signs and symptoms into pathological states. Physicians can try to understand patients' systems of disease classification, but many systems have not been carefully delineated and many change as groups interact with other groups and individuals with other individuals.

Application to the case: The Hmong disease classification system for headache seems straightforward, as there is one main word for headache (*mob taub hau*), but there are multiple types of headaches based on etiology. One recognized type of headache is associated with stroke. Contact with biomedicine has altered the concept of stroke for some Hmong people in the United States.

C. THEORIES OF DISEASE CAUSATION

Every system of health and disease considers causation, linking events in the social, natural, and supernatural realms with recognized sicknesses. The finding of a cause serves multiple purposes. It can guide therapy prospectively, confirm actions retrospectively, and affirm actions that were not taken. Perhaps most importantly, etiologies can explain bodily dysfunction, render meaning to catastrophe, and thus give solace to human suffering.

Delineating etiologies can be a complex process, depending on many factors, such as the signs and symptoms of the sickness, responses to various therapies, the stature and reputation of the person who is sick, and historical events that occurred to the individual, the family, and the community. Multiple etiologies may surface during a sickness episode, and multiple etiologies, even seemingly contradictory etiologies, may remain after the event.

Cecil Helman organized disease etiologies into four categories: (1) individual, (2) natural, (3) social, and (4) supernatural. In any given ethnic group the four categories likely overlap.

1. Individual types of etiologies include behaviors that allopathic medicine perceives as risk factors for disease: poor diet and life-style, lack of exercise, use of tobacco and alcohol, not using seat belts, nonsafe sexual practices, etc. This category is associated with blaming the victim ("He got what was coming to him"), feelings of guilt ("I shouldn't have done *x* all those years"), and taking individual responsibility ("If you want to be healthy, then you need to do *x, y,* and *z*").

2. Etiologies that come from the natural world include germs, environmental factors (temperature, wind, barometric pressure, chemical pollutants), humoral factors (ether and hot/cold elements), and the universe (stars, planets, and constellations). In this type of etiology, there is less personal responsibility for an illness, as factors out of human control often cause the problem.

3. Social etiologies are a result of interactions or conflicts between people, such as family or community members. Examples include stressed social relations: when people are not getting along well, their general "unhappiness" or lack of harmony can cause one or more people to be sick. Also, the "evil eye," a curse, or a spell can cause illness.

4. Finally, the types of disease caused by supernatural powers are influenced by the culture's religious beliefs. For some Christians, sinful actions or thoughts may be punished by an angry or judgmental God. Preventive actions to avoid these disasters depend on the specific religious perspectives and are included in the religious values of righteous behaviors.

Whereas physicians' allopathic system of healing focuses on finding cause in the individual and natural realms, patients may consider other types of causes. Respectfully inquiring into patients' perception of etiology may decrease miscommunication and decrease conflict about the optimal treatment approach and may also strengthen relationships.

Application to the case: The Hmong concept of etiology includes any or all four categories, depending on the type and seriousness of the illness. Multiple etiologies can be investigated concurrently and can coexist to cause one person's problem.

D. TREATMENT OPTIONS

Multiple treatment options are available throughout the world. In the United States allopathic medicine is well established, alternative-complementary healing methods are growing, and traditional healing approaches of many people from around the globe are available. Kleinman has divided types of healers into three sectors that are overlapping and interconnected rather than mutually exclusive.

First, the Popular or Lay Sector consists of sick people, their family, friends, neighbors, and local community members. These people have acquired authority through experience, either from their own illnesses or from working with others' illnesses. Their knowledge and wisdom come from generations of people like themselves, but they have been influenced by folk or professional healers in their own societies. Their range of therapies is broad, working with medicines of various origins, herbs, amulets, rituals, massage, food, and other remedies to treat ailments and restore health. This sector is pervasive; in addition to offering therapies, it also teaches the principles of disease prevention and health promotion.

Second, the Folk Sector consists of sacred and secular healers who have acquired authority via inheritance, apprenticeship, religious position, or divine choice. Their favor is affirmed by their reputation in the community, performance of healing power, or signs and revelations. A large category, it encompasses herbalists, bonesetters, traditional midwives, spiritual healers, shamans, and injectionists. Their approach tends to be holistic, dealing with whatever identified natural elements, psychological concerns, social conflicts, and supernatural forces may be related to the sickness within the context of family and community members.

Third, the Professional Sector consists of health care providers whose authority is achieved by schooling and by licensure, both determined by the profession's organizations and sanctioned by the government. This sector includes physicians, nurses, chiropractors, and physical therapists.

These three sectors operate continuously and concurrently. The vast majority of illnesses are treated in the lay sector, as self-therapy and home therapy deal with all ailments; often it is only when this sector is unable to respond adequately to a sickness that help is sought from other sources.

Physicians must understand that a wide range of healers and healing ideas in the community influences patients and their families. Asking what other assistance patients have sought, what advice they have received, and whom else they intend to consult can broaden the physician's understanding of patients' healing networks. This understanding can help physicians ascertain their place in patients' pursuits of assistance.

Application to the case: The Hmong traditional system of healing included well-developed lay and folk sectors. In extended families there were men and women who knew about diseases and treatments, grandparents who knew about maintaining health and preventing disease, and heads of households who had the responsibility to maintain relationships with the spirits. In villages there were experts in diagnosis and herbal medicines, in rituals, and in shaman ceremonies. Access to professionals was limited.

E. INTERPRETATION OF BODILY SIGNS AND SYMPTOMS

The four preceding sections focus on an ethnic group's general understanding of health and disease. The ensuing two sections focus on how individual patients and families deal with particular sickness within the context of their cultural beliefs and behaviors.

Initially, individuals sense a symptom or other people perceive a sign. Questions arise: "Is this normal or abnormal? If it is abnormal, what does it signify? Is it serious or mild? What caused it? What should be done about it?" The answers to these questions are influenced by people's understandings of their culture's general approach to bodily functions and malfunctions, disease classification, etiology, and seriousness, but also may be influenced by other individual factors. Together the answers constitute what Arthur Kleinman has called an explanatory model.

According to Kleinman individuals' "explanatory models" (EMs) of their sickness have five aspects (Table 54–1) and providers need to ask questions to pursue people's perspectives about their sickness (Table 54–2). The sick person, family members, social network, and providers have different EMs about the sickness event, which may be complementary or contradictory. More agreement among the EMS facilitates smoother interactions among people, whereas more disagreement leads to more conflict.

Whereas individuals feel sick when they interpret their signs or symptoms as abnormal, their family members and/or healers must agree for them to assume the "sick role." Parsons describes the sick role as legitimizing a withdrawal from regular responsibilities and as obligating others to give assistance. Without others' agreement, which is influenced by cultural beliefs of health and disease, individuals are not given permission to withdraw and to receive special care. In some cultures, runny noses, or fluid coming from ears, or frequent loose bowel movements are normal, and hence do not result in someone seeking care. In other cultures, being frightened by a near accident or having a disagreement with a relative may be reason to miss work.

Learning about patients' EMs can provide physicians with a deeper understanding of their patients' illness experiences and struggles. Physicians can work with this information to address fears and concerns, to plan health educational needs, and to develop a care plan. This communication may improve overall health care delivery, health care outcomes, and satisfaction between providers and patients.

Application to the case: The patient's EM was not known, as she was too sick to communicate; information came from her husband and sons. Also, her tradi-

Table 54–1. Kleinman's explanatory models.

1. Etiology of the condition
2. Timing and mode of onset of symptoms
3. Pathophysiological processes
4. Natural history and severity of illness
5. Appropriate treatments

Table 54–2. Kleinman's questions to explore explanatory models.

1. What do you call your problem?
2. What do you think has caused your problem?
3. Why do you think it started when it did?
4. What does your sickness do to you?
5. How severe is it? Will it have a long or short course?
6. What do you fear most about your sickness?
7. What chief problems has your sickness caused for you?
8. What kind of treatment do you think you should receive?

Five alternative questions:
1. What do you think is wrong?
2. What are you afraid of?
3. What do you think has caused the problem?
4. What have you tried to relieve the problem?
5. What do you think would help you?

tional sick role meant that she should be passive and allow her family members to take care of her. At home, MT had had a severe headache for which her husband gave her Tylenol, a Thai pharmaceutical preparation (probably aspirin or acetaminophen), and a Hmong herbal medication. As the headache worsened, the husband called her sons; the whole family became alarmed about the serious nature of the problem as the gait instability developed, and they decided to seek assistance from the hospital.

Her husband and sons believed the doctor's interpretation of bleeding in the brain, but they were concerned about the invasive and potentially harmful nature of the proposed operation. Hoping to find a less dangerous treatment, they sought a shaman's assistance. During a trance, the shaman discovered that one of the patient's souls had left her body and was going to be reincarnated. The necessary treatment was to return the soul to the body in a shaman ritual, which required that she return home from the hospital, or face imminent death. Other family members' EMs were different; some did not agree with the pathophysiology of the doctors and others were skeptical about the spiritual problem. During the ceremony to retrieve the soul, the shaman discovered a long-standing intrafamilial conflict that had contributed to the soul loss.

F. MEDICAL DECISION MAKING

Once sick individuals have determined the need for therapeutic assistance, how do they choose, given the lay, folk, and professional sectors, which group to consult? The decision-making process is complex, and includes cultural and social influences.

Cultural beliefs about health, sickness, and etiology influence which healers are deemed appropriate to treat the problem. After the healer has been chosen and the healing method completed, cultural factors continue to influence the healing process as sick individuals and family members evaluate the method's effectiveness, discern the etiologies, learn from the experience, and consider the need for further assistance.

Social factors also influence the process, as sick individuals' social networks express approval or disapproval for certain healers and healing methods. Generally, lay healers and folk healers more than professional healers bond with patients by sharing the same ethnicity, language, medical terminology, socioeconomic class, and worldview.

Ethnic identity, the extent to which individuals and families identify with a particular ethnic group, also influences the choice of healers. Although ethnic identity may be strong when people initially arrive in another country, that identity changes over time by the process of acculturation. Because acculturation is an irregular, dynamic, bidirectional process that results in considerable variation within individuals, families, and communities, intrafamilial conflicts can arise about appropriate treatments.

Although an ideal provider may be identified by cultural and social factors, the presence of physical, economic, or structural factors also influences choice. Where is the healer? Is transportation available when needed? Are others free to accompany the sick person? How expensive is the healer and the potential therapies? These factors are often referred to as "structural barriers to care."

In pluralistic societies such as those in the United States, where multiple systems of healing coexist and therapies from multiple traditions are available, sick people and their family members may seek assistance from different healing traditions concurrently or sequentially. They may use one type of practice after another, depending on their interpretation of the situation, on the fit between the sickness and the healing approach, as well as on the efficacy of the therapies. Or they may use several different types of healing methods at the same time, not waiting to evaluate the efficacy of one treatment before seeking another.

In the United States complementary and alternative medical approaches are becoming common and mainstream. It has been estimated that one-third of all Americans use some kind of "unconventional medicine," whether relaxation, massage, chiropractic manipulation, herbal medicines, acupuncture, vitamins, or traditional ethnic medical systems. The vast majority of these people do not inform their physicians about their actions.

Sensitivity to the multiple issues that influence decision making for a given ailment—including inquiring about patients' historical roots, ethnic identity, acculturation, social networks, transportation needs, and ability to pay—will allow physicians to work with patients more effectively and serve the interests and needs for which they seek assistance. An awareness of patients' practices aligns physicians with their healing efforts.

Application to the case: MT and her husband had been in the United States for 10 years, were living in a Hmong community, and had not learned English. Their traditional spiritual beliefs were extremely important to the couple, and to their sons. From a spiritual perspective, MT needed the shaman's ceremony to retrieve her soul and return her to spiritual health. From a physical perspective, she would not have been able to survive an operation without all of her souls intact. The family decision-making process included a discussion of the pros and cons, with the younger more acculturated members wanting the surgery and the older sons and her husband choosing the traditional ceremony. The morning after the shaman ceremony the family met again, determined that her souls were intact, realized that her physical condition had continued to deteriorate, and decided that she needed the operation to get well. Spiritually intact, she might be able to survive the operation.

G. HEALER–SICK PERSON RELATIONS

Every cultural system has expectations about the healer–sick person–family relationship. The rules of this relationship—such as the appropriate styles of communication, the approaches to relevant topics, the boundaries concerning who shares what with whom, the cultural values, and the amount of the power that the healer exerts over the patient and family—are culturally influenced. Physicians in the United States learn the presently preferred manner of physician–patient relationships. However, patients from different ethnic groups may perceive some of these approaches as foreign, rude, mean, or unacceptable.

Cultural values are always present in the clinical encounter. The biomedical and western values of physicians may conflict with the values of patients from other cultures. For instance, physicians may believe in their ability to conquer problems and exert control over nature, whereas patients may trust their ability to live in harmony with nature. Physicians may value direct and precise communication whereas patients may value indirect and polite communication. Doctors may emphasize the importance of the individual whereas patients may emphasize the group. Doctors may look to the future and exalt the young whereas patients may look to the past and revere their elders. And physicians may focus on the physical and psychological aspects of personhood whereas patients may expect to pursue the social and spiritual aspects of personhood.

There is a power differential between healers and patients that can be both helpful and harmful to patients. Biomedical physicians generally are from middle and upper socioeconomic classes, have high incomes, and are often from the dominant society. In addition to their personal status, they have the status granted to physicians, giving them access to and an understanding of a complicated and privileged body of knowledge. Although this power differential can be helpful to the healing relationship, in cross-cultural situations it can also be abused, intentionally or unintentionally, to the detriment of patients and their health status. People have long expressed their feelings of powerlessness in relationships with health care providers in biomedical institutions. Add the dimensions of different expectations of healer–sick person and extended family relations and verbal and nonverbal language barriers and the situation is ripe for patients to feel disempowered in getting their needs met.

It is important that physicians acknowledge culture as an important force in patients' lives, embrace a patient-focused approach, and work to empower patients and their families.

Application to the case: When the family had decided to take MT home, they felt the neurologist's frustration and anger at their decision, which perplexed them. "Why should he be angry with our taking care of our mother? After all, it is up to us, her family, to make the appropriate decisions for her. We are responsible, not the physicians." However, they felt support from the neurosurgeon who had accepted their decision, stating "I don't know everything. Do what you need to do." He then offered to be available should they want the operation later. His accepting and respectful attitude toward their beliefs probably made it easy for them to return the next morning for the operation. It may have been harder to return if they had had to face the angry neurologist. Their decision to return for the operation was probably buttressed by the shaman, who, after the ritual, reassured the family that MT was spiritually strong enough to survive the operation.

Culhane-Pera KA et al: *Healing by Heart: Clinical and Ethical Case Stories of Hmong Families and Western Providers.* Vanderbilt University Press, 2003.

Helman CG: *Culture, Health and Illness: An Introduction for Health Professionals,* ed 4. Butterworth-Heinemann, 2000.

Kleinman A: Concepts and a model for the comparison of medical systems as cultural systems. Social Sci Med 1978;12(2B):85.

Kleinman A: *Patients and Healers in the Context of Culture: An Exploration of the Borderland Between Anthropology, Medicine, and Psychiatry.* University of California Press, 1980.

Parsons T: *The Social System.* Free Press, 1951.

How to Provide Culturally Competent Care

How can family physicians deal with cultural influences successfully, and thus empower diverse communities of patients to optimize health and reduce disability? We have six recommendations.

1. Learn about ourselves as cultural beings.
2. Learn about patients as cultural beings.
3. Learn culturally appropriate communication skills.
4. Apply cultural information in medical interactions.
5. Do not abuse power.
6. Create and work within culturally competent institutions.

A. LEARN ABOUT OURSELVES AS CULTURAL BEINGS

"Culture" isn't a factor that influences only "others," "ethnic groups," or "minority peoples," it is an important aspect of every human being. Physicians need to learn about how culture influences their views of health, disease, and treatment, and their reactions to others, both positively and negatively. Essential elements of culturally competent care are self-awareness and cultural humility: "Cultural humility incorporates a lifelong commitment to self-evaluation and self-critique, to redressing the power imbalances in the patient-physician dynamic, and to developing mutually beneficial and non-paternalistic clinical and advocacy partnerships with communities on behalf of individuals and defined populations."

Biomedicine is also a cultural system, influenced by historical, social, economic, political, religious, and scientific events. It has its own language, which can make it difficult for physicians to translate concepts into lay terms. It also has its own values; exposed to these values, physicians may give up personal values that conflict with the mainstream biomedical perspective or they may continue to experience personal dissonance within their work. Each professional group within medicine has variations on these themes and therefore unique variations of beliefs, values, and behaviors toward health and disease.

B. LEARN ABOUT PATIENTS AS CULTURAL BEINGS

Physicians need to familiarize themselves with the prevailing beliefs, values, ethics, healing practices, community resources, and traditional healers for the communities they serve. In addition to understanding about health, disease, and treatment, life-cycle concepts are important, including pregnancy, birth, death, and end-of-life decision making. Difficulties delivering multicultural care may arise from differences in beliefs, communication styles, ethical concepts, and moral values.

Cross-cultural ethical conflicts can be particularly challenging. For example, whereas many North Americans expect to be told the truth about hopeless medical conditions and consider a focus on the patient as respecting individuality, patients from other cultures may believe that family members should decide whether patients can handle tragic news and would prefer to have the family members involved in every step of the sick person's care.

Deciding how to respond to these conflicts—acting on the ethical values of biomedicine, bowing to patients' value systems, or finding a creative compromise—is not an easy process for physicians. But understanding how different cultural beliefs and values contribute to the situation is a first step in being prepared to respond to specific patients in clinical encounters or to specific situations in community settings. The more physicians know, the more they can be prepared to deal with potential areas of congruity and incongruity between biomedical perspectives and patients' general beliefs and values. And they can be better prepared to create partnerships with community resources for addressing community health problems.

C. Learn Culturally Appropriate Communication Skills

For optimal communication with patients, physicians must learn culturally appropriate patient-centered communication skills. And to be effective in cross-cultural settings, they need to be proficient in multiple languages and/or learn to work with interpreters (Table 54–3).

Knowing what verbal and nonverbal communication style to use is a challenge. Clues can be obtained from prior information, familiarity with the cultural group, and the individual patients and their family members, and by asking medical experts, such as medical interpreters.

Table 54–3. Recommendations for working with interpreters.

Working with a medically trained interpreter, personally if at all possible or via telephone services:

1. Greet patients in their language
2. Introduce yourself and everyone present
3. Arrange seats in a triad and address the patient
4. Speak clearly in a normal voice
5. Use common terms and simple language structure
6. Express one idea at a time, and pause for interpretation
7. Expect the interpreter to use the first person singular, verbatim translation
8. Consider multiple meanings to nonverbal gestures
9. Ask the same questions in different ways if you get inconsistent or unconnected responses
10. Ask the interpreter to explain issues, but do not place the interpreter in the middle of conflicts

Verbal communication styles are different for people from different cultural perspectives. For many Native Americans, not talking about social connections conveys a sense of being rude and uncivilized. To many Chinese, asking direct questions about sensitive issues can cause loss of face. To many Islamic patients, speaking about future blessings may mean that they won't occur, unless we say "God willing." Using first names or family titles (such as grandmother or uncle) can be insulting to many African-Americans, but using first names can be experienced as caring by many Hispanic patients, and using family titles can be experienced as respectful by many Africans and Asians. To many ethnic groups who value speaking indirectly, a direct assertive approach by a physician is experienced as shocking and rude; and although physicians may expect patients to answer directly, politeness may demand that they not directly question or challenge authority figures.

Nonverbal expressions are also replete with multiple, even opposite meanings. For many Asians, making "sincere" constant eye contact is experienced as invasive and disrespectful, like a child who stares, and speaking loudly is experienced as an expression of anger. For Islamic patients, giving things in the left hand is revolting because the left hand is symbolically dirty whereas the right hand is symbolically clean. To Native Americans, asking questions without waiting an appropriate amount of time for a reply is an indication of lack of interest in the response. And whereas smiles and laughter usually mean enjoyment, in certain cultures they are used at moments of embarrassment and shyness, particularly at moments of conflict; thus, even smiles can be misinterpreted.

D. Apply Cultural Information in Medical Interactions

Understanding general information about the communities in which they work, physicians are ready to apply that cultural information to specific medical encounters. One multicultural patient-centered approach to the clinical encounter physicians can use is Berlin and Fowkes's LEARN model.

- **Listen** to patients' perspectives. The most important first step is to listen to the stories of patients and their families about the illness experiences. Before listening, physicians must ask about and display a genuine desire to hear the patients' perspectives. To elicit their perspectives of their illness, disease, or EMs, physicians can try Kleinman's questions or modifications thereof (Table 54–2). Physicians must remember, though, that asking directly may not be the optimal method of obtaining information and gaining understanding for all patients.

- **Explain** our views. After gathering information from patients' stories and physical findings, physicians need to explain their views of the patient's condition. They can explain the biomedical assessment by building upon patients' ideas, beliefs, and values and by addressing their fears and concerns. Using principles of patient education and knowledge of patients, physicians can empower patients so they can use biomedical information in whatever manner they determine is best.

- **Acknowledge** similarities and differences. Physicians can acknowledge similarities and differences in multiple perspectives concerning normal or abnormal bodily functions, disease classification, etiology, projected course, and preferred treatment. It may be important to emphasize commonalties (ie, "We both want your child's fever to come down") as well as differences (ie, "I believe this is not a serious condition").

- **Recommend** a course of action. As recommendations for diagnostic or therapeutic plans are made, physicians can ask permission of ("I would like to draw blood from your arm to....; is that OK with you?") and lay out options for patients, as well as asking what options patients would like to pursue.

- **Negotiate** plans. Depending upon how much disagreement there is between patients' desires and physicians' recommendations, physicians may need to negotiate a plan. Remembering that the intent is to empower patients to lead healthy lives, physicians need to work with patients' perspectives about their bodies, illnesses, and desired treatments. Patients who have had input into creating plans are more likely to adhere to the specifics.

E. Do Not Abuse Power

In the context of multicultural care, physicians have to be aware of power differences between patients and providers and of power struggles that can arise, and must avoid abuse of their power. To these ends, doctors need to know about their personal and professional biases and prejudices and need to monitor their actions and emotional reactions to patients. Balint groups, physician support groups, ethical committees, and religious societies are multiple ways for physicians to examine their personal struggles. Physicians can consider "caring-in-relation" and "power-in-relation" as ways to avoid abuse of power.

F. Create and Work within Culturally Competent Institutions

Physicians need to be active members in clinics, hospitals, and medical societies so as to create culturally competent institutions. Physicians can be powerful advocates for hiring bilingual–bicultural workers, employing trained interpreters, obtaining reimbursement for interpreter services, creating health education practices for patients with limited English proficiency, and engaging institutions in caring for diverse patients. The more systems are constructed to empower patients and avoid societal prejudices and biases, the more physicians can provide culturally competent care and improve the health of all patients.

Berlin EA, Fowkes WC: A teaching framework for cross-cultural health care. West J Med 1983;139:934.

Candib L: *Medicine and the Family: A Feminist Perspective.* Basic Books, 1995.

Kleinman A: *Writing at the Margin: Discourse Between Anthropology and Medicine.* University of California Press, 1995.

Loustaunau MO, Sobo EJ: *The Cultural Context of Health, Illness, and Medicine.* Bergin & Garvey, 1997.

Luckman J, Nobles ST: *Transcultural Communication in Health Care.* Delmar/Thompson Learning Press, 2001.

Salimbene S: *What Language Does Your Patient Hurt In?: A Practical Guide to Culturally Competent Patient Care.* Amherst Educational Publishing, 2001.

Spector RE: *Cultural Diversity in Health and Illness,* ed 5. Prentice-Hall, 2000.

Tervalon M, Murray-Garcia J: Cultural humility versus cultural competence: a critical distinction in defining physician training outcomes in multicultural education. J Health Care Poor Underserved 1998;9(2):117.

WEB SITES

Asian and Pacific Islander American Health Forum
http://www. apiahf.org

Association for Asian Pacific Community Health Organizations
http://www.aapcho.org

Bayer Institute for Health Care Communication
www.bayerinstitute.org

Center for Cross-Cultural Health
www.crosshealth.com

Cross Cultural Health Care Program
www.xculture.org

National Council on Interpretation in Health Care
www.diversityrx.org

National Health Law Program
http://www.healthlaw.org

Provider's Guide to Quality and Culture
http://erc.msh.org

Resources for Cross-Cultural Health
www.diversityrx.org

U.S. Department of Health and Human Services: *Healthy People 2010*
http://www.health.gov/healthypeople/

U.S. Department of Health and Human Services: *Initiative to Eliminate Racial and Ethnic Disparities of Health*

http://www.raceandhealth.hhs.gov/

U.S. Department of Health and Human Services: *National Standards on Culturally and Linguistically Appropriate Services (CLAS) in Health Care*

http://www.omhrc.gov/clas/

U.S. Department of Health and Human Services, Office for Civil Rights, Policy Guidance

http://www.hhs.gov/ocr/lep/guide.html

Health Disparities

Jeannette E. South-Paul, MD

General Considerations

The population physicians serve has changed dramatically in the past two decades; between 1980 and 2000 the white non-Hispanic population of the United States increased 7.9% as compared to an 88% increase in the aggregated minority (people of races other than white or people of Hispanic origin) population. An estimated 25% of Americans (almost 70 million persons) are classified as a member of one of the four major racial or ethnic minority groups—African-American, Latino/Hispanic, Native American, or Asian/Pacific Islander. By the year 2050, the U.S. Census estimates that people of color will represent one in three Americans. Much of this change will be due to higher birth rates and immigration among racial and ethnic minority populations. The number of states with a 30% or more minority population doubled from 8 in 1980 to 17 in 2000. During this same time, in California and New Mexico the minority became the majority, and Texas came close at 48% (Hawaii and the District of Columbia remained majority–minority as they had been in 1980).

These populations bear a disproportionate burden of illness and disease relative to their percentage distribution in the population. The explanations for this disparate health status are extensive. Understanding the factors that contribute to poor health among these populations and the strategies that have resulted in improved health can inform and promote the delivery of quality health care.

Little evidence is available to support the contention that the principal causes of these overall inequalities in health are genetic factors operating at the population level. Attempts have been made to use social status, as measured by proxy variables such as income and education, to provide epidemiological information about the black–white differential in health status. What is neglected in many of these analyses, however, is an appreciation of the interaction between underlying patho/physiological mechanisms and social processes. Explanations that take into consideration how social relations impact health offer a framework for understanding these inequalities in health status.

Historical Factors

Original American citizens of color bear a historical legacy that affects all aspects of their integration into society today. American Indians make up a fraction of today's citizens (0.7% in the 2000 census) but exhibit significant disparities in health. The prevalence of diabetes mellitus, obesity, alcoholism, and suicide is substantially greater in this population than in other American population groups. They are the one population with a health system established to help meet their medical needs. The availability of these services, however, is limited by distance when located in the rural areas inhabited by many American Indians, or they are completely inaccessible to those living in urban areas.

African-Americans encompass several groups that came to this country at different times and under different circumstances. The impact of slavery on the original Africans cannot be minimized. Residual effects of this historical tragedy have been associated with residential practices that favor segregation, educational disadvantage, and less favored treatment in health care facilities. Later immigrants of African origin came to the United States from the West Indies. These islands also received many slaves during the early to mid nineteenth century, but abolished slavery before the Emancipation Proclamation did so in the United States in 1865. These differing experiences have influenced the views of Caribbean-Americans and result in differences between them and African-Americans who descended directly from slaves on the North American continent. The final group of immigrants from African countries chose to come to the United States in recent years for both educational and economic reasons. Cultural differences often exist among these three groups in custom, dress, family roles, and religious preferences.

In spite of the fact that the foundation of this nation was a union of indigenous groups and immigrants, the above groups—plus new immigrants—bear much of the burden of disease in the nation today. The number of immigrants entering the United States during the past 15 years has increased dramatically compared to the numbers seen in the previous four decades. Political crises, natural disasters, poverty, and hunger have forced population groups of significant size to leave their homes. These migrations have resulted in loss of homes and support systems, overcrowding and overexposure, decreased access to food and medical services, and contact with new infectious agents and other toxins.

The term "immigrant" has been applied to legal and illegal (undocumented) refugees and international adopted children. Most of these immigrants reside in "linguistically isolated" households (those in which no one over the age of 14 speaks English), which were identified for the first time in the 1990 U.S. Census. Four percent of U.S. households are in this category. This includes 30% of Asian households, 23% of Hispanic households, and 28% of all immigrant households with school-age children. This is not surprising since more than 500,000 illegal immigrants, the majority of whom are from Mexico, are thought to enter the United States every year. There is less health care and fewer preventive services for a population whose first language is not English. Furthermore, these migrations and population shifts have severely taxed the municipal, educational, and health care resources of many American communities, especially those in the most affected states—California, Texas, and Florida.

Refugees tend to settle in communities in which fellow countrymen already live. In recent years East African refugees have gravitated toward the north central United States (specifically Minnesota), Afghan refugees have settled in the San Francisco Bay Area, and citizens of the former Yugoslavia have migrated to specific areas of the United Kingdom and the United States.

Weitzman M et al: Health care for children of immigrant families. Peds 1997;100:153.

Poverty

The percentage of African-Americans and Latinos who are below the 100% poverty level is three times that of non-Hispanic white Americans across the life span (28%, 29%, and 9%, respectively). Financial disadvantage impacts health in that mortality rates around the world decline with increasing social class and access to financial resources.

Poor, minority, and uninsured children are twice as likely as other children to lack the usual sources of care, nearly twice as likely to wait 60 min or more at their sites of care, and use only about half as many physician services after adjusting for health status. Poverty, minority status, and absence of insurance exert independent effects on access to and use of primary care.

Homelessness results in poor health status and high service use among children. Homeless children were reported to experience a higher number of acute illness symptoms, including fever, ear infection, diarrhea, and asthma. Emergency department and outpatient medical visits are higher among the homeless group.

Newacheck PW et al: Children's access to primary care: differences by race, income, and insurance status. Peds 1996;97(1):26.

Weinreb L et al: Determinants of health and service use patterns in homeless and low-income housed children. Peds 1998;102 (3):554.

Medical Insurance

A substantial portion of the U.S. population is medically uninsured or underinsured. A greater percentage of racial and ethnic minorities and immigrants are in this category. These numbers increase if they include those who are without health insurance for 3 months or more in a given year. Underinsurance is the inability to pay out-of-pocket expenses despite having insurance, and usually implies inability to use preventive services as well. The underinsured category includes unemployed persons aged 55—64 years of age and those not provided with health insurance coverage with their jobs. They are not eligible for Medicare and must pay high individual health premiums when they can obtain some form of group coverage. Lack of health insurance is associated with delayed health care and a higher mortality rate. Underinsurance also may result in adverse health consequences. An estimated 8 million children from diverse groups in the United States are uninsured. Substantial differences in both sources of care and utilization of medical services exist between insured and uninsured children.

In 1993, one-third of all nonelderly adult Hispanics living in the United States lacked health insurance coverage (either private or public) compared to 8% of the entire nonelderly population. Because Hispanics are more likely to be uninsured than any other ethnic group and because they are the fastest growing minority group in the United States, it is likely that the total number of uninsured people in the United States will steadily increase.

Persons with Medicare and Medicaid have twice the mortality rate of those with employer-provided insurance, and the working uninsured show a higher mortality rate than the working insured. The higher mortality rate in those with public insurance (Medicaid) or with no insurance probably reflects the combined effect of poor existing health status, exposure to illness, trauma, and disease, and lack of access to medical care. Although the general health and mental health of the uninsured are slightly worse in comparison to the privately insured, the uninsured have fewer chronic health problems. This may reflect the fact that many uninsured regularly work in physically demanding, low-wage jobs that provide few benefits. Those with chronic debilitating illnesses are unable to work. Those with chronic, less serious illnesses persist in working in spite of mild to moderate symptoms (eg, arthritis, fatigue) because they have no alternative sources of income.

There are marked discrepancies in access to and utilization of medical services, including preventive services, between uninsured and insured children, although both groups have similar rates of chronic health conditions and limitations of activity (evidence of the general health of the children being seen). Expansions in Medicaid coverage and tax credits have had little impact on the overall problem. At least 2.3 million Medicaid-eligible children were unenrolled in 1993. These children were more likely to have a working parent than children on Medicaid. Children eligible for Medicaid but who remain unenrolled are often less than 6 years of age, live in female-headed single-parent families, or are African-American or Hispanic. Not only do uninsured children lack routine medical and sick care, they also lack appropriate well-child care compared with insured children. Children who have a chronic disease, such as asthma, face difficulties in access to care and utilize substantially fewer outpatient and inpatient health services. Even if all children were universally insured, parents' utilization of health care would remain a key determinant in their children's use of services. Neglecting financial access to care for adults may have the unintended effect of diminishing the impact of targeted health insurance programs for children.

The uninsured can manifest psychopathology similar to that seen in refugees. Rates of current psychiatric disorders in ethnically diverse women on public medical assistance or uninsured are extremely high, including major depression, anxiety disorders, and history of sexual trauma. These women also engage in behaviors that pose serious health risks, including smoking (32%) and illicit drug use (2%). Fewer than 50% of them have access to comprehensive primary medical care. Young, poor women who seek care in public-sector clinics would benefit from comprehensive medical care addressing their psychosocial needs.

In the United States, the cost of health care services is a major barrier to health care access. In addition, 75% of persons in the United States who have difficulties paying their medical bills have some type of health insurance. Although the affordability of health care among persons without health insurance has been described, few details regarding affordability among persons who are underinsured exist.

There has always been concern that previously uninsured patients would overutilize the system if granted access to health care. However, a study of utilization of health care services by previously uninsured low-income patients provided with comprehensive health maintenance organization (HMO) insurance indicated no differences between the study and control groups in hospital admissions, hospital days, and outpatient laboratory, pharmacy, and radiology use. Compared with an insured commercial group of the same age and sex, the patterns of utilization were similar and the financial costs of care were only moderately more for the previously uninsured group. With the growth of managed care, these data should be beneficial in the development of health care programs for the growing number of uninsured Americans.

When looking at state programs offering subsidized health coverage in commercial managed care organizations to low-income and previously uninsured people, there was no evidence of greater initial demand for service or an unusual level of chronic illness between people enrolled through large employer-benefit plans and previously uninsured patients. Similarly, there was little evidence of underutilization, although dissatisfaction and reported barriers to service were more frequent among nonwhite enrollees. Of patients admitted to a hospital, undocumented immigrants had more complicated and serious diagnoses on admission, but a lower adjusted average length of stay than native-born populations and those with permanent residency status (insured by Medicaid or of uninsured status).

Although physicians who are generalists appear to be more likely than physicians who are specialists to provide care for poor adult patients, they may still perceive barriers, both financial and nonfinancial, to providing such care. Nonwhite physicians were more likely to care for uninsured and Medicaid patients than were white physicians. In addition to poor reimbursement, nonfinancial factors such as perceived risks of litigation were cited by 60–90% of physicians as important in the decision not to care for Medicaid and uninsured patients (Table 55–1).

Bograd H et al: Extending health maintenance organization insurance to the uninsured. A controlled measure of health care utilization. JAMA 1997;277(13):1067.

Centers for Disease Control and Prevention: Age- and state-specific prevalence estimates of insured and uninsured persons—United States 1995–1996. MMWR 1998;47(25):529.

Table 55–1. Barriers to care for uninsured.

Cost of care/poor reimbursement
Few willing providers
Litigation risk
Nonadherence to therapy
Perceived patient ingratitude

Hanson KL: Is insurance for children enough? The link between parents' and children's health care use revisited. Inquiry (US) 1998;35(3):294.

Kilbreth EH et al: State-sponsored programs for the uninsured: is there adverse selection? Inquiry (US) 1998;35(3):250.

Miranda JAF, Komaromy M, Golding JM: Unmet mental health needs of women in public-sector gynecologic clinics. Am J Obstet Gynecol 1998;178(2):212.

Housing

Young to middle-aged residents of impoverished urban areas manifest excess mortality from a number of causes—both acute and chronic. African-American youth in some urban areas faced lower probabilities of surviving to 45 years of age than white youths nationwide faced of surviving to 65 years.

Minorities comprise 80% of the residents of high-poverty, urban areas in the United States and more than 90% of the residents in the largest metropolitan areas. The lower their socioeconomic position, the less ability people have to gain access to information, services, or technologies that could provide protection from or modify risks.

It has been suggested that residential segregation based on race is a fundamental cause of racial disparities in health. Although legislation exists to eliminate discrimination in this area, the degree of residential segregation in the United States grew dramatically from 1860 to 1940 and has remained extremely high for most African-Americans since then. It has been argued that segregation is a primary cause of racial differences in socioeconomic status (SES) by limiting access to education and employment opportunities. Furthermore, segregation creates conditions that hamper a healthy social and physical environment.

For most Americans, housing equity is a major source of wealth. Because the value of housing tends to be lower in segregated areas, residential segregation directly impacts socioeconomic status. Although income is directly correlated with health for both whites and African-Americans, African-Americans report poorer health than whites at all levels of income. People residing in disadvantaged neighborhoods have a higher incidence of heart disease than people who live in more advantaged neighborhoods. The quality of housing is also likely to be poorer in highly segregated areas, and poor housing conditions also adversely affect health. For example, research reveals that a lack of residential facilities and concerns about personal safety can discourage leisure-time physical exercise.

A strong correlation exists between the percentage of poor students in a school and the percentage of African-American and Hispanic students in the same school. Although there are millions of poor whites in the United States, poor white families tend to be dispersed throughout communities, with some residing in more desirable areas. Compared to schools in middle-class areas, segregated schools have lower average test scores, fewer students in advanced placement courses, more limited curricula, less qualified teachers, less access to good academic counseling, fewer connections with colleges and employers, older deteriorated buildings, higher levels of teen pregnancy, and higher dropout rates.

Jargowsky P: *Poverty and Place: Ghettos, Barrios, and the American City.* Russell Sage Foundation, 1997.

Williams DR, Collins C: Racial residential segregation: a fundamental cause of racial disparities in health. Public Health Rep 2001;116(5):404.

Health Status & Risk

Racial and ethnic groups differ greatly both among and within themselves with respect to health status. Because mortality rates in general decline with increasing social class, there is a strong interaction between race and ethnicity and rates of mortality in the United States (Table 55–2). In addition to socioeconomic influences, variations in comparisons of health status are often related to biological differences among different racial and ethnic groups. Well-described genetic abnormalities account for conditions such as sickle cell disease in persons of African and Mediterranean origin and Tay-Sachs disease in Semitic people. Physiological differences account for the predisposition of certain populations to hypertension, the influence of this hypertension on the heart and kidney, and sensitivity and response to alcohol ingestion.

Certain disease manifestations probably result from more than one factor. For example, differences in body composition between black and white women have been well established and probably relate to genetic and behavioral factors. Black women have more bone and muscle mass, but less fat, as a percentage of body weight than white women. However, black women have more upper body fat than white women. The greater skeletal and muscle mass in black women compared to white women appears to protect them from osteoporosis. These ethnic differences in body composi-

Table 55–2. Minority health status indicators.

Higher infant mortality
Lower life expectancy
Lower immunization rates
Toxic environmental exposures
Higher morbidity and mortality from chronic disease
    (hypertension, diabetes mellitus, cancer, coronary artery disease)

tion appear to be associated with disease risk in women, such that black and Hispanic women have increased risk for diabetes mellitus. Genetic and behavioral factors are also thought to influence the overwhelming prevalence of diabetes mellitus in the Pima Indians in the southwestern United States.

Higher rates of neurovascular complications are seen in minorities with diabetes mellitus. These disparities in complications are usually attributed to disparate access to quality health care. Studies of manifestations of diabetes among diverse patients in a nonprofit, group practice, prepaid health plan (Kaiser Permanente) confirmed an elevated incidence of end-stage renal disease among ethnic minorities despite uniform medical coverage. These persistent disparities suggest a possible genetic origin, the contribution of unmeasured environmental factors, or a combination of these.

Mortality from all causes is higher for those who have fewer years of education and for African-Americans. A study of data from the National Health Interview Survey conducted from 1986 to 1994 demonstrated that although many conditions contribute to socioeconomic and racial disparities in potential life-years lost, a few conditions account for most of the disparities—smoking-related diseases in the case of mortality among persons with fewer years of education and hypertension, human immunodeficiency virus (HIV), diabetes mellitus (as noted above), and trauma in the case of mortality among African-Americans.

Life expectancy of white and African-American men shows wide geographic variation in the United States. White men in the 10 "healthiest" counties have a life expectancy above 76.4 years. African-American men in the 10 "least healthy" counties have a shorter life expectancy: 61 years in Philadelphia, 60 years in Baltimore and New York, and 57.9 years in the District of Columbia. This 20-year gap in life expectancy is as great as differences between countries at widely different stages of economic development: the best off are like Japan, whereas the worst are similar to Bangladesh and Kazakhstan.

Environmental exposures are known to vary dramatically between minority and majority communities. Minority communities are more than three times more likely to be exposed to unacceptably high levels of lead, toxic wastes, and violence with all the associated consequences. Furthermore, there are specific and devastating risks to health from behaviors involving the use of pharmacologically active substances such as tobacco in cigarettes, cigars, and snuff, and other recreational drugs.

Environmental pollution and poor occupational safety in the countries of origin are common and contribute to the health problems of many immigrant populations. Other health problems identified include obe-

sity and various dental conditions requiring treatment. The absence of basic health screening measures such as cholesterol testing, high blood pressure screening, Pap smears, and mammograms also has a devastating impact on health.

At each age of the life span until age 44, African-Americans, Latinos, and Native Americans, have, on average, higher mortality rates than non-Hispanic white Americans. Only Asians in the aggregate average lower mortality rates than whites, although Vietnamese Americans manifest higher mortalities when evaluated as a separate subpopulation. When overall mortality is examined relative to socioeconomic status, differences between African-Americans and whites are reduced but not eliminated. For example, infant mortality rate, one of the most sensitive indicators of the health and well-being of a population, is twice as high among African-American infants as whites. Yet infant mortality rates among Mexican Americans, the third largest minority group and one of the poorest groups in the United States, are equivalent to that of whites, signifying a previously unacknowledged protective effect.

Some immigrants, especially those from non-European countries, have a longer life expectancy and more years of life free of disability and dependency than do native-born citizens. This longevity is likely related to the "healthy immigrant effect," ie, that those who migrate abroad represent a healthier and more motivated segment of the population of origin.

However, life-style in the country of origin impacts immigrant health. Life expectancy and infant mortality rates among new Soviet refugees compare poorly with those of the general population in the United States. In spite of reported universal health care coverage, there were wide variations between communities, access to care was dependent on Communist party membership, and there was little emphasis on promoting a healthy life-style. Heavy cigarette use, high alcohol intake, poor dietary intake, little attention to physical fitness, and crowded living conditions contributed to poor health in this population.

Recent research on access to medical care suggests that although minorities may have achieved improved equity of access during the 1980s, this may no longer be the case. The Institute of Medicine defines access as the timely use of personal health services to achieve the best possible health outcomes. This definition requires considering both the use of services and the outcome of services as indicators of access. It also implies availability of preventive services. Although less than 5% of the U.S. population regularly use hospital emergency departments, 10% of Hispanic Americans and 16% of African-Americans regularly use these hospital-based facilities for their medical needs. African-Americans and Hispanic Americans are more likely to be uninsured

(21% and 32%, respectively, versus 14% of the general population) and less likely to see a physician than majority members of the population (63% and 59%, respectively, versus 71% of the general population). Even when controlling for health status, disparities remain in the use of services for uninsured Americans regardless of race and ethnicity (Table 55–3).

Migrant farm workers and their families have restricted access to health and human services because of their frequent relocation between states, language and cultural barriers, and limited economic and political resources. Living and working in substandard environments, these families are at greater risk for developing chronic and communicable diseases. Primary and secondary prevention are almost nonexistent because funds for these services are not readily available. Childhood immunization rates are improving, but dental caries and head lice are epidemic. Among adults, almost one-third test positive for tuberculosis exposure. Urinary tract infections are the most common health problem among women in these groups.

Pregnant women are of major concern because of risk for poor pregnancy outcomes. In spite of these concerns, evidence suggests that infants of Mexican immigrants have favorable birth outcomes despite their high socioeconomic risks. These favorable outcomes have been associated with a protective sociocultural orientation among this immigrant group including a strong family unit. Yet, 25% of infants of immigrants in predominantly Spanish-speaking households are at high risk for serious infectious disease despite using preventive care. As these children mature beyond the neonatal period, factors predisposing to illness are large households, poor access to care, and maternal characteristics including smoking, complications of pregnancy, and employment.

Lack of understanding of traditional remedies for common ailments by health care workers can result in negative interactions between patient and clinician and misdiagnosis—both of which hinder health care utilization. Health care workers and the population of Vietnamese immigrants for whom they cared both identified misinterpretation of patient symptoms and health care provider recommendations as major issues. The special problems of unemployment, depression, surviving torture, and getting assistance are all made more difficult for refugees living in small communities that lack sufficiently large ethnic populations to facilitate culturally sensitive provision of health care.

With the exception of Southeast Asian refugees, there are few clinical studies on the health problems of refugees after arrival in the United States. For example, in Southeast Asian households, hepatitis B (HBV) transmission occurs throughout childhood, even in U.S.-born children, and the prevalence of chronic HBV infection approaches that of the country of origin. More information is needed regarding the incidence and progression of this disease in other racial and ethnic groups (Table 55–4). Tuberculosis, nutritional deficiencies, intestinal parasites, chronic hepatitis B infection, lack of immunization, and depression are major problems in many groups. There is great variation in health and psychosocial issues, as well as cultural beliefs, among the refugees that requires careful attention during the medical encounter. In addition to a complete history and physical examination, tests for tuberculosis, hepatitis B surface antigen, and ova and parasites, as well as a hemoglobin measurement, are advised for most groups (Table 55–5).

Ackerman LK: Health problems of refugees. J Am Board Fam Pract 1997;10(5):337.

Cornelius LJ: Ethnic minorities and access to medical care: where do they stand? J Assoc Acad Minor Phys 1993;4(1):15.

Institute of Medicine (IOM): *Access to Health Care in America.* Millman M (editor). National Academy Press, 1993.

Lillie-Blanton ML: Race/ethnicity, the social environment, and health. Soc Sci Med 1996;43(1):83.

Marmot M: Inequalities in health. New Engl J Med 2001;345:134.

Nickens HW: The role of race/ethnicity and social class in minority health status. Health Serv Res 1995;30(1, Pt 2):151.

Mental Health Issues

Disparities in mental health services have been known to exist among diverse communities for decades. The practice of psychiatry is heavily influenced by culture. The cultural identity of patients as well as providers, their perceptions of mental illness and appropriate treatment, and their background and current environment potentially all have an impact on the psychiatric

Table 55–3. Health care utilization issues.

Access through urgent care facilities
Poor continuity of care
Shortage of like-ethnic providers
Uninsured and underinsured (eg, Medicaid)

Table 55–4. Common immigrant/refugee health problems.

Tuberculosis
Nutritional deficiencies
Intestinal parasites
Chronic hepatitis B infection
Lack of immunizations
Depression and stress-related disorders

Table 55–5. Recommended evaluation of immigrants/refugees.

History
Psychosocial assessment
Physical examination
Purified protein derivative ± chest x-ray
Hepatitis B surface antigen
Stool for ova and parasites
Hemoglobin/hematocrit

diagnosis made, the therapy selected, and the therapeutic outcome. Mental illness has been diagnosed more frequently in African-Americans and Hispanics than in non-Hispanic white Americans for more than 100 years (Table 55–6). Many of the studies reporting these data have been criticized for faulty methodology, cultural bias, and suspect racial theories.

There is some evidence that appropriate research and mental health care delivery for these populations are influenced by factors such as poor cultural validation of the *Diagnostic and Statistical Manual of Mental Disorders,* fourth edition (*DSM-IV*), misdiagnosis of minority patients, and the unwillingness of many psychiatrists to acknowledge culturally defined syndromes and folk-healing systems.

General mental health screening is difficult in part because assessment of psychological health in non-English-speaking populations is impeded by lack of instruments that are language and population specific. Patients whose first language is not English most often undergo psychiatric evaluation and treatment in English. Cultural nuances are encoded in language in ways that are often not readily conveyed in translation, even when equivalent words in the second language are used. An appropriately trained interpreter will routinely identify these nuances for the monolingual clinician. When such an interpreter is not available, these nuances can be clarified through consultation with a clinician who shares the patient's first language and culture to maximize delivery of quality health care.

Distress is often expressed as somatic symptoms in many cultural groups. For example, values traditional to Hispanic culture, such as respeto, allocentrism, and familialism, are important to Hispanic elders in the

Table 55–6. Mental health issues.

High rate of misdiagnosis
Lack of linguistically competent therapists
Culturally insensitive diagnostic measures
Exposure to abuse

United States, many of whom were born in rural Mexico. Our knowledge of determinants of healthy aging in this population is still preliminary, but rapidly expanding, in part because of increased attention to ethnicity in health reporting.

Immigrants and refugees are exposed to a different set of emotional stressors. Those experiencing physical privation recover more rapidly and completely than those suffering from emotional trauma and loss. Children may show minimal distress when faced with armed conflict until the violence reaches their nuclear family. Then the psychological effects are more serious. Even when the nuclear family escapes injury, growing up in a war-affected community can promote aggression in children. Of newly immigrated Chilean children (mean age 6 years) whose parents had been tortured or persecuted, 75% had sleep disturbances, anxiety, defiance, depression, concentration failures, and aggressiveness. Children whose families had escaped persecution had significantly lower symptom levels. After a period of time, if the family remains intact, children and parents can heal from the effects of political abuse and the impact of war. The longer the time elapsed since resettlement or exposure to traumatic events the less the amount and severity of symptoms.

When Cambodian high school students living in the United States who had witnessed violence were studied, almost 50% met the criteria for posttraumatic stress disorder (PTSD) and half met the criteria for other clinical problems—most notably anxiety and depression. Rather than problems with conduct, the most commonly reported symptoms in adolescent Cambodian refugees were somatic complaints, social withdrawal, attention problems, anxiety, and depression.

Much of the vulnerability of Latino children to mental health problems stems from the numerous challenges faced by their families with respect to acculturation and poverty. Most of the problems these children face relate to depression and social withdrawal. Experiences subsequent to immigration such as discrimination, loneliness, unemployment, and isolation from mainstream society negatively affect levels of anxiety and depressive symptoms.

Feeling accepted by the host society, being involved with Americans and U.S. culture, and increased acculturation promote better mental health. Greater resistance to the dominant culture results in poorer mental health; a better transition to the new culture results in improved mental health.

Collins JL et al: Ethnic and cultural factors in psychiatric diagnosis and treatment. In: *Handbook of Mental Health and Mental Disorders among Black Americans.* Greenwood Press, 1990.

Kirmayer LJ et al: Affective disorders in cultural context. Psychiatr Clin North Am 2001;24.

Lewis-Fernandez R et al: Cultural psychiatry: theoretical, clinical and research issues. Psychiatr Clin North Am 1995;18:433.

Mehta S: Relationship between acculturation and mental health for Asian Indian immigrants in the United States. Genet Soc Gen Psychol Monogr (US) 1998;124(1):61.

Pernice R et al: Refugees' and immigrants' mental health: association of demographic and post-immigration factors. J Soc Psychol (US) 1996;136(4):511.

Discrimination

In addition to cost, the minority status of the patient creates significant differences in how physicians make therapeutic decisions. Women, ethnic minorities, and uninsured persons receive fewer procedures than do affluent white male patients. Furthermore, the race and sex of a patient independently influence how physicians manage acute conditions such as chest pain. Women and minorities were less likely to be diagnosed with angina when presenting with risk factors and symptoms comparable to those exhibited by white men.

Illegal immigrants underutilize health services, especially preventive services such as prenatal care, dental care, and immunizations due to cost, language and cultural barriers, and fear of apprehension by immigration authorities. Further complicating efforts to provide access to health care for this group is fear for the well-being of family members who may be undocumented, even when the patient is here legally. The increasing number of immigrants entering the United States in recent years has resulted in more legislation seeking to restrict access of various refugee and immigrant groups to public services. Legislation such as Proposition 187, passed in California in 1994, prohibits people lacking legal residency status from obtaining all but emergency medical care at any health care facility receiving public funds.

This legislation has encouraged further obstacles to health care access for countless other people residing in the United States. For example, minorities who were born in the United States find that they are pressured to produce immigration documentation to receive care. Family physicians seeking to care for immigrants and refugees must recognize and effectively deal with problems in communication, establish trust regarding immigration concerns, understand cultural mores influencing the encounter, find the resources to provide necessary services, make an accurate diagnosis, and negotiate a treatment. Unfortunately, fear of restrictive immigration laws and socioeconomic hardships combine to delay both seeking and obtaining curative care for these populations.

Current federal mandates ensuring access to emergency medical services and new restrictions on financing health care for immigrants under federal programs such as Medicaid and Medicare appear to be in direct conflict. The Personal Responsibility and Work Opportunity Reconciliation Act and the Illegal Immigration Reform and Immigrant Responsibility Act specifically reaffirm federal law on the delivery of emergency services without addressing the financing of that care. Unfunded mandates in an era of diminished ability to shift costs onto insured patients create a major dilemma for the institutions that provide uncompensated care. Medicaid is considered one form of insurance, although the level of reimbursement to providers has been so low that many providers will not treat patients with that coverage.

Ivey SL et al: Immigrant women and the emergency department: the juncture with welfare and immigration reform. J Am Med Women's Assoc 1998;53(2):94.

Schulman KA et al: The effect of race and sex on physicians' recommendations for cardiac catheterization. New Engl J Med 1999;340:618.

Health Care Needs of Gay, Lesbian, Bisexual, & Transgender Patients

Peter J. Katsufrakis, MD, MBA

Introduction

Factors unique or common to gay, lesbian, bisexual, and transgender (GLBT) patients are identified and the resulting health care needs of this population are assessed. When not specified otherwise, "gay" will refer to both gay men and lesbians. Although GLBT individuals comprise a very diverse group, they share the burden of inadequate research documenting their health needs.

The basis for many problems faced by lesbian and gay patients is not sexual orientation per se, but society's response to this minority population. Stigmatization, differential treatment, and past diagnosis of homosexuality as a psychiatric disease by the American Psychiatric Association contribute to problems of credibility and access to health care for gay and lesbian patients. Homophobia is prevalent in medical schools and health care settings, and contributes to the differences observed in health and in the differential health care treatment received by lesbians and gay men.

There may also be health effects directly due to delayed or declined reproduction and to behaviors common or unique to gay patients. Thus although differences in various health parameters exist, determining causality can be problematic, and ultimately of limited importance in a clinical setting. Our understanding of many aspects of gay men's and lesbians' health needs is in its infancy; however, what is known can be used to enhance GLBT patients' health care. The information presented here summarizes what is currently known, identifies deficiencies in existing knowledge, and presents suggestions to improve care.

AMA Council on Scientific Affairs: Health care needs of gay men and lesbians in the United States. JAMA 1996;275:1354.

Saunders J: Health problems of lesbian women. Nurs Clin North Am 1999;34:381.

Ungvarski P, Grossman A: Health problems of gay and bisexual men. Nurs Clin North Am 1999;34:313.

Problems with Existing Research

Research and the resulting knowledge of GLBT health needs are increasing. However, most existing health research is troubled by a failure to identify differences due to sexual orientation. Additionally, research focusing on GLBT patients frequently suffers from a small sample size, potential sampling errors, and other significant shortcomings. The population studied must be precisely defined to allow accurate interpretation of results. Prevailing homophobic attitudes may even prevent such research from being conducted.

Even though gay men and lesbians will certainly be included among a population cross-sectional sample, the vast majority of published biomedical research to date has failed to assess the sexual orientation or behavior of study populations. This leads to at least two problems: (1) not inquiring about sexual orientation precludes the collection of information about the distinctive characteristics of lesbians and gay men, and (2) the unique attributes of these populations may be ascribed erroneously to the larger population. Failure to assess study participants' sexual orientation prevents us from advancing our knowledge of gay men's and lesbians' special health needs. Furthermore, where differences exist between heterosexual and homosexual populations, failure to assess sexual orientation incorrectly attributes a broader range of results than would otherwise be true, to the extent that populations not characterized with regard to sexual orientation are erroneously assumed to be heterosexual (Figure 56–1).

Many studies of gay and lesbian patients suffer from small sample size, thus limiting their power and generalizability. Although a study of 10–15 patients may achieve statistical significance, its applicability to the larger lesbian and gay male populations could be questioned. Convenience sampling has been used frequently in the past. Study participants drawn from gay bars, bathhouses, gay community centers, and other areas known to have concentrations of lesbian and gay people are not likely to be representative of the larger lesbian and gay male populations. Empiric evidence demonstrates that differences exist between such convenience samples and samples drawn using random sampling techniques. Problems defining and identifying transgender and bisexual populations pose even greater challenges.

The existing body of GLBT research may not be representative of the population. Because social stigma-

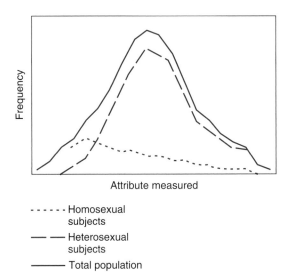

- - - - - Homosexual
          subjects
——— Heterosexual
          subjects
——— Total population

Figure 56–1. Failed recognition of sexual orientation: impact on reported results.

tization and societal discrimination against homosexuals may cause individuals to conceal their sexual orientation, individuals who are likely to identify themselves politically or socially with the gay community and are thus willing to disclose their sexual orientation to researchers may be overrepresented. Furthermore, inconsistent definitions of the populations studied contribute to difficulty in comparing across studies, and thus in advancing our knowledge about gay and lesbian patients' health care needs. Fortunately, these problems have been identified nationally and are being addressed by increased attention to GLBT health within academic communities and by the U.S. government. Increased attention and enhanced research methodologies should improve the quality and amount of information available.

Kinsey's original reports that 10% of men were predominantly gay and 6% of women were lesbians have been supplanted by more recent studies using probability sampling methods that estimate 5–9% of men are gay and 4% of women are lesbians. For the purposes of this chapter and in the interest of simplicity, we will refer to gay men and lesbians as if they were single populations. However, this is a gross oversimplification of very complex and diverse human behavior.

Who Is Gay? What Is "Bisexual"?

A person's sexual orientation can be categorized on the basis of fantasies or desires, actual behavior, or self-identified label. For example, a man could think of

himself and describe himself as heterosexual, engage in sex with men more frequently than with women, and in his sexual fantasies focus almost exclusively on male images; a simple label or categorization would fail to capture the reality of his sexuality. Even when limiting discussion to sexual behaviors and ignoring labels and fantasies, differences may exist between actual versus desired, past versus present, admitted versus practiced, and consensual versus forced.

Just as in formulating research studies, this distinction is important in the medical setting because asking about a patient's label (eg, "Are you gay or bisexual?") may fail to obtain the desired information, as many individuals who engage in same-gender sexual behavior do not self-identify as gay or bisexual, despite engaging in high-risk sexual behaviors.

Another example of the importance of this distinction comes from research into women's risk of acquiring sexually transmitted diseases (STDs). Women who have sex with men and women (WSMW) may have an increased risk for STDs and substance abuse compared with women who have sex with women (WSW) only. Differentiation would not be possible by asking a patient only if she identifies herself as lesbian, as both WSMW and WSW may identify themselves as lesbian.

Little specific literature analyzing the characteristics of bisexual men and women as distinct from either strictly heterosexual or strictly homosexual persons exists. Again, the question of definitions arises: What amount of sexual activity with partners of both sexes is sufficient to "qualify" as bisexual? Some researchers analyze bisexual patients separately, others group bisexual patients with gay or lesbian patients, and others choose not to distinguish. Given that there is a range of human sexual behavior, the label "bisexual" will necessarily be arbitrary, and perhaps not even useful in the context of clinical care, but it is impossible to be certain of this conclusion until the question has been asked and answered.

Clearly, labels are insufficient. An understanding of patients' sexuality is needed to provide the best health care possible.

Discrimination & Homophobia

Homophobia has been defined as the irrational fear of, aversion to, or discrimination against homosexuality or homosexuals. Reading newspapers or monitoring other media is sufficient to realize that discrimination on the basis of sexual orientation pervades virtually all aspects of our society. In its most extreme manifestation, homophobia results in physical violence and murder. In countless less dramatic ways, discrimination against lesbians and gay men causes problems, including negative effects on health.

Despite beliefs we may hold about beneficence, nonmaleficence, equal access, and other humanitarian ideals, in many ways our health care system mirrors and responds to society's values. In the health care setting, homophobia is present from medical school onward. In a recent study of students at a U.S. medical school, 25% of students reported believing homosexuality is immoral and dangerous to the institution of the family, and expressed aversion to socializing with homosexuals, and 9% believed that homosexuality was a mental disorder. Of 543 internal medicine house staff surveyed in Canada, respondents reported witnessing homophobic remarks directed toward lesbians or gay men by more than 50% of all attending physicians, peers, patients, nurses, or other health care workers.

One survey of physicians found that 52% had observed colleagues providing substandard care to patients because of sexual orientation. The Women Physicians' Health Study surveyed a probability sample of 10,000 women physicians and found that lesbian physicians are four times more likely to experience sexual orientation-based harassment than heterosexual physicians, and 32% of lesbian physicians report sexual orientation harassment in the work setting after medical school. Of 501 respondents in a study of Canadian general internal medicine practices, approximately 40% of general internists report homophobic remarks by both health care team members and patients. Furthermore, homophobic attitudes and experiences affect medical students' training, residency choices, and subsequent career decisions.

The evidence is overwhelming that homophobia pervades health care. But what are its consequences? Limited access to health care due to actual or perceived discrimination results in the reluctance of patients to disclose information about their sexuality and sexual orientation in health care settings. This can lead to delayed diagnosis and can prevent physicians from pursuing optimal courses of evaluation and treatment.

The perceived need of patients to hide their sexual orientation leads to measurable adverse health effects. Among 80 human immunodeficiency virus (HIV)-seropositive gay men who were otherwise healthy, HIV infection advanced more rapidly, exhibiting a dose–response relationship, in participants who concealed their homosexual identity. Homosexual and bisexual individuals report discrimination more frequently than heterosexual persons, and perceived discrimination has been associated with harmful effects on both quality of life and psychiatric health. A study of 1067 lesbians and gay men found that feelings of victimization resulting from perceived social stigma were a significant contributor to depression, and another study of 912 Latino men found that experiences of social discrimination were strong predictors of suicidal ideation, anxiety, and depressed mood (80%). Discrimination against gay and lesbian individuals produces needless human suffering.

Brogan D et al: Harassment of lesbians as medical students and physicians. MSJAMA 1999;282:1290.

Cole SW et al: Accelerated course of human immunodeficiency virus infection in gay men who conceal their homosexual identity [see comments]. Psychosom Med 1996;58:219.

Klamen DL, Grossman LS, Kopacz DR: Medical student homophobia. J Homosexuality 1999;37:53.

Mays VM, Cochran SD: Mental health correlates of perceived discrimination among lesbian, gay, and bisexual adults in the United States. Am J Public Health 2001;91:1869.

Health Concerns of Gay Men

A. HIV/AIDS

Men who have sex with men (MSM) continue to account for the largest number of new acquired immunodeficiency syndrome (AIDS) diagnoses in the United States, 16,944 in 2002. Discussion of HIV risk and transmission should be a routine part of the care for all sexually active patients, especially MSM. In addition to a discussion of routes of transmission and means to reduce risk, physicians wishing to provide optimal care should also investigate other conditions that may increase the patient's risk of acquiring HIV. In one study of risk factors for HIV infection, 116 of 327 (35.5%) homosexual and bisexual men reported being sexually abused as children. Those who were abused were more likely to have had unprotected receptive anal intercourse in the past 6 months. Sexual abuse remained a significant predictor of unprotected receptive anal intercourse in a logistic model adjusting for potential confounding variables. Substance abuse also plays a role in HIV risk, and is discussed below.

From the standpoint of preventing new HIV infections, both HIV-positive and HIV-negative patients would ideally never engage in unprotected intercourse or other risk behaviors. However, risk reduction messages such as "Condoms every time with every partner" are increasingly recognized as unrealistic and ineffective. Effective interventions to change behavior should consider the patient's knowledge, cultural context, and different behavior with "primary" versus casual or anonymous partners. Counseling to reduce risk may effect greater behavior change than counseling to eliminate HIV risk behaviors completely.

Patients infected with HIV require a comprehensive care plan that involves skilled physicians, ancillary health services, pharmacological therapy, and access to social and other support services. Excellent resources exist to guide physicians in the detailed management and care of patients with HIV/AIDS (see Bartlett and

Gallant as well as web-based resources such as the *Guidelines for the Use of Antiretroviral Agents in HIV-Infected Adults and Adolescents* published by the U.S. Public Health Service and available at http://www.aidsinfo.nih.gov or the *HIV InSite Knowledge Base* available at http://hivinsite.ucsf.edu/InSite.jsp?page=KB).

B. Sexually Transmitted Diseases

Hepatitis A and hepatitis B are both sexually transmissible. Hepatitis B is transmissible via sexual intercourse in both men and women, but its increased prevalence in the gay male population makes it a particular risk for MSM. Because hepatitis A is transmissible via fecal–oral contact, persons who engage in anilingus, or "rimming," are particularly at risk. MSM should receive vaccination for both hepatitis A and B.

Gonorrhea, chlamydia, and nonchlamydial nongonococcal urethritis (NGU) are common problems in sexually active gay men. As each of these may cause asymptomatic infection, periodic screening may be useful to detect clinically silent disease. Organisms that commonly cause enteritis and proctocolitis may be sexually transmitted, and even organisms not commonly thought to be pathogenic such as *Endolimax nana* and *Blastocystis hominis* should be treated in the symptomatic patient lacking other causes of abdominal symptoms. Fellatio, commonly thought to be a "safe" sexual practice, may be an independent risk factor for urethral gonorrhea and nonchlamydial NGU and has been recently associated with localized syphilis epidemics in gay men. Syphilis epidemics have also been associated with high-risk sexual activity among HIV-positive men.

Kaposi sarcoma (KS) poses another health risk for gay men. Although generally associated with HIV infection, KS seems to be the result of infection with a separate herpes virus, KSHV/HHV-8. Furthermore, it appears that this virus is sexually transmitted, probably by receptive anal intercourse, and may be carried in saliva. Although cases of KS among gay men in the absence of coexisting HIV infection are rare and even in HIV-infected patients the incidence has decreased significantly from the early period of the AIDS epidemic, physicians should be suspicious of red or purple patches or nodules on the skin or mucous membranes, and should evaluate and/or refer patients for treatment when indicated.

C. Anal Dysplasia

Human papillomavirus (HPV) infection and dysplastic changes occur commonly in the anal mucosa of both HIV-positive and HIV-negative gay men. Anal HPV DNA in one study was detected initially in 91.6% of HIV-positive and 65.9% of HIV-negative men. HIV exacerbates HPV effects, and is associated with more prevalent HPV infection and higher-grade squamous intraepithelial lesions (SILs). Anoscopy and anal cytology show that anal intraepithelial neoplasia (AIN) and infection with multiple oncogenic HPV types are very common among immunosuppressed HIV-positive homosexual men. Apparent progression from low-grade to high-grade cytological changes occurs rapidly. HIV-positive men were more likely to develop high-grade squamous intraepithelial lesions (HSILs) than HIV-negative men, although high rates were found at all CD4 levels among HIV-positive and HIV-negative men. Screening HIV-positive homosexual and bisexual men for anal SILs and anal squamous cell carcinomas with anal Papanicolau (Pap) tests offers quality-adjusted life expectancy benefits at a cost comparable with other accepted clinical preventive interventions. Because the observed increased incidence of anal cancer does not appear to be solely due to HIV infection, high-resolution anoscopy and cytological screening for all MSM with anal condyloma and other benign noncondylomatous anal disorders is supported by current knowledge.

D. Substance Abuse

Both alcohol and psychoactive drug use appear more widespread in gay men than in the general heterosexual population and in some venues the prevalence of illicit drug use and associated high-risk sexual activity is dramatic, with use of substances such as methylenedioxymethamphetamine (MDMA or ecstasy) approaching 80% of the population. Men who attend "circuit parties"—a series of dances or parties held over a weekend that are attended by hundreds to thousands of gay and bisexual men—should be considered at high risk for concurrent illicit substance use and should be counseled accordingly. Interestingly, it appears that alcohol and drug use may be decreasing among younger gay and bisexual men, although still existing at levels greater than among the general heterosexual population.

Alcohol use has been associated with high-risk sexual behavior, ie, unprotected anal and oral intercourse. Gay men who have unprotected anal intercourse are more likely to have a drinking problem and to drink more than gay men who do not have unprotected intercourse, and unprotected intercourse after drinking is more common with nonsteady sexual partners. Drug use is also associated with increased high-risk sexual behaviors. Drugs for which this association has been demonstrated include hallucinogens, nitrate inhalants, and cocaine and other stimulants. Drug use during high-risk sex is common. However, associations between drug use and high-risk sexual behavior exist only for current, not past, drug or alcohol use. This finding lends further support to and justification for efforts to provide adequate treatment to patients with substance abuse problems.

Increased substance abuse by gay men has been described as a coping method for dealing with stresses such as fear of HIV infection, lack of social supports, fear of discrimination in housing or employment, rejection by family or friends on the basis of sexual orientation, and antigay verbal or physical assaults. For some patients, substance abuse can be thought of as one more symptom of the social disease homophobia.

The literature dealing specifically with anabolic steroid use by gay men is limited, focusing primarily on steroid use in treating HIV-associated wasting. Anecdotal observations of physicians treating large numbers of gay men indicate that illicit anabolic steroid use in weight training and bodybuilding regimens is not uncommon. One British study of over 1000 gay men recruited from five gymnasiums found that 13.5% of the study population used anabolic steroids. Of the 8.1% who injected their steroids, none reported needle sharing. Although shared needles did not appear to pose significant HIV risk, anabolic steroid users were more likely than never users (21% versus 13%) to report engaging in unprotected anal intercourse, increasing their risk for HIV infection.

Steroid use also has been associated with numerous adverse effects, including acne, testicular atrophy, heightened aggression, atherogenic blood lipid changes, and development of peliosis hepatis, liver tumors, and liver failure. Patients should be apprised of these adverse health effects and provided with the support and treatment needed to discontinue illicit steroid use. Significant social pressures may cause patients to resort to steroids as a means to achieve an idealized masculine physique; for these patients substantial support and counseling may be required to overcome steroid abuse.

E. DEPRESSION

Feelings of being stigmatized, internalized homophobia (the direction of society's negative attitudes toward gay men to the self), and actual experiences of discrimination or violence contribute to gay men's distress. In a study of HIV-infected men that may have relevance for all gay men, it was found that men who did not demonstrate traditional gender identity were more likely to have current symptoms of anxiety and depression and to have had a lifetime history of depression. Depression has also been linked to the AIDS epidemic, and particularly to being a caregiver for someone with AIDS, regardless of whether the caregiver is HIV positive or HIV negative. Interestingly, low levels of vitamin B_{12} have been correlated with increased depression and anxiety in men, independent of HIV serostatus, although the potential response to vitamin B_{12} therapy has yet to be investigated.

F. SUICIDE

Well-designed studies with valid sampling techniques have demonstrated that suicidal ideation, attempts at suicide, and completed acts of suicide are more common in gay, lesbian, and bisexual youth than in their heterosexual counterparts. Population-based research demonstrates significantly higher rates of suicidal symptoms and suicide attempts among men who reported same-sex than among men who reported exclusively opposite-sex sexual partners, and other investigators have demonstrated similar findings in a study of twins in which one brother reported same-sex partners after age 18 and the other did not. Suicidality has been linked to the process of "coming out," or revealing one's homosexual orientation to others. Thus, physicians caring for gay adolescents or adults disclosing their sexual orientation to others should be especially sensitive to symptoms or signs suggesting any increase in suicide risk.

Bartlett J, Gallant J: *Medical Management of HIV Infection.* Johns Hopkins University, 2001.

Cochran SD, Mays VM: Lifetime prevalence of suicide symptoms and affective disorders among men reporting same-sex sexual partners: results from NHANES III. Am J Public Health 2000;90:573.

Friedman HB et al: Human papillomavirus, anal squamous intraepithelial lesions, and human immunodeficiency virus in a cohort of gay men. J Infect Dis 1998;178:45.

Lafferty WE, Hughes JP, Handsfield HH: Sexually transmitted diseases in men who have sex with men. Acquisition of gonorrhea and nongonococcal urethritis by fellatio and implications for STD/HIV prevention. Sex Transmit Dis 1997;24:272.

Meyer IH: Minority stress and mental health in gay men. J Health Social Behav 1995;36:38.

Skinner WF, Otis MD: Drug and alcohol use among lesbian and gay people in a southern U.S. sample: epidemiological, comparative, and methodological findings from the Trilogy Project. J Homosexuality 1996;30:59.

Common Health Concerns of Lesbians

The body of research documenting the health needs of lesbians is even more limited than that for gay men. Some past studies suggest that lesbians do not seek health care as often as heterosexual women, although results from a national community-based sample show that lesbians have healthy behaviors in general and utilize routine health screening. This difference may reflect study methodology or may reflect real changes in lesbian behavior, perhaps in part as a consequence of evolving societal attitudes toward lesbians and gay men. Fortunately, a recent National Institute of Medicine report provides valuable guidance in formulating a lesbian research agenda.

One area of concern relates to health risks that remain undetected because they are a consequence of behaviors that occurred in the patient's past. For example, because risk of cervical dysplasia and cervical cancer is associated with age at first intercourse with a male, an adult woman who is now exclusively sexually active with a female partner may not be identified as being at risk without considering her entire sexual history.

A. Sexually Transmitted Diseases

Generally, lesbians are felt to be at less risk for STDs than heterosexual women. However, women who deny having any prior male sexual partners have been shown to have trichomoniasis, anogenital warts, and abnormal Pap smears. Some studies have shown comparable rates of sexually transmitted infection between lesbians and heterosexual women, although the types of infections varied; genital herpes and genital warts were more common in heterosexual women and bacterial vaginosis (BV) was more common in lesbians. Other research indicates a different prevalence of BV and warts, but not herpes, although the nature of the inner city population studied may preclude generalizing these findings to all lesbians. Generally, the risk of acquiring an STD seems to be different in WSW than in WSM.

There is a mistaken belief that lesbians are at no or small risk for acquiring HIV. Clearly lesbians are still at risk from injection drug use. It has also been shown that sexually active lesbians have a *higher* prevalence of HIV infection than women who have sex exclusively with men. Additionally, sexual transmission of HIV from woman to woman is possible, although prevalence is unknown.

B. Cancer

Breast cancer may be more common in nulliparous or uniparous women and thus may be more common in lesbians, but well-designed, prospective studies are lacking. One study compiling survey data from almost 12,000 women found greater prevalence rates of obesity and alcohol and tobacco use and lower rates of parity and birth control pill use, but reported rates of breast cancer did not differ from adjusted U.S. female population estimates. Interestingly, these women were also less likely to have health insurance coverage or to have had a recent pelvic examination or mammogram. Data for ovarian or endometrial cancers are even more limited than for breast cancer.

Cervical cancer may be less prevalent in women who never engage in heterosexual vaginal intercourse. However, dysplasia and cervical cancer are very real problems for lesbians. Many lesbians who have engaged in sex with men may not be detected as being at risk of cervical cancer if their physicians erroneously conclude that they do not need routine Pap smears and thus fail to screen. Lesbian patients may concur with this mistaken belief, perceiving themselves to be less susceptible to cervical cancer than heterosexuals or bisexuals, even though one study showed 79% reported previous sexual intercourse with a male. Even in women reporting no prior sex with men, HPV DNA and SILs may be found in up to 20% of patients.

In another study of health care practices among lesbians, 25% of respondents had not had a Pap test within the past 3 years, and 7.6% had never had a Pap test. However, these effects can be ameliorated by the physician, as women who reported that their health care providers were more knowledgeable and sensitive to lesbians' issues were significantly more likely to have had a Pap test within the past year, even when controlling for age, education, income, and insurance status. Women who have sex with women should receive Pap smear screening in accordance with current guidelines for all women.

C. Substance Abuse

The population-based 1996 National Household Survey on Drug Abuse suggested that lesbians consume more alcohol than heterosexual women. Others have reported few differences between lesbians and heterosexual women in heavy alcohol consumption, although lesbians did show increased use of other psychoactive substances. A recent review of tobacco use found that smoking rates among adolescent and adult lesbians, gays, and bisexuals are higher than in the general population.

D. Depression

Research on lesbians' mental health is limited. One study considered predictors of depression and looked at relationship status, relationship satisfaction, social support from friends, social support from family, "outness" (degree to which the woman publicly shared her sexual orientation), and relationship status satisfaction. It was found that lack of social support from friends, poor relationship status satisfaction, and lack of perceived social support from family were significant predictors of depression.

E. Contraception and Reproductive Health

Physicians who assume that all women of reproductive age need contraception risk alienating lesbian patients, who may consequently decline to disclose their sexual orientation. However, lesbians who are sexually active with men may be interested in obtaining contraceptives.

Lesbian patients may also be, or wish to become, mothers and so may welcome a discussion of reproductive options. Lesbians and gay men may choose to become parents via adoption, artificial insemination, surrogacy, or heterosexual intercourse. Existing evidence suggests that gay men and lesbians have parenting skills comparable to heterosexual parents. When compared with children of heterosexual parents, children of gay men and lesbians seem to be no different in significant variables measured, including their sexual or gender identity, personality traits, and intelligence. Despite this, gay men and lesbians may face unjustified barriers in their attempts to become foster and adoptive parents. Issues that warrant physician awareness include parental legal rights and durable power of attorney; gestation and pregnancy; choice of surrogate, sperm, and/or egg donor; possible HIV risk; and routine preconception and prenatal care. Physicians caring for lesbians and gay men wishing to become parents should maintain information about appropriate referrals to facilitate this process.

Cochran SD et al: Estimates of alcohol use and clinical treatment needs among homosexually active men and women in the U.S. population. J Consult Clin Psychol 2000;68:1062.

Cochran SD et al: Cancer-related risk indicators and preventive screening behaviors among lesbians and bisexual women. Am J Public Health 2001;91:591.

Institute of Medicine Committee on Lesbian Health Research Priorities: *Lesbian Health: Current Assessment and Directions for the Future.* National Academy Press, 1999.

Oetjen H, Rothblum ED: When lesbians aren't gay: factors affecting depression among lesbians. J Homosexuality 2000;39:49.

Rankow EJ, Tessaro I: Cervical cancer risk and Papanicolaou screening in a sample of lesbian and bisexual women. J Fam Pract 1998;47:139.

Roberts SJ, Sorensen L: Health related behaviors and cancer screening of lesbians: results from the Boston Lesbian Health Project. Women Health 1999;28:1.

Skinner CJ et al: A case-controlled study of the sexual health needs of lesbians. Genitourinary Med 1996;72:277.

Transgender Patients

The Diagnostic and Statistical Manual of Mental Disorders (*DSM*) defines Gender Identity Disorder (GID) as "A strong and persistent cross-gender identification" with "persistent discomfort with [one's] sex or sense of inappropriateness in the gender role of that sex." This definition and the alternate *DSM* diagnoses (Transvestic Fetishism and Gender Identity Disorder Not Otherwise Specified) attempt to classify conditions in which an individual may experience discordance between his or her perceived and observed gender, but fail to capture the full spectrum of experiences of individuals who do not fit traditional gender roles. The *DSM* characterization considers transgender individuals as suffering

pathology, and in this manner is similar to the treatment of homosexuality prior to the American Psychiatric Association's revision of the *DSM* in 1973. Although the *DSM* reflects current societal attitudes toward transgender individuals and the limits of our understanding, increased awareness of the etiology of gender discordance and appreciation of the needs of transgender individuals may result in a different characterization in the future.

Prevalence seems to vary from country to country, with the ratio of male(-to-female) to female(-to-male) patients consistently showing a male preponderance ranging from approximately 2:1 to more than 4:1. Culture influences these patients' experience, as some cultures do not recognize a transsexual identity and may assign a mystical or religious significance to transgender individuals.

A. Terminology

Terminology can be problematic when describing transgender individuals, reflecting our evolving knowledge and remaining uncertainty. "Transgender" (TG) can be used as an umbrella term for a diverse group of individuals who cross or transcend culturally defined categories of gender in some way. "Transsexual" (TS) is often used in reference to an individual who has undergone partial or complete sex reassignment surgery (SRS).

Considering gender-discordant individuals born with male genitalia, one classification system characterizes *transvestites* as men who never wished to change their sex and become a woman, had never taken female hormones, and had never seriously considered sex change surgery. This classification is consistent with the *DSM-IV* diagnostic criteria of transvestic fetishism, which occurs only in heterosexual males.

Transsexuals, who differ from transvestites, wish to change their sex and become a woman, have taken female hormones, and have seriously considered (or undertaken) SRS. *Transgender* individuals have been described as men who generally cross-dress more frequently, possibly daily, and often have a more stable sense of feminine identification than transvestites, although not necessarily to the point that they desire SRS. In this schema, "transgender" falls on a continuum between transvestite (TV) and transsexual. In other settings, the term "transgender" serves as an umbrella for patients experiencing discordance between their physical gender and their gender identity.

The term "male-to-female" (MTF) describes individuals born with male genitalia who may undergo treatment to create a female-appearing body; the reverse is true for "female-to-male" (FTM) individuals. Additional ways to characterize the biological, social, psychological, and legal identity of TG individuals have been described. In caring for an individual patient, the best approach for physicians is to determine how patients wish to be addressed and to understand how they conceptualize their gender.

In the spectrum of GID, individuals who experience the strongest feelings of dissonance between their gender identity and their physical appearance believe the quest for full hormonal and surgical sex reassignment is vital because they actually feel "trapped" in an anatomically wrong body. Currently, the transgender movement includes cross-dressers, female and male impersonators, transgenderists and bigender persons (who identify as both man and woman), as well as transsexuals who have undergone or desire to undergo sex reassignment therapy. Limited research into the etiology of GID suggests that it may be multifactorial; there may be anatomic brain differences between TS and non-TS individuals, as well as differences in parental rearing. Regardless of the etiology or classification, the needs of transgender patients are increasingly recognized as valid, authentic, and deserving of attention from health care educators, researchers, policymakers, and clinicians of all types.

B. TREATMENT

Some patients choose partial medical and/or surgical treatment of their gender dysphoria, finding that a physical existence with components of both genders best addresses the emotional dysphoria caused by their birth physiognomy. Others wish to use surgery and hormonal treatment to manifest physically their "internal" gender as fully as possible. The literature describing the health needs of transgender patients focuses principally upon psychological and psychiatric evaluation and treatment, surgical modification or SRS, and hormonal therapy. Although common practice is to delay initiating sex reassignment therapy until the patient is at least 18 or 21 years of age, it appears that for carefully selected individuals treatment in adolescence is well tolerated, does not lead to postoperative regret, and may forestall psychopathology seen in transgender individuals forced to delay therapy.

The psychiatric literature historically has indicated that TS patients suffer from increased Axis I psychopathology. TS men experienced less sexual drive, more psychiatric symptoms, and a greater feminine gender role than TV or TG men. However, a population of TV, TG, and TS men not seen for clinical reasons was virtually indistinguishable from non-cross-dressing men using a measure of personality traits, a sexual functioning inventory, and measures of psychological distress. Another study of 137 TS individuals completing the Minnesota Multiphasic Personality Inventory found that transsexualism is usually an isolated diagnosis and is not part of any general psychopathological disorder. Initial treatment of a patient consider-

ing SRS should include a complete psychological evaluation by a therapist experienced in working with this population.

Intensive psychological counseling, hormonal treatment, and living in the role of the desired gender for a period of at least 1 year should precede surgical treatment. Surgical treatment can involve the breasts, genitalia, and larynx. Breast surgery includes reduction, removal, and implant placement. One survey of male-to-female transsexual patients found that 75% were satisfied with breast surgery results, although 15% opted to undergo additional mammaplasty. Genital surgery may include penile skin inversion and/or sigmoido-colpoplasty for male-to-female transsexuals and meta-idioplasties and neophalloplasties for female-to-male transsexuals; careful attention to technique can result in >90% patient satisfaction with cosmetic and functional results that endures years after surgery. Cricothyroid approximation surgery has been employed to raise the vocal pitch of MTF patients. Interestingly, even in health systems funded by government support, courts have found that transsexuals have the right to SRS. Because of individual psychological and anatomic variations, surgical approaches must be tailored to individual patients, and patients seeking SRS should be referred to teams experienced with these procedures.

Hormonal treatment is often employed in both genders. Hormones induce feminization or virilization and suppress the hypothalamic–pituitary–gonadal axis. Cross-sex hormonal treatment may have substantial medical side effects, so the smallest doses needed to achieve the desired result should be used. Treatment with ethinyl estradiol in MTF transsexuals causes an increase in subcutaneous and visceral fat and a decrease in the thigh muscle area, whereas administration of testosterone in FTM transsexuals markedly increases the thigh muscle area, reduces subcutaneous fat at all levels measured, but slightly increases the visceral fat area. Outcome studies suggest that known complications of hormonal therapy such as galactorrhea and thromboembolic events occur, but that the incidence of complications can be held to acceptable levels with careful attention to regimens used. Extensive experience with hormonal therapies in transsexual patients indicates that hormonal therapy, particularly if transdermal formulations are used, does not cause increased morbidity or mortality; monitoring luteinizing hormone levels in MTF transsexuals may increase the benefit-to-risk ratio by limiting hormone-related bone loss.

American Psychiatric Association: *Diagnostic and Statistical Manual of Mental Disorders.* American Psychiatric Association, 1994.

Lombardi E: Enhancing transgender health care. Am J Public Health 2001;91:869.

Michel A, Mormont C, Legros JJ: A psycho-endocrinological overview of transsexualism. Eur J Endocrinol 2001;145:365.

Schlatterer K, von Werder K, Stalla GK: Multistep treatment concept of transsexual patients. Exp Clin Endocrinol Diabetes 1996;104:413.

Special Populations within the Gay & Lesbian Community

A. ADOLESCENTS

Lesbian and gay adolescents are vulnerable to parental wrath and withdrawal of support upon disclosure or suspicion of their homosexual orientation. This can initiate a chain of events that leaves the youth homeless. Lacking employable skills, homeless gay youths may resort to prostitution or "survival sex" to support themselves.

Gay youths have an increased risk for suicide compared to their heterosexual peers and gender nonconformity may be particularly detrimental to boys. Despite this, homosexual adolescents are generally more similar to than different from their heterosexual peers, face many of the same challenges, and mostly grow up healthy and happy.

Physicians caring for families need to be aware of the possibility that the normal adolescent struggle to establish identity may be compounded when a teen in a potentially hostile environment recognizes his or her gay or lesbian identity. Parental acceptance and support can dramatically reduce the adverse effects of coming out and the potential risk for suicide, and can increase the likelihood of healthy psychological development and maturation.

B. OLDER LESBIANS AND GAY MEN

Older lesbians and gay men developed and matured in a different social milieu, when society was less tolerant of homosexuality and the consequences of being gay or lesbian included even greater threats to the individual's social and family relationships, housing, and livelihood than exist today. Thus, older patients may be even less willing to disclose their homosexual orientation to physicians, and may have special health care needs.

Although not extensive, research suggests that many lesbians and gay men successfully navigate the aging process and remain connected and involved in life. In fact, the demands of being gay may cause individuals to face the challenges associated with aging more successfully than their heterosexual counterparts.

C. FAMILY AND COMMUNITY

One aspect of being gay or lesbian that may be overlooked in caring for a patient's medical needs is the role of family and social networks in providing support and sustenance to the GLBT patient. In this context, family often includes individuals unrelated by biological ties.

A sometimes useful concept is that of "family of origin," which consists of parents, siblings, and others with whom one shares a blood relation, contrasted with "family of choice," which includes those close friendship relationships that endure over time and incorporate the same types of support and emotions often associated with idealized views of the traditional family. The family of a lesbian or gay patient, just as with heterosexual patients, is a vital part of the individual's health and can serve as a source of both stress and support. Physicians caring for gay men and lesbians need to assess the resources and stressors that exist within the family, as defined by the patient.

Garofalo R, Katz E: Health care issues of gay and lesbian youth. Curr Opin Pediatr 2001;13:298.

Stronski Huwiler S, Remafedi G: Adolescent homosexuality. In: *Advances in Pediatrics,* Vol. 45. Barness L (editor). Mosby, 1998.

Wojciechowski C: Issues in caring for older lesbians. J Gerontol Nurs 1998;24:28.

Reparative Therapy & "Treatments" for Homosexuality

Efforts to pathologize homosexuality by claiming that it can be cured result not from rigorous scientific or psychiatric research, but from religious and political forces opposed to full civil rights for gay men and lesbians. Previous ignorance contributed to the medical profession's treatment of homosexual patients in ascribing psychiatric pathology to normal homosexual patients. This situation improved in 1973 when the American Psychiatric Association (APA) removed homosexuality as a diagnosis in the *DSM*. In 1998, the APA joined the American Psychological Association, the National Association of Social Workers, and the American Academy of Pediatrics, which had previously made statements against "reparative therapy" because of concerns for the harm caused to patients, in stating that the "APA opposes any psychiatric treatment, such as 'reparative' or 'conversion' therapy, that is based on the assumption that homosexuality per se is a mental disorder or is based on the a priori assumption that the patient should change his or her homosexual orientation."

APA Commission of Psychotherapy by Psychiatrists: Position statement on therapies focused on attempts to change sexual orientation (reparative or conversion therapies). Am J Psychiatry 2000;157:1719.

Recommendations

Table 56–1 outlines recommendations for physicians caring for gay and lesbian patients. Table 56–2 describes some of the potential pitfalls physicians may face, and offers suggestions for avoiding problems.

Table 56–1. Physician recommendations when caring for gay and lesbian patients.

Create a positive, supportive office environment for lesbian and gay patients. Ensure that reading matter, educational materials, and even office artwork represent the interests of homosexual patients in a manner comparable to heterosexual patients.

Incorporate a complete assessment of development and social history into the database for gay and lesbian patients. Include an assessment of any problems arising from sexual orientation, and of relations with family of origin and family of choice.

Assess problems with substance abuse and provide appropriate treatment and/or referral.

Assess HIV risk for *all* patients: gay men, lesbians, *and* heterosexuals. Revisit the topic periodically for patients at risk, and educate all patients to reduce risk of acquiring or transmitting HIV.

For sexually active gay men not in a mutually monogamous relationship, consider periodic screening for gonorrhea, chlamydia, and syphilis if warranted by local epidemiology.

For men, especially those with evidence of anal or genital warts, consider periodic anal cytology to screen for anal dysplasia.

Inquire about plans for reproduction with gay and lesbian patients, and be prepared to discuss options and/or refer for additional care.

Provide regular, age-appropriate screening (eg, mammography, fecal occult blood, etc) as recommended for all patients.

Provide routine Pap surveillance to *all* women; screen for other sexually transmitted diseases as indicated by patient behavior.

Provide leadership in your local community to counter inaccurate portrayals and beliefs about lesbians and gay men, and combat homophobia and its deleterious health effects.

Physicians with biases that prevent them from delivering optimal care to gay and lesbian patients should recognize their limitations and take steps to correct these deficiencies. Physicians unable or unwilling to change should seek appropriate referral sources for their gay and lesbian patients, just as they would for any patient whose medical needs fall outside the scope of their practice.

Table 56–2. Pitfalls in caring for gay and lesbian patients.

Assumption	Solution
Assumption about sexual orientation: Many patients are neither exclusively heterosexual nor exclusively homosexual.	Learn to inquire about sexual orientation in a nonjudgmental manner that recognizes the range of human diversity and apply this learning to all patients.
Assumptions about sexual activity: Lesbian and gay male patients may have numerous different sexual partners, be in a monogamous relationship, be celibate, or vary in patterns of activity over time.	Take a specific, sensitive sexual history from all patients.
Assumptions about contraception: The need for contraception arises from a wish to prevent pregnancy from heterosexual intercourse, *regardless* of the patient's gender identity, sexual orientation or label.	Inquire about need (rather than assuming need) or lack of need for all patients. Tailor recommendations to patient's needs.
Assumptions about marriage: Lesbians and gay men may have been, and may still be, married to persons of the opposite sex. Additionally, individuals in same-sex relationships may refer to themselves as married, and physicians doing otherwise risk alienating their patients.	Inquire about significant relationships for all patients. Use the terminology that your patients choose.
Assumptions about parenting: Lesbian and gay male couples are often interested in and choose to bear and raise children.	Inquire about parenting wishes and choices, and be prepared to discuss options.

Complementary & Alternative Medicine[1]

Wayne B. Jonas, MD, & Ronald A. Chez, MD

Background

Practices that lie outside the mainstream of "official" medicine have always been an important part of the public's health care. Recently these practices have become more prominent in the west and are frequently called complementary and alternative medicine (CAM). In April 1995 a panel of experts convened at the National Institutes of Health defined complementary and alternative medicine as "a broad domain of healing resources that encompasses all health systems, modalities, practices and their accompanying theories and beliefs, other than those intrinsic to the politically dominant health system of a particular society or culture in a given historical period." Surveys of CAM use have defined it as those practices used for the prevention and treatment of disease that are neither taught widely in medical schools nor generally available in hospitals. Complementary and alternative medicine is that subset of practices that is not an integral part of conventional care but is still used by patients in their health care management. Table 57–1 list some of the categories of CAM defined by the White House Commission on CAM Policy.

A. USE OF COMPLEMENTARY AND ALTERNATIVE MEDICINE

Complementary, alternative, and unconventional medicine is becoming increasingly popular in the United States. Two identical surveys of unconventional medicine use in the United States, done in 1990 and 1996, showed a 45% increase in use of CAM by the public. Visits to CAM practitioners increased from 400 million to over 600 million per year. The amount spent on these practices rose from $14 billion to $27 billion—most of it not reimbursed. Professional organizations are now beginning the "integration" of these practices into mainstream medicine. Seventy-five medical schools teach something about CAM practices, many hospitals have developed complementary and integrated medicine programs, and some health management organiza-

tions are offering "expanded" benefits packages that include alternative practitioners and services. Biomedical research organizations are also investing more into the investigation of these practices. For example, the budget of the Office of Alternative Medicine at the U.S. National Institutes of Health rose from $5 million to $100 million in 5 years and changed from a coordination office to a National Center for Complementary and Alternative Medicine (NCCAM).

Multiple surveys have now been conducted on populations with cancer, human immunodeficiency virus (HIV), children, minorities, and women on CAM use. Rates of use are significant in all these populations. Women, for example, are consistently more likely to explore and use CAM. Frequently central in health care decisions for a family, women seek out health care options in a pragmatic way. In the survey by Eisenberg 49% of women used CAM. Emigrant populations often use traditional medicines not commonly used in the west. According to the World Health Organization, between 65% and 80% of the world's health care services are classified as traditional medicine. Much of this health care is also delivered by women. These become complementary, alternative, or unconventional when used in Western countries. Even in countries in which modern Western biomedicine dominates, the public (and more women than men) makes extensive use of unconventional practices. In Western Europe and Australia, for example, regular use of complementary and alternative practices ranges from 20% to 70%.

The public uses these practices for both minor and major problems. Surveys show 50% of patients with cancer and HIV will use unconventional practices at some point during the course of their illness. Complementary medicine is an area of great public interest and activity, both nationally and worldwide. It appears that CAM has again "come of age" in the west.

B. CONVENTIONAL PHYSICIAN USE OF CAM

Conventional physicians are not only frequently faced with questions about CAM but also refer patients for CAM treatment and, to a lesser extent, provide CAM services. A review of 25 surveys of conventional physi-

---

[1]This chapter was submitted for publication April 26, 2002.

Table 57–1. CAM systems of health care, therapies, or products.[1]

Major Domains of CAM	Examples under Each Domain
Alternative health care systems	Ayurvedic medicine Chiropractic Homeopathic medicine Native American medicine (eg, sweat lodge, medicine wheel) Naturopathic medicine Traditional Chinese medicine (eg, acupuncture, Chinese herbal medicine)
Mind–body interventions	Meditation Hypnosis Guided imagery Dance therapy Music therapy Art therapy Prayer and mental healing
Biological based therapies	Herbal therapies Special diets (eg, macrobiotics, extremely low-fat or high-carbohydrate diets) Orthomolecular medicine (eg, megavitamin therapy) Individual biological therapies (eg, shark cartilage, bee pollen)
Therapeutic massage, body work, and somatic movement therapies	Massage Feldenkrais Alexander method
Energy therapies	Qigong Reiki Therapeutic touch
Bioelectromagnetics	Magnet therapy

[1]This table was adapted from the major domains of CAM and examples of each developed by the National Center for Complementary and Alternative Medicine, National Institutes of Health.

cian referral and use of CAM found that 43% of physicians had referred patients for acupuncture, 40% for chiropractic services, and 21% for massage. The majority believed in the efficacy of these three practices. Rates of use of CAM practices ranged from 9% (homeopathy) to 19% (chiropractic and massage). National surveys have confirmed that many physicians refer for and fewer incorporate CAM practices into their health care management.

C. RISKS OF CAM

The amount of research on CAM systems and practices is small compared to research on conventional medicine. There are over 1000 times more citations in the National Library of Medicine's bibliographic database, MEDLINE, on conventional cancer treatments than on alternative cancer treatments. With increasing public use of CAM, poor communication between patients and physicians about it, and few studies on the safety and efficacy of most CAM treatments, a situation exists for misuse and harm from these treatments. Many practices, such as acupuncture, homeopathy, and meditation, are low risk but require practitioner competence to avoid inappropriate use. Botanical preparations can be toxic and produce herb–drug interactions. Contamination and poor quality control also exist with these products, especially if shipped from Asia and India.

D. POTENTIAL BENEFITS OF CAM

CAM practices have value for the way we manage health and disease. In botanical medicine, for example, there is research showing the benefit of herbal products such as ginkgo biloba for improving dementia due to circulation problems and possibly Alzheimer's disease, benign prostatic hypertrophy with saw palmetto and other herbal preparations, and the prevention of heart disease with garlic. A number of placebo-controlled trials have been done showing that *Hypericum* (St. John's wort) is effective in the treatment of depression, although recent studies in the United States have cast doubt on the generalizability of those studies. Additional studies report that *Hypericum* is as effective as some conventional antidepressants, but produces fewer side effects and costs less. The quality of many of these trials is poor, however, so physicians need to have basic skills in the evaluation of clinical literature.

Astin JA: Why patients use alternative medicine: results of a national study. JAMA 1998;279(19):1548.

Description PoDa: Defining and describing complementary and alternative medicine. Alt Ther Health Med 1997;3(2):49.

Federation of State Medical Boards: *Report on Health Care Fraud from the Special Committee on Health Care Fraud.* Federation of State Medical Boards of the United States, Inc., 1997.

Le Bars PL et al: A placebo-controlled, double-blind, randomized trial of an extract of ginkgo biloba for dementia. JAMA 1997; 278(8):1327.

Marwick C: Alterations are ahead at the OAM. JAMA 1998;280: 1553.

Role of the Family Physician

What is the role of the family physician in the management of CAM? The goal is to help patients make informed choices about CAM as they do in conventional medicine. Specifically, physicians can protect, permit, promote, and partner with patients about CAM practices as appropriate.

A. PROTECTING PATIENTS FROM RISKS OF CAM

Many practices, such as acupuncture, biofeedback, homeopathy, and meditation, are low risk if used by competent practitioners, but if used in place of more effective treatments they can result in harm. Practitioners should be qualified to help patients avoid inappropriate use. Many herbal preparations contain powerful pharmacological substances with direct toxicity and herb–drug interactions. Contamination and poor quality control occur more often than with conventional drugs, especially if preparations are obtained from overseas. The family physician can help distinguish between CAM practices with little or no risk of direct toxicity (eg, homeopathy, acupuncture) and those with greater risk of toxicity (eg, megavitamins and herbal supplements). Physicians should be especially cautious about those products that can produce toxicity, work with patients so they do not abandon proven care, and alert patients to signs of possible fraud or abuse. "Secret" formulas, cures for multiple conditions, slick advertising for mail order products, pyramid marketing schemes, and any recommendation to abandon conventional medicine are "red flags" and should be suspect.

B. PERMITTING USE OF NONSPECIFIC THERAPIES

Spontaneous healing and placebo effects account for the improvement seen in many illnesses. Science attempts to separate these factors from those that are specific aspects of a therapy. Physicians, however, are interested in how to combine both specific and nonspecific factors for maximum benefit. Many medical systems emphasize high-touch, personalized approaches for the management of chronic disease. The physician can permit the integration of selected CAM approaches that are not harmful or expensive but that may enhance these nonspecific factors.

C. PROMOTING CAM USE

Proven therapies that are safe and effective should be available to the public. As research continues, expanded options for managing clinical conditions will arise. Gradually the physician and patients will have more options for management of disease. In arthritis, for example, there are studies suggesting improvements with homeopathy, acupuncture, vitamin and nutritional supplements, botanical products, diet therapies, mind–body approaches, and manipulation. A similar collection of small studies exists for other conditions such as heart disease, depression, asthma, and addictions. The Cochrane Collaboration conducts systematic reviews of randomized controlled trials on both conventional and complementary medicine and is an excellent source for evidence-based evaluation of such studies. As research accumulates, rational therapeutic options can be developed in these areas.

D. PARTNERING WITH PATIENTS ABOUT CAM USE

Over 70% of patients who use CAM practices do not reveal this information to their conventional physicians. Thus, there is a major communication gap between physicians and the public about CAM. Patients use alternative practices for a variety of reasons. This includes because it is part of their social network, because they are not satisfied with the result of their conventional care, or because they have an attraction to CAM philosophies and health beliefs. The overwhelming majority of patients use CAM practices as an adjunct to conventional medicine. Less than 5% use CAM exclusively. Patients who use alternative medicine do not foster antiscience or anticonventional medicine sentiments, or represent a disproportionate number of the uneducated, poor, seriously ill, or neurotic. Often patients do not understand the role of science in medicine and will accept anecdotal evidence or slick marketing as sufficient justification for use. The conventional practitioner can play a role in examining the research base of these medical claims and working with patients to incorporate more evidence into their health care decisions. Quality research on these practices can help to provide this evidence and the physician can help interpret that evidence with patients.

Other social factors have also influenced the rise in prominence of CAM. These include the prevalence of chronic disease, increasing access to health information, the "consumerization" of medical decision making, a declining faith that scientific breakthroughs will have relevant benefits for personal health, and an increased interest in spiritualism. In addition, the public and professionals are increasingly concerned over side effects and escalating costs of conventional health care. Ignorance about CAM practices by physicians and scientists can broaden the communication gap between the public and the profession that serves them. All physicians should learn about these practices and discuss them with patients.

Chez RA, Jonas WB: The challenge of complementary and alternative medicine. Am J Obstet Gynecol 1997;177(5):1156.

Eisenberg DM et al: Trends in alternative medicine use in the United States 1990–1997: results of a follow-up national survey. JAMA 1998;280:1569.

Lewith G et al: *Clinical Research in Complementary Therapies: Principles, Problems and Solutions.* Churchill Livingston, 2002.

WEB SITE

Cochrane Collaboration
www.cochrane.de

Evidence Hierarchy or Evidence House?

We all need good evidence to make medical decisions. Evidence comes in a variety of forms and what may be good for one purpose may not be good for another. The term "evidence-based medicine" (EBM) has become a synonym for "good" medicine recently and is often used to support and deny the value of complementary medicine. EBM uses the "hierarchy of evidence" (Figure 57–1). In this hierachary, systematic reviews (SR) are seen as the "best" evidence, then individual randomized controlled trials (RCT), then nonrandomized trials, then observational studies, and finally case series. All efforts are focused on approximating evidence at the top of the pyramid and lower levels are considered inferior. Clinical experiments on causal links between an intervention and outcomes become the "gold standard" when this model is used.

All family physicians have seen patients who recover from disease because of complex factors many of which are not additive and cannot be isolated in controlled experiments. Under these circumstances observational data from clinical practice may offer the best evidence rather than controlled trials. Patients' illnesses are complex, and holistic phenomena cannot be reduced to single, objective measures. Often highly subjective judgments about life quality may be the best information on which to make a decision on a case. Such experiences may be captured only with qualitative research,

not with scans or blood tests. In that case the meaning patients have of their illness and recovery is the "best" evidence for medical decisions. Sometimes the "best" evidence comes from laboratory tests. For example, the most crucial evidence for management of St. John's wort in patients on immunosuppressive medications comes from a laboratory finding that it accelerates drug metabolism via cytochrome P-450. Arranging evidence in a "hierarchy" obscures the fact that the "best" evidence may not be about cause and effect, may not be objective, and may not be clinical.

We suggest that family physicians not use an evidence hierarchy, rather that they build an evidence "house" (Figure 57–2). On the left side of this house is evidence for causal attributions, for mechanisms of action, and for "proof." However, if physicians confine themselves to the left side of the house they will never know about the relevance of a treatment for patients or what happens in the real world of clinical practice. They will also not know if proven treatments can be generalized to populations such as the ones they see or the health care delivery system in which they practice. The "rooms" on the right side of the house provide evidence about patient relevance and usefulness, in practices both proven and unproven.

How evidence is approached has ethical implications. Different groups prefer different types of evidence. Regulatory authorities are most interested in randomized controlled trials or systematic reviews (left side), which may never be done. Health care practitioners usually want to know the likelihood of benefit or harm from a treatment (right side) Patients are intensely interested in stories and descriptions of cures (right side). Rationalists want to know how things work

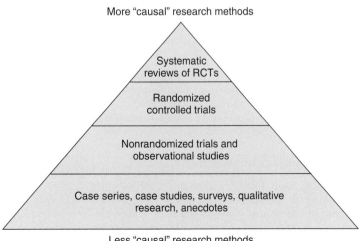

Figure 57–1. The evidence hierachy.

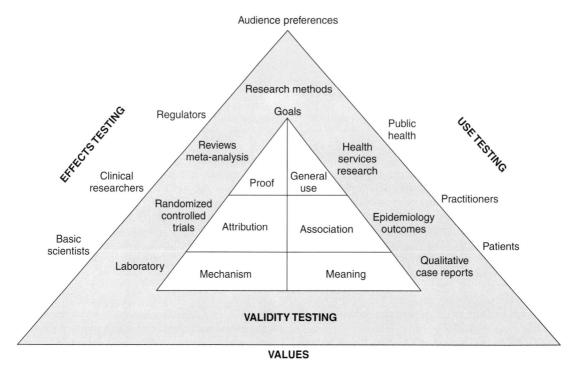

Figure 57–2. The evidence house.

and so need laboratory evidence (left side). If one type of evidence is selected to the exclusion of others science will not allow for full public input into clinical decisions. A livable house needs both a kitchen and a bathroom, a place to sleep and play. Each type of evidence has different functions and all need to be high quality.

Jonas W: Evidence, ethics and evaluation of global medicine. In: *Ethical Issues in Complementary and Alternative Medicine.* Callahan D (editor). Hastings Center Report, 2001.

Kelner M, Wellman B: *Complementary and Alternative Medicine: Challenge and Change.* Gordon & Breach, 2000.

Linde K, Jonas WB: Evaluating complementary and alternative medicine: the balance of rigor and relevance. In: *Essentials of Complementary and Alternative Medicine.* Jonas WB, Levin J (editors). Lippincott Williams & Wilkins, 1999.

Norquist G, Lebowitz B: Expanding the frontier of treatment research. Prevent Treat 1999;2.

An Evidence-Based Approach

Fortunately, most treatment decisions need information on whether a practice has a specific effect and on the magnitude of that effect in practice. This is evidence from randomized controlled trials and outcomes research, respectively. An evidence-based practice would then involve clinical expertise, informed patient com-

munication, and quality research. This presumes that the physician has good clinical and communication skills. Medical training and experience address these, but evaluation of the research evidence may not be something the physician feels fully prepared for in CAM. Obtaining research, selecting appropriate research for clinical situations, and then evaluating the quality of that research in CAM are essential for a fully evidence-based practice that addresses these topics.

A. FINDING AND SELECTING GOOD INFORMATION

Where can the family physician obtain research on CAM? A number of groups have collated and produced a CAM-specific database, although central, comprehensive, and easily accessed sources for quality CAM literature are not yet available. Table 57–2 lists some good sources of clinical information on CAM and what they provide. When searching these databases look for the following key terms: (1) meta-analyses, (2) randomized controlled trials, and (3) observational or prospective outcomes data. Although there are many other types of studies, it is necessary to be cautious about using these for problem-oriented decision making in practice. If no research information is found from the databases listed, it is likely that there is little relevant evidence for the practice on that clinical condition. A search for this in-

Table 57–2. Sources of quality medical information on CAM.

Literature	Web Site	Source and Use
Primary		
MEDLINE	www.nlm.nih.gov/hinfo.html or	National Library of Medicine
	www.ncbi.nlm.nih.gov/PubMed	PubMed (free internet access to MEDLINE)
EMBASE	www.embase.com	Excerpta Medica
CAM Citation Index	http://NCCAM.nih.gov	National Center for Complementary and Alternative Medicine, NIH
CISCOM	www.gn.apc.org/rccm	Research Council for Complementary Medicine
Secondary		
The Cochrane Library	www.cochrane.org www.cochrane.de	Cochrane has a field group in CAM CD-ROM available
Best Evidence Selection	www.webcom.com/mjljweb/jrnl clb/index.html	ACP Journal Club and Evidence-Based Medicine CD-ROM available
Agency for Healthcare Research and Quality	Text.nlm.nih.gov/ www.guideline.gov	Evidence-Based Practice Guidelines
Focus on Alternative and Complementary Therapies	www.exeter.ac.uk/FACT/	Quarterly Journal Club for CAM

formation need not take up a lot of time. A trained office assistant can often do the search, streamlining time spent on this process. After a literature search, the physician can have confidence knowing the quantity of evidence on the therapy. Patients are usually grateful for this effort as they will come to their physician in the hopes of obtaining science-based information they can trust

B. RISKS AND TYPES OF EVIDENCE FOR PRACTICE

If there are studies on a specific type of CAM practice, then the risk of toxicity and the cost of the therapy indicate which types of data are needed. Low-risk practices include counter homeopathic medications, acupuncture and gentle massage or manipulation, meditation, relaxation and biofeedback, other mind–body methods, and vitamin and mineral supplementation below toxic doses. Low-cost therapies involving self-care are also often low risk. High-risk practices include herbal therapies, high dosage vitamins and minerals, vaccine products, colonics, and intravenous administration of substances. Some otherwise harmless therapies can produce considerable cost if they require major lifestyle changes. Herbal therapies can produce serious adverse effects. Because patients frequently take herbal products along with prescription medications, physicians should specifically inquire about their use. High-risk or high-cost practices and products require randomized controlled trial data.

Under some circumstances observational (outcomes) data are more important and in other circumstances randomized controlled trial (RCT) data are more im-

portant. Outcomes research provides the probability of an effect and the absolute magnitude of effects in the context of normal clinical care. It is more similar to clinical practice and usually involves a wide variety of patients and variations of care to fit the patient's circumstances. It does not provide information on whether a treatment is specific or better than another treatment. With low-risk practices, the physician wants to know the probability of benefit from the therapy. Quality outcomes data from practices are preferable to RCT data if the data are collected from actual practice on populations similar to the practitioner's patient. This may be sufficient evidence for making clinical decisions. Often it will be the only useful information available for chronic conditions. For example, if quality outcomes studies report a 75% probability of improving allergic rhinitis using a nontoxic, low-cost, homeopathic remedy this information can assist in deciding on its use.

For high-risk, high-cost interventions the physician should use randomized controlled trials (or meta-analyses of those trials). RCTs address the relative benefit of one therapy over another (or no therapy). RCTs can determine if the treatment is the cause of improvement and how much the treatment adds to either no treatment or placebo treatment. RCTs provide relative (not absolute) information effects between a CAM and control practice. They are difficult to do properly for more than short periods and difficult if the therapy being tested is complex and individualized or if there are marked patient preferences. In addition, RCTs remove any choice about therapy and, if blinded, blunt expectations—

both of which exist in clinical practice. They are largely dependent on the control group, which requires careful selection and management. Strong patient preference for CAM, differing cultural groups, and informed consent may also alter RCT results. RCTs are more important the more we need to know about specific benefit–harm comparisons, such as with high-risk high-cost interventions.

The more a CAM practice addresses chronic disease, depends on self-care (eg, meditation, yoga, biofeedback), or involves a complex system (eg, classical homeopathy, traditional Chinese medicine, Unani-Tibb), the more outcomes data are important. The more a CAM practice involves high risk or high cost the more essential RCT data become.

C. Evaluating Study Quality

Once data are found and the preferred type of study is selected the practitioner should apply some minimum quality criteria to these studies (Table 57–3). Three items can be quickly checked: (1) blind and random allocation of subjects to comparison groups (in RCTs) or blind outcome assessments (in outcomes research), (2) the clinical relevance and reliability of the outcome measures, and (3) the number of subjects that could be fully analyzed at the end of the study compared to the number entered. These same minimum quality criteria apply to RCTs or observational studies, except that blinded, random allocation to treatment and comparison groups does not apply in the latter. However, evaluation of effects before and after treatment can be blinded to the treatment given. Detailed descriptions of patients, interventions, and drop outs are hallmarks of a quality outcomes trial.

Finally one can ask if the probability of benefits reported in the outcomes study is worth the inconvenience, risk of side effects, and costs of the treatment and, in addition, whether confidence intervals were reported. Confidence intervals are the range of minimum to maximum benefit expected in 95% of similar studies. If confidence intervals are narrow the physician can be confident that similar benefits will occur with other patients. If confidence intervals are broad the chance of benefits from treatment in other patients will be unpredictable.

Quality screening questions that show there are marked quality flaws in the studies retrieved indicate that the evidence for the CAT is insufficient and so should not be used as a basis for clinical decisions.

D. The Population Studied

Even if good evidence is found for a practice, physicians should determine whether the population in the studies is similar to the patient being seen. Although this matching is largely subjective, the physician can compare five areas: determine if the study was done (1) in a primary, secondary, or tertiary referral center, (2) in a Western, Eastern, developing, or industrialized country, and (3) with diagnostic criteria similar to the patient (eg, the same criteria were used to diagnose osteoarthritis or congestive heart failure); and determine if (4) the age and (5) the gender of the study population were similar. If the study population is not similar to the patient being seen, then the data, even though valid, cannot be applied to the situation. The study country may be especially important for some CAM practices. For example, data on use of acupuncture to treat chronic pain derives largely from China. Pain percep-

Table 57–3. Minimum guidelines for assessment of study quality.

Study Type	Guidelines			
Randomized controlled trials	Was there concealed random allocation to comparison groups?	Were outcome measures of known or probable clinical importance?	Were there few lost to follow-up compared with the number of bad outcomes (<20%)?	
Observational and outcomes studies	Were outcome measures assessed blind to patient treatment?	Were outcome measures of known or probable clinical importance?	Were there few lost to follow-up compared with the number of bad outcomes (<20%)?	Were confidence intervals reported and were they narrow or broad?
Reviews	Were explicit criteria for selecting articles and rating their quality used?	Was there a comprehensive search for all relevant articles?	Were negative and unpublished articles found?	

Adapted from Haynes RB et al: Transferring evidence from research into practice: 2. getting the evidence straight. ACP J Club 1997;126:A14.

tion may be different in China than in the United States. Results from a study done in one country may not be applicable in another. If the study and clinic population match, an appropriate body of evidence for moving forward with a therapeutic trial exists.

E. BALANCING BELIEFS

Belief in the treatment by the physician and the patient needs to be explicitly considered in CAM. In conventional medicine both patient and physician accept the plausibility of treatment. Belief has long been known to affect outcome. Strong belief enhances positive outcomes and weak belief interferes with them. A physician may feel that a CAM practice has incredibly low plausibility although the patient may have a strong belief in the therapy. This so-called "prior probability" (or belief) by the physician and patient should be considered in the decision to allow or not allow the patient to

use a CAT. If physician and patient have similar beliefs, then a decision is easily made. Sometimes, however, the patient has a strong belief in the therapy but the physician finds it unbelievable. In such situations, the physician should work with the patient to decide the best action—including referral elsewhere as an option.

F. ALTERNATIVE DIAGNOSES

Some diagnoses are not very useful for management of a patient's illness. If the family physician's conventional diagnosis is not helping a patient the clinician may want to consider an evaluation by an alternative system. Chinese medicine uses energy diagnosis, for example, and homeopathy as a remedy classification. Sometimes obtaining an assessment from a CAM system may prove useful. For example, a 51-year-old woman with several years of idiopathic urticaria has obtained no relief from several conventional physicians. A homeo-

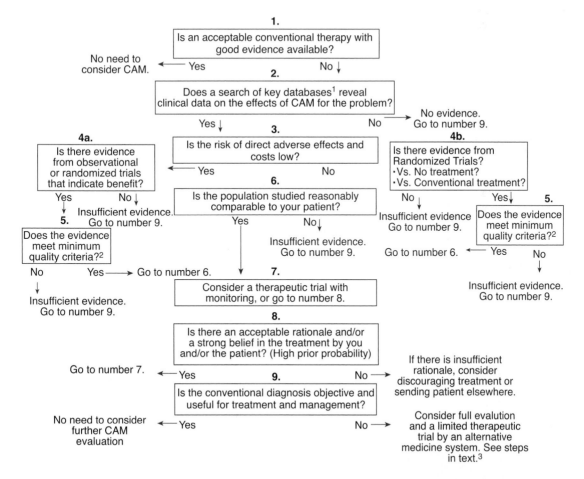

Figure 57–3. Decision tree for evidence-based complementary and alternative medicine.

pathic assessment shows that she may benefit from the remedy Mercurius. She is given several small doses and the urticaria clears. The physician should also be alert to practitioners who pursue CAM diagnoses that are not useful. A complicated CAM evaluation and treatment with little effect might be managed simply and effectively by conventional medicine. For example, a 57-year-old man with cardiovascular disease and recurrent bouts of angina was treated by a CAM practitioner for 3 years with special diets and nutritional supplements without help. Consultation with a conventional practitioner shows that he has myxedema. A thyroid supplement clears his angina rapidly. In cases in which the diagnostic approach of the medical system fails, a professional consultation may be needed. In situations in which the alternative system's diagnostic and treatment approach is clear, a limited therapeutic trial with specific treatment goals and follow-up can be attempted. Of course quality products and qualified practitioners must be located. In situations of serious disease, such as cancer, anxiety-ridden patients may seek out CAM treatments. Under these circumstances good training and clinical experience and protection of patients from harm (even from themselves) should prevail.

Evidence-based medicine can be applied to complementary and alternative medicine. Figure 57–3 summarizes the steps involved and Table 57–4 summarizes questions for CAM management. Although evidence-based CAM may initially seem like a large task, appropriate data-driven clinical decisions can be made with complementary and alternative medicine as with all medical care.

Eisenberg DM: Advising patients who seek alternative medical therapies. Ann Intern Med 1997;127:61.

Gatchel RJ, Maddrey AM: Clinical outcome research in complementary and alternative medicine: an overview of experimental design and analysis. Alt Ther Health Med 1998;4(5):36.

Jonas WB: Clinical trials for chronic disease: randomized, controlled clinical trials are essential. J NIH Res 1997;9:33.

Table 57–4. Summary of questions for evidence-based CAMT management.

A patient is using a complementary and alternative medicine therapy (CAMT) or an alternative treatment is sought. The following questions should be answered.

1. Has the patient received proper conventional medical care?
2. Is the CAMT likely to produce direct toxic or adverse effects or is it high cost?
3. Are there clinical data from randomized trials or outcomes research on the CAMT?
4. Do the studies meet minimum quality criteria? (Table 57–3)
5. Is the study population similar to the patient using or seeking the CAMT?
6. Is the plausibility of the therapy acceptable to both patient and physician?
7. Can a quality product or a qualified practitioner be accessed?
8. Can the patient be monitored while undergoing the CAMT?
9. Is a full diagnostic assessment by a conventional or CAM system in order?

Jonas WB et al: How to practice evidence-based complementary and alternative medicine. In: *Essentials of Complementary and Alternative Medicine.* Jonas WB, Levin JS (editors). Lippincott Williams & Wilkins, 1999.

Kirsch I: *How Expectancies Shape Experience.* American Psychological Association, 1999.

WEB SITES

Clinical Pearls News: Current Research on Nutrition and Preventive Medicine

www.clinicalpearls.com

National Center for Complementary and Alternative Medicine (NCCAM)

www.altmed.od.nih.gov/NCCAM

Chronic Pain Management

58

Ronald M. Glick, MD, & Dawn A. Marcus, MD

General Considerations

Pain, as defined by the International Association for the Study of Pain, is *an unpleasant sensory or emotional experience associated with actual or potential tissue damage or described in terms of such damage.* This definition emphasizes that the pain experience is multidimensional and may include sensory, cognitive, and emotional components. Additionally, the latter part of the definition allows for the possibility, as in chronic pain states, that the overt tissue damage may no longer be present. Pain persisting longer than 3–6 months is defined as chronic pain. Pain persisting for 3 months, however, is unlikely to resolve spontaneously and will continue to be reported by patients after 12 months. In addition, many of the secondary problems associated with chronic pain, such as deconditioning, depression, sleep disturbance, and disability, begin within the first few months of the onset of symptoms of pain. Studies indicate that early patient identification and treatment are essential to reduce pain chronicity and prevent further disability.

Chronic pain has been associated with significant disability and economic costs. Nearly 50% of primary care patients report some type of chronic pain; in family practice 64% of patients with chronic pain continue to report persistent pain 2 years later. Chronic pain is experienced by about one-third of Americans, resulting in $85–$90 billion in annual economic costs. Consequently, it is crucial to focus on early identification and intervention as well as on prompt involvement in rehabilitation. The subacute period, between 3 weeks and 3 months, affords the opportunity to have the greatest impact.

Clark JD: Chronic pain prevalence and analgesic prescribing in a general medical population. J Pain Symptom Manage 2002; 23:131.

Croft PR et al: Outcome of low back pain in general practice: a prospective study. Br Med J 1998;316:1356.

Elliott AM et al: The epidemiology of chronic pain in the community. Lancet 1999;354:1248.

Pathogenesis

Acute pain occurs following some form of tissue injury (eg, ankle sprain), and is treated with RICE (rest, immobilization, compression, and elevation) and pain-soothing treatments, such as heat, ice, and massage. During the acute period of tissue injury and healing, patients appropriately limit activity to reduce risks of further injury, such as developing a Charcot joint in a patient with neuropathy who risks aggravation of the injury because of impaired sensation. Studies show that patients improve best after acute injury when they reduce activities to what can be tolerated and allow healing to occur, compared with patients treated with either bed rest or acute physical therapy.

Chronic pain occurs after the acute healing period has been completed or in the context of chronic degenerative changes (eg, neuropathy or arthritis). Restriction of activity in patients with chronic pain leads to deconditioning, with muscle and bone loss that increases pain and the risk for reinjury, and also promotes psychological sluggishness, if not depression. Consequently, the RICE approach will actually aggravate the symptoms of chronic pain. The natural response of restricting activities when experiencing pain is appropriate for acute injury pain, but aggravates chronic pain. Patients with chronic pain require an active, progressive exercise program. They must learn appropriate strategies for treating pain, must avoid a tendency to restrict activity excessively, and must resume more normal activity levels through a stepwise, progressive activity program.

Clinical Findings

The most common chronic pain conditions in young and middle adulthood are low back pain, neck pain, and headaches. Musculoskeletal diseases rank fifth in generating hospital expenses and first in generating expenses related to work absenteeism and disability. The most common cause for chronic pain in older adults is degenerative joint and disc diseases, with arthritis causing chronic pain in over 80% of elderly patients with pain. Other causes of chronic pain that occur more frequently with increasing age are pain related to cancer, vascular disease, and neuropathy (eg, postherpetic neuralgia). Throughout the life cycle, pain can be associated with a variety of general medical conditions, such as Crohn's disease or sickle cell anemia.

The overall pain experience includes primary pain-generating signals, along with common secondary problems that develop regardless of pain etiology and that complicate pain management (Figure 58–1). Both physical (eg, joint restrictions and deconditioning) and psychological (eg, depression and anxiety) changes frequently accompany chronic pain. Depression or anxiety is diagnosed in 58% of chronic pain patients, and comorbid psychological distress predicts more recalcitrant chronic pain complaints. Psychosocial stress may result from difficulties related to school or work, family relationships, social isolation, and legal and financial areas. Although the possibility of secondary gain (eg, litigation) may increase pain complaints, true malingering and factitious disorders are uncommon, occurring in only 1–10% of patients. The *Diagnostic and Statistical Manual of Mental Disorders,* 4th edition (*DSM-IV*), appropriately recognizes the ability of psychological variables to impact complaints of pain and offers the designation of a Pain Disorder, reflecting the coexistence of both physical dysfunction and psychological factors, both of which impact patients' overall presentation and function. The family physician is in a unique position to identify and treat the physical and psychosocial factors influencing complaints of pain.

Croft PR et al: Psychological distress and low back pain. Evidence from a prospective study in the general population. Spine 1995;20:2731.

Macfarlane GJ et al: Predictors of early improvement in low back pain amongst consulters to general practice: the influence of premorbid and episode-related factors. Pain 1999;80:113.

Nahit ES et al: The influence of work related psychological factors and psychological distress on regional musculoskeletal pain: a study of newly employed workers. J Rheumatol 2001;28:1378.

Treatment

Management of chronic pain focuses on reduction in symptoms and improvement of function rather than on disease cure. It often includes utilization of a variety of medication and nonmedication treatment modalities to effectively address both primary and secondary symptoms of chronic pain (Table 58–1). Both doctors and patients must accept that complete resolution of complaints of pain may not be possible and they need to work toward rehabilitative goals of reducing symptoms and minimizing disability. Although modern medicine

and rehabilitation techniques can be beneficial, the patient's mindset must shift from the search for a medical cure to engaging in collaborative rehabilitation, geared toward decreasing pain and optimizing function. Goals of chronic pain rehabilitation include improvement in both pain and secondary symptoms, including deconditioning, depression, and disability (Table 58–2). Early identification and treatment should reduce the severity of secondary symptoms.

A. Psychological

Cognitive–behavioral therapy (CBT) is an effective psychological treatment technique that challenges a dysfunctional perception of pain ("My pain must be cured. I can't do anything if I have pain.") and replaces it with one that is more conducive to change ("Pain limits me from lifting 25 pounds, but I can still carry a bag of groceries."). CBT helps change patients' perceptions or locus of control from external control (believing pain is not controllable by the patient) to internal control (believing the patient can positively impact symptoms). When patients endorse an external locus of control, they see themselves as victims of the pain and as powerless to improve their situation. This results in the expectation that only fate or the doctor can help when pain becomes severe. When expectations are not met, these patients seek alternative evaluations and treatments (eg, another physician, a different diagnostic test, or surgical procedures) that may not be in their best interest. The clinician must help patients to move into a pain self-management, internal locus of control belief system, in which patients see themselves as the agent for change. Greater perceived self-control of pain decreases both pain and secondary symptoms. Although CBT is typically the purview of psychologists, the family physician can reinforce these concepts through interactions with the patient.

B. Physical and Occupational Therapy

Identification and treatment of musculoskeletal dysfunctions and decisions concerning limitations on activity often require consultation with physical or occupational therapists. Reconditioning, active stretching and strengthening exercise, and graded activity programs are effective for managing chronic pain. Physical therapists should instruct patients in a daily exercise routine as well as flare management techniques (eg, trigger point massage, oscillatory movements, and use of heat and ice). Exercise therapy is most effective when initiated through a supervised physical therapy program rather than through self-exercise. Occupational therapists will address work simplification, body mechanics, and pacing skills.

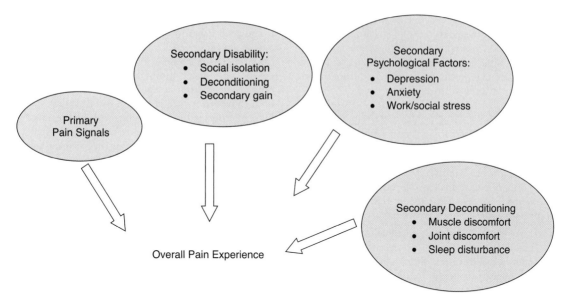

Figure 58–1. Primary and secondary features of chronic pain.

The secondary problems, as noted above, can develop rapidly after a problem with pain starts and should be addressed early in the course of treatment of pain. The most important intervention is reinforcing the need to resume more normal activity schedules, eg, returning to work or school, even on a modified basis. Prolonged absence from normal activities increases the difficulty of reducing disability. Return to normal activity as soon as possible, however, should be the primary goal of pain management and the physician should work to expedite that return, with modifications if needed. Conflicts with the employer, fear of losing one's job and benefits, or other intervening factors need

to be identified and addressed to facilitate a successful return to work. In addition, the longer the patient with pain has avoided employment or school, the more difficult and emotionally stressful a return to work or school becomes. In the case of a child or adolescent, anxiety around return to school may actually increase complaints of pain. Migraines and abdominal pain, for

Table 58–1. Comprehensive treatment of chronic pain.

Specialist	Treatment Modalities
Physician	Analgesics, adjunctive medications, nerve blocks
Physical/occupational therapist	Musculoskeletal dysfunction, deconditioning, work simplification
Psychology/psychiatry	Adjust locus of control, depression therapy, anxiety therapy
Complementary/ alternative therapist	Acupuncture, yoga/Tai Chi, meditation, chiropractic therapy

Table 58–2. Appropriate treatment goals.

General Goal	Specific Treatment Target
Decreased pain	Pain reduction to moderate levels; reduced frequency and duration of flares
Improved function	Return to school/work; increased number of household chores; increased participation in leisure activities
Improved sleep	Reduced number of wake-ups; improved overall sleep to 5 h per night
Improved mood	Increased participation in social activities; reduced time in bed/inactive; improved nutrition intake
Reduced use of medical resources	Reduced emergency room visits; reduced use of excessive analgesics

example, are particularly reactive to anxiety and the associated avoidant behavior, creating a vicious cycle.

Additionally, counseling should be directed toward issues concerning mood, sleep, and other psychosocial factors. Severe symptoms of depression or anxiety or significant psychosocial stressors may necessitate a psychiatric referral.

C. MEDICATIONS

Medications are prescribed to treat an underlying medical condition (eg, disease-modifying medications in rheumatoid arthritis), relieve symptoms of pain, and relieve secondary symptoms (eg, depression, anxiety, and/or sleep disturbance). Most medications used to treat chronic pain address the latter two factors (Table 58–3).

1. Pain relievers—Analgesics rarely eliminate pain entirely, and may result in either significant adverse effects or habituation. Treatment should begin with simple analgesics, such as acetaminophen or nonsteroidal antiinflammatory drugs (NSAIDs). Daily doses of acetaminophen should not exceed 4 g and patients need to consider the cumulative dosage from both over-the-counter and prescription pain relievers. Acetaminophen may be restricted in patients with significant alcohol intake or liver disease. A variety of available NSAIDs share similar efficacy and tolerability. Patients with gastrointestinal disease may tolerate cyclooxygenase-II inhibitors (COX-II drugs) better.

Table 58–3. Medication management of chronic pain.

Symptom Treated	Medication Class	Examples
Pain	Analgesics Long-acting opioids	Acetaminophen NSAIDs[1] Sustained-release morphine, oxycodone, or fentanyl
Neuropathic pain	Antidepressants Anticonvulsants	Nortriptyline 25–100 mg at bedtime Gabapentin 300–1200 mg three times a day
Muscle spasm	Muscle relaxants	Tizanidine 2–4 mg at bedtime to three times a day
Sleep disturbance	Antidepressants	Nortriptyline 25–100 mg at bedtime
Depression	Antidepressants	Nortriptyline 25–150 mg at bedtime

[1]NSAIDs, nonsteroidal antiinflammatory drugs.

The use of opioids for management of chronic pain is controversial. Although isolated treatment with opioids is not effective for managing chronic pain, opioids can provide a safe, cost-effective adjunctive pain therapy because of reduced morbidity and cost associated with organ toxicity from analgesics. Chronic opioid use has been shown to reduce both pain and disability. Opioids may be considered in patients with severe, disabling chronic pain that is unrelieved with simple analgesics and is associated with significant impairment in daily functioning and quality of life. Relative contraindications include a history of substance abuse, serious psychopathology, and lack of motivation to engage in an appropriate therapy program or to improve functioning. Patients with no history of substance abuse are at low risk for abuse with prescribed medications. Patients with current addiction problems should be referred to a drug rehabilitation facility before pain management is initiated. Patients with recent problems with substance abuse or addiction should be managed by a pain specialist, ideally in conjunction with a counselor specializing in treating patients with these types of problems.

Patients with constantly present, severe chronic pain are best managed with long-acting medication rather than frequent dosing with immediate-release agents. Short-acting medications are best used infrequently for intermittent, short-lived pain flares. Long-acting opioids include sustained-release morphine sulfate, sustained-release oxycodone, transdermal fentanyl, and methadone. Methadone is the least expensive (about one-tenth the cost of brand name opioids); however, titration is difficult because of individual variability in metabolism. Opioid equivalence charts may be helpful when converting patients from one medication to another (Table 58–4). For example, the amount of opioid administered from a 100-μg/h fentanyl patch is roughly equivalent to 240 mg morphine sulfate daily. In general, musculoskeletal pain is more responsive to opioids than neuropathic pain or chronic headache. Opioids may be a useful adjunctive treatment to other neuropathic medications in patients with neuropathic pain.

2. Adjunctive medications—Adjunctive medications supplement the benefits from analgesics, treat neuropathic or central pain, and treat secondary complaints. In addition, effective use of adjunctive agents often reduces the need for analgesic medications. Adjunctive agents interact with the mechanism of neuropathic or central pain and chronic headache by reducing nervous system wind-up, the process by which the nervous system amplifies and eventually perpetuates pain signals in the absence of ongoing nociceptive input from the periphery.

The two primary categories of adjunctive analgesics are antidepressants and anticonvulsants. Tricyclic antide-

Table 58–4. Opioid conversion chart.[1]

	Oral Dose (mg)	Transdermal Dose (μg/h)	Intravenous Dose (mg)	Brand Names
Morphine sulfate	15		5	MSContin, Kadian, Oramorph
Hydromorphone	4		0.8	Dilaudid
Oxycodone	10			Percocet, Roxicet, Oxycontin
Hydrocodone	15			Vicodin, Lorcet, Norco
Meperidine	150		35	Demerol
Fentanyl		6.25		Duragesic

[1]Dose conversions are approximate, with variation based on both individual patients and drug preparations.

pressants (TCAs) are effective as once daily, nighttime medications for treating neuropathic pain, myofascial pain, fibromyalgia, and tension-type and migraine headaches. Nortriptyline may be particularly suited for treating chronic pain because it provides moderate sedation, which helps with sleep, and low anticholinergic effects (eg, orthostasis). Selective serotonin reuptake inhibitors (SSRIs) are used to treat headaches and neuropathic pain, although their efficacy is generally less than TCAs. Newer antidepressants, particularly venlafaxine and bupropion, have been reported to be helpful for treating neuropathic and myofascial pain. Augmenting both noradrenergic and serotonergic pathways, which influence descending neural inhibition, is important for treating chronic pain with TCAs and venlafaxine.

Anticonvulsants, particularly gabapentin, have become a mainstay for the treatment of neuropathic pain. They are also beneficial for treating chronic headaches and may be beneficial for treating fibromyalgia. Newer anticonvulsant drugs that show promise for the treatment of neuropathic pain include topirimate, oxcarbazine, and zonisamide. Some have multiple mechanisms of action including membrane stabilization involving sodium and calcium channels, N-methyl-D-aspartate blockade, and gabaergic effects.

Most muscle relaxants (eg, carisoprosol and cyclobenzaprine) used to treat acute musculoskeletal pain are associated with significant sedation, reducing their usefulness as a treatment for chronic pain, where the primary focus is reducing disability and time spent in bed. Tizanidine, a unique muscle relaxant with both antispasticity and α-adrenergic effects, results in reduced spasticity and reduced pain perception with both acute and chronic use. In addition to reducing spasticity related to neurological conditions, eg, multiple sclerosis, stroke, or spinal cord injury, tizanidine can also reduce symptoms associated with myofascial pain, fibromyalgia, and headaches, with some evidence of benefit for neuropathic pain. Tizanidine is often used in low doses (2–8 mg daily) given at bedtime or divided into three daily doses. Tizanidine is mildly sedating, which can assist with associated sleep disturbance.

3. Adverse events with chronic pain medications—
The annual costs associated with toxicity from nonopioid analgesics approach $1.9 billion, with $1.35 billion caused by NSAID toxicity. Gastric ulcers occur in 15–30% of chronic NSAIDs users. In addition, renal impairment occurs in 24% and renal papillary necrosis in 12% of arthritic patients using chronic NSAIDs. Fortunately, renal insufficiency is often improved when the drugs are discontinued. NSAIDs must be used with particular caution in the elderly, as their use reduces the effectiveness of diuretics and doubles the risk for hospitalization from congestive heart failure.

Opioids are not associated with organ toxicity. Practitioners must monitor for evidence of the development of tolerance (reduced effectiveness of the medication over time) or abuse (failure to identify prescribed opioids on random urine testing or repeated lost or overused medications). In either circumstance, patients will likely need a change in treatment.

Newer anticonvulsants used to treat neuropathic pain do not require the frequent laboratory monitoring that is common with older anticonvulsants, eg, carbamazepine and sodium valproate. Gabapentin is cleared by the kidneys, requiring dose adjustment of reduced frequency of administration in patients with renal insufficiency. Dialysis patients receive gabapentin dosing after each treatment with hemodialysis.

TCAs, typically prescribed in low to moderate doses to treat neuropathic pain, are still associated with a small risk for cardiac arrhythmia. All prepubertal children treated with TCAs should receive a baseline electrocardiogram (ECG), followed by regular assessments of heart rate and blood pressure, periodic testing of antidepressant drug levels, and repeat ECGs. Similarly, older adults or individuals with a history of cardiac disease should also be monitored with blood tests and ECGs when TCA doses approach the low therapeutic range. SSRIs and bupropion have been associated with seizures in higher doses and should be used with caution in individuals with tendencies to seizure. Venlafaxine can have a cardiac stimulatory effect at higher doses and blood pressure should be watched.

Tizanidine has been associated with hepatotoxicity and should be avoided in individuals with a history of liver problems. Periodic liver enzyme screening should be obtained in patients taking tizanidine chronically.

4. Medication management in pediatric patients and in older patients—Chronically administered opioids are generally avoided in pediatric patients, although there are certainly exceptions with chronic disease states such as hemophilia and sickle cell disease. Acetaminophen and nonsteroidal agents should be considered first-line therapy for pediatric patients with pain. TCAs and gabapentin have been extensively utilized for neuropathic pain in pediatric patients, and pediatric dosing guidelines are available. As noted, caution must be taken regarding the potential for cardiac conduction disturbance with the use of TCAs in prepubertal children.

When selecting medication for older adults physicians need to strongly consider the side effect profiles, particularly for agents that have central nervous system effects—including opioids, antidepressants, and anticonvulsants. As opposed to the mild sedation or dizziness experienced by younger individuals, geriatric patients may experience more profound drowsiness, confusion, delirium, and increased risk for falls. Medical comorbidities and medications for these conditions increase the risk for adverse events in geriatric patients. The potential for activation or inhibition of cytochrome P-450 pathways is problematic in patients taking multiple medications, particularly agents with a narrow therapeutic index, such as digoxin and warfarin. With the exception of gabapentin, the dosing of adjunctive analgesics typically is lower for older adults.

Low to modest doses of opioids may be a very useful part of the treatment regimen for geriatric patients with pain, particularly because of good tolerability at low doses. It is common to see older patients with arthritis who are unable to tolerate even the COX-II agents. Additionally, as the degree of degenerative disease progresses, benefits from NSAIDs may be limited, necessitating stronger analgesia. When used judiciously, opioids typically are well tolerated and can allow individuals to retain a level of functioning sufficient to maintain their independence.

D. INTERVENTIONAL PAIN MANAGEMENT

Interventional techniques are considered for patients failing conservative therapy or when specific nervous system pathology has been identified. Lumbar epidural steroid injections are effective for treating herniated discs or spinal stenosis. Sympathetic blocks reduce the burning pain of complex regional pain syndrome or reflex sympathetic dystrophy that may develop after acute extremity injury or surgery. Trigger point injections are useful for localized muscle pain. The benefit from injections is often transient, so these techniques are often used in conjunction with physical therapy and medication management. Radiofrequency ablation may be considered for recalcitrant symptoms of facet, disc, sympathetic, or neural pain.

Implantable devices, including intrathecal pumps and dorsal column stimulators, can be used to treat individuals with cancer-related pain or severe incapacitating pain resulting from nonmalignant conditions. Intrathecal medications are considered for patients requiring high medication doses when side effects from oral medications become intolerable. Dorsal column stimulators are considered when pain is limited to a single extremity. For the treatment of pain resulting from nonmalignant conditions, it is essential to obtain psychological consultation prior to the surgery.

Nerve blocks may be particularly beneficial for postherpetic neuralgia (PHN), which can be quite difficult to treat. The early use of antiviral agents, eg, valacyclovir, is important in attenuating the initial infection and decreasing the acute pain as well as chronic symptoms. In addition, early treatment of zoster with TCAs (25 mg amitriptyline daily for 90 days) reduces chronicity of symptoms of PHN. Nerve blocks, particularly thoracic epidural local anesthetics or intercostal blocks, can be used in the acute or chronic stage. Early use of nerve blocks, especially within the first 2 months of onset of symptoms, greatly decreases the incidence and severity of PHN.

E. COMPLEMENTARY AND ALTERNATIVE MEDICINE

Complementary and alternative treatments are used by 40% of chronic pain sufferers. Acupuncture reduces pain for a variety of painful conditions, including fibromyalgia. In clinical trials, acupuncture is as effective as transcutaneous electrical nerve stimulation or trigger point injections. Chiropractic treatment is recommended during the first month of symptoms for acute low back pain without radiculopathy. There is no clear consensus on the effectiveness of chiropractic manipulation for chronic pain, and controlled studies are needed to provide efficacy data. Exercise therapy with Tai Chi does effectively reduce pain in geriatric populations. Mind–body medicine (eg, meditation, guided imagery, and yoga) engages the patient actively in treatment, changing the locus of control and encouraging use of health-promoting behaviors. Mind–body techniques are also effective in reducing pain.

Ansari A: The efficacy of newer antidepressants in the treatment of chronic pain: a review of current literature. Harv Rev Psychiatry 2000;7:257.

Attal N et al: Effects of IV morphine in central pain: a randomized placebo-controlled study. Neurology 2002;26:554.

Bowsher D: The effects of pre-emptive treatment of postherpetic neuralgia with amitriptyline: a randomized, double-blind, placebo-controlled trial. J Pain Symptom Manage 1997;13: 327.

Ernst E, Assendelft WJJ: Chiropractic for low back pain. Br Med J 1998;317:160.

Faas A: Exercises: which ones are worth trying, for which patients, and when? Spine 1996;21:2877.

Gray CM et al: Complementary and alternative medicine use among health plan members. A cross-sectional survey. Eff Clin Pract 2002;5:17.

Jensen MP, Turner JA, Romano JM: Changes in beliefs, catastrophizing, and coping are associated with improvement in multidisciplinary pain treatment. J Consult Clin Psychol 2001; 69:655.

Kapural L, Mekhail N: Radiofrequency ablation for chronic pain control. Curr Pain Headache Rep 2001;5:517.

Mathew NT: Antiepileptic drugs in migraine prevention. Headache 2001;41(Suppl 1):18.

Portenoy RK: Opioid therapy for chronic nonmalignant pain: a review of the critical issues. J Pain Symptom Manage 1996;11: 203.

Rainov NG, Heidecke V, Burkert W: Long-term intrathecal infusion of drug combinations for chronic back and leg pain. J Pain Symptom Manage 2001;22:862.

Ross MC et al: The effects of a short-term program on movement, pain, and mood in the elderly. J Holist Nurs

Schofferman J: Long-term opioid analgesic therapy for refractory lumbar spine pain. Clin J Pain 1999;15:136.

Tortensen TA et al: Efficiency and costs of medical exercise therapy, conventional physiotherapy, and self-exercise in patients with chronic low back pain. A pragmatic, randomized, single-blinded, controlled trial with 1-year follow-up. Spine 1998; 23:2616.

Van Tulder MW et al: The effectiveness of acupuncture in the management of acute and chronic low back pain. A systematic review with the framework of the Cochrane Collaboration Back Review Group. Spine 1999;24:1113.

Hospice & Palliative Medicine

Terence L. Gutgsell, MD, Steven D. Passik, PhD, Hahn X. Pham, MD, Sherrie Weisenfluh, MSW, Billie May, RN, David Hilton, Mdiv, & Kenneth Kirsch, PhD

HOSPICE

Homes for the dying or, as they were soon to be called, hospices, were established in Ireland and France almost simultaneously by two separate religious orders of nuns in the nineteenth century. By the mid-twentieth century, the Irish Sisters of Charity established Saint Joseph Hospice in London, England, and there a nurse turned social worker, Cicely Saunders, determined that her life work was to be dedicated to the care of the terminally ill and dying. She earned her medical degree in 1957, and in 1967 helped to establish the first truly modern hospice, Saint Christopher's Hospice in London. At Saint Christopher's, Dr. Saunders helped to establish the underlying philosophy of hospice and palliative medicine. She emphasized excellence in pain and symptom management; care of the whole person including their physical, emotional, social, and spiritual needs; and the need for research in this newly developing field of medicine. Interdisciplinary team care became the norm, as it became clear that not any one physician, nurse, social worker, or chaplain could address all the needs of the terminally ill person. Further, although the focus of care was clearly on the dying individual, the needs of the family were also addressed.

Florence Wald, RN, Ph.D., Dean of the Yale School of Nursing, invited Dr. Saunders to lecture to medical, nursing, and social work students at Yale in 1963 on the care of the terminally ill. In 1965, Dr. Saunders returned to Yale as a visiting scholar. Dr. Wald spent 1968 at Saint Christopher's on sabbatical and, on returning to the United States, helped establish in 1974 the first hospice in the United States, the Connecticut Hospice.

In 1968, Dr. Elizabeth Kuebler-Ross, a psychiatrist working closely with the terminally ill in the United States, published her seminal work, *On Death and Dying*. This book, for the first time, described the psychological crisis of the terminally ill person in terms of defined stages—denial, anger, bargaining, depression, and acceptance. This book has since become essential reading for clinicians who care for the terminally ill. In 1972 Dr. Kuebler-Ross testified before the Congress of the United States about the needs of the dying, stressing the need for personal autonomy, death with dignity, and the benefit of death in the home versus a health care facility.

In 1974, several United States congressmen, recognizing the rapidly growing field of hospice and palliative medicine, introduced legislation to establish hospice as a government-funded program. The legislation failed but, nonetheless, the Connecticut Hospice was founded that year. Five years later, in 1979, the Health Care Financing Administration (HCFA) funded 26 demonstration projects to develop hospice programs throughout the country in an effort to answer the following questions: (1) What is a hospice? (2) What should a hospice provide? and (3) Is hospice cost effective?

From those demonstration projects came enough information for congressmen to craft legislation to support hospice programs throughout the country. In 1982, the Congress created the Medicare Hospice Benefit (MHB), and in 1986, the benefit was made permanent. By the year 2002, 3100 hospice programs were providing health care services to the terminally ill and their families throughout the United States.

Eligibility criteria for hospice enrollment through the MHB require that patients waive traditional Medicare coverage for curative and life-prolonging care related to the terminal diagnosis and be certified by their physician and the hospice medical director as having a life expectancy of 6 months or less if the disease runs its usual course. Recertification periods within the MHB allow for reexamination of hospice eligibility. If the hospice medical director, using his or her best medical judgment, believes the patient has a prognosis of 6 months or less if the disease runs its usual course, the patient may be recertified as eligible for the MHB, even if the patient has already been on the benefit for 6 months or longer.

The philosophy and structure of hospice care in the United States have been defined through the work of its early clinical pioneers as well as its unique funding source, the Medicare Hospice Benefit. In many parts of the world hospice has come to be defined primarily as a place, such as Saint Christopher's Hospice in England. In the United States, however, hospice is defined as a philosophy of care. Regarding place of care, most American hospice care is delivered in the patient's home and "home" is defined by the patient, whether it be the patient's own house, the home of a loved one, an assisted living facility, or a long-term care center.

The goal of hospice care is the relief of suffering and the improvement of the patient's and family's quality of daily life. To achieve those goals, care has come to be defined as holistic, person, and family centered rather than disease centered. The complex goal of relief of suffering cannot be unidimensional but must include the four dimensions of human experience: the physical (pain, dyspnea, cough, nausea, vomiting, constipation, agitation, delirium, etc), the emotional (anxiety, depression, grief, etc), the social (unfinished business with family members, financial concerns, caregiving issues, child care, etc), and the spiritual (guilt, worthlessness, meaning, etc). Hospice provides a team (a medical director, hospice nurse, social worker, chaplain, bereavement counselor, nursing assistant, and volunteer) that is composed of members trained to care for problems in these four areas. The hospice team meets weekly, under the direction of the hospice medical director, to review the care plans of all patients.

The hospice program is charged with providing (purchasing and bringing to the patient) (1) medications for the relief of physical distress, such as analgesics, antiemetics, anticholinergics, antidiarrheals, laxatives, sedatives, antidepressants, and other symptom-directed medications; (2) durable medical equipment, such as hospital beds, oxygen, bedside commodes, and walkers; and (3) supplies, such as dressings, urinary catheters, adult diapers, and pads. The hospice nurse visits the patient at least weekly, but more often if needed. The nurse is available by telephone 24 h/day, 7 days/week. The nursing assistant may go to the home daily to provide assistance with daily care needs. The social worker attends to practical needs and emotional support of the patient and family. The hospice chaplain provides spiritual support, often in conjunction with the family's own minister, priest, rabbi, or imam. Hospice volunteers provide companionship and practical help to the patients and families.

Upon the death of the patient, hospice provides a variety of bereavement services to the grieving family members. These may include individual counseling, groups, weekend camps for bereaved children and teens, books, pamphlets, videotapes, and audiotapes. Bereavement counseling may begin even before the death of the patient. Bereavement services are provided for at least a year after the death of the patient, but may continue as long as the family member is in need. Many hospice organizations do not restrict their bereavement services just to families of hospice patients, but extend this service to the entire community. A recent example has been the grief experienced after the World Trade Towers tragedy. Many hospices provided emotional and bereavement support for grieving people throughout their local communities.

The length of time patients remain in hospice programs has steadily decreased over time. There are many factors that contribute to this trend, including better treatments for advanced illnesses, physician and patient desire for aggressive treatments, misunderstandings about hospice and palliative care, and physician and hospice fears of regulatory scrutiny and punishment if patients are improperly labeled as "terminal."

PALLIATIVE MEDICINE

Palliative medicine has been developing as a subspecialty in the United States for over 10 years in partial response to the declining length of stays in hospice programs as well as a desire to bring a "hospice-like" approach to the patient with a terminal or life-limiting illness but with a much better prognosis than 6 months. The goals of palliative care programs now developing across the country are much the same as those of hospice: excellence in pain and symptom management; emotional, social, and spiritual support of patients and families; and facilitation of clear and compassionate communication regarding goals of treatment. A major difference between hospice and palliative medicine is that palliative care, although delivered to patients with life-threatening or terminal illnesses, may also be delivered to patients with chronic illnesses who may continue to live for many more years. For many practitioners of palliative medicine the primary goal is the relief of suffering, not just to the terminally ill but to any patient with a chronic illness.

Many models of palliative care are under development. There are palliative care consultation teams in hospitals, nursing homes, and clinics. These teams are generally multidisciplinary and include physicians, nurses, social workers, chaplains, pharmacists, and psychologists in various permutations and combinations. Because there is, as yet, no funding mechanism for palliative care teams, collaborative arrangements between hospices, hospitals, academic centers, and nursing homes are supporting this work. Multiple granting agencies are also providing support for these pioneering programs.

Palliative medicine fellowships are in the process of development as well. In the mid-1990s there was only one fellowship program in the United States. By 2002 there were 17 programs offering advanced training. The American Association of Hospice and Palliative Medicine (AAHPM) is a professional society composed of physicians and other clinicians working in the hospice and palliative medicine field. The AAHPM has initiated a board examination and certification process in palliative medicine. A goal of the AAHPM is to have palliative medicine recognized as a bona fide medical subspecialty by the American Board of Medical Specialties in the next 5 years.

Pain & Symptom Management

Good symptom control is the cornerstone of palliative medicine. Distressing symptoms can consume patients and rob them of their will to live. Uncontrolled symptoms detract from patients' quality of life, their interactions with loved ones, and their ability to attend to issues important at the end of life. Multiple studies have documented the high frequency of symptoms and the tendency for symptoms to increase in intensity as the disease progresses. As with most medical problems, successful management of symptoms starts with a careful history and physical examination with therapy directed at the underlying etiology whenever possible.

A. PAIN

Pain can be classified into somatic, visceral, neuropathic, or mixed types of pain. Pain can occur from direct tumor involvement, as a consequence of cancer therapy, or from unrelated pathology. It is important to remember that pain is a subjective experience that can be influenced by psychosocial and spiritual issues.

The WHO published guidelines on pain control in 1996 (Figure 59–1). These guidelines have proven effective in large-scale studies in cancer patients and for the majority of patients their application will lead to effective pain control. Based initially on the severity of the patient's pain, different medications can be utilized and adjustments made depending on the patient's response.

General principles of opioid administration include the following:

- Equianalgesic tables for opioids are available in most general pharmacology texts; these tables may differ slightly.
- Morphine is the most commonly used opioid and is the most versatile in terms of available formulations.
- Opioid-naive patients should be started with 5 mg morphine sulfate immediate release orally every 4 h scheduled and every 2 h as needed. This should be converted to morphine sulfate sustained release based on the previous 24-h dose and titrated based on pain control.
- Chronic pain deserves around the clock pain medication, not just as needed.

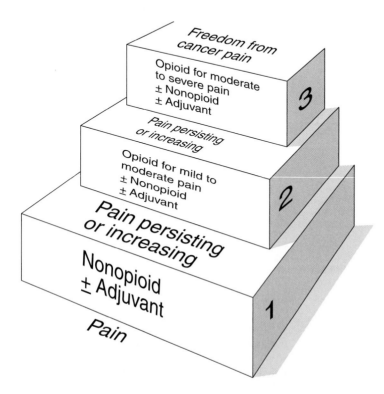

Figure 59–1. WHO three-step pain control guidelines.

- As needed medications should always be provided for breakthrough pain.
- Breakthrough doses are generally 10–15% of the 24-h dose.
- Breakthrough medications can be given as frequently as the time to peak onset of action, 1.5–2 h for oral immediate release formulations and 5–10 min for intravenous formulations.
- When pain control is inadequate, the scheduled dose should be increased by 30–50% after 24 h (after 48 h for fentanyl patches). The amount of breakthrough medications used must be taken into consideration; patients can tolerate at least this much additional.
- There is no specific limit to the opioid dose; opioids should be titrated to pain control or development of side effects.
- Fentanyl patches should not be used *alone* for acute severe pain as its onset of effect is 12 h and, because of its long half-life, it cannot be titrated quickly for rapid pain control.
- The lowest available fentanyl patch may be excessive in patients who are opioid naive (25 μg/h fentanyl patch is approximately equivalent to 50 mg of morphine sulfate).
- Morphine sulfate, hydromorphone, and fentanyl can be administered subcutaneously for patients unable to take them orally and who do not have intravenous access. Subcutaneous doses are equivalent to intravenous doses.
- When pain is severe, parenteral opioids are preferable because of their quicker onset of action and ease of titration. Conversion to oral formulations can occur after pain is controlled.
- With patient-controlled analgesia (PCA), opioids can be infused at a continuous basal rate and patients can control the amount of bolus doses. The total hourly dose and lockout interval between boluses are preprogrammed. PCA can be administered intravenously or subcutaneously at home with specialized syringe drivers or infusion pumps.
- With most opioids, oral and parenteral doses are not equal; parenteral morphine sulfate is one-third oral morphine sulfate and parenteral hydromorphone is one-quarter oral hydromorphone; care should be taken when converting from oral to parenteral forms.
- When side effects develop and are not easily controlled, options include decreasing the opioid dose if the pain is well controlled, opioid rotation, or decreasing the opioid dose and adding adjuvant pain medication.
- Because nausea and vomiting are common transient side effects of opioid therapy, metoclopramide or haloperidol is sometimes started prophylactically for the first several days of opioid therapy.
- Tolerance to the respiratory depressant effects occurs rapidly; opioids can be used safely when titrated to pain control.
- Constipation is a side effect of opioids to which patients do not become tolerant; laxatives should be included whenever patients are on opioids.
- Because methadone has a biphasic and variable half-life, administration can be difficult and should be attempted carefully and probably by those experienced in its use.
- Psychostimulants, methylphenidate and amphetamine, can be prescribed for some patients troubled by persistent opioid-induced sedation.

Unlike opioids, nonsteroidal antiinflammatory drugs (NSAIDs) and acetaminophen have a ceiling effect to their analgesia. The use of opioid/nonopioid combinations therefore is limited by the dose of the NSAIDs or acetaminophen. Despite this fact, NSAIDs are effective pain medication, especially for inflammatory conditions. Their use can decrease the amount of opioids required and hence decrease the incidence of opioid side effects. Unless contraindicated, all pain protocols should include NSAIDs.

Neuropathic pain results from nerve injury. Often described as sharp, electric shock-like, or burning in nature, neuropathic pain generally occurs along specific dermatomes. Patients with neuropathic pain occasionally respond to opioids alone; many require the addition of adjuvant pain medications. Commonly used adjuvants for neuropathic pain include tricyclic antidepressants, anticonvulsants, and antiarrhythmics. The choice of an adjuvant is usually dictated by the individual drug side effect profile, the potential for drug interactions, and the previous drug therapy. The secondary amines, nortryptyline and desipramine, tend to be more tolerable than amitriptyline. The analgesic effects of tricyclic antidepressants occur at lower doses and usually within several days, as compared to the antidepressant effects. The data on selective serotonin reuptake inhibitors (SSRIs) for neuropathic pain are not convincing. Of the anticonvulsants, carbamazepine, valproic acid, and gabapentin are commonly used for neuropathic pain. Carbamazepine and valproic acid are cost effective but have a higher risk for drug interactions and toxicity compared to gabapentin. Gabapentin requires more frequent dosing, slower titration secondary to sedation, and dose adjustments for renal insufficiency. Antiarrhythmics, topical lidocaine, and oral mexilitine have also been used successfully for neuropathic pain. For adjuvant pain medications, standard initial dosing and titration guidelines should be followed, although lower than usual doses have been effective for pain control. For the elderly, it is generally safer to start at low doses and titrate at a slower rate.

Corticosteroids, benzodiazepines, and anticholinergics are also used as adjuvant pain medication. Corticosteroids, by decreasing peritumor edema and by their antiinflammatory effects, are useful for pain due to multiple pathologies, including bone metastasis, liver capsule distention from metastasis, and conditions in which the tumor is compressing sensitive structures. Benzodiazepines and baclofen are indicated for pain from spasticity. Anticholinergics can relieve colic due to intestinal obstruction.

In addition to drug therapy for pain control, interventions such as palliative radiation therapy for bone metastasis, nerve blocks (celiac plexus block for pancreatic cancer), palliative surgical resection, and immobilization of fractures should be considered. Before undertaking such interventions, the patient's overall prognosis and the effectiveness of less invasive measures need to be taken into account.

Fear of addiction should not hinder the use of opioids for pain control. Addiction is a rare occurrence in patients with terminal illness and in patients without prior history of drug abuse. Psychological addiction should be differentiated from physical dependence. Patient with physical dependence develop withdrawal symptoms with the abrupt cessation of a drug or significant reduction of dosage. If the need arises for a rapid decrease in the opioid dose, administering 25% of the stable dose can prevent withdrawal symptoms. In patients previously on steady opioid doses, dose escalation portends disease progression rather than tolerance to opioid analgesic effects. Tolerance, like addiction, is rarely seen.

B. NAUSEA/VOMITING

Nausea and vomiting entail a complex physiological process. Several discrete afferent neural pathways terminate at the "vomiting center" (Figure 59–2). Stimulation of the vomiting center leads to the efferent emetic reflex. Multiple receptors and neurotransmitters are involved with each pathway. Patients can experience nausea without vomiting and vice versa.

The list of possible etiologies of nausea and vomiting is extensive. Treatment should be directed at correcting the underlying pathology when possible. The choice of antiemetics is based primarily on the suspected afferent pathway involved. Other factors to consider include the route of administration, patient's previous antiemetic drug experience, drug side effect profile, and cost of therapy.

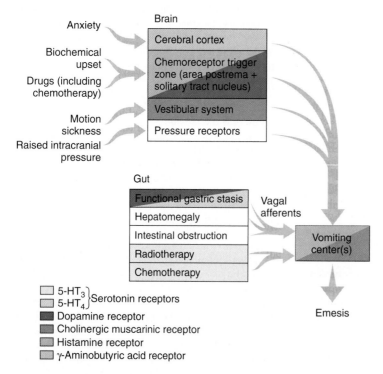

Figure 59–2. Vomiting pathways.

Classes of antiemetics include the following:

- Butyrophenones: haloperidol, droperidol (narrow-spectrum dopamine-2 antagonists)
- Phenothiazines: promethazine, prochlorperazine, chlorpromazine (broad-spectrum anticholinergic, antihistamine, and antidopaminergic)
- Benzamide: metoclopramide [antidopaminergic, cholinergic, and at high doses 5-hydroxytryptamine-3 (5-HT$_3$) antagonist]
- 5-HT$_3$ receptor antagonists: ondansetron, granisetron, dolasetron
- Anticholinergics: scopolamine, hyoscyamine, glycopyrrolate
- Antihistamines: meclizine, diphenhydramine
- Cannabinoids: dronabinol
- Corticosteroids: dexamethasone

Drug therapy for specific causes of nausea and vomiting includes the following:

- Vestibular dysfunction (motion induced): antihistamines and/or anticholinergics
- Delayed gastric emptying or squashed stomach syndrome (hepatomegaly, ascites): metoclopramide
- Drug-induced and metabolic causes (hypercalcemia, uremia): selective antidopaminergic agents, haloperidol or dronabinol
- Increased intracranial pressure: steroids, specifically dexamethasone
- Chemotherapy and radiation induced: 5-HT$_3$ receptor antagonists
- Anticipatory nausea associated with chemotherapy: benzodiazepines

Dronabinol has an unknown antiemetic mechanism. Dronabinol's psychomimetic effects limit its use to refractory nausea. About one-third of patients will require more than one antiemetic for symptom control. A combination of high-potency specific receptor antagonists is recommended before reverting to broad-spectrum low-affinity drugs. Antiemetics that can be administered by several different routes, including the subcutaneous route, can prove extremely useful. Such versatile drugs include haloperidol, metoclopramide, glycopyrrolate, ondansetron, and dexamethasone.

Nausea and vomiting may be presenting symptoms of malignant gastrointestinal obstruction. If the patient's situation is not amenable to invasive procedures such as venting gastrostomy, intraluminal stent, or surgical diversion, palliative medications can help relieve symptoms. With partial obstruction, the use of metoclopramide and dexamethasone along with a low-fiber diet can provide significant relief of symptoms for several weeks or longer. When obstruction becomes complete, therapy is geared at decreasing intestinal motility and secretions. Anticholinergics and somatostatin analogs are both effective for this purpose. The combination of haloperidol, an anticholinergic, and octreotide can preclude the use of nasogastric tube decompression for many patients with complete intestinal obstruction.

C. DYSPNEA

Dyspnea is described as breathlessness or difficult breathing. Like pain, it is a subjective experience. Dyspnea can be present in the absence of hypoxia. With a broad differential existing for dyspnea, reversible causes should always be considered first. The optimal therapy is aimed at the presumed etiology. Palliative therapy can involve chemotherapy, radiotherapy, thoracentesis, pericardiocentesis, and bronchial stent placement. Minor adjustments in the environment, such as providing a fan and keeping the room temperature cool or a careful trial of supplemental oxygen, can help dyspneic patients. Available palliative drug therapy includes steroids, opioids, bronchodilators, diuretics, anxiolytics, antibiotics, and anticoagulants. All these drugs can be used in combination depending on the etiology of dyspnea.

Opioids can relieve breathlessness associated with advanced cancer. The mechanism is unclear. Opioid administration, dose, frequency, and titration are the same as for pain control. The use of nebulized morphine sulfate is not more effective than placebo. Patients with end-stage pulmonary or cardiac conditions with dyspnea at rest show variable benefits from the use of opioids. Opioids can increase exercise tolerance in patients with chronic obstructive airways. Fear of addiction or fear of respiratory depression should not preclude a trial of opioids in this population. Starting at low doses, carefully titrating the dose to symptom control, and close monitoring allow for safe effective use.

Steroids are useful for dyspnea caused by bronchospasm and peritumor edema. Specific indications include malignant bronchial obstruction, carcinomatous lymphangitis, and superior vena cava syndrome. Dexamethasone can be started at 8 mg twice a day and subsequently reduced to the lowest effective dose. Compared to other steroids, dexamethasone is more potent and has low mineralocorticoid activity, resulting in less fluid retention.

Some patients with dyspnea express disturbing fears of suffocation and choking. Understandably, anxiety often coexists with chronic dyspnea, which can heighten breathlessness, making symptom control more difficult. The use of anxiolytics such as benzodiazepines and buspirone can help treat dyspnea associated with a high component of anxiety. Lorazepam 0.5–1 mg can be tried initially. If patients show benefit, long-acting diazepam or clonazepam can then be prescribed.

D. ANOREXIA AND CACHEXIA

Anorexia (poor appetite) and cachexia (severe weight loss) are prevalent distressing symptoms in patients with advanced cancer. Factors released either by the tumor or by the host response appear to produce the anorexia/cachexia syndrome. Cytokines implicated include tumor necrosis factor, interferon-γ, and interleukins-1 and -6. The syndrome is characterized by impaired carbohydrate, protein, and lipid metabolism. A perpetual catabolic state ensues with loss of protein and lipid stores. Patients lose weight and appear malnourished despite adequate nutrient intake. There is an abundant amount of research in this field, but little effective drug therapy available. Medications prescribed for the anorexia/cachexia syndrome include megestrol acetate, corticosteroids, dronabinol, and anabolic steroids. Megestrol acetate, a progestin, has been shown to increase appetite and result in weight gain. Doses start at 160 mg/day and can be titrated to 800 mg/day if required. Corticosteroids, such as dexamethasone, can be prescribed as an appetite stimulant for patients in whom long-term steroid side effects are of less concern. Beneficial effects tend to be limited to several weeks. Significant weight gain is not seen with corticosteroids in this population. Dexamethasone can be started at 2–4 mg daily with titration to 16 mg daily as needed. The lowest effective steroid dose should always be used. Androgens and dronabinol have been effective for human immunodeficiency virus (HIV) patients with acquired immune deficiency syndrome (AIDS)-associated anorexia and cachexia. Investigations are ongoing with respect to the use of omega-3 fatty acids and melatonin.

Anorexia can be provoked by conditions such as delayed gastric emptying, constipation, mucositis/thrush, or ill-fitting dentures. Metoclopramide, a prokinetic agent, can improve anorexia with concurrent symptoms of early satiety or nausea. It is important not to overlook reversible causes of anorexia.

Nutritional support, parenteral and enteral, has not been shown to prolong survival in patients with advanced cancer who are not candidates for disease-specific therapy. Regardless, a role for palliative nutritional support exists. Patients who suffer from concurrent malnutrition, for example, patients with dysphagia from head and neck cancer or patients with gastrointestinal dysfunction from radiation toxicity or neuromuscular disorders, can potentially benefit from nutritional support. Consideration of artificial nutrition should be on an individual basis.

E. ASTHENIA

Asthenia is generally described as excessive fatigue. Patients with asthenia feel tired after minimal activity or lack the energy to perform daily activities. As a result they become increasingly dependent on others for basic needs. Feelings of helplessness can lead to mood disturbances and depression, symptoms that often accompany asthenia. Asthenia is pervasive in advanced disease. Asthenia can result from direct tumor effects, such as cancer cachexia, paraneoplastic neuropathy/myopathy, and tumor involvement of the central nervous system or spine, or can be a consequence of therapy, steroid myopathy, chemotherapy, or radiation or drug toxicity. Unfortunately, when disease-specific therapy is not effective, asthenia is difficult to palliate.

Nondrug therapies include a trial of transfusion for anemia, optimizing fluid and nutritional status, aggressive treatment of nausea/vomiting/constipation, oxygen supplementation for hypoxia, moderate physical therapy to improve mobility, providing appropriate assistive devices, and providing psychosocial support. Symptomatic drug therapy includes corticosteroids and psychostimulants. A short course of dexamethasone or methylphenidate can increase patients' energy levels and improve their mood. The usual starting dose of dexamethasone is 2–4 mg once or twice daily and of methylphenidate is 2.5–5 mg twice daily. To lessen potential insomnia at night, these drugs should be administered early in the day, ie, 0800 and 1200 h.

Psychiatric Dimensions

A. DEPRESSION

There is a common assumption that all patients with cancer are and should be depressed. This minimizes the degree of suffering that can be associated with comorbid depression and its impact on a person's quality of life and also promotes the underdiagnosis of depression and in turn its undertreatment. Health professionals may underestimate the morbidity caused by depression because they tend to believe they would feel depressed if the roles were reversed. Depressive states exist on a continuum from normal sadness that accompanies life-limiting disease to major affective disorders. It is important for physicians to differentiate these levels of distress. Using screening tools and raising awareness about depression are important steps. Physicians and nurses often do not recognize levels of depressive symptoms, particularly when the symptoms are more severe.

Diagnosing depression in physically healthy patients depends heavily on the presence of somatic symptoms such as decreased appetite, loss of energy, insomnia, loss of sexual drive, and psychomotor retardation. These neurovegetative symptoms of depression are very compelling when present in the absence of physical illness but are somewhat less reliable for diagnosing depression in patients with advanced disease. Loss of appetite can be due to chemotherapy, fatigue can be due to cancer, and lack of sleep can be due to unrelieved pain. Thus it is difficult to determine whether certain somatic symptoms are an indication of depression or simply the result of other medical causes. Physical symptoms must be carefully evaluated to clarify their etiology and target them for intervention. However, due to the correlation between higher levels of symptom distress and the other more reliable cognitive or ideational symptoms, they should not be discounted and indeed may be a useful tool for beginning discussion with the patient. Assessing these symptoms can be a way to open a dialogue with patients who might otherwise resist discussions of emotional issues (ie, those who are not psychologically minded). Moreover, antidepressants can be chosen to target the physical symptoms that are most distressing to the patient.

Persistently depressed mood and sadness can be an appropriate response for a patient with a life-threatening disease, so the diagnosis of depression in advanced cancer patients relies more on other psychological or "cognitive symptoms." Anhedonia is a useful, if not the most reliable, symptom of depression to monitor. Cancer patients who are not depressed, although periodically sad, maintain the capacity for experiencing pleasure. Such patients react positively to opportunities to engage in the activities that they enjoy, even though the range of activities available to them may be diminished. Indeed, some patients with far advanced disease experience exhilaration in things such as intimacies with family or friends, knowing that the experiences are among the last they might have. The knowledge that death is near can increase the poignancy and emotion in such contacts. Feelings of hopelessness and worthlessness, excessive guilt, loss of self-esteem, and wishes to die are also among the most diagnostically reliable symptoms of depression in patients with cancer.

The interpretation of even these more reliable symptoms can be difficult. For example, feelings of hopelessness in dying patients who have no hope for recovery can be normal. Although many cancer patients have no hope of a cure, they are able to maintain hope that life can be extended, symptoms can be controlled, and/or quality of life can be maintained. Hopelessness that is pervasive and is accompanied by a sense of despair or despondency is more likely to represent a symptom of a depressive disorder. Similarly, patients often state that they feel they are burdening their families unfairly, causing them great pain and inconvenience. These beliefs can be addressed through counseling by helping patients come to see that the care they need is something their family needs to provide as part of the mourning process. Patients with such beliefs are less likely to be depressed than patients who suffer with guilty recrimination, feel that their life has never had any worth, or that they are being punished for evil things they have done. Suicidal ideation, even if mild and passive, is very likely associated with significant degrees of depression in patients with advanced disease. Recognizing the difficulties in applying traditional *Diagnostic and Statistical Manual of Mental Disorders,* fourth edition (*DSM-IV*), diagnoses of depression in these settings, several groups have tried to define more relevant variables responsive to a range of interventions, such as loss of meaning, hopelessness, loss of dignity, boredom, and demoralization.

B. ANXIETY

Patients with advanced disease may present with a complex mixture of physical and psychological symptoms in the context of their frightening reality. Thus, recognizing symptoms of anxiety that require treatment can be challenging. Patients with anxiety complain of tension or restlessness, or they exhibit jitteriness, autonomic hyperactivity, vigilance, insomnia, distractibility, shortness of breath, numbness, apprehension, worry, or rumination. Often the physical or somatic manifestations of anxiety overshadow the psychological or cognitive ones. These symptoms are a cue to further inquiry about the patient's psychological state, which is commonly one of fear, worry, or apprehension. In deciding whether to treat anxiety, the patient's subjective level of distress is the primary impetus for the initiation of treatment rather than qualifying for a psychiatric diagnosis. Other considerations include problematic patient behavior such as noncompliance, family and staff reactions to the patient's distress, and the balancing of the risks and benefits of treatment.

In this population anxiety is a symptom that can have many etiologies. It may be encountered as a component of an adjustment disorder, panic disorder, generalized anxiety disorder, phobia, or agitated depression. Additionally, in patients with advanced disease, symptoms of anxiety are most likely to arise from some medical complication of the illness or treatment such as organic anxiety disorder, delirium, or other organic mental disorders. Hypoxia, sepsis, poorly controlled pain, and adverse drug reactions such as akathisia, or withdrawal states are specific entities that often present as anxiety. Withdrawal from benzodiazepines, for example, can present first as agitation or anxiety, although the diagnosis is often missed in cancer patients with advanced disease, and especially the elderly, in whom physiological dependence on these medications is often unrecognized.

Although anxiety in patients with advanced disease commonly results from medical complications, psychological factors related to existential issues equally often cause anxiety, particularly in patients who are alert and not confused. Patients frequently fear isolation and estrangement from others, and may have a general sense of feeling like an outcast. Also, financial burdens and changes in family role are common stressors.

C. DELIRIUM AND DEMENTIA

Delirium has been characterized as an etiologically nonspecific, global, cerebral dysfunction, characterized by concurrent disturbances of level of consciousness, attention, thinking, perception, memory, psychomotor behavior, emotion, and the sleep–wake cycle. Disorientation, fluctuation, or waxing and waning of the above symptoms, as well as acute or abrupt onset of such disturbances are other critical features of delirium. Delirium is also conceptualized as a reversible process as compared to dementia. At times it is difficult to differentiate delirium from dementia as they frequently share common clinical features such as impaired memory, thinking, and judgment as well as disorientation. Dementia appears in relatively alert individuals with little or no clouding of consciousness. The temporal onset of symptoms in dementia is more insidious or chronically progressive, and the patient's sleep–wake cycle is generally not impaired. Most prominent in dementia are difficulties in short- and long-term memory, impaired judgment and abstract thinking, as well as disturbed higher cortical functions (ie, aphasia, apraxia, etc). Occasionally delirium is superimposed on an underlying dementia such as in the case of an elderly patient, a patient with AIDS, or a patient with a paraneoplastic syndrome.

Delirium is most common in patients with far advanced disease. Between 15% and 20% of hospitalized cancer patients have organic mental disorders and more than 75% of terminally ill cancer patients were found to have delirium. Delirium can be due either to the direct effects of cancer on the central nervous system (CNS) or to indirect CNS effects of the disease or treatments (medications, electrolyte imbalance, failure of a vital organ or system, infection, vascular complications, and preexisting cognitive impairment or dementia). Early symptoms of delirium can be misdiagnosed as anxiety, anger, depression, psychosis, or unreasonable or uncooperative attitudes toward rehabilitative efforts or other treatments. In any patient showing acute onset of agitation, impaired cognitive function, altered attention span, or a fluctuating level of consciousness, a diagnosis of delirium should be considered.

A common error among medical and nursing staff is to conclude that a new psychological symptom is functional without completely ruling out all possible organic etiologies. For example, given the large numbers of drugs patients with advanced disease require, and the fragile state of their physiological functioning, even routinely ordered hypnotics are enough to create an organic mental syndrome. Opioid analgesics such as levorphanol, morphine sulfate, and meperidine are common causes of confusional states, particularly in the elderly and in patients with advanced disease. Most patients receiving these agents will not develop prominent CNS effects. Exceptions involve steroids and biological response modifiers. The spectrum of mental disturbances related to steroids includes minor mood lability, affective disorders (mania or depression), cognitive impairment (reversible dementia), and delirium (steroid psychosis). The incidence of these disorders ranges from 3% to 57% in noncancer populations, and they occur most commonly on higher doses. Symptoms usually develop within the first 2 weeks of treatment, but in fact can occur at any time and on any dose, even during the tapering phase. Prior psychiatric illness or prior disturbance on steroids is a poor to fair predictor of susceptibility to, or the nature of, mental disturbances during subsequent steroid treatments. These disorders are often rapidly reversible upon dose reduction or discontinuation.

Breitbart W, Passik SD: Psychiatric aspects of palliative care. In: *Oxford Textbook of Palliative Care.* Oxford University Press, 1990.

Byock L: *Dying Well: The Prospect for Growth at the End of Life.* Riverhead Books, 1997.

Chocinov HM: Dignity-conserving care—a new model for palliative care: helping the patient feel valued. JAMA 2002;287 (17):2253.

Dugan W et al: Use of the zung self-rating depression scale in cancer patients: feasibility as a screening tool. Psycho-Oncology 1998;7:483.

Katon W, Sullivan MD: Depression and chronic medical illness. J Clin Psychiatry 1990;51(Suppl 6):3.

Passik SD et al: Depression in cancer patients: recognition and treatment. Medscape 1998;2(5):1.

COMPLEMENTARY & ALTERNATIVE MEDICINE

Complementary and alternative medicine (CAM) is a growing trend in American health care. CAM has been defined in the past as therapies that are not taught in medical schools and are not reimbursed by health insurance. A study reported in 1998 in the *Journal of the American Medical Association (JAMA)* found that in 1997, 42% of people in the United States had used alternative therapies. The majority of these people had not discussed the use of these therapies with their physicians and had paid most of the cost out of pocket.

In 1993, the National Institutes of Health created the Office of Alternative Medicine (OAM), which expanded into the National Center for Complementary and Alternative Medicine (NCCAM) in 1998. This center focuses on the scientific research of CAM therapies and the dissemination of information to the public and health care professionals. As a result of the tremendous growth of CAM over the past decade, more than 50% of medical schools in the United States now offer courses in CAM, and a growing number of hospital systems are developing programs to include complementary approaches. In addition, most major insurers are beginning to integrate CAM into their benefits.

Complementary therapies focus on the whole person and treatment of symptoms, with the emphasis on healing rather than cure. Most CAM therapies encourage active participation, thus giving the person more control of the symptoms being treated. Palliative medicine focuses on the integrative care of the patient to relieve suffering and improve quality of life. Attention is given to the patient and family in a holistic approach instead of focusing on treatment of the disease. Psychological, social, cultural, and spiritual approaches are used to treat the individual's mind, body, and spirit. These approaches are consistent with the philosophy of most CAM therapies. Although there is little evidence to support the use of CAM as a curative treatment, CAM modalities can be useful in the supportive care of the patient.

Conducting rigorous research of use of CAM in palliative medicine is challenging for several reasons. Overall, there is a lack of funding for large-scale studies in this area. Many palliative care patients may be reluctant to participate in a study because of the severity of their illness. Because many of the CAM therapies involve hands-on treatment, it is difficult to maintain blinding during research studies. In spite of these challenges, there are small numbers of controlled trials that support the use of CAM therapies in improving the comfort of patients in the late stages of illness. The CAM therapies listed in Table 59–1 have been shown to be helpful in palliative care and are examples of strategies that may be used. They should be used complementary to biomedicine and individualized to the patient being treated.

CAM has a growing role in palliative medicine. Even though CAM therapies have not received the usual scientific validation, there is evidence to support the use of some CAM modalities to provide comfort and improve the quality of life of terminally ill patients. Many CAM therapies are easy to use with minimal side effects. They offer patients a sense of control over the symptoms that accompany the disease process. Physician education on the use of CAM in palliative medicine will benefit the patients as it allows physicians, patients, and complementary medicine practitioners to work as a team to help manage patients' symptoms and enhance their quality of life.

CARE OF THE DYING PATIENT

At some point in a person's illness, whether it be progressive cancer or an end-stage medical illness, it becomes clear that further attempts to treat the underlying condition are not only futile but harmful in that it exposes the patient to treatments that do more harm than good, delays the important conversations that must occur around the issues of death and dying, and reduces the likelihood of good symptom control because of the focus on disease management. Family practitioners, because of their long-term patient-centered relationships, are in the best position to have conversations about goals of care, treatment options with attendant benefits and burdens, the use of hospice or palliative care services, and prognosis issues.

Cary interviewed 84 terminally ill patients to understand what factors predict who will best cope with dying and what can be done by physicians and other professionals to make life more meaningful. His findings were as follows:

1. Most people want to hear the truth from their physicians. Patients with a limited life expectancy prefer to be told in person, with time allowed to express feelings and ask questions.

2. Patients want to be assured that their physician will not abandon them.

3. If the physician feels that he or she does not have the time or training to provide effective counseling for the patient or family, it is best to refer the patient elsewhere for care.

4. The proper administration of pain medication is a major factor in emotional adjustment to the terminal illness. Patients will have greater peace if they know that suffering will be kept at a minimum.

5. Because of the patient's many needs, physicians should be willing to seek and accept the help of other professionals, including clergy, social workers, and nurses.

An essential first step in facilitating the shift from the curative to the palliative mode is communicating the terminal diagnosis. Buckman describes a six-step protocol to be used by physicians for such a conversation:

1. Getting started: patients and their support person should attend. Ensure a comfortable environment. Allot adequate time and prevent interruptions. Know the facts of the illness and treatment to date.

2. Ask what the patient knows and assess the patient's ability to comprehend the information.

Table 59–1. Definitions of modalities and recommendations for use in palliative medicine.

Therapy	Brief Description	Recommendations
Acupuncture	Stimulation of defined points on the skin using a needle, electrical current (electroacupuncture), or pressure (acupressure). These points correspond to meridians, or pathways of energy flow with the intent to correct energy imbalances and restore a normal, healthy flow of energy in the body.	1. Acupuncture may provide pain relief in terminally ill patients with cancer pain. 2. Acupuncture may provide relief from breathlessness. 3. Acupressure may reduce chemotherapy-and radiation-induced nausea and vomiting.
Aromatherapy	Therapeutic use of essential oils, which are applied to the skin or inhaled. The impact on the emotional and psychological state is mediated through the olfactory nerve and the limbic system in the brain.	1. Aromatherapy may be used in conjunction with other complementary therapies, such as massage. 2. Aromatherapy may provide reduction in anxiety.
Massage therapy	Manipulation of the muscles and soft tissues of the body for therapeutic purposes.	1. Massage might provide short-term reduction in cancer pain. 2. Massage has been shown to reduce stress and anxiety and enhance feelings of relaxation.
Hypnosis	A state of increased receptivity of suggestion and direction.	1. Hypnotherapy may reduce nausea and vomiting in persons receiving chemotherapy. 2. Hypnotherapy can enhance pain relief.
Relaxation	The use of muscular relaxation techniques to release tension. These techniques are often used in conjunction with meditation, biofeedback, and guided imagery techniques	1. Relaxation can reduce stress and tension. 2. Relaxation techniques can improve pain control in advanced cancer patients.
Therapeutic touch	A technique performed by physical touch and/or the use of hand movements to balance any disturbances in a person's energy flow.	1. Therapeutic touch may increase hemoglobin levels. 2. Therapeutic touch may relieve anxiety and tension and reduce the effects of stress on the immune system.
Music therapy	The use of music as a therapy to influence mental, behavioral, or physiological disorders.	1. Music therapy may assist in the reduction of pain perception. 2. Music therapy may reduce anxiety and help persons cope with grief and loss.
Support group	The use of groups and psychosocial interventions to help persons learn how to cope better with their disease.	1. Support groups can enhance the quality of life. 2. Support group therapy can improve pain management and coping skills. 3. Support group therapy can reduce anxiety and depression.

3. Find out how much the patient wants to know, taking into account cultural, religious, social, and personal issues.

4. Share the information in small bits using simple language. Avoid technical terms, jargon, and euphemisms. Pause frequently. Check for patient understanding.

5. Respond to feelings. Listen. Empathize. Reflect. Be aware of nonverbal communication.

6. Next steps: treat symptoms, make referrals, plan for support, and schedule a timely follow-up visit.

Similarly, predicting the course of the illness and the patient's life expectancy is an essential component of good end-of-life care. Most patients and family members want to know for emotional, spiritual, and practical reasons. Loprinzi suggests that these discussions should contain the following elements:

1. Acknowledge uncertainty.

2. Foretell a general, realistic time frame.

3. Recommend "doing the things that should be done."

4. Provide realistic assurance that you will be available to help the patient through the dying process.

5. Refer the patient to other professionals for emotional and spiritual support in "dying well."

6. Ask the patients what they want to accomplish.

7. Encourage additional questions.

As death approaches the patient will develop a series of signs that predict its closeness (Table 59–2).

It is important to recognize that death is approaching and share this information compassionately with the patient, if desired, and the family. Medical care should be simplified as much as possible. Laboratory tests, radiological procedures, and other interventions should be done only if they will result in improvement of the patient's comfort. Nonessential medicines should be discontinued. Blood pressure medicines, for example, may be safely reduced in dosage or stopped as the patient becomes bed bound, reduces his or her activity, and reduces oral intake. Artificially provided hydration and nutrition are seldom necessary or helpful for the dying person. More often than not, these fluids result in progressive edema, lung congestion, oral secretions, and frequent urination with attendant discomfort and distress. Experienced hospice professionals note no increase in discomfort or suffering with the naturally occurring dehydration that accompanies the dying process. However, some authorities suggest that modest intravenous or subcutaneous fluids may be helpful for the delirious dying patient not responding to neuroleptics. A brief trial of fluids in this circumstance may be warranted. Family members frequently are concerned that not providing food by some route will result in increased suffering and "starvation" of their loved one. Confronting this

misconception with care and compassion but directly will usually provide reassurance for the concerned family that food is not necessary at the "time of dying."

Certain medicines are important to manage the symptoms that may occur during the dying process (Table 59–3). Additionally, of great importance are the following nursing interventions that should not be forgotten:

1. Daily bathing with application of a lubricating lotion and/or talcum powder to the entire body.

2. Frequent cleaning of the mouth with application of lip balm.

3. Application of artificial tears and lubricating ointment to the eyes.

4. Comfortable positioning in the bed with pillows placed under the calves or for other areas of support.

5. An open window for fresh air if possible; if not, then a fan at the bedside.

6. A calm and peaceful environment.

Family members may be instructed in these nursing interventions and participate in the care of their loved one. This often is very meaningful and comforting to both the patient and family member. As the patient becomes minimally responsive or nonresponsive, family members are encouraged to gently talk to and touch their loved one. Hospice experience teaches that patients are able to hear and recognize touch until the very moment of death.

Buckman R: *How to Break Bad News: A Guide for Health Care Professionals.* The Johns Hopkins University Press, 1992.

Cary RG: Living until death: A program of service and research for the terminally ill. In: *Death: The Final Stages of Growth.* Kubler-Ross E (editor). Simon and Schuster, 1975.

Loprinzi CL, Johnson ME, Steer G: "Doc, how much time do I have?" J Clin Oncol 2000;18(3):699.

Nelson A et al: The dying cancer patient. Semin Oncol 2000;27: 84.

ADVANCE CARE PLANNING

Advance directives are legal documents that allow patients to make their health care choices known. Terms for advance directive documents are not standardized from state to state but usually encompass one or more of the following options:

1. Patients appoint someone to make health care decisions (surrogate or proxy) for them.

2. Patients specify their own choices regarding various life-sustaining treatments (often called a Living Will).

3. Patients sign a form alerting emergency medical workers (EMS) that they have signed an advance directive.

Table 59–2. Signs of impending death.

1. Bed bound
2. Confusion
3. Cool/mottled extremities
4. Death rattle
5. Decreased hearing and vision
6. Decreased urinary output
7. Difficulty swallowing
8. Diminished interest in conversation
9. Diminished interest in oral intake
10. Disoriented to time
11. Drowsiness progressing to extended periods of somnolence
12. Dry mouth
13. Hallucination
14. Increasing distancing from all but a few intimate others
15. Limited attention span
16. Profound weakness

Table 59–3. Drugs used to control symptoms in the dying process.

Symptom	Drug Class	Drug	Route[1]	Dose
Pain	Nonopioid NSAID[2]	Ketorolac	IV/SC	15–30 mg every 6 h
	Opioid	Morphine	IV/SC	10 mg every 4 h
			PR	30 mg every 4 h
"Death rattle"	Anticholinergic	Scopolamine	TD	1 patch every 3 days
		Atropine	IV/SC	0.2–0.4 mg every 2 h
		Glycopyrrolate	IV/SC	0.2 mg every 4 h
		Hyoscyamine	SL	0.125–0.25 mg every 4 h
Dyspnea	Opioid	Morphine	IV/SC	10 mg every 4 h
			PR	30 mg every 4 h
Restlessness/anxiety	Benzodiazepine	Midazolam	SC	2.5 mg every 2 h
		Lorazepam	SC/SL	0.5–1.0 every 4 h
Agitation/hallucinations	Antipsychotic	Haloperidol	IV/SC	5–10 mg every 30 min to effect
		Thorazine	IV	12.5–25 mg every 6 h
			PR	25–50 every 6 h

[1]The oral route is not listed as it is often not a viable choice in the last 48 h. IV, intravenous; SC, subcutaneous; PR, rectal; SL, sublingual; TD, transdermal.
[2]NSAID, nonsteroidal antiinflammatory drug.

4. The American Bar Association Commission on Legal Problems of the Elderly (www.abanet.org) suggests that patients are best served by selecting a trusted individual to serve as a surrogate or proxy and executing a Living Will to provide guidance on treatment choices.

Advance directive documents typically go into effect when a patient loses decision-making capability. Most states, through law, require the document to be witnessed and/or notarized.

Patients, families, and the health care system benefit from advance directives and from the decision-making process patients and their families go through to create a written document. Advance care planning (the process of arriving at an end-of-life care decision) is important to patients because they can "direct" and inform the health care system when they are no longer able to speak for themselves. Families benefit from advance directives, as they are relieved from making extremely difficult decisions that often lead to family disagreements over the patient's wishes. Advance care planning is important to physicians because they can be assured they are following the patient's wishes. Given the importance of advance care directives it is hard to understand why fewer than 20% of Americans have signed an advance directive.

How to Start the Process

The advance care planning process should begin with physicians educating themselves on what legal statutes exist for advance directive documents and where to direct patients for further education. Hospices, senior citizen centers, and hospital social service departments are all good resources for obtaining documents and education materials.

The ideal time to discuss an advance care directive is when a patient is still healthy. A discussion should become a part of routine health care. Although advance directive documents are important, advance care planning is a process that allows for adequate time to reflect, educate, and involve family members. A physician can initiate an end-of-life care discussion with a patient, direct the patient on where to obtain information, and encourage the patient to seek additional guidance from religious or legal advisors. Patients should also be encouraged to have a discussion with their family members so that the family can be made aware of their loved ones' health care preferences. Ideally, the physician should follow up with the patient at a latter date to address questions or concerns and obtain a copy of a signed advance directive document for inclusion in the patient's medical record. Physicians who follow a patient for several years may want to have further discussions to ensure that the documents still reflect the patient's choices. Advance directives can and should be updated. States may or may not outline specific processes for changing an advance directive.

Numerous articles and studies have shown that the avoidance of planning for end of life results in families agonizing over difficult health care decisions, costly futile care, and time-consuming lawsuits to sort out the results. Hammes and Briggs give the following common reasons why health care professionals avoid having end-of-life conversations:

1. A belief that the person is not sick enough, may become upset, is not able to understand, and will be robbed of hope.
2. Professionals often lack confidence in skills related to delivering bad news.
3. A perceived lack of time.
4. A belief that there are simply too many contingencies for individuals to consider regarding their future potential medical conditions.

Patients may also wish to avoid end-of-life conversations. Fear and a lack of understanding of medical technology prevent patients from initiating discussions with their physician. A study conducted in 2000 by the National Hospice and Palliative Care Organization found that adult children would have an easier time discussing sex and/or drugs with their teenage children than having end-of-life care discussions with their aging parents. That so few individuals have signed advance care directives may in large part be a result of a combination of health care professional and patient avoidance. The need for conversation, however, could not be more critical.

Talking to the Palliative Care Patient

As the change from curative care to palliative care begins, opportunities to engage in meaningful compassionate discussions with patients will appear. Asking patients what they understand about their disease can inform physicians of patients' perceptions and possible gaps in knowledge about the disease progression. When discussing new palliative care options, the discussion should include the goal of each treatment. Patients and their families should have a clear understanding of the benefits and the burdens of any proposed treatment.

Patients, when asked about end-of-life care choices, often use vague phrases such as "I don't want to be a vegetable" or "I don't want to be hooked up to machines." Such phrases, although descriptive, if not further explored leave gaps in making concrete treatment decisions. End-of-life care discussions are often difficult because the conversation is based on patients' and their family members' values and beliefs. Some individuals believe that removing a loved one from a ventilator constitutes an act of murder. Others, when asked about feeding tubes, wonder about "starving their loved one to death." Such beliefs are often difficult to address and are clearly emotionally laden. Additionally, when the patient dies, the loved one, having been forced to make a difficult decision, may face a longer and more complicated bereavement period.

One approach to helping patients with advance directives is to guide the conversation to what would constitute a "good day" for the patient. By focusing on living each day to the best extent possible the physician can learn what is important to the patient and can help the patient weigh treatment options against the patient's measure of a good day. Several documents exist to help patients think about what is important to them. *Five Wishes* produced by Aging with Dignity provides an excellent format to assist patients and their families. *Five Wishes* and other resources lead patients and their families through a series of questions designed to stimulate thought and conversation about quality of life issues.

Hammes BJ, Briggs L: *Respecting Choices.* Gundersen Lutheran Medical Foundation, 2001.

Hopp F: Preferences for surrogate decision makers, informal communication, and advance directives among community-dwelling elders: results from a national study. Gerontologist 2000;40(4):449.

National Hospice Foundation: *Baby Boomers Fear Talking to Parents About Death.* National Hospice Foundation, 1999.

Sabatino CF: End-of-life care legal trends. Internal memorandum. American Bar Association Commission on Legal Problems of the Elderly, April 2000. www.abanet.org.

Sabatino CF: 10 Legal myths about advance medical directives. American Bar Association Commission on Legal Problems of the Elderly, March 13, 2002. www.abanet.org.

WEB SITES

Aging with Dignity: *Five Wishes*
www.agingwithdignity.org
American Association of Retired Persons
www.aarp.org
Partnership for Caring
www.partnershipforcaring.org

SPIRITUAL DIMENSIONS

A growing body of evidence suggests that attention to spiritual issues is important in relief from pain and suffering related to terminal illness.

Increased interest in the relationship between spirituality and medicine is growing. In 1992 only one medical school had a course in spirituality and medicine. Today, more than 70 medical schools in the United States offer these courses.

National surveys and polls document the desire of patients to have their physicians address their spiritual concerns. A 1990 Gallup Poll reveals that religion plays an important part in the lives of many Americans. In a 1996 *USA Today Weekend* health survey, 63% of patients indicated that it was good for doctors to talk with patients about spiritual beliefs. Only 10% reported that their doctors had discussed spiritual issues with them.

Spirituality includes religious practices but is more inclusive. The search for meaning and purpose, transcendence, connectedness, and values involves spiritual dimensions. Attention to this dimension necessitates the physician's willingness to stay with patients in the midst of their pain and suffering. This transition from dominant authority to caring presence provides an environment for spiritual exploration. Being present, attentive, and supportive invites patients to share the physical, emotional, and spiritual aspects of their suffering.

Victor Frankl, a psychiatrist writing from a Nazi concentration camp, observed: "Man is not destroyed by suffering; he is destroyed by suffering without meaning." The following existential or spiritual questions are often raised: Why is this happening to me now? What will happen to me when I die? What will my family do without me? Will I be missed or even remembered? Is there a God? Will I be able to finish my life's work? These are real spiritual questions that relate to healing when physical cure may not be possible. Spiritual healing and comfort can be experienced as acceptance of illness and peace with one's life.

Research indicates that patients want to explore and utilize spiritual resources at the time of illness and suffering. They often need permission and assistance from their health care providers. This requires active listening and attention to patients' fears, hopes, pain, and dreams. This exploration is aided by recording a spiritual history or spiritual assessment. Spiritual assessment questions invite patients to identify beliefs and values that assist in comfort and healing. One model, the **FICA** method of taking a spiritual history, follows.

F *Faith and belief.* Ask: Are there spiritual beliefs that help you cope with stress or difficult times? What gives your life meaning?

I *Importance and influence.* Ask: Is spirituality important in your life? What influence does it have on how you take care of yourself? Are there any particular decisions regarding your health that might be affected by these beliefs?

C *Community.* Ask: Are you part of a spiritual or religious community?

A *Address/action.* Think about what you as the health care provider need to do with the information the patient shared, eg, refer the patient to a chaplain, meditation, yoga classes, or another spiritual resource. It helps to talk with the chaplain in your hospital to familiarize yourself with available resources.

Examples of spiritual suffering will emerge as patients tell their stories. These include **spiritual anger** ("I'm mad at God. " "I blame God for this."), **spiritual loss** ("I feel empty." "I don't care anymore."), **spiritual despair** ("There is no way God could ever care for me." "I'm just a corpse waiting to happen."), **spiritual alien-**

ation ("Where is God when I need God most?" "Why isn't God listening?"), **spiritual anxiety** ("Will I ever be forgiven?" "Am I going to die a horrible death?"), and **spiritual guilt** ("I deserve this." "I didn't pray hard enough.").

Attention and response to patients' spiritual issues encourage health care professionals to be aware of and attentive to their own spirituality. The opportunity to share personal insights, experiences, and resources must be acted upon with sensitivity and acceptance of patients' faith, traditions, and practices.

Consultation with and referral to a chaplain or other faith community leader is often helpful. However, not all religious leaders are able to respond with insight and understanding.

FICA: Copyright Christina M. Puchalski, MD, 1996.

Frankle V: *Man's Search for Meaning.* Simon and Schuster, 1984.

Plotnikoff MD: Should medicine reach out to the spirit? Postgrad Med 2000;108:19.

RESOURCES

Books

Dickerson E et al: *Palliative Care Pocket Consultant, a Reference Guide for Symptom Management in Palliative Care,* ed 2. Kendal/Hunt Publishing Company, 2001.

Doka K: *Living with Life-Threatening Illness: A Guide for Patients, Their Families, and Caregivers.* Jossey-Bass, 1998.

Doyle D, Hanks GWC, MacDonald N (editors): *Oxford Textbook of Palliative Medicine,* ed 2. Oxford University Press, 1998.

Lynn J, Harrold J: *Handbook for Mortals: Guidance for People Facing Serious Illness.* Oxford University Press, 1999.

Participant's Handbook and Trainer's Guide for Education for Physicians on End-of-Life Care (EPEC). Download from American Medical Association, Chicago, IL: www.ama-assn.org/catalog/.

Journals

American Journal of Hospice & Palliative Care. Enck RE (editor). Prime National Publishing Corporation, Weston, MA.

Hospice Journal. Lind DL (editor). The Haworth Press Inc., Binghamton, NY.

Journal of Pain and Symptom Management. Portenoy RK (editor). Elsevier Science Publishers, New York.

Journal of Palliative Medicine. Weissman DE (editor). Mary Ann Liebert, Inc., Larchmont, NY.

Supportive Care in Cancer. Senn HJ (editor). Springer-Verlag, Heidelburg, Germany.

WEB SITES

ACP-ASIM End-of-Life Care Consensus Panel

www.acponline. org/ethics/eolc.htm

(Consensus statements in journal articles on critical arenas of medical practice, including terminal sedation, pain management, and communication.)

AMA: Education for Physicians in End-of-Life Care

www.ama-assn.org/ethic/epec/epec.htm

(The EPEC Project provides materials designed to educate all U.S. physicians on the essential clinical competencies required to provide quality end-of-life care.)

American Academy of Hospice and Palliative Medicine

www. aahpm.org

(AAHPM is dedicated to the advancement of practice, research, and education about hospice and palliative medicine.)

American Alliance of Cancer Pain Initiatives

www.aacpi.org

(Materials to support efforts to reduce pain, both through changes in practitioner behavior and in regulatory matters.)

American Board of Hospice and Palliative Medicine

www.abhpm.org

(The ABHPM promotes the development of standards for training and practice in palliative medicine.)

Center for the Advancement of Palliative Medicine

www. capcmssm.org

[The Center to Advance Palliative Care (CAPC) is a resource for hospitals and health systems interested in developing palliative care programs. The Center serves a broad constituency of providers and interested groups in an effort to improve the availability and quality of palliative care.]

End-of-Life Physician Education Resource Center

www.iago.lib. mcw.edu/pallmed/

[EPERC provides online peer-reviewed information about instructional and evaluation materials (eg, lectures, small group exercises, slide sets, videotapes, self-study guides, and assessment tools) focused on end of life.]

Growth House

www.growthhouse.org

(Growth House contains resources for life-threatening illness and end-of-life care such as hospice and home care, palliative care, and pain management.)

Last Acts

www.lastacts.org

(Last Acts is a national campaign to engage both health professionals and the public in efforts to improve care at the end of life. Offerings include peer-reviewed examples of promising practices, a weekly e-mail newsletter, and current information on end-of-life issues.)

National Hospice and Palliative Care Organization

www.nhpco.org

(The National Hospice and Palliative Care Organization is the industry's largest association and leading resource for professionals and volunteers committed to providing service to patients and their families during end of life.)

Project on Death in America

www.soros.org/death

(PDIA's mission is to understand and transform the culture and experience of dying and bereavement through initiatives in research, scholarship, the humanities, and the arts, and to foster innovations in the provision of care, public education, professional education, and public policy.)

Supportive Care of the Dying

www.careofdying.org

(Collaboration of Catholic health systems that has created resources to support improvement activities, including a newsletter and assessment tools.)

Index